D1605039

Electrophysiology and Pharmacology of the Heart

Electrophysiology and Pharmacology of the Heart

A Clinical Guide

edited by
Kenneth H. Dangman

College of Physicians and Surgeons
Columbia University
New York, New York

Dennis S. Miura

Albert Einstein College of Medicine
Bronx, New York

Marcel Dekker, Inc.   **New York • Basel • Hong Kong**

Library of Congress Cataloging-in-Publication Data

Basic and clinical electrophysiology and pharmacology of the heart: a clinical
    guide / edited by Kenneth H. Dangman, Dennis S. Miura. -- 1st ed.
        p.   cm.
    Includes bibliographical references and index.
    ISBN 0-8247-8449-9 (alk. paper)
    1. Arrhythmia--Pathogenesis. 2. Arrhythmia--Animal models.
3. Heart--Electric properties. 4. Myocardial depressants--Mechanism of
action. I. Dangman, Kenneth H. II. Miura, Dennis Senji.
    [DNLM: 1. Anti-Arrhythmia Agents--therapeutic use. 2. Cardiotonic Agents
--therapeutic use. 3. Electrophysiology. 4. Heart--drug effects. 5. Heart
--physiology. WG 202 B311]
    RC685.A65B35   1991
    616.1'28--dc20
    DNLM/DLC
    For Library of Congress   91-20052
                                                                 CIP

This book is printed on acid-free paper.

Marcel Dekker, Inc.
270 Madison Avenue, New York, New York 10016

Current printing (last digit):
10 9 8 7 6 5 4 3 2 1

PRINTED IN THE UNITED STATES OF AMERICA

Preface

Electrophysiology and Pharmacology of the Heart is designed to provide an introduction to the essential topics in cardiac electrophysiology and pharmacology. We enlisted a diverse group of qualified scientists and clinicians to write chapters in their areas of expertise. The joint effort of the editors and contributors has resulted in a relatively comprehensive review of cardiac electrophysiology.

The text is divided into four parts. Part I discusses the four major techniques that can be used to investigate the electrical behavior of the heart, cardiac cells, and the ion channels of those cells. Part II discusses the electrophysiology of the five major types of excitable tissue in the heart: the sinus node, the atrioventricular node, the Purkinje fibers, and the atrial and ventricular myocardium. Part III discusses the common laboratory models of cardiac arrhythmias, and Part IV discusses the pharmacology of positive inotropic agents and antiarrhythmic drugs.

As such, the audience for this book should be fairly broad. One group that should find it useful includes graduate students, medical students, and many postdoctoral fellows and clinicians who are seeking basic information about cardiac electrophysiology and pharmacology. Although some background in general physiology is helpful, the various chapters included here should be helpful to this audience. A second group who should find this book helpful are basic scientists and clinicians involved in cardiovascular research or medicine, who may find this volume to be a useful reference source. To these readers, many points raised in these chapters may suggest new avenues for research.

Kenneth H. Dangman
Dennis S. Miura

Contents

Preface   iii

Contributors   ix

Introduction: Contributions of Research in Cardiac Electrophysiology
and Pharmacology to Improvement of Therapy of Clinical Arrhythmias   xiii

I. TECHNIQUES FOR STUDY OF CARDIAC ELECTROPHYSIOLOGY   1

1. Extracellular Recording Techniques   3
Karen J. Beckman and Robert J. Hariman

2. Standard and Ion-Selective Microelectrodes   19
Karl P. Dresdner, Jr.

3. The Multicellular Cardiac Voltage Clamp: Approaches and Problems   33
Ira S. Cohen and Nicholas B. Datyner

4. Single-Channel Recording as Applied to Cardiac Electrophysiology   41
Steven A. Siegelbaum

II. ELECTROPHYSIOLOGY OF THE HEART: ANATOMY, PHYSIOLOGY, AND PATHOPHYSIOLOGY   57

5. Electrophysiology of the Sinus Node: Ionic and Cellular Mechanisms Underlying Primary Cardiac Pacemaker Activity   59
Donald L. Campbell, Randall L. Rasmusson, and Harold C. Strauss

6. Electrophysiology of the Atrial Myocardium   109
Steve Sorota and Penelope A. Boyden

7. Electrophysiology of the Atrioventricular Node: Conduction,
Refractoriness, and Ionic Currents   141
   Jacques Billette and Wayne R. Giles

8. Electrophysiology of the Purkinje Fiber   161
   Kenneth H. Dangman

9. Electrophysiology of Mammalian Ventricular Muscle   199
   J. Andrew Wasserstrom and Robert E. Ten Eick

III. MODELS AND MECHANISMS OF CARDIAC ARRHYTHMIAS   235

10. Reentrant Excitation in the Atrium   239
    Penelope A. Boyden

11. Reflection and Circus Movement Reentry in Isolated Atrial
and Ventricular Tissues   251
    Charles Antzelevitch and Anton Lukas

12. Digitalis Toxicity   277
    Gregory R. Ferrier

13. Arrhythmias in the Canine Heart Two to Twenty-Four Hours
After Myocardial Infarction   301
    Eugene Patterson, Benjamin J. Scherlag, and Ralph Lazzara

14. Reentrant Ventricular Rhythms in the Three- to-Five-Day-Old
Canine Postinfarction Heart   331
    Nabil El-Sherif, Mark Restivo, and William B. Gough

15. Arrhythmias in the Cat Heart with Chronic Myocardial Infarction   351
    Shinichi Kimura, Arthur L. Bassett, and Robert J. Myerburg

16. Proarrhythmic Effects of Antiarrhythmic Drugs   375
    Kenneth H. Dangman and Dennis S. Miura

17. Cellular Basis for Arrhythmias in Cardiac Hypertrophy
and Cardiomyopathy   397
    Ronald S. Aronson

18. Animal Models of Naturally Occurring Arrhythmias   413
    Philip R. Fox

IV. MECHANISMS AND APPLICATIONS OF CARDIOVASCULAR
PHARMACOLOGY: CARDIOTONIC AND ANTIARRHYTHMIC AGENTS   431

19. α-Adrenergic Receptor-Effector Coupling   433
    Susan F. Steinberg and Micahel R. Rosen

20. Positive Inotropic Drugs. Part I. Principles of Action   443
    Eduardo Marban and Stefan Herzig

21. Positive Inotropic Drugs. Part II. Specific Therapeutic Agents 463
Stefan Herzig

22. Characteristic Local Anesthetic Actions of Antiarrhythmic Drugs 477
Gary A. Gintant

23. Quinidine 493
Dan M. Roden

24. Procainamide 517
Elsa-Grace V. Giardina

25. Disopyramide 537
Betty I. Sasyniuk and Teresa Kus

26. Lidocaine 561
Jonathan C. Makielski and Morton F. Arnsdorf

27. Mexiletine and Tocainide 585
Lawrence H. Frame

28. Propafenone 603
Hrayr S. Karagueuzian

29. Cibenzoline 627
Dennis S. Miura and Kenneth H. Dangman

30. Amiodarone 637
Bertram G. Katzung, Michael A. Lee, and Jonathan J. Langberg

31. Moricizine 655
Dennis S. Miura and Kenneth H. Dangman

32. Class II Drugs 665
Dennis S. Miura, William H. Frishman, and Kenneth H. Dangman

33. Class III Antiarrhythmic Agents 677
Thomas M. Argentieri, Mark E. Sullivan, and Jay R. Wiggins

34. Class IV Antiarrhythmic Drugs 697
Elliott M. Antman and James D. Marsh

35. Antifibrillatory Drugs 723
Andrew C. G. Uprichard and Benedict R. Lucchesi

Index 741

Contributors

Elliott M. Antman Samuel A. Levine Cardiac Unit, Cardiovascular Division, Department of Medicine, Brigham and Women's Hospital and Harvard Medical School, Boston, Massachusetts

Charles Antzelevitch Masonic Medical Research Laboratory, Utica, New York

Thomas M. Argentieri Department of Pharmacology, Berlex Laboratories, Inc., Cedar Knolls, New Jersey

Morton F. Arnsdorf Section of Cardiology, Department of Medicine, The University of Chicago, Chicago, Illinois

Ronald S. Aronson Department of Medicine, Albert Einstein College of Medicine, Bronx, New York

Arthur L. Bassett Department of Molecular and Cellular Pharmacology, University of Miami School of Medicine, Miami, Florida

Karen J. Beckman Department of Medicine, University of Illinois, Chicago, Illinois

Jacques Billette Department of Physiology, Faculty of Medicine, University of Montreal, Montreal, Quebec, Canada

Penelope A. Boyden Department of Pharmacology, College of Physicians and Surgeons, Columbia University, New York, New York

Donald L. Campbell Department of Pharmacology, Duke University Medical Center, Durham, North Carolina

Ira S. Cohen Department of Physiology and Biophysics, Health Sciences Center, State University of New York at Stony Brook, Stony Brook, New York

Kenneth H. Dangman Department of Pharmacology, College of Physicians and Surgeons, Columbia University, New York, New York

Nicholas B. Datyner Department of Physiology and Biophysics, Health Sciences Center, State University of New York at Stony Brook, Stony Brook, New York

Karl P. Dresdner, Jr.* Department of Pharmacology, College of Physicians and Surgeons, Columbia University, New York, New York

Nabil El-Sherif Departments of Medicine and Physiology, Health Sciences Center, State University of New York Health Sciences Center and the Veterans Administration Medical Center, Brooklyn, New York

Gregory R. Ferrier Department of Pharmacology, Dalhousie University, Halifax, Nova Scotia, Canada

Philip R. Fox Department of Medicine, The Animal Medical Center, Speyer Hospital, and Caspary Research Institute, New York, New York

Lawrence H. Frame Department of Medicine, University of Pennsylvania School of Medicine, Philadelphia, Pennsylvania

William H. Frishman Department of Medicine, Jack Wiler Hospital, Albert Einstein College of Medicine, Bronx, New York

Elsa-Grace V. Giardina Cardiovascular Clinical Pharmacology Laboratory, Department of Medicine, College of Physicians and Surgeons, Columbia University, New York, New York

Wayne R. Giles Department of Medical Physiology, University of Calgary Health Science Centre, Calgary, Alberta, Canada

Gary A. Gintant Masonic Medical Research Laboratory, Utica, New York

William B. Gough Division of Cardiology, Department of Medicine, State University of New York Health Sciences Center and the Veterans Administration Medical Center, Brooklyn, New York

Robert J. Hariman Department of Medicine, University of Illinois, Chicago, Illinois

Stefan Herzig Department of Pharmacology, University of Kiel, Kiel, Germany

Hrayr S. Karagueuzian Division of Cardiology, Cedars-Sinai Medical Center and UCLA School of Medicine, Los Angeles, California

Bertram G. Katzung Department of Pharmacology, University of California, San Francisco, California

Shinichi Kimura Division of Cardiology, Department of Medicine, University of Miami School of Medicine, Miami, Florida

Teresa Kus Centre de recherche, Hôpital du Sacre-Coeur de Montréal, Montreal, Quebec, Canada

Jonathan J. Langberg Department of Internal Medicine, University of Michigan Medical Center, Ann Arbor, Michigan

Ralph Lazzara Department of Medicine, University of Oklahoma Health Sciences Center and Veterans Administration Medical Center, Oklahoma City, Oklahoma

Michael A. Lee Department of Cardiology, University of California, San Francisco, California

Benedict R. Lucchesi Department of Pharmacology, The University of Michigan Medical School, Ann Arbor, Michigan

Anton Lukas Masonic Medical Research Laboratory, Utica, New York

Jonathan C. Makielski Department of Medicine, The University of Chicago, Chicago, Illinois

Eduardo Marban Department of Medicine, The Johns Hopkins University School of Medicine, Baltimore, Maryland

---

Present affiliation: Pennie & Edmonds, New York, New York.

James D. Marsh Cardiovascular Division, Department of Medicine, Brigham and Women's Hospital and Harvard Medical School, Boston, Massachusetts

Dennis S. Miura Division of Cardiology, Department of Medicine, Albert Einstein College of Medicine, Bronx, New York

Robert J. Myerburg University of Miami School of Medicine, Miami, Florida

Eugene Patterson Departments of Pharmacology and Medicine, University of Oklahoma Health Sciences Center and Veterans Administration Medical Center, Oklahoma City, Oklahoma

Randall L. Rasmusson Department of Biomedical Engineering, Duke University Medical Center, Durham, North Carolina

Mark Restivo Cardiology Division, State University of New York Health Sciences Center and the Veterans Administration Medical Center, Brooklyn, New York

Dan M. Roden Departments of Medicine and Pharmacology, Vanderbilt University School of Medicine, Nashville, Tennessee

Michael R. Rosen Department of Pharmacology, College of Physicians and Surgeons, Columbia University, New York, New York

Betty I. Sasyniuk Department of Pharmacology and Therapeutics, McGill University Faculty of Medicine, Montreal, Quebec, Canada

Benjamin J. Scherlag Department of Medicine, University of Oklahoma Health Sciences Center and Veterans Administration Medical Center, Oklahoma City, Oklahoma

Steven A. Siegelbaum Department of Pharmacology, College of Physicians and Surgeons, Columbia University, New York, New York

Steve Sorota Department of Pharmacology, College of Physicians and Surgeons, Columbia University, New York, New York

Susan F. Steinberg Departments of Medicine and Pharmacology, College of Physicians and Surgeons, Columbia University, New York, New York

Harold C. Strauss Departments of Medicine and Pharmacology, Duke University Medical Center, Durham, North Carolina

Mark E. Sullivan Department of Pharmacology, Berlex Laboratories, Inc., Cedar Knolls, New Jersey

Robert E. Ten Eick Department of Cellular and Molecular Pharmacology, Northwestern University, Chicago, Illinois

Andrew C. G. Uprichard* The University of Michigan Medical School, Ann Arbor, Michigan

J. Andrew Wasserstrom Department of Medicine/Reingold ECG Center, Northwestern University, Chicago, Illinois

Jay R. Wiggins Department of Diagnostic Imaging, Berlex Laboratories, Inc., Cedar Knolls, New Jersey

*Present affiliation: Parke-Davis Clinical Research, Ann Arbor, Michigan.

Introduction
Contributions of Research in Cardiac Electrophysiology and Pharmacology to Improvement of Therapy of Clinical Arrhythmias

Present-day knowledge of cardiac electrophysiology is based on cumulative insights obtained from experiments done over many decades in many laboratories. Starting in the 1850s, a series of studies by Michael Foster, Hermann Stannius, and Walter Gaskell suggested the myogenic theory (as opposed to the neurogenic theory) of the origin of the cardiac impulse in the vertebrate heart. By 1855, Rudolph von Kolliker had demonstrated that the cardiac impulse produced with each beat in the frog heart was associated with an electrical current. In 1880, J. Burdon-Sanderson was the first to record directly the electrical activity of the heart using a capillary electrometer, and by 1887, Augustus Waller used this device to record the heartbeat using limb leads. Subsequently (in 1903), Wilhelm Einthoven used the string galvanometer to record the surface electrocardiogram in a brilliant series of experiments. This device avoided the inertia inherent in the capillary electrometer, and this produced a more accurate recording of the electrical activity of the heart. These experiments were the basis for the modern electrocardiogram. The development of the electrocardiogram allowed novel studies re-

garding the mechanisms of the origin of the heartbeat, of ventricular hypertrophy, conduction block, arrhythmias, and myocardial infarction during the first decades of this century.

Sir Thomas Lewis was a prominent investigator during this period. Capitalizing on the availability of the electrocardiogram and the polygraph, he studied mechanisms of both regular sinus rhythms and many abnormal ectopic rhythms. These studies laid the foundations for various electrocardiographic tests of cardiac function. In addition, Lewis started the journal *Heart* in 1909. For the next 24 years, *Heart* was an important publication for reports of studies in clinical cardiology and cardiovascular science. In 1933, Lewis ended publication of *Heart*. Lewis published his rationale for this step in the "Final Editorial Note" to Volume 16. He wrote that when he began the journal, "cardiac problems were being studied with unusual intensity, and a journal specially designed to publish original work dealing with the physiology and pathology of the cardiovascular system had become a necessity to workers in this field. It [*Heart*] served this purpose. It was understood, however, even at its conception, that such a journal might not always be required." By 1926, the number of important new contributions to the journal was declining precipitously. Lewis thus replaced *Heart* with a new journal, *Clinical Science*. It was clear that Lewis felt that a publication with a broader scope was necessary, because only limited progress would be made on problems in cardiovascular science and medicine in the future.

Although, in retrospect, the termination of *Heart* may appear to have been premature, from Lewis' perspective it was almost certainly necessary. By the late 1920s, many of the insights that could be obtained using simple surface electrocardiograms and extracellular electrograms had been obtained. Further progress in cardiac physiology therefore would be slow until the next advance in technology. Lewis' action was justified by Burton-Sanderson's idea (1900) that the rate of progress in cardiac electrophysiology would be tied to development of the technology for detecting and recording electrical signals from the heart.

Critical advances in electronic instrumentation occurred 10–15 years after Lewis closed *Heart*. After World War II, voltage clamp techniques were developed by Hodgkin and Huxley in squid axons that allowed study of transmembrane sodium and potassium ion currents, and intracellular microelectrodes were developed by Ling and Gerard that allowed the recording of transmembrane action potentials from single cardiac cells.

Electrophysiologic research on isolated tissue preparations made tremendous progress after these techniques became available. Microelectrode techniques allowed detailed study of the putative mechanisms of ectopic arrhythmias in normal and pathological cardiac tissues starting in the early 1950s. In the 1960s, much effort was devoted to studies using voltage clamp techniques in multicellular cardiac tissue preparations. These efforts continued until the early 1980s despite the significant limitations of the whole-tissue approaches pointed out by Johnson and Lieberman in 1971.

Today, efforts in basic cardiac electrophysiology are increasing based on patch clamp techniques in single cells or the function of ion channels in reconstituted membrane preparations. Advances in the understanding of the biophysics of the various types and interrelationships of sodium, potassium, calcium, and chloride channels and "pumps" are of great interest.

The present volume is organized in view of this background. This book not only reviews the electrophysiology of the intact heart and isolated cardiac tissues, but also presents the recent developments that have occurred on membrane biophysics of cardiac cell membranes. Both topics should be of importance to interested students of cardiovascular physiology, pharmacology, and disease.

Many books dealing with cardiovascular physiology and medicine are published every year. These are often symposia or anthologies in which the individual chapters deal with specialized topics or emphasize recent advances in the field. As such, these books speak to experts and advanced students in the field. These works unquestionably fill important needs and function as valuable reference sources for an increasingly experienced and sophisticated scientific and clinical audience.

The idea for the present book developed as a result of a series of courses on cardiac electrophysiology taught biannually by Dr. Brian Hoffman and others in the Department of Pharmacology at Columbia University. The courses, given as part of a postdoctoral training grant to introduce the incoming fellows to elementary concepts of cardiac electrophysiology, used existing texts in the field. Although these books were often quite stimulating and useful, discussions over the course of several years led to the conclusion that essentially what was needed was an updated and expanded version of Hoffman and Cranefield's 1960 classic *Electrophysiology of the Heart*.

When we were invited to organize a book by Marcel Dekker, Inc., in late 1987, we chose to try to achieve this ambitious goal. Specifically, we wanted to produce a book that would present a series of critical reviews that would be useful to a fairly broad audience, including graduate and medical students, postdoctoral and cardiology fellows, and interested clinicians. We quickly decided to make this a multiauthored text, because the ever-growing cardiology literature would have made it difficult or impossible for us to cover even just the essential topics in a comprehensive and critical way. We selected a group of respected scientists and clinicians as primary authors and invited them to contribute a review in an area of their expertise. The resulting chapters review the assigned topics and critically evaluate the literature, pointing out major advances that have been achieved.

TECHNIQUES FOR STUDY OF CARDIAC ELECTROPHYSIOLOGY

This section consists of four chapters, which progress from the most physiologic to the most biophysical techniques utilized in cardiac electrophysiology.

The first chapter by Beckman and Hariman discusses the use of extracellular recording techniques in cardiac research. Although these techniques have been available, in some form, for many decades, they still have a role in modern cardiology and cardiovascular physiology. In particular these techniques are essential for identifying the specific cause of arrhythmias in the in situ heart. Today, one can only speculate on the cause of most clinically significant ventricular arrhythmias. A given tachycardia can result from reentrant activity, enhanced automaticity, or triggered activity. Definitive proof that a specific arrhythmia is caused by one or more of these mechanisms cannot be derived from studies on isolated cells or tissues. Although this evidence from in vitro preparations may provide useful insights, proof requires demonstration of (1) circus movement derived from "mapping" studies of the activation sequences of reentrant beats, or (2) demonstration of waveforms characteristic of automaticity or triggered activity from ectopic foci by recording of high-gain unipolar electrograms.

The second chapter, by Dresdner, discusses the use of standard and ion-selective microelectrodes. These valuable techniques are used in both tissue preparations and isolated myocytes. Limitations of the method include (1) selectivity of the resins for ion sensitivity; (2) response times of the electrodes compared to physiologic events, such as the action potential and; (3) sensitivity of the electrodes to bound cations versus unbound cations in the intracellular millieau.

The third chapter, by Cohen and Datyner, discusses the use of the voltage clamp technique in multicellular tissue preparations. This technique may still provide important insights into basic phenomena in cardiac electrophysiology, but one must be aware of the limitations and complications that may be involved.

In the fourth chapter of this section Siegelbaum discusses the use of the newest technique in cardiac electrophysiology, the patch clamp. In the future patch clamp no doubt will be applied to provide much more detailed information about net ionic currents in single cells as well as unitary currents in single channels in membrane preparations.

Extracellular Recording Techniques

Karen J. Beckman and Robert J. Hariman

University of Illinois
Chicago, Illinois

INTRODUCTION

Extracellular recording of electrical activity of the heart possesses one distinct advantage over intracellular recording in that extracellular recording can be performed in the in vivo heart under neurohormonal control. Although extracellular recording is subject to certain limitations, it provides information that has been correlated to intracellular electrical events.

GENERAL CONCEPTS

Voltage potential changes recorded extracellularly result from current flowing across the membrane of excitable cells (i_m). The simple electrical model for an excitable membrane consists of capacitors C_m in parallel with resistors r_m (1). Action potential changes that occur across the membrane (V) over time t result in i_m that can be calculated using the equation

$$i_m = 2\frac{V}{r_m}5 + C_m 2\frac{dV}{dt}$$

From this equation it is clear that cells that generate large action potential amplitude and high dV/dt also generate larger i_m and larger extracellular potential changes. In this context the His-Purkinje potential is larger and more easily recorded extracellularly than the sinus node or atrioventricular (AV) node potential. The equation is an oversimplification of what is actually occurring in the heart because impulse propagation, activation of neighboring cells, and the resulting changes in extracellular current flow are not taken into account. We refer readers interested in the cable theory to a comprehensive discussion of the subject (2).

Propagation of the cardiac electrical impulses may be viewed as a series of dipoles moving through a cardiac fiber (3,4). A dipole is a positive and negative charge separated by a small distance. At rest there exists uniform charge on either side of the cell membrane (Fig. 1A), with the inside of the cells negative with respect to the outside. When the cell is stimulated, electrical current flows across the membrane, depolarizing it and changing its polarity. A dipole then exists between the barrier between excited and nonexcited tissue (Fig. 1B). This dipole is then propagated across the length of the fiber (Fig. 1). The

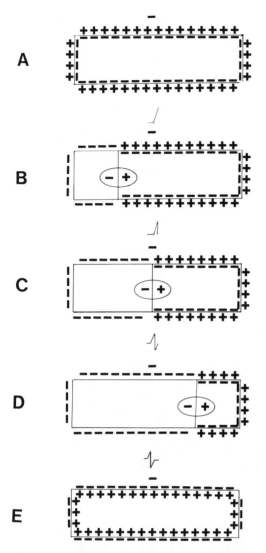

Figure 1 Depolarization as a series of moving dipoles: (A) resting membrane; (B, C, D) progressive depolarization; (E) completely depolarized cell. − and + represent the equivalent dipole between areas of polarized and depolarized tissue.

Complete depolarization of the fiber results in another return to baseline (Fig. 1E).

The spread of electrical impulses in the heart is not uniform in all directions (5). In myocardial tissues where the fibers are oriented in the same direction, conduction down the long axis of myocardial fibers (and parallel to the orientation of the fibers) is faster than conduction perpendicular to the long axis, a property known as uniform anisotropy. Slower conduction in the short axis is due to higher effective axial resistivity, which may stem in part from fewer intercalated disks connecting fibers side to side than end to end. The size and shape of electrograms may be affected by whether the electrode configuration is parallel or perpendicular to the long axis of the myocardial fibers. In diseased myocardium the fibers may be disorganized with altered orientation with respect to each other (non-uniform anisotropy), which may add to the complexities of analyzing the electrograms recorded (6).

The voltage potential generated at a particular site decreases exponentially with distance, so that the closer the electrode to the source of the potential the larger the potential recorded. The electrodes mainly reflect current generated directly below them, but they also to some extent reflect the current generated by the heart as a whole.

TECHNIQUES OF EXTRACELLULAR RECORDING

Electrodes

Electrodes are transducers that transform a biologic event, cellular depolarization and repolarization, into an electrical event. When a metal electrode is placed in an electrolyte solution, there is a tendency for metal ions to be released into solution and for ions in solution to attach to the electrode. As a result of the redistribution of ions that occurs when the metal electrode enters solution, the electrode develops a double layer of charge. It is not possible to measure the actual charge potential generated at a single electrode, since voltage potential at one point must always be measured in reference to some other point. If a

extracellular electrode in Figure 1 records a progressively positive deflection as the positive end of the dipole approaches the electrode. When the dipole is directly underneath the electrode, the positive and negative ends of the dipole result in a return of the deflection to baseline (Fig. 1C). As the dipole moves away from the recording site, a progressively larger negative deflection is recorded through the electrode (Fig. 1D).

second electrode identical to the first is placed in the same solution, the same potential is generated at this electrode as the first, and the net difference between the two is zero. In this system any voltage charges above zero that are recorded must result from an external event, not the electrodes themselves. If the second electrode is of a different material from the first, the difference between them is not zero, and in fact, a galvanic cell is created; however, there is a stable potential over which an external electrical event can be superimposed.

In biologic systems, body fluids such as blood and interstitial fluid serve as the electrolyte solution into which extracellular electrodes are placed. Recording from a beating heart imposes a number of limitations concerning the electrode/tissue interface that must be addressed when selecting an appropriate electrode system.

Random ionic reactions between metal electrodes and tissue electrolytes disturb the layer of electric charges at the electrode/tissue interface and are recorded as noise and drift. Electrodes should be constructed from materials with stable electrode to electrolyte properties and thus less liable to polarization. Some electrode systems require time to equilibrate with the tissue electrolytes. Silver, platinum, and silver/silver chloride have all been found to be excellent materials. Disruption of the electrode/electrolyte connection as a result of motion can cause artifacts. Local injury due to tissue damage and inflammation at the site of electrode contact may predominate or overwhelm whatever changes in voltage potential are taking place from the biologic event.

Electrode impedance is a function of both resistance and capacitance at the electrode/electrolyte interface. The impedance of the electrode depends not only on the material from which it is made but also the size of the electrode: the larger the electrode area, the smaller the impedance.

Bipolar Versus Unipolar

Electrograms can be recorded in either a bipolar or a unipolar fashion. Bipolar electrodes

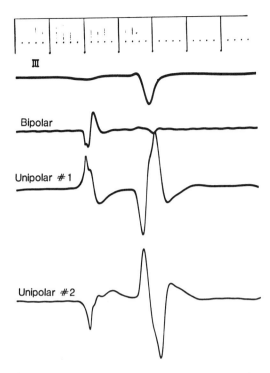

Figure 2 Comparison of bipolar and unipolar electrograms. Unipolar electrogram 1 was recorded from the positive terminal. Unipolar electrogram 2 was recorded from the negative terminal. The bipolar electrogram was recorded from the active poles of the two unipolar electrodes. The bipolar electrogram is narrower and shorter than the unipolar electrograms, suggesting that there is some canceling out of potential changes between them.

are closely spaced with respect to each other, usually 1–20 mm in distance. The electrograms recorded reflect the difference between the potential changes recorded by both poles. Unipolar electrograms also reflect the potential differences between two electrodes, but in this case only one of the electrodes is close to the source of biopotential. The other electrode, the "indifferent" electrode, is far from the source of biopotential and is considered to have a stable potential. As can be seen in Figure 2, a bipolar recording is essentially the sum of the two unipolar recordings.

The electrograms generated by unipolar and bipolar methods have different characteristics, and either may be useful in specific conditions. Since bipolar electrodes reflect mainly the electrical activity of the tissue between them and little far-field activity, the electrograms tend to be small and discrete. The size and shape of electrograms depends on the orientation of the bipolar electrodes with respect to the direction of conduction. Because they represent local electrical activity, bipolar electrograms are most useful to measure local activation times, sequence of activation in mapping studies, and local electrical events, such as bundle of His depolarization. Unipolar electrograms, in contrast, reflect not only potential generated under the active electrode but also to some extent the electrical activity of the whole heart; therefore, unipolar electrograms are larger and wider. The direction of propagation relative to the electrode can be assessed by its polarity; that is, with the active electrode connected to the positive input of the amplifier, positive deflection indicates impulse propagation toward the recording site and negative deflection, away from it. Unipolar recordings are most useful for measurements of QRS duration, T wave analysis, and isopotential distribution (7).

Examples of Specific Electrode Designs and Their Uses

Multipolar Endocardial Catheters

This electrode design provides an advantage in that it can be percutaneously inserted into a peripheral blood vessel and passed to the heart. The electrodes, variable in number, are usually made of platinum. The rest of the catheter consists of an insulated multifilar metal lead with multiple terminals corresponding to the electrodes. These catheters can be used for unipolar or bipolar recording.

Suction Electrodes

The major use of suction electrodes is for recording monophasic action potentials. Negative pressure from suction brings the electrode into contact with the myocardium, causing injury to cell membranes. The injured cells are no longer excitable, but membrane potential changes in the adjacent normal tissue can still be recorded. These potential changes produce an electrogram that corresponds to a proportion of the transmembrane action potential and

accurately reflect repolarization phenomena as recorded with intracellular electrodes (8,9).

Needle Electrodes

Stable intracardiac extracellular recordings can be obtained with plunge electrodes inserted directly into the myocardium, usually through a small needle. Recordings may be bipolar or unipolar. These electrodes can be used to record subendocardial or intramyocardial electrical activity.

Wick Electrodes

Wick electrodes are called nonpolarizable because the metal electrode is not in direct contact with the tissue (10). Instead, a thread or a string is in contact with the biologic system and an electrolyte solution connects the string and the electrode wire. This electrode is nontraumatic since the only part in contact with myocardial tissue is a piece of cotton soaked in electrolyte solution. For this reason wick electrodes are ideal for evaluation of repolarization phenomena.

Other Technical Considerations in Extracellular Recordings

Even with stable electrodes constructed from ideal material, optimal recordings depend on appropriate attention to the amplifiers, gains, or filters used. Since the biopotentials generated by biologic events are quite small, of the order of a few millivolts, amplifiers are necessary to enlarge the signal. Amplifiers are designed to record and amplify desired signals while eliminating other extraneous electrical events, such as 60 cycle interference. Capacitor-coupled (AC) amplifiers are more widely used for extracellular recordings than direct-coupled (DC) amplifiers, because capacitor-coupled amplifiers allow different filterings, higher gains, and neutralization of potential changes due to electrode-tissue interaction. Amplifiers used to record low voltage potential need to have high-input impedance. A high-input impedance is necessary to attenuate the noise that would otherwise result from the current drawn into the amplifier system. Additionally, common mode rejection allows the amplifier to disregard identical sig-

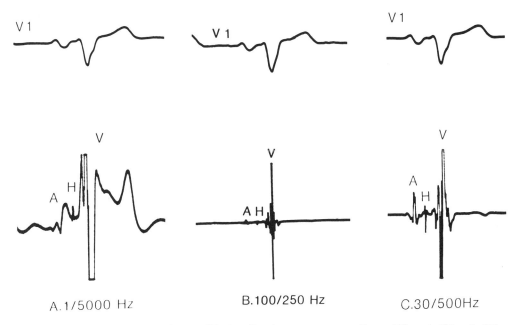

Figure 3 Effect of filter setting on His bundle electrograms recordings: (A) underfiltered; (B) over-filtered; (C) optimum filter settings.

nals, such as 60 cycle interference, picked up from all electrode sources. Variable gain settings allow the size of the generated potential to be enlarged by increasing the voltage output of the amplifier by a multiple of the input voltage. The ideal gain setting is that which allows the biopotential to be clearly seen with a minimal amount of noise.

Although gain settings increase or decrease the amplitude of the entire signal, filter settings allow the investigator to attenuate aspects of the signal based on frequency. Filters help minimize the effects of drift, motion artifacts, and electronic noise on extracellular recordings. The high-frequency (low-pass) filter attenuates signals above a given frequency. The low-frequency (high-pass) filter attenuates signals below a certain frequency. Notch filters are used to help eliminate 60 cycle interference. An example of the dramatic effect filters can have on His bundle recording is illustrated in Figure 3. At extremely low, low-frequency and high, high-frequency filter settings (Fig. 3A) the channel is essentially open (i.e., the signal is relatively unfiltered) and the resulting recording has an excess of unwanted electrical activity. On the other

hand, hand, high, low-frequency and low, high-frequency filter settings attenuate the tracings to such a degree that valuable information is lost (Fig. 3B). For extracellular His bundle recordings, the optimal settings have been found to be a low-frequency setting of 30 Hz and a high-frequency setting of 500 Hz (Fig. 3C). Proper grounding, in addition to being necessary for safety reasons, also helps to eliminate 60 cycle interference by shielding the electrodes from electrical noise from outside sources.

EXTRACELLULAR RECORDING OF SPECIFIC STRUCTURES

The Sinus Node

Studies carried out in dogs and humans have reported various deflections preceding the P wave (11–15). Later studies by Cramer et al. demonstrate conclusively the characteristics of pacemaker activity in the rabbit and canine sinus node (16,17). The pacemaker activity of the sinus node consists of two slow negative-going deflections, a diastolic slope corresponding to phase 4 and an upstroke slope corresponding to phase 0 of the sinus nodal

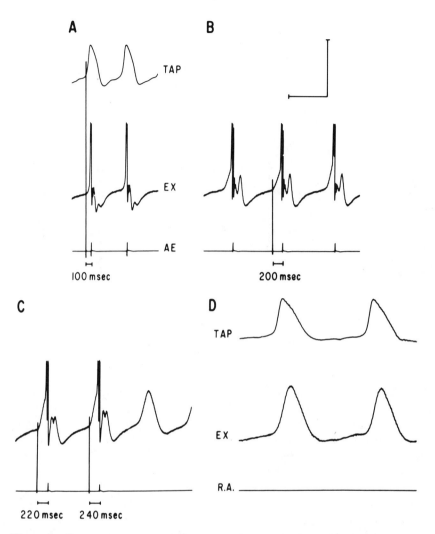

Figure 4 Sinus nodal electrogram recorded in the in vitro canine preparation of the sinus node. During control (A) and during tetrodotoxin superfusion (B, C, and D) transmembrane action potentials of the sinus node (TAP), extracellular electrograms (EX), and a reference right atrial electrogram (AE and RA) are recorded simultaneously. Diastolic and upstroke slopes in EX correspond to phase 4 and phase 0 in TAP. Tetrodotoxin gradually prolongs the sinoatrial interval (100 msec in A and 220–240 msec in C) measured from the beginning of the upstroke slope (vertical cursor) to the beginning of atrial activity in AE. TAP was not recorded in B and C because of microelectrode dislodgment. When atrial activity is completely suppressed by tetrodotoxin (D), synchronous sinus nodal activity can be seen in both TAP and EX. The vertical bar is 80 mV in TAP and 100 μV in EX. The horizontal bar is 200 msec in A, B, and C and 400 msec in D. Polarity of unipolar recording in EX is reversed. (Reproduced from Ref. 7 with the permission of Technical Publishing Co.)

pacemaker activity (Fig. 4). These slow negative-going deflections precede the primary negativity due to conduction of atrial impulses moving away from the recording site (18). In Figure 4, tetrodotoxin prolongs the sinoatrial interval before completely abolish-

ing the atrial activity and thereby resulting in synchronous deflections recorded in the extracellular and intracellular tracings.

Application of the unipolar recording technique using reversed-polarity, low-pass filters (0.1–30 Hz or DC recording) and high ampli-

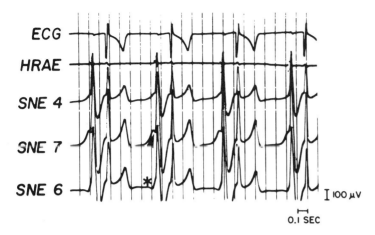

Figure 5 Electrograms recorded from three adjacent sites in the sinus node region of a conscious dog. Diastolic slope, upstroke slope, and primary negativity are recorded from site 4 (SNE 4). Diastolic slope, upstroke slope, a slow positive deflection (arrowhead), and primary negativity are recorded from site 7 (SNE 7). Diastolic slope, a slow positive deflection (asterisk), a slow negative deflection, and primary negativity are recorded from site 6 (SNE 6). ECG = electrocardiogram, HRAE = high right atrial electrogram, SNE = sinus nodal electrogram. Voltage calibration is for SNE. See text for details. (Reproduced from Ref. 10 with the permission of the American Heart Association, Inc.)

fication (100 μV/cm) in dogs and humans using probe, plaque, and catheter electrodes further proves that the deflections are specific for sinus nodal pacemakers (17,19,20). In addition to the negative-going diastolic and upstroke slopes seen preceding the primary negativity in vitro (16,17), two other types of slow positive-going deflections preceding the primary negativity are seen in the conscious dog model for sinus node studies (20). The first type follows the negative-going upstroke slope and precedes the primary negativity (Fig. 5, arrowhead). This type of slow positive-going deflection is frequently seen in association with a relative long sinoatrial interval and most likely represents phase 3 of sinus nodal action potential. The second type of slow positive-going deflection follows the negative-going diastolic slope and precedes a slow negative-going upstroke slope or primary negativity (Fig. 5, asterisk). This type of slow positive-going deflection, typically recorded from an area adjacent to sites from which both diastolic and upstroke slopes are recorded, most likely represents conduction through the sinus node toward the recording site.

Figure 6 shows a diagram that explains the origin of various deflections recorded from the sinus node region. The diagram shows a cross section through the sinus node and the right atrium, four terminals on the epicardial surface, the local changes in transmembrane potential, the extracellular current caused by local differences in transmembrane potential, and also the extracellular potential differences caused by the currents. In the diagram, each box represents a group of automatic cells in the sinus node. Early during the diastolic interval of the automatic cells, there is a potential gradient between automatic cells (−50 mV) and atrial cells (−90 mV) that causes current to flow extracellularly to the automatic cells. This current increases in magnitude as the potential gradient increases during phase 4 depolarization of the automatic cells and is responsible for the negative-going diastolic slope in the sinus electrograms. Thus, in Figure 6A, all four electrograms show a diastolic slope. In Figure 6B, the automatic cells under terminal 1 develop early phase 0 of the action potential, which causes a gradient in intracellular potential between this group of cells and the adjacent cells, a more intense local current, and the beginning of upstroke slope in sinus electrogram recorded through terminal 1. The next extracellular current at any point

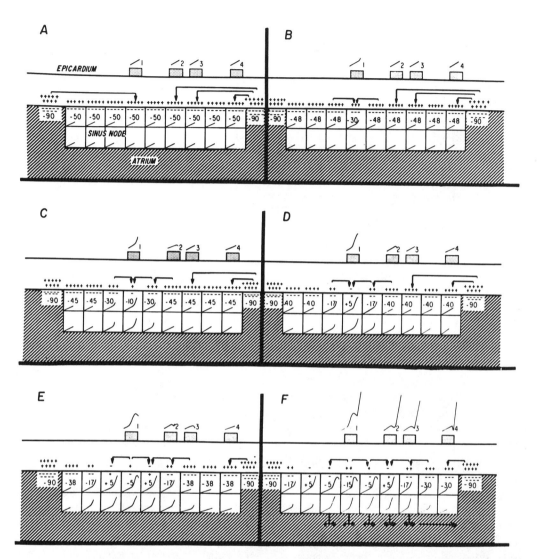

Figure 6 A diagram showing how various deflections recorded from the sinus nodal region can be related to changes in transmembrane potentials. The square indicates groups of automatic cells within the sinus node, and the shaded area, the right atrium. The numbers in the squares and in the shaded area indicate the magnitude of transmembrane potentials. The + and − signs are estimates of the positivity and negativity outside and inside these cells. Arrows in the clear area indicate extracellular current flow; arrows in the shaded area, impulse propagation in the right atrium. Deflections inside the square indicate transmembrane action potentials of the automatic cells; deflections above electrode bars 1–4 indicate the recorded extracellular potentials from these sites. See text for details. (Reproduced from Ref. 10 with the permission of the American Heart Association, Inc.)

depends on the current still engendered by phase 4 depolarization in groups of automatic cells that have not reached the threshold and the current caused by the coupling of adjacent groups, some of which have initiated regenerative response and some have not. In Figure 6C, extracellular current flows from the automatic cells under terminal 2 to the automatic

cells under terminal 1, and as a result, the electrogram from site 2 shows the second type of slow positive-going deflection already described. In Figure 6D, both the negative-going deflection from site 1 and the positive-going deflection from site 2 are larger as a result of increasing net currents flowing into site 1 and out of site 2. In Figure 6E, repolarization of sinus nodal cells under terminal 1 causes a more negative intracellular potential than the adjacent groups, which have more positive intracellular potentials as a result of the action potential upstroke. Thus, extracellular current flows away from the automatic cells of site 1, resulting in the first type of slow positive-going deflection from site 1. At this time, the automatic cells under terminal 2 start a regenerative response that causes a decrease in net extracellular current flowing away from it. The decrease in net current results in reversal of the extracellular deflection recorded from site 2 from positive to negative going. At this time, also, the automatic cells under terminal 3 have a more negative intracellular potential than the adjacent cells, which have undergone partial or complete regenerative excitation; this causes extracellular current to flow away from the automatic cells under terminal 3 to the adjacent cells, resulting in the second type of positive deflection recorded from site 3. In Figure 6F, the net extracellular current flows to automatic cells under terminal 2 because the cells are at the peak of the action potential and are intracellularly more positive than the adjacent cells. The atrium is depolarized as a result of impulse propagation from sites 1, 2, and 3. Therefore, primary negativity is recorded from these sites. The electrogram from site 4 shows a rapid positive-going deflection as a result of atrial impulse propagation toward this site.

Recordings of sinus electrograms have provided better understanding of the physiology of the sinus node in intact hearts. For example, it is now known that sinus arrhythmia is the result of variation not only in sinus cycle length but also variation in sinoatrial intervals and sinus pacemaker location (20). The responses of the sinus node pacemakers of intact hearts to atrial stimulation, vagal stimulation, ouabain, and potassium changes are now better understood as a result of this method (21–23).

The Bundle of His

Extracellular recording of His bundle (H) potential using needle electrodes in intact animal hearts was reported by Alanis et al. in 1958 (24). The biphasic H potential, typically recorded between atrial (A) and ventricular (V) electrograms, was independent of these electrograms. The investigators used atrial pacing, vagal stimulation, and injection of acetylcholine or epinephrine to vary the A-H and H-V intervals and to prove that the H potential indeed represented electrical activity of the His bundle. Other investigators have used plaque electrodes, plunge electrodes, probe electrodes, and catheter electrodes placed in the region of the His bundle and showed high success rates in recording His bundle potential in animals (25–27).

Applications of those recording techniques clinically have not only proved useful for patient management but have also provided better understanding of the anatomy, physiology, and pathology of normal and diseased hearts. During open heart surgery, recording of the His bundle potential is achieved by the use of a probe containing close bipolar electrodes placed in the septal area (28). The technique is useful in aiding cardiac surgeons to localize the His bundle during repair of hearts with complex congenital anomalies or during ablation of septal accessory tracts in patients with Wolff-Parkinson-White syndrome to prevent the occurrence of postsurgical atrioventricular block (29). Significant contributions to the cardiac electrophysiology of the human heart have been made as a result of the ability to record His bundle activity using a catheter electrode inserted transvenously (30). His bundle potential in humans has been recorded using unipolar, close bipolar (interelectrode space 5 mm), or distant bipolar (interelectrode space 5–20 mm) electrodes. Although His bundle potential can be recorded using a wide range of filter settings, the optimal high-pass filters are usually set between 30 and 500 Hz. Catheter recording of the His bundle has proved useful in the diagnosis and treatment of various types of atrioventricular blocks, differentiation of supraventricular and ventricular arrhythmias, and localization of the His bundle before catheter ablative procedures of the atrioventricular conduction system (31,32). In addition, other advances in the understanding of the physiology of the conduction system have resulted from the catheter recording technique.

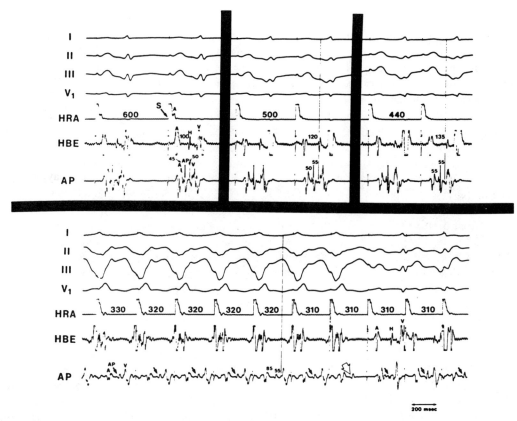

Figure 7   Effect of incremental atrial pacing on conduction through the atrioventricular bypass tract (AP). Recorded are leads I, II, III, and V_1 of the ECG, high right atrial electrogram (HRA), His bundle electrogram (HBE), and AP located in the right posteroseptal area. Note that during incremental atrial pacing the A to AP interval increases from 45 to 85 msec whereas the AP to V interval remains relatively constant at 50–55 msec until block (open arrow) occurs distal to the AP recording site. S = stimulus artifact. AP potentials are labeled as AP or indicated by small arrows. (Reproduced from Ref. 1 with the permission of the American Heart Association, Inc.)

Atrioventricular Bypass Tracts

Using close bipolar electrodes it is possible to record deflections between atrial and ventricular electrograms believed to represent electrical activity from atrioventricular bypass tracts (33–35). Jackman et al. have suggested the use of orthogonal location of the electrodes on the catheter (36), to line up to the direction of impulse propagation to the electrode position and by doing so optimize the recording yield; however, recording of these tracts is also possible using a standard bipolar catheter electrode with 5 mm interelectrode spacing (35). The ability to record the electrical activity of atrioventricular bypass tracts has improved our understanding of characteristics of these tracts:

their refractory periods, patterns of conductions and blocks, and more detailed anatomic location; the last may increase the success rate in transcatheter ablation of these tracts (33–36). Figure 7 shows a recording of electrical activity of an atrioventricular (AP) bypass tract localized to the right posterior septal area of the atrioventricular junction. This AP deflection precedes the onset of the delta wave on the surface ECG by 15 msec. Atrial pacing at gradually decreasing cycle length results in lengthening of the A to AP intervals from 45 to 85 msec and relatively constant AP to V intervals of about 50–55 msec. A conduction block below the site of AP recording is also noted during atrial pacing (33).

Recording of Other Areas of the Heart

Recording of electrical activity from the atria, the ventricles, the atrioventricular junction, and the coronary sinus has contributed to our knowledge of the arrhythmias arising from or supported by changes in the electrical properties of this area. The information obtained depends to a large extent on the technique used for recording and can be summarized as follows.

Site of Earliest Activation

Recording the sequence of activation using bipolar or unipolar electrodes has been used in electrical mapping to identify the earliest site of activation in the atria or ventricles. Most commonly, high-pass filters are used for this type of recording to achieve a stable baseline in a multitrace recording. Computerized methods using a multiplexer sampling each channel at high frequency (in the range of 1.0 kHz) allow recording from up to a few hundred sites simultaneously.

Continuous/Fractionated Electrical Activity

This type of electrical activity was initially described in ischemic myocardium in dogs (37–39) and later in humans with ventricular arrhythmias (40). Fractionated electrical activity represents slow conduction in the region recorded by the bipolar electrode (40). Continuous electrical activity bridging two consecutive ventricular electrograms during ventricular tachycardia suggests that macroreentry is responsible for the arrhythmia. The continuous activity is due to temporally different activation times recorded through the bipolar electrode. Therefore, the ability to record fractionated or continuous activity is a function of the size of the electrodes and the interterminal distance: that is, the bigger the electrode or the larger the interelectrode distance covering the macroreentry circuit, the greater the ability to record fractionation. The use of composite electrodes to record this type of electrical activity is an example (41). The use of a multiplexer and the construction of isochronal maps provide a more precise definition of the reentrant activity (42,43).

Monophasic Action Potential

Recording of the monophasic action potential allows measurement of the local action potential duration and determination of the onset of depolarization (8). Using Ag/AgCl catheter electrodes it is possible to obtain stable recording the monophasic action potentials in humans (44). Other possible utilizations of the recording of monophasic action potentials include the recording of early and delayed afterdepolarization. This technique may provide more conclusive evidence that early or delayed afterdepolarizations are responsible for clinical arrhythmias (45).

Recording of Phase 4 Depolarization and Delayed Afterdepolarization

Using the unipolar recording technique described for the sinus node (see the Sinus Node), low-pass filters, high amplification in the range of 100 μV/cm, and reversed polarity, it is possible to record diastolic slope from the coronary sinus ostium, atrioventricular junction, or ventricles when these sites become the primary pacemaker of the heart (46–48). The site from which the diastolic slope representing phase 4 depolarization can be recorded is usually small. Figure 8 shows such an example (47). Two unipolar tracing (UE1 and UE2) are recorded through two terminals of plunge electrodes placed in the His bundle area of a dog with junctional rhythm. UE2 shows a large His bundle deflection and a strong diastolic slope. In contrast, UE1 shows no diastolic slope, because terminal 1 is slightly remote from the His bundle area and therefore does not record His bundle activity. During infusion of isoproterenol (Fig. 8B and C) the diastolic slope in UE2 becomes stronger, whereas no diastolic slope is recorded in UE1.

In dogs that underwent ligation of the distal branches of left anterior descending diagonal branches and left circumflex coronary arteries converging at the apex, unipolar recording from the surviving endocardial tissue 24 h postligation shows a negative-going diastolic slope preceding the ventricular beat arising from areas that show the earliest activation. These areas show slow deflections during interectopic pauses and during cessation of the ventricular arrhythmia (Fig. 9). It is likely

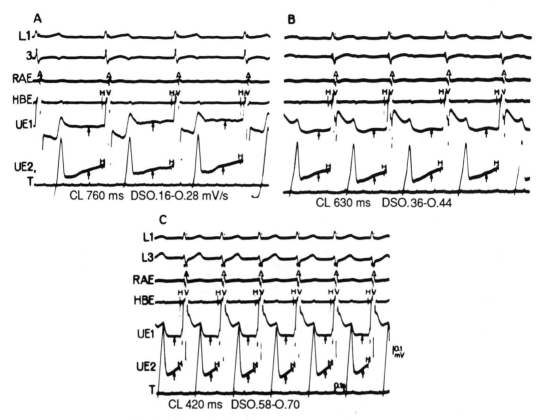

Figure 8 Effect of isoproterenol infusion on two unipolar electrograms recorded from the junctional area in a dog with junctional rhythm. Diastolic slope is noted only in UE2, which shows a His bundle deflection, but not in UE1, which shows no His bundle deflection. Isoproterenol infusion, 0.5 μg/min in B and 2 1g/min in C, decreases the junctional cycle length (CL) and increases the diastolic slope (DS) in UE2 (arrows). No slope is observed during diastole in UE1 throughout isoproterenol infusion. L1 and L3 = two leads to ECG, RAE = right atrial electrograms, HBE = His bundle electrogram recorded bipolarly. Amplification of UE is indicated by vertical bar to the right of C. (Reproduced from Ref. 12 with the permission of the American Heart Association)

that the diastolic depolarization recorded during cessation of the ventricular rhythm represents subthreshold delayed afterdepolarizations (49). Recording of junctional pacemaker activity in the human heart with junctional rhythm has also been reported (50). Because the recording technique is applicable only to rhythm during which there is a clear diastolic separation between cardiac complexes, clinical application of the technique may be limited to slower automatic or triggered rhythms.

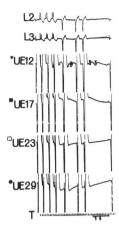
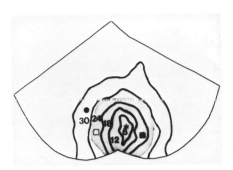

Figure 9   Slow negative-going potentials (arrowheads) recorded from the area of earliest activity during pauses of ventricular ectopic rhythm initiated by stimulated ventricular beats in a dog with a small 1-day-old infarction. The first three beats are stimulated beats. L2 and L3 are surface electrocardiograms. Four unipolar electrograms recorded with high amplifications (UE12, 17, 23, and 29) are displayed with the ECG and time lines (T). The right diagram shows the locations of the electrodes on the endocardial surface of the heart (asterisk for UE12, black square for UE17, open square for UE23, and dot for UE29). The infarction is indicated by the shaded area. Numbers in the diagram indicate 6 msec isochrones. Negative-going diastolic slopes precede the major ventricular deflections in the area of the earliest activation (UE12 and 17). Positive-going slopes precede the major ventricular deflection in unipolar electrograms recorded from areas remote to the area of earliest activity (UE23 and 29). Regular polarity was used for this experiment.

REFERENCES

1. Aidley DG. Electrical properties of the nerve axon. In: The Physiology of excitable cells. Cambridge University Press, 1971:47–52.
2. Jack JJB, Noble D, Tsien RW. Electric current flow in excitable cells. Oxford: Clarendon Press, 1975.
3. Wilson FN, Johnston FD, Rosenbaum FF, Barker PS. On Einhovens triangle, the theory of unipolar electrocardiographic leads, and the interpretation of the precordial electrogram. Am Heart J 1946; 32:277–310.
4. Geselowitz DB. Dipole theory in electrocardiography. Am J Cardiol 1964; 14:301–6.
5. Spach MS, Miller WT, Geselowitz DB, et al. The discontinuous nature of propagation in normal canine cardiac muscle: evidence of recurrent discontinuities of intracellular resistance that affect the membrane currents. Circ Res 1981; 48:39–54.
6. Gardner PI, Ursell PC, Fenoglio JJ, Wit AL. Electrophysiologic and anatomic basis for fractionated electrograms recorded from healed myocardial infarcts. Circulation 1985; 72:596–611.
7. Kupersmith J. Electrophysiologic mapping during open heart surgery. Prog Cardiovasc Dis 1976; 19:167–202.
8. Olsson B, Varnauskas E, Korsgren M. Further improved method for measuring monophasic action potentials of the intact human heart. J Electrocardiol 1971; 4:19–23.
9. Hoffman BF, Cranefield PF, Lepeschkin E, Surawicz B, Herrlich HC. Comparison of cardiac monophasic action potentials recorded by intracellular and suction electrodes. Am J Physiol 1959; 196:1297–1301.
10. Geddes LA. Subintegumental electrodes. In: Electrodes and the measurement of bioelectric events. New York: John Wiley and Sons, 1972:107–37.
11. Hecht HH. Potential variations of the right auricular and ventricular cavities in man. Am Heart J 1946; 32:39–51.
12. Battro A, Bidoggia H. Endocardiac electrocardiogram obtained by heart catheterization in the man. Am Heart J 1947; 33: 604–32.
13. Van der Kooi MW, Durrer D, Van Dam RT, Van der Tweel LH. Electrical activity in sinus node and atrioventricular node. Am Heart J 1956; 51:684–700.

14. Ramlau RA. Electrograms of the sinu-atrial node in dogs following surgical implantations of electrodes on the epicardium. J Electrocardiol 1974; 7:137–48.

15. Thery CL, Lekieffre J, Lemaire P, Asseman P, Dupuis B, Warembourg H. L'activite electrique de la region du noeud sinusal. Arch Mal Coeur 1976; 69:661–9.

16. Cramer M, Siegal M, Bigger JT, Hoffman BF. Characteristics of extracellular potentials recorded from the sinoatrial pacemaker of the rabbit. Circ Res 1977; 41:292–300.

17. Cramer M, Hariman RJ, Boxer R, Hoffman BF. Electrograms from the canine sinoatrial pacemaker recorded in-vitro and in situ. Am J Cardiol 1978; 42:939–46.

18. Lewis T, Oppenheimer BS, Oppenheimer A. The site of origin of the mammalian heartbeat, the pacemaker in the dog. Heart 1910; 2:147–69.

19. Hariman RJ, Krongrad E, Boxer RA, Weiss MB, Steeg CN, Hoffman BF. Method for recording electrical activity of the sino-atrial node and automatic atrial foci during cardiac catheterization in humans subjects. Am J Cardiol 1980; 45:775–81.

20. Hariman RJ, Hoffman BF, Naylor RE. Electrical activity from the sinus node region in conscious dogs. Circ Res 1980; 47:775–91

21. Hariman RJ, Hoffman BF. Sinus node function in conscious dogs. Effects of atrial stimulation (Abstract). Am J Cardiol 1979; 43:373.

22. Hariman RJ, Hoffman BF. Effects of ouabian and vagal stimulation on sinus nodal function in conscious dogs. Circ Res 1982; 51:760–8.

23. Hariman RJ, Chen CM. Effects of hyperkalemia on sinus nodal function in dogs: sinoventricular conduction. Cardiovasc Res 1983; 17:509–17.

24. Alanis J, Gonzalez H, Lopez E. The electrical activity of the bundle of His. J Physiol (Lond) 1958; 142:127–40.

25. Hoffman BF, Cranefield PF, Stuckey JH, Bagdonas AA. Electrical activity during the P-R interval. Circ Res 1960; 8:1200–11.

26. Amer NS, Stuckey JH, Hoffman BF, Cappelleti RR, Domingo RT. Activation of the interventricular septal myocardium studied during cardiopulmonary bypass. Am Heart J 1960; 59:224–37.

27. Scherlag BJ, Helfant RH, Damato AN. A catheterization technique for His bundle stimulation and recording in the intact dog. J Appl Physiol 1968; 25:425–8.

28. Stuckey JH, Hoffman BF. Open heart surgery. The prevention of injury to the specialized conducting system. Arch Surg 1962; 85:224–9.

29. Kaiser GA, Waldo AL, Beach PM, Bowman FO, Hoffman BF, Malm JR. Specialized cardiac conduction system. Improved electrophysiologic identification technique at surgery. Arch Surg 1970; 101:673–6.

30. Scherlag BJ, Lau SH, Helfant RH, Berkowitz WD, Stein E, Damato AN. Catheter technique for recording His bundle activity in man. Circulation 1969; 39:13–8.

31. Damato AN, Gallagher JJ, Lau SH. Application of His bundle recordings in diagnosing conduction disorders. Prog Cardiovasc Dis 1972; 14:601–20.

32. Scheinman MM, Evans-Bell T. Catheter ablation of the atrioventricular junction: a report of the percutaneous mapping and ablation registry. Circulation 1984; 70:1024–9.

33. Jackman WM, Friday KJ, Scherlag BJ, Dehning MM, Schechter E, Reynolds DW, Olson EG, Berbari EJ, Harrison LA, Lazzara R. Direct endocardial recording from accessory atrioventricular pathway: localization of the site of block, effect of antiarrhythmic drugs, and attempt at nonsurgical ablation. Circulation 1983; 906.

34. Prystowsky EN, Browne KF, Zipes DP. Intracardiac recording by catheter electrode of accessory pathway depolarization. J Am Coll Cardiol 1983; 1:468–70.

35. Winters SL, Gomes JA. Intracardiac electrode catheter recordings of atrioventricular bypass tracts in Wolff-Parkinson-White Syndrome: techniques, electrophysiologic characteristics and demonstration of concealed and decremental propagation. J Am Coll Cardiol 1986; 7:1392–403.

36. Jackman W, Beck B, Aliot F, Friday K, Lazzara R. Basis for concealed accessory AV pathways (abstract). Circulation 1984; 70(Suppl.II):II-1348.

37. Waldo AL, Kaiser GA. A study of ventricular arrhythmias associated with acute myocardial infarction in the canine heart. Circulation 1973; 47:1222–8.

38. Boineau JP, Cox JL. Slow ventricular activation in acute myocardial infarction. A source of re-entrant premature ventricular contractions. Circulation 1973; 48:702–13.

39. El-Sherif N, Schlerlag BJ, Lazzara R. Electrode catheter recordings during malignant

ventricular arrhythmia following experimental acute myocardial ischemia. Circulation 1975; 51:1003–14.

40. Josephson ME, Horowitz LN, Farshidi A, Kastor JA. Recurrent sustained ventricular tachycardia. 1. Mechanisms. Circulation 1978; 57:431–40.

41. El-Sherif N, Scherlag BJ, Lazzara R, Hope RR. Re-entrant ventricular arrhythmias in the late myocardial infarction period. I. Conduction characteristics in the infarction zone. Circulation 1977; 55:686–702.

42. El-Sherif N, Smith RA, Evans K. Canine ventricular arrhythmias in the late myocardial infarction period. Epicardial mapping of reentrant circuits. Circ Res 1981; 49:255–65.

43. Wit AL, Allessie MA, Bonke FIM, Lammas W, Smeets J, Fenoglio JJ, Jr. Electrophysiologic mapping to determine the mechanism of experimental ventricular tachycardia initiated by premature impulses: experimental approach and initial results demonstrating reentrant excitation. Am J Cardiol 1982; 49:166–85.

44. Hoffman BF, Cranefield PF, Lepeschkin E, Surawicz B, Herrlich HC. Comparison of cardiac monophasic action potentials recorded by intracellular and suction electrodes. Am J Physiol 1959; 196:1297–1301.

45. Franz MR. Long-term recording of monophasic action potentials from human endocardium. Am J Cardiol 1983; 51:1629–34.

46. Ben-David J, Zipes DP. Differential response to right and left ansae subclaviae stimulation of early afterdepolarizations and ventricular tachycardia induced by cesium in dogs. Circulation 1988; 78:1241–50.

46. Hariman RJ, Cramer M, Naylor RE, Hoffman BF. Coronary sinus rhythm in dogs. Induction, recording and characteristics (abstract). Am J Cardiol 1980; 45:492.

47. Hariman RJ, Chen CM. Recording of diastolic slope from the junctional area in dogs with junctional rhythm. Circulation 1983; 68:636–43.

48. Hariman RJ, Gough WB, Gomes JAC, El-Sherif N. Recording of diastolic slope in a canine model of automatic and unifocal ventricular tachycardia (abstract). J Am Cardiol 1983; 1:731.

49. Hariman RJ, Holtzman R, Gough WB, Mehra R, Gomes JAC, El-Sherif N. In vivo demonstration of delayed afterdepolarization as a cause of ventricular rhythms in a day old infarction (abstract). J Am Coll Cardiol 1984; 3:478.

50. Hariman RJ, Gomes JAC, El-Sherif N. Recording of diastolic slope with catheters during junctional rhythm in humans. Circulation 1984; 69:485–91.

2

Standard and Ion-Selective Microelectrodes

Karl P. Dresdner, Jr.*

College of Physicians and Surgeons, Columbia University
New York, New York

INTRODUCTION

The objective of this chapter is to provide an introductory view of the practical details of making and using standard and ion-selective microelectrodes (ISE). For additional details note that a complete treatise on standard microelectrodes was written by Purves in 1981: *Microelectrode Methods for Intracellular Recordings and Iontophoresis* (1). Likewise for additional details note that the most complete treatise on ISE was written by Ammann in 1986: *Ion-Selective Microelectrodes* (2).

First, this chapter describes the basics of the standard microelectrode technique as needed to obtain cardiac cell transmembrane potentials. Second, the chapter describes some of the practical ion-selective microelectrode methods used to measure intracellular ions in cardiac cells.

STANDARD MICROELECTRODE METHODOLOGY: CARDIAC CELL TRANSMEMBRANE POTENTIAL MEASUREMENT USING STANDARD INTRACELLULAR GLASS MICROELECTRODES

Standard Intracellular Glass Microelectrodes

The invention of the microelectrode 40 years ago was an important stimulus to basic cellular electrophysiology. Ling and Gerard in 1949 were among the first to use a glass microelectrode to measure the action potential of the cell (3). The standard intracellular glass microelectrode was subsequently used quite advantageously to study the cellular mechanisms of cardiac arrhythmias (4).

Before machines became available to heat and pull micropipettes from glass tubing, microelectrodes had to be heated and pulled

---

**Present affiliation:* Pennie & Edmonds, New York, New York.

by hand. This manual process required great skill. First a glass capillary tube was twisted over a gas flame, and once it softened it was rapidly pulled in a straight line. Micropipettes with a straight needle and a submicrometer tip were sought (3). The micropipette was then filled with an aqueous salt solution so that it could function as a microelectrode.

The microelectrode is usually attached to a mechanical micromanipulator so that one can precisely control the advancement of the microelectrode tip into the cell. When the microelectrode pierces the cell membrane the microelectrode's potential shifts rapidly negatively to the resting membrane potential. In cardiac cells, which fire action potentials continuously, the most negative potential observed during diastole is frequently studied as one might study a resting potential. This is termed the "maximum diastolic potential."

Selection and Treatment of Glass Tubing

Before pulling micropipettes glass tubing may have to be cleaned. This cleaning is done by placing the tubing in boiling water, acid, or organic solvents and then drying it at 150°C.

Generally, only one piece of approximately 4 inch long glass tubing is electrically heated and mechanically pulled on a commercial microelectrode puller at a time. This forms two micropipettes. It is important to use a microscope to view the tip shape of freshly pulled micropipettes and establish visual criteria at $\times 400$ magnification.

Standard microelectrodes are made most often from borosilicate glass tubing (Corning Brand 7740). This glass softens at 820°C and has a relatively high specific resisitivity (10^{16} Ω-cm). Alternatively, aluminosilicate glass tubing may be used. Such glass has a 10- to 100-fold higher resistance than No. 7740 borosilicate glass and must be heated to a higher temperature, 915°C, to soften it before pulling. This higher softening temperature may be a disadvantage because it means that a hotter puller temperature is required, and this can greatly increase puller wear.

It used to be a chore to coax the salt solution down into the micropipette tip. It is now standard practice for the electrophysiologist to buy glass capillary tubing that is made with a fine inner filament. This inner filament lowers the filling solution surface tension inside the micropippete. The micropipette tip now automatically fills when exposed to an aqueous salt solution (5).

Selection of a Micropipette Puller

The three most common machines used to pull microelectrodes are (1) the David Kopf 700C vertical puller, (2) the Narishige PE-2 vertical puller, and (3) the Brown & Flaming microprocessor-controlled horizontal puller. The Kopf 700C vertical puller (Tujunga, CA) is the least expensive of the three, but it can make quality microelectrodes from 1–2 mm borosilicate glass tubing.

The Narashige PE-2 vertical puller (Narashige Co., Tokyo, Japan) costs more but can pull thicker types of single-barreled glass, double-barreled glass, and aluminosilicate glass. Finally, the Brown & Flaming model (Sutter Instruments, San Rafael, CA) is an expensive, horizontal puller specialized for the construction of high-resistance microelectrodes used to impale disaggregated single cells. The Brown & Flaming puller has many adjustments to optimize micropipette characteristics. Also, the adjustments are stored in computer memory in the puller.

Selection of Microelectrode Electrical, Tip, and Taper Characteristics

Selection of intracellular glass microelectrode electrical, tip, and taper characteristics are designed to obtain fast cardiac action potential upstroke characteristics. Studies indicate that the transmembrane potential during diastole is -100 to -50 mV negative to the bulk extracellular fluid (6). When an action potential fires the transmembrane potential rapidly depolarizes to 0–40 mV in only 1–2 msec. In the mammalian heart the action potential repolarizes in 20–500 msec.

If one is to accurately record the rapid cardiac action potential upstroke transient, then the responsiveness of the intracellular microelectrode should better than 10 times faster than the rate of action potential depolarization. Since the upstroke occurs in 2 msec, this means that the microelectrode should equilibrate in 0.2 msec. Assuming the equilibration is exponential, then the equilibration time equals approximately five time-constant periods, known as RC times. In this case the intracellular microelectrode RC time is less than 0.2 divided by 5, or less than 0.040 msec (1).

The intracellular microelectrode RC time is the product of the intracellular microelectrode circuit resistance (R in ohms) and the intracellular microelectrode circuit capacitance (C in farads). The largest contributor to R and C is generally the microelectrode tip. RC is varied by altering the configuration of the microelectrode tip through changes in puller settings. The amount of heating to soften glass tubing and the strength of the pull are the basic settings that are changed.

Basically how the puller setting influences the microelectrode R and C values is now described. For cardiac cells intracellular microelectrodes usually require that R be between 10 and 20 $m\Omega$. For single cells R must be higher (7). The intracellular microelectrode capacitance C is usually less than 2 pF (1). C is largest at the microelectrode tip, where the glass tubing has the thinnest walls. The walls act as a dielectric for the capacitor. The thinner the dielectric between two conducting solutions, the larger is the capacitor. Thus one can try to not have microelectrodes taper too slowly. During tissue bath experiments a minimum depth of solution over the tissue also helps to diminish C. This is important if the goal of the experiment is to measure the maximum upstroke velocity of the cell (dV/dt_{max}).

Thus RC is 0.02–0.04 msec when R is 10–20 $M\Omega$ and C is 2 pF, and 5 RC is 0.1–0.2 msec. The RC time constant can be further reduced by fine-tuning the circuit capacitance. This is explained further in the section on minimizing circuit capacitance. However, let us first consider how to make a microelectrode that has a good tip shape.

Good Tip Shape: The Value of Proper Puller Settings

Heat Setting

An important step in the art of making a microelectrode is choosing optimal puller settings. Proper selection of the heating coil current (H) and the puller solenoid strength (P) are important. Extreme H values cause distortion of the micropipette tip taper and shape. Low heat during the pull produces a short micropipette that may break prematurely during the operation. Such micropipettes cannot be used to make intracellular measurements. Alternatively, high heat oversoftens the glass, and the formed micropipettes have too long a taper. These tapers are too flexible for successful cell membrane penetration.

Puller Setting

If the puller setting on the softened glass tubing is too weak, then the micropipette tip is too large. On the other hand, a strong puller setting causes the micropipette tip to be too small and its R value too high. High-resistance microelectrodes produce noisy measurements and respond too slowly during the upstroke. The noise may interfere with resolution of the cardiac action potential. Thus trial-and-error studies are required to find suitable micropipette settings for the heat and pull. In this regard room temperature should be kept stable. For long-term storage micropipettes should be stored in a low-humidity container, such as a desiccator, to avoid tip damage and dust.

Selection of the Microelectrode Electrolyte Filling Solution

Aqueous 3 M potassium chloride solution is the standard internal filling solution for intracellular microelectrodes (8,9). The filling solution is delivered by a syringe with a long wire needle (22–26 gauge). Batches of microelectrodes are best immersed in the filling solution for at least several hours before their use. This allows the air bubbles trapped in their tips to dissolve. It is commonly believed that the storage of microelectrodes in the filling solution for more than a few days is undesirable because this may erode the sharp edges of the microelectrode tip.

A 3 M KCl filling solution is not physiologic. The concentration of cytoplasmic potassium is 150 mM in heart cells (10). Adrian reported in 1956 that 3 M KCl was a useful microelectrode filling because it greatly suppressed a microelectrode tip potential artifact (8,9). The artifact was as much as 10–30 mV if 150 mM KCl or NaCl was the filling solution. The tip potential artifact disappeared after the microelectrode tip was broken to a large diameter.

According to theory a microelectrode tip potential artifact occurs if the free diffusion of the filling solution cations or anions out of the microelectrode tip is impaired (9). The inner glass walls of the microelectrode, being negatively charged, may bind cations, thus slowing the rate of free diffusion of the cations out of the microelectrode tip. When the KCl filling solution is concentrated the tip potential artifact is smaller, apparently because the average ionic diffusion rate is less impaired. When the intrinsic rates of free diffusion of the cation and anion in the filling solution are different, as with NaCl, then employing a high salt concentration does not adequately reduce the tip potential artifact (8). KCl solutions are preferred over most other salt solutions for the simple reason that the intrinsic rates of diffusion of K^+ and Cl^- are nearly the same. Lithium acetate (1 M) is a filling solution that can be used when a Cl^-- or K^+-free solution is sought, since lithium and acetate have similar rates of free diffusion (2).

If a filling solution other than 3 M KCl or 1 M lithium acetate is to be used, then the tip potential error should be estimated. Note the approach in Reference 10, where 1 M KCl and the mixture of 0.150 M KCl and 0.850 M NaCl were used instead of 3 M KCl. Double-barreled microelectrodes were used in experiments on cardiac Purkinje cells. One barrel was filled with aqueous 3 M aqueous KCl, and the other barrel was filled with 1 M KCl or a mixture of 150 mM KCl and 850 mM NaCl solution. In these tests the double-barreled microelectrode measured the transmembrane potential twice in the same cell.

The mean difference in the potentials of the two microelectrode barrels was the difference in the tip potentials of the two barrels (10).

Plugging the Microelectrode Tip

Microelectrode tips frequently plug with cell debris during attempts to make cell punctures. This is commonly seen during experiments as a sudden shift in the microelectrode baseline potential and constitutes an increase in the tip potential. It may also occur spontaneously. Plugging of the microelectrode tip also increases the microelectrode resistance R and the noise.

Microelectrode resistance should be monitored. A resistance measuring circuit is included in most standard microelectrode amplifiers. Usually by a switch one passes a 1 nA pulse through the microelectrode circuit to determine R. A 1 nA pulse generates a 10 mV baseline signal deflection (V = IR by Ohm's law) for every 10 MΩ of microelectrode resistance. Microelectrodes should be discarded when microelectrode resistance has increased or decreased significantly. A reduced microelectrode resistance indicates that the microelectrode tip has broken and may be too large to insert into cells.

Other Precautions

Several other precautions are noteworthy. Because the microelectrode is electrically connected to the microelectrode amplifier via a silver/silver chloride (Ag/AgCl) wire or pellet electrode, KCl evaporation at the Ag/AgCl electrode causes an unstable voltage offset. This can be avoided by preventing evaporation by sealing the end of the microelectrode. In addition, all filling solutions should always contain several millimolar Cl⁻ ions to stabilize the potential at the Ag/AgCl electrode junction.

Another common problem arises when the outside of the microelectrode shaft is contaminated by dried filling solution salt. This short-circuits the microelectrode. It is easily avoided by washing the microelectrode shaft (by dipping) in a beaker of distilled water, followed by drying the glass shaft with a paper towel.

Minimizing Circuit Capacitance

To enhance microelectrode response time (RC product), microelectrode capacitance C should be minimized as much as possible. To reduce C use a shallow bath so that the microelectrode tip is immersed only 2 mm. Second, shorten the length of wire running from the microelectrode to the amplifier to less than 2 inches. This is automatically done with most commercial microelectrode equipment, which positions the preamplifier stage immediately behind the microelectrode.

The capacitance of the microelectrode circuit under experimental conditions may be reduced by *tuning* a capacitance neutralization circuit. This is a standard feature with most commercial microelectrode amplifier systems. The tuning must be carefully accomplished, or damage to circuits, microelectrode, and cell results. The end point for circuit capacitance neutralization is determined using a circuit square-pulse signal.

Use a triangle ramp voltage pulse, which is differentiated by a 1 pF capacitor in parallel with the bath ground wire. This delivers a square pulse to the microelectrode circuit. Through adjustments of the capacitance neutralization at the preamplifier stage the square pulse *leaving* the amplifier is squared as well as possible. Capacitance is slightly underneutralized when the pulse out remains slightly rounded. This is preferred to overneutralized capacitance, however, as indicated by a rippled square-pulse output. This latter situation is more likely to oscillate out of control.

Standard Microelectrode Cell Impalement Criteria

The standard intracellular glass microelectrode should have an outer tip diameter less than 1 μm to minimize damage to the cell during impalement (6,10). The microelectrode tip size should puncture the cell membrane of the cardiac cell without causing excessive damage. The degree to which one meets the criteria for a quality cell membrane impalement is easily determined (10).

First, acceptable impalement of a cell should cause a nearly instantaneous change in microelectrode output potential from the baseline value in the extracellular fluid to the cell's value.

Second, clean impalements should result in stable resting potentials in quiescent cardiac cells, and in repetitively firing cardiac cells the action potential waveform should be artifact free, reproducible, and stable from one action potential to the next. It should be comparable to published data on such action potentials.

Third, upon withdrawal of the microelectrode from the cell into the tissue bath the potential observed in the extracellular fluid should be the same (or within 1 or 2 mV) as the value before the cell impalement. An example meeting these three criteria is the record of the heart cell impalement ($V_1 = V_m$ in Fig. 1) by the reference barrel of a double-barreled K^+-sensitive microelectrode shown in Figure 1.

ION-SELECTIVE MICROELECTRODE METHODOLOGY

Transmembrane ion gradients are known to have important roles in cell and organ function. Transcellular gradients for K^+ (potassium ion), Na^+ (sodium ion), Ca^{2+} (calcium ion), Mg^{2+} (magnesium ion), pH, and Cl^- (chloride ion) have been studied using ion-selective microelectrodes. Walker was among the first to successfully make K^+-sensitive microelectrodes (K-ISE) and measure the free concentration of K^+ in the cardiac extracellular and intracellular space (11). This required placing both a K-ISE and a standard microelectrode in the cell cytoplasm. The transmembrane potential had to be subtracted from the K-ISE to obtain the potential due to K^+ changes alone. This subtraction is required for all intracellular ISE ion measurements.

Only the open tip of an ion-selective microelectrode is ion sensitive. The tip normally contains a small column of an ion-selective organic liquid. Fluka Chemical Co. and Corning Chemical Co. (Corning, NY) sell ion-selective organic liquid membranes (''resins'') that

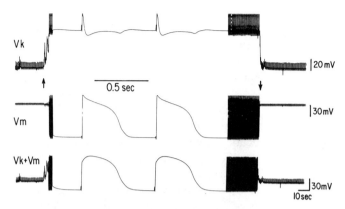

Figure 1 Using a double-barreled potassium-sensitive microelectrode the intracellular potassium ion activity and transmembrane potential of a canine subendocardial Purkinje cell was studied. The separate outputs of the two barrels of the K-ISE are shown, and the differential ouput E_{2-1} is labeled V_k. The reference barrel V_2 is labeled V_m. V_m displays a normal resting and action potential. The action potential measured by the ISE electrode $E_{2-1} + V_2$ is labeled $V_k + V_m$ and is slightly rounded owing to diminished electrode response time. The upward arrow indicates the impalement, and the downward arrow withdrawal of the double-barreled microelectrode. The chart recorder speed is briefly increased to show two action potentials. The intracellular potassium activity is calculated from the increase in V_k, the difference trace. V_k is free of artifacts only between action potentials. The figure was obtained using a Gould chart recorder with 60 Hz frequency response.

measure K^+, Na^+, Ca^2, Mg^{2+}, H^+, or Cl^- (free ion concentration or ion activities). The ion-selective membrane forms an equilibrium *potential* E across the ion-selective liquid membrane. The equilibrium potential can be correlated with the chemical gradient across the ISE membrane by using the Nicolsky-Eisenmann equation, an extended form of the Nernst equation. The ISE potential is calibrated in solutions of different ion concentration having a constant ionic strength. Once an ISE has been fabricated and calibrated it is usually used without delay because its function usually lasts less than 12 hr.

Role of the Reference Electrode

It is usually assumed that the extracellular fluid (ECF) is at a ground potential equal to 0 mV. If it is not, then the ISE (ion-selective microelectrode) amplifier offset controls are used to make the ECF potential equal to zero.

An intracellular ISE measures the transmembrane potential of the cell. Let us call its potential V_1. Also, ISEs measure an intracellular equilibrium chemical potential. Let us call the extracellular equilibrium potential of the ISE E_1 and the intracellular equilibrium

potential of the ISE E_2. Assuming the net ISE potential in the extracellular fluid is set to zero potential, the intracellular ISE potential is the sum of the transmembrane potential and the ISE transmembrane chemical equilibrium potential (V_1 plus E_{2-1}). To determine E_{2-1} the experimenter *must* measure the transmembrane potential a second time by using a intracellular reference microelectrode. Let us call its potential V_2. It is assumed that $V_1 = V_2$. This assumption is accurate if a double-barreled ISE is used but is less accurate when the intracellular ISE and intracellular reference microelectrodes are separate (see subsequent discussion and Ref. 10). To calculate E_{2-1} the reference potential V_2 is subtracted from the ISE potential ($E_{2-1} + V_1$).

Figure 1 presents a record of an automated method that uses a θ-style double barreled ISE (DB-ISE). With θ tubing the ISE and reference microelectrode barrels are combined and have a common impalement tip that enters only one cell at a time. Thus a DB-ISE obtains a measurement of V_1 and V_2 in the same cell at the same time. When double-barreled microelectrodes contain 3 M aqueous KCl in both barrels, V_1 and V_2 agree within 1 mV (10).

Because the adjacent barrel contains an ion-selective liquid membrane, leakage of reference barrel electrolyte from the tip is one problem to avoid with DB-ISE. This is because the leaking reference barrel ions may alter the extracellular or intracellular chemical potential, E_1 or E_2, of the ISE. If so, the standard 3 M aqueous KCl filling solution must be replaced by an electrolyte that generates negligible chemical potential on the ISE barrel (10).

Many laboratories have measured intracellular ion levels by the two separate microelectrode technique. This approach requires two simultaneous cell impalements in separate, nearby cells. When V_1 and V_2 are measured in separate cells an error may be produced (7,10,12). Note also that this method assumes good electrical coupling between the cells and that the cells have the same transmembrane potentials.

Which Is the Correct Formalism: Free Ion Concentration or Ion Activity?

Intracellular or extracellular ion levels can be presented as the free ion concentration or as the ion activity. These are interchangeable values, as is explained later. Calibration solutions for ISE use salts that ionize well in solution, and calculation of the free ion concentration in an ISE calibration solution is straightforward.

There is a simple relation between the free ion concentration in a calibration solution and ion activity (13). The ion activity of ion x is A_x. A_x equals the product of the free ion concentration of x, $[C_x]$, and the ion activity coefficient of x. When the activity coefficients are approximated by the Debye-Hückel equation, *monovalent* ions have similar estimated ion activity coefficients, between 0.75 and 0.78 at *constant* physiologic ionic strengths of 0.15–0.16 M (10, 11, 13). By the same equation the *divalent* cations also have similar estimated ion activity coefficients, between 0.30 and 0.35 at *constant* physiologic ionic strengths of 0.15–0.16 M (7,9–13).

In mammalian heart experiments the tissue is superfused by a 0.15–0.16 M solution of salts. Ion activities are easily determined, regardless of the complexity of the aqueous environment. It is often stated that the ISE chemical potential E more exactly reflects ion activities than free ion concentrations (11). When an ISE enters a cell, a different set of ion activities are measured. It is also true that E_{2-1} reflects the ratio between the extracellular and intracellular activities of ion x. As mentioned earlier, the ECF chemical potential of the ISE, E_1, is sometimes set to zero. With E_{2-1} and the extracellular ion activity one may calculate the intracellular ion level (see Fundamental form of the Nicolsky-Eisenmann equation for more details). Sometimes the impetus for using ion activity is that no assumptions need to be made about the cytoplasmic activity coefficient, which is unknown anyway. *It generally agreed that it is a mistake to attempt to calculate an actual intracellular activity coefficient. Apparent cytoplasmic activity coefficients have been calculated from the ratio of the intracellular ion activity to the total cell ion concentration (14).* However, these numbers have merely confirmed the expectation that total cell ion concentrations need not be the same as cytoplasmic ion concentrations. Some of the cell's ions are sequestered in the intracellular organelles (i.e., mitochondria, sarcoplasmic reticulum, and nucleus) at concentrations quite different from those than in the cytoplasm (14).

A second reason ion activity may be used is that the selectivity coefficients used in calculations of the Nicolsky-Eisenmann equation (see later) employ the ion activity rather than free ion concentration values (13).

Electrical Circuitry and Experimental Apparatus Requirements

ISE have high electrical resistance (between 100 and 10,000 mΩ). Changes in E_{2-1} voltages range from 0.5 V maximum to 0.25 mV minimum. These changes must be resolved over baseline noise. A 4% change in monovalent ion activity occurs when E_{2-1} changes by about 1 mV. One uses amplifiers (ISE electrometers) with high-input impedances (at least 1000-fold higher than the resistance of the ISE).

Two suppliers of ISE electrometers in the United States are World Precision Instruments (New Haven, CN) and Bloom Associates (Narbeth, PA). The electrometers have capacitance neutralization and low-pass filters to match the response times of the ISE and reference microelectrodes. In this regard it should be noted that when two separate microelectrodes are used it is seldom possible to obtain a action potential on the ISE barrel. When DB-ISE are used capacitive coupling between barrels occurs. Surprisingly, this helps barrel matching. Only a slight adjustment of the capacitive neutralization on the ISE barrel is required to optimally tune both barrels. The action potential on the barrels of the DB-ISE then become distinct. DB-ISE can distinguish between the action potential waveforms of ventricular muscle and Purkinje cells.

To avoid loss of signal or pickup of noise, wires to the ISE amplifier from the ISE should pass through the air without touching surfaces. The entire electrical system must be isolated inside a metal screen enclosure (Faraday cage) to shield the microelectrode from ac electrical noise. A Narishige hydraulic micromanipulator system (MO-10 or MO-22) can be used by remote control to drive the ISE into cells while the Faraday cage remains closed. The tissue chamber should be electrically insulated. All equipment in the cage must be grounded to to the cage. Obviously no ac electrical equipment should be operative inside the Faraday cage. The entire apparatus can be mounted on an air suspension table to minimize the effects of floor vibrations during cell impalements.

The tissue bath for cardiac tissue superfusion experiments should be grounded to the Faraday cage. There should be only one ground. A good stable ground is made using 6 inches of 1 mm (inner diameter) polyethylene (PE) tubing containing 2 M aqueous KCl congealed in 2% agar. One end of the PE tubing can sit in a well at the downstream end of the tissue superfusion bath while the other end sits in a light- and air-tight 50 ml vial containing 2 M aqueous KCl and a thick wire Ag/AgCl electrode. The Ag/AgCl electrode post is connected to the Faraday cage. If needed an ad-

justable battery can be placed in between the Faraday cage and ground to calibrate the ISE-electrometer circuit. The battery and the electrometer outputs can be quantitatively tested using Fluke LCD digital voltmeters. The use of digital voltmeters to test and precisely calibrate the electrical system is a good way to guarantee experimental accuracy.

Flow of physiologic saline into the tissue bath and flow out to the waste bottle must be carefully designed to avoid noise. Fluid can exit the bath as a drip to reduce this noise problem. The physiologic saline coming into the cage should be delivered by gravity rather than electric pump. Flow of water in the perfusate heat exchanger must be arranged to avoid carrying 60 cycle noise into the Faraday cage. The water pumps for heat exchange are grounded.

Outside the Faraday cage an equipment rack is used to hold the ISE electrometer, oscilloscope, Fluke voltmeters, and other equipment (cell stimulator, strip chart recorder, and personal computer for data files). Illumination should be delivered from an external light source using a fibreoptic light source. This allows illumination of the bath without local heating artifacts or 60 Hz interference.

Choice of Glass Tubing for ISE

Borosilicate glass tubing, 1 or 2 mm Corning 7740) or aluminosilicate glass tubing (Corning 1720) without an internal filament is recommended for construction of single-barreled ISE. ISE are less prone to artifacts when using aluminosilicate glass because of its higher wall resistance (2). However, this glass is more difficult than borosilicate glass to use in the micropipette puller owing to its 95° C higher softening point of 915° C.

Currently, θ-style, double-barreled aluminasilicate glass is not available. Only double-barreled shotgun-style aluminosilicate glass tubing is available. The barrels are poorly bonded, and it makes unsuitable DB-ISE micropipettes. These lack a single common point and thus are not appropriate for cardiac cell impalements.

The 2.2–2.7 mm OD θ-style, double-barreled borosilicate glass tubing (William

Dehn-R&D Optical, Bethesda, MD) was found to make suitable DB-ISE micropipettes on the Narishige PE-2 puller. The puller heating coil should have two full turns and have a diameter twice that of the widest aspect of the θ-style glass tubing. The tapering portion of the ISE micropipette should be short.

Silanization of the Glass Micropipette

Glass is intrinsically hydrophilic. For ISE the glass must be made hydrophobic because the micropipette tip must retain a short column of organic, ion-selective liquid resin. The tip is therefore silanized to render the inner micropipette wall hydrophobic. The silanizing chemical is a silicon-based molecule with alkyl side chains (typically one to four carbons), such as monochlorotrimethylsilane (MCTMS) (15). Silanes have a silyl chloride group that reacts with hydroxyl groups of the glass surface.

It generally thought that having multiple reactive sites per silanizing molecule permits silane molecules to form polymers that could plug the micropipette tip. To avoid this possibility monoreactive silanes are used. Silanization applies a monolayer of hydrophobic silane to the glass surface of the micropipette.

Because silanes react with glass hydroxyl groups and water hydroxyl groups equally well, the glass micropipette must be dry for silanization to be effective. Immediately after glass tubing is electrically heated to 850–950°C to make a micropipette, the tapered region and micropipette tip are dry. Thus micropipettes should be silanized as soon as the micropipettes are pulled. It is desirable to keep the laboratory room humidity low and the glass tubing as dry as possible. Many methods of silanization have been described (2,3,10–15). All depend upon the presence of glass hydroxyl groups for the silanizing chemical reaction. Work in a ventilated hood, and avoid inhalation of the fumes because they are toxic.

To silanize the microelectrode tips place single-barreled micropipettes horizontally in a 10 cm diameter covered Pyrex petri dish and heat by electric hot plate to 200°C. Expose to several small drops of silane, and cover the dish. Allow about 30 min for silane gas to react fully with the glass micropipettes. Then vent the dish by removing its lid, and allow it to cool.

A more controlled method is required to silanize θ-style double-barreled micropipettes. This is because silanization of the reference barrel must be avoided. Otherwise, during the experiment the silanized reference barrel may attract ion-selective resin from the ISE barrel and become ion sensitive.

After the double-barreled micropipette has been pulled it is tightly capped at its back end with Parafilm (American Can Co., Greenwich, CT). Then one barrel is selected for silanization and labeled. The Parafilm at the back of the barrel to be silanized is punctured using a large-gauge syringe needle.

About 5 ml MCTMS is stored in a 10 ml volumetric flask (with a ground glass stopper). The 10 ml flask is mounted on a rod stand by a strong clamp. Using large forceps the double-barreled micropipette is held upside down in the gas portion of the flask after the stopper is removed. About 1 inch of the double-barreled micropipette is held inside the neck of the flask over the MCTMS liquid. The critical aspect here is the duration of MCTMS gas exposure. The optimal duration of MCTMS exposure is about 12 sec.

The micropipette is then withdrawn and capped with Parafilm. This is done for batches of 6–20 micropipettes. The electrodes are capped for 1 hr to allow diffusion of MCTMS. The Parafilm capping is then removed. Micropipettes were placed horizontally in an open Pyrex petri dish and baked at 120–200° C for several hours. Silanized micropipettes are stored in dry, stable, dust-free containers and used within 2 days to avoid contamination and blockage of the tip by dust. DB-ISE for potassium and pH require more silanization than those for sodium. The reason is not known.

Filling the Silanized Micropipette Tip with Ion-Selective Liquid Membrane

A 5 ml plastic syringe with a 3–4 inch long 28 gauge stainless steel needle is used to deliver a small drop of ion-selective resin into the inner tapering portion of the silanized barrel. Generally the resin runs down into the tip within a few hours. The resin can also be delivered into the tip using a combination of vacuum and pressure perturbations. Pressure changes of several atmospheres are usually needed. Such pressures are easily delivered using a 50 ml syringe via a tightly fitting plastic or elastic rubber tubing on the micropipette. For efficiency the process should be monitored by observation under a microscope at ×100 to ×400.

The resin should not be allowed to enter the tip of the reference barrel of the DB-ISE because this converts the reference barrel into an ISE. Obviously it is also bad if resin does not fill the tip of the ISE barrel. If this happens consistently it suggests that the tips are plugged. The problem may be corrected by shortening the exposure time to MCTMS.

Sometimes filling the reference barrel of the DB-ISE with aqueous filling solution causes the resin to retract from the tip. This makes the ISE effectively nonfunctional. When this problem occurs the micropipette must be discarded.

Use an Internal Ujec Micropipette to Enhance ISE Electrical Response Time

The impedance of the ISE is between 10- and 1000-fold higher than the impedance of the reference microelectrode barrel. This is because the ion-selective resin has a very high resistivity. If the resistance of the resin column in the tip of the ISE can be reduced, it can improve the electrical response time of the electrode. It also reduces ISE drift and lowers noise. Resistance may be minimized by reducing the height of the resin column in the tip to less than 500 μm. However, this causes two new problems. First, the tendency of the resin to float out of the tip is increased. Second, the electrical potential of the ISE may dissipate significantly if the silanized shunt path is shortened. This silanized shunt path is a narrow film space between the ISLM and the walls of the micropipette, and ideally it is composed of only silane molecules. It may contain aqueous fluid as well, however, and

have substantially lower resistance. A long silanized shunt path has higher resistance and reduces ISE failure. Thus it is best to have a resin column height of about 2 mm.

Ujec et al. found an easy method to reduce resistance of single-barreled ISE (16). Ujec inserted an electrolyte-filled micropipette into the barrel of the ISE and advanced it toward the tip as far as possible. This shortened the effective length of the resin column and thus lowered the ISE resistance. For DB-ISE good results are obtained if the internal Ujec pipette is brought to within 500 μm of the ISE tip (10). Also, the ISE backfill solution should be placed in advance of insertion of the Ujec pipette for a distance of about 1 cm behind the resin in the ISE barrel to wash the Ujec pipette.

Fundamental Form of the Nicolsky-Eisenmann Equation

ISE are not perfectly selective for one ion, but particular ISE are relatively selective for one ion of interest in the physiologic environment. If ISE were perfectly selective, the Nernst equation could be used to translate the ISE voltages into ion concentrations, and vice versa. The Nicolsky-Eisenmann equation should be used because it corrects for interfering ions that increase the ISE signal for the primary ion of interest. This equation, by subtracting interfering ion input, allows a proper equation between the ISE electrical signal and the primary ion concentration in the test solution.

For example, to an ISE for ion A 100 mM of an interfering ion B might look like 10 mM of ion A. Thus, if there is 10 mM of ion A present, the addition of 100 mM of B could change the ISE signal to suggest 20 mM of A is present. We could calculate a selectivity coefficient k_{AB} of an A-type ISE for interfering ion B. If A and B are monovalents then k_{AB} is 0.1.

Now let us look at the Nicolsky-Eisenmann equation. The potential of the ISE in the bath is denoted E_1 and is E_2 in the cell or a second salt solution. The general forms of these two equations for ions A, B, . . . , X with valences zA, zB, . . . , zX and selectivity co-efficients k_{AB}, . . ., k_{AX} are as follows:

$$E_1 = \text{slope} \times [\log (A_o + k_{AB}B_o^{zA/zB} + \ldots + k_{AX}X_o^{zA/zX})] \tag{1}$$

and

$$E_2 = \text{slope} \times [\log (A_i + k_{AB}B_i^{zA/zB} + \ldots + k_{AX}X_i^{zA/zX})] \tag{2}$$

$$E_{2-1} = E_2 - E_1 \tag{3}$$

The slope is determined by ISE calibration. The selectivity coefficients are known or calculated. By taking the difference of the ISE chemical potential outside the cell E_1 and the intracellular ISE chemical potential E_2, the change in ion activity from outside to inside the cell is obtained. One can then solve for the intracellular ion activity from E_{2-1} and the extracellular ion activity.

Fundamental Calibration Considerations

Each ISE must be calibrated before it is used to confirm that it is working properly. The calibration data allow the ISE slope and selectivity to be determined. There are different calibration solutions for each kind of ISE. It is beyond the scope of this chapter to define them all. In general, at least six different calibration solutions should be used to encompass the range of ion levels expected to be encountered in the experiments. ISE should be tested repeatedly in calibration solutions for about 1 hr after their construction and before their experimental use. This approach eliminates ISE that will fail prematurely.

A useful calibration system involves using a circular arrangement of six 15 ml plastic cups embedded in ½ inch of paraffin wax in a plastic petri dish. Solutions should be used only a few times during the day and then replaced. This diminishes effects of contamination by the KCl ground electrode. Calibration can be done inside the Faraday cage with the DB-ISE mounted on the manipulator used for experimental measurements.

ISE that can measure intracellular sodium (10,11,13,14), intracellular calcium (11,12, 14,17), intracellular magnesium (11), intra-cellular pH (11,13,18), and intracellular chloride (11,13,14,19–21) in heart cells have been described.

Each kind of intracellular ion measurement has specific features and problems. These features and problems are exemplified in the results that have been obtained for potassium ISE. Thus, the remainder of the chapter focuses on how potassium-selective microelectrodes are used to measure intracellular K^+ in heart cells (3,7,10,11,13,14,18,22–25).

INTRACELLULAR POTASSIUM ION MEASUREMENT BY K-ISE

Normal Cardiac Intracellular K^+ Activity

Cardiac intracellular K^+ activity (aK_i) in mammals (rat, guinea pig, dog, sheep, and baboon) generally ranges between 101 and 125 mM (10,11,14,22,28). The published levels indicate that aK_i is low (83–91 mM) in the rabbit and cat (22). Assuming an activity coefficient of 0.74–0.77 for aK_i, the corresponding free K^+ ion concentration $[K^+]$ ranges between 140 and 170 mM (excluding the known values for the rabbit and cat).

K^+ Liquid Ion-Exchanger Resin Selectivity

Corning liquid ion exchanger 477317 (LIE) contains the lipophilic salt potassium tetrakis (p-chlorophenyl)borate dissolved in 2,3-dimethylnitrobenzene (3,11). For this resin the major interfering ion is the sodium ion. Extracellular $[Na^+]$ is a significant factor because extracellular $[K^+]$ is relatively low, usually between 2 and 6 mM (3,10). The selectivity of the K-ISE to Na^+ (k_{KNa}) averages 0.030

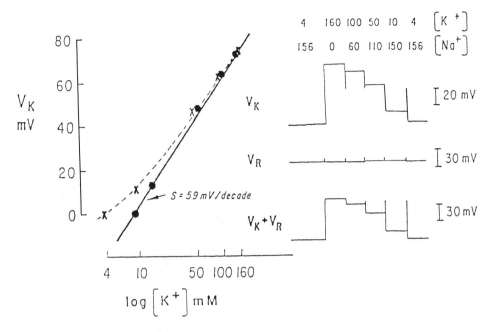

Figure 2 Double-barreled K^+-sensitive microelectrodes are calibrated in 160 mM constant ionic strength mixture solutions of KCl and NaCl. On the right side are records of the steady-state potentials of ion-sensitive barrel output ($E_{2-1} + V_2$), labeled ($V_k + V_r$), the reference barrel output V_1, labeled V_R, and the differential output E_{2-1}, labeled V_k. The graph (left) shows a plot (dashed line) of V_K versus the logarithm of the calibration solution $[K+]$. After correction for Na^+ interference the linear plot (solid line) with slope 59 mV per decade $[K^+]$ at 23°C is obtained.

(3,7,10,11,13,14,18,22–24). Therefore the extracellular $[Na^+]$, typically about 105 mM, adds about 5 mM K^+ to the K-ISE signal. In other words, a K-ISE in a solution of 4 mM $[K^+]$ and 150 mM $[Na^+]$ behaves as though it were in a solution of 9 mM $[K^+]$ (at 0.154 M ionic strength). Other ions, such as the divalents (Ca^{2+} and Mg^{2+}) and H^+, do not interfere with the K-ISE under normal physiologic conditions. However, there is significant interference from essentially all lipophilic cations, such as ammonium, tetramethyl- and tetrabutylammonium, acetylcholine, and procaine. Simple cations, such as Cs^+ and Rb^+, also interfere strongly (2,13).

Backfill Solution for the K-ISE

A typical ISE barrel backfill solution is an aqueous mixture of 4 mM KCl and 156 mM NaCl. The backfill solution behind K^+ LIE should have the same $[K^+]$ as the superfusion bath. This minimizes the sensitivity of the ISE to thermal changes because the electrode's equilibrium potential equals essentially zero. It does not matter then that the electrode's slope is temperature sensitive. To minimize temperature effects it is also helpful to immerse the ISE so that the resin column is below the surface of the bath and thus isothermal (9,26).

The Nicolsky-Eisenmann Equation for the K-ISE

For the K-ISE the form of the Nicolsky-Eisenmann equation needs to deal with a term for extracellular $[Na^+]$ interference:

$$E_1 = \text{slope} \times [\log (aK_o + k_{KNa} \, aNa_o)] \quad (4)$$

$$E_2 = \text{slope} \times \log [aK_i] \quad (5)$$

and

$$E_{2-1} = E_2 - E_1 \quad (6)$$

Here aK_o and aK_i are the extracellular and intracellular K^+ activities and aNa_o is the extracellular sodium ion activity.

K-ISE Calibration

The K-ISE is calibrated in mixtures of KCl and NaCl having a constant ionic strength of 160 mM (2,13). The six recommended aqueous solutions (in millimolar) are

1. 160 KCl
2. 100 KCl + 60 NaCl
3. 20 KCl + 140 NaCl
4. 10 KCl + 150 NaCl
5. 4 KCl + 156 NaCl
6. 4KCl + 125 NaCl + 24 NaHCO$_3$ +
    1 NaH$_2$PO$_4$ + 2.7 CaCl$_2$ + 1 MgCl$_2$

Solution 6 is a mammalian physiologic saline (Tyrode's solution) and should give a calibration potential similar to that of solution 5. When interference for aNa_o is taken into account the K-ISE potential, V_k in Figure 2, becomes linear as a function of the calibration $[K^+]$.

Note that the slope of the K-ISE can be estimated using Equations #4–6 and the change in ISE potential from solution 1 to 2 as evident from Figure 2. The Nernst slope at 24 and 37° C for a perfectly cation-selective membrane is 59.0 and 61.6 mV, respectively, per decade ion concentration change. Slopes within 1 mV of these values have been reported for the K-ISE (2,10,13,14).

Algebraically solving Equation (#4) for k_{KNa} then allows one to determine the selectivity coefficient k_{KNa} from the change in ISE potential between solutions 1 and solution 5. The equation for solving k_{KNa} is

$$k_{KNa} = \frac{\{_{10}[(-E2-E1) / \text{slope}] \times 0.16\} - 0.004}{0.156} \quad (7)$$

Here using Equations (4) through (6) let V_x be the negative change in K-ISE potential seen upon changing from a 160 mM KCl calibration solution (solution 1) to a 4 mM KCl + 156 mM NaCl calibration solution (solution 5). The k_{KNa} averages about 0.030 as mentioned.

Using equations (4) through (6) one can algebraically solve for aK_i (from the values for the K-ISE slope, k_{KNa}, V_x, aK_o, and aNa_o) as follows:

$$aK_i = 10^{(V_x / \text{slope})} (aK_o + K_{KNa} \, aNa_o) \quad (8)$$

Technical Limitations of Intracellular K-ISE Measurements

K-ISE electrochemical response is adequately linear over the biologic range of K^+ encountered, provided one avoids contamination of the K-ISE resin by lipophilic cations.

Once inside a cardiac cell, a K-ISE cannot be used to detect the small changes in K^+ (less than 5 mM) due to changes in membrane Na, K-ATPase activity changes. This is because each millivolt of K-ISE response in the intracellular compartment corresponds to a 4% change in aK_1, which is 101–125 mM (see earlier discussion). In addition, noise may add 0.3 mV to the system. Variations in impalement quality and significant cellular variations in aK_i can lead one to observe substantial cell-to-cell variations in aK_i (10,11,18,22,23). Changes in intracellular Mg^{2+}, Ca^{2+}, pH, and Na^+ do not cause errors when levels of aK_i are normal, but see Chapman et al. (1987) for the K-ISE correction procedures to follow should enormous decreases in aK_i occur with large increases in aNa_i (intracellular sodium activity) (24).

REFERENCES

1. Purves R D. Microelectrode methods for intracellular recordings and iontphoresis. New York: Academic Press, 1981.
2. Ammann D. Ion selective microelectrodes—principals, design and applications. New York: Springer-Verlag, 1986.
3. Ling G, Gerard R W. The normal membrane potential of frog sartorius muscles. J Cell Comp Physiol 1949; 34:383–96.
4. Weidman S. The microelectrode and the heart 1950–1970. In: Kao F F, Koizumi K, Vasalle M, eds. McCusky Brooks—Bologna: Aulo Gaggi, 1971; 3–25.
5. Thomas R C. Intracellular sodium activity and the sodium pump in sail neurones. J Physiol, (Lond) 1972; 220:55–71.

6. Tranum-Jensen J, Janse M J. Fine structural identification of individual cells subjected to microelectrode recordings in perfused cardiac preparations. J Mol Cell Cardiol 1982; 14:233–47.

7. Boyden P A, Albalba A, Dresdner K P. Electrophysiology and ultrastructure of canine subendocardial Purkinje cells isolated from control and 24 hour infarcted hearts. Circ Res 1989; 65:955–70.

8. Adrian R H. The effect of internal and external potassium concentration on the membrane potential of frog muscle. J Physiol (Lond) 1956; 133:631–58.

9. Hironaka T, Morimoto S. The resting potential of frog sartorius muscle. J Physiol (Lond) 1979; 297:1–8

10. Dresdner K P, Kline R P, Wit A L. Cytoplasmic K^+ and Na^+ activity in subendocardial canine Purkinje fibers from one day old infarcts using double barrel ion selective microelectrodes: comparison with maximum diastolic potential. Circ Res 1987; 60:122–32.

11. Walker JL. Ion specific liquid ion exchanger microelectrodes. Anal Chem 1971; 43:89–92A.

12. Lee C O, Uhm D Y, Dresdner K P. Sodium-calcium exchange in rabbit heart cells: direct measurement of sarcoplasmic Ca^{++} activity. Science 1980; 209:699–701.

13. Meier F, Lanter F, Ammann D, Steiner R A, Simon W. Applicability of available ion-selective liquid membrane microelectrodes in intracellular ion-activity measurements. Pflugers Arch 1982; 393:23–30.

14. Lee C O. Ionic activities in cardiac muscle cells and application of ion-selective microelectrodes. Am J Physiol 1981; 241:H459–78.

15. Munoz J L, Deyhimi F, Coles J A. Silanization of glass in the making of ion sensitive microelectrodes. J Neurosci Methods 1983; 8:231–47.

16. Ujec E, Keller O, Machek J, Pavlik V. Low impedance coaxial K^+ selective microelectrodes. Pflugers Arch 1979; 382:189–92.

17. Ammann D, Buhrer T, Schefer U, Muller M, Simon W. Intracellular neutral carrier-based Ca^{++} microelectrode with subanomolar detection limit. Pflugers Arch 1987; 409:223–8.

18. Walker J L. Intracellular potassium and chloride measurements in sheep cardiac Purkinje fibers. In: Sykova E, Hnik P, Vyklicky L, eds. Ion selective microelectrodes and their use in excitable tissues. New York, Plenum Press, 1981.

19. Spitzer K W, Walker J L. Intracellular chloride activity in quiescent cat papillary muscle. Am J Physiol 1980; 238:H487–93.

20. Chao A C, Armstrong W M D. Cl-selective microelectrodes: sensitivity to anionic Cl^- transport inhibitors. Am J Physiol 1987; 253:C343–C347.

21. Kondo Y, Buhrer T, Seiler K, Fromter E, Simon W. A new double-barreled, ionophore-based microelectrode for chloride ions. Pflugers Arch 1989; 414:663–8.

22. Dangman K H, Dresdner K P, Michler R E. Transmembrane action potentials and intracellular K^+ activity of baboon cardiac tissues. Cardiovasc Res 1986; 32:204–12.

23. Sheu S, Korth M, Lathrop D A, Fozzard H A. Intra- and extracellular K^+ and Na^+ activities and resting membrane potential in sheep cardiac Purkinje strands. Circ Res 1980; 47:692–700.

24. Chapman R A, Fozzard H A, Friedlander I R, January J T. Effects of Ca^{++}/Mg^{++} removal on aNa_i aK_i, and tension in cardiac Purkinje fibers. Am J Physiol 1987; 251:C920–7.

25. Miura D S, Hoffman B F, Rosen M R. The effect of extracellular potassium on the intracellular potassium ion activity and transmembrane potentials of beating canine cardiac Purkinje fibers. J Gen Physio 1977; 69:463–74.

26. Vaughan-Jones R D, Kaila K. The sensitivity of liquid sensor, ion-selective microelectrodes to changes in temperature and solution level. Pflugers Arch 1986; 406:641–4.

3

The Multicellular Cardiac Voltage Clamp
Approaches and Problems

Ira S. Cohen and Nicholas B. Datyner

State University of New York at Stony Brook
Stony Brook, New York

INTRODUCTION

The heart is an electrical syncytium, and as such its physiologic properties depend on both the cardiac cell membrane and its extracellular space. The study of the ionic conductances in the cardiac cell membrane began in 1964 when the voltage clamp was applied to the multicellular Purkinje fiber (1). This study, performed a quarter of a century ago, ushered in an era of great advances in understanding and also many false starts, not at all a surprise considering the complicated geometry of the cardiac preparations under study. In this chapter we briefly review the approaches to the voltage clamp of the cardiac syncytium and describe the advantages and disadvantages of each approach. We also consider a general difficulty in any multicellular voltage clamp: extracellular ion concentration changes. It is undoubtedly true that the patch clamp technique and the isolated cardiac myocyte have removed much of the justification for voltage clamping a syncytium. Nevertheless the syncytium remains the more physiologic preparation, which should be employed continuously in conjunction with the simpler preparations to test the physiologic relevance of the experimental results.

TWO-MICROELECTRODE VOLTAGE CLAMP TECHNIQUE

One of the simplest of the multicellular cardiac preparations on which to employ the voltage clamp is the Purkinje fiber. This preparation has a core of myocytes electrically connected by gap junctions. When the cable properties of the fibers are analyzed it is found that the best electrical model is a simple one-dimensional cable with sealed ends (2,3).

In such an electrical analog when a current passing electrode is placed at the center of the Purkinje fiber then the voltage at any point a normalized distance X from the center of the fiber is related to the voltage at $X = 0$ by

$$V_X = V_{X=0} \frac{\cosh(L - X)}{\cosh(L)} \qquad (1)$$

where L is the length of half the fiber divided by the length constant λ, and X is the distance x along the cable divided by the length constant λ (4). Typically the length constant of a

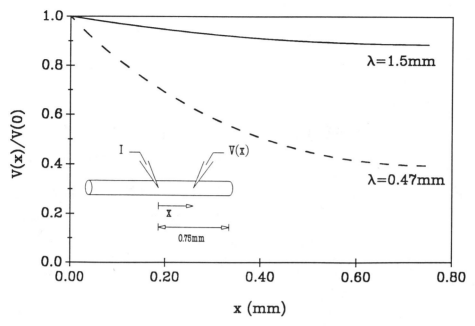

Figure 1 Normalized potential along a Purkinje fiber. For a Purkinje fiber with half-length of 0.75 mm and length constant of 1.5 mm the normalized potential along the fiber is shown by the solid line. The dashed line demonstrates the deterioration in voltage uniformity when the membrane resistance is reduced to one-tenth of its resting value.

Purkinje fiber is about 1.5 mm and the normalized half-length L is about 0.5 (i.e., $\lambda = 1.5$ mm). This means that the fraction of nonuniformity at the edge of the cable when $X = L$ (in this case at the end of the fiber) is roughly 10% (see Fig. 1).

$$\frac{V_{X=L}}{V_{X=0}} = \frac{\cosh(0)}{\cosh(0.5)} = 0.89 \qquad (2)$$

It is worth pointing out that this relatively rosy picture applies only in the diastolic range of potentials near rest. If sodium current is activated the membrane resistance can drop from the resting value of 20 kΩ/cm^2 to less than a tenth of that value. Now consider the Purkinje fiber with one-tenth the membrane resistance; then $\lambda = 1.5$ mm$/\sqrt{10} = 0.47$ mm.

The same estimate of the voltage decrement from the center to the edge is

$$\frac{V_{X=L}}{V_{X=0}} = \frac{\cosh(0)}{\cosh(0.5 \times \sqrt{10})} = 0.39 \qquad (3)$$

The voltage gradient as a function of distance along a Purkinje fiber with these properties is illustrated in Figure 1.

This simple calculation points to a major problem when clamping time-dependent currents: the turn on of membrane conductances may reduce the length constant λ and increase voltage nonuniformity to an unacceptable degree. Obviously this problem is markedly reduced in the isolated Purkinje myocyte. In this case the length of the myocyte is less than 200 μm (5,6).

When applying the voltage clamp to study rapidly activating membrane conductances it is necessary to consider not only the steady level of voltage nonuniformity but also the speed with which the voltage clamp settles. Even under optimal circumstances with negligible series resistance external to the preparation the speed of the Purkinje fiber voltage clamp is limited. The limitation arises because the membrane capacitance at a distance from the center of the fiber is charged by current flow down the fiber through an axial resistance. This "axial charging time constant" can be estimated from Equation (4):

$$\tau_a = R_i \left(C_m \frac{8h^2}{\pi^2 a} \right) \qquad (4)$$

where R_i ($\Omega \cdot$cm) is the internal resistance, C_m (μF/cm^2) is the membrane capacitance, h (μm) is the distance from a centrally placed electrode to either end of the preparation, and a is the radius of the fiber (μm). This τ_a is typically about a millisecond (2,3). This means for roughly 3 msec (three time constants represent 95% of the relaxation) *after* the measured voltage on the voltage electrode has settled the membrane capacity continues to be charged. Thus the membrane voltage continues to change even after the voltage measured by the voltage electrode has settled. One approach to this problem has been to lower the temperature to slow the gating of the membrane conductances. This can extend the period of activation sufficiently to allow its study after axial charging has occurred (7,8).

An additional approach is to subtract the capacity current from the total membrane current. This subtraction allows one to observe ionic current exclusively. However, since the ionic current that occurs during the axial charging is not at a constant voltage, the dependence of the kinetics on membrane voltage cannot be accurately analyzed.

A third difficulty in this preparation is the restricted extracellular space. This is discussed later in the section on ion accumulation.

Thus, although the Purkinje fiber has a simple one-dimensional cable geometry, application of the voltage clamp is fraught with difficulty. There are both steady-state difficulties when studying large membrane conductances as well as transient difficulties in studying fast conductances. Nevertheless it has been a useful tool in initial attempts to define the membrane conductances of the Purkinje membrane. Experimenters employing this technique have examined many cardiac currents, including those underlying pacemaker activity (9), delayed rectification (10), and the Na/K pump (11). In each of these cases, however, some errors in interpretation were caused by the complicated geometry of the preparation under study.

THE SUCROSE GAP

The myocytes within the Purkinje fiber are of large diameter (30–50 μm); those of atrium and sinus node are much narrower. ($<$10 μm). This difference in diameter has a number of significant consequences. First, the smaller diameter implies a larger surface-to-volume ratio (which for a cylindrical cell is proportional to 1/radius). Thus for a preparation of a given physical size, one with smaller diameter myocytes requires more current to voltage clamp if membrane conductances are similar. As a consequence more current is injected into a smaller cell, leading to a much higher current density; as a result the cell into which the current is injected frequently uncouples from its neighbors, contracts, and ejects the microelectrode.

Therefore, investigators interested in atrial membrane properties developed an alternative approach: the double-sucrose gap (12). This approach was modeled on the successful investigations of myelinated nerve by Stampfli (13). However, there are several important differences between the experimental preparations. First, and foremost, the myelinated nerve is one cell with no restricted intercellular spaces. In contrast, atrial trabeculae have narrow intercellular spaces. As illustrated in Figure 2, the chamber contains five compartments. Two outside KCl compartments, two sucrose compartments, with a central Ringer's (or test solution) compartment. The sucrose/Ringer's interface may be well defined at the preparation surface, but both sucrose and Ringer's diffuse beneath the preparation surface, creating a large region of poorly defined ion concentrations. The net result is that current collected from this area of membrane is bathed in a nonhomogeneous solution (14).

A second difficulty also exists. Current is injected in one end compartment and is supposed to travel through the compartment insulated by extracellular sucrose without leaving the cells. Low concentrations of ions are sometimes added to the sucrose solution to prevent cell uncoupling (15). This reduces the resistance of the extracellular pathway and leads to a leakage current collected in the center compartment, but *not* passing through the membranes in this center compartment. This leakage current distorts the membrane current and makes it difficult to estimate true mem-

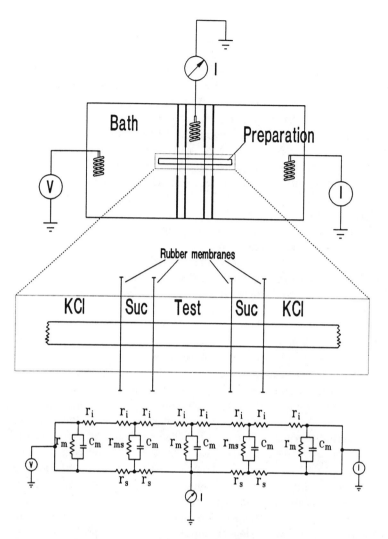

Figure 2 The double-sucrose gap. The upper panel illustrates the five compartments in a double-sucrose gap chamber. The central chamber, where membrane properties are measured, has adjacent sucrose-containing chambers to insulate the test membrane. Adjacent to the sucrose chambers are those containing KCl and providing access to the intracellular side of the preparation. To minimize solution flow between chambers petroleum jelly or silicon grease is used to seal the area surrounding the preparation at each interface, or as in the diagram the preparation is passed through small holes in rubber membranes (middle panel). Current is passed through one end of the preparation and potential measured at the opposing end. In this case current is shown being monitored using a virtual ground in the central chamber. The simplified electrical circuit model is shown in the lower panel. Although the circuit elements are represented in lumped form the preparation should be viewed as a cable structure. r_i = resistivity of intracellular fluid per unit length (Ω/cm); r_m = membrane resistivity per unit length (Ω/cm) in the test region; c_m = membrane capacitance per unit length (μF/cm); r_{ms} = membrane resistivity per unit length (Ω/cm) in the sucrose region; r_s = external resistivity in the sucrose region. The external resistivity in the KCl regions has been neglected. If r_s is considered infinite then it is clear that the membrane of the central region can be electrically isolated.

brane conductances (16). Further, if the length constant in the sucrose region is not much longer than the compartment itself, voltage is also not accurately recorded.

Results from this method provided the first insights into the actions of the autonomic transmitters on frog atrium (17,18). Nevertheless, the results of these studies were contaminated by the problems already described.

THE HYBRID GAP

Ventricle was studied with a hybrid gap method (19). In this case voltage was recorded with an internal microelectrode and current was passed via a conventional sucrose gap. This technique had the advantage that one end of the cable in the test region was sealed, providing better uniformity. Further, the microelectrode allowed more accurate recordings of membrane potential. The preparation had at least one significant additional deficit. It was usually of larger diameter (up to 0.7 mm), leading to larger problems of radial series resistance, voltage escape, and ion accumulation.

ION ACCUMULATION AND DEPLETION

A common aspect to all cardiac preparations is narrow intercellular spaces (see Fig. 3 A and B). This geometric factor adds radial series resistance and creates small extracellular volumes facing much of the membrane surface area, which are in restricted diffusional equilibrium with the bulk solution (14,20,21).

Experimentally these narrow extracellular spaces have two important consequences for the voltage clamp: (1) ion concentrations in these extracellular spaces differ from those in the bulk solution, and (2) membrane at the center of the preparation has a different transmembrane voltage than surface membrane. These difficulties have been treated at some length in a number of important reviews (20,21). At best the measured ion currents allow a distorted estimate of membrane con-

ductances, selectivity, and kinetics; at worst completely artifactual conclusions can be reached. Figure 4 shows sample records from a Purkinje fiber with a two-microelectrode voltage clamp and an extracellular K^+ electrode. The cleft $[K^+]$ can drop to a fraction of the value in the bulk solution on hyperpolarization. This $[K^+]$ depletion was a significant factor in the original misinterpretation of the ion selectivity and gating of the pacemaker current i_f in Purkinje fibers (22,23).

ADVANTAGES

Given these major disadvantages, why are multicellular cardiac preparations not abandoned for voltage clamp studies on isolated myocytes? The simple answer is that cardiac muscle is a syncytium whose physiologic properties depend on the cell membrane, on cell-to-cell coupling, and on the properties of the extracellular space. Any technique that studies the isolated cell cannot answer all relevant physiologic questions. Further, the most common approach to voltage clamping the single cell, the whole-cell patch clamp technique, relies on an abnormal intracellular milieu in which the Ca^{2+} is buffered with EGTA and other ions are buffered by the proximity of the patch pipette. Second messengers and enzymes are frequently lost. The voltage dependences of many currents are abnormal and shift during the course of the experiment (24,25).

Thus, in conclusion, complete understanding of physiologic function must include a reconstruction of syncytial properties. This can only occur following study of multicellular cardiac preparations with the voltage clamp technique.

ACKNOWLEDGMENTS

We thank Judy Samarel for help in manuscript preparation. This work was supported by HL20558 and PPG HL28958.

(A)

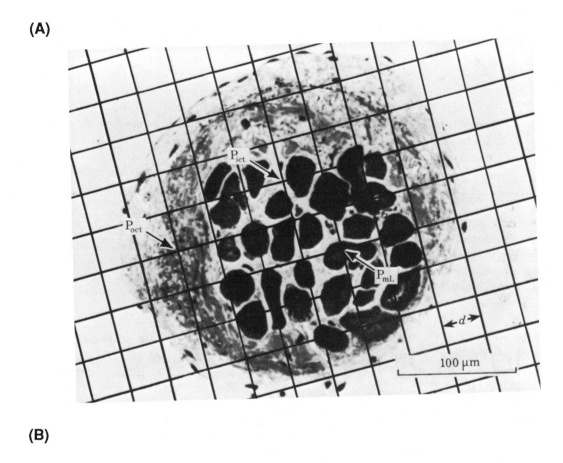

(B)

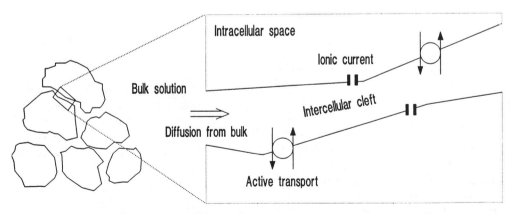

Figure 3 Ion accumulation and depletion. (A) Cross section of the Purkinje fiber illustrating the inter-cellular spaces. P_{ict} is the inner connective tissue, P_{oct} is the outer connective tissue. P_{mL} is a point on a myocyte and small unseen extracellular spaces. $d = 33.3$ μm. (Reproduced from Ref. 26.) (B) Accumulation or depletion of ions in the intercellular cleft is controlled by the balance between the factors illustrated. Ions enter or leave the cell via ionic channels, are actively transported across the membrane, or move to or from the bulk solution.

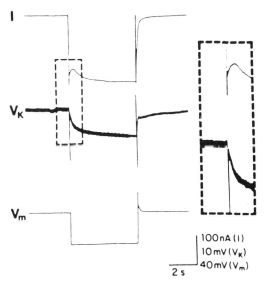

100 nA (I)
10 mV (V_K)
40 mV (V_m)
2 s

Figure 4 From a holding potential of -40 mV the membrane is stepped to -86 mV for 5 sec. The current I, membrane voltage V_m, and extracellular cleft $[K^+]$ V_K are shown. The $[K^+]$ depletes from a starting value of 8.0 mM to 4.7 mM during the voltage step. The inset shows enlargements of the first second of the current and $[K^+]$ traces. About two-thirds of the $[K^+]$ depletion occurs in the first 500 msec. (Reproduced from Ref. 27.)

REFERENCES

1. Deck KA, Kern R, Trautwein W. Voltage clamp technique in mammalian cardiac fibres. Pflugers Arch Ges Physiol 1964; 280:50–62.
2. Colatsky TJ, Tsien RW. Electrical properties associated with wide intercellular clefts in rabbit Purkinje fibers. J Physiol (Lond) 1979; 290:227–52.
3. Cohen I, Falk R, Kline R. Voltage clamp studies on the canine Purkinje strand. Proc R Soc [Biol] 1983; 217:215–36.
4. Jack J, Noble D, Tsien RW. Electrical current flow in excitable cells, Oxford: Clarendon Press, 1975.
5. Callewaert G, Carmeliet E, Vereecke J. Single cardiac Purkinje cells: general electrophysiology and voltage clamp analysis of the pacemaker current. J Physiol (Lond) 1984; 349:643–61.
6. Cohen I, Datyner N, Gintant G, Mulrine N, Pennefather P. Properties of an electrogenic Na/K pump in isolated canine Purkinje myocytes. J Physiol (Lond) 1987; 383:251–67.
7. Dudel J, Rudel R. Voltage and time dependence of excitatory sodium current in cooled sheep Purkinje fibres. Pflugers Arch Ges Physiol 1971; 315:136–58.
8. Colatsky TJ, Tsien RW. Sodium channels in rabbit cardiac Purkinje fibres. Nature 1979; 278:265–8.
9. Noble D, Tsien RW. The kinetics and rectifier properties of the slow potassium current in cardiac Purkinje fibres. J Physiol (Lond) 1968; 195:185–214.
10. Noble D, Tsien RW. Outward membrane currents activated in the plateau range of potentials in cardiac Purkinje fibres. J Physiol (Lond) 1969; 200:205–31.
11. Eisner DA, Lederer J. Characterization of the electrogenic sodium pump in cardiac Purkinje fibres. J Physiol (Lond) 1980; 303:441–74.
12. Rougier O, Vassort G, Stampfli R. Voltage clamp experiments on frog atrial heart muscle fibres with the sucrose gap technique. Pflugers Arch Ges Physiol 1968; 301:91–108.
13. Stampfli R. A new method for measuring membrane potentials with external electrodes. Experientia 1954; 10:508.
14. Attwell D, Cohen I. The voltage clamp of multicellular preparations. Prog Biophys Mol Biol 1977; 31:201–45.
15. Kleber A. Effects of sucrose solution on the longitudinal tissue restivity of trabecular muscle from mammalian heart. Pflugers Arch Ges Physiol 1973; 345:195–205.
16. McGuigan JAS. Some limitations of the double sucrose gap and its use in the study of slow outward current in mammalian ventricular muscle. J Physiol (Lond) 1974; 240: 795–806.
17. Brown RH, Noble S. Effects of adrenaline on membrane currents underlying pacemaker activity in frog atrial muscle. J Physiol (Lond) 1974; 238:51–53.
18. Giles WR, Noble SJ. Changes in membrane currents in bullfrog atrium produced by acetylcholine. J Physiol (Lond) 1976; 261: 103–23.
19. Beeler CW Jr, Reuter H. Voltage clamp experiments on ventricular myocardial fibres. J Physiol (Lond) 1970; 207:165–90.
20. Attwell D, Eisner DA, Cohen I. Voltage clamp and tracer flux data: effects of a restricted extracellular space. Q Rev Biophys 1979; 12:213–61.
21. Cohen I, Kline R. K^+ fluctuations in the extracellular spaces of cardiac muscle: evidence

from the voltage clamp and K^+ selective microelectrodes. Circ Res 1982: 50:1–16.

22. DiFrancesco D. A new interpretation of the pacemaker current in calf Purkinje fibres. J Physiol (Lond) 1981; 314:359–76.

23. DiFrancesco D. A study of the ionic nature of the pacemaker current in calf fibres. J Physiol (Lond) 1981; 314:377–93.

24. Makielski JC, Sheets MF, Hanck DA, January CT, Fozzard HA. Sodium current in voltage clamped internally perfused canine cardiac Purkinje cells. Biophys J 1987; 52:1–11.

25. DiFrancesco D, Ferroni A, Mazzanti M, Tromba C. Properties of the hyperpolarizing-activated current (i_f) in cells isolated from the rabbit sino-atrial node. J Physiol (Lond) 1986; 377:61–88.

26. Eisenberg в, Cohen I. The ultrastructure of the canine Purkinje strand: a morphometric analysis. Proc R Soc [Biol] 1983; 217: 191–213.

27. Kline R, Cohen I. Extracellular $[K^+]$ fluctuations in voltage-clamped canine cardiac Purkinje fibers. Biophys J 1984; 46:663–8.

4

Single-Channel Recording as Applied to Cardiac Electrophysiology

Steven A. Siegelbaum

College of Physicians and Surgeons, Columbia University
New York, New York

INTRODUCTION

With the combined advances of the patch clamp technique introduced by Neher, Sakmann, and their colleagues (Neher and Sakmann, 1976; Hamill et al. 1981; Sakmann and Neher, 1983a) and techniques for dissociation of single cardiac myocytes (Powell and Twist, 1976; Trube, 1983), our understanding of the ionic channels, pumps, and transporters responsible for cardiac electrical excitability has rapidly grown over the past 10 years. As the technical aspects of amplifier design, patch pipette construction, and statistical analyses have been thoroughly described and reviewed (Hamill et al., 1981; Sakmann and Neher, 1983), here we focus on the application of the patch clamp to cardiac electrophysiology.

Figure 1 summarizes the four basic patch clamp configurations: the cell-attached patch, cell-free inside-out and outside-out patches, and the whole-cell recording mode (Hamill et al., 1981). These configurations are discussed here, followed by a brief review of some of the classes of cardiac ion channels that have been identified and characterized using single-channel recording.

Cell-Attached Patches

The basic patch clamp configuration is the cell-attached patch. It is obtained by first pressing a fire-polished glass patch pipette (tip diameter of 0.5–5 µM) against the surface of an enzymatically cleaned cell. After obtaining a mechanical seal, gentle suction is applied to the pipette, causing a variable amount of membrane to enter the pipette and resulting in the formation of an omega-shaped intrusion of membrane (Fig. 1). Under favorable conditions, the membrane and glass form a tight bond, resulting in a high-resistance gigaohm seal between pipette and membrane (1–100 GΩ) that is mechanically stable. This configuration provides a very low inherent electrical noise due to the high impedance of the small patch and permits the recording of the small unitary currents that flow through single open channels. Cell-attached patches have been used to characterize at the single-channel level a number of cardiac ion channels that had been previously identified at the macroscopic level of voltage-clamped ionic currents. In addition, single-channel recording has resulted in the identification of several types of previously unrecognized classes of ion channels.

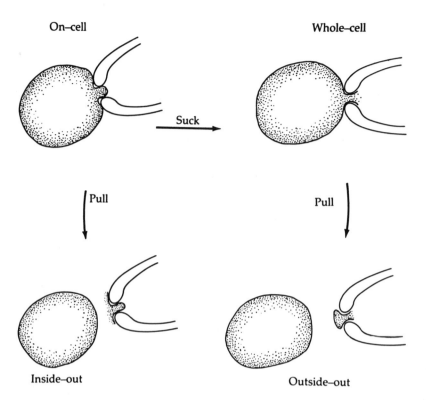

Figure 1 Different patch clamp recording configurations. Top left, cell-attached patch configuration. Bottom left, inside-out patch configuration obtained by pulling pipette away from cell. Top right, whole-cell recording obtained by applying suction to rupture patch after obtaining cell-attached patch. Bottom right, outside-out patch obtained by withdrawing pipette from cell in whole-cell recording mode. (From Hille, 1984.)

Cell-attached patch recordings have also provided important information about how neurotransmitters and hormones regulate channel activity in that they can be exploited to study the modulation of ion channel function through the action of various hormones and second messenger systems. For example, application of β-adrenergic agonists to the bath solution (outside the patch pipette) leads to an increase in opening of the L-type calcium channels in cell-attached patches (see Fig. 3) (Brum et al., 1984). This type of result provides evidence that the β-adrenergic agonists must act through an intracellular second messenger since the seal between the pipette and membrane is tight enough to prevent substances applied to the bath from directly reaching receptors in the membrane under the patch pipette. Conversely, the inability of bath-applied muscarinic cholinergic agonists

to open acetylcholine-activated K channels in cell-attached patches suggests that the action of acetylcholine is not mediated by a freely diffusible second messenger (see Fig. 5) (Soejima and Noma, 1984).

Inside-out Patches

After obtaining a cell-attached patch, an inside-out patch can be formed by withdrawing the pipette from the cell. Because of the mechanical stability of the seal the patch remains intact, with the inside surface of the membrane facing the bathing solution (Fig. 1). After pulling the patch off the cell, the torn edges of membrane often seal over to form a small vesicle. The high-input impedance of the vesicle reduces the amplitude of the single-channel currents and can lead to significant distortion in the time course of single-channel currents owing to the resistive and capacitative properties of the vesicle (Hamill et al., 1981). However, by passing the pipette through the air/water interface, the outer surface of the vesicle can be ruptured, re-establishing the inside-out configuration. Inside-out patches have proved useful in studying the actions of various intracellular ions and metabolites on channel function, yielding some rather surprising results. In particular, two K channels have been identified whose gating is not regulated by voltage or by an extracellular hormone; rather, the channels are controlled by the concentrations of intracellular ligands (see Fig. 6).

One problem often encountered with inside-out patches is that many types of channels stop functioning within a few minutes after formation of the cell-free patch (washout) or display altered gating properties. Thus, the L-type calcium channel stops opening within a few minutes upon patch excision. The fast voltage-dependent sodium channels can remain active for hours in inside-out patches, but there is a shift in the voltage dependence of steady-state inactivation of these channels by as much as 30 mV in the hyperpolarizing direction (e.g. Cachelin et al., 1983) and a three- to four-fold prolongation in single-channel open time (Kirsch and Brown, 1989). Some of these changes may be due to the loss of some intracellular metabolic factor in the cell-free conditions. Thus, Kameyama et al. (1988) have reported that a tissue extract from cardiac muscle is capable of rescuing Ca channels from rundown in inside-out patches. In the pituitary GH3 cell line, Armstrong and his colleagues (1989) have shown that addition of cAMP-dependent protein kinase to inside-out patches prevents rundown of calcium channel function. So far the factors regulating sodium channel gating have not been identified.

Whole-Cell Recording

After obtaining a cell-attached patch, application of strong suction to the pipette ruptures the patch membrane under the pipette while leaving the seal between the pipette and the rest of the membrane intact. In this whole-cell recording mode (Fig. 1), the inside of the pipette is coupled to the inside of the cell through the relatively low access resistance of the patch pipette (1–10 MΩ), providing for the faithful recording of either the cell membrane potential under current clamp or the whole-cell membrane current under voltage clamp. The high seal resistance ensures a low-leakage conductance around the recording pipette, in contrast to recordings using microelectrodes. The whole-cell recording technique is an extension of earlier techniques for recording from single cells pioneered by Kostyuk and his colleagues (Kostyuk, 1984).

Another advantage of the whole-cell recording mode is that the inside of the cell is dialyzed with the contents of the pipette. This allows control of internal ionic conditions as well as introduction of small metabolites and even enzymes. Soejima and Noma (1984) introduced a convenient method for changing the solution in the patch pipette during a continuous recording. By altering the concentrations of internal Na and Ca, Kimura, Noma and Irisawa (1986) were able to identify a membrane current associated with the Na-Ca exchange mechanism (see also Mechmann and Pott, 1986), and Gadsby, Kimura and Noma (1985) were able to characterize the voltage dependence of the Na/K pump. Of course, intracellular dialysis can also be a disadvantage in that the normal intracellular environment is altered. As for the inside-out patches, washout of channels and changes in voltage dependence have been reported in the whole-cell mode, although the effects are generally not as pronounced as for the inside-out patches.

Recently, Horn and Marty (1988) have introduced a modification of the whole-cell recording mode, the perforated patch, that circumvents cell dialysis. In this technique the patch pipette is filled with the pore-forming antibiotic nystatin. Upon formation of a cell-attached patch, nystatin inserts into the patch membrane, forming ion channels selective for monovalent cations. This leads to a relatively low access resistance (10–20 MΩ) between the interior of the pipette and the inside of the cell. Since nystatin is impermeant to divalent cations as well as metabolites and enzymes, the perforated patch technique maintains the normal intracellular milieu and internal calcium buffering at normal levels. Using this technique, Horn and Marty were able to record stable responses to acetylcholine (ACh) in salivary gland acinar cells that quickly run down under normal whole-cell recording conditions.

As the access resistance obtained with both normal and perforated patch whole-cell recording conditions ranges from 1 to 20 mΩ, care must be taken to compensate for this series resistance using an appropriate electronic circuit (e.g., Sigworth, 1983), especially when measuring large currents of several nanoamperes or more.

Outside-out Patch

After obtaining a whole-cell recording, if the patch pipette is pulled away from the cell the torn edges of membrane seal over to form an outside-out patch, where the external surface of the patch pipette faces the bath solution (Fig. 1). This configuration has proven especially useful in studying transmitter-activated channels in muscle and nerve cells that do not depend on second messengers. Outside-out patches have been used less frequently in studying cardiac ionic channels and currents.

LIMITATIONS AND SOURCES OF ERROR

Sources of Noise

Limitations on the types of ion channels that can be measured are largely due to the electrical noise in the recordings (Colquhoun and Sigworth, 1983). In recordings with low seal resistances (<1 GΩ), the dominant noise source is due to the thermal current noise associated with the seal resistance. The standard deviation (or rms) of the voltage noise s_V associated with an ideal resistor due to normal fluctuations of the charge carriers in the resistor (Johnson noise) is given by $s_V = \sqrt{4kTRf}$, where k is Boltzmann's constant, T absolute temperature, R resistance, and f the upper frequency limit of the measurements (in Hz). At room temperature $4kT = 1.6 \times 10^{-20}$

J. Since we are interested in measuring single-channel current, not voltage, it is the standard deviation of the current noise s_I that is relevant. The magnitude of the current noise is related to the voltage noise through Ohm's law:

$$s_I = \frac{s_V}{R} = \sqrt{\frac{4kTf}{R}}$$

For a bandwidth of 1 kHz and a seal resistance of 400 MΩ, $s_I = 0.2$ pA.

What does this magnitude of background current noise mean in terms of detecting a channel opening or closing? Often channel openings and closings are defined in terms of a threshold that falls halfway between the closed- and open-channel current levels. For example, if a channel has a unit current amplitude of 1.6 pA, the threshold for defining an opening is at 0.8 pA, which equals four times the standard deviation of the background current noise s_I just considered (for a 400 MΩ seal at 1 kHz bandwidth). If the background current noise has standard Gaussian characteristics, we can expect that for this signal-to-noise ratio of 4, the background noise level exceeds the threshold level for channel detection at a rate of 0.2–0.3 times sec^{-1} (Colquhoun and Sigworth, 1983). If the signal-to-noise ratio is increased to 5 (i.e., 0.16 pA rms noise and 0.8 pA threshold), the rate of false events falls to around 0.002–0.003 times sec^{-1}. The tolerable limit for false events depends on the rate of true channel openings. Thus for an active patch, where channels may open 10 times or more sec^{-1}, a false event rate of 0.1 sec^{-1} may be tolerable. However, for a patch where channels open only once every few seconds, this false event rate is too high.

The background noise can be reduced by decreasing the bandwidth (i.e., reducing f) using a low-pass electronic filter. The low-pass filtering, however, distorts the time course of the event. For a Gaussian filter, which approximates the properties of commercially available analog Bessel filters, the 10–90% rise time is given by approximately $0.34/f_c$. where f_c is the cutoff frequency. Thus for a 1 kHz filter frequency, the rise time is 0.34 msec. Since the background noise decreases as the square root of the resistance, it is preferable to increase the signal-to-noise ratio by simply increasing the seal resistance. However, once the seal resistance reaches 10 GΩ, other noise sources become limiting. The most serious of these is an inherent voltage noise associated with the input of the patch clamp amplifier. This voltage noise source is coupled to the patch pipette and leads to a current noise as it drives an electrical current across the pipette capacitance. Since the current through a capacitor C is given by $I = CdV/dt$, this noise source becomes significant at higher frequencies where dV/dt is large (above 500–1000 Hz). To reduce this noise it is important to minimize pipette capacitance by ensuring that the electrode holder is dry and by coating the shank of the pipette that is immersed in the bath solution with a hydrophobic resin, such as Sylgard (Dow Corning, 184).

Sources of Error

Although the patch clamp technique has alleviated many of the technical problems associated with the study of cardiac membrane conductances, several potential sources of error need to be considered.

The voltage across the patch membrane is given by the difference between the intracellular voltage and the extracellular voltage within the patch pipette. By controlling the patch pipette potential, one can rapidly change the potential across the patch and study voltage-dependent channels. However, without knowledge of the intracellular potential one can only measure potential changes relative to an unknown resting potential. If the resting potential varies from one cell to another or changes during the course of an experiment, a change of unknown magnitude is introduced in the true patch potential. This problem can be circumvented by bathing cells in an isotonic potassium solution, which depolarizes the cell membrane to near 0 mV. However, this prolonged depolarization can alter the normal electrophysiologic properties of the cell. For example, in cell-attached recordings of voltage-dependent sodium channels, we find that the position of the steady-state inactivation curve is often shifted 20–30 mV in the hyperpolarizing direction under such conditions.

Another potential problem with cell-attached patches that has received little attention results from possible series resistance errors. For channels present in high density, such as the sodium channel, the magnitude of the patch clamp current in a cell-attached patch can exceed 10 pA, sometimes reaching currents as large as 50 pA. With a patch pipette resistance of 10 MΩ or less, even this large a current causes a negligible voltage error (<0.5 mV). However, the series resistance could be rather higher than this estimate for two reasons. First, as membrane is sucked up into the neck of the pipette during gigaohm seal formation, a narrow constriction can form at the neck of the pipette, often introducing a large series resistance, of the order of several hundred megaohms. This constriction often forms after initial seal establishment during a recording. It can show up in the recording as a decrease in single-channel amplitude and as a rounding of the normally square single-channel current waveform. Second, the rest of the cell membrane is also in series with the patch, and this whole-cell input resistance can reach values above 100 MΩ, especially for smaller cells. Thus voltage errors of the order of 10 mV or more can be expected to occur. One possible effect of such series resistance errors is to make the apparent time course of a given ionic current dependent on the magnitude of the current.

TYPES OF CARDIAC ION CHANNELS

A brief survey of the types of cardiac ion channels that have been identified and characterized using single-channel recording follows.

Sodium Channels

Several groups have used single-channel recording to study voltage-dependent sodium conductance. Since an initial report by Cachelin et al. (1983), there has been general agreement concerning single sodium channel conductance and kinetics. In response to step depolarizations, the channel opens rapidly and then rapidly inactivates, giving rise to brief

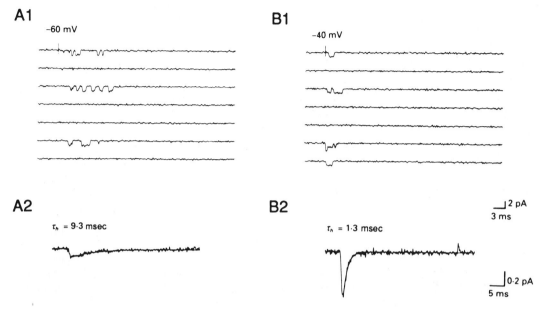

Figure 2 Single cardiac sodium channels in cell-attached patch. (A) Single-channel records in response to step depolarizations from -100 to -60 mV. Records show seven consecutive sweeps. Bottom trace is ensemble-averaged current obtained by averaging currents from 50 sweeps. (B) Sodium channel currents evoked by step from -100 to -40 mV. Note that channels open more rapidly and open only once during depolarization. Bottom trace is ensemble-averaged current. Records obtained from adult dog ventricular myocytes. (From Berman et al., 1989.)

rectangular pulses of inward current (Fig. 2). Under normal ionic conditions (i.e., 140 mM Na, 2 mM Ca, and 1 mM Mg in the bath) the major type of sodium channel has a single-channel conductance of around 10–15 pS. Upon lowering external Ca^{2+} to 0.1 mM, the single-channel conductance increases to 26 pS (Nilius, 1988a), suggesting that external calcium ions can block the channel. The sodium channel is also blocked by external TTX but not by internal TTX (Cachelin et al., 1983). Single-channel recordings have further shown that local anesthetics can decrease channel open time (Nilius et al., 1987; McDonald et al., 1989) with no change in single-channel conductance.

From analyzing single sodium channel currents from neuroblastoma, Aldrich and colleagues (1983,1987) concluded that, contrary to the original model proposed by Hodgkin and Huxley for the squid giant axon, activation or opening of the sodium channels is relatively slow compared to the rate of inactivation. As a result, the time course of the ap-

parent rate of inactivation of the macroscopic sodium current is dominated by the kinetics of activation. Moreover, Aldrich et al. (1983) reported that the rate of open-channel inactivation is largely voltage independent and concluded that the apparent voltage-dependent inactivation of the macroscopic sodium current results from the coupling of inactivation to the voltage-dependent activation process.

In cardiac muscle, a number of studies have recently shown that the behavior of the sodium channels is more in accord with the Hodgkin-Huxley model (Grant and Starmer, 1987; Yue et al., 1989; Berman et al., 1989). Thus, in response to step depolarizations positive to -40 mV, activation is rapid relative to inactivation and inactivation from the open state is inherently voltage dependent. As studies in squid (Armstrong, 1981), neuroblastoma (Aldrich et al., 1983) and GH_3 cells (Cota and Armstrong, 1989) all indicate that inactivation is voltage independent (but cf. Horn and Vandenberg, 1984), there is apparently a true heterogeneity in the inactivation process that may reflect underlying structural differences among the different sodium channel genes that have been cloned from rat brain (Noda et al., 1986) and rat cardiac muscle (Rogart et al., 1989).

One novel property of cardiac sodium channels, reported by Patlak and Ortiz (1985), is that these channels can occasionally enter a mode of gating in which the channels open normally in response to a depolarization but only inactivate very slowly if at all. This gating mode is characterized by prolonged bursts of openings that can last for several hundred milliseconds. Normally these prolonged bursts are seen rarely, in less than 1% of all openings. However, the appearance of prolonged bursts is promoted upon formation of cell-free inside-out patches (Nilius, 1988b). The prolonged gating mode of sodium channels may underlie the slowly inactivating component of sodium current seen under voltage clamp conditions, which contributes to maintaining the action potential plateau (Carmeliet, 1987; Kiyosue and Arita, 1989).

Several groups have also reported the presence of a second class of sodium channels that have a single-channel conductance that is 50% smaller than the main class of sodium channels (Cachelin et al., 1983; Kunze et al., 1985; Scanley and Fozzard, 1987). The physiologic or pharmacologic significance of this second class of channels is not clear.

Recently it has been shown that sodium channels are subject to modulatory control by neurotransmitters acting through G proteins and second messengers (Schubert et al., 1989; Ono et al., 1989). Thus, Schubert et al. (1989) report that isoproterenol inhibits cardiac sodium current by shifting the voltage dependence of steady-state inactivation toward more negative potentials. This effect of isoproterenol is mediated by a GTP binding protein (G protein), most likely the stimulatory G protein G_S (Gilman, 1987). G_S appears to control sodium channel activity through two independent actions. First, it stimulates adenylate cyclase, leading to the production of cyclic AMP and activation of the cyclic AMP-dependent protein kinase. Second, G_S may directly interact with and inhibit the sodium channel, independently of second messenger production. Thus, Schubert et al. found that 8-bromo cyclic AMP, a membrane-permeant cAMP analog, simulated the isoproterenol-induced inhibition of the sodium current. Ono et al. (1989) also report that dibutyryl-cAMP and forskolin, an activator of adenylate cyclase, inhibit the sodium current. Further, Schubert et al. (1989) found that activated purified G_S from human erythrocytes also inhibited sodium channel function in inside-out patches. Since these patches lack ATP, the inhibition with purified G_S cannot be due to either cAMP production or protein phosphorylation. It will be of interest to see whether other second messenger systems are also capable of modulating cardiac sodium channel function.

Calcium Channels

Two types of voltage-dependent calcium channels have been identified in heart cells, the L-type and T-type calcium channels (Nilius et al., 1985). The L-type channel is a high-voltage activated calcium channel that is activated by depolarizations positive to around -30 mV. With isotonic Ba (110 mM) in the external solution, the channel has a conductance of around 25 pS. The L-type channel shows little voltage-dependent inactivation during a depolarizing pulse but may show calcium-mediated inactivation (Kass and Sanguinetti, 1984; Lee, Marban and Tsien, 1985). Steady-state inactivation of the L-type calcium channel requires depolarizations positive to -40 mV to produce significant inactivation. The L-type channel is very sensitive to block by various organic calcium antagonists, including benzothiazipines (diltiazem), phenylalkylamines (verapamil), and dihydropyridines (nifedipine) (Lee and Tsien, 1983). In addition, dihydropyridine calcium agonists, such as Bay K 8644, increase current flow through the L-type calcium channel by promoting a gating mode of the channel characterized by prolonged openings (Hess, Lansman and Tsien, 1984). Finally, the L-type channel is regulated by β-adrenergic agents, which lead to an increase in channel open probability

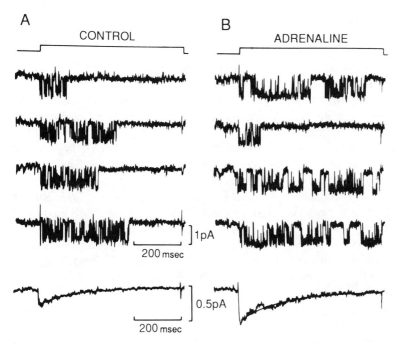

Figure 3 Modulation of L-type calcium channels by epinephrine (adrenaline) in cell-attached patches. (A) Control records of single calcium channel currents (top traces) and ensemble-averaged current. (B) After addition of epinephrine (adrenaline) to the bath there is an increase in channel opening during the depolarization. (From Kameyama et al., 1985.)

(Fig. 3) (Cachelin et al., 1983; Brum et al., 1984). The action of β-adrenergic agonists is mediated through the stimulatory guanine nucleotide binding protein G_S (Gilman, 1987), which stimulates adenylate cyclase, leading to an activation of the cAMP-dependent protein kinase and phosphorylation of the calcium channel (Trautwein et al., 1987). Recently, Brown and his colleagues have shown that G_S may also directly modulate the L-type calcium channel without the need for protein phosphorylation (Yatani et al., 1987). These dual modulatory processes produce temporally distinct actions: the direct G protein effect is rapid in onset and offset, and the phosphorylation-dependent effect has a slower onset and provides a longer lasting modulation (Yatani and Brown, 1989).

The T-type calcium channel is a low voltage-activated channel that turns on at negative potentials and shows rapid, voltage-dependent inactivation. Steady-state inactivation occurs at voltages positive to -70 mV. The T-type channel has a small ("tiny") single-channel

conductance of around 8 pS in isotonic Ba. The T-type channels are also pharmacologically distinguishable from the L-type channels in that they are not blocked by the organic calcium antagonists nor are they enhanced by Bay K 8644 or β-adrenergic agonists. The T-type channels are blocked by inorganic calcium antagonists. One important physiologic role for the T-type channels was suggested by Hagiwara et al. (1988), who showed that current carried by the T-type channels contributes to the late phase of the pacemaker depolarization in SA node cells.

Potassium Channels

Voltage-Dependent Channels

Inward Rectifier. The inward rectifier potassium channel has been analyzed in some detail (Kameyama et al., 1983; Sakmann and Trube, 1984a,b; Payet et al., 1985; Josephson and Brown, 1986; Tourneur et al., 1987; Biermans et al., 1987; Harvey and Ten Eick, 1988;). Under normal ionic conditions (high internal

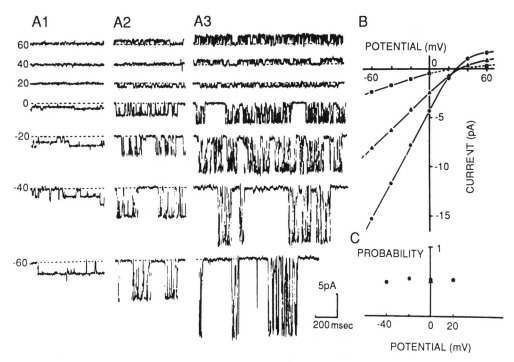

Figure 4 Different K channels in cardiac guinea pig ventricular cells. (A1) Inward rectifier K channel (squares in B). (A2) ATP-sensitive channel (triangles in B). (A3) Na^+-activated channel (circles in B). Currents shown at different patch potentials (given at left). (B) *I-V* curves for three channel types. (C) Open probability of Na^+-activated channel is voltage independent. (From Kameyama et al., 1984.)

K^+ and low external K^+), the channel conducts K^+ readily in the inward direction but passes no detectable outward K^+ current (Fig. 4A1). With symmetrical concentrations of 145 mM KCl bathing the patch, the channel has a conductance of 27 pS. Recently, the rectifying properties of the channel were shown to be due to channel block by internal Mg^{2+} (Matsuda et al., 1987; Vandenberg, 1987). At negative potentials, internal Mg^{2+} is swept out of the channel by K^+ influx. At depolarized potentials, Mg^{2+} enters and blocks the channel, preventing K^+ efflux.

The inward rectifier channel also exhibits a slower voltage-dependent gating in addition to the Mg^{2+}-induced inward rectification. Hyperpolarizing pulses cause the channel to inactivate in a voltage-dependent manner with a relatively slow time course (Sakmann and Trube, 1984b). This effect may be due to voltage-dependent block of the channel by external sodium and/or calcium ions (Biermans et al., 1987; Harvey and Ten Eick, 1989).

Delayed Rectifier. Relatively less is known about the cardiac delayed rectifier K^+ channel. Clapham and Logothetis (1988) have described a 15 pS K channel in embryonic chick ventricle that activates slowly in response to a step depolarization with a time constant of several hundred milliseconds. Ensemble-averaged current from this channel resembles the whole-cell macroscopic delayed rectifier current. Shibasaki (1987) has reported a similar K channel in rabbit sinoatrial (SA) node cells with a conductance of 11 pS. More recently, Yue and Marban (1989) have described a rapidly activating voltage-dependent K channel from guinea pig ventricular myocytes. This channel has a conductance of 14 pS, opens within 10 msec following a voltage step depolarization, and shows little inactivation.

Transient Outward Channels. Several types of rapidly inactivating or transient outward K^+ channel currents have been described. Callewaert et al. (1986) characterized a 120 pS K^+ channel from cow Purkinje fiber myocytes that is both voltage and Ca^{2+}_i dependent, corresponding to the Ca^{2+}_i-dependent transient outward current originally described with microelectrode voltage clamp (Siegelbaum and Tsien, 1980). Several groups have also reported one or more types of voltage-dependent but Ca^{2+}_i-independent transient outward K channels in sheep Purkinje fibers (Callewaert et al., 1986), mouse ventricular muscle (Benndorf et al., 1987; Benndorf, 1988) and rabbit atrioventricular (AV) node (Nakayama and Irisawa, 1985).

Ligand-Gated Channels

Muscarinic Activated Channel. The muscarinic ACh-activated K current was one of the first conductances to be described in cardiac cells (Hutter, 1957). However, for many years it was unclear whether ACh directly gated a K channel (KACh), similar to the activation of the nicotinic ACh receptor channel at the end plate, or whether ACh modulated channel activity via a second messenger. Over the past several years, a series of elegant experiments have now elucidated the basic aspects of KACh channel activation.

Sakmann et al. (1983) first identified a 25 pS K^+ channel activated by ACh in cell-attached patch recordings from rabbit SA and AV node cells. The channel shows inward rectification and has a mean open time of around 1 msec. Later, Soejima and Noma (1984) showed that this channel could only be activated in cell-attached patches if ACh was present in the pipette; application of ACh to the bath solution had no effect (Fig. 5). This suggested a tight coupling between the muscarinic ACh receptor (mAChR) the K channel. Next, several groups demonstrated that activation of a pertussis toxin-sensitive G protein was required for activation of KACh (Pfaffinger et al., 1985; Breitweiser and Szabo, 1985). Taken together with the results of Soejima and Noma, these findings suggested a novel mechanism of ion channel regulation: the direct gating of channels by G proteins. Further evidence for this hypothesis was provided by an experiment of Kurachi et al. (1986), who showed that ACh (in the patch pipette) could activate KACh in cell-free inside-out patches

as long as GTP was present in the bath. Finally, work by Brown and Birnbaumer and their colleagues has shown that purified activated α_i G protein subunits activate KACh in inside-out patches (Codina et al., 1987). Moreover, antibodies to α_i block the action of ACh (Yatani et al., 1988). The work of Clapham and Neer and their colleagues also implicates a role for the $\beta\gamma$ subunits of G proteins in activating KACh (Logothetis et al., 1987). This effect appears to be due to activation of phospholipase A_2 and the production of 5-lipoxygenase metabolites of arachidonic acid (Kurachi et al., 1989; Kim et al., 1989). Although the lipoxygenase pathway does not mediate the response to ACh, it does appear involved in K channel activation in response to α_2-agonists (Kurachi et al., 1989).

ATP-Gated Channel. Noma (1983; Kakei and Noma, 1984) and Trube and Hechsler (1983, 1984) first identified a novel K^+ channel that is regulated by intracellular ATP (Figs. 4A2 and 6B). The channel has a conductance of around 30–40 pS and is voltage independent. In cell-free patches, the channel is open in the absence of ATP and shows little voltage dependence. Raising ATP levels in the bath cause a dose-dependent decrease in channel open probability (with half-maximal activation at 0.5 mM and a Hill coefficient of 3–4). In an intact cell this channel is normally closed. However, during anoxia or metabolic poisoning, as ATP levels fall the channel opens, leading to a hyperpolarization and decrease in action potential duration (Kakei and Noma, 1984). These effects are thought to be important in protecting metabolically compromised muscle from damage by reducing Ca entry.

Na+-Gated Channel. A second novel K^+ channel, identified by Kameyama et al. (1984), is activated by high levels of intracellular Na^+ (>20 mM; Figs. 4A3 and 6A). This channel has a very large single-channel conductance (200 pS with 150 mM K^+) and shows little voltage dependence. Presumably this channel serves a role similar to that of the ATP-sensitive K^+ channel, protecting ischemic myocardium from Ca^{2+} overload by hyperpolarizing the muscle and reducing action potential duration.

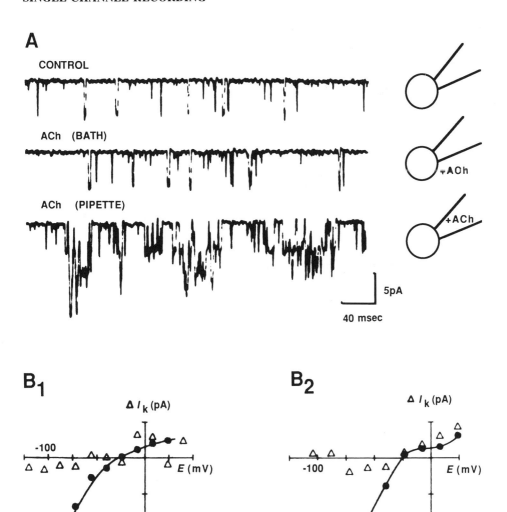

Figure 5 The ACh-activated K channel. (A) ACh activates a K channel in SA node cells only when applied inside the pipette. (From Soejima and Noma, 1984). (B) Role of G proteins in action of ACh in chick atrial cells. (B1) Activation of K current by ACh requires GTP in whole-cell recording pipette. Circles, + 100 μM GTP; triangles, no GTP. (B2) Pertussis toxin (PTX) pretreatment blocks K current activation by ACh. Circles, no PTX; triangles, after PTX.

Cationic Channels

Calcium-Activated Cation Channel

In response to conditions of calcium overload, cardiac cells display a delayed afterdepolarization (Hoffman and Rosen, 1981) that is due to a transient inward current (Lederer and Tsien, 1976). This inward current has been identified as a calcium-activated cation conductance (Kass et al., 1978) and/or as an electrogenic sodium-calcium exchange current (Mullins, 1979; Lipp and Pott, 1988). Although the controversy has not yet been resolved, two groups have reported the presence of calcium-

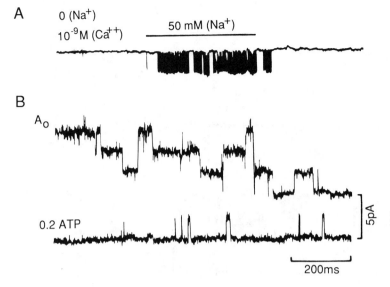

Figure 6 Internal ligand gated K$^+$ channels. (A) Internal Na$^+$ (50 mM) activates a K$^+$ channel in guinea pig ventricular cells (From Kameyama et al., 1984.) (B) Internal ATP (0.2 mM) closes a K$^+$ channel from guinea pig heart cells (from Noma, 1983).

activated cationic channels in heart cells. Colquhoun et al. (1981) first described a cation channel with a single-channel conductance of 30 pS in embryonic rat ventricular cells in culture. The channel was activated by high concentrations of internal calcium. In a more recent study, Ehara et al. (1988) described a cationic channel in adult guinea pig ventricular myocytes that has a conductance of 15 pS. This channel is permeable to monovalent cations and shows a steep dependence on intracellular calcium, with half-activation occurring at 1.2 μM Ca^{2+}$_i$ and a Hill coefficient for activation by Ca^{2+}$_i$ of 3. The opening of the channel is not affected by voltage.

Pacemaker Channel

The pacemaker depolarization in Purkinje fibers was initially thought to result from the turning off of a voltage-dependent K conductance (Vassalle, 1966), termed I_{K2} (Noble and Tsien, 1968), following repolarization. However, subsequent voltage clamp experiments showed that the pacemaker current is in fact an inward cationic current carried by Na$^+$ and K$^+$, termed I_f, which activates upon repolarization negative to -50 mV (DiFrancesco et al., 1986). Using cell-attached patches from rabbit SA node, DiFrancesco (1986) identified

single I_f channels using hyperpolarizing voltage steps. The channel has a very small unitary conductance of around 1 pS and activates in a voltage-dependent manner in response to hyperpolarizing pulses. Epinephrine increases the probability of channel opening without changing single-channel conductance.

SUMMARY

Single-channel recording has greatly expanded our understanding of both the variety of cardiac ion channels as well as their basic biophysical properties. An understanding of the molecular properties of cardiac ion channels is now at hand with the recent molecular cloning and sequencing of genes coding for the cardiac L-type calcium channel (Mikami et al., 1989), voltage-dependent sodium channel (Rogart et al., 1989) and transient potassium channels (Tseng-Crank and Tanouye, 1989). With such information it is now possible to address questions about the relation of structure to function. In the future, the combination of molecular biologic approaches with patch clamp studies offers the promise of achieving further insight into the molecular mechanism of cardiac ion channel function and drug-channel interaction. Such information should provide at last a rational basis for designing drugs that interact with cardiac ion channels as well as permit a better understanding of the role that channels play in various cardiac diseases.

REFERENCES

1. Aldrich RW, Corey DP, Stevens CF. A reinterpretation of mammalian sodium channel gating based on single channel recording. Nature 1983; 306:436–41.

2. Aldrich RW, Stevens CF. Voltage-dependent gating of single sodium channels from mammalian neuroblastoma cells. J Neurosci 1987; 7:418–31.

3. Armstrong CM. Sodium channels and gating currents. Physiol Rev 1981; 61:644–83.

4. Armstrong DL. Calcium channel regulation by calcineurin, a Ca^{2+} activated phosphatase in mammalian brain. Trends Neurosci 1989; 12:117–22.

5. Benndorf K. Three types of single K channels contribute to the transient outward current in myocardial mouse cells. Biomed Biochim Acta 1988; 47:401–16.

6. Benndorf K, Markwardt R, Nilius B. Two types of transient outward currents in cardiac ventricular cells of mice. Pflugers Arch 1987; 409:641–3.

7. Berman MF, Camardo JS, Robinson RB, Siegelbaum SA. Single sodium channel currents from canine ventricular myocytes: voltage-dependence and relative rates of activation and inactivation. J Physiol (Lond) 1989; 415:503–31.

8. Biermans G, Vereecke J, Carmeliet E. The mechanism of the inactivation of the inward-rectifying K current during hyperpolarizing steps in guinea-pig ventricular myocytes. Pflugers Arch 1987; 410:604–13.

9. Breitweiser GE, Szabo G. Uncoupling of cardiac muscarinic and β-adrenergic receptors from ion channels by a guanine nucleotide analogue. Nature 1985; 317:538–40.

10. Brum G, Osterrieder W, Trautwein W. Beta-adrenergic increase in the calcium conductance of cardiac myocytes studied with the patch clamp. Pflugers Arch 1984; 401:111–8.

11. Cachelin AB, De Peyer JE, Kokubun S, Reuter H. Sodium channels in cultured cardiac cells. J Physiol (Lond) 1983; 340:389–401.

12. Cachelin AB, de Peyer JE, Kokubun S, Reuter H. Ca^{2+} channel modulation by 8-bromcyclic AMP in cultured heart cells. Nature 1983; 304:462–4.

13. Callewaert G, Vereecke J, Carmeliet E. Existence of a calcium-dependent potassium channel in the membrane of cow cardiac Purkinje cells. Pflugers Arch 1986; 406: 424–6.

14. Carmeliet E. Slow inactivation of the sodium current in rabbit cardiac Purkinje fibres. Pflugers Arch 1987; 408:18–26.

15. Cavalie A, Pelzer D, Trautwein W. Fast and slow gating behaviour of single calcium channels in cardiac cells. Relation to activation and inactivation of calcium-channel current. Pflugers Arch 1986; 406:241–58.

16. Cavalie A, Ochi R, Pelzer D, Trautwein W. Elementary currents through Ca^{2+} channels in guinea pig myocytes. Pflugers Arch 1983; 398:284–97.

17. Clapham DE, Logothetis DE. Delayed rectifier K^+ current in embryonic chick heart ventricle. Am J Physiol 1988; 254:H192–7.

18. Codina J, Yatani A, Grenet D, Brown AM, Birnbaumer L. The α subunit of the GTP binding protein G_k opens atrial potassium channels. Science 1987; 236:442–5.

19. Colquhoun D, Sigworth FJ. Fitting and statistical analysis of single-channel records. In: Sakmann B, Neher E, eds. Single channel recording. New York, Plenum, 1983:191–264.

20. Colquhoun D, Neher E, Reuter H, Stevens CF. Inward current channels activated by intracellular Ca in cultured cardiac cells. Nature 1981; 294:752–4.

21. Cota G, Armstrong CM. Sodium channel gating in clonal pituitary cells. J Gen Physiol 1989; 94:213–32.

22. DiFrancesco D. Characterization of single pacemaker channels in cardiac sino-atrial node cells. Nature 1986; 324:470–3.

23. DiFrancesco D, Ferroni A, Mazzanti M, Tromba C. Properties of the hyperpolarizing-activated current (i_f) in cells isolated from the rabbit sino-atrial node. J Physiol (Lond) 1986; 377:61–88.

24. Ehara T, Noma A, Ono K. Calcium-activated non-selective cation channel in ventricular cells isolated from adult guinea-pig hearts. J Physiol (Lond) 1988; 403:117–33.

25. Findlay I. Effects of ADP upon the ATP-sensitive K^+ channel in rat ventricular myocytes. J Membr Biol 1988; 101:83–92.

26. Gadsby DC, Kimura J, Noma A. Voltage dependence of Na/K pump current in isolated heart cells. Nature 1985; 315:63–5.

27. Gilman AG. G proteins: transducers of receptor generated signals. Annu Rev Biochem 1987; 56:615–49.

28. Grant AO, Starmer CF. Mechanisms of closure of cardiac sodium channels in rabbit ventricular myocytes: single-channel analysis. Circ Res 1987; 60:897–913.

29. Grant AO, Starmer CF, Strauss HC. Unitary sodium channels in isolated cardiac myocytes of rabbit. Circ Res 1983; 53:823–9.

30. Hagiwara N, Irisawa H, Kameyama M. Contribution of two types of calcium currents to the pacemaker potentials of rabbit sino-atrial node cells. J Physiol (Lond) 1988; 395: 233–53.

31. Hamill OP, Marty A, Neher E, Sakmann B, Sigworth FJ. Improved patch-clamp techniques for recording from cells and cell-free membrane patches. Pflugers Arch 1981; 391:85–100.

32. Harvey R, Ten Eick R. Characterization of an inward rectifying potassium current in cat ventricular myocytes. J Gen Physiol 1988; 91:593–615.

33. Hille B. Ionic channels of excitable membranes. Sunderland, MA: Sinauer, 1984.

34. Hescheler J, Belles B, Trube G. ATP-dependent potassium channels in cardiac cells. Biomed Biochim Acta 1987; 46:S677–81.

35. Hess P, Lansman JB, Tsien RW. Different modes of calcium channel gating behavior favoured by dihydropyridine Ca agonists and antagonists. Nature 1984; 311:538–44.

36. Hoffman BF, Rosen MR. Cellular mechanisms for cardiac arrhythmias. Circ Res 1981; 49:1–15.

37. Horn R, Marty A. Muscarinic activation of ionic currents measured by a new whole-cell recording method. J Gen Physiol 1988; 92:145–59.

38. Horn R, Vandenberg CA. Statistical properties of single sodium channels. J Gen Physiol 1984; 84:505–34.

39. Hutter OF. Mode of action of automatic transmitters on the heart. Br Med Bull 1957; 13:176–80.

40. Johnson EA, Lieberman M. Heart: excitation and contraction. Annu Rev Physiol 1971; 33:479–532.

41. Josephson IR, Brown AM. Inwardly rectifying single-channel and whole cell K$^+$ currents in rat ventricular myocytes. J Membr Biol 1986; 94:19–35.

42. Kakei M, Noma A. Adenosine-5'-triphosphate-sensitive single potassium channel in the atrioventricular node cell of the rabbit heart. J Physiol (Lond) 1984; 352:265–84.

43. Kameyama M, Kiyosue T, Soejima M. Single channel analysis of the inward rectifier K current in rabbit ventricular cells. J Physiol 1983; 33:1039–56.

44. Kameyama M, Kakei M, Sato R, Shibasaki T, Matsuda H, Irisawa H. Intracellular Na$^+$ activates a K$^+$ channel in mammalian cardiac cells. Nature 1984; 309:354–6.

45. Kameyama M, Kameyama A, Nakayama T, Kaibara M. Tissue extract recovers cardiac calcium channels from 'run-down'. Pflugers Arch 1988; 412:328–30.

46. Kameyama M, Hoffman F, Trautwein W. On the mechanism of beta-adrenergic regulation of the Ca channel in the guinea-pig heart. Pflugers Arch 1985; 405:285–93.

47. Kass RS, Sanguinetti MC. Calcium channel inactivation in the calf cardiac Purkinje fiber: evidence for voltage- and calcium-mediated mechanisms. J Gen Physiol 1984; 84:705–26.

48. Kass RS, Lederer WJ, Tsien RW, Weingart R. Role of calcium ions in transient inward currents and after-contractions induced by strophanthidin in cardiac Purkinje fibres. J Physiol (Lond) 1978; 281:187–208.

49. Kim D, Lewis DL, Graziadei L, Neer EJ, Bar-Sagi D, Clapham DE. G-protein βγ subunits activate the cardiac muscarinic K$^+$ channel via phospholipase A$_2$. Nature 1989; 337:557–60.

50. Kimura J, Noma A, Irisawa H. Na-Ca exchange current in mammalian heart cells. Nature 1986; 319:596–7.

51. Kirsch GE, Brown AM. Kinetic properties of single sodium channels in rat heart and rat brain. J Gen Physiol 1989; 93:85–99.

52. Kiyosue T, Arita M. Late sodium current and its contribution to action potential configuration in guinea pig ventricular myocytes. Circ Res 1989; 64:389–97.

53. Kostyuk PG. Metabolic control of ionic channels in the neuronal membrane. Neuroscience 1984; 13:983–9.

54. Kunze DL, Lacerda AE, Wilson DL, Brown AM. Cardiac Na currents and the inactivating, reopening, and waiting properties of

single cardiac Na channels. J Gen Physiol 1985; 86:691–719.

55. Kurachi Y, Nakajima T, Sugimoto T. On the mechanism of activation of muscarinic K^+ channels by adenosine in isolated atrial cells: involvement of GTP-binding proteins. Pflugers Arch 1986; 407:264–74.

56. Kurachi Y, Nakajima T, Sugimoto T. Acetylcholine activation of K^+ channels in cell-free membrane of atrial cells. Am J Physiol 1986; 251:H681–4.

57. Kurachi Y, Ito H, Sugimoto T, Shimuzu T, Miki I, Ui M. Arachidonic acid metabolites as intracellular modulators of the G protein-gated cardiac K^+ channel. Nature 1989; 337:555–7.

58. Kurachi Y, Ito H, Sugimoto T, Shimuzu T, Miki I, Ui M. Alpha-adrenergic activation of the muscarinic K^+ channel is mediated by arachidonic acid metabolites. Pflugers Arch 1989; 414:102–4.

59. Lederer WJ, Tsien RW. Transient inward current underlying arrhythmogenic effects of cardiotonic steroids in Purkinje fibres. J Physiol (Lond) 1976; 263:73–100.

60. Lee KS, Marban E, Tsien RW. Inactivation of calcium channels in mammalian heart cells: joint dependence on membrane potential and intracellular Ca^{2+}. J Physiol (Lond) 1985; 364:395–411.

61. Lee KS, Tsien RW. Mechanism of calcium channel blockade by verapamil, D600, diltiazem and nitrendipine in single dialyzed heart cells. Nature 1983; 302:790–4.

62. Lipp P, Pott L. Transient inward current in guinea-pig atrial myocytes reflects a change of sodium-calcium exchange current. J Physiol (Lond) 1988; 397:601–30.

63. Logothetis DE, Kurachi Y, Galper J, Neer EJ, Clapham DE. The $\beta\gamma$ subunits of GTP-binding proteins activate the muscarinic K^+ channel in heart. Nature 1987; 325:321–6.

64. MacDonald TV, Courtney KR, Clusin WT. Use-dependent block of single sodium channels by lidocaine in guinea pig ventricular myocytes. Biophys J 1989; 55:1261–6.

65. Matsuda H, Saigusa A, Irisawa H. Ohmic conductance through the inwardly rectifying K channel and blocking by internal Mg^{2+}. Nature 1987; 325:156–9.

66. Mechmann S, Pott L. Identification of Na-Ca exchange current in single cardiac myocytes. Nature 1986; 319:597–9.

67. Mikami A, Imoto K, Tanabe T, Niidome T, Mori Y, Takeshima H, Narumiya S, Numa S. Primary structure and functional expression of the cardiac dihydropyridine-sensitive calcium channel. Nature 1989; 340:230–3.

68. Mullins LJ. The generation of electric currents in cardiac fibers by Na/Ca exchange. Am J Physiol 1979; 236:C103–10.

69. Nakayama T, Irisawa H. Circ Res 1985; 57:65–76.

70. Neher E, Sakmann B. Single-channel currents recorded from membrane of denervated frog muscle fibres. Nature 1976; 260:799–802.

71. Nilius B, Hess P, Lansman JB, Tsien RW. A novel type of cardiac calcium channel in ventricular cells. Nature 1985; 316:443–6.

72. Nilius B, Benndorf K, Markwardt F. Effects of lidocaine on single cardiac sodium channels. J Mol Cell Cardiol 1987; 19:865–74.

73. Nilius B. Calcium block of guinea-pig heart sodium channels with and without modification by the piperazinylindole DPI 201-106. J Physiol (Lond) 1988; 399:537–58.

74. Nilius B. Modal gating behavior of cardiac Na channels in cell-free membrane patches. Biophys J 1988; 53:857–62.

75. Noble D, Tsien RW. The kinetics and rectifier properties of the slow potassium current in cardiac Purkinje fibres. J Physiol (Lond) 1968; 195:185–214.

76. Noma A. ATP-regulated K^+ channels in cardiac muscle. Nature 1983; 305:147–8.

77. Ono K, Kiyosue T, Arita M. Isoproterenol, DBcAMP, and forskolin inhibit cardiac sodium current. Am J Physiol 1989; 256:C1131–7.

78. Patlak JB, Ortiz M. Slow currents through single sodium channels of the adult rat heart. J Gen Physiol 1985; 86:89–104.

79. Payet MD, Rousseau E, Sauve R. Single channel analysis of a potassium inward rectifier in myocytes of newborn rat heart. J Membr Biol 1985; 53:143–56.

80. Pfaffinger PJ, Martin JM, Hunter DD, Nathanson NM, Hille B. GTP-binding proteins couple cardiac muscarinic receptors to a K^+ channel. Nature 1985; 317:536–8.

81. Powell T, Twist VW. A rapid technique for the isolation and purification of adult cardiac muscle cells having respiratory control and a tolerance to calcium. Biochem Biophys Res Commun 1976; 72:327–33.

82. Rogart RB, Cribbs LL, Muglia LK, Kephart DD, Kaiser MW. Molecular cloning of a putative tetrodotoxin-resistant rat heart Na^+

channel isoform. Proc Natl Acad Sci USA 1989; 86:8170–4.

83. Sakmann B, Neher E, eds. Single channel recording. New York: Plenum, 1983.

84. Sakmann B, Neher E. Geometric parameters of pipettes and membrane patches. In: Sakmann B, Neher E, eds. Single channel recording. New York: Plenum, 1983:37–51.

85. Sakmann B, Noma A, Trautwein W. Acetylcholine activation of single muscarinic K^+ channels in isolated pacemaker cells of the mammalian heart. Nature 1983; 303:250–3.

86. Sakmann B, Trube G. Voltage-dependent inactivation of inward-rectifying single-channel currents in the guinea-pig heart cell membrane. J Physiol (Lond) 1984; 347:659–83.

87. Sakmann B, Trube G. Conductance properties of single inwardly rectifying potassium channels in ventricular cells from guinea-pig heart. J Physiol (Lond) 1984; 347:641–57.

88. Scanley BE, Fozzard HA. Low conductance sodium channels in canine cardiac Purkinje cells. Biophys J 1987; 52:489–95.

89. Schubert B, VanDongen AMJ, Kirsch GE, Brown AM. Beta-adrenergic inhibition of cardiac sodium channels by dual G-protein pathways. Science 1989; 245:516–9.

90. Shibasaki T. Conductance and kinetics of delayed rectifier potassium channels in nodal cells of the rabbit heart. J Physiol (Lond) 1987; 387:227–50.

91. Siegelbaum SA, Tsien RW. Calcium-activated transient outward current in calf cardiac Purkinje fibers. J Physiol (Lond) 1980; 299:585–606.

92. Soejima M, Noma A. Mode of regulation of the ACh-sensitive K-channel by the muscarinic receptor in rabbit atrial cells. Pflugers Arch 1984; 400:424–31.

93. Trautwein W, Cavalie A, Flockerzi V, Hoffmann F, Pelzer D. Modulation of calcium channel function by phosphorylation in guinea pig ventricular cells and phospholipid bilayer membranes. Circ Res 1987; I:17–23.

94. Trautwein W, Cavalie A. Cardiac calcium channels and their control by neurotransmitters and drugs. J Am Coll Cardiol 1985; 6:1409–16.

95. Trube G. Enzymatic dispersion of heart and other tissues. In: Sakmann B, Neher E, eds. Single channel recording. New York: Plenum, 1983:69–76.

96. Trube G, Hescheler J. Inward-rectifying channels in isolated patches of the heart cell membrane: ATP-dependence and comparison with cell-attached patches. Pflugers Arch 1984; 401:178–84.

97. Tseng-Crank JC-L, Tanouye MA. Molecular cloning of a rat heart potassium channel cDNA. Soc Neurosci Abstr 1989; 15:540.

98. Vandenberg, CA. Inward rectification of a potassium channel in cardiac ventricular cells depends on internal magnesium ions. Proc Natl Acad Sci USA 1987; 84:2560–4.

99. Vassalle M. Analysis of cardiac pacemaker potential using a 'voltage-clamp' technique. Am J Physiol 1966; 210:1335–41.

100. Yatani A, Codina J, Imoto Y, Reeves JP, Birnbaumer L, Brown AM. A G protein directly regulates mammalian cardiac calcium channels. Science 1987; 238:1288–92.

101. Yatani A, Hamm H, Codina J, Mazzoni MR, Birnbaumer L, Brown AM. A monoclonal antibody to the α subunit of Gk blocks muscarinic activation of atrial K^+ channels. Science 1988; 241:828–31.

102. Yatani A, Mattera R, Codina J, Graf R, Okabe K, Padrell E, Iyengar R, Brown AM, Birnbaumer L. The G protein-gated atrial K^+ channel is stimulated by three distinct Gi α-subunits. Nature 1988; 336:680–2.

103. Yue DT, Marban E. A novel cardiac potassium channel that is active and conductive at depolarized potentials. Pflugers Arch 1989; 413:127–33.

104. Yue DT, Lawrence JH, Marban E. Two molecular transitions influence cardiac sodium channel gating. Science 1989; 244:349–52.

ELECTROPHYSIOLOGY OF THE HEART: ANATOMY, PHYSIOLOGY, AND PATHOPHYSIOLOGY

This section consists of five chapters. Each discusses the electrophysiology of one of the five major categories of tissue in the heart. The first chapter, by Campbell, Rasmusson, and Strauss, discusses the electrophysiology of the primary pacemaker of the heart, the sinoatrial node. The next chapter, by Sorota and Boyden, discusses the electrophysiology of the ordinary working myocardium of the atria. Next, the electrophysiology of the atrioventricular node is discussed by Billette and Giles. In the fourth chapter we discuss the electrophysiology of the His-Purkinje system. And finally, Wasserstrom and Ten Eick discuss the electrophysiology of the working myocardium of the ventricle. Each chapter is intended to allow the student to gain insight into the basic form and function of the different cardiac cell types.

Much of basic science research today on the electrophysiology of sinus and atrioventricular node cells, atrial muscle cells, and ventricular muscle cells utilizes patch clamp techniques in enzymatically isolated myocytes. Few studies have been reported on the electrophysiology of single Purkinje fibers. The reported studies of collagenase-isolated single cells from any tissue of the heart makes many assumptions, including (1) single-cell preparations that are patch clamped or impaled with microelectrodes are assumed to be representative of the cells of that specific type in the heart; and (2) isolation of cardiac cells using a collagenase with exposure to zero or micromolar calcium concentrations and ''gentle'' physical separation of the individual myocytes has not damaged the properties of these single cells.

Collagenase is obtained from cultures of the gram-negative anaerobic bacteria *Clostridium*. These enzyme preparations are generally contaminated by a variety of proteolytic enzymes. These proteolytic enzymes may be important constituents for successful myocardial cell isolates. This variation in contaminants may explain why certain batches of collagenase from one source may be better for cell isolation than are other batches from the same vendor with nominally the same reported enzyme activity. Are cell preparations the same, therefore, from one study to the next? Disaggregation of tissue from cells is typically done in zero calcium media to control the action of the enzyme: physical separation is done using gentle trituration by repeatedly drawing and expelling a slurry of tissue softened by enzyme treatment into a pipette. Are isolated cells after physical separation the same as those in tissues?

Each step of the single-cell isolation procedure is almost certainly traumatic, both individually and collectively. Many cells are disrupted and die during the isolation procedure. Only a few of the cells from an entire heart can be studied extensively. It is therefore possible that the reports of single-cell studies in fact represent data from only robust cells that survived the isolation procedure. That is, these results are obtained from a small subgroup of cells that may or may not be representative of the entire population. In preparations made from normal tissues this may not be an overwhelming problem since we assume that the physiology of the individual cells is generally similar. In damaged or pathologic tissues, such as ventricular muscle or Purkinje tissue exposed to acute or chronic ischemic damage, this assumption may not be correct. In these tissues the rigors of the preparation technique may lead to selection for the more robust cells and elimination of the more highly damaged cells. This could introduce an important bias, in that the more highly damaged cells are probably those of most interest to the electrophysiologist investigating the arrhythmogenic mechanisms that occur during ischemia or infarction.

Obviously, the various patch clamp techniques in single cardiac myocytes provides a useful method to study net transmembrane and single-channel currents. Until other technical advances are introduced in the study of tissues in the normal or pathologic medium, the student should be aware of these present limitations.

5

Electrophysiology of the Sinus Node
Ionic and Cellular Mechanisms Underlying Primary Cardiac Pacemaker Activity

Donald L. Campbell, Randall L. Rasmusson, and Harold C. Strauss

Duke University Medical Center
Durham, North Carolina

INTRODUCTION

Understanding the mechanisms underlying spontaneous cardiac pacemaker activity has kindled the interest of basic scientists and clinicians alike. In part this is due to the specialized function of the sinus node in the heart and the role that it plays in initiating the heart beat, as well as the functional implications resulting from its malfunction. As a result efforts designed to unravel its mechanisms have spanned a variety of disciplines and are reviewed in this chapter. What distinguishes the sinus node from adjacent atrial tissue is its intrinsic rhythmicity. As a result, the first two sections review the basic ionic mechanisms underlying the generation of spontaneous diastolic depolarization and the action potential at the cellular level. The pacemaker cell does not function in isolation, however, and as a result the intrinsic rhythmicity is determined not only by the properties of individual cells but also by the interactions between cells. In addition, the excitation that results from diastolic depolarization must propagate in an orderly fashion to the rest of the atrium to initiate atrial systole. The third section therefore reviews

both how the sinus node functions in the multicellular preparation and the progress that has been made in our ability to understand sinus node function in humans. Finally, the last section reviews progress made in our ability to understand what functional derangements underlie sinus node dysfunction in patients.

BASIC IONIC MECHANISMS GENERATING SPONTANEOUS PACEMAKER ACTIVITY AT THE CELLULAR LEVEL

The spontaneous pacemaker activity of the vertebrate heart results from the intrinsic sarcolemmal properties of specialized myocardial cells in anatomically distinct regions of the heart. The location of these primary pacemaker cells depends upon species: in fish and amphibians they are located in the sinus venosus (SV); in birds and mammals they are in the sinoatrial (SA) node. The electrical characteristics of these primary pacemaker cells differ markedly from working (i.e., atrial and ventricular) myocardial cells in that they display a slow and spontaneous diastolic depolar-

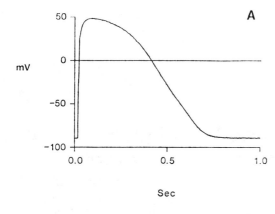

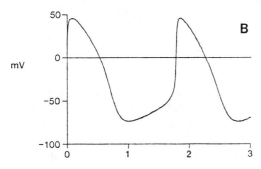

Figure 1 Differences in the basic electrical characteristics of primary pacemaking versus working myocardial cells. (A) A typical action potential recorded from an enzymatically isolated single bullfrog atrial myocyte in response to a small depolarizing current pulse. (B) Typical spontaneous activity in a single isolated bullfrog sinus venosus myocyte. Both recordings were made in normal 110 mM $[Na^+]_o$, 2.5 mM $[K^+]_o$, and 2.5 mM $[Ca^{2+}]_o$ Ringer's solution. *(From 162, 175.)*

ization (or "pacemaker potential") that brings the membrane potential to the threshold for action potential generation (Fig. 1). Upon completion of the action potential the cycle is reinitiated. Since the rate of the diastolic depolarization is usually greatest in the cells within the small regions of the SV or SA node, these regions serve as the natural pacemakers of the vertebrate heart.

To understand the mechanisms responsible for the generation of cardiac primary pacemaking one must understand the basis of the origin of the spontaneous diastolic depolarization as well as the action potential of the pri-

mary pacemaking cells. As in other excitable cells the electrical behavior of myocardial pacemaker cells is determined by the complement of different ionic currents present in their sarcolemmal membranes. These transarcolemmal currents can be mediated by channels (e.g., for Ca^{2+} and K^+), ATP-dependent carriers (e.g., the electrogenic Na^+/K^+ pump), and various co- and countertransporters (e.g., the electrogenic Na^+-Ca^{2+} exchanger). That SV and SA node cells beat spontaneously and atrial and ventricular cells display stable resting potentials indicates a significant difference between ionic currents expressed in the sarcolemma of pacemaking versus working myocardial cells.

The *dV/dt* of the spontaneous diastolic depolarization is relatively small, and consequently very small changes in net membrane current can produce substantial alternations in pacemaker rate. Modulation of any individual current (e.g., by neurotransmitters, such as acetylcholine or norepinephrine) can significantly affect the heart rate. However, as is demonstrated here, alteration of only one current system can produce rather complex results in a spontaneous pacemaking cell, results that at first may seem counterintuitive or paradoxical. Therefore, understanding the influence of the ionic currents underlying the generation of primary pacemaker activity is not only of biophysical interest but is also a prerequisite for realistically understanding neuromodulation, pharmacologic manipulations, metabolic control, and therapeutic interventions on heart rate.

Numerous excellent recent review articles have been published on the electrophysiology of cardiac pacemaker cells, their morphology, neuromodulation, and pharmacology (e.g., 11, 23, 32, 62, 80, 85, 96, 106–108, 138, 151, 153, 193, 194). The first two sections of this chapter are intended to focus on what we believe to be the most important basic transarcolemmal ionic mechanisms underlying generation of both the spontaneous diastolic depolarization and the action potential of cardiac primary pacemaking cells. As such, it is hoped that these first two sections are of use not only to beginning students in the field and specialized cardiac electrophysiologists, but also to practicing cardiologists and general physiologists interested in pacemaking activity in excitable cells. Emphasis is placed upon discussion of a new model of pacemaking activity in single bullfrog sinus venosus myocytes (163, 164). We have chosen to emphasize the amphibian SV since the most complete voltage clamp data to date in a single cardiac pacemaking cell have been obtained from this preparation (83, 175, 176). The SV model of Rasmusson et al. (164) is therefore the most complete and realistic model of primary pacemaking activity available at present and as such is the most physiologically instructive.

There are differences between amphibian and mammalian pacemaker cells, possibly the most notable being the presence of an additional current system in the mammal, the so-called current I_f, which is activated by hyperpolarization (58–62). Work from a number of laboratories (summarized in 62, 85, 107, 108, 149, 202) has demonstrated that I_f is present in single mammalian SA node myocytes but is absent in single bullfrog SV myocytes (83, 175, 176). Nonetheless, isolated SV myocytes display spontaneous pacemaker activity identical to that observed in the intact SV. Furthermore, it has been experimentally demonstrated that pharmacologic blockade of I_f (e.g., by 1–5 mM external Cs^+) slows (by approximately 10–20%) but does not block spontaneous activity in isolated SA node myocytes (see, e.g., 62, 85, 151). These results indicate that (1) I_f is not a universal current involved in pacemaking, and (2) when I_f is present it acts as a *modulator* of pacemaker activity, not as the primary current underlying its generation. Therefore, we believe it is important to emphasize that, with the exception of I_f, all the other currents that have been found to date in isolated bullfrog SV myocytes have their analogs in the mammalian SA node. [Recent work has indicated that there is an additional "T-type" calcium current [see 12, 198] in SA node myocytes (92); however, the presence or absence of such a T-type calcium current in SV myocytes has yet to be adequately addressed, and as such this issue is not

further addressed in this chapter; see Campbell and Giles (37) for discussion.]

The results of the basic model underlying SV pacemaker activity is presented first. The results of simulations involving simple increases and decreases in the various individual current components are then presented. In addition, an "interspecies" simulation is also presented in which the current I_f is introduced into the SV model to demonstrate its probable role as a modulator of pacemaker activity in the mammalian SA node. It is hoped that these simulations give the reader a basic understanding of (1) the roles that the different ionic currents, both channel mediated and carrier mediated, play in normal pacemaking, (2) the effects of alterations of these currents, and (3) the overall complexity of the mechanisms underlying pacemaker activity. The major message that we wish to convey is that pacemaking is a rather complex process resulting from the interactions of several nonlinear current systems and that the generation of pacemaking activity *"cannot"* be attributed to any one current system alone; that is, there is no one "pacemaker current."

At this point, mainly for those unfamiliar with voltage clamp terminology, a few important key terms used in the kinetic analysis of voltage-dependent current systems should be briefly defined (see 16, 17, 37, 101, 102, 163, 164). First, the general term "gating" refers to the underlying molecular processes that determine whether a channel responsible for the generation of a given current is either open (i.e., conducting) or closed (i.e., nonconducting). The gating processes of voltage-dependent channel-mediated currents generally are highly nonlinear and extremely sensitive to the transmembrane potential (although neurotransmitters and ions can also control or alter gating). Second, voltage-dependent ionic channels can exist in a least three different gating states: resting, activated, and inactivated. There may, in turn, be more than one subset of any one of these three main states. When the channel enters the activated state it conducts ions for which it is selective; in the resting and inactivated states the channel is nonconductive. It is important not to confuse the resting state with the inactivated state: they are separate and distinct. Finally, the processes governing the macroscopic kinetics describing the transitions into and out of these various states are usually referred to by the following terms. *Activation* is the process(es) in which the channel enters the activated state from the resting state. *Deactivation* is the reverse process, that is, the process(es) in which an activated channel returns back to the resting state. *Inactivation* refers to the process(es) underlying the entry of the channel into either (1) a nonconducting state once it has been activated or (2) a nonconducting state in which it is no longer available for activation (i.e., the inactivated state may also be reached from the resting state without previous activation). The processes of deactivation and inactivation are frequently confused, but it is very important to understand the difference. For example, not all voltage-gated channels that activate upon depolarization subsequently inactivate; however, all such channels deactivate back to the resting state upon hyperpolarization. Finally, *recovery* refers to the process(es) that determine the return of an inactivated channel back to the resting state, thereby making it available again for activation.

In summary, activation is the process that opens (or "turns on") the channel in response to a stimulus (e.g., a voltage change away from the resting membrane potential or application of a neurotransmitter). Inactivation "turns off" the channel in response to the same stimulus. Deactivation is the reversal of the activation process in response to removal of the stimulus; recovery is the reversal of inactivation in response to removal of the stimulus. Channel behavior can be extremely complex, and the interested reader is referred to the excellent discussions of gating processes given in Hille (101), Bezanilla (16), and Bezanilla and White (17).

Background: Modeling of Voltage Clamp Results from Single Bullfrog SV Myocytes

Mathematical models of cardiac cellular electrophysiology have been quite influential and are often referenced in textbooks (e.g., Purkinje fiber; 53, 61, 74, 140, 150; atrium: 100; ventricle: 13; SA node: 28, 34, 154, 206). Most of these models are of the Hodgkin-Huxley (HH) type (102). However, it is important to note that these cardiac models were based largely on voltage clamp data obtained from multicellular preparations. The interpretation of such multicellular current data is fraught with many difficulties, which can be briefly summarized as follows (for more thorough discussions see 8, 9, 37, 163, 164). First, intact cardiac tissue behaves as an electrical syncytium, that is, the cells are electrically connected with each other via gap junctions. Such a complex morphology leads to spatial nonuniformity of potential. Since the gating kinetics of the channel-mediated currents are highly sensitive nonlinear functions of membrane potential adequate spatial control of membrane potential (isopotentiality) is a prerequisite for their analysis and interpretation. Second, multicellular cardiac preparations contain small restricted extracellular spaces (ECS). The presence of such ECS can produce significant diffusion barriers, which in turn can lead to either accumulation or depletion of cations. Furthermore, both the ECS clefts and endothelial sheath can produce a significant and variable "cleft resistance" in series with the sarcolemmal membrane resistance, which can contribute to nonuniformities in potential. Such phenomena make the isolation of individual current components, measurements of their kinetics, and determination of their ion transfer characteristics very unreliable. Finally, there is the possibility of intrinsic neurotransmitter release in multicellular preparations, the neuromodulatory effects of which can greatly complicate analysis.

The use of single enzymatically isolated cardiac myocytes (e.g., 31, 37, 47, 85, 106, 155, 160, 161, 167, 168, 195, 197, 204) eliminates or greatly minimizes many of the inherent problems associated with multicellular preparations. The membrane potential can be directly measured and controlled using either conventional microelectrode or patch clamp techniques. The cable properties often reduce to or closely approximate a single one-dimensional "short cable" (see Jack et al., 110). Since the ECS is eliminated diffusion barriers are minimized and the series resistance is greatly reduced and more easily compensated. Finally, both intrinsic neurotransmitter release and changes in gap junction resistance are eliminated. As such, isolated cardiac myocytes allow much more accurate separation and measurement of sarcolemmal current densities. (However, single myocytes are still far from ideal, particularly when attempting to reliably record and analyze large and very rapid transient currents; see discussions in 37, 48, 50).

Work with which two of the authors have been involved with while in the laboratory of Dr. Wayne Giles has been devoted to quantitative voltage clamp analysis and computer modeling of the ionic currents underlying electrical activity in single myocytes enzymatically isolated from the bullfrog sinus venosus and atrium. The single SV myocyte model that has arisen from this work is unique (compared to previous models of cardiac pacemaking) in that it is based as closely as possible upon voltage clamp data obtained from individual primary pacemaking SV myocytes. Thus, this model represents a comprehensive summary of data from a single laboratory with a sustained commitment to furthering our understanding of the physiologic basis of primary cardiac pacemaker activity. Given the considerable commitment required for a comprehensive characterization of this sort, as well as the relative uniformity and simplicity of the frog sinus venosus, it is unlikely that a comparable model based on the accurate characterization of the mammalian sinoatrial node will be available for many years (see the third section for a discussion of the complexity of fiber types between the pacemaker site in the sinus node and the atrium).

The isolated myocyte voltage clamp data out of the Giles laboratory was obtained using the whole-cell "ruptured patch" variation of the single microelectrode voltage clamp technique (93, 103, 104, 136). This data indicates the presence of the following three channel-mediated current systems in SV myocytes.

I_B is an inward background current carried mainly by sodium ions. The measured current-voltage (I-V) relationship for the total I_B in single SV myocytes (162–164, 175) is approximately linear and displays no obvious kinetic behavior; that is, it appears to act as a simple ohmic background "leak" current (Fig. 2A). However, although we have described I_B as a channel-mediated current, it must be pointed out that this has not yet been rigorously demonstrated: the exact sarcolemmal mechanism(s) responsible for I_B (e.g., carrier versus channel, or both) has not yet been determined. This is an important question that remains to be resolved in cardiac pacemaking, since (as is demonstrated here) I_B is an extremely important determinant of the rate of the diastolic depolarization.

I_K is an outward time- and voltage-dependent "delayed rectifier" potassium current (Fig. 3). I_K is highly selective for K^+ ions, its activation-deactivation kinetics are slow (with activation displaying a significant sigmoidicity) and are not dependent upon calcium influx, and it does not display any significant inactivation (83; see also 105, 178). The activation of I_K can be well described using a single Hodgkin-Huxley type of activation gating variable n raised to the second power (i.e., n^2).

I_{Ca} is an inward time- and voltage-dependent calcium current (Fig. 4). I_{Ca} in SV myocytes appears to be largely an "L-type" calcium channel-mediated current (see 12, 37, 198). I_{Ca} is TTX insensitive and extremely selective for Ca^{2+} ions over monovalent cations (permeability ratio under control conditions of $P_{Ca}/P_K > 1000:1$; 38, 41). The channel mechanisms underlying this high Ca^{2+} selectivity are complex functions of both potential and concentration (for details see 5, 37, 43, 76, 97, 200). I_{Ca} is an essentially pure calcium ion current; that is, Na^+ and K^+ are not significant charge carriers of this current.

I_{Ca} displays both rapid activation and inactivation kinetics. Activation is quite rapid (e.g., I_{Ca} reaches peak amplitude under 5 msec at potentials around 0 mV, indicating that I_{Ca} is far from a "slow" current; see, e.g., 31, 37–41, 109, 117, 176, 199). Activation can be

A

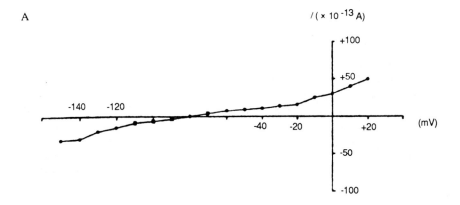

B

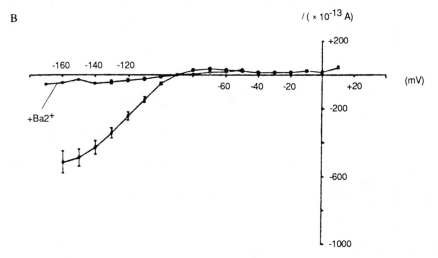

Figure 2 Background current-voltage (I-V) relationships of isolated bullfrog (A) sinus venosus and (B) atrial myocytes. The background I-V relationship in both cell types was measured using 100 msec voltage clamp pulses applied from a holding potential of -80 mV in normal Ringer's solution to which was added 10^{-5} M $LaCl_3$ (to block I_{Ca}) and 3×10^{-6} M tetrodotoxin (to block I_{Na} in the atrial myocytes). Notice the essentially linear background I-V in SV myocytes compared to the pronounced inward rectification in atrial myocytes. This is due to the presence of the background inwardly rectifying potassium current I_{K1} in atrial myocytes and its absence in SV myocytes. As a result of the lack of I_{K1} the input resistance of SV myocytes during the diastolic depolarization is very high (approximately 1–5 GΩ) compared to the input resistance in the same range of potentials for atrial myocytes (approximately 300 MΩ). (B) The background I-V in atrial myocytes after I_{K1} has been blocked by applying 50×10^{-6} M $BaCl_2$ ($+Ba^{2+}$). After blocking I_{K1} the background I-V curves for both cell types look very similar. (From 83.) *Technical note:* The background I-V curves illustrated may be a bit confusing in light of the fact that we have stated that the net background current I_B is an inward depolarizing current. It is therefore important to note that these I-V curves have not been "leakage corrected" for reference to an absolute zero-current level. SV myocytes are spontaneously active; that is, they do not have a stable resting (i.e., zero current) potential. As a result, the holding potential in these experiments was set at -80 mV (i.e., close to the maximum diastolic potential) and the currents were measured *relative* to the -80 mV holding current. Net I_B in these particular figures therefore appears to be an outward current with a reversal potential of -80 mV; however, net I_B is actually an inward current with a reversal potential lying in the depolarized range of potentials close to the sodium equilibrium potential E_{Na}.

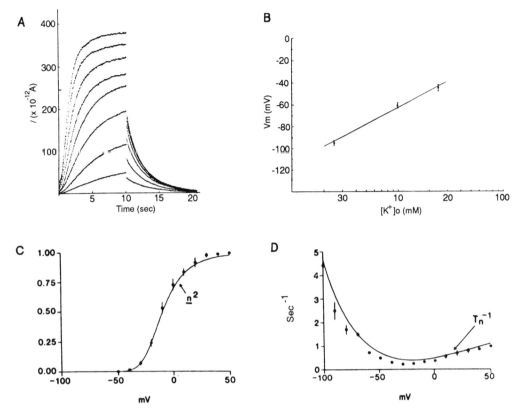

Figure 3 Characteristics of the delayed rectifier potassium current I_K in isolated bullfrog SV myocytes. (A) Representative I_K recordings elicited in response to 10 sec voltage clamp pulses applied from -30 to +50 mV in 10 mV increments. Control Ringer's solution. Note both the sigmoid activation and slow activation-deactivation kinetics of I_K. (From 83.) (B) Reversal potential of I_K as a function of $[K^+]_o$. The slope of the line is 51 mV per decade change in $[K^+]_o$, indicating that I_K is selective for K^+ ions over other monovalent cations (from Ref. 176). (C, D) SV model description of the potential dependence of the I_K activation variable n and rate constants of activation $(1/\tau_n)$ based upon voltage clamp measurements of I_K in single SV myocytes. The n curve was constructed by normalizing the value of peak I_K tail currents (i.e., the initial size of the deactivating I_K current generated upon repolarization back to the holding potential; e.g., see A) and plotting these normalized tail current amplitudes as a function of the depolarizing clamp pulse potential. The sigmoid activation of I_K is described by raising n to the second power, n^2. (From 83, 164)

described by a conventional HH-type activation variable d, which in the present SV model is raised to the first power (Fig. 4D). However, the mechanisms governing inactivation of I_{Ca} are clearly "non-Hodgkin-Huxley" in nature (Fig. 5). Briefly, the I_{Ca} inactivation process appears to possess both voltage-dependent and so-called current-dependent components (e.g., 37, 39, 68, 69, 91, 96, 117–119, 197). The term "current-dependent" refers to the experimental observation that both the rate and extent of inactivation of I_{Ca}

depend upon both (1) the size of the current and (2) the species of cation carrying the current through the calcium channel. For example, inactivation is reduced if either Sr^{2+} or Ba^{2+} carries the current in the place of Ca^{2+}; conversely, inactivation is increased if there is a greater influx of Ca^{2+} ions through the channel (see 37).

At present the exact intracellular biochemical mechanisms governing current-dependent inactivation are not understood and are the subject of much research and debate. Possi-

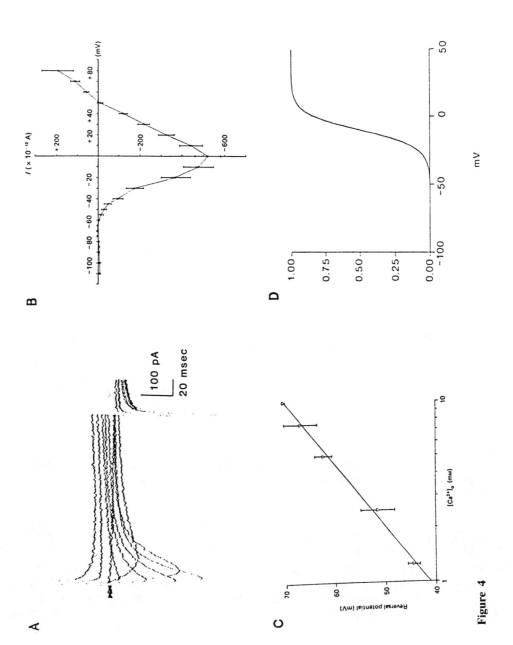

Figure 4

bilities include an enzymatic mechanism in which activation of a Ca-dependent phosphatase during the flow of I_{Ca} leads to dephosphorylation of the channel (thus promoting inactivation; e.g. 69; but see 96), or a Ca-dependent modulation of the kinetics of either the inherent voltage-dependent or a second Ca^{2+}-dependent inactivation "gate" (see discussions in 37, 96, 119, 160). Regardless of what the exact mechanisms of inactivation of I_{Ca} turn out to be, two very important properties of the macroscopic I_{Ca} result (Fig. 5).

The inactivation curve (or f curve, f being the inactivation gating variable in the SV model) is not a conventional Boltzmann relation (see 16, 17, 101, 102). Instead, the inactivation f curve is a nonmonotonic, "U-shaped" function of membrane potential; that is, the degree of inactivation of I_{Ca} as a function of membrane potential closely parallels the I_{Ca} current-voltage (I-V) relationship (Figs. 4B and 5A–C). This presumably reflects modulation of the current-dependent component of inactivation by the magnitude of Ca^{2+} influx. An important consequence of this behavior is that at depolarized potentials (e.g., those corresponding to the action potential plateau) I_{Ca} does not completely inactivate.

The rate of inactivation of I_{Ca} as a function of membrane potential (i.e., the τ_f-membrane potential curve) is also U-shaped, again presumably reflecting modulation of the current-dependent component. [As a result of the U-shaped τ_f curve the voltage dependence of the rate constants of inactivation (i.e., the $1/\tau_f$-membrane potential curve) is bell-shaped; Fig. 5D.] As a consequence, I_{Ca} inactivates more slowly at depolarized (e.g., plateau) potentials.

These two properties of I_{Ca}, which to date have been underappreciated in the less biophysically oriented (i.e., multicellular) cardiac electrophysiology literature dealing with propagation and conduction processes, are extremely important, especially during generation of the action potential plateau and early phases of repolarization.

The following transporter-mediated currents have also been identified in either bullfrog SV or atrial myocytes.

I_{NaK} is the electrogenic ATP-dependent Na^+/K^+ pump current. I_{NaK} has been found and well-characterized in many preparations (e.g., 18, 51, 52, 57, 70, 77, 78, 181, 182, 189). I_{NaK} is an outward (hyperpolarizing) current that maintains the gradients for Na^+ and K^+ across the sarcolemma. Currents attributable to I_{NaK} have been measured in single bullfrog atrial myocytes (177). The coupling ratio of Na^+/K^+ exchanged per transport cycle is 3:2. I_{NaK} is inhibited by various therapeutically useful cardiac glycosides, such as ouabain, strophanthidin, and digitalis (see 135). Further quantitative details on the formulation of I_{NaK} in the SV model [including both its voltage dependence [e.g. 78] and sigmoidicity of activation by Na^+ and K^+ [51, 52] are given in Rasmusson et al. (163, 164).

I_{NaCa} is the electrogenic Na^+-Ca^{2+} exchanger current. I_{NaCa} is the major mechanism for intracellular Ca^{2+} extrusion in both bullfrog SV and atrial myocytes and, as such, is an extremely important current system involved in Ca^{2+} homeostasis (36, 37, 40, 42, 162). Currents attributable to I_{NaCa} have been measured in single bullfrog atrial myocytes (40, 42; Fig. 6). In contrast to I_{NaK}, I_{NaCa}

Figure 4   Potential dependence and selectivity characteristics of inward I_{Ca} in single bullfrog SV and atrial myocytes. (A) Representative I_{Ca} recordings in a single bullfrog SV myocyte in normal 2.5 mM $[Ca^{2+}]_o$ Ringer's solution. The 200 msec voltage clamp pulses from -60 to 60 mV were applied from a holding potential of -65 mV. Note that under voltage clamp conditions I_{Ca} displays both (1) rapid activation and inactivation kinetics and (2) a genuine reversal potential at depolarized potentials. (From Ref. 20.) (B) Mean peak I-V relationship of I_{Ca} in single SV myocytes in normal 2.5 mM $[Ca^{2+}]_o$ Ringer's solution. (From 33.) (C) Reversal potential of I_{Ca} as a function of $[Ca^{2+}]_o$ in single bullfrog atrial myocytes. The slope of the line is 29 mV per decade change in $[Ca^{2+}]_o$, indicating that I_{Ca} is extremely selective for Ca^{2+} ions over external monovalent cations, such as Na^+ or K^+. I_{Ca} is therefore not either (1) a "slow" current or (2) a "mixed Na^+-Ca^{2+}" current (from Ref. 38). (D) Potential dependence of the I_{Ca} activation variable d used in the SV model based upon the measured I_{Ca} I-V relationship in single SV myocytes. In the SV model in its present form d is raised only to the first power. (From 162.)

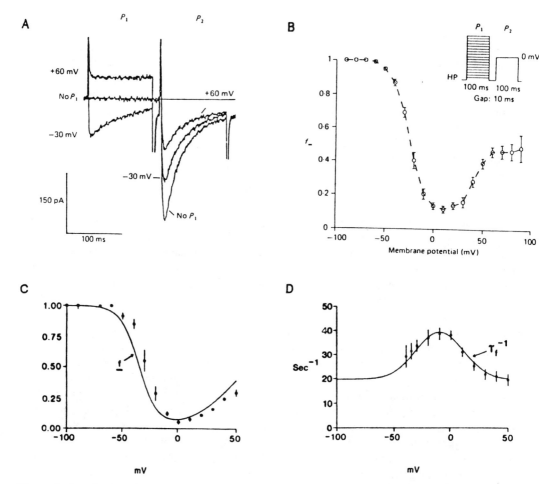

Figure 5 Inactivation characteristics of I_{Ca} in single bullfrog SV and atrial myocytes. (A) Voltage clamp protocol for the measurement of the nonmonotonic U-shaped inactivation relationship of I_{Ca} in single bullfrog atrial myocytes in normal 2.5 mM $[Ca^{2+}]_o$ Ringer's solution. A double-pulse (P_1-P_2) protocol (see inset in B) was applied from a holding potential of -90 mV. Selected I_{Ca} currents elicited for the indicated P_1-P_2 pulse potentials are illustrated. Note the "regrowth" of the P_2 I_{Ca} when P_1 is made more positive (+60 mV trace). This behavior presumably reflects modulation of the current-dependent component of inactivation by the size of the P_1 I_{Ca}. (From 39.) (B) Mean inactivation relationship (f curve) obtained using the P_1-P_2 protocol from a total of eight single atrial cells. This inactivation curve was obtained by (1) normalizing each peak I_{Ca} elicited by P_2 following a variable P_1 to the peak I_{Ca} elicited by P_2 in the absence of a P_1 (no P_1 in A) and (2) plotting the normalized peak P_2 I_{Ca} as a function of the P_1 potential. Because of the "regrowth" of the P_2 I_{Ca} the f curve "bends up" (i.e., the f variable increases) at potentials depolarized to approximately +20 mV. (From 39.) (C) SV model fit to the I_{Ca} f curve measured in single SV myocytes in control Ringer's solution. (From 164, 175.) (D) Kinetics of I_{Ca} inactivation. Model fit to measured rate constants ($1/\tau_f$). I_{Ca} inactivates more slowly at plateau potentials than it does at less depolarized potentials. (From 164, 175.)

is not directly dependent upon ATP per se; instead, the influx of Na^+ ions down their electrochemical gradient (which is maintained by I_{NaK}) is coupled to countertransport of Ca^{2+} ions out of the myoplasm. The gen-erally accepted coupling ratio for Na^+-Ca^{2+} ions exchanged per transport cycle is $r = 3:1$. Therefore, I_{NaCa} is electrogenic and as such is capable of influencing membrane potential. For a coupling ratio of $r = 3:1$, I_{NaCa} has a

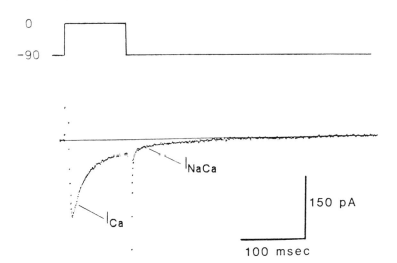

Figure 6 Representative recording of current generated by the electrogenic sodium-calcium exchanger I_{NaCa} in a single bullfrog atrial myocyte. The figure shows a I_{Ca} (control 110 mM $[Na^+]_o$ and 2.5 mM $[Ca^+]_o$ Ringer's solution) elicited by a 100 msec voltage clamp pulse to 0 mV. Upon repolarization back to -90 mV an inward "slow tail" is generated. This slow tail observed upon repolarization is due to activation of I_{NaCa} produced by the calcium influx via I_{Ca} elicited during the preceding 100 msec depolarizing pulse. Notice both (1) the small magnitude and (2) very slow time course of decay of I_{NaCa}. (From 40; see 40, 163, and 165 for details.)

reversal potential E_{NaCa} given by $E_{NaCa} = 3E_{Na} - 2E_{Ca}$, where E_{Na} and E_{Ca} are the Nernst equilibrium potentials for Na^+ and Ca^{2+}, respectively (see 37, 40, 42, 46, 61, 71, 72, 145, 152). Since (1) E_{NaCa} depends upon both E_{Na} and E_{Ca}, and (2) intracellular Ca^{2+} concentration changes during the flow of I_{Ca}, E_{NaCa} is not a fixed value but varies during the pacemaking cycle. Therefore, assuming that E_{Na} remains constant, at any given membrane potential both the magnitude and polarity of I_{NaCa} depend upon E_{Ca}. For these reasons the possible electrophysiologic influences of I_{NaCa} have recently received much theoretical and experimental attention in the cardiac field. In the SV model simulations presented here the DiFrancesco-Noble (61) formulation of I_{NaCa} has been used, with a coupling ratio of $r = 3:1$. Further details on the formulation of I_{NaCa} in the SV model are given in Rasmusson et al. (163, 164) and Campbell et al. (40, 42). Recent excellent discussions of I_{NaCa} include Hilgemann (98, 99) and the collected chapters in Allen et al. (4).

There is also good biochemical evidence for the presence of an ATP-dependent sar-

colemmal calcium "pump" current I_{CaP} in bullfrog myocardial tissue (see 36, 162). However, this current has not yet been directly measured in either single amphibian SV or atrial myocytes. A formulation of I_{CaP} has been incorporated into the SV model, but the possible influence of this very small membrane current is not further discussed in this chapter. An excellent discussion of calcium pumps has recently been given by Schatzmann (171) and of intracellular Ca^{2+} homeostatic mechanisms by Carafoli (44).

In addition to these identified current systems, it is just as important to note that single SV myocytes do *not* have the following currents: (1) a voltage-dependent, TTX-sensitive sodium current I_{Na}, (2) an inwardly rectifying background potassium current I_{K1} (see Fig. 2B), (3) a hyperpolarization activated Na^+/K^+ current I_f, (4) a voltage-dependent inactivating transient outward potassium current I_A, or (5) calcium-activated potassium or nonspecific cation currents.

The absence of both I_{Na} and I_{K1} has also been noted in isolated primary pacemaking cells from mammalian SA node cells (see 85,

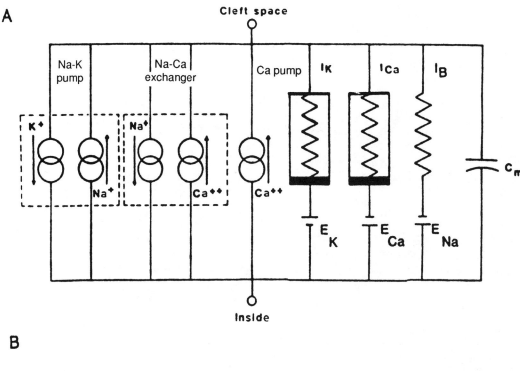

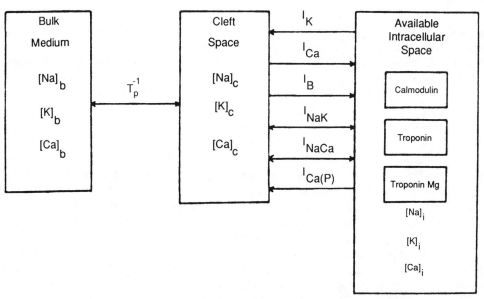

Figure 7 Single bullfrog sinus venosus myocyte model. (A) Equivalent circuit of the sarcolemma of the model bullfrog SV myocyte and (B) associated intracellular and extracellular fluid compartments. The model SV myocyte sarcolemma includes the channel-mediated currents I_K, I_{Ca}, and I_B and the transporter-mediated currents I_{NaK}, I_{NaCa}, and I_{CaP}. Note that there is no I_{Na}, I_{K1}, or I_f. Also note that the intracellular compartment includes the two myoplasmic Ca^{2+} binding proteins calmodulin and troponin. For further quantitative details see Rasmusson et al. (163, 164). In all simulations to be presented the following initial values were used: 111 mM $[Na^+]_o$, 2.5 mM $[K^+]_o$, 2.25 mM $[Ca^{2+}]_o$, 7.5 mM $[Na^+]_i$, 130 mM $[K^+]_i$, and 0.3×10^{-6} M $[Ca^{2+}]_i$. All results (with the exceptions of Figs. 14.B and 20) were obtained from simulations that were run for a sufficiently long time to allow attainment of steady-state conditions.

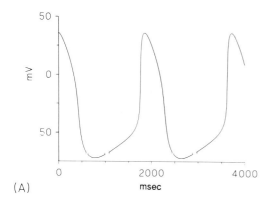

(A)

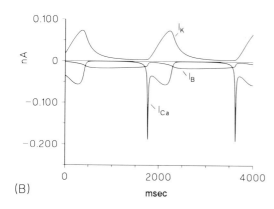

(B)

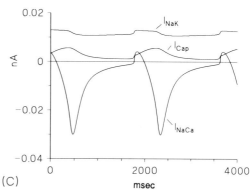

(C)

Figure 8 Control simulations of the currents underlying generation of primary SV pacemaking activity. In this and all subsequent current figures inward (depolarizing) currents are shown as negative and outward (hyperpolarizing) currents as positive. (A) Model-generated SV spontaneous diastolic depolarization and action potential cycle (compare to Fig. 1B). (B) Kinetic behavior of the channel-mediated currents I_{Ca}, I_K, and I_B. In particular, note the complex inactivation sequence displayed by I_{Ca} during the action potential plateau and early repolarization. (C) Behavior of the transporter-mediated currents I_{NaK}, I_{NaCa}, and I_{CaP}. Note that although I_{NaCa} displays dynamic behavior, I_{NaK} remains a relatively constant small outward current. Also note the difference in current scales between B and C.

149). The single-cell voltage clamp data available at present from amphibians and mammals are therefore in agreement in indicating that primary pacemaking cells lack both I_{Na} and I_{K1}. It is very important to note that the inwardly rectifying background potassium current I_{K1} is the major current responsible for generation of the stable resting potential of both atrial and ventricular cells (143, 163; Fig. 2B). Therefore, an important point that we wish to make is that it is the absence of a stabilizing background I_{K1} in primary pacemaking cells that allows spontaneous pacemaking to develop (see Fig. 16).

Using these data, the SV model developed consists of two parts (Fig. 7): (1) a cell membrane consisting of membrane capacitance C_m, gated ionic channel currents I_K, I_{Ca}, and I_B, and pump I_{NaK} (and I_{CaP}) and exchanger I_{NaCa} currents; and (2) a lumped fluid compartment that describes changes in the concentrations of Na^+, K^+, and Ca^{2+}. The specific details of

the model, the formulations used, and the mathematical techniques employed are given in Rasmusson et al. (163, 164). Two points about the SV model of Rasmusson et al. (164) should be emphasized. First, in contrast to previous models of cardiac electrical activity, the SV model of Rasmusson et al. (164) uses mathematical characterizations of the various sarcolemmal currents that are based as closely as possible upon experimental voltage clamp data obtained from single cells (36, 38–41, 83, 175–177). As such, possible biases in the model's predictions have been avoided by not having to introduce questionable correction factors for the effects of the ECS. Second, the model accounts for changes in intra- and extracellular concentrations of cations. In particular, the effects of two physiologically important myoplasmic Ca^{2+} binding proteins, calmodulin and troponin, are included. [It should be noted that troponin has two classes of Ca^{2+} binding sites: a Ca^{2+}-specific site (denoted Tn_{Ca} in the SV model) and a competitive Ca^{2+}-Mg^{2+} site (denoted Tn_{MgCa}; see Fig. 9). There are two Ca^{2+}-Mg^{2+} sites per troponin molecule; for details see 40, 42, 163, 164, 169). Simulations of intracellular Ca^{2+} homeostasis are not emphasized here, but the effects of these two proteins are extremely important for modulating intracellular Ca^{2+} transients during the flow of I_{Ca} and therefore the predicted behavior of I_{NaCa}. Although the contribution of troponin to the bullfrog myoplasmic Ca^{2+} buffering capacity is important, the magnitude of its contribution compared with that of mammalian SA node myocytes may be considerably more. Cells of the mammalian primary pacemaking tissue and the specialized conduction system have sparse and poorly developed myofibrils (e.g. 191, 192). This does not mean, however, that Ca^{2+} is poorly buffered in these cells: in addition to calmodulin there are other substantial Ca^{2+} regulatory and binding systems within the myoplasm of both pacemaking and working myocardial cells (see, e.g. 15, 44). The model of Rasmusson et al. (164) is therefore unique in the cardiac electrophysiology literature in terms of its physiologic plausibility. (Indeed, the model is still somewhat "conservative" in its present form in that it considers only the effects of calmodulin and troponin.)

Control Simulations: Behavior of Ionic Currents During Normal Pacemaking in Single SV Myocytes

Figure 8 shows the model-generated normal spontaneous electrical activity of a single SV myocyte under control conditions (Fig. 8A) and the underlying channel-mediated (Fig. 8B) and transporter-mediated (Fig. 8C) currents. The generation of the spontaneous diastolic depolarization is first discussed, then the generation of the action potential.

Diastolic Depolarization

The SV model demonstrates that a dynamic interaction of several current systems underlies generation of the spontaneous pacemaker potential (Fig. 8B and C). The earliest phase of the diastolic depolarization (i.e., that immediately following the maximum diastolic

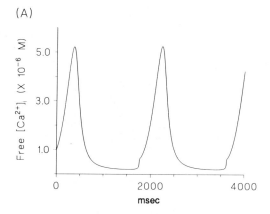

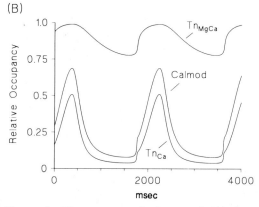

Figure 9 Time course of change of (A) *free* $[Ca^{2+}]_i$ and (B) Ca^{2+} binding by calmodulin and troponin during the control simulations presented in Figure 8. Ca^{2+} binding is represented as relative occupancy (i.e., fraction of sites occupied by Ca^{2+} relative to the total number of available sites) of the different Ca^{2+} binding sites on calmodulin (calmod) and troponin (Tn_{Ca}, Ca^{2+}-specific site; Tn_{MgCa}, competitive Ca^{2+}-Mg^{2+} site; see 40, 163, 164, 169). Note the significant Ca^{2+} buffering capacity provided by calmodulin and troponin (compare to Fig. 10).

potential) arises from an interaction between the inward background I_B, an inward I_{NaCa}, an outward I_{NaK}, and deactivation of the outward I_K. As I_K progressively deactivates (reversing the residual activation from the preceding action potential) its hyperpolarizing influence declines with time. Since there is no I_{K1} to dominate the membrane conductance and stabilize the membrane potential the influence of the small background currents becomes very important during this phase. As a result, as I_K

progressively deactivates the combined depolarizing influences of I_B and I_{NaCa} become more prominent, halting repolarization and allowing the diastolic depolarization to proceed. However, as diastolic depolarization continues the inward I_{Ca} becomes activated during approximately the last one-third of the pacemaker potential. I_{Ca} therefore also makes a significant contribution to the last phase of the pacemaker depolarization. Finally, although I_B, I_{NaCa}, I_{Ca}, and I_K all display dynamic behavior during the diastolic depolarization the Na^+/K^+ pump current I_{NaK} remains a relatively constant outward current during the entire process. However, it should be noted that I_{NaK} is of a similar magnitude to I_B; therefore, as is demonstrated here, I_{NaK} can significantly influence the rate of diastolic depolarization.

In summary, the spontaneous diastolic depolarization arises from a complex dynamic interaction between (1) a deactivating outward I_K, (2) the inward currents I_B and I_{NaCa}, (3) a relatively constant outward I_{NaK}, and (4) activation of the inward I_{Ca} during the final one-third of the depolarization. In working myocardium these depolarizing interactions are dominated by the high conductance of I_{K1}. Basic primary pacemaking therefore arises from a combination of a lack of I_{K1} and an interaction of five different current systems: no one current is solely responsible for generating pacemaking activity.

Action Potential: Upstroke and Plateau

As noted earlier, primary pacemaking cells lack a fast inward sodium current I_{Na}. Instead, the upstroke of the SV action potential is generated by activation of I_{Ca}, which occurs during the latter one third of the diastolic depolarization. During generation of the upstroke I_{Ca} activates quite rapidly. I_{Ca} then displays rapid but incomplete inactivation during the early plateau phase. Instead of progressively declining during the subsequent plateau phase, however, I_{Ca} displays quite complex behavior. In particular, a secondary inward "hump" of I_{Ca} develops during the later phases of the plateau and early repolarization (see 65, 139).

This predicted incomplete inactivation sequence of I_{Ca} is due to the complex inactiva-

tion processes previously discussed, that is, the nonmonotonic U-shaped inactivation f curve and the slowed inactivation kinetics at depolarized potentials (Fig. 5). During the plateau the membrane potential is in the range in which the f curve "bends up": as a result the net I_{Ca} only very slowly and incompletely inactivates. As the plateau progresses and the membrane begins to repolarize (due to activation of I_K; see later) the driving force for Ca^{2+} flow through the calcium channel progressively increases. As a result I_{Ca} increases again, producing the secondary inward hump. However, as repolarization proceeds further, the membrane potential enters the region in which both (1) the inactivation f variable is minimal and (2) I_{Ca} inactivation kinetics are the fastest. I_{Ca} therefore begins to decline again. Finally, as repolarization progresses further the remaining noninactivated I_{Ca} rapidly deactivates. The SV model therefore suggests that the incomplete inactivation phenomena displayed by I_{Ca} produces the maintained inward component of current that sustains the action potential plateau.

Action Potential: Repolarization

The ionic current mechanisms underlying the initiation of repolarization of the cardiac action potential have been an area of much confusion and controversy. For example, at various times all three of the individual hyperpolarizing currents I_{K1}, I_{NaK}, and I_K have been proposed as the current responsible for initiating repolarization (see discussion in 105).

The results of the SV model of Rasmusson et al. (164) clarify the mechanism(s) of repolarization in cardiac pacemaker tissue. First, as we have repeatedly emphasized, I_{K1} is not responsible for repolarization in pacemaking myocytes (although I_{K1} does play a role in the final phase of repolarization in working myocardial cells; see 105). Second, the SV model does repolarize in the absence of the Na^+/K^+ pump current I_{NaK}, suggesting that I_{NaK} is not the primary current underlying repolarization (see 163; however, I_{NaK} may be importantly involved in modulation of repolarization in Purkinje fibers; e.g., 111). Rather, the SV model indicates that the delayed rectifier current I_K slowly but progressively activates during the action potential plateau. Repolarization occurs as the result of a complex interaction between the delayed rectifier I_K and the maintained (incompletely inactivated) inward component of I_{Ca}. Once the activated I_K "wins out" over the small and incompletely inactivated I_{Ca} repolarization rapidly progresses. I_K then deactivates, allowing the next diastolic depolarization to begin. The duration of the plateau and initiation of repolarization are therefore determined by a fine balance between I_{Ca} and I_K: alteration of the behavior of either one of these currents can have quite significant effects on pacemaking.

The role of the delayed rectifying current I_K in SV in initiating repolarization of the action potential is thus very similar to the role of the delayed rectifying potassium current in squid giant axon (102). However, the activation-deactivation kinetics of I_K in the amphibian SV are approximately 1000 times slower than those of the squid axon. It is these slow gating kinetics that allow I_K to exert its effects on both the action potential and the diastolic depolarization.

Action Potential: Transporter-Mediated Currents

As can be seen by a comparison of the current scales in Fig. 8B and C, the sizes of the various transporter-mediated currents are all small compared to I_{Ca} and I_K. As during the diastolic depolarization, I_{NaK} remains a small and relatively constant outward current during the action potential. In contrast, I_{NaCa} displays complex dynamic behavior, changing polarity during the action potential (outward during the upstroke and early plateau; inward during the later plateau and repolarization). However, despite its complex dynamic behavior, I_{NaCa} is still always a small net current during all phases of the action potential. As such, neither I_{NaK} or I_{NaCa} exerts significant influence on the SV action potential under control conditions.

The predicted behavior of I_{NaCa} in this SV model warrants a little more discussion. It has been quite frequently hypothesized in the cardiac electrophysiology literature that $[Ca^{2+}]_i$

increases significantly during each action potential as a result of activation of I_{Ca}. Indeed, the SV model indicates that in the *absence* of intracellular Ca^{2+} binding proteins or other intracellular Ca^{2+} sequestration mechanisms $[Ca^{2+}]_i$ rapidly increases during the action potential (see also 40). The time course of the transient change in $[Ca^{2+}]_i$ during the flow of I_{Ca} has a number of very important electrophysiologic consequences, since it can both (1) significantly alter E_{Ca} (i.e., shift it in the hyperpolarizing direction) and (2) strongly activate the Na^+-Ca^{2+} exchanger (e.g., without myoplasmic Ca^{2+} binding and buffering processes the increase in $[Ca^{2+}]_i$ would be nearly instantaneous, and I_{NaCa} would therefore be a large and net inward current during all phases of the action potential; e.g., 61, 51, 152, 154).

The predicted behavior of I_{NaCa} in the SV model of Rasmusson et al. (164) therefore seems to be at odds with hypotheses currently popular in the cardiac electrophysiology literature regarding the interactions between I_{Ca} and I_{NaCa}. However, it must be pointed out that all these hypotheses regarding large I_{Ca}-mediated transient increases in $[Ca^{2+}]_i$ have not considered the known effects of physiologically important cardiac myoplasmic Ca^{2+} binding proteins. However, as stated, the SV model of Rasmusson et al. (164) has incorporated into the intracellular space two such important proteins, calmodulin and troponin. All simulations that have been presented have included the effects of these two proteins. Figure 9 shows the predicted magnitude and time course of change in free $[Ca^{2+}]_i$ and Ca^{2+} binding to the various sites on calmodulin and troponin during the corresponding simulations presented in Figure 8 (for details, see 37, 40, 42, 163, 164).

It is not the purpose of this chapter to emphasize intracellular Ca^{2+} homeostatic mechanisms (see, e.g., 44), but the simulations illustrated in Figure 9 have two important implications for basic mechanisms involved in primary pacemaking.

First, because of the significant buffer capacity provided by calmodulin and troponin, over 95% of the free Ca^{2+} that enters during

(A)

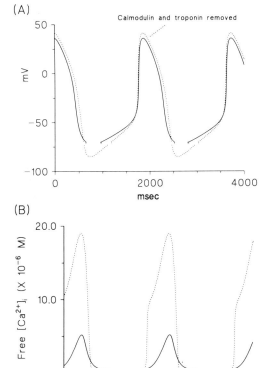

(B)

(C)

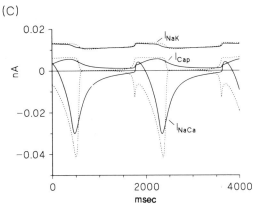

Figure 10 Effects of removing calmodulin and troponin on the $[Ca^{2+}]_i$ transient and behavior of I_{NaCa}. (A) Solid curve, control pacemaking activity (i.e., calmodulin and troponin included; see Fig. 8A); dashed curve, control pacemaking activity in the *absence* of calmodulin and troponin. (B) Associated $[Ca^{2+}]_i$ transients. Solid curve, control; dashed curve, calmodulin and troponin removed. (C) Behavior of the transporter-mediated currents I_{NaK}, I_{CaP}, and I_{NaCa}. Solid curves, control; dashed curves, calmodulin and troponin removed. Note that in the absence of calmodulin and troponin I_{NaCa} is always a large net inward current, which rapidly declines during repolarization. In the presence of these proteins I_{NaCa} is reduced and flows during both the action potential and the diastolic depolarization. These results should be compared to the voltage clamp results illustrated in Figure 6.

activation of I_{Ca} is buffered. Therefore, instead of a large maximal $[Ca^{2+}]_i$ transient occurring during the upstroke and the early plateau phase of the action potential the Ca^{2+} binding proteins both reduce and delay this peak in $[Ca^{2+}]_i$ until late repolarization. E_{NaCa} ($= 3E_{Na} - 2E_{Ca}$; $r = 3:1$) is therefore still a dynamic reversal potential that changes during the pacemaking cycle. However, the maximal change in E_{Ca} and thus E_{NaCa} occurs at a much later time in the action potential plateau than would be predicted without considering the effects of myoplasmic Ca^{2+} binding proteins. In essence, calmodulin and troponin effectively delay the large $[Ca^{2+}]_i$ transients that would otherwise be produced by I_{Ca}; as a result I_{NaCa} extrudes Ca^{2+} over a much longer portion of the pacemaker cycle.

Second, both the buffering capacity and the kinetics of Ca^{2+} binding to the various sites on the proteins largely determine the magnitude and time course of the I_{Ca}-mediated $[Ca^{2+}]_i$ transient. As a result, the magnitude,

polarity, and kinetics of I_{NaCa} are largely determined and modulated by the myoplasmic Ca^{2+} binding proteins and interactions between them (see also 15).

These effects are illustrated in Figure 10, which compares the time course of the $[Ca^{2+}]_i$ transient and I_{NaCa} from the previous control simulations (Figs. 8 and 9) to that predicted when the same simulations are run in the absence of calmodulin and troponin. As can be seen the combined effects of calmodulin and troponin are significant. Such myoplasmic protein-mediated effects could be very important in the intact cell in determining the effects of I_{NaCa} on both the diastolic depolarization and the action potential. It seems clear that such effects must be taken into account in the assessment of the normal roles of any calcium-mediated current system; otherwise, incorrect conclusions about the influences of such current systems may be reached. This is an area of research that deserves much careful future attention.

In summary, (1) the upstroke of the SV action potential is produced by rapid activation of I_{Ca}, (2) the plateau is maintained by a small inward I_{Ca} that is produced by a complex incomplete inactivation sequence, and (3) repolarization is initiated by activation of I_K. The subsequent deactivation of I_K then sets the stage for the next diastolic depolarization. (4) Finally, the SV model suggests that under control conditions both I_{NaK} and I_{NaCa} are small currents that are not significantly involved either in generation of the action potential plateau or initiation of repolarization.

EFFECTS OF SIMPLE ALTERATIONS IN THE MAGNITUDE OF MEMBRANE CURRENTS

In this section we briefly describe the effects of selectively increasing and decreasing the magnitude of each of the various current systems on spontaneous SV pacemaking. The available magnitude of one current at a time is altered by a simple multiplicative scaling factor. The voltage dependence of gating is not altered—only the possible available size of the current. This is analogous to changing the total number of transporter molecules or ionic channels available for activation. We hope this provides insight into both the roles and important modulatory influences that each current system can exert in pacemaking, as well as illustrates the sometimes very complex interactions between the many nonlinear current systems that can result from selectively altering only one current system.

Channel-Mediated Currents I_K and I_{Ca}

The effects of increasing by twice and decreasing by one-half the available sizes of I_K and I_{Ca} are shown in Figure 11. As can be seen, selectively altering the available size of either one of these channel-mediated currents pro-

duces significant effects on both the rate of pacemaking and the action potential configuration.

The effects of these maneuvers on the action potential are relatively straightforward and expected. (1) Increasing I_K reduces the overshoot and shortens the plateau; decreasing I_K heightens the overshoot and broadens the plateau. (2) Increasing I_{Ca} increases the overshoot and broadens the plateau; decreasing I_{Ca} reduces the overshoot and shortens the plateau.

However, what may seem somewhat counterintuitive or paradoxical are the effects of these selective maneuvers on the pacemaking rate. One might conclude that a selective increase in I_K (a hyperpolarizing current) would slow pacemaking rate or that a selective increase in I_{Ca} (a depolarizing current) would increase it. However, pacemaking is the result of a complex interaction of several nonlinear voltage-dependent current systems. As a result, selectively altering the characteristics of only one current system in the "freely pacing" cell also affects the behavior of all the other current systems.

This very important point is illustrated in Figure 12, which shows a comparison of the previously illustrated channel-mediated currents activated during normal SV pacemaking to the predicted behavior of these currents when the available size of I_K has been increased twofold. As can be seen, making more I_K available during the action potential not only affects the size of I_K but also alters I_{Ca} and the time course of I_B. Through its increased hyperpolarizing influence the larger I_K produces shortening of the plateau, a slight increase in the rate of repolarization, and a slight increase in the maximum diastolic potential. However, these effects in turn have three important consequences: (1) the total degree of inactivation of I_{Ca} developed during its plateau incomplete inactivation sequence is lessened, (2) I_{Ca} deactivates sooner owing to the more rapid repolarization, and (3) I_K deactivates slightly faster. As a result, (4) I_B is able to exert its depolarizing influence sooner in the cycle, and (5) more I_{Ca} is available for activation during both the final phase of the

(A)

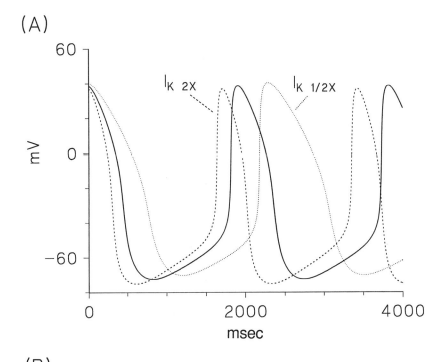

(B)

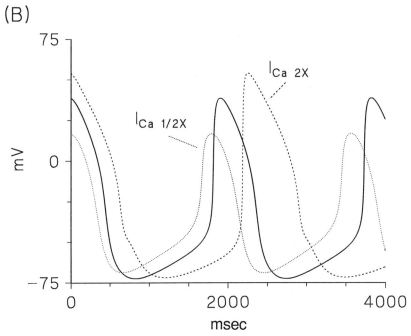

Figure 11 Effects of selectively altering the channel-mediated currents I_K (A) and I_{Ca} (B) on basic SV pacemaking. Solid curves, control simulations (Fig. 8A); dashed curves, available I_K or I_{Ca} increased two times; dotted curves, available I_K or I_{Ca} decreased by one-half.

(A)

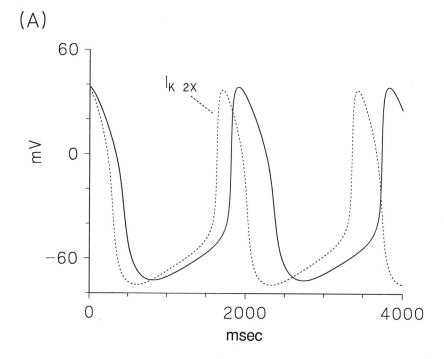

(B)

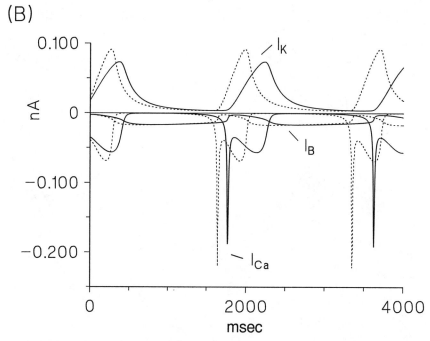

diastolic depolarization and the action potential because the threshold potential is reached more rapidly. There are also slight changes in the pump and exchanger currents (Fig. 12C), the effects of which should also be kept in mind.

The results of the example "increased I_K" simulation just discussed point out the extreme importance of having both action potential and voltage clamp current data when attempting to analyze the effects of either drugs or neuromodulatory compounds on pacemaking activ-

(C)

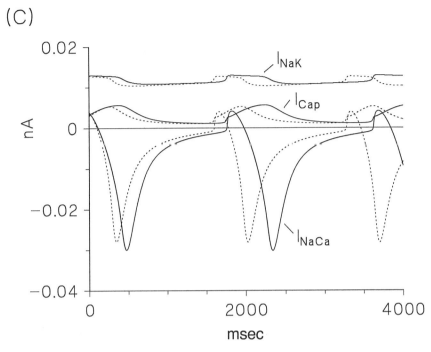

Figure 12 Complex interactions between the various nonlinear sarcolemmal current systems. This figure illustrates the alterations in all the other sarcolemmal currents produced by selectively increasing the available I_K two times (Fig. 11A). The solid curves are the control action potential and currents previously illustrated in Fig. 8A and B. The dashed curves show the resulting changes in the (A) diastolic depolarization and action potential, (B) channel-mediated currents, and (C) transporter-mediated currents when the available I_K is selectively increased two times.

ity. Looking at action potential parameters alone does not allow one to unequivocally determine which particular current system(s) is affected by a given pharmacologic compound. Indeed, if a given compound is extremely specific but one does not understand the basic current systems involved in generation of the electrical activity under study, one could be quite easily led astray by studying only action potentials. Furthermore, it is now recognized that many neuromodulatory compounds exert their effects in cardiac muscle by altering more than one current system (96). For example, it is now known that β-adrenergic compounds both increase I_{Ca} and shift the activation kinetics of I_K to more hyperpolarized potentials (the net effect is that I_K is also increased; e.g., 66, 82, 203). It is by altering both I_{Ca} and I_K that these compounds probably exert their well-known and much studied effects on the heart rate. Conversely, it is very

difficult to extrapolate from voltage clamp data the dynamic behavior of the currents during generation of the action potential (e.g., the behavior displayed by I_{Ca}) and the effects produced by altering the currents without resorting to both mathematical computer modeling and basic action potential measurements. These considerations point out the extreme value of having a realistic mathematical model of cellular electrical activity based as closely as possible upon a reliable and consistent set of both action potential and voltage clamp data obtained from a single cell type: such models are of use not only to theoretical membrane biophysicists but are also of extreme practical and instructional value to both pharmacologists and clinicians.

Therefore, in the remaining simulations to be presented only the net effects of alterations of individual currents are discussed; however, the complex interactions produced by such ap-

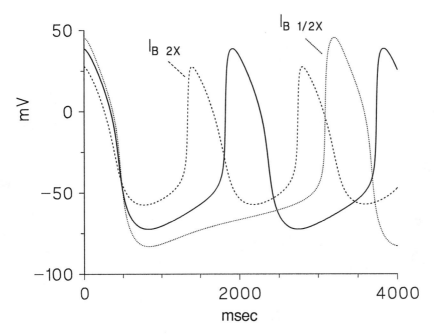

Figure 13 Effects of selectively altering the inward background current I_B on basic SV pacemaking activity. Solid curve, control; dashed curve, available I_B increased two times; dotted curve, available I_B decreased by one-half.

parently simple maneuvers on all the current systems must be kept in mind when evaluating the end results.

I_B

Figure 13 shows the predicted effects of selectively increasing by twice and decreasing by one-half the available inward background current I_B. Both maneuvers have a profound effect on the rate of pacemaking. Any drug or neurotransmitter that selectively modulates or affects I_B significantly affects heart rate. However, as previously pointed out, the exact biophysical mechanisms underlying generation of I_B are still unclear.

I_{NaK}

Figure 14A shows the predicted effects of a short-term (after 10 sec) increase in I_{NaK} two times above its available control level. Increasing I_{NaK} both increases the maximum diastolic potential and slows the pacemaker rate.

Figure 14B shows the effects of reducing I_{NaK} by one-half. Both the immediate (after 10 sec) and long-term (after 30 min) effects are

illustrated. The immediate effect of reducing I_{NaK} is to reduce the maximum diastolic potential and increase the pacemaking rate. However, by 30 min the system readjusts, such that (1) the maximum diastolic depolarization returns nearly to control levels and (2) the rate of pacemaking is reduced. This is due to an increase in the levels of $[Na^+]_i$ (entering the cell via I_B and I_{NaCa}) during prolonged reduction of I_{NaK}. Elevated $[Na^+]_i$ stimulates I_{NaK}, so that although maximal pump capacity has been diminished the normal current level is reestablished. Therefore, a long-term reduction in I_{NaK} produces a counterintuitive reduction in SV pacemaking rate. Clinically, patients being treated with cardiac glycosides display bradycardia. However, this bradycardia is attributable to an increase in vagal tone (e.g., 45, 188), the neuromodulatory effects of which may obscure those produced by the direct involvement of I_{NaK} at the cellular level.

The results illustrated in Figure 14 demonstrate that although I_{NaK} is not importantly involved in the action potential it can play a very important role in modulation of the pacemaker rate.

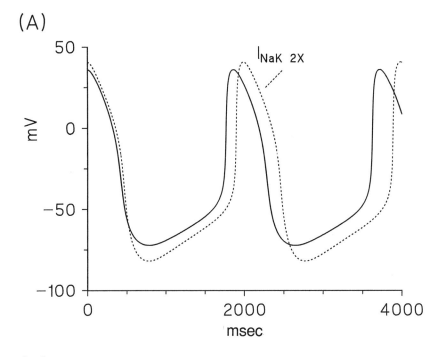

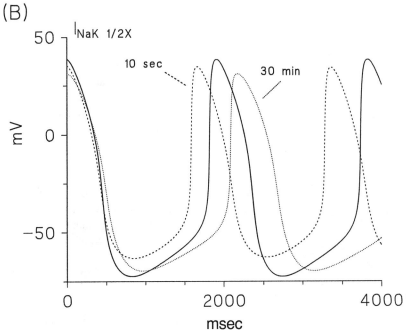

Figure 14 Effects of selectively altering the electrogenic Na^+/K^+ pump current I_{NaK}. (A) Effects of increasing I_{NaK}. Solid curve, control; dashed curve, available I_{NaK} increased two times. (B) Short-term (10 sec, dashed curve) and long-term (30 min, dotted curve) effects of decreasing the available I_{NaK} by one-half. Note that upon reduction of I_{NaK} by one-half the pacemaking rate is initially increased, but by 30 min pacemaking is reduced compared to control (solid curve) levels. This is because even though the available I_{NaK} has been reduced, the increase in $[Na^+]_i$ (via I_B and I_{NaCa}) stimulates I_{NaK} to return nearly back to control levels by 30 min.

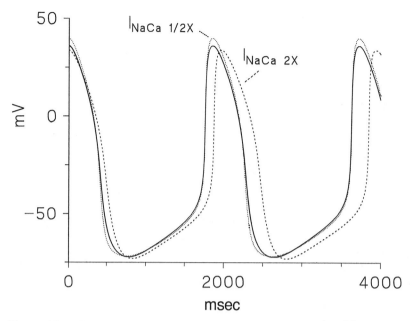

Figure 15 Effects of selectively altering the electrogenic Na^+/Ca^{2+} exchanger current I_{NaCa}. Solid curve, control; dashed curve, available I_{NaCa} increased two times; dotted curve, available I_{NaCa} decreased by one-half.

I_{NaCa}

Figure 15 shows the effects of both increasing by two times and decreasing by one-half the available magnitude of the electrogenic Na^+-Ca^{2+} exchanger current I_{NaCa}. Interestingly, although a 50% reduction of I_{NaCa} produces subtle effects, selective reduction of this current does not significantly alter pacemaking activity. However, doubling I_{NaCa} does lead to a somewhat counterintuitive slight reduction in pacemaking rate. These results reflect the importance of the probable roles that calmodulin and troponin play in modulating the behavior of I_{NaCa}; that is, its behavior is largely determined by the Ca^{2+} binding kinetics of these two proteins (see also 15). Therefore, under certain conditions I_{NaCa} could also act as a modulator of pacemaking rate.

Effect of Introducing I_f

Figure 16 shows an "interspecific" simulation on the effects of introducing the mammalian current I_f into the SV model. The formulation used for I_f was that given in DiFrancesco and Noble (61), to which readers are referred for

details. Figure 16 shows the effects of introducing I_f at 10, 40, and 60% of the maximum value obtainable in the DiFrancesco-Noble formulation. The quantitative aspects of this simulation are clearly not to be taken too literally, but the qualitative result is important: introduction of I_f causes both a reduction in the maximum diastolic potential and a significant increase in pacemaking rate. Therefore, as a result of the very slow activation-deactivation kinetics of I_f (for quantitative details see 60–62) this current behaves very much like a simple background "leak" current; that is, its effects are very similar to those produced by I_B. This simulation points out the very important modulatory role that I_f probably plays in mammalian SA node cells. However, we emphasize that I_f is a prominent and well-characterized current that is probably activated in the potential range of the diastolic depolarization of mammalian SA node cells (e.g., 33, 62, 85, 107, 149, 201, 202). As such, I_f displays both the voltage dependence and pharmacologic sensitivity to make it an extremely important current system for the study of future clinical interventions on heart rate.

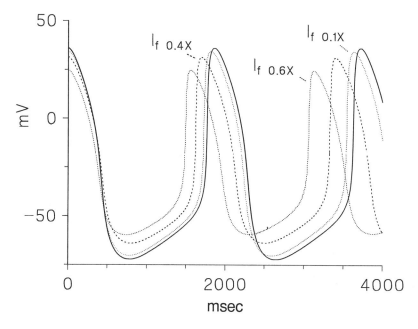

Figure 16 Effects of introducing the current I_f into the SV model myocyte. Solid curves, control; dashed curves, I_f introduced. I_f values of 10% ($I_f \times 0.1$), 40% ($I_f \times 0.4$), and 60% ($I_f \times 0.6$) of that available from the DiFrancesco-Noble formulation were used. As can be seen, introduction of I_f into the SV model leads to a significant modulation of pacemaking activity.

Effects of Introducing I_{K1}

As repeatedly emphasized, I_{K1} is not present in primary pacemaking cells. To illustrate the importance of this finding, Figure 17A shows the effect of introducing I_{K1} into the SV model. I_{K1} was formulated according to the measured properties of I_{K1} in single bullfrog atrial myocytes (see 163). As can be seen, introduction of an I_{K1} of only 10% of its value in a bullfrog atrial myocyte greatly slows the rate of SV pacemaking. Further increasing I_{K1} to only 40% of the atrial value completely stops pacing and produces a stabilized resting potential.

The simulations presented in Figure 17A clearly point out that it is the absence of I_{K1} that allows I_B and I_{NaCa} to exert their depolarizing influences in generation of the diastolic depolarization. This point has been elegantly demonstrated experimentally by Moore et al. (143), who have shown that block of I_{K1} in single bullfrog atrial myocytes by 50 µm extracellular Ba^{2+} induces spontaneous pacemaker activity in these normally quiescent myocytes (Fig. 17B). The same Ba^{2+} concen-

tration had no effect on the spontaneous activity of isolated SV myocytes. The absence of I_{K1} in primary pacemaking cells has been recognized for some time, but the important functional significance of its absence has frequently been overlooked or underappreciated in many discussions of mechanisms of pacemaking. Finally, it is also of interest to briefly note that the vagally released neurotransmitter acetylcholine slows pacemaking rate. The effects of ACh are complex (96), but one important effect is activation of an "I_{K1}-like" potassium current "I_{KACh}" (e.g., 27, 142). The probable effects of I_{KACh} are likely very similar to those illustrated here by the addition of I_{K1} into the SV model.

SINUS NODE FUNCTION IN MULTICELLULAR PREPARATIONS

Functional and Morphologic Organization of the Rabbit Sinus Node

The experimental data and simulations presented in the first two sections were designed

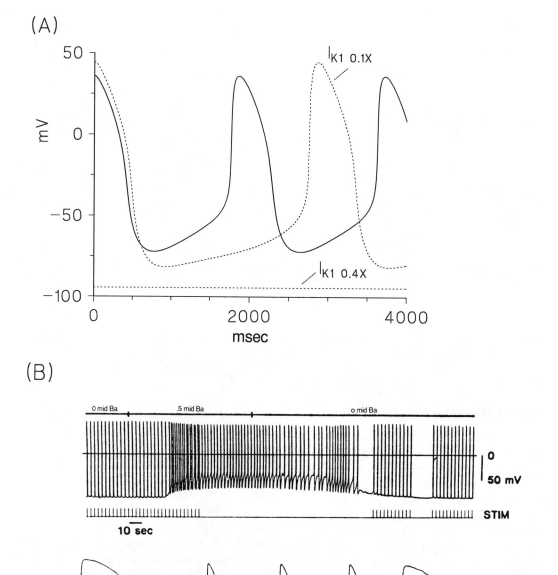

Figure 17 (A) Effects of introducing the background inwardly rectifying potassium current I_{K1} into the SV model myocyte. Solid curves, control; dashed curves, I_{K1} introduced. I_{K1} values of 10% (I_{K1} ×0.1) and 40% (I_{K1} ×0.4) of the available I_{K1} in a single bullfrog atrial myocyte were used (16). Introducing an I_{K1} of only 40% of the atrial value completely suppresses spontaneous pacemaking activity. (B) Induction of spontaneous pacemaking activity in a single bullfrog atrial myocyte by block of I_{K1} with 50×10^{-6} M $BaCl_2$. Atrial action potentials were elicited with a stimulus train before and during initial application of Ba^{2+}; the train was then discontinued. Notice that block of I_{K1} by Ba^{2+} causes the normally quiescent atrial cell to begin to spontaneously pace. The lower panel shows the results on an expanded time scale. [From Moore et al. (143).]

to elucidate at the cellular level the basic ionic mechanisms underlying generation of spontaneous diastolic depolarization and action potential. Studies designed to evaluate sinus node function in multicellular preparations not only assess the sum of ionic currents that underlie the action potential at the cellular level but also the currents that flow between cells that result from cell-to-cell interactions via gap junctions. The most complete story to date about the functional organization in the mammalian heart has been deduced from experiments on the isolated rabbit right atrial preparation.

These experiments have identified a group of cells whose activation preceded other cells in the atrium, whose diastolic depolarization was the steepest, whose upstroke velocity was the slowest, and in which there was a gradual transition from diastolic depolarization to the upstroke (158, 170, 183, 196, 205). Early studies (183) recognized that action potential morphology gradually changed between an impalement site in the sinus node and another in the crista terminalis. Bleeker et al. (19) were the first to extensively map the endocardial surface of the rabbit right atrial preparation to establish the activation sequence as well as the transmembrane action potential characteristics from different regions of the endocardial surface (Fig. 18). The site of earliest discharge was found to be located in the intercaval region, 0.5–2 mm away from the medial border of the crista terminalis. From this site the excitation wave propagated preferentially in an oblique cranial direction toward the crista terminalis. The conduction velocity increased markedly as the activation front left the central portion of the node. As seen in Figure 18 the spread in excitation resulted in an activation front that simultaneously reached a broad part of the crista terminalis. Several investigators have suggested that sodium channels do not contribute to the upstroke of the action potential in the central part of the node (see discussion in the first section), whereas they do in the surrounding latent pacemaker cells (149). Using the criterion that cells displaying the highest rate of diastolic depolarization at the end of diastole represent activity

arising from the dominant pacemaker site, the highest rates were observed in a rather large but not sharply delineated area (about 0.3 mm^2) consisting of approximately 5000 cells.

Synchronization of pacemaker activity within the dominant pacemaker site is mediated through electrical coupling between cells. Although gap junctions are relatively sparse in the sinus node (approximately one-tenth of that in working myocardial cells) there is ample experimental evidence indicating appreciable electrical coupling between nodal cells (22, 35, 137, 156, 174, 191, 192). However, the effective electrical coupling and synchronization between primary pacemaker cells in the face of a relatively high intercellular resistance is not entirely unexpected. As noted earlier, primary pacemaker cells lack an inwardly rectifying background potassium current I_{K1} (83, 85, 143, 176). Thus the membrane resistance in the range of diastolic depolarization is approximately an order of magnitude higher than in working myocardium (see Fig. 2). As a result very little current flow between pacemaker cells is required for their synchronization during diastole. In the absence of a dissipative I_{K1} conductance a high level of spatial homogeneity of potential can be maintained in primary pacemaker tissue despite a relatively high intercellular resistance. [For a rigorous discussion of the effects of intercellular and transmembrane resistance in the spatial distribution of electrical activity see Jack et al. (110)]. This is an important illustration of the fact that morphology (e.g., gap junctional density, restricted extracellular space, and myocyte orientation) interacts with the spatial heterogeneity of the biophysical properties of cardiac cells (e.g., the presence or absence of I_{K1}) to produce the complex and still poorly understood phenomenon associated with propagated electrical activity in the heart.

A variety of interventions, including autonomic agonists, have been shown to induce chronotropic responses. These chronotropic responses have been frequently associated with a shift in pacemaker site away from the central part of the node (25, 129, 131, 180). For example, both epinephrine and low concentrations of acetylcholine induce a pacemaker shift

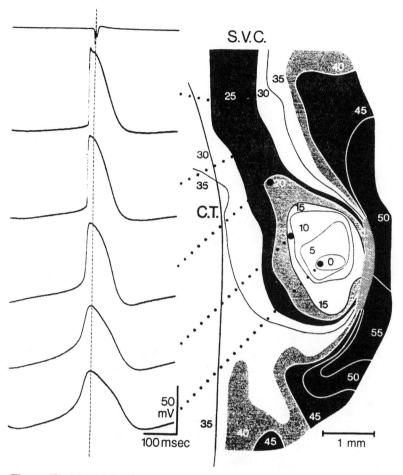

Figure 18 Map of the sinoatrial activation pattern from the endocardial surface of the rabbit right atrial preparation. The isochrones are groups in 5 msec increments. The dashed line corresponding to the steepest deflection in surface electrogram recording from the crista terminalis serves as the time reference. Action potential configuration is shown for representative microelectrode impalements along the path of preferential excitation. Note the gradual transition in all components of the action potential as the impalement site moves from the pacemaker center to the crista terminalis. The numbers in the map give the activation time in msec. CT = crista terminalis, SVC = superior vena cava. [Reproduced from Bleeker et al. (19) with permission of the American Heart Association.]

toward the inferior part of the node, whereas higher concentrations of acetylcholine induce a pacemaker shift toward cells near the upper part of the crista terminalis (131). Shifts in pacemaker site also occur following electrical stimulation, indicating that the activation patterns depicted in Figure 18 cannot be assumed to be fixed but are dynamic and changeable in response to a variety of interventions (141, 179, 180).

Although the isolated rabbit right atrial preparation has been used extensively to in-

vestigate the electrophysiology of the sinus node and results obtained from this preparation have been extrapolated to other animal species and humans, recent studies from Boineau's laboratory have suggested that a more complicated picture may exist (20, 21). These studies in the intact dog heart have demonstrated that the atrial depolarization sequence at the superior vena caval-right atrial junction is multicentric in origin. The conclusion drawn from these studies was that this reflected either an uneven spread of activity from a single focus or multiple distributed pacemaker sites.

Although bradyarrhythmias associated with sinus node dysfunction were initially thought to be due to a depression of sinus node automaticity, closer examination of the ECG recordings in patients with this disorder suggested that conduction disturbances could also contribute to the excessively slow heart rate in these patients. As a result interest grew in examining the functional behavior of the sinus node. The functional variables that were examined therefore included automaticity, conduction, and refractoriness. As discussed in the first two sections, diastolic depolarization reflects a very fine balance between different ionic currents. It should therefore be noted that a depression of automaticity cannot simply be attributed to a change in the value of a particular conductance, pump or exchanger current, or intercellular resistance. Instead, what one attempts to assess is an aggregate property of the pacemaker site, namely its rhythmicity. Similarly, measures of conduction and refractoriness provide information about aggregate properties of the sinus node but limited information about the underlying ionic mechanisms. Nonetheless, such approaches still represent an important first step in elucidating the underlying pathophysiology of sinus node dysfunction.

Disturbance in any or all of these three variables, that is, automaticity, conduction, and refractoriness, could be responsible for the abnormally slow heart rate seen in patients with sinus node dysfunction (207). Because electrical activity within the sinus node is not manifest in the surface ECG, measures of different electrophysiologic variables in the sinus node have by necessity been indirect and deduced from analysis of atrial responses to programmed stimulation. The assumptions underlying interpretation of these indirect tests have been examined in electrophysiologic studies in vitro on the sinus node performed in the isolated rabbit right atrial preparation.

Assessment of Sinus Node Automaticity

Although measurement of spontaneous heart rate provides a measure of sinus node automa-

ticity, the intermittent nature of the slowing implied that more provocative tests were required to unmask latent or episodic sinus node dysfunction. As automaticity is sensitive to autonomic tone, any measure of sinus node automaticity is distorted by a change in the balance and/or absolute magnitude of parasympathetic and sympathetic tone. As a consequence, automaticity has been measured following autonomic blockade as well as under basal conditions. Early investigations suggested that assessment of the chronotropic response to a β-agonist would be a useful adjunct in this regard (1, 2, 63, 64, 112, 113, 116, 133, 134). Unfortunately, implementation of this technique is not readily applicable to in vivo experiments because of (1) the need to establish the agonist concentration in vivo and (2) the inability to differentiate a change in functional properties of the receptor from an abnormality in electrophysiologic properties of the sinus node.

It was widely appreciated that transient suppression of rhythmicity usually followed cessation of a rapid heart beat (30, 83, 126, 130, 132). Microelectrode studies in the isolated rabbit right atrial preparation subsequently demonstrated suppression of spontaneous diastolic depolarization in the sinus node following cessation of rapid stimulation of the atrium (130, 180). Further, the magnitude of such "overdrive suppression" was altered by autonomic agents in a manner that paralleled their effect on the spontaneous heart rate; for example, atropine and isoproterenol reduced the degree of overdrive suppression (30, 130). As a result it was thought that studying the phenomenon of overdrive suppression in vivo might prove useful in identifying abnormalities of automaticity.

At the cellular level induction of overdrive suppression attempts to stress the sinus node by increasing its rate of excitation. How quickly the sinus node recovers its normal pacemaker function is then taken as an index of the degree of normal automatic function (Figs. 19 and 20). The mechanisms underlying overdrive suppression are not yet fully elucidated, but experimental as well as modeling studies have indicated that it is dependent on

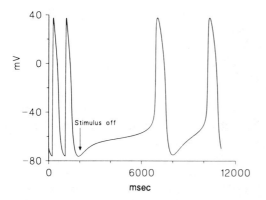

Figure 19 Simulated "overdrive suppression" in a single isolated bullfrog SV myocyte. The model SV cell (164) was rapidly paced once every 800 msec (i.e., 2.5 times above its normal level) by a 5 msec depolarizing current pulse for a total of 60 sec. The last two paced action potentials of this sequence are shown. The stimulus train was then stopped (indicated by the "stimulus off" arrow), and the SV myocyte was allowed to "free run." Notice that after cessation of the rapid stimulus train there is a marked slowing (i.e., suppression) of the rate of pacemaking.

sodium loading of the cell, mediated mainly by an increase in activity of the electrogenic Na^+-Ca^{2+} exchanger. As a result of the sigmoid dependence of I_{NaK} activation on $[Na^+]_i$ [i.e., $[Na^+]_i^3$; e.g. Cohen et al. (51, 52)], an increase in $[Na^+]_i$ above its control level can appreciably increase I_{NaK}. The corresponding increase in outward I_{NaK} then slows the rate of pacemaking until normal intracellular sodium levels are reestablished (see Figs. 14A and 19).

Investigators have therefore applied the technique of rapid atrial pacing to the study of sinus node automaticity in patients in an attempt to verify the usefulness of overdrive suppression as a method for identifying abnormalities in automaticity in these patients (132, 133, 146, 184). A train of rapid stimuli applied to the atrium near the sinus node should theoretically be conducted retrogradely into the sinus node. This should prevent spontaneous diastolic depolarization from attaining a threshold. Experimentally it is observed that after abruptly stopping rapid atrial pacing the interval between the last driven and first spontaneous depolarization in the sinus node is longer than the cycle length of the spontane-

ous cycles that precede the pacing train (Fig. 20); regular rhythmicity is then usually reestablished within the next 5–10 depolarizations. Action potential recordings show that the slope of diastolic depolarization is not the only variable altered. Changes in (1) the transition between the terminal part of diastolic depolarization and excitation and (2) the time interval between the sinus node and atrial depolarizations also occur, implying that restoration of spontaneous impulse formation may be associated with a shift in primary pacemaker site (180). It is important to note that all these changes impact on the duration of the atrial escape cycle, as this is determined by (1) the retrograde conduction time of the paced impulse into the sinus node, (2) the spontaneous sinus node cycle, and (3) the conduction time of the impulse from the pacemaker site back to the atrium. The duration of the first return cycle, which is termed the sinus node recovery time (SNRT), is thus only an estimate of the degree of sinus node suppression (112, 120, 122, 207). In general, the duration of SNRT increases as the pacing rate increases.

The magnitude of sinus node suppression depends on (1) the inherent automaticity of the sinus node, (2) the number of impulses entering the node, and (3) the autonomic tone during the course of the experiment (112, 207). The actual number of impulses entering the node in turn depends on the duration and frequency of pacing and the degree of entrance block into the sinus node. Development of entrance block as the atrial pacing rate increases has been demonstrated to occur and explains why SNRT, after reaching a maximum value, shortens with further increases in pacing rate (122, 180) (see Fig. 21). Shortening of SNRT after attainment of a maximal value coincided with the development of a 2:1 atriosinus block (122). Using repeated microelectrode impalements to determine the activation sequences for the different paced beats, the site of atriosinus block was identified as the point at which action potential amplitude fell rapidly. With progressively faster pacing rates the site of block moved progressively farther from the pacemaker site in the sinus node. Conduction failure may be a manifestation of a combina-

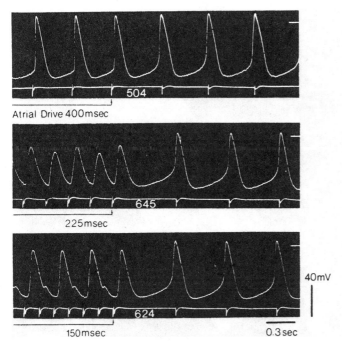

Figure 20   Effects of atrial pacing cycle length on atriosinus conduction and sinus node recovery time in the rabbit right atrial preparation. Pacing periods of 30 sec were used. The end of the train is marked by the arrow. The pacing cycle length was 400, 225, and 150 msec. A transmembrane action potential recording from the same cell in the primary pacemaker area is shown along with a surface electrogram recording from the crista terminalis of the rabbit right atrial preparation. Note the increase in sinus node recovery time from 504 to 645 msec as the pacing cycle length decreases from 400 to 225 msec. At the shorter pacing cycle length (150 msec) a 2:1 block occurs during the pacing train and the SNRT decreases from 645 to 624 msec. At the pacing cycle lengths of 400 and 225 msec, note the time difference between activation of the sinus node and the crista terminalis for the first escape cycle. In addition, at a pacing cycle length of 225 msec this time interval progressively increased from 4 to 20 msec by the third activation after termination of the pacing train. [From Steinbeck et al. (180) with permission of the American Heart Association.)

tion of basic cellular phenomena (i.e., the relative refractory period during which I_{Ca} has not yet recovered from inactivation and I_K has not fully deactivated) coupled with a multicellular phenomenon (i.e., the high coupling resistance in the SA node). The presence of disease may compound this problem through increases in the tortuosity of intercellular connections (e.g., due to scar tissue) or an increase in intercellular resistance (e.g., due to changes in gap junctions). Thus an increase in intercellular resistance as well as an increase in refractory period due to basic sarcolemmal mechanisms at the cellular level all probably play a role in the development of 2:1 atriosinus block and of deceptively low SNRT. Thus

a proper understanding of sinus node function must include evaluation of the conduction of the primary pacemaking impulse to the atrium.

Assessment of Sinoatrial Conduction

The interval between activation of the dominant pacemaker site in the sinus node and the crista terminalis represents the sinoatrial conduction time (SACT). The crista terminalis is that portion of the atrium that is responsible for the beginning of the inscription of the P wave; as a result, only certain degrees of conduction disturbance (second degree) can be detected in the surface ECG. More advanced

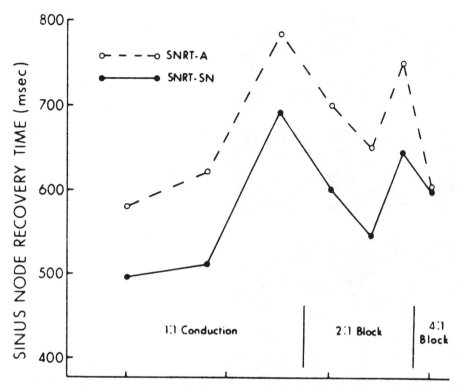

Figure 21 The relationship between sinus node recovery time determined from action potential recordings from the sinus node (SNRT-SN) and from electrogram recordings from the atrium (SNRT-A) and pacing cycle length. SNRT increases as pacing cycle length decreases until the 2:1 atriosinus block develops. A second peak of SNRT occurs just before development of the 4:1 block. The basic cycle length for this preparation was 490 msec. [From Kerr and Strauss (122) with permission of the American Heart Association.]

degrees of conduction disturbance, in particular lesser degrees of conduction disturbance, elude detection in the surface ECG. Because of the limited information about conduction that could be deduced from the ECG, two indirect methods (premature atrial stimulation and constant atrial pacing) and one direct recording method were developed to measure sinoatrial conduction time.

Premature Atrial Stimulation

Figure 22 diagrammatically depicts the principle underlying the estimation of the sinoatrial conduction time using this indirect technique (186). Activation sequences and atrial and sinus cycle length are illustrated for three representative atrial premature depolarizations (APD) introduced at different coupling intervals during diastole. When a premature depolarization is followed by a compensatory

response (see Fig. 22) this was taken to mean that this depolarization did not alter the pacemaker cycle in the sinus node, presumably because it falls too late in the cycle and instead "collides" with the emerging sinus node impulse. An earlier premature depolarization followed by a return cycle that is less than compensatory (point 3 in Fig. 22) is early enough to enter and reset the sinus node. In this case, however, the return cycle is longer than the spontaneous sinus cycle. The reason for this disparity in cycle length has been assumed to reflect the time taken for the APD to conduct retrogradely into the sinus node (A_2SAN_2), the sinus node return cycle (SAN_2SAN_3), and the antegrade conduction time of the recovery impulse (SAN_3A_3). If one assumes that the sinus node return cycle (SAN_2SAN_3) equals the spontaneous cycle (SAN_1SAN_1 or A_1A_1), then the sum of retro-

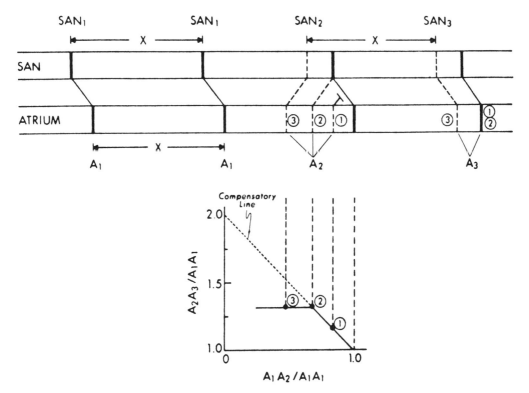

Figure 22 Principle underlying estimation of the sinoatrial conduction time. (Top) Three premature atrial depolarizations (A_2) falling at different points during the cardiac cycle. Electrical events within the sinus node, atrium, and intervening tissue are depicted in the ladder diagram. SAN_1 = sinus node depolarization, A_1 = atrial depolarization, A_1A_1 = spontaneous cycle length, A_1A_2 = Premature interval, and A_2A_3 = atrial return cycle. The two late atrial premature depolarizations (1 and 2) are followed by compensatory return cycles, where $A_2A_3 + A_1A_2 = 2 \times A_1A_1$. The earliest A_2 is followed by a less than compensatory response, and the difference between A_2A_3 (dashed line) and A_1A_1 is then the retrograde and antegrade conduction time between the atrium and sinus node. In the bottom panel A_2A_3 is plotted against A_1A_2, both normalized by the spontaneous sinus cycle length (A_1A_2). [From Strauss et al. (187) with permission.]

grade plus antegrade sinoatrial conduction time may be calculated by taking the difference between A_2A_3 and A_1A_1. If it is further assumed that antegrade and retrograde conduction are equal, then $A_2A_3 - A_1A_1$ should equal twice the antegrade sinoatrial conduction time (SAN_1A_1). Experiments have indicated, however, that the assumptions underlying the premature atrial stimulation technique can be only partly verified, meaning that the technique can provide only an approximate measure of the sinoatrial conduction time (141, 179). As mentioned, the analysis assumes an invariant sinus node return cycle length following each premature depolarization. This assumption is not fulfilled, as

changes in sinus node repolarization and slope of diastolic depolarization that follow each premature depolarization lead to a sinus node return cycle length that is different from SAN_1SAN_1. In other words, $A_2A_3 - A_1A_1$ does not always reliably track conduction time because of changes in SAN_2SAN_3 cycle length.

Continuous Atrial Pacing

This indirect technique employs analysis of the atrial return cycle following a short period of atrial pacing (147). The atrium is paced for eight beats at a rate slightly faster than the sinus rate. SACT is then calculated as the difference between the first return cycle and the mean spontaneous cycle. The mean of four or five determinations is taken as the SACT. Problems similar to those already discussed for the premature atrial stimulation technique affect the accuracy of the measurement of SACT using this technique (89).

Direct Recording of Sinus Node Electrical Activity

Attempts have been made to record the electrical activity of the sinus node directly. The small anatomic size of the sinus node and the slow rate of depolarization during diastole and the upstroke, as well as the interference produced by higher frequency electrical activity from neighboring atrial tissue, have all combined to make this task technically difficult. However, a technique for obtaining extracellular electrogram recordings of sinus node depolarization using extracellular electrodes placed near the sinus node has been developed. The technique developed by Cramer et al. (55) takes advantage of the absence of diastolic depolarization in atrial myocardium as well as the delay between the upstroke of the action potentials recorded in the sinus node and in the atrium. Unipolar extracellular electrograms are recorded at high gain with one electrode placed in proximity to the pacemaker site and the indifferent electrode placed some distance away yielding information concerning diastolic depolarization and excitation in the sinus node and in the atrium (Fig. 23). Since the initial reports demonstrating the feasibility of recording sinus node electrograms from the epicardial or endocardial surfaces of rabbit and dog hearts, the technique has been extended to humans using a catheter electrode (54, 88, 90, 94, 95, 166). Technical limitations can interfere with the success rate of the recording, but another concern relates to the need for proper catheter localization to accurately measure the sinoatrial conduction time. This technique offers the advantage of being able to measure sinoatrial conduction time on a beat-to-beat basis as opposed to a measurement that represents an average of many beats. Hence, the ability of this technique to assess dynamic changes in conduction, such as those occurring during intermittent conduction failure or during the postpacing period, is readily apparent.

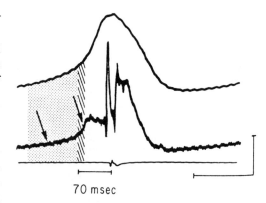

70 msec

Figure 23. Transmembrane potential (top trace) and a unipolar extracellular electrogram recording (middle trace) from the primary pacemaker area of the sinus node of the rabbit right atrial preparation recorded simultaneously with a bipolar atrial electrogram (bottom trace). Diastolic depolarization and the early component of the transition to excitation are indicated by the two arrows and shaded areas. Horizontal bar is 150 msec, and vertical bar corresponds to 35 mV for the transmembrane potential recording and 25 μV for the unipolar electrogram recording. [From Cramer et al. (55) with permission of the American Heart Association.]

Assessment of Sinus Node Refractoriness

To measure refractoriness in most regions of the heart, electrical activity proximal and distal to that tissue is recorded in response to premature stimulation. Depolarizations arising as a result of atrial stimulation are conducted retrogradely toward the sinus node, which is engulfed by the approaching wavefront and is depolarized last (170). Electrical activity cannot be measured distal to the node, and therefore the conventional method used to measure refractoriness elsewhere in the heart cannot be applied to the sinus node.

Examination of atrial return cycles following premature atrial stimulation may, however, provide insight into refractoriness of the sinus node (121). Analysis of recovery cycles following premature atrial stimulation introduced during atrial pacing fall into different categories (see Fig. 24). These include (1) "reset", in which the return cycle (A_2A_3) approximates the cycle length seen after termination of the pacing train (A_1A_1), and (2) "interpolation", when a premature depolarization is followed by a return cycle (A_2A_3) whose cycle length is shorter than a reset response. Complete interpolation occurs when the recovery depolarization is unaffected by A_2 and the encompassing interval (A_1A_3) approximates the spontaneous recovery cycle length without a premature depolarization.

A variety of investigators who have observed interpolation in both animals and humans postulated that interpolation is due to encroachment of the premature impulse on the refractory period of the sinus node, thereby precluding premature excitation (67, 127, 146). Kerr et al. (121) examined the distribution of refractoriness in the sinus node and the site of block of premature impulses. Using previously accepted criteria to identify the primary pacemaker site within the sinus node, incompletely interpolated responses were associated with low-voltage depolarizations in the primary pacemaker site that delayed diastolic depolarization and excitation (Fig. 24). During complete interpolation these low-voltage depolarizations were not seen (121). In fact, the transition from a reset to an incompletely interpolated response paralleled the abrupt reduction in action potential amplitude, rendering the action potential response in the pacemaker site incapable of resetting diastolic depolarization (Fig. 25). By examining relative action potential amplitude at various sites between the pacemaker site and the atrium at the same premature interval the pattern of block of premature impulses was identified (Fig. 26). Progressively earlier premature responses were blocked at progressively greater distances from the node, indicating that a gradation in refractoriness exists between the sinus node and atrium. A possible cellular basis for this observed gradation in refractoriness lies in the difference in channel-mediated current systems between primary pacemaker cells versus secondary pacemaker, crista terminalis, and atrial cells. In particular, many of the secondary pacemaker cells possess I_{Na}, but crista terminalis and atrial cells possess both I_{Na} and a transient inactivating outward potassium current (I_A or I_{to}) (49, 81, 84, 85, 149) The inactivation and recovery

characteristics of I_{to}, in particular, are very complex (49). Hence, the measurement of refractoriness does not solely reflect recovery of excitability in the sinus node pacemaker site but also includes the complex recovery characteristics of the intermediate cells in the pathway.

SINUS NODE FUNCTION IN THE HUMAN

As mentioned earlier, sinus node dysfunction in the human is an important clinical problem, as this disorder is capable of causing appreciable morbidity and mortality. In an attempt to establish the underlying pathophysiology, investigators set out to quantitate the underlying disturbance and developed a series of noninvasive and invasive techniques designed to assess sinus node function in the patient under a variety of conditions. These techniques were first established experimentally using animals before being applied to patients. Thus the techniques presented in this section represent a recapitulation of the experimental approaches outlined in the third section. Obviously these approaches are much more constrained because of safety considerations, with limits placed on the duration of study and the number of stimulating and recording sites. In addition, placing a value on a particular test result in managing a patient depends on a variety of factors, including the magnitude of disturbance of sinus node function, automaticity of infranodal pacemaker tissue, degree of contractile impairment of the left ventricle, and the degree of vascular insufficiency (207). The methods as applied to humans are briefly described, followed by a discussion of the utility and limitations of each.

Definition of Sinus Node Dysfunction

Electrocardiographic criteria used to define sinus node dysfunction have been established by Ferrer (73). The dominant disturbance is too slow a heart rate. More specifically, these criteria include (1) persistent, severe, and inappropriate bradycardia; (2) cessation of sinus rhythm for short or long intervals (sinus pause

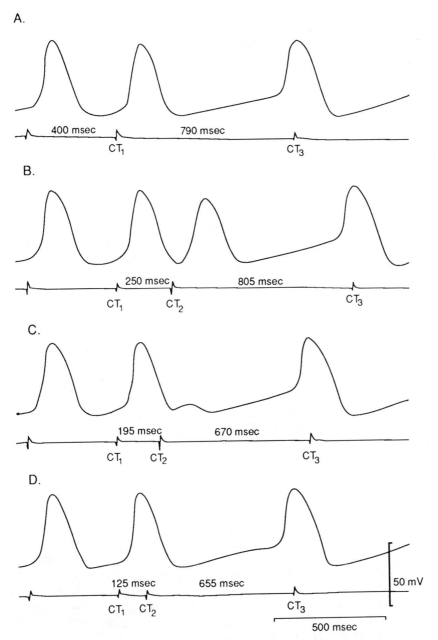

Figure 24 Examples of three types of responses following premature depolarizations compared to a spontaneous return cycle without a premature depolarization. The last beat of a 400 msec pacing train is shown in each panel. (A) Spontaneous recovery without a premature depolarization. (B) A reset response in which the atrial recovery cycle CT_2CT_3 is slightly longer than spontaneous recovery cycle in A. (C) Incomplete interpolation in which the atrial return cycle (CT_2CT_3) is slightly longer than in D. (D) Complete interpolation in which the atrial return cycle (CT_2CT_3) is such that the sum of it and the premature cycle ($CT_1CT_2 + CT_2CT_3$) is similar to the spontaneous recovery cycle in A. Note the low-voltage depolarization associated with incomplete interpolation in C. [From Kerr et al. (121) with permission of the American Heart Association.]

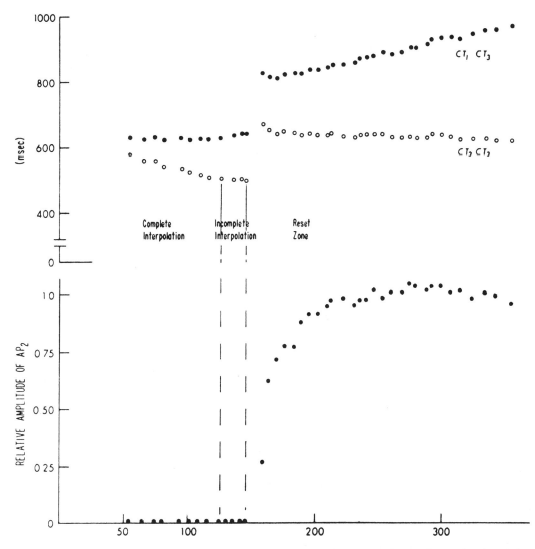

Figure 25 Comparison of the relative action potential amplitude to zones of reset, incomplete interpolation, and complete interpolation. The encompassing interval (CT_1CT_3) and the recovery interval (CT_2CT_3) are plotted as a function of prematurity (CT_1CT_2). The sudden fall in relative action potential amplitude recorded from a typical pacemaker cell in the sinus node occurred immediately before the transition from reset to incomplete interpolation. [From Kerr et al. (121) with permission of the American Heart Association.]

or sinus arrest) with or without the appearance of an ectopic escape rhythm; (3) episodes of sinoatrial exit block; (4) chronic atrial fibrillation with a slow ventricular response in a non-digitalized patient; and (5) inability of the heart to resume sinus rhythm following dc cardioversion of atrial fibrillation. Several authors (120, 207) have also described alternating bradycardia and supraventricular tachycardia (bradycardia-tachycardia syndrome),

which has now become a sixth criterion of sinus node dysfunction.

Noninvasive Evaluation of Sinus Node Function

The most definitive way to relate the diagnosis of sinus node disease to a symptom is to record an ECG during such an episode. Routine 12-lead electrocardiograms may display one or more of the ECG manifestations of

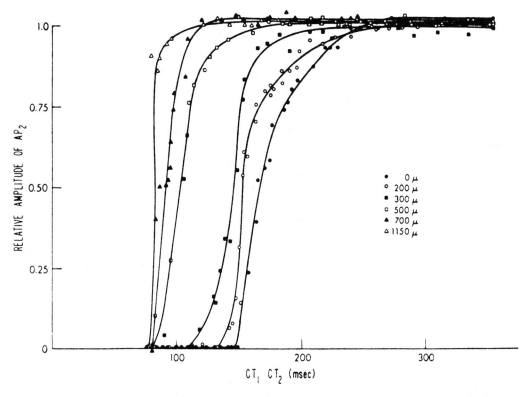

Figure 26 Relative amplitude of the premature action potential (AP$_2$) as a function of distance from the pacemaker site. Six different impalements were obtained between the sinus node pacemaker site and the crista terminalis as shown in the key (total distance from the node to the crista terminalis = 1150 μm). As the microelectrode was moved farther from the node, the curve relating relative amplitude to prematurity moved to the left, that is, closer to the crista terminalis. The range of prematurity over which the decrease in relative amplitude occurred became shorter. [From Kerr et al. (121) with permission of the American Heart Association.]

sinus node dysfunction. Because the abnormalities are often intermittent, longer periods of observation (24 hr) are often necessary to document abnormal function. However, differentiating a pathologically slow heart rate from a physiologically slow heart rate can be difficult. For example, a study (29) of young volunteers without heart disease reported minimum heart rates (53 ± 5 beats/min while awake and 43 ± 5 while asleep) that could easily be mislabeled as abnormal. Pauses as long as 1.7 sec during waking hours and 2.0 sec during sleeping hours may be observed in normal young subjects. Hence, more rigorous means are needed to identify an abnormal slowing of the heart rate.

The autonomic nervous system exerts a profound influence on sinus node function (190). The effects of autonomic agonists and antagonists, Valsalva and tilt maneuvers, and exercise on sinus node function in patients with sinus node dysfunction have been extensively analyzed (1, 2, 63, 64, 115, 116, 133, 134, 147, 185). An abnormal response can be elicited by these manipulations in many patients with sinus node dysfunction. However, the utility of these techniques for selecting therapy has never been established (120, 207). Atropine and propranolol have been used in combination in an attempt to isolate intrinsic sinus node activity from extrinsic neuromodulatory influences (3, 56, 112, 113, 116). The sinus rate (or intrinsic heart rate, IHR_0) that follows administration of atropine and propranolol can then be compared with predicted values (IHR_p) derived from an empirically determined relationship between intrinsic heart rate and age of control subjects (75, 114). Studies suggest that patients with abnormal intrinsic heart rates are more likely to respond abnormally to electrophysiologic testing than patients with normal intrinsic heart rates (207). Although these studies have provided additional information, definitive proof concerning the utility of these results to independently select therapy and predict outcome for patients with sinus node dysfunction is lacking.

Invasive Evaluation of Sinus Node Function

The techniques described in the third section were designed to assess indirectly the effects of the three electrophysiologic variables automaticity, conduction, and refractoriness to establish which mechanism(s) underlie sinus node dysfunction. Although one may wish to obtain accurate or independent assessment of each of these variables, in fact each of the different techniques described in the previous section is not able to dissect apart coexisting disturbances in function. Nevertheless they have been employed in humans, and consequently we discuss their findings, utility, and limitations below.

Determination of SNRT continues to be the mainstay of invasive evaluation of sinus node function. The rapid atrial pacing technique is also usually performed following exposure to a variety of drugs. Because the SNRT depends on the prepacing cycle length, the following method of correction has been employed (112, 146). The basic cycle length is subtracted from SNRT to derive the "corrected sinus node recovery time" (CSNRT). The reported percentage of patients with suspected sinoatrial node dysfunction who demonstrated an abnormal response to rapid atrial pacing varies greatly (207). This variability undoubtedly reflects differences in the sample population of each study, but outcomes from this test do

help to guide therapy. For example, a mildly symptomatic patient with a minimally prolonged CSNRT is much less likely to receive an artificial pacemaker than a symptomatic patient with a markedly prolonged CSNRT.

Estimation of the sinoatrial conduction time using either the premature atrial stimulation or constant atrial pacing techniques has proved to be of limited value (207). Apart from the limited contribution of this measurement to the evaluation of the patient, the need to repeatedly assess the return cycle response to atrial premature depolarizations to obtain an average value precludes its use in assessing conduction.

The ability of the sinus node electrogram recording technique to evaluate conduction in patients for each beat means that this technique can be used to establish whether sudden prolongations in rhythm or sinus pauses reflect a disturbance of automaticity or conduction. Further episodes of sinoatrial block that appeared following termination of rapid atrial pacing suggest that sinoatrial conduction abnormalities may also become manifest after a period of rapid atrial pacing (14). Asseman et al. (6, 7) have documented the occurrence of sinoatrial exit block after cessation of rapid atrial pacing, with conduction block persisting beyond the first postpacing cycle. Gomes et al. (87) have recently provided direct evidence that impaired conduction may be the prime factor responsible for the prolongation of postpacing responses.

Determination of sinus node refractoriness appears to be the most promising of the techniques described previously. Several studies have demonstrated a large difference in the values of sinoatrial refractory period between patients with and without sinus node dysfunction (123, 157).

Formerly, attempts to elucidate the extent to which exaggerated vagal or sympathetic tone might exacerbate or mask abnormalities in sinus node function have yielded highly variable results. For example, the effects of atropine on CSNRT are variable in patients with sick sinus syndrome, shortening it in some, having no effect in others, and paradox-

ically prolonging it in a small number (10, 56, 165). The reduction in magnitude of overdrive suppression after parasympathetic blockade may be more than offset by facilitation of retrograde atriosinus conduction during the period
of rapid atrial pacing. Which effect of atropine predominates determines the effect of atropine sulfate on CSNRT. Propranolol has effects comparable to those seen with atropine for opposing reasons (56, 148, 185). Propranolol increases the magnitude of overdrive suppression and tends to inhibit atriosinus conduction.

Estimation of intrinsic sinus node function was performed in 93 patients with sinus node dysfunction and was reported in four separate articles (56, 115, 116, 173). Of these patients, 43% had an abnormal intrinsic heart rate; a strikingly large number of these patients with an abnormal intrinsic heart rate (98%) had an abnormal CSNRT either before or after autonomic blockade. Moreover, in those patients with a markedly abnormal CSNRT (>1 sec) seen either before or after autonomic blockade, the intrinsic heart rate was abnormally low in 89%. These data argue that patients with an abnormal intrinsic heart rate have a high likelihood of having a markedly abnormal response to rapid atrial pacing. The functional significance of such an abnormality is appreciable, since it appears that patients with prolonged CSNRT values are more likely to be symptomatic than those with minimally abnormal values (207).

Assessment of Mechanism

Invasive electrophysiologic techniques for the indirect assessment of sinoatrial automaticity and conduction have proved rather limited in their capacity to identify and separate distinct pathophysiologic mechanisms underlying the various manifestations of sinus node dysfunction. In patients with sinus bradycardia alone, CSNRT may frequently be normal (207), contrary to the expectation that this technique would be able to detect the underlying disturbance in automaticity. In the subgroup of patients with sinoatrial pauses, exit block, or bradycardia-tachycardia syndrome, early stud-

ies (26) suggested that there was a high prevalence of conduction disturbances that were also manifest during the postpacing period. However, the strong association between conduction disturbance and sinus pauses, exit block, or bradycardia-tachycardia syndrome reported in the early studies has not been confirmed in more recent studies (207).

There are several possible reasons that the estimates of CSNRT and SACT either fail or do not appear to elucidate the underlying mechanisms. The technique for using CSNRT as a measure of sinus node automaticity is predicated on the assumption that sinoatrial conduction is unchanged during the postpacing period. The results of studies involving direct recording of sinus node electrograms clearly demonstrate that conduction may be perturbed, therefore affecting the ability of rapid atrial pacing techniques to assess automaticity (207). Furthermore, pacemaker shifts within the sinus node toward the crista terminalis could present a shorter conduction path to pacemaker impulses, thereby affecting the usefulness of the SACT measurement in the assessment of the conduction disturbance.

Conclusion

Clinical usefulness of the different testing procedures that have been discussed in the last two sections goes beyond establishing the diagnosis of sick sinus syndrome. Their usefulness in predicting the outcome of pacemaker therapy or in predicting adverse drug responses has been demonstrated in only a limited number of studies (207). Although these different testing procedures have made major inroads in improving our understanding of the underlying pathophysiology of sick sinus syndrome, at present they have proved to be of limited clinical value, and the mainstay of diagnosis remains electrocardiographic monitoring, determination of sinus recovery times in selected patients, and assessment of intrinsic autonomic function.

FUTURE PERSPECTIVES

To date there have been four major lines of investigation into the origin and control of myogenic primary cardiac pacemaking. At the molecular level, several investigators using the patch clamp technique have looked at the unitary currents mediated by a single-channel protein molecule. These molecular single-channel studies have provided significant information about the role of membrane potential, neurotransmitters, and second messenger systems in the cellular basis of excitation. Similarly, whole-cell macroscopic current studies on single isolated cardiac myocytes have provided significant insights into the effects of membrane potential, neurotransmitters, and physiologic state on the various sarcolemmal ionic pathways and their role in normal physiologic and pathophysiologic activity of the heart. Unfortunately, only occasionally are attempts made to realistically correlate results obtained under the more extreme recording conditions routinely used in single-channel recording (e.g., nonphysiologically high ionic concentrations in the patch pipette, large electrochemical potential gradients, and high drug concentrations to alter channel gating kinetics) with macroscopic (whole-cell) voltage clamp results obtained under more physiologic conditions. An almost overwhelming amount of data obtained from various multicellular preparations from the heart exists at present. Again, very few attempts have been made to correlate this vast amount of multicellular data and phenomena with the rapidly expanding data base being generated by the isolated myocyte groups. It is now clear that the effects of surrounding cells on the electrical activity of any individual cell are not negligible and must be accounted for (e.g., 144). However, as we have discussed, realistically sorting out such complex multicellular effects on the electrical activity of a single cell is fraught with many difficulties, if not close to impossible. Furthermore, much interest has recently been generated in the possible applications of nonlinear dynamics theory (referred to by many as "chaos theory"; e.g., 86) as a framework for explaining both normal and pathophysiologic behavior of cardiac tissue. The application of nonlinear dynamic theory to cardiac function could be a fruitful and exciting area of future research.

However, we hope that we have conveyed in this chapter that it is the sarcolemmal properties of the individual cells that are highly nonlinear; that is, the heart is an electrical syncytium consisting of many individual and heterogeneous active nonlinear elements (channels, pumps, and so on) "wired up" within an essentially linear network (i.e., the passive "RC" network of membrane capacitance and intra- and intercellular resistances). The physiologic significance of any particular model of whole-tissue cardiac function is therefore greatly enhanced by the incorporation of both the biophysical properties of single myocyte cell types and the heterogeneity existing between cell types in different regions of the heart. The development of such whole-tissue cardiac models will require much closer interaction and communication between the various biophysical, isolated myocyte, and multicellular groups than exists at present; however, such interaction could be extremely fruitful. Finally, clinical observations of sick sinus syndrome, although extensively studied in vivo, await a more complete integration of biophysical, cellular, and multicellular information to yield further understanding of the underlying pathophysiology and, ultimately, more effective pharmacologic treatment.

In this chapter we have attempted to provide an integrative approach to the electrophysiology of cardiac primary pacemaking. All the basic mechanisms discussed have been extensively studied at many different levels (molecular, cellular, multicellular, and whole heart), but integration of all this information as it realistically relates to the heart as a physiologically functioning system remains one of the greatest challenges facing cardiac electrophysiologists in the next decade. Such an integration will ultimately require a closer interaction between all the different groups studying the many different levels of cardiac electrical activity than exists at present.

ACKNOWLEDGMENTS

Supported in part by Grant HL 19216 from the National Heart, Lung and Blood Institute. Campbell and Rasmusson gratefully acknowledge both the support and intellectual inspiration provided by their respective thesis advisors Dr. Wayne R. Giles (Department of Medical Physiology, University of Calgary School of Medicine, Calgary, Alberta, Canada) and Dr. John Clark (Department of Electrical Engineering, Rice University, Houston, Texas). We are also very grateful to Yusheng Qu, Anne Crews, and Steffani Webb for much needed help in final preparation of the manuscript.

NOTE ADDED IN PROOF

During final preparation of this manuscript a paper was published indicating that the current I_f could be recorded in single myocytes isolated from the sinus venosus of the frog *Rana esculenta* (Bois P., Lenfant J. Pflugers Arch 1990; 416:339–346).

REFERENCES

1. Abbott JA, Hirschfeld DS, Kunkel FW, Scheinman MM. Graded exercise testing in patients with sinus node dysfunction. Am J Med 1977; 62:330–8.
2. Agruss NS, Rosin EY, Adolf RJ, Fowler NO. Significance of chronic sinus bradycardia in elderly people. Circulation 1972; 46:924–30.
3. Alboni P, Malcarne C, Pedroni P, Masoni A, Narula OS. Electrophysiology of normal sinus node with and without autonomic blockade. Circulation 1982; 66:1236–42.
4. Allen TJA, Noble D, Reuter H, eds. Sodium-calcium exchange. London: Oxford University Press, 1989.
5. Almers W, McCleskey EW. The non-selective conductance in calcium channels of frog muscle: calcium selectivity in a single file pore. J Physiol (Lond) 1984; 353: 585–608.
6. Asseman P, Berzin B, Desry D, Vilarem D, Durand P, Delmotte C, Sarkis EH, Lekieffre J, Thery C. Persistent sinus nodal electrograms during abnormally prolonged fast pacing atrial pauses in sick sinus syndrome in humans: sinoatrial block vs. overdrive suppression. Circulation 1983; 68:33–41.
7. Asseman P, Berzin B, Desry D, Vilarem D, Durand P, Sarkis EH, Thery L, Lekieffre J. Sinus region electrograms. Circulation 1983; 67:1159–60.
8. Atwell D, Cohen I. The voltage clamp of multicellular preparations. Prog Biophys Mol Biol 1977; 31:201–45.
9. Atwell D, Eisner D, Cohen I. Voltage clamp and tracer flux data: effects of a restricted extracellular space. Q Rev Biophys 1979; 12:213–61.
10. Bashour T, Hemb R, Wickramesekaran R. An unusual effect of atropine on overdrive suppression. Circulation 1973; 48:911–3.
11. Baumgarten C M, Fozzard HA. The resting and pacemaker potentials. In: Fozzard HA, Haber E, Jennings RB, Katz AM, Morgan HE, eds. The heart and cardiovascular system: scientific foundations. New York: Raven Press, 1986:601–26.
12. Bean BP. Classes of calcium channels in vertebrate cells. Annu Rev Physiol 1989; 51: 367–84.
13. Beeler GW, Reuter H. Reconstruction of the action potential of ventricular myocardial fibers. J Physiol (Lond) 1977; 68:177–210.
14. Benditt DG, Strauss HC, Scheinman MM, Behar VS, Wallace AG. Analysis of secondary pauses following termination of rapid atrial pacing in man. Circulation 1976; 54:436–41.
15. Beuckelmann DJ, Wier WG. Sodium-calcium exchange in guinea-pig cardiac cells: exchange current and changes in intracellular Ca^{2+}. J Physiol (Lond) 1989; 414:499–520.
16. Bezanilla F. Gating of sodium and potassium channels. J Membr Biol 1985; 88:97–111.
17. Bezanilla F, White MM. Properties of ionic channels in excitable membranes. In: Andreoli TE, Hoffman JF, Fanestil DD, Schultz SG, eds. Membrane transport processes in organized systems. New York: Plenum Medical, 1987:53–64.
18. Blaustein MP, Lieberman M, eds. Electrogenic transport: fundamental principles and physiological implications. Society of General Physiologists Series, Vol. 38. New York: Raven Press, 1984.
19. Bleeker WK, Mackaay AJC, Masson-Pévet M, Bouman LN, Becker AE. Functional and morphological organization of the rabbit sinus node. Circ Res 1980; 46:11–22.
20. Boineau JP, Schuessler RB, Mooney CR, Wylds AC, Miller CB, Hudson RD, Borremans JM, Brockus CW. Multicentric origin of the atrial depolarization wave: the pacemaker complex. Relation to dynamics of atrial conduction, P-wave changes and heart rate control. Circulation 1978; 58:1036–48.

21. Boineau JP, Schuessler RB, Roeske WR, Autry LJ, Miller CB, Wylds AC. Quantitative relation between sites of atrial impulse origin and cycle length. Am J Physiol 1983; 245:H781–9.

22. Bonke FIM. Electrotonic spread in the sinoatrial node of the rabbit heart. Pflugers Arch 1973; 339:17–23.

23. Bonke FIM, ed. The sinus node: structure, function, and clinical relevance. Boston: Martinus Nijhoff, 1978.

24. Bouman LN, Gerlings ED, Biersteker PA, Bonke FIM. Pacemaker shift in the sinoatrial node during vagal stimulation. Pflugers Arch 1968; 302:255–67.

25. Bouman LN, Mackaay AJC, Bleeker WK, Becker AE. Pacemaker shifts in the sinus node: effects of vagal stimulation, temperature, and reduction of extracellular calcium. In: Bonke FIM, ed. The sinus node. Boston: Martinus Nijhoff, 1978:245–57.

26. Breithardt G, Seipel L, Loogen F. Sinus node recovery time and calculated sinoatrial conduction time in normal subjects and patients with sinus node dysfunction. Circulation 1977; 56:43–50.

27. Breitwieser GE, Szabo G. Mechanism of muscarinic receptor-induced K^+ channel activation as revealed by hydrolysis-resistant GTP analogues. J Gen Physiol 1988; 91: 469–93.

28. Bristow D, Clark JW. A mathematical model of primary pacemaking cell in S-A node of the heart. Am J Physiol 1982; 243:H207–18.

29. Brodsky M, Wu D, Denes P, Kanakis C, Rosen KM. Arrhythmias documented by 24 hour continuous electrocardiographic monitoring in 50 male medical students without apparent heart disease. Am J Cardiol 1977; 39:390–95.

30. Brooks C, Lu HH. The sinoatrial pacemaker of the heart. Springfield, IL: Charles C. Thomas, 1972.

31. Brown AM, Yatani Y. Ca and Na channels in the heart. In: Fozzard HA, Haber E, Jennings RB, Katz AM, Morgan HE, eds. The heart and cardiovascular system: scientific foundations. New York: Raven Press, 1986: 627–36.

32. Brown HF. Electrophysiology of the sinoatrial node. Physiol Rev 1982; 62:505–30.

33. Brown HF, Campbell DL, Clark RB, Denyer JC. Isolated sino-atrial node cells of rabbit: long, thin cells which are calcium-tolerant. J Physiol (Lond) 1987; 390: 60p.

34. Brown HF, Kimura J, Noble D, Noble SJ, Taupignon A. The ionic currents underlying pacemaker activity in rabbit sino-atrial node: experimental results and computer simulations. Proc Soc Lond [Biol] 1984; 222: 329–47.

35. Bukauskas FF, Veteikis RP, Gutman AM, Mutskus KS. Intracellular coupling in the sinus node of the rabbit heart. Biofizika 1977; 22:108–12.

36. Campbell DL. Calcium current and calcium homeostasis in bullfrog atrial cells. Ph.D. Dissertation, University of Texas Medical Branch, Galveston, Texas, 1986.

37. Campbell DL, Giles WR. Calcium currents. In: Langer GA, ed. Calcium and the heart. New York: Raven Press, 1990:27–83.

38. Campbell DL, Giles WR, Hume JR, Noble D, Shibata EF. Reversal potential of the calcium current in bull-frog atrial myocytes. J Physiol (Lond) 1988; 403:267–86.

39. Campbell DL, Giles WR, Hume JR, Shibata EF. Inactivation of calcium current in bullfrog atrial myocytes. J Physiol (Lond) 1988; 403:287–315.

40. Campbell DL, Giles WR, Robinson K, Shibata EF. Studies of the sodium-calcium exchanger in bull-frog atrial myocytes. J Physiol (Lond) 1988; 403:317–40.

41. Campbell DL, Giles WR, Shibata EF. Ion transfer characteristics of the calcium current in bullfrog atrial myocytes. J Physiol (Lond) 1988; 403:239–66.

42. Campbell DL, Rasmusson RL, Robinson K, Clark JW, Giles WR. Are the "slow tails" in single bullfrog atrial cells due to the electrogenic Na^+/Ca^{2+} exchanger? In: Giles WR, ed. Recent studies of ion transport and impulse propagation in cardiac muscle. New York: Alan R. Liss, 1990 (in press).

43. Campbell DL, Rasmusson RL, Strauss HC. Theoretical study of the voltage and concentration dependence of the anomalous mole fraction effect in single calcium channels. Biophys J 1988; 54:945–54.

44. Carafoli E. Intracellular calcium homeostasis. Annu Rev Biochem 1987; 56:235–65.

45. Chai CY, Wang HH, Hoffman BF, Wang SC. Mechanisms of bradycardia induced by digitalis substances. Am J Physiol 1967; 212:26–34.

46. Chapman RA, Noble D. Sodium-calcium exchange in the heart. In: Allen TJA, Noble

D, Reuter H, eds. Sodium-calcium exchange. London: Oxford University Press, 1989: 102–25.

47. Clapham DE. A brief review of single channel measurements from isolated heart cells. In: Pinson A, ed. The heart in cell culture. Boca Raton, FL: CRC Reviews, 1986:159–68.

48. Clark RB, Giles WR. Sodium current in single cells from bullfrog atrium: voltage dependence and ion transfer properties. J Physiol (Lond) 1987; 391:235–65.

49. Clark RB, Giles WR, Imaizumi Y. Properties of the transient outward current in rabbit atrial cells. J Physiol (Lond) 1988; 405: 147–68.

50. Clark RB, Rasmusson R, Giles WR. Na$^+$ currents in single cells from bullfrog atrium: a computer simulation study. In: Recent studies of ion transport and impulse propagation in cardiac muscle. New York: Alan R. Liss, 1990 (In press).

51. Cohen IS, Daytner NB, Gintant GA, Mulrine NK, Pennefather P. Properties of an electrogenic sodium-potassium pump in isolated canine Purkinje myocytes. J Physiol (Lond) 1987; 383:251–67.

52. Cohen IS, Kline RP, Pennefather P, Mulrine NK. Models of the Na/K pump in cardiac muscle predict the wrong intracellular Na$^+$ activity. Proc Soc Lond [Biol] 1987; 231:371–82.

53. Coulombe A, Coraboeuf E. Simulation of potassium accumulation in clefts of Purkinje fibres: effect on membrane electrical activity. J Theor Biol 1983; 104:211–29.

54. Cramer M, Hariman RJ, Boxer R, Hoffman BF. Electrograms from the canine sinoatrial pacemaker recorded in vitro and in situ. Am J Cardiol 1978; 42:939–46.

55. Cramer M, Siegel M, Bigger JT Jr, Hoffman BF. Characteristics of extracellular potentials recorded from the sinoatrial pacemaker of the rabbit. Circ Res 1977; 41:292–300.

56. Desai J, Scheinman MM, Strauss HC, Massie B, O'Young J. Electrophysiological effects of combined autonomic blockade in patients with sinus node disease. Circulation 1981; 63:953–60.

57. De Weer P, Gadsby DC, Rakowski RF. Voltage dependence of the Na-K pump. Annu Rev Physiol 1988; 50:225–41.

58. DiFrancesco D. A new interpretation of the pacemaker current in calf Purkinje fibers. J Physiol (Lond) 1981; 314:359–76.

59. DiFrancesco D. A study of the ionic nature of the pacemaker current in calf Purkinje fibres. J Physiol (Lond) 1981; 314:377–93.

60. DiFrancesco D. The cardiac hyperpolarizing-activated current, i_f: origins and developments. Prog Biophys Mol Biol 1985; 46: 163–83.

61. DiFrancesco D, Noble D. Model of cardiac electrical activity incorporating ionic pumps and concentration changes. Philos Trans R Soc Lond [Biol] 1985; 307:353–98.

62. DiFrancesco D, Noble D. Current I_f and its contribution to cardiac pacemaking. In: Jacklet JW, ed. Neuronal and cellular oscillators. New York: Marcel Dekker, 1989: 31–58.

63. Dighton DH: Sinus bradycardia: autonomic influences and clinical assessment. Br Heart J 1974; 36:791–7.

64. Dighton DH. Sinoatrial block: autonomic influences and clinical assessment. Br Heart J 1975; 37:321–5.

65. Doerr T, Denger R, Trautwein W. Calcium currents in single SA nodal cells of the rabbit heart studied with action potential clamp. Pflugers Arch 1989; 413:599–603.

66. Duchatelle-Gourdon I, Hartzell HC, Lagrutta AA. Modulation of the delayed rectifier potassium current in frog cardiomyocytes by beta-adrenergic agonists and magnesium. J Physiol (Lond) 1989; 415:251–74.

67. Eccles JC, Hoff HE. The rhythm of the heart. III. Disturbances of rhythm produced by early premature beats. Proc R Soc Lond [Biol] 1934; 115:352–68.

68. Eckert R, Chad JE. Inactivation of Ca channels. Prog Biophys Mol Biol 1984; 44:215–67.

69. Eckert R, Chad JE. Mechanism for calcium-dependent inactivation of Ca current. In: Heinemann U, Klee M, Neher E, Singer W, eds. Calcium electrogenesis and neuronal functioning. Berlin: Springer-Verlag, 1986: 35–50.

70. Eisner DA. The Na-K pump in cardiac muscle. In: Fozzard HA, Haber E, Jennings RB, Katz AM, Morgan HE, eds. The heart and cardiovascular system: scientific foundations. New York: Raven Press, 1986: 489–508.

71. Eisner DA, Lederer WJ. Na-Ca exchange: stoichiometry and electrogenicity. Am J Physiol 1985; 248:C198–202.

72. Eisner DA, Lederer WJ. The electrogenic sodium-calcium exchange. In: Allen TJA,

Noble D, Reuter H, eds. Sodium-calcium exchange. London: Oxford University Press, 1989:178–207.

73. Ferrer MI. The sick sinus syndrome in atrial disease. JAMA 1968; 206:645–6.

74. Fischmeister R, Vassort G. The electrogenic Na^+/Ca^{2+} exchange and the cardiac electrical activity. 1. Simulation on Purkinje fibre action potential. J Physiol (Paris) 1981; 77:705–9.

75. Frick MH, Heikkila J, Kahanpaa A. Combined parasympathetic and beta-receptor blockade as a clinical test. Acta Med Scand 1967; 182:621–8.

76. Friel DD, Tsien RW. Voltage-gated calcium channels: direct observation of the anomalous mole fraction effect at the single-channel level. Proc Natl Acad Sci USA 1989; 86:5207–11.

77. Gadsby DC. The Na/K pump of cardiac cells. Annu Rev Biophys Bioeng 1984; 13: 373–98.

78. Gadsby DC, Kimura J, Noma A. Voltage dependence of Na/K pump current in isolated heart cells. Nature 1985; 315:63–5.

79. Gaskell WH. On the innervation of the heart with especial reference to the heart of tortoise. J Physiol (Lond) 1883; 4:43–127.

80. Giles W, Eisner DA, Lederer WJ. Sinus pacemaker activity in the heart. In: Carpenter DO, ed. Cellular pacemakers. New York: John Wiley & Sons, 1982:91–126.

81. Giles WR, Imaizumi Y. Comparison of potassium currents in rabbit atrial and ventricular cells. J Physiol (Lond) 1988; 405: 123–45.

82. Giles W, Nakajima T, Ono K, Shibata EF. Modulation of the delayed rectifier K^+ current by isoprenaline in bull-frog atrial myocytes. J Physiol (Lond) 1989; 415:233–49.

83. Giles WR, Shibata EF. Voltage clamp of bull-frog cardiac pacemaker cells: a quantitative analysis of potassium currents. J Physiol (Lond) 1985; 368:265–92.

84. Giles WR, van Ginneken A. A transient outward current in isolated cells from the crista terminalis of rabbit heart. J Physiol (Lond) 1985; 368:243–64.

85. Giles WR, van Ginneken ACG, Shibata EF. Ionic currents underlying pacemaker activity: a summary of voltage clamp data from single cells. In: Nathan R, ed. Cardiac muscle: the regulation of excitation and contraction. Orlando, FL: Academic Press, 1986:1–28.

86. Glass L, Mackey MC. From clocks to chaos: the rhythms of life. Princeton, NJ: Princeton University Press, 1988.

87. Gomes JAC, Hariman RI, Chowdry IA. New application of direct sinus node recordings in man: assessment of sinus node recovery time. Circulation 1984; 70:663–71.

88. Gomes JA, Kang PS, El-Sherif N. The sinus node electrogram in patients with and without sick sinus syndrome: technique and correlation between directly measured and indirectly estimated sinoatrial conduction time. Circulation 1982; 66:864–73.

89. Grant AO, Kirkorian G, Benditt DG, Strauss HC. The estimation of sinoatrial conduction time in rabbit heart by the constant atrial pacing technique. Circulation 1979; 60: 597–604.

90. Haberl R, Steinbeck G, Lüderitz B. Comparison between intracellular and extracellular direct current recordings of sinus node activity for evaluation of sinoatrial conduction time. Circulation 1984; 70:760–7.

91. Hadley RW, Hume JR. An intrinsic potential-dependent inactivation mechanism associated with calcium channels in guinea-pig myocytes. J Physiol (Lond) 1987; 389:205–22.

92. Hagiwara N, Irisawa H, Kameyama M. Contribution of two types of calcium currents to the pacemaker potentials of rabbit sinoatrial node cells. J Physiol (Lond) 1988; 396: 233–53.

93. Hamill OP, Marty A, Neher E, Sakmann B, Sigworth FJ. Improved patch clamp techniques for high-resolution current recording from cell and cell-free membrane patches. Pflugers Arch 1981; 391:85–100.

94. Hariman RJ, Krongard E, Boxer RA, Weiss MB, Steeg CN, Hoffman BF. Method for recording electrical activity of the sinoatrial node and automatic atrial foci during cardiac catheterization in human subjects. Am J Cardiol 1980; 45:775–81.

95. Hariman RJ, Krongard E, Boxer RA, Bowman FO Jr, Malm JR, Hoffman BF. Methods for recording electrograms of the sinoatrial node during cardiac surgery in man. Circulation 1980; 61:1024–9.

96. Hartzell HC. Regulation of cardiac ion channels by catecholamines, acetylcholine and second messenger systems. Prog Biophys Mol Biol 1988; 52:165–247.

97. Hess P, Tsien RW. Mechanism of ion permeation through calcium channels. Nature 1984; 309:453–6.

98. Hilgemann DW. Numerical approximations of sodium-calcium exchange. Prog Biophys Mol Biol 1988; 51:1–45.

99. Hilgemann DW. Regulation and deregulation of cardiac Na^+-Ca^{2+} exchange in giant excised sarcolemmal membrane patches. Nature 1990; 344:242–5.

100. Hilgemann DW, Noble D. Excitation-contraction coupling and extracellular calcium transients in rabbit atrium: reconstruction of basic cellular mechanisms. Proc R Soc Lond [Biol] 1988; 230:163–205.

101. Hille B. Ionic channels of excitable membranes. Sunderland, MA: Sinauer Associates, 1984.

102. Hodgkin AL, Huxley AF. A quantitative description of membrane current and its application to conduction and excitation in nerve. J Physiol (Lond) 1952; 117:500–44.

103. Hume JR, Giles WR. Active and passive electrical properties of single bullfrog atrial cells. J Gen Physiol 1981; 78:18–43.

104. Hume JR, Giles WR. Ionic currents in single isolated bullfrog atrial cells. J Gen Physiol 1983; 81:153–94.

105. Hume JR, Giles W, Robinson K, Shibata EF, Nathan RD, Kanai K, Rasmusson R. A time- and voltage-dependent K current in single cardiac cells from bullfrog atrium. J Gen Physiol 1986; 88:777–98.

106. Irisawa H. Electrophysiology of single cardiac cells. Jpn J Physiol 1984; 34:375–88.

107. Irisawa H, Hagiwara N. Pacemaker mechanism of mammalian sinoatrial node cells. In: Mazgalev T, Dreifus LS, Michelson EL, eds. Electrophysiology of the sinoatrial and atrioventricular nodes. Progress in Clinical and Biological Research, Vol. 275. New York: Alan R. Liss, 1988:33–52.

108. Irisawa H, Nakayama T, Noma A. Membrane currents of single pacemaker cells from rabbit S-A and A-V nodes. In: Noble D, Powell T, eds. Electrophysiology of single cardiac cells. Orlando, FL: Academic Press, 1987:167–86.

109. Isenberg G, Klockner U. Calcium currents of isolated bovine ventricular myocytes are fast and of large amplitude. Pflugers Arch 1982; 395:30–41.

110. Jack JJB, Noble D, Tsien RW. Electric current flow in excitable cells. Oxford: Clarendon Press, 1975.

111. Johnson EA, Chapman JB, Kootsey JM. Some electrophysiological consequences of electrogenic sodium and potassium transport in cardiac muscle: a theoretical study. J Theor Biol 1980; 87:737–56.

112. Jordan JL, Yamaguchi I, Mandel WJ. Function and dysfunction of the sinus node: clinical studies in the evaluation of sinus node function. In: Bonke FIM, ed. The sinus node: structure, function, and clinical relevance. Boston: Martinus Nijhoff, 1978:3–22.

113. Jordan J, Yamaguchi I, Mandel WJ. Studies on the mechanism of sinus node dysfunction in the sick sinus syndrome. Circulation 1978; 57:217–23.

114. Jose AD, Collison D. The normal range and determinants of the intrinsic heart rate in man. Cardiovasc Res 1970; 4:160–7.

115. Kang PS, Gomes JAC, El-Sherif N. Differential effects of functional autonomic blockade of the variables of sinus node automaticity in sick sinus syndrome. Am J Cardiol 1982; 49:273–82.

116. Kang PS, Gomes JAC, Kelen G, El-Sherif N. Role of autonomic regulatory mechanisms in sinoatrial conduction and sinus node automaticity in sick sinus syndrome. Circulation 1981; 64:832–8.

117. Kass RS, Krafte DS. Electrophysiology of the Ca channels in excitable cells. In: Venter JC, Triggle D, eds. Structure and physiology of the slow inward calcium channel. New York, Alan R. Liss, 1987:71–88.

118. Kass RS, Sanguinetti MC. Inactivation of Ca channel current in the calf cardiac Purkinje fiber: evidence for voltage and Ca-mediated mechanisms. J Gen Physiol 1984; 84:705–26.

119. Kass RS, Sanguinetti MC, Krafte DS. Inactivation and modulation of calcium channels. In: Nathan R, ed. Cardiac muscle: the regulation of excitation and contraction. Orlando, FL: Academic Press, 1986:29–54.

120. Kerr CR, Grant AO, Wenger TL, Strauss HC. Sinus node dysfunction. In: Zipes DP, ed. Cardiology clinics: arrhythmias II, Vol. 1, No. 2. Philadelphia: W. B. Saunders, 1983:187–207.

121. Kerr CR, Prystowsky EN, Browning DJ, Strauss HC. Characterization of refractoriness in the sinus node of the rabbit. Circ Res 1980; 47:742–56.

122. Kerr CR, Strauss HC. The nature of atrio-sinus conduction during rapid atrial pacing in the rabbit heart. Circulation 1981; 63: 1149–57.

123. Kerr CR, Strauss HC. The measurement of sinus node refractoriness in man. Circulation 1984; 68:1231–7.

124. Kodama I, Boyett MR. Regional differences in the electrical activity of the rabbit sinus node. Pflugers Arch 1985; 404:214–26.

125. Kodama I, Goto J, Ando S, Toyama J, Yamada K. Effect of rapid stimulation on the transmembrane action potentials of rabbit sinus node pacemaker cells. Circ Res 1980; 46:90–9.

126. Lange G. Action of driving stimuli from intrinsic and extrinsic sources on in situ cardiac pacemaker tissues. Circ Res 1965; 17:449–59.

127. Langendorf R, Lesser ME, Plotkin P, Levin BD. Atrial parasystole with interpolation. Observations on prolonged sinoatrial conduction. Am Heart J 1962; 63:649–58.

128. Lee KS, Marban E, Tsien RW. Inactivation of calcium channels in mammalian heart cells: joint dependence on membrane potential and intracellular calcium. J Physiol (Lond) 1985; 364:395–411.

129. Lu H-H. Shifts in pacemaker dominance within the sinoatrial region of cat and rabbit hearts resulting from increase of extracellular potassium. Circ Res 1970; 26:339–46.

130. Lu H-H, Lange G, Brooks CM. Factors controlling pacemaker action in cells of the sinoatrial node. Circ Res 1965; 17:460–71.

131. Mackaay AJC, Hof TO, Bleeker WK, Jongsma HJ, Bouman LN. Interaction of adrenaline and acteylcholine on cardiac pacemaker function. Functional inhomogeneity of the rabbit sinus node. J Pharmacol Exp Ther 1980; 214:417–22.

132. Mandel WJ, Hayakawa H, Danzig R, Marcus HS. Evaluation of sino-atrial node function in man by overdrive suppression. Circulation 1971; 44:59–66.

133. Mandel WJ, Hayakawa H, Danzig R, Marcus HS. Assessment of sinus node function in patients with the sick sinus syndrome. Circulation 1972; 46:761–9.

134. Mandel WJ, Lalis MM, Obayashi K. Sinus node function. Evaluation in patients with and without sinus node disease. Arch Intern Med 1975; 135:388–94.

135. Marban E, Smith TW. Digitalis. In: Fozzard HA, Haber E, Jennings RB, Katz AM, Morgan HE, eds. The heart and cardiovascular system: scientific foundations. New York: Raven Press, 1986:1573–96.

136. Marty A, Neher E. Tight-seal whole-cell recording. In: Sakmann B, Neher E, eds. Single-channel recording. Plenum Press, New York, 1983:107–22.

137. Masson-Pévet M, Bleeker WK, Gros D. The plasma membrane of leading pacemaker cells in the rabbit sinus node. A qualitative and quantitative ultrastructural analysis. Circ Res 1979; 45:621–9.

138. Mazgalev T, Dreifus LS, Michelson EL (eds). Electrophysiology of the sinoatrial and atrioventricular nodes. Progress in Clinical and Biological Research, Vol. 257. New York: Alan R. Liss, 1988.

139. Mazzanti M, DeFelice LJ. Regulation of the Na-conducting Ca channel during the cardiac action potential. Biophys J 1987; 51:115–21.

140. McAllister RE, Noble D, Tsien RW. Reconstruction of the electrical activity of cardiac Purkinje fibres. J Physiol (Lond) 1975; 251:1–59.

141. Miller HC, Strauss HC. Measurement of sinoatrial conduction time by premature atrial stimulation in the rabbit. Circ Res 1974; 35:935–47.

142. Momose Y, Giles W, Szabo G Acetylcholine-induced K^+ current in amphibian atrial cells. Biophys J (Biophysical Discussions: Ionic Channels in Membranes) 1984; 45:20–2.

143. Moore LE, Clark RB, Shibata EF, Giles WR. Comparison of steady-state electrophysiological properties of isolated cells from bullfrog atrium and sinus venosus. J Membr Biol 1986; 89:131–8.

144. Morad M. Physiological implications of K accumulation in heart muscle. Fed Proc 1980; 39:1533–9.

145. Mullins LJ. Ion transport in heart. New York: Raven Press, 1981.

146. Narula OS, Samet P, Xavier RP. Significance of the sinus-node recovery time. Circulation 1972; 45:140–58.

147. Narula OS, Shantha N, Vazquez M, Towne WD, Linhart JW. A new method for measurement of sinoatrial conduction time. Circulation 1978; 58:706–14.

148. Narula OS, Vasquez M, Shantha N, Chuquimia R, Towne WD, Linhart JW. Effect of propranolol on normal and abnormal sinus node function. In: Bonke FIM, ed. The sinus node: structure, function, and clinical relevance. The Hague: Martinus Nijhoff, 1978:112–28.

149. Nathan RD. Two electrophysiologically distinct types of cultured pacemaker cells from rabbit sinoatrial node. Am J Physiol 1986; 250:H325–9.

150. Noble D. A modification of the Hodgkin Huxley equations applicable to Purkinje fibre action and pacemaker potentials. J Physiol (Lond) 1962; 160:317–52.

151. Noble D. The surprising heart: a review of recent progress in cardiac electrophysiology. J Physiol (Lond) 1984; 353:1–50.

152. Noble D. Sodium-calcium exchange and its role in generating electric current. In: Nathan R, ed. Cardiac muscle: the regulation of excitation and contraction. New York: Academic Press, 1986:171–200.

153. Noble D, DiFrancesco D, Denyer J. Ionic mechanisms in normal and abnormal cardiac pacemaking activity. In: Jacklet JW, ed. Neuronal and cellular oscillators. New York: Marcel Dekker, 1989:59–86.

154. Noble D, Noble S. A model of s-a node electrical activity using a modification of the DiFrancesco-Noble (1984) equations. Proc R Soc Lond [Biol] 1984; 222:295–304.

155. Noble D, Powell T (eds.). Electrophysiology of single cardiac cells. Orlando, FL: Academic Press, 1987.

156. Noma A, Irisawa H. Membrane currents in the rabbit sinoatrial node cell as studied by the double microelectrode method. Pflugers Arch 1976; 364:45–52.

157. Omori I, Inoue D, Shirayama T, Asayama J, Katsume H, Nakagawa M. Effect of paced cycle length on sinus node effective refractory period before and after autonomic blockade in patients with sick sinus syndrome. Eur Heart J 1989; 10:409–16.

158. Paes de Carvalho A. Cellular electrophysiology of the atrial specialized tissues. In: Paes de Carvalho A, de Mello WC, Hoffman BF, eds. The specialized tissues of the heart. New York: Elsevier, 1961:115–33.

159. Paes de Carvalho A, DeMello WC, Hoffman BF. Electrophysiologic types in rabbit atrium. Am J Physiol 1959; 196:483–8.

160. Pelzer D, Cavalie S, Trautwein W. Activation and inactivation of single calcium channels in cardiac cells. In: Heinemann U, Klee M, Neher E, Singer W, eds. Calcium electrogenesis and neuronal functioning. Berlin: Springer-Verlag, 1986:17–34.

161. Powell T. Methods for the isolation and preparation of single adult myocytes. In: Clark WA, Decker RS, Borge TK, eds. Biology of isolated adult cardiac myocytes. New York: Elsevier, 1988:9–13.

162. Rasmusson RL. A model of frog atrial and sinus electrical activity. Master's Thesis, Department of Electrical Engineering, Rice University, Houston, Texas, 1986.

163. Rasmusson RL, Clark JW, Giles WR, Robinson K, Clark RB, Shibata EF, Campbell DL. A mathematical model of electrophysiological activity in a bullfrog atrial cell. Am J Physiol 1990; 259:H370–H389.

164. Rasmusson RL, Clark JW, Giles WR, Shibata EF, Campbell DL. A mathematical model of a bullfrog cardiac pacemaker cell. Am J Physiol 1990; 259:H352–H369.

165. Reiffel JA, Bigger JT Jr, Giardina EGV. Paradoxical prolongation of sinus node recovery time after atropine in the sick sinus syndrome. Am J Cardiol 1975; 36:98–104.

166. Reiffel JA, Gang E, Gliklich J, Weiss MB, Davis JC, Patton JN, Bigger JT Jr. The human sinus node electrogram: a transvenous catheter technique and a comparison of directly measured and indirectly estimated sinoatrial conduction time in adults. Circulation 1980; 62:1324–34.

167. Reuter H. Calcium channel modulation by neurostransmitters, enzymes, and drugs. Nature 1983; 301:569–74.

168. Reuter H, Porzig H, Kokubun S, Prod'hom B. Voltage-dependent binding and action of 1,4-dihydropyridine enantiomers in intact cardiac cells. In: Hille B, Fambrough DM, eds. Proteins of excitable membranes. New York: Society of General Physiologists, Wiley Interscience, 1987:189–99.

169. Robertson S, Johnson D, Potter J. The time-course of Ca^{2+} exchange with calmodulin, troponin, parvalbumin, and myosin in response to transient increases in Ca^{2+}. Biophys J 1981; 34:559–69.

170. Sano T, Yamaguchi S. Spread of excitation from the sinus node. Circ Res 1965; 26:423–30.

171. Schatzman HJ. The calcium pump of the surface membrane and of the sarcoplasmic reticulum. Annu Rev Physiol 1989; 51:473–85.

172. Scheinman MM, Strauss HC, Abbott JA, Evans GT, Peters RW, Benditt DG, Wallace AG. Electrophysiologic testing in patients with sinus pauses and/or sinoatrial block. Eur J Cardiol 1978; 8:51–60.

173. Sethi KK, Jaishanker S, Balachander J, Bahl VK, Gupta MP. Sinus node function after

autonomic blockade in normals and in sick sinus syndrome. Int J Cardiol 1984; 5: 707–19.

174. Seyama I. Characteristics of the rectifying properties of the sino-atrial node cell of the rabbit. J Physiol (Lond) 1976; 255:379–97.

175. Shibata EF. Ionic currents in isolated cardiac pacemaker cells. Ph.D. Dissertation, University of Texas Medical Branch, Galveston, 1984.

176. Shibata EF, Giles WR. Ionic currents that generate the spontaneous depolarization in individual cardiac pacemaker cells. Proc Natl Acad Sci USA 1985; 82:7796–800.

177. Shibata EF, Momose Y, Giles WR. An electrogenic Na^+/K^+ pump current in individual bullfrog atrial myocytes. Biophys J 1984; 45:136a.

178. Simmons M, Creazzo T, Hartzell HC. A time-dependent and voltage-sensitive K current in single cells from frog atrium. J Gen Physiol 1986; 88:739–55.

179. Steinbeck G, Allessie MA, Bonke FIM, Lammers WJEP. Sinus node response to premature atrial stimulation in the rabbit studied with multiple microelectrode impalements. Circ Res 1978; 43:695–704.

180. Steinbeck G, Haberl R, Lüderitz B. Effects of atrial pacing on atrio-sinus conduction and overdrive suppression in the isolated rabbit sinus node. Circ Res 1980; 46: 859–69.

181. Stimers JR, Lobaugh LA, Liu S, Shigeto N, Lieberman M. Intracellular sodium affects ouabain interaction with the Na/K pump in cultured chick cardiac myocytes. J Gen Physiol 1990; 95:77–95.

182. Stimers JR, Shigeto N, Lieberman M. Na/K pump current in aggregates of cultured chick cardiac myocytes. J Gen Physiol 1990; 95:61–76.

183. Strauss HC, Bigger JT Jr. Electrophysiological properties of the rabbit sinoatrial perinodal fibers. Circ Res 1972; 31:490–505.

184. Strauss HC, Bigger JT JR, Saroff AL, Giardina EGV. Electrophysiologic evaluation of sinus node dysfunction. Circulation 1976; 53:763–76.

185. Strauss HC, Gilbert M, Svenson RH, Miller HC, Wallace AG. Electrophysiologic effects of propranolol on sinus node function in patients with sinus node dysfunction. Circulation 1976; 54:452–9.

186. Strauss HC, Saroff AL, Bigger JT Jr, Giardina EGV. Premature atrial stimulation as a key to the understanding of sinoatrial conduction in man: presentation of data and critical review of the literature. Circulation 1973; 47:86–93.

187. Strauss HC, Scheinman MM, LaBarre A, Browning DJ, Wenger TL, Wallace AG. Programmed atrial stimulation and rapid atrial pacing in patients with sinus pauses and sinoatrial exit block. In: Bonke FIM, ed. The sinus node. Boston: Martinus Nijhoff, 1978:56–64.

188. Ten Eick RE, Hoffman BF. Chronotropic effect of cardiac glycosides in cats, dogs, and rabbits. Circ Res 1969; 25:365–78.

189. Thomas RC. Electrogenic sodium pump in nerve and muscle cells. Physiol Rev 1972; 52:563–94.

190. Thormann J, Schwartz F, Ensslen R, Sesto M. Vagal tone, significances of electrophysiologic findings and clinical course in symptomatic sinus node dysfunction. Am Heart J 1978; 95:725–31.

191. Tranum-Jensen J. The fine structure of the atrial and atrioventricular (AV) junctional specialized tissues of the rabbit heart. In: Wellens HJJ, Lie KI, Janse MJ, eds. The conduction system of the heart. Leiden: Stenfert Kroese VF, 1976:55–81.

192. Tranum-Jensen J. The fine structure of the sinus node: a survey. In: Bonke FIM, ed. The sinus node: structure, function, and clinical relevance. Boston: Martinus Nijhoff, 1978:149–65.

193. Trautwein W. Effect of acetylcholine on the S-A node of the heart. In: Carpenter DO, ed. Cellular pacemakers. New York: John Wiley & Sons, 1982:127–62.

194. Trautwein W, Kameyama M. The mechanism of beta-adrenergic regulation of calcium channels: intracellular injections and patch-clamp studies. In: Noble D, Powell T, eds. Electrophysiology of single cardiac cells. Orlando, FL: Academic Press, 1987:105–23.

195. Trautwein W, Pelzer D. Voltage-dependent gating of single calcium channels in the cardiac cell membrane and its modulation by drugs. In: Marme D, ed. Calcium and cell physiology. Berlin: Springer Verlag, 1985:53–93.

196. Trautwein W, Uchizono K. Electron microscopic and electrophysiologic study of the pacemaker in the sinoatrial node of the rabbit heart. Z Zellforsch Mikrosk Anat 61:96–109.

197. Tsien RW. Calcium channels in excitable cell membranes. Annu Rev Physiol 1983; 45:341–58.

198. Tsien RW, Fox AP, Hess P, McCleskey EW, Nilius B, Nowycky MC, Rosenberg RL. Multiple types of calcium channel in excitable cells. In: Hille B, Fambrough DM, eds. Proteins of excitable membranes. Society of General Physiologists, Wiley Interscience, 1987:167–87.

199. Tsien RW, Hess P, Lansman JB, Lee K. Current views of cardiac calcium channels and their response to calcium antagonists and agonists. In: Zipes D, Jalife J, eds. Cardiac electrophysiology and arrhythmias. Orlando, FL: Grune and Stratton 1985:19–29.

200. Tsien RW, Hess P, McCleskey EW, Rosenberg RL. Calcium channels: mechanisms of selectivity, permeation, and block. Annu Rev Biophys Chem 1987; 16:265–90.

201. van Ginneken A, Giles W. I_f in isolated cells from the rabbit S-A node. Biophys J 1985; 47:496a.

202. van Ginneken ACG, Giles WR. Voltage clamp analysis of i_f in single cells from rabbit sino-atrial node. In: van Ginneken ACG, ed. Membrane currents in mammalian cardiac pacemaker cells. Doctoral Thesis, Amsterdam, 1987.

203. Walsh KB, Begenisich TB, Kass RS. Beta-adrenergic modulation in the heart: independent regulation of K and Ca channels. Pflugers Arch 1988; 411:232–4.

204. Watanabe AM, Green FJ, Farmer BB. Preparation and use of cardiac myocytes in experimental cardiology. In: Fozzard HA, Haber E, Jennings RB, Katz AM, Morgan HE, eds. The heart and cardiovascular system: scientific foundations. New York: Raven Press, 1986:241–52.

205. West TC. Ultramicroelectrode recording from the cardiac pacemaker. J Pharmacol Exp Ther 1955; 115:283–90.

206. Yanigihara K, Noma A, Irisawa H. Reconstruction of sino-atrial node pacemaker potential based on voltage clamp experiments. Jpn J Physiol 1980; 30:841–57.

207. Yee R, Strauss HC. Electrophysiologic mechanisms: Sinus node dysfunction. Circulation 1987; 75 (Suppl. III):12–8.

6

Electrophysiology of the Atrial Myocardium

Steve Sorota and Penelope A. Boyden

College of Physicians and Surgeons, Columbia University
New York, New York

RECORDS OF TRANSMEMBRANE ACTION POTENTIALS

With fine-tipped glass microelectrodes, intracellular recordings can be obtained from cells of the atrial chambers. The configuration of the action potential elicited by stimulation can vary considerably within the same chamber and even between species. Rabbit, canine, and human atrial cells have been studied extensively (1–5). Recently, single-cell models have been developed using rabbit, canine, human, guinea pig, and frog atrial cells. These have allowed a more complete understanding of the nature of the ionic currents that underly the various action potential configurations (see later).

Ordinary atrial muscle fibers, commonly referred to as contractile fibers, show a uniformly configured action potential. The cell remains quiescent at a stable negative potential until stimulation. At that point there is a rapid depolarization of the membrane, a rapid phase of repolarization (phase 1) with little or no maintained potential level during the plateau phase (phase 2), and then a slowly occurring terminal phase of repolarization (phase 3). Action potentials elicited from single atrial myocytes from the guinea pig and rabbit atrium show resting potentials in the range of -67 to -73 mV. Total action potential amplitudes of these action potentials range from 92 to 109 mV (6,7). Human atrial cells, on the other hand, have resting potentials in -83 mV range (2).

Electrophysiologically, another type of atrial fiber has been identified. Controversy remains about whether this type of cell exists in anatomically defined specialized tracts of conduction (8,9). Recent evidence suggests that although the cells are present in atria, the specialized pathways of conduction do not have an anatomic basis (10). Nevertheless, this second type of fiber has been characterized as having a high resting potential, total action potential amplitude, and maximum upstroke velocity, These "specialized" or "plateau" atrial fibers are commonly found when recording from sites within the large atrial bundles, such as the crista terminalis and Bachmann's bundle (4). Importantly, unlike the ordinary contractile fibers already described these fibers have a prominent phase 1 but phase 2 is more like a plateau. Phase 3 is

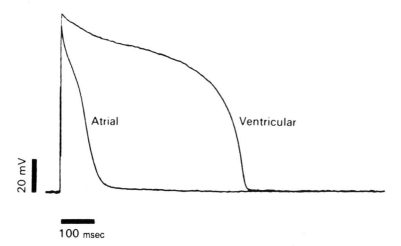

Figure 1   Superimposed tracings of action potentials of atrial and ventricular myocytes. Action potentials were elicited using a single-suction micropipette technique and a current clamp. (From Hume and Uehara, 1985, Ref.6.)

the terminal phase of repolarization. Plateau fibers can demonstrate phase 4 membrane depolarization at slow drive rates or after cessation of drive (2).

Other cell types are in functional continuity with these fibers of the atrial myocardium. The electrophysiology of cells of the sinoatrial node and the cells of the atrioventricular node are discussed in other chapters.

BASIS FOR ATRIAL TRANSMEMBRANE POTENTIAL: PASSIVE AND ACTIVE PROPERTIES

Atrial and ventricular muscle cells differ with respect to their action potential configuration. The dissimilar action potentials have been demonstrated in multicellular preparations (11, 12) as well as in single cardiac myocyte preparations (6,7). Atrial action potentials have a lower plateau amplitude and a shorter duration than those seen in the ventricle (Fig. 1). The atrial action potential tends to be more triangular with a steeper phase 2 compared to the relatively rectangular action potentials in ventricular muscle. Dissimilarities in both passive and active properties contribute to the nonidentical action potential configurations.

Passive Properties

The passive electrical behavior of the cell membrane is like that of a resistor and a capacitor in parallel. The decay of electrical potential across such a circuit over time can be described by the equation

$$E_t = E_0 e^{-t/R_m C_m} = E_0 e^{-t/\tau_m}$$

where E_t = potential at time = t (V)
E_0 = potential at time = 0 (V)
R_m = membrane resistance for a unit area of membrane ($\Omega \ast cm^2$)
C_m = membrane capacitance per unit area of membrane (F/cm^2)
τ_m = membrane time constant (sec)

The membrane time constant is the time required for the transmembrane potential to reach approximately 63% of the steady-state value in a short fiber (13,14). The equation refers to the special case in which the value of E decays to zero. When the steady-state value of E differs from zero (i.e., injection of a constant current across the RC circuit, or a cell with a resting potential), the equation becomes

$$E_t = (E_0 - E_\infty)\, e^{-t/\tau} + E_\infty$$

where E_∞ = the steady state value for E.

Cable theory provides a description of the decay of potential over space. The membrane length constant is the distance at which poten-

Table 1 Comparison of Atrial and Ventricular Cardiac Myocytes[a]

Species	Cell type	R_m (kΩ/cm^2)	τ_m (msec)	SA 10^{-5} cm^2	RP (mV)
Guinea pig	Atrial	4.6[b]	5.5	4.2	-73
	Ventricular	2.3[b]	2.3	7.1	-74
Rabbit	Atrial	29.1	33.5[c]	5.4	-67
	Ventricular	1.8	2.5[c]	7.3	-74

[a]R_m = specific membrane resistance, τ_m = membrane time constant, SA = average capacitative surface area, RP = average resting potential. Guinea pig data from Hume and Uehara (6). Rabbit data from Giles and Imaizumi (7).
[b]Calculated from $R_m = R_{in}/C_{in}$.
[c]Calculated from $\tau_m = R_m C_m$.

tial has decayed to $1/e$ ($\approx 37\%$) of the value at the source of current application. The following equation defines the membrane length constant:

$$\lambda_m = \sqrt{\frac{r_m}{r_i + r_o}}$$

where λ_m = membrane length constant (cm)
r_m = membrane resistance for a unit length of membrane (Ω*cm)
($r_m = R_m/2\pi$ radius)
r_i = internal resistance of the fiber per unit length (Ω/cm)
r_0 = external resistance per unit length (Ω/cm)

Because r_0 is small compared to r_i, the following approximation is often used:

$$\lambda_m = \sqrt{\frac{r_m}{r_i}}$$

The decay of potential over distance can be calculated using

$$E_x = E_0 e^{-x/\lambda_m}$$

where E_x = potential at distance = x
E_0 = potential at distance = 0

Four variables can be used to determine τ_m and λ_m. These are R_m, r_m, r_i, and C_m. r_i is proportional to $1/\text{radius}^2$. As cross-sectional area decreases, r_i increases. Because atrial cells tend to be smaller in diameter than ventricular cells (6), r_i is higher in atrial cells, assuming the cytoplasm of atrial and ventricular cells has a similar conductivity. This effect tends to make λ_m shorter in atrial compared to ventricular myocytes. On the other hand, under conditions in which chemically sensitive

potassium channels would not be expected to be open, R_m at the resting potential is higher in atrial myocytes than in ventricular myocytes (Table 1) (6,7). The higher R_m in atrial cells causes λ_m to be longer in atrial cells compared to ventricular cells. The membrane resistance effect on λ_m probably predominates; however, no direct comparisons of λ_m measurements in single atrial and ventricular cells have been reported. In single frog and guinea pig atrial cells values of 921 and 850 mm, respectively, have been reported for λ_m at the resting potential (15,16). The high R_m in atrial cells also affects τ_m. The membrane time constant is longer in atrial cells than in ventricular cells (Table 1) (6).

The factors that influence R_m at the resting potential of the cell are the number of opened ion channels and leaks of ions across the membrane. The reason for a high R_m in atrial muscle is probably a reflection of fewer open ion channels.

Although R_m in single atrial muscle cells is higher than in single ventricular muscle cells in vitro, the atrium possesses a chemically regulated potassium channel that can be opened by acetylcholine or adenosine (17–19). In situ, the R_m of atrial muscle may be closer to that seen in ventricular muscle because of the influence of endogenous adenosine and acetylcholine on atrial membrane resistance.

Background Potassium Conductance

Inward Rectifying Background Potassium Current

The predominant background potassium channel in atrial cells appears to differ from that

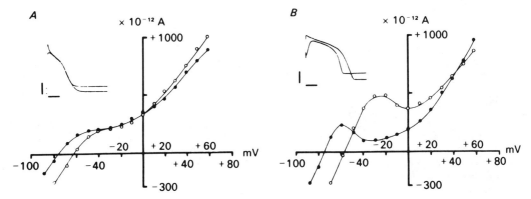

Figure 2 Action potentials and steady-state current-voltage relationships in $[K^+]_o$ = 6 mM (filled circles) and 11 mM (open circles) for an atrial myocyte (A) and a ventricular myocyte (B). Note the prominent negative slope conductance region present in the curve of the ventricular myocyte and absent in the curve of the atrial myocyte. (From Hume and Uehera, 1985, Ref. 6.)

seen in the ventricle. In this chapter the abbreviation i_{K1} is used to refer to the predominant background potassium current found in ventricular and Purkinje cells. The properties of i_{K1} are discussed to allow comparison to the predominant background potassium current in atrial cell. Mammalian atrial cells have been reported to have less i_{K1} than ventricular cells (6,7,20,21).

The ventricular i_{K1} channel is sensitive to both the potassium equilibrium potential E_K and the transmembrane potential (22,23). Little outward current flows positive to the potassium equilibrium potential because of the inward rectifying properties of the channel (22–27). The inward rectification has been attributed to the blocking effects of either intracellular magnesium (28) or calcium ion (29). The conductance of the i_{K1} channel is increased by extracellular potassium K_0 (22,26,30). As K_0 is raised, the inward and outward current through i_{K1} channels increases and the reversal potential becomes less negative. In ventricular cells there is a crossover in the steady-state current-voltage relationships with elevation of K_0 (Fig. 2) (6,22,24,27).

Inward rectification and regulation by K_0 are also properties of the background potassium current in atrial cells (6,7,18,31). However, atrial and ventricular cells differ in the amount of crossover of the steady-state current-voltage relationship when K_0 is elevated (6).

In ventricular and Purkinje cells there is an N-shaped steady-state current-voltage relationship with a region of negative slope conductance (24). In some cases the negative slope region has been attributed to an extracellular calcium-dependent steady-state inward current (32,33). However, the negative slope region is a property of the i_{K1} channel itself and not entirely due to contaminating inward currents for the following reasons. First, calcium channel blockade does not always eliminate the negative slope conductance (34). Second, the background potassium current is blocked by barium and cesium ions (25,35–38) and Cs^+- and Ba^{2+}- sensitive steady-state currents also show a region of negative slope conductance (7,36). Finally, K^+ accumulation in intercellular clefts of frog ventricular muscle decreases at potentials at which the negative slope conductance is seen (24,36).

In contrast to the ventricle, steady-state current-voltage relationships show little or no negative slope conductance in the atrium (Fig. 2) (6,7,18,31). Barium-sensitive steady-state current has a region of negative slope conductance in rabbit ventricle that is less apparent in rabbit atrium (7). The lack of a negative slope conductance region contributes to the faster initial repolarization seen in atrium compared to ventricle (6).

At one time i_{K1} was thought to be a time-independent current. However, patch clamp experiments have demonstrated that i_{K1} decays in a time-dependent manner during depolarizing voltage clamp steps from (E_K -30 mV) and increases in a time-dependent manner during hyperpolarizing voltage clamp steps to (E_K -30 mV) (28,39,40). At physiological K_O, the channels are believed to be optimally activated at approximately -110 mV and nonconducting at approximately -40 mV (28,39,40). The decrease in conductance seen at potentials positive to E_K appears to be due to both a time-dependent closing of a channel gate and to an instantaneous rectification (28,39).

Another voltage- and time-dependent conductance change in i_{K1} occurs with hyperpolarizations negative to approximately (E_K -40 mV). These strong hyperpolarizations lead to a time-dependent decrease in the inward current through i_{K1} channels (25,37,39–42). This decay of the inward current during strong hyperpolarizing voltage clamp steps has been attributed to block of the channels by extracellular sodium ion (40).

The background potassium current in the atrium does not have the same kinetics as i_{K1}. The inward current response to hyperpolarizing voltage clamp steps from a holding potential of -50 mV decays over time in the ventricle but not in the atrium (6).

Single-channel recordings also indicate that the main background potassium channel reported in guinea pig atrial cells is an inward rectifying current that differs from i_{K1} (6). Guinea pig and rabbit atrial cells have a background potassium channel with conductance and mean channel open time similar to that of the acetylcholine-induced potassium channel (mean channel open time of ~1 msec; single-channel conductance at 25°C in elevated K^+ of ~30–40 pS) (6,21,43).

Single-channel conductance measurements of inward current through i_{K1} channels in symmetrical 145 mM potassium range from 21 to 32 pS (6,26,28) at room temperature. A single-channel conductance of 40–47 pS has been reported at higher temperatures (30–36°C) (25,39). The mean channel open time of these channels is voltage dependent (37,39). The range of mean channel open times reported for the i_{K1} channel under various conditions is from 10 to 223 msec (6,20,25,37,39).

The mean channel open time of the main background potassium channel in atrium is much shorter than is seen for ventricular i_{K1} channels. In guinea pig atrial cells, i_{K1} channel activity was rarely detected (6). However, rabbit atrial cells have some ventricular-type i_{K1} channels in addition to the short open time background potassium channels (20,21). It is not clear at this time if the short open time background potassium channel in the atrium is the same channel that can be activated by ACh. The absence of a time-dependent relaxation of background K^+ current in guinea pig atrial cells (6) suggests that the background K current differs kinetically from the acetylcholine-activated K^+ current (44).

Surface Receptor-Regulated Inward Rectifying Potassium Current

Acetylcholine (ACh) hyperpolarizes atrial muscle (45) by increasing the permeability of atrial muscle to potassium (17). The potassium current induced by ACh (i_{KACh}) is an inward rectifier, like i_{K1}, but does not exhibit a region of negative slope conductance (Fig. 3) (18). The amplitude of the current is increased by elevated K_O (46). The acetylcholine-induced current increases with time after a hyperpolarizing voltage clamp step and decreases with time after depolarizing voltage clamp steps (44,47,48). The acetylcholine-induced current also differs from i_{K1} by its slower kinetics after hyperpolarizing voltage clamp steps and weaker sensitivity to block by barium (48). Adenosine can also activate i_{KACh} (18,19), albeit with lower efficacy than full muscarinic agonists. The effects of adenosine are inhibited by the adenosine receptor antagonist theophylline but not by the muscarinic antagonist atropine (19). The current desensitizes with prolonged exposure to high concentrations of either agonist (19,47–49). Single-channel records reveal a channel with a mean open time of ~1 msec and a conductance for inward currents of 40–50 pS with 150 mM KCl on both sides of the membrane (43,50–52).

Acetylcholine and adenosine receptors are linked to i_{KACh} channels by a pertussis toxin-

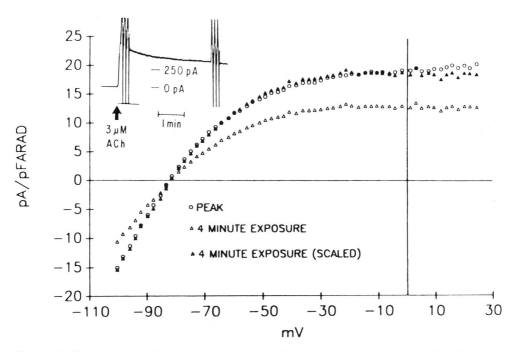

Figure 3 Outward ACh-induced current during prolonged exposure to 3 μM ACh. Voltage ramps generated these current-voltage relationships at various times after the beginning of the ACh superfusion. Inset shows the time course of the ACh-induced current recorded from the canine atrial myocyte after 2 days in culture. (From Sorota and Hoffman, 1989, Ref. 49.)

sensitive GTP binding protein (G protein) (19,46,53–55). Hydrolysis-resistant GTP analogs can activate i_{KACh} independently of receptor activation (19,47,49,50,52,56). The activated α subunits of several GTP binding proteins have been shown to activate i_{KACh} (51,52,57). Further evidence that a G protein α subunit is the physiologic link between muscarinic receptors and i_{KACh} channels is that antibody raised against the α subunit of transducin cross-reacts with α subunits of other G proteins and inhibits the activation of i_{KACh} channels by agonist (58). There are several different pertussis toxin-sensitive GTP binding proteins in atrial muscle (59–63). Although at least three distinct GTP binding proteins can activate i_{KACh} (57), the GTP binding protein(s) responsible for the physiologic coupling of the receptors to i_{KACh} has not been determined.

Voltage-Dependent Sodium Current

The sodium dependence of the upstroke of the cardiac action potential in non-nodal cells was demonstrated in the early 1950s (64–66). Cardiac sodium channels, like those found in the squid axon (67–70), appear to open rapidly in response to depolarization of the transmembrane potential and then inactivate during maintained depolarization. The result is a brief inward current that generates the initial spike of the action potential in cardiac muscle. On return to hyperpolarized potentials, channels recover to the resting state either by recovery from inactivation (inactivated state to resting state) or deactivation (open state to resting state). The Hodgkin-Huxley model predicts single exponential time courses for inactivation and recovery from inactivation and a sigmoidal time course for activation of the sodium current.

Sodium channels appear to be identical in ventricular muscle, Purkinje fibers, and atrial muscle (71–80). Few studies have been done on the sodium current in atrium (75,78–82). For this reason results from ventricle and Purkinje preparations are combined with those from atrial preparations. Estimates of sodium

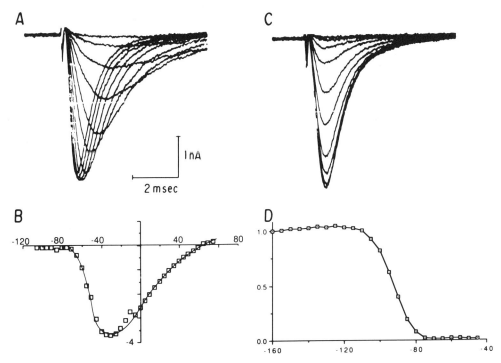

Figure 4 Tracings and plots showing characteristics of the Na$^+$ current in a voltage-clamped rabbit atrial myocyte. (A) The current tracings obtained with a holding potential of -120 mV and depolarizing clamp steps to positive potentials. (B) The peak *I-V* resulting from the protocol illustrated in A. (C) The current obtained during the protocol designed to determine the inactivation curve. (D) The normalized steady-state inactivation curve for traces shown in C. (From Gilliam et al, 1989, Ref. 80.)

current amplitude from maximum change in voltage over time during the upstroke of the action potential $\dot{V}_{max}$ indicate that there are more sodium channels per unit membrane area in Purkinje cells than in ventricular or atrial cells.

Initial studies on the cardiac sodium current used $\dot{V}_{max}$ to monitor the amplitude of the current. This practice was adopted because it was difficult to reliably voltage clamp intact cardiac muscle preparations owing to the large amplitude and rapid kinetics of the cardiac sodium current at physiologic temperatures and normal extracellular sodium concentrations (83,84). The main assumption made in using $\dot{V}_{max}$ as a reflection of sodium current amplitude is that the sodium current is much larger than other ionic currents flowing during the upstroke of the action potential. The use of $\dot{V}_{max}$ as a measure of sodium current in cardiac muscle is controversial (85–88). There is a nonlinear relationship between $\dot{V}_{max}$ and so-

dium current amplitude (89). However, this technique is still useful for estimating sodium current under physiologic conditions. Although there are reports of successful voltage clamp measurements of sodium current in mammalian myocardium, none have been done with a normal extracellular sodium concentration at 37°C.

Weidmann (66) used sheep or calf Purkinje fibers and measured steady-state inactivation using $\dot{V}_{max}$ as an indicator of sodium current amplitude. The permeability to sodium appeared greatest when the membrane potential, just before eliciting an action potential, was -90 mV or more negative. The sodium permeability was reduced to half its maximum value by depolarizing the conditioning membrane potential to -71 mV and changed *e*-fold per 5 mV change in transmembrane potential (slope factor = 5) at the steepest portion of the curve (66). Similar steady-state inactivation curves have been observed in canine atrial muscle (90), canine ventricle (91), and frog atrial muscle (81).

The voltage dependence of activation and the rapid kinetics of the sodium channel were not studied until adequate voltage clamp methods could be developed. Early attempts at measuring the cardiac sodium current (81,91,92) were hindered by imperfect spatial and temporal control of the transmembrane potential as well as problems with the series resistance resulting from narrow intracellular clefts (83,84). However, short segments of rabbit Purkinje fibers, which have wide intracellular clefts, were reliably voltage clamped with time resolution adequate to measure the peak inward sodium current with low temperature and reduced extracellular sodium concentrations (72,93). Successful measurements of sodium current have also been made in spherical clusters of chick embryonic heart cells with normal extracellular sodium at 37°C (73).

Some of the difficulties involved in voltage clamping intact myocardial preparations can be circumvented by measurements of sodium currents using isolated single cardiac myocytes. Macroscopic sodium current measurements have been reported from isolated myocytes from adult rat and mouse ventricular cells, human, cat, rabbit, and frog atrial cells, canine Purkinje cells, and neonatal rat ventricular myocytes in culture (71,74–80,82,94–98). The average peak Na^+ current density in rabbit atrial cells is 0.125 nA/pF (80).

Studies on the activation of cardiac sodium channels show a threshold for activation of the sodium channel around -65 to -50 mV and a peak sodium current between -40 and -5 mV (Fig. 4). The steady-state activation and inactivation curves measured in experiments in which the cytoplasm is either exchanged for or mixed with the solution in the recording pipette are more negative than the curves reported from intact preparations. There are at least two reasons for the discrepant results. First there is a shift in the steady-state inactivation curves over time after membrane rupture (76,99–101). In addition, the steady-state inactivation curve is shifted to hyperpolarized potentials with cooling (72,92,102). Most

voltage clamp measurements of sodium currents have been made at room temperature or cooler.

The activation of the sodium current is rapid, with a time to peak of a millisecond or less (71–73). Activation can be explained using the Hodgkin and Huxley model (103). However, cardiac sodium channel inactivation kinetics appear to require a model that is more complex than that proposed for squid axon by Hodgkin and Huxley (70). Inactivation has been reported to occur with a time course requiring two exponentials for an adequate description in atrial (78,79) and other myocardial cells (74,77,92,93,104). Estimates for these time constants depend on the voltage and temperature at which they are measured. Estimates of the fast time constant for inactivation range from less than 1 msec to as much as 240 msec. Values reported for the slow time constant for inactivation are between 2 and 1270 msec. In contrast, a recent study on cultured atrial cells suggests that inactivation develops with a single exponential time course at subthreshold and threshold levels of potential (80).

The recovery from inactivation also requires more than one exponential to describe the time course accurately (74,79,95,105–108). The longer time constant is between 10 and 100 msec under physiologic conditions after short conditioning pulses (66,105,109). A time constant for recovery from inactivation of the order of 1 sec can be observed after long conditioning depolarizations or in the presence of drugs (105–107,110)

Single-channel recordings of cardiac sodium channels have shown that the predominant sodium channel has at least two rates of inactivation, suggesting multiple inactivated states (100,111,112). Other possibilities for the two rates of inactivation are repetitive openings of sodium channels (reopenings) or return from inactivated state during prolonged test pulses (111,112). Mean open times around 1 msec and single-channel conductances between 7.8 and 20 pS have been reported for cardiac sodium channels (76,78,100,111,113,114). Estimates of sodium channel density range from as low as 1–2 channels per μm^2 in neonatal rat ventricle to as high as 260 channels per μm^2 in canine Purkinje cells (76,77,100,115). In frog atrial cells the density of sodium channels has been estimated to be 2–3 channels per μm^2 (78).

Tetrodotoxin blocks the sodium current in mammalian cardiac muscle with a higher dissociation constant than the sodium channels from nerve or muscle ($K_d \simeq 1 \, \mu M$) (74,116,117). The effects of tetrodotoxin are independent of conditioning voltage or frequency of stimulation in nerve and skeletal muscle. In contrast, the reduction of the cardiac sodium current by tetrodotoxin is dependent on the frequency of stimulation (106,118,119). Controversy exists about whether the block of cardiac sodium channels by tetrodotoxin is voltage dependent (106,116–119). Tetrodotoxin shortens the action potential in Purkinje fibers without affecting $\dot{V}_{max}$ (120). A slow inward tetrodotoxin-sensitive sodium current, which is important during the plateau of the action potential, has been measured in Purkinje fibers (119,121). This current could be a steady-state current resulting from overlap of the voltage dependence of activation and inactivation, a slowly inactivating component of the sodium current, or a current through a sodium channel that is distinct from the channel that is open during the upstroke of the action potential. The late sodium current has not been demonstrated in atrial cells.

Voltage-Dependent Calcium Currents

L-Type Calcium Current

This current, originally called the slow inward current, was first demonstrated in a two-microelectrode voltage clamp study on short Purkinje fiber segments (122). The existence of a slow inward calcium current i_{Ca} was subsequently confirmed and shown to occur in atrial and ventricular muscle (32,34,123,124). Like the fast inward sodium current, the slow inward current activated upon depolarization and then inactivated with maintained depolarization.

Atrial L-type calcium channels are similar to those observed in the ventricle or Purkinje cells (6,16,125–127). I_{Ca-L} density normalized

with respect to cell capacitance is lower in frog atrium than ventricle, but in guinea pig atrium and ventricle the current density appears to be similar (6,125). Because the properties of the L-type calcium current are similar in atrium and other cardiac cells, results from ventricle and atrium are combined in this section.

In single-sucrose gap experiments on bovine papillary muscle, the threshold for activation was approximately $\sim$ -40 mV and the current was optimally activated at 0 mV (Fig. 5) (128). The peak inward current-voltage relationship was biphasic, with the largest inward current at 0 mV. The curve for the voltage dependence of activation was sigmoidal, with a midpoint of approximately $\sim$ -24 mV and an e-fold change per 7 mV at its steepest part (128). The midpoint of the sigmoidal steady-state inactivation curve was approximately $\sim$ -20 mV with a slope factor of 7 mV (128). The steady-state activation and inactivation curves overlapped (128). As a result a portion of the slow inward current is not expected to inactivate at plateau potentials and could be important for maintaining the plateau of the cardiac action potential. In single-cell experiments using ventricle (129–133), the voltage dependencies of activation and inactivation are in good agreement with the results of Reuter and Scholz (128,134). In human atrial cells, the results agree qualitatively with those of Reuter and Scholz. The threshold for activation of i_{Ca-L} was positive to -30 mV, the steady-state activation curve had a midpoint of 0 mV with a slope factor of 3.9, and the maximum inward current was observed at 8 mV (127). The steady-state inactivation curve overlapped the activation curve and had a midpoint of -15 mV with a slope factor of 3.

For reasons already discussed (see Voltage-Dependent Sodium Channel), the kinetics of the L-type i_{Ca} are better resolved in single-cell voltage clamp experiments than in multicellular preparations. In these types of experiments peak inward L-type i_{Ca} occurs within several milliseconds (129–131,135). A time to peak of 2–3 msec has been reported for guinea pig atrial L-type i_{Ca} (16). Activation of L-type i_{Ca}

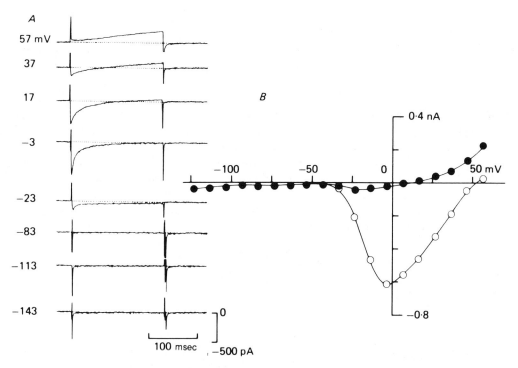

Figure 5 (A) The current in response to depolarizing steps to various potentials in a single atrial myocyte under conditions designed to isolate the L-type Ca current. (B) The current-voltage relationships for the peak inward current (open circles) and current at the level of a 200 msec step (filled symbols). (From Iijima et al. 1985, Ref. 16.)

occurs with a sigmoidal time course thus suggesting that activation is a multistep process (135).

Inactivation of cardiac L-type i_{Ca} has generally been described as the sum of two exponentials with time constants of 5–10 ms (τ_{fast}) and 30–100 msec (τ_{slow}) at 0 mV (16,127,129,131,133). Comparable results have been reported for guinea pig atrial cells (τ_1 = 6 msec and τ_2 = 48 msec at -6 mV) (16). The value of the fast time constant increased with depolarization, but the slow time constant had a U-shaped voltage dependence with its lowest value near 0 mV. Similar results were found in human atrial cells (127).

Inactivation of L-type calcium channels occurs through two distinct mechanisms. When strontium or barium are the charge carriers the degree of inactivation is slowed (130), suggesting that inactivation of L-type i_{Ca} occurs through both a voltage-dependent and a calcium-dependent mechanism (130,136). Recovery from inactivation is slower than the de-

velopment of inactivation (128,131) and occurs with a fast and a slow phase (131). The time constants for inactivation and recovery from inactivation have been shown to be species dependent (131).

Single-channel recordings of barium currents through single L-type calcium channels show the complex kinetics of this channel (133,137,138). Brief openings are separated by rapid closures. Longer closures separate bursts of channel openings. The results are consistent with a single open state with a mean open time of 0.6–1.4 msec and two closed states with time constants of approximately 0.2 and 1.8 msec at membrane potentials that result in maximal inward current (133,137,138). Channel density has been estimated at 3–5 per μm^2 (132,133).

A cardiac L-type calcium channel can be regulated by both β -adrenoceptor agonists and muscarinic agonists. β-Adrenoceptor agonists increase the current amplitude through a cyclic AMP-dependent phosophorylation that results in an increased probability of channel opening (134,137,139–142). Recent evidence also suggests that the L channel can be directly gated by a G protein (52). Muscarinic agonists can induce a direct inhibition of i_{Ca-L} under conditions in which cyclic AMP levels are not elevated or an indirect inhibition of i_{Ca-L} that only occurs after cyclic AMP levels have been elevated (143). This indirect effect has been referred to as accentuated antagonism (144).

In contrast to mammalian ventricle, the direct effect of muscarinic agonists on i_{Ca-L} is reported to occur in adult atrium (16,145–147). The maximum direct reduction of L-type i_{Ca} produced by the agonist is approximately 25–30% of control current amplitude. However, this direct effect on L-type i_{Ca-L} requires a higher concentration of muscarinic agonist than that needed to induce i_{KACh} in mammalian atrium (16,146). In amphibian atrium, lower concentrations of muscarinic agonist inhibit L-type i_{Ca} directly (145,147). The occurrence of the direct inhibition in amphibian atrium has recently been challenged (125). ACh was shown to have no effect on the cadmium-sensitive current in frog atrial cells. In contrast, muscarinic agonists can reduce the amplitude of the cobalt-sensitive inward current in guinea pig atrial cells (16) and cadmium-sensitive current in canine atrial cells (Sorota, unpublished observation). In mammals, this direct effect on i_{Ca-L} occurs only in supraventricular tissues. The indirect effect on i_{Ca-L} occurs in cells of both the atrium and the ventricle (143,148,149).

T-Type Calcium Current

A barium current through a cardiac calcium channel that activates and inactivates at more negative voltages than the L-type i_{Ca} was first described in canine atrial cells (Fig. 6), (126). Subsequently this current (referred to as the T-type i_{Ca}) has been identified in ventricular, sinoatrial node, and Purkinje cells (150–156). The T-type Ca current has much faster kinetics of activation and inactivation than the L-type i_{Ca} (126). Unlike the L-type current the inactivation kinetics of the T-type i_{Ca} are not slowed when barium is used as the charge carrier. T-type i_{Ca} can to be selectively blocked by 40

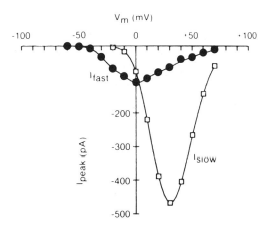

Figure 6 Peak current-voltage relationships for two components of inward currents carried by barium in a single canine atrial cell. I_{fast} (T-type Ca current) and I_{slow} (L-type Ca current) were elicited using the same clamp steps but from different holding potentials. (From Bean, 1985, Ref. 126.)

μM nickel in the cells of the sinoatrial node (153). The current density of the T-type i_{Ca} appears to be greatest in sinoatrial node cells and Purkinje myocytes and lowest in the ventricle (126,153,156) (also reviewed in Ref. 157). The T-type i_{Ca} has been reported to contribute to the later portion of phase 4 depolarization in the sinoatrial node potentials (153). There are conflicting reports regarding the regulation of T-type i_{Ca} by isoproterenol (126,151,154). A possible source of the discrepancy is the difficulty in resolving i_{Ca-T} and i_{Ca-L} when calcium is used as the charge carrier (154,157).

Transient Outward Current

An outward current displaying activation followed by inactivation during depolarizing voltage clamp steps positive to -20 mV was first observed in sheep Purkinje fibers (158,159). This transient outward current has been related to the presence of a notch between phase 1 and phase 2 of some cardiac action potentials (160,161).

Results from chloride substitution experiments led to this current initially being identified as a chloride current (162,163). In the past the names dynamic chloride current (162), positive dynamic current (164), i_{qr} (165), or early outward current (166) have

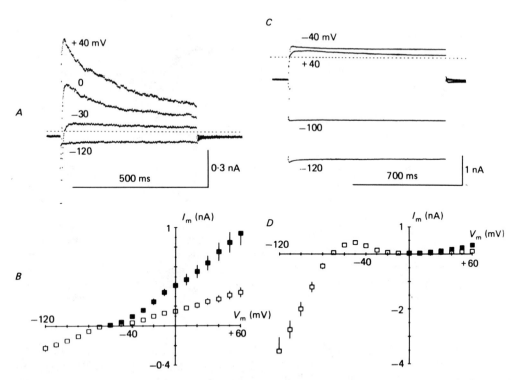

Figure 7 Ionic currents recorded from a rabbit atrial myocyte (A and B) and a rabbit ventricular myocyte (C and D) under conditions needed to "isolate" outward K currents. Note the large transient outward current recorded in the atrial myocyte and the absence of a transient outward current in the ventricular myocyte. Current-voltage relationships (B and D) of current 30 msec after the beginning of the clamp step (filled symbols) and at the end of the clamp step (open symbols) show marked differences. (From Giles and Imaizumi, 1988, Ref. 7.)

been used to refer to the transient outward current i_{to}. Reexamination of chloride substitution experiments under conditions in which the activity of calcium ion was kept constant demonstrated that the majority of i_{to} was not carried by chloride ion. The current was subsequently characterized as a 4-aminopyridine-sensitive potassium current (166,167). A problem with the interpretation of this current as a pure potassium current is that computed or measured reversal potentials are always positive to the potassium equilibrium potential. The most negative value for the reversal potential for this current (-70 mV, 5 mM K_o) was reported in a study on rabbit crista terminalis cells (168).

Transient outward currents have been identified in rabbit, rat, dog, and mouse ventricle, from rabbit, elephant seal, and human atrium, and from cells of the rabbit crista terminalis (7,131,168–175).

In calf Purkinje fibers a calcium-dependent transient outward current has been recorded (176–178). The transient outward current of sheep Purkinje fibers can be pharmacologically dissected into two components, a long-lasting 4-aminopyridine-sensitive component and a briefer calcium-activated component similar to that seen in calf Purkinje fibers (179). Two components of transient outward current in the same cell type have been identified in atrial and ventricular cells (171,172,175).

Although the specific characteristics of transient outward currents may vary from one report to the next, the generalization can be made that there are at least two types of transient outward currents in the heart. One is a current displaying voltage-dependent kinetics that is blocked by 4-aminopyridine. The other is a calcium-dependent outward current that is blocked by caffeine and ryanodine. The transient nature of this current is a result of the intracellular calcium transient.

Voltage-Dependent Transient Outward Current

The voltage-dependent transient outward current is the larger of the two components of the transient outward current in sheep Purkinje fibers, human atrial cells, and canine ventricle cells (167,171,175,179). In addition, a 4-aminopyridine-sensitive transient outward current has been studied in rat ventricle cells and rabbit atrial and ventricular cells (Fig. 7) (7,168,173,180). The voltage-dependent transient outward current has been referred to as i_{to1}, i_{to}, or i_t by various investigators (171,173,175,179).

The threshold for activation of this current is between -40 and -20 mV in all these preparations except human atrial cells, where a threshold for activation of -6 mV was reported (167,168,171,173,179,180). Full activation of the voltage-dependent transient outward current occurs by + 10 mV and + 30 mV in rabbit crista terminalis and atrial cells, respectively (168,173).

Steady-state inactivation of i_{to1} appears to differ in ventricle and atrium. In the ventricle of dogs and rats the curve is sigmoidal with midpoints of -47 and -60 mV, respectively (171,180). Currents were fully inactivated between -40 and -30 mV. In contrast, the midpoints of the steady-state inactivation curves in atrial cells are between -32 and -23 mV, with full inactivation not occurring until 0 mV (173,175). The steady-state inactivation curve in crista terminalis cells of the rabbit was similar to that seen in rabbit atrial cells, with a midpoint at -27 mV and full inactivation by -10 mV (168). It seems then that the voltage dependence of inactivation is shifted to more positive transmembrane potentials in atrial cells compared to ventricular cells.

The voltage-dependent transient outward current reaches its peak amplitude in approximately 10 msec (168,171,173,175,179). The exact time to peak depends on the test potential. Time to peak is reduced at more depolarized potentials (168,171,173,175).

The time course of decay of this current is not similar among tissues. A rapid decay of i_{to1} (time constants between 10 and 40 msec) has been reported for rat and canine ventricle and for human atrial cells (170,171,175,180). In contrast, in rabbit crista terminalis cells the time constant for decay of outward current is 300 msec (168). Two exponentials have been used to describe the decay of this outward current in sheep Purkinje fibers and rabbit atrial cells, with the fast time constants between 30 and 100 msec and slow time constants in the range 250–470 msec.

Recovery from inactivation is slow for the voltage-sensitive transient outward current. Although there is no agreement about whether recovery is mono- or biexponential, a time constant with a value between 350 msec and 1 sec is required (161,170,171,179). The slowest values for recovery from inactivation are from rabbit atrial cells (7). In these cells recovery from inactivation occurred in two phases. The fast phase had a time constant of 5 sec; the slower phase had a time constant greater than 15 sec. However, the low temperature (23°C) used in the studies on rabbit atrial cells may have slowed the kinetics. When recovery of the voltage-dependent transient outward current from inactivation was estimated from the size of the notch in the canine ventricular action potential, a fast and slow phase of recovery were seen (τ_{fast} = 41–85 msec; τ_{slow} = 350–500 msec) (161). A fast monoexponential recovery from inactivation has been reported in rat ventricle cells (time constant = 35 msec) (180).

A consequence of the slow recovery from inactivation of the voltage-dependent transient outward current is that as the cycle length decreases the plateau amplitude and/or the action potential duration increase as a result of the loss of hyperpolarizing current flow. A profound effect of cycle length on action potential configuration has been demonstrated in rabbit atrial cells and correlated with rate-dependent changes in voltage-dependent transient outward current (7).

Rabbit atrial cells have been reported to have a much larger voltage-dependent transient outward current than rabbit ventricle (7). This is also true for canine atrium and ventricle (Sorota, unpublished). A possible explanation for the differences in action potential configuration between atrial and ventricular cells is the difference in the size of the transient outward current (7). Although no data from human ventricle have been published, human atrial cells also have a prominent transient outward current (48,175). Not all mammalian atrial cells have a large transient outward current (6). In contrast to most other mammalian species, millimolar concentrations of 4-aminopyridine have no effects on action potential or background current-voltage relationship in guinea pig atrial cells (6).

Human atrial cells differ from rabbit atrial cells in that the former have a calcium-dependent transient outward current in addition to a voltage-dependent outward current (7,175). Results of experiments studying the effects of 4-aminopyridine and caffeine on human atrial action potential configuration suggest that with age there is an increase in the density of voltage-dependent transient outward current in human atrial fibers. The action potentials of adult atrial fibers exhibit a more prominent notch and a lower plateau amplitude than the action potentials of neonatal atrial fibers (181).

Stimulation of myocardial α-adrenoceptors causes a rate-dependent increase in the force of contraction associated with an increase in the action potential duration. Transient outward current i_{to1} in rat ventricular myocytes and rabbit atrial myocytes is inhibited by α-adrenoceptor agonists (182,183), and this finding may provide insight into the α-agonist positive inotropic effect. Protein kinase C activators also inhibit the transient outward current in rat ventricular cells, suggesting that α-adrenoceptor agonist may inhibit transient outward current by activating protein kinase C (182). Transient outward current is reduced by low concentrations (3–10 μM) of quinidine (184). This block probably contributes to the quinidine-induced action potential prolongation.

Calcium-Dependent Transient Outward Current

The calcium-dependent transient outward current has been difficult to study because it is dependent on the influx of calcium ions through voltage-sensitive calcium channels, which then trigger the release of calcium from the sarcoplasmic reticulum. This current is inhibited by removal of extracellular calcium, calcium channel blockers, intracellular calcium chelator (EGTA), replacement of extracellular calcium with strontium, and inhibitors of calcium release from the sarcoplasmic reticulum (171,175,176,178,179). A calcium-dependent transient outward current has been reported in elephant seal (174) and human atrial cells (175). In the latter study, the calcium-dependent transient outward current had faster kinetics than the voltage-dependent transient outward current (175). The current peaked in 5.5 msec and decayed with a time constant of 9.1 msec. The transient nature of this current is a reflection of the intracellular calcium transient rather than a voltage-dependent activation and inactivation.

Delayed Rectifier

During depolarizing steps to plateau potentials, a slowly developing outward current can be recorded. Although the details are variable from one report to another, similar slowly developing outward currents have been recorded in multicellular preparations of the mammalian ventricle and sinoatrial node and the frog atrium and sinus venosus (185–194). The delayed rectifier current has also been demonstrated in single cells from mammalian ventricle and atrium and frog and chick atrium (6,31,195–202). In contrast to the original observations, the delayed rectifier current was thought to be relatively selective for potassium, with a reversal potential at or slightly positive to the potassium equilibrium potential in ventricular muscle and Purkinje fibers (187,188,203). Thus the abbreviation i_K is used to represent this current.

A delayed rectifier current appears to be a consistent finding in frog atrial fibers and myocytes (31,191–193,201–202) and chick atrial cells (200). In mammalian atrial cells a significant delayed rectifier current is not always detected. In fact, in rabbit atrial cells i_K has been reported to be too small and slow to be

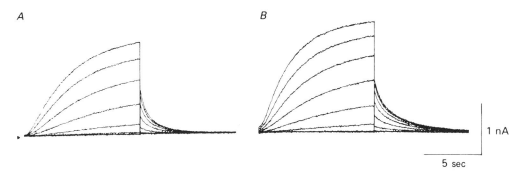

Figure 8 The effect of isoproterenol (10^{-6} M) on i_K after blockade of i_{Ca-L}. The membrane currents in response to depolarizing clamp steps before (A) and after isoproterenol application (B) are shown. Note that isoproterenol increased i_K even after i_{Ca} was blocked. (From Giles et al, 1989, Ref. 201.)

important for repolarization (7). In contrast, in guinea pig atrial cells there is a relatively large delayed rectifier current (6,198). The mammalian delayed rectifier current appears to be similar in atrium and ventricle (6,198).

The reported voltage dependence for i_K is variable. Some of the variability may be due to species and tissue differences. Reports for the threshold for activation are between -80 and -20 mV, with full activation between -10 and 50 mV (188,192,195,199,200,204,205).

The reports on the kinetics of i_K are variable. The activation has been reported to be either sigmoidal or monoexponential. The decay of current on repolarization has been reported to be either monoexponential or biexponential. The parallel conductance mechanism for the delayed rectifier is not the only model that can explain the biexponential decay of i_K on repolarization (203,205). A model with a single conducting state and two closed states has been proposed for Purkinje fibers and single Purkinje cells. In guinea pig ventricle, activation of isoproterenol-stimulated i_K followed a sigmoidal time course (195). The time course of the decaying current was monoexponential at potentials negative to -50 mV. A Hodgkin-Huxley type of model with second-order activation was fit to the data (195).

The delayed rectifier current is enhanced by β-adrenoceptor agonists in a cyclic AMP-dependent manner (139,197,201,202, 206–210). Experiments on frog cardiac myocytes demonstrated that the voltage dependence of activation is shifted slightly to more

negative potentials with β-adrenoceptor stimulation (Fig. 8) (201,202). The shortening of the action potential that usually occurs with β-adrenoceptor stimulation can be explained by the enhancement of i_K. Activation of protein kinase C also enhances i_K with no apparent effect on the kinetics (196,199). The enhancement of i_K by β-adrenoceptor agonists or activators of protein kinase C is temperature sensitive (196,197). The delayed rectifier current is enhanced by either mechanism at 32°C but not at 22°C (196).

Sodium/Potassium Pump Current

The sodium/potassium pump utilizes energy from ATP to extrude three sodium ions from the cell while moving two potassium ions into the cell (reviewed in Refs. 211 and 212). The result is a net outward (hyperpolarizing) current. Sodium loading of cardiac tissue results in a transient hyperpolarization of the muscle that has been attributed to an electrogenic sodium/potassium pump current (213–220). Hyperpolarizations induced by internal sodium loading has been observed in mammalian atrial cells (215,217,218). Brief exposures to dihydro-ouabain, an inhibitor of the sodium/potassium pump, prolonged the action potential in Purkinje fibers through inhibition of an outward background current (221). The sodium/potassium pump current has been directly measured in sodium-loaded cardiac preparations (219,220,222–224), including frog atrium (225). The electrogenic sodium/potassium pump is present in all cardiac tissue and is required for maintenance of the normal electrochemical gradients for sodium and potassium across the cell membrane.

Sodium-Calcium Exchange Current

Early evidence for a sodium-calcium exchange mechanism came from experiments that showed an effect of extracellular sodium on tension development in amphibian and mammalian heart (226–230). Ion flux measurements confirmed the existence of a sodium-calcium exchange process in guinea pig atrium and sheep ventricle (231).

Sodium-calcium exchange is an electrogenic counterporter that utilizes the electrochemical gradient of these ions as the energy source for ion movement. (reviewed in Refs. 232–235). The stoichiometry of the sodium-calcium exchanger appears to be $3Na^+$ to $1Ca^{2+}$ (232,236). The exchanger is reversible, generating an inward current when calcium is extruded and an outward current when sodium is pumped out. The current-voltage relationship for sodium-calcium exchange current is variable and dependent on the intracellular and extracellular concentration of sodium and calcium (236).

Currents attributable to electrogenic sodium-calcium exchange have been measured in embryonic chick heart cultures, frog atrium, and guinea pig atrium and ventricle (236–245). Because of the lack of evidence to the contrary, it can probably be assumed that the sodium-calcium exchange current and its functional significance are similar in atrium and other cardiac cell types. However, the role of sodium-calcium exchange current in cardiac electrical activity has not been unequivocally demonstrated.

Assuming that the exchanger operates near equilibrium with a 3:1 stoichiometry, the sodium-calcium exchanger could theoretically carry an inward current in resting cells that could account for at least part of the deviation of the resting potential from the potassium equilibrium potential [reviewed in Noble (246)]. Some of the inward current responsible for the plateau of the guinea pig ventricle action potential appears to be sodium-calcium exchange current (245). In guinea pig atrial cells sodium-calcium exchange has been implicated in the generation of a transient inward current (241,243).

Hyperpolarization-Activated Inward Current i_f

A time-dependent net inward current that is activated by hyperpolarization has been described in Purkinje and sinoatrial node fibers (158,247,248). The current in sinoatrial node was shown to be an activating inward current (249). Although the current in Purkinje fibers was initially considered a decaying outward current, it was subsequently demonstrated to be an activating inward current carried by sodium and potassium and blocked by cesium (250,251).

A role in the generation of spontaneous activity has been proposed for the hyperpolarization-activated inward current. Stimulation of β-adrenoceptors causes a shift in the voltage dependence of activation to less negative potentials but stimulation of muscarinic receptors has the opposite effect (252–254). In sinoatrial node i_f is activated between -50 and -100 mV (255). A similar current has been reported in sucrose gap experiments on sheep atrial trabeculae (256). In some but not all isolated cat right atrial and human myocytes i_f has been detected (48,257). The pacemaker activity found in some atrial preparations may be attributable to the presence of a small population of cells with morphology similar to those seen in the sinoatrial node region (258).

Calcium-Activated Nonspecific Cation Current

A cation-selective current that can be carried by sodium, potassium and calcium has been demonstrated in cultured neonatal rat heart cells and adult guinea pig ventricular myocytes (259,260). This current has a linear current-voltage relationship. Delayed afterdepolarizations and aftercontractions occur in calcium-overloaded cardiac preparations, including atrial muscle (reviewed in Ref. 261). A transient inward current related to aftercontractions and delayed afterdepolarizations can be measured (262). There may be a relationship between the calcium-activated nonspecific cation current and the transient inward current (259,263). As mentioned, an alternative explanation for the transient inward current is activation of the inward sodium-calcium exchange current (264,265).

ATP-Sensitive Potassium Current

A large-conductance single-channel current that was inhibited by intracellular adenosine-5'-triphosphate (ATP) was first observed in isolated inside-out membrane patches of guinea pig and rabbit atrial and ventricular cells (266). No difference was noted between the channel properties in atrium or ventricle. The existence of this channel was soon confirmed in guinea pig ventricular myocytes (267). With potassium-rich solutions on both sides of the membrane, both inward and outward current flow through the ATP-sensitive potassium channel can be measured. The current voltage relationship is linear until it rectifies inwardly approximately 60 mV positive to the reversal potential (266–269). When there is potassium-rich solution on the inner side of the membrane and a sodium-rich solution on the extracellular side of the membrane, only outward current flows through the channel and the current-voltage relationship is no longer linear (Fig. 9) (269). This current was blocked by 1–10 mM barium in a voltage-dependent manner (269,270). The block by barium was increased by depolarization (269).

The ATP-sensitive current in heart cells can be activated by pinacidil and BRL-34915 (cromakalim), but glybenclamide and tolbutamide inhibit the current (271–273). Activation of the ATP-sensitive potassium channel causes a decrease in the action potential plateau amplitude and duration without a significant effect on the resting membrane potential (267,273, 274). The resting potential is not affected because of the outward rectification of the ATP-sensitive potassium channel in physiologic salt solutions (269). The function of this channel is unknown. It may help to reduce energy utilization of cardiac muscle during periods of hypoxia (266). The channel may be partly

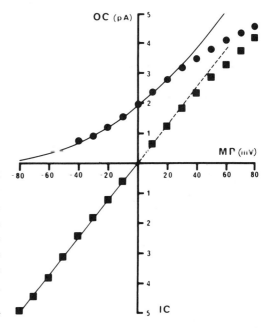

Figure 9 Current-voltage relationships for the K⁺ ATP channels recorded in Na⁺-rich solution bathing the external and K⁺-rich solution bathing the internal surfaces of the patch membrane (circles) or with K⁺-rich solution bathing both sides of the patch membrane (squares). Note that when Na⁺ is present on the external side of the membrane only outward current flows through this channel. (From Findlay, 1987, Ref. 269.)

responsible for the increase in extracellular potassium at the expense of intracellular potassium that occurs in hypoxic myocardium.

Summary

The action potential in mammalian atrial muscle is characterized by its triangular shape and lower plateau compared to ventricular muscle or Purkinje fibers. No significant differences have been reported in inward currents that could account for the dissimilar action potential configurations, although atrial cells appear to have a higher density of T-type calcium current than the ventricular cells. The lack of a negative slope conductance region in the background potassium current-voltage relationship contributes to the low plateau amplitude and the slow terminal repolarization phase seen in atrial cells. There is more background outward current in atrial cells at plateau potentials. As the cells repolarize toward the resting potential the ventricular cell has a large outward current because of the negative slope conductance. The higher density of the 4-aminopyridine-sensitive transient outward current in rabbit atrial cells is a major factor in the lower plateau amplitude when compared to ventricular cells. In addition to the background potassium current in the atrium, there is also an important chemically activated potassium current. This current is activated by adenosine and muscarinic agonists and lacks a region of negative slope conductance. Some endogenous activator of this current is probably always present in situ. The activation of i_{KACh} by adenosine or muscarinic agonist further shortens the action potential.

IN SITU ATRIUM

Monophasic Potentials

Since it is very difficult to record using fine-tipped microelectrodes from the intact beating atrial chambers, recording techniques have been developed that allow the investigator to record from several fibers in the endocardium or epicardial surface of the chamber. An action potential recorded with the monophasic recording technique closely resembles the action potential recorded through an intracellular microelectrode (11). The original discussion of this technique and its disadvantages has been described (275). A disadvantage is that despite the similarities between the intracellular action potential and the monophasic action potential (MAP), the MAP has lower total amplitude than the action potential and the upstroke velocity of the MAP is a measure of the rate of depolarization of several cells and therefore is not a precise measure of cell velocity. Generally, measurements of the time course of repolarization of the action potential are valid using this method.

Recently, monophasic action potential recording catheters were fabricated in such a way that a central recording electrode protrudes from the catheter and is connected to the positive input of a directly coupled amplifier (276). The protrusion of the electrode

from the catheter end is essential so that when pressed lightly against the epicardial or endocardial surface some tissue injury occurs. The negative input of the amplifier must be connected to a laterally placed indifferent electrode. In some cases suction is used to produce a slight change in the membrane surface to record the MAP.

MAP recordings have provided information on the time course of atrial repolarization in diseased and arrhythmic atria (277–279) as well as during antiarrhythmic drug action (280–282).

Extracellular Recordings of Atrial Activity

Unipolar and bipolar extracellular electrodes attached to different sites on the atrium have been used to determine the precise pattern of atrial activation during a normal sinus impulse and during abnormal impulses. The important differences between these two types of extracellular recording techniques have been discussed elsewhere (275).

Much has been learned by using these techniques to record conduction patterns in atrial tissue. For instance, the configuration of the P wave on a surface ECG of a normal person can show variation, and this may be due to a change in the pattern of atrial activation during normal sinus rhythm (see Ref. 283). A series of studies in which a P wave's polarity and morphology were related to a precise sequence of atrial activation suggests that in the atrial chambers there are functionally preferential pathways for atrial conduction (284).

As mentioned, controversy still exists about the underlying mechanism providing one atrial tissue bundle preferential conduction and another none. For instance, conduction along a specific tract composed of specific atrial cells with specialized membrane properties could lead to specialized preferential conduction (285). On the other hand, different membrane properties cannot account for the different conduction velocities measured at the same atrial site when the direction of the propagating wavefront changes. Therefore, the preferential conduction of an impulse evident in most maps of atrial activation during a sinus impulse can be explained on the basis of the anisotropic properties of the three-dimensional atrial tissue.

If a multidimensional structure is isotropic, then the structure has the same passive properties along any given axis of the preparation. A large flat atrial muscle bundle,such as the crista terminalis of the atrium of a young dog, is considered a structure exhibiting uniform anisotropy (275). In this structure rates of propagation are dependent on the direction of propagation. That is, propagation along the longitudinal axis of the bundle (parallel to fiber orientation) is rapid, but propagation along the transverse axis (perpendicular to fiber orientation) is slow. This type of directional difference in conduction velocity has also been described for other parts of the myocardium (286–288).

It now appears that variation in the distribution of connection between fibers and muscle bundles can cause the uniform anisotropic nature of conduction of the impulse to become nonuniform. Nonuniform anisotropic conduction is similar to uniform anisotropic conduction in that it maintains the directional differences in conduction velocity, but in addition, when propagation occurs in the transverse direction, the extracellular waveforms recorded are not smooth but are irregular and fractionated as a result of the superimposition of several smaller deflections. For instance, the anisotropic properties of human atrial tissue change with age (289). These age-related changes in conduction have been correlated with the progressive increase and interpositioning of extensive collagen septa between longitudinally oriented atrial bundles. It may be that such anatomic discontinuities provide a substrate for a barrier to impulse propagation (289). Uniform anisotropic conduction in the atrial chamber may lead to nonuniform anisotropic conduction in other situations in which increased fibrosis is secondary to a disease process (e.g., in mitral valvular fibrosis).

The functional significance of uniformly anisotropic tissue that becomes nonuniformly anisotropic with age or atrial disease is in the role that this change could play in setting up conduction nonuniformities that could initiate or perpetuate a reentrant type of arrhythmia. In a nonuniformly anisotropic structure in which effective transverse conduction is very slow, reentrant excitation could occur in a smaller region of tissue than that required in the uniformly anisotropic tissue (289).

ABNORMAL ELECTROPHYSIOLOGY OF THE ATRIUM

Automatic Rhythms: Abnormal Automaticity, Normal Pacemakers (Subsidiary)

When the function of the primary pacemaker of the heart (the sinoatrial node) is altered, pacemaker cells from the inferior right atrium can assume control of the heart (290–292). These subsidiary pacemaker cells of the heart generate slow upstroke action potentials and marked diastolic depolarization that exhibits two distinct slopes; the initial slope is steeper than the secondary, more gradual slope (293). Cells of this type have also been recorded from the tricuspid valve leaflet of rabbit (294).

Abnormal automaticity is a form of impulse initiation that occurs in atrial fibers when the maximum diastolic potential is no longer -85 to -90 mV but is between -40 and -60 mV. The resting potential of atrial fibers can be easily shifted toward zero as a result of cardiac disease. For instance, depolarization of atrial fibers has been reported in diseased human and feline atria (2,295,296).

Triggered Activity

Sustained nondriven rhythmic activity can also occur in atrial fibers immediately after a single stimulated beat. When this type of abnormal electrical activity is associated with "afterpotential" it is referred to as "triggered activity." A recent monograph by Cranefield and Aronson (297) reviews the experimental literature on afterpotentials as they occur in all tissue types.

Normal atrial muscle fibers in various locations within the atrial chamber have been shown to elicit afterpotentials, particularly the delayed afterdepolarization (DAD). DADs have been described in electrical activity of atrial fibers that extend into the midsection of the valve leaflet of the canine, simian, rabbit, and human mitral and tricuspid valves (298–300). Atrial fibers in the coronary sinus region of the canine heart readily give rise to DADs in the presence of catecholamines (301). Several studies in isolated rabbit atrial preparations have shown that DADs are present in transmembrane potentials of fibers of the upper pectinate muscles and crista terminalis (302–305). In normal dog atrium DADs can occur in some fibers in the absence of catecholamines (292).

In general, the occurrence of afterpotentials is associated with atrial fibers from diseased hearts or fibers exposed to toxic concentrations of ouabain.

Reentrant Excitation

A discussion of abnormal electrical activity in the atria resulting from different types of atrial reentrant excitation is found in Chapter 10.

REFERENCES

1. Paes de Carvalho A, deMello WC, Hoffman BF. Electrophysiological evidence for specialized fiber types in rabbit atrium. Am J Physiol 1959; 196:483–8.
2. Gelband H, Bush HL, Rosen MR, Myerburg RJ, Hoffman BF. Electrophysiologic properties of isolated preparations of human atrial myocardium. Circ Res 1972; 30:293–300.
3. Mary-Rabine L, Hordof AJ, Danilo P Jr, Malm JR, Rosen MR. Mechanisms for impulse initiation in isolated human atrial fibers. Circ Res 1980; 47:267–277.
4. Wagner ML, Lazzara R, Weiss RM, Hoffman BF. Specialized conducting fibers in the interatrial band. Circ Res 1966; 18:502–18.
5. Hogan P, Davis LD. Evidence for specialized fibers in the canine right atrium. Circ Res 1968; 23:387–96.
6. Hume JR, Uehara A. Ionic basis of the different action potential configuration of single guinea-pig atrial and ventricular myocytes. J. Physiol (Lond) 1985; 368:525–44.
7. Giles WR, Imaizumi Y. Comparison of potassium currents in rabbit atrial and ventricular cells. J. Physiol (Lond) 1988; 405:123–45.
8. Janse MJ, Anderson RH. Specialized internodal pathways—fact or fiction?. Eur J Cardiol 1974; 212:117–36.
9. James TN, Sherf L. Specialized tissues and preferential conduction in the atria of the heart. Am J Cardiol 1971; 28:414–27.
10. Spach MS, Miller WT III, Dolber PC, Kootsey JM, Sommer JR, Mosher CE Jr. The functional role of structural complexities in the propagation of depolarization in the atrium of the dog. Cardiac conduction disturbances due to discontinuities of effective axial resistivity. Circ Res 1982; 50:175–91.
11. Hoffman BF, Cranefield PF. Recording techniques. In: Hoffman BF, Cranefield PF, eds. Electrophysiology of the heart. New York: McGraw-Hill, 1960:1–19.
12. Nawrath H. Action potential, membrane currents and force of contraction in mammalian heart muscle fibers treated with quinidine. J Pharmacol Exp Ther 1981; 216:176–82.
13. Hodgkin AL, Rushton WAH. The electrical constants of a crustacean nerve fiber. Proc R Soc Lond [Biol] 1946; 133:444–79.
14. Fozzard HA, Arnsdorf MF. Cardiac electrophysiology. In: Fozzard HA, Haber E, Jennings RB, Katz AM, Morgan HE, eds. The heart and cardiovascular system. Scientific foundations. New York: Raven Press, 1986: 1–30.
15. Hume JR, Giles W. Active and passive electrical properties of single bullfrog atrial cells. J Gen Physiol 1981; 78:19–42.
16. Iijima T, Irisawa H, Kameyama M. Membrane currents and their modification by acetylcholine in isolated single atrial cells of the guinea-pig. J Physiol (Lond) 1985; 359:485–501.
17. Trautwein W, Dudel J. Zum mechanismus der membranwirkung des acetylcholin an der herzmuskelfaser. Pflügers Arch 1958; 266:324–34.
18. Belardinelli L, Isenberg G. Isolated atrial myocytes: adenosine and acetylcholine increase potassium conductance. Am J Physiol 1983; 244:H734–7.
19. Kurachi Y, Nakajima T, Sugimoto T. On the mechanism of activation of muscarinic K^+ channels by adenosine in isolated atrial cells: involvement of GTP-binding proteins. Pflügers Arch 1986; 407:264–274.

20. Sakmann B, Noma A, Trautwein W. Acetylcholine activation of single muscarinic K $^+$ channels in isolated pacemaker cells of the mammalian heart. Nature 1983; 303:250–3.

21. Noma A, Nakayama T, Kurachi Y, Irisawa H. Resting K conductances in pacemaker and non-pacemaker heart cells of the rabbit. Jpn J Physiol 1984; 34:245–54.

22. Hall AE, Hutter OF, Noble D. Current-voltage relations of Purkinje fibers in sodium-deficient solutions. J Physiol (Lond) 1963; 166:225–40.

23. Noble D. Electrical properties of cardiac muscle attributable to inward going (anomalous) rectification. J Cell Comp Physiol 1965; 66:127–36.

24. Cleeman L, Morad M. Potassium currents in frog ventricular muscle: evidence from voltage clamp currents and extracellular K accumulation. J Physiol (Lond) 1979; 286: 113–43.

25. Kameyama M, Kiyosue T, Soejima M. Single channel analysis of the inward rectifier K current in the rabbit ventricular cells. Jpn J Physiol 1983; 33:1039–56.

26. Sakmann B, Trube G. Conductance properties of single inwardly rectifying potassium channels in ventricular cells from guinea-pig heart. J Physiol (Lond) 1984; 347:641–57.

27. Carmeliet E, Vereecke J. Electrogenesis of the action potential and automaticity. In: Berne RM, Sperelakis N, Geiger SR, eds. Handbook of physiology. Section 2. The cardiovascular system. Vol. 1. The heart. Baltimore: Waverly Press, 1979:269–334.

28. Matsuda H, Saigusa A, Irisawa H. Ohmic conductance through the inwardly rectifying K channel and blocking by internal Mg^{2+}. Nature 1987; 325:156–9.

29. Mazzanti M, DiFrancesco D. Intracellular Ca modulates K-inward rectification in cardiac myocytes. Pflügers Arch 1989; 413: 322–4.

30. Daut J. The passive electrical properties of guinea-pig ventricular muscle as examined with a voltage-clamp technique. J Physiol (Lond) 1982; 330:221–42.

31. Hume JR, Giles W. Ionic currents in single isolated bullfrog atrial cells. J Gen Physiol 1983; 81:153–94.

32. Rougier O, Vassort G, Garnier D, Gargouil YM, Coraboeuf E. Esistence and role of a slow inward current during the frog atrial action poetential. Pflügers Arch 1969; 308: 91–110.

33. Kass RS, Tsien RW. Multiple effects of calcium antagonists on plateau currents in cardiac Purkinje fibers. J Gen Physiol 1975; 66:169–92.

34. Vitek M, Trautwein W. Slow inward current and action potential in cardiac Purkinje fibers. The effects of Mn^{++}-ions. Pflügers Arch 1971; 323:204–18.

35. Isenberg G. Cardiac Purkinje fibers: cesium as a tool to block inward rectifying potassium currents. Pflügers Arch 1976; 365: 99–106.

36. Cleeman L, Morad M. Extracellular potassium accumulation in voltage-clamped frog ventricular muscle. J Physiol (Lond) 1978; 286:83–111.

37. Sakmann B, Trube G. Voltage-dependent inactivation of the inward-rectifying single-channel currents in the guinea-pig heart cell membrane. J Physiol (Lond) 1984; 347: 659–83.

38. Carmeliet E, Mubagwa K. Characterization of the acetylcholine-induced potassium current in rabbit cardiac Purkinje fibers. J Physiol (Lond) 1985; 371:219–37.

39. Kurachi Y. Voltage-dependent activation of the inward-rectifier potassium channel in the ventricular cell membrane of guinea-pig heart. J Physiol (Lond) 1985; 366:365–85.

40. Biermans G, Vereecke J, Carmeliet E. The mechanism of the inactivation of the inward-rectifying K current during hyperpolarizing steps in guinea-pig ventricular myocytes. Pflügers Arch 1987; 410:604–13.

41. Ehara T. Rectifier properties of canine papillary muscle. Jpn J Physiol 1971; 21:49–69.

42. DeHemptinne A. The current voltage relationship of the delayed outward current in the heart of the frog *(Rana esculenta)* and the tortoise *(Testudo germani)*. Pflügers Arch 1978; 377:235–43.

43. Soejima M, Noma A. Mode of regulation of the ACh-sensitive K-channel by the muscarinic receptor in atrial cells. Pflügers Arch 1984; 400:424–31.

44. Noma A, Trautwein W. Relaxation of the ACh-induced potassium current in the rabbit sinoatrial node cell. Pflügers Arch 1978; 377:193–200.

45. Hoffman BF, Suckling EE. Cardiac cellular potentials: effect of vagal stimulation and acetylcholine. Am J Physiol 1953; 173:312–20.

46. Pfaffinger PJ, Martin JM, Hunter DD, Nathanson NM, Hille B. GTP-binding pro-

teins couple cardiac muscarinic receptors to a K channel. Nature 1985; 317:536–8.

47. Breitwieser GE, Szabo G. Mechanism of muscarinic receptor-induced K$^+$ channel activation as revealed by hydrolysis-resistant GTP analogues. J Gen Physiol 1988; 91: 469–93.

48. Heidbüchel H, Vereecke J, Carmeliet E. The electrophysiological effects of acetylcholine in single human atrial cells. J Mol Cell Cardiol 1987; 19:1207–19.

49. Sorota S, Hoffman BF. Role of G-proteins in the ACh-induced potassium current of canine atrial cells. Am J Physiol 1989; 257: H1516–22.

50. Logothetis DE, Kurachi Y, Galper J, Neer EJ, Clapham DE. The beta gamma subunits of GTP-binding proteins activate the muscarinic K$^+$ channel in heart. Nature 1987; 325:321–6.

51. Cerbai E, Klockner U, Isenberg G. The alpha subunit of the GTP binding protein activates muscarinic potassium channels of the atrium. Science 1988; 240:1782–3.

52. Yatani A, Codina J, Imoto Y, Reeves JP, Birnbaumer L, Brown AM. A G protein directly regulates mammalian cardiac calcium channels. Science 1987; 238:1288–92.

53. Sorota S, Tsuji Y, Pappano AJ. Pertussis toxin blocks muscarinic hyperpolarization and action potential shortening in chick atrium. Fed Proc 1985; 44:1861.

54. Sorota S, Tsuji Y, Tajima T, Pappano AJ. Pertussin toxin treatment blocks hyperpolarization by muscarinic agonists in chick atrium. Circ Res 1985; 57:748–58.

55. Endoh M, Maruyama M, Iijima T. Attenuation of muscarinic cholinergic inhibition by islet-activating protein in the heart. Am J Physiol 1985; 249:H309–20.

56. Breitwieser GE, Szabo G. Uncoupling of the cardiac muscarinic and beta-adrenergic receptors from ion channels by a guanine nucleotide analogue. Nature 1985; 317:538–40.

57. Yatani A, Mattera R, Codina J, et al. The G protein-gated atrial K$^+$ channel is stimulated by three distinct Giα-subunits. Nature 1988; 336:680–2.

58. Yatani A, Hamm H, Codina J, Mazzoni MR, Birnbaumer L, Brown AM. A monoclonal antibody to the alpha subunit of G$_k$ blocks muscarinic activation of atrial K$^+$ channels. Science 1988; 241:828–31.

59. Halvorsen SW, Nathanson NM. Ontogenesis of physiological responsiveness and guanine nucleotide sensitivity of cardiac muscarinic receptors during chick embryonic development. Biochemistry 1984; 23:5813–21.

60. Malbon CC, Rapiejko PJ, Sainz JAG. Pertussis toxin catalyzes the ADP-ribosylation of two distinct peptides, 40 and 41 kDa, in rat fat cell membranes. FEBS 1984; 176(2): 302–6.

61. Malbon CC, Mangano TJ, Watkins DC. Heart contains two substrates ($M_r = 40,000$ and 41,000) for pertussis toxin-catalyzed ADP-ribosylation that co-purify with N$_s$. Biochem Biophys Res Commun 1985; 128: 809–15.

62. Tajima T, Tsuji Y, Sorota S, Pappano AJ. Positive vs. negative inotropic effects of carbachol in avian atrial muscle: role of N$_i$-like protein. Circ Res 1987; 61(Suppl. I):I–105.

63. Scherer NM, Toro M-J, Entman ML, Birnbaumer L. G-protein distribution in canine cardiac sarcoplasmic reticulum and sarcolemma: comparison to rabbit skeletal muscle membranes and to brain and erythrocyte G-proteins. Arch Biochem Biophys 1987; 259: 431–40.

64. Cranefield PF, Eyster JAE, Gilson WE. The effects of reduction of external sodium chloride on the injury potentials of cardiac muscle. Am J Physiol 1951; 166:269–72.

65. Draper MH, Weidmann S. Cardiac resting and action potentials recorded with an intracellular microelectrode. J Physiol (Lond) 1951; 115:74–94.

66. Weidmann S. The effect of the cardiac membrane potential on the rapid availability of the sodium-carrying system. J Physiol (Lond) 1955; 127:213–24.

67. Hodgkin AL, Huxley AF. Currents carried by sodium and potassium ions through the membrane of the giant axon of Loligo. J Physiol (Lond) 1952; 116:449–72.

68. Hodgkin AL, Huxley AF. The components of membrane conductance in the giant axon of Loligo. J Physiol (Lond) 1952; 116: 473–96.

69. Hodgkin AL, Huxley AF. The dual effects of membrane potential on sodium conductance in the giant axon of Loligo. J Physiol (Lond) 1952; 116:497–506.

70. Hodgkin AL, Huxley AF. A quantitative description of membrane current and its application to conduction and excitation in nerve. J Physiol (Lond) 1952; 117:500–44.

71. Lee KS, Weeks TA, Kao RL, Akaike N, Brown AM. Sodium current in single heart muscle cells. Nature 1979; 278:269–71.

72. Colatsky TJ. Voltage clamp measurements of sodium channel properties in rabbit cardiac Purkinje fibers. J Physiol (Lond) 1980; 305: 215–34.

73. Ebihara L, Johnson EA. Fast sodium current in cardiac muscle. A quantitative description. Biophys J 1980; 32:779–90.

74. Brown AM, Lee KS, Powell T. Sodium current in single rat heart muscle cells. J Physiol (Lond) 1981; 318:479–500.

75. Bustamante JO, McDonald TF. Sodium currents in segments of human heart cells. Science 1982; 220:320–1.

76. Cachelin AB, DePeyer JE, Kokubun S, Reuter H. Sodium channels in cultured cardiac cells. J Physiol (Lond) 1983; 340:389–401.

77. Makielski JC, Sheets MF, Hanck DA, January CT, Fozzard HA. Sodium current in voltage clamped internally perfused canine cardiac Purkinje cells. Biophys J 1987; 52: 1–11.

78. Clark RB, Giles WR. Sodium current in single cells from bullfrog atrium: voltage dependence and ion transfer properties. J Physiol (Lond) 1987; 391:235–65.

79. Follmer CH, Ten Eick RE, Yeh, JZ. Sodium current kinetics in cat atrial myocytes. J Physiol (Lond) 1987; 384:169–97.

80. Gilliam FR III, Starmer CF, Grant AO. Blockade of rabbit atrial sodium channels by lidocaine. Characterization of continuous and frequency dependent blocking. Circ Res 1989; 65:723–39.

81. Haas HG, Kern R, Einwachter HM, Tarr M. Kinetics of Na inactivation in frog atria. Pflügers Arch 1971; 323:141–57.

82. Gatlin MR, Follmer CH, Yeh JZ, Hartz RS, Ten Eick RE. Atrial Na^+ currents: human and cat compared. Circulation 1985; 72(suppl III):229.

83. Johnson EA, Lieberman M. Heart: excitation and contraction. Annu Rev Physiol 1971; 33:479–532.

84. Fozzard HA, Beeler GW Jr. The voltage clamp and cardiac electrophysiology. Circ Res 1975; 37:403–13.

85. Cohen IS, Strichartz GR. On the voltage dependent action of tetrodotoxin. Biophys J 1977; 17:275–9.

86. Hondeghem LM. Validity of V_{max} as a measure of the sodium current in cardiac and nervous tissues. Biophys J 147–52.

87. Strichartz GR, Cohen IS. $\dot{V}_{max}$ as a measure of G_{Na} in nerve and cardiac membranes. Biophys J 1978; 23:153–6.

88. Walton M, Fozzard HA. The relation of $\dot{V}_{max}$ to I_{Na}. G_{Na} and h in a model of the cardiac Purkinje fiber. Biophs J 1979; 25:407–420.

89. Fozzard HA, Hanck DA, Sheets MF. Nonlinear relationship of maximal upstroke velocity to sodium current in single canine cardiac Purkinje cells. J Physiol (Lond) 1987; 382.

90. Trautwein W, Schmidt RF. Zur membranwirkung des adrenalins an der herzmuskelfaser. Pflügers Arch 1960; 271:715–26.

91. Beeler GW Jr, Reuter H. Voltage clamp experiments on ventricular myocardial fibers. J Physiol (Lond) 1970; 207:165–90.

92. Dudel J, Rudel R. Voltage and time dependence of excitatory sodium current cooled sheep Purkinje fibers. Pflügers Arch 1970; 315:136–58.

93. Colatsky TJ, Tsien RW. Electrical properties associated with wide intercellular clefts in rabbit Purkinje fibers. J physiol (Lond) 1979; 290:227–52.

94. Brown AM, Lee KS, Powell T. Voltage clamp and internal perfusion of single rat heart muscle cells. J Physiol (Lond) 1981; 318:455–77.

95. Payet MD. Effect of lidocaine on fast and slow inactivation of sodium current in rat ventricular cells. J Pharmacol Exp Ther 1982; 223:235–40.

96. Bodewei R, Hering S, Lemke B, Rosenshtraukh LV, Undrovinas AI, Wollenberger A. Characterization of the fast sodium current in isolated rat myocardial cells: simulation of the clamped membrane potential. J Physiol (Lond) 1982; 325:301–15.

97. Benndorf K, Boldt W, Nilius B. Sodium current in single myocardial mouse cells. Pflügers Arch 1985; 404:190–6.

98. Sheets MF, Scanley BE, Hanck DA, Makielski JC, Fozzard HA. Open sodium channel properties of single canine cardiac Purkinje cells. Biophys J 1987; 52:13–22.

99. Sachs F, Specht P. Sodium current in single cardiac Purkinje cells. Biophys J. 1981; 33:123a.

100. Kunze DL, Lacerda AE, Wilson DL, Brown AM. Cardiac Na currents and the inactivating, reopening and waiting properties of single cardiac Na channels. J Gen Physiol 1985; 86:691–719.

101. Fozzard HA, Hanck DA, Makielski JC, Sheets MF. Shift in inactivation and activation parameters of Na$^+$ current in internally dialyzed canine cardiac Purkinje cells. J Physiol (Lond) 1986; 371.

102. Iijima T, Pappano AJ. Ontogenetic increase of the maximal rate of rise of the chick embryonic heart action potential: relationship to voltage, time and tetrodotoxin. Circ Res 1979; 44:358–67.

103. Kunze DL, Brown AM. Cardiac sodium channels. In: Piper HM, Isenberg G, eds. Isolated adult cardiomyocytes, Vol. II. Boca Raton, FL: CRC Press, 1989;15–28.

104. Fozzard HA, Friedlander I, January CT, Makielski JC, Sheets MF. Second-order kinetics of Na$^+$ channel inactivation in internally dialysed canine cardiac Purkinje cells. J Physiol (Lond) 1984; 353.

105. Weld FM, Bigger JT Jr. Effect of lidocaine on the early inward transient current in sheep cardiac Purkinje fibers. Circ Res 1975; 37:630–9.

106. Cohen CJ, Bean BP, Colatsky TJ, Tsien RW. Tetrodotoxin block of sodium channels in rabbit Purkinje fibers. J Gen Physiol 1981; 78:383–411.

107. Saikawa T, Carmeliet E. Slow recovery of the maximal rate of rise ($\dot{V}_{max}$) of the action potential in sheep cardiac Purkinje fibers. Pflügers Arch 1982; 390:90–3.

108. Ebihara L, Shigeto N, Lieberman M, Johnson EA. A note on the reactivation of the fast sodium current in spherical clusters of embryonic chick heart cells. Biophys J 1983; 42:191–4.

109. Gettes LS, Reuter H. Slow recovery from inactivation of inward currents in mammalian myocardial fibers. J Physiol (Lond) 1974; 240:703–24.

110. Clarkson CW, Matsubara T, Hondeghem LM. Slow inactivation of $\dot{V}_{max}$ in guinea pig ventricular myocardium Am J Physiol 1984; 247:H645–54.

111. Patlak JB, Ortiz M. Slow currents through single sodium channels of the adult rat heart. J Gen Physiol 1985; 86:89–104.

112. Grant AO, Starmer CF. Mechanism of closure of cardiac sodium channels in rabbit ventricular myocytes: single-channel analysis. Circ Res 1987; 60:897–913.

113. Grant AO, Starmer CF, Strauss HC. Unitary sodium channels in isolated cardiac myocytes of rabbit. Circ Res 1983; 53:823–9.

114. Ten Eick R, Yeh J, Matsuki N. Two types of voltage dependent Na channels suggested by differential sensitivity of single channels to tetrodotoxin. Biophys J 1984; 45:70a.

115. Fozzard HA, January CT, Makielski JC. New studies of the excitatory sodium currents in heart muscle. Circ Res 1985; 56:475–85.

116. Baer M, Best PM, Reuter H. Voltage-dependent action of tetrdodtoxin in mammalian cardiac muscle. Nature 1976; 263: 344–5.

117. Reuter H, Baer M, Best PM. Voltage dependence of tetrodotoxin action in mammalian cardiac muscle. In: Morad M, ed. Biophysical aspects of cardiac muscle. London: Academic Press, 1978:129–42.

118. Inoue D, Pappano AJ. Block of avian cardiac fast sodium channels by tetrodotoxin is enhanced by repetitive depolarization but not by steady depolarization. J Mol Cell Cardiol 1984; 16:943–52.

119. Carmeliet E. Voltage-dependent block by tetrodotoxin of the sodium channel in rabbit cardiac Purkinje fibers. Biophys J 1987; 51: 109–14.

120. Coraboeuf E, Deroubaix E, Coulombe A. Effect of tetrodotoxin on action potentials of the conducting system in the dog heart. Am J Physiol 1979; 236:H561–7.

121. Gintant GA, Daytner NB, Cohen IS. Slow inactivation of a tetrodotoxin-sensitive current in canine cardiac Purkinje fibers. Biophys J 1984; 45:509–12.

122. Reuter H. The dependence of slow inward current in Purkinje fibers on the extracellular calcium-concentration. J Physiol (Lond) 1967; 192:479–92.

123. Tarr M. Two inward currents in frog atrial muscle. J Gen Physiol 1971; 58:523–43.

124. Ochi R. The slow inward current and the action of manganese ions in guinea-pig's myocardium. Pflügers Arch 1970; 316:81–94.

125. Hartzell HC, Simmons MA. Comparison of effects of acetylcholine on calcium and potassium currents in frog atrium and ventricle. J Physiol (Lond) 1987; 389:411–22.

126. Bean BP. Two kinds of calcium channels in canine atrial cells. J Gen Physiol 1985; 86: 1–30.

127. Escande D, Coulombe A, Faivre JF, Coraboeuf E. Characteristics of the time-dependent slow inward current in adult human atrial single myocytes. J Mol Cell Cardiol 1986; 18:547–51.

128. Reuter H, Scholz H. A study of the ion slectivity and the kinetic properties of the calcium-dependent slow inward current in mammalian cardiac muscle. J Physiol (Lond) 1977; 264:17–47.

129. Isenberg G, Klöckner U. Calcium currents of isolated bovine ventricular myocytes are fast and of large amplitude. Pflügers Arch 1982; 395:30–41.

130. Mitchell MR, Powell T, Terrar DA, Twist VW. Characteristics of the second inward current in cells isolated from rat ventricular muscle. Proc R Soc Lond [Biol] 1983; 219:447–69.

131. Josephson IR, Sanchez-Chapula J, Brown AM. A comparison of calcium currents in rat and guinea pig single ventricular cells. Circ Res 1984; 54:144–56.

132. McDonald TF, Cavalie A, Trautwein W, Pelzer D. Voltage-dependent properties of macroscopic and elementary calcium channel currents in guinea pig ventricular myocytes. Pflügers Arch 1986; 406:437–48.

133. Pelzer D, Cavalie A, McDonald TF, Trautwein W. Calcium channels in single heart cells. In: Piper HM, Isenberg G, eds. Isolated adult cardiomyocytes, Vol. II. Boca Raton, FL: CRC Press, 1989:29–73.

134. Reuter H, Scholz H. The regulation of the calcium conductance of cardiac muscle by adrenaline. J Physiol (Lond) 1977; 264:49–62.

135. Lee KS, Tsien RW. High selectivity of calcium channels in single dialysed heart cells of the guinea-pig. J Physiol (Lond) 1984; 354:253–72.

136. Lee KS, Marban E, Tsien RW. Inactivation of calcium channels in mammalian heart cells: joint dependence on membrane potential and intracellular calcium. J Physiol (Lond) 1985; 364:395–411.

137. Reuter H, Stevens CF, Tsien RW, Yellen G. Properties of single calcium channels in cardiac cell culture. Nature 1982; 297:501–4.

138. Cavalie A, Pelzer D, Trautwein W. Fast and slow gating behaviour of single calcium channels in cardiac cells. Pflügers Arch 1986; 406:241–58.

139. Tsien RW, Giles W, Greengard P. Cyclic AMP mediates the effects of adrenaline on cardiac Purkinje fibers. Nature New Biol 1972; 240:181–3.

140. Trautwein W, Taniguchi J, Noma A. The effect of intracellular cyclic nucleotides and calcium on the action potential and acetylcholine response of isolated cardiac cells. Pflügers Arch 1982; 392:307–14.

141. Osterrieder W, Brum G, Hescheler J, Trautwein W, Flockerzi V, Hofmann F. Injection of subunits of cyclic AMP-dependent protein kinase into cardiac myocytes modulates Ca^{2+} current. Nature 1982; 298:576–8.

142. Kameyama M, Hofmann F, Trautwein W. On the mechanism of beta-adrenergic regulation of the Ca channel in the guinea-pig heart. Pflügers Arch 1985; 405:285–93.

143. Biegon RL, Pappano AJ. Dual mechanism for inhibition of calcium-dependent action potentials by acetylcholine in avian ventricular muscle. Circ Res 1980; 46:353–62.

144. Levy MN. Parasympathetic control of the heart. In: Randall WC, ed. Neural regulation of the heart. New York: Oxford University Press, 1977:95–129.

145. Giles W, Noble SJ. Changes in membrane currents in bullfrog atrium produced by acetylcholine. J Physiol (Lond) 1976; 261:103–23.

146. Ten Eick R, Nawrath H, McDonald TF, Trautwein W. On the mechanism of the negative inotropic effect of acetylcholine. Pflügers Arch 1976; 361:207–13.

147. Garnier D, Nargeot J, Ojeda C, Rougier O. Action of carbachol on atrial fibers: induced extra current and slow inward current inhibition. J Physiol (Lond) 1978; 276:27–8.

148. Josephson I, Sperelakis N. On the ionic mechanisms underlying adrenergic-cholinergic antagonism in ventricular muscle. J Gen Physiol 1982; 79:69–86.

149. Hescheler J, Kameyama M, Trautwein W. On the mechanism of muscarinic inhibition of the cardiac Ca current. Pflügers Arch 1986; 407:182–9.

150. Nilius B, Hess P, Lansman JB, Tsien RW. A novel type of cardiac calcium current in ventricular cells. Nature 1985; 316:443–63.

151. Mitra R, Morad M. Two types of calcium channels in guinea pig ventricular myocytes. Proc Natl Acad Sci USA 1986; 83:5340–4.

152. Bonvallet R. A low threshold calcium current recorded at physiological Ca concentrations in single frog atrial cells. Pflügers Arch 1987; 408:540–2.

153. Hagiwara N, Irisawa H, Kameyama M. Contribution of two types of calcium currents to the pacemaker potentials of rabbit sino-atrial node cells. J Physiol (Lond) 1988; 395:223–53.

154. Tytgat J, Nilius B, Vereecke J, Carmeliet E. The T-type Ca channel in guinea-pig ventricular myocytes is insensitive to isoproterenol. Pflügers Arch 1988; 411:704–6.

155. Hirano Y, Fozzard HA, January CT. Characteristics of L- and T-type Ca^{2+} currents in canine cardiac Purkinje cells. Am J Physiol 1989; 256:H1478–92.

156. Tseng GN, Boyden PA. Multiple types of Ca currents in single canine Purkinje cells. Circ Res 1989; 65:1735–50.

157. Bean BP. Classes of calcium channels in vertebrate cells. Annu Rev Physiol 1989; 51:367–84.

158. Deck KA, Trautwein W. Ionic currents in cardiac excitation. Pflügers Arch 1964; 280: 63–80.

159. Hecht HH, Hutter OF. Action of pH on cardiac Purkinje fibers. In: Taccardi B, Marchetti G, eds. Electrophysiology of the heart. Oxford: Pergamon Press, 1964:105–23.

160. Coraboeuf E, Vassort G. Effects of some inhibitors of ionic permeabilities on ventricular action potential and contraction of rat and guinea-pig hearts. J Electrocardiol 1968; 1:19–30.

161. Litovsky SH, Antzelevitch C. Transient outward current prominent in canine ventricular epicardium but not endocardium. Circ Res 1988; 62:116–26.

162. Dudel J, Peper K, Rudel R, Trautwein W. The dynamic chloride component of membrane current in Purkinje fibers. Pflügers Arch 1967; 295:197–212.

163. Fozzard HA, Hiroaka M. The positive dynamic current and its inactivation properties in cardiac Purkinje fibers. J Physiol (Lond) 1973; 234:569–86.

164. Peper K, Trautwein W. A membrane current related to the plateau of the action potential of Purkinje fibers. Pflügers Arch 1968; 303:108–23.

165. McAllister RE, Noble D, Tsien RW Reconstruction of the electrical activity of cardiac Purkinje fibers. J Physiol (Lond) 1975; 251: 1–59.

166. Kenyon JL, Gibbons WR. Influence of chloride, potassium and tetraethylammonium on the early outward current of sheep cardiac Purkinje fibers. J Gen Physiol 1979; 73:117–138.

167. Kenyon JL, Gibbons WR. 4-Aminopyridine and the early outward current of sheep cardiac Purkinje fibers. J Gen Physiol 1979; 73:139–57.

168. Giles WR, van Ginneken ACG. A transient outward current in isolated cells from the crista terminalis of rabbit heart. J Physiol (Lond) 1985; 368:243–64.

169. Kukushkin NI, Gainullin RZ, Sosunov EA. Transient outward current and rate dependence of action potential duration in rabbit cardiac ventricular muscle. Pflügers Arch 1983; 399:87–92.

170. Simurda J, Simurdova M, Cupera P. 4-Aminopyridine sensitive transient outward current in dog ventricular fibers. Pflügers Arch 1988; 411:442–9.

171. Tseng G-N, Hoffman BF. Two components of transient outward current in canine ventricular myocytes. Circ Res 1989; 64:633–47.

172. Benndorf K, Markwardt F, Nilius B. Two types of transient outward currents in cardiac ventricular cells of mice. Pflügers Arch 1987; 409:641–3.

173. Clark RB, Giles WR, Imaizumi Y. Properties of the transient outward current in rabbit atrial cells. J Physiol (Lond) 1988; 405: 147–68.

174. Maylie J, Morad M. A transient outward current related to calcium release and development of tension in elephant seal atrial fibres. J Physiol (Lond) 1984; 357:267–92.

175. Escande D, Coulombe A, Faivre J-F, Deroubaix E, Coraboeuf E. Two types of transient outward currents in adult human atrial cells. Am J Physiol 1987; 252:H142–8.

176. Siegelbaum SA, Tsien RW, Kass RS. Role of intracellular calcium in the transient outward current of calf Purkinje fibres. Nature 1977; 269:611–3.

177. Siegelbaum SA, Tsien RW. Calcium-activated transient outward current in cardiac Purkinje fibres. J Physiol (Lond) 1979; 287: 36P–37P.

178. Siegelbaum SA, Tsien RW. Calcium-activated transient outward current in calf cardiac Purkinje fibers. J Physiol (Lond) 1980; 299:485–506.

179. Coraboeuf E, Carmeliet E. Existence of two transient outward currents in sheep cardiac Purkinje fibers. Pflügers Arch 1982; 392: 352–9.

180. Josephson IR, Sanchez-Chapula J, Brown AM. Early outward current in rat single ventricular cells. Circ Res 1984; 54:157–62.

181. Escande D, Loisance D, Planche C, Coraboeuf E. Age-related changes of action po-

tential plateau shape in isolated human atrial fibers. Am J Physiol 1985; 249:H843–50.

182. Apkon M, Nerbonne JM. Alpha$_1$-adrenergic agonists selectively suppress voltage-dependent K$^+$ currents in rat ventricular myocytes. Proc Natl Acad Sci USA 1988; 85:8756–60.

183. Fedida D, Shimoni Y, Giles WR. A novel effect of noradrenaline on cardiac cells is mediated by alpha$_1$-adrenoceptors. Am J Physiol 1989; 256:H1500–4.

184. Imaizumi Y, Giles WR. Quinidine-induced inhibition of transient outward current in cardiac muscle. Am J Physiol 1987; 253: H704–8.

185. Giebisch G, Weidmann S. Membrane currents in mammalian ventricular heart muscle fibers using a voltage-clamp technique. J Gen Physiol 1971; 57:290–6.

186. McGuigan JAS. Some limitations of the double sucrose gap, and its use in a study of the slow outward current in mammalian ventricular muscle. J Physiol (Lond) 1974; 240:775–806.

187. Katzung BG, Morgenstern JA. Effects of extracellular potassium on ventricular automaticity and evidence for a pacemaker current in mammalian ventricular myocardium. Circ Res 1977; 40:105–11.

188. McDonald TF, Trautwein W. The potassium current underlying delayed rectification in cat ventricular muscle. J Physiol (Lond) 1978; 274:217–46.

189. Noma A, Yanagihara K, Irisawa H. Inward current of the rabbit sinoatrial node cell. Pflügers Arch 1977; 372:43–51.

190. DiFrancesco D, Noma A, Trautwein W. Kinetics and magnitude of the time-dependent potassium current in the rabbit sinoatrial node. Pflügers Arch 1979; 381:271–9.

191. DeHemptine A. Properties of the outward currents in frog atrial muscle. Pflügers Arch 1971; 329:321–31.

192. Ojeda C, Rougier O. Kinetic analysis of the delayed outward currents in frog atrium, existence of two types of preparation. J Physiol (Lond) 1974; 239:51–73.

193. Brown HF, Clark A, Noble SJ. Analysis of pacemaker and repolarization currents in frog atrial muscle. J Physiol (Lond) 1976; 258:547–77.

194. Brown HF, Giles W, Noble SJ. Membrane currents underlying activity in frog sinus venosus. J Physiol (Lond) 1977; 271:783–816.

195. Matsuura H, Ehara T, Imoto Y. An analysis of the delayed outward current in single ventricular cells of the guinea-pig. Pflügers Arch 1987; 410:596–603.

196. Walsh KB, Kass RS. Regulation of a heart potassium channel by protein kinase A and C. Science 1988; 242:67–9.

197. Walsh KB, Begenisich TB, Kass RS. Beta-adrenergic modulation of cardiac ion channels. J Gen Physiol 1989; 93:841–54.

198. Hume JR. Time-dependent outward current in isolated guinea-pig atrial and ventricular myocytes. Biophys J 1983; 41:311a.

199. Tohse N, Kameyama M, Irisawa H. Intracellular Ca^{2+} and protein kinase C modulate K$^+$ current in guinea pig heart cells. Am J Physiol 1987; 253:H1321–4.

200. Clay JR, Hill CE, Roitman D, Shrier A. Repolarization current in embryonic chick atrial heart cells. J Physiol (Lond) 1988; 403:525–37.

201. Giles W, Nakajima T, Ono K, Shibata EF. Modulation of the delayed rectifier K$^+$ current by isoprenaline in bull-frog atrial myocytes. J Physiol (Lond) 1989; 415:233–49.

202. Duchatelle-Gourdon I, Hartzell HC, Lagrutta AA. Modulation of the delayed rectifier potassium current in frog cardiomyocytes by beta-adrenergic agonists and magnesium. J Physiol (Lond) 1989; 415: 251–74.

203. Bennett PB, McKinney LC, Kass RS, Begenisich T. Delayed rectification in the calf cardiac Purkinje fiber. Biophys J 1985; 48:553–67.

204. Noble D, Tsien RW. Outward membrane currents activated in the plateau range of potentials in cardiac Purkinje fibres. J Physiol (Lond) 1969; 200:205–31.

205. Gintant GA, Daytner NB, Cohen IS. Gating of delayed rectification in acutely isolated canine cardiac Purkinje myocytes. Biophys J 1985; 48:1059–64.

206. Brown HF, Noble SJ. Effects of adrenaline on membrane currents underlying pacemaker activity in frog atrial muscle. J Physiol (Lond) 1974; 238:51P–53P.

207. Pappano AJ, Carmeliet EE. Epinephrine and the pacemaking mechanism at plateau potentials in sheep cardiac Purkinje fibers. Pflügers Arch 1979; 382:17–26.

208. Brown H, DeFrancesco D. Voltage-clamp investigations of membrane currents underlying pace-maker activity in rabbit sinoatrial node. J Physiol (Lond) 1980; 308:331–51.

209. Noma A, Kotake H, Irisawa H. Slow inward current and its role mediating the chronotropic effect of epinephrine in the rabbit sinoatrial node. Pflügers Arch 1980; 388:1–9.

210. Kass RS, Wiegers SE. The ionic basis of concentration-related effects of noradrenaline on the action potential of calf cardiac Purkinje fibres. J Physiol (Lond) 1982; 322:541–58.

211. Gadsby DC. The Na/K pump of cardiac cells. Annu Rev Biophys Bioeng 1984; 13: 373–98.

212. Eisner DA. The Na-K pump in cardiac muscle. In: Fozzard HA, Haber E, Jennings RB, Katz AM, Morgan HE, eds. The heart and cardiovascular system. Scientific foundations, Vol. 1. New York: Raven Press, 1986: 489–507.

213. Page E, Storm S. Cat heart muscle in vitro. VIII. Active transport of sodium in papillary muscle. J Gen Physiol 1965; 48:957–72.

214. Vassalle M. Electrogenic suppression of automaticity in sheep and dog Purkinje fibers. Circ Res 1970; 27:361–77.

215. Glitsch HG. Activation of the electrogenic sodium pump in guinea-pig auricles by internal sodium ions. J Physiol (Lond) 1972; 220: 565–82.

216. Noma A, Irisawa H. Electrogenic sodium pump in rabbit sinoatrial node cell. Pflügers Arch 1974; 351:177–82.

217. Glitsch HG, Grabowski W, Thielen J. Activation of the electrogenic sodium pump in guinea-pig atria by external potassium ions. J Physiol (Lond) 1978; 276:515–25.

218. Glitsch HG. Characteristics of active Na transport in intact cardiac cells. Am J Physiol 1979; 236:H189–99.

219. Eisner DA, Lederer WJ. The role of sodium pump in the effects of potassium depleted solutions on mammalian cardiac muscle. J Physiol (Lond) 1979; 294:279–301.

220. Gadsby DC, Cranefield PF. Direct measurement of changes in sodium pump current in canine cardiac Purkinje fibers. Proc Natl Acad Sci USA 1979; 76:1783–7.

221. Isenberg G, Trautwein W. The effect of dihydro-ouabain and lithium ions on the outward current in cardiac Purkinje fibers. Pflügers Arch 1974; 350:41–54.

222. Eisner DA, Lederer WJ. Characterization of the electrogenic sodium pump in cardiac Purkinje fibres. J Physiol (Lond) 1980; 303: 441–74.

223. Gadsby DC, Kimura J, Noma A. Voltage dependence of Na/K pump current in isolated heart cells. Nature 1985; 315:63–5.

224. Boyett MR, Fredida D. Changes in the electrical activity of dog cardiac Purkinje fibres at high heart rates. J Physiol (Lond) 1984; 350:361–91.

225. Akaou T, Ohta Y, Koketsu K. The effect of adrenaline on the electrogenic Na^+ pump in cardiac muscle cells. Experientia 1978; 34: 488–90.

226. Wilbrandt W, Koller H. Die calciumwirkung am froschherzen als funktion des ionengleichgewichts zwischen zellmembran und umbegung. Helv Physiol Pharmakol Acta 1948; 6:208–21.

227. Luttgau HA, Niedergerke R. The antagonism between Ca and Na ions on the frog's heart. J Physiol (Lond) 1958; 143:486–505.

228. Reiter M. Die beziehung von calcium und natrium zur inotropen glykosidwirkung. Arch Exp Pathol Pharmacol 1961; 245:487–9.

229. Scholz H. Uber die wirkung von calcium und natrium auf die katliumkontrakur isolierter meerschweinchenvorhofe. Pflügers Arch 1969; 308:315–32.

230. Glitsch HG, Reuter H, Scholz H. The effect of the internal sodium concentration on calcium fluxes in isolated guinea-pig auricles. J Physiol (Lond) 1970; 209:25–43.

231. Reuter H, Seitz H. The dependence of calcium efflux from cardiac muscle on temperature and external ion composition. J Physiol (Lond) 1968; 195:451–70.

232. Sheu SS, Blaustein MP. Sodium/calcium exchange and regulation of cell calcium and contractility in cardiac muscle, with a note about vascular smooth muscle. In: Fozzard HA, Haber E, Jennings RB, Katz AM, Morgan HE, eds. The heart and cardiovascular system. Scientific foundations, Vol. 1. New York: Raven Press, 1986:509–35.

233. Eisner DA, Lederer WJ. Na-Ca exchange. Stoichiometry and electrogenicity. Am J Physiol 1985; 236:C189–202.

234. Langer GA. Sodium-calcium exchange in the heart. Annu Rev Physiol 1982; 44:435–449.

235. Mullins LJ. The generation of electric currents in cardiac fibers by Na/Ca exchange. Am J Physiol 1979; 236:C103–10.

236. Kimura J, Miyamae S, Noma A. Identification of sodium-calcium exchange current in single ventricular cells of guinea-pig. J Physiol (Lond) 1987; 384:199–222.

237. Clusin WT, Fischmeister R, DeHaan RL. Caffeine-induced current in embryonic heart cells: time course and voltage dependence. Am J Physiol 1983; 245:H528–32.

238. Hume JR, Uehara A. Properties of "creep currents" in single frog atrial cells. J Gen Physiol 1986; 87:833–55.

239. Hume JR, Uehara A. "Creep currents" in single frog atrial cells may be generated by electrogenic Na/Ca exchange. J Gen Physiol 1986; 87:857–84.

240. Kimura J, Noma A, Irisawa H. Na-Ca exchange current in mammalian heart cells. Nature 1986; 319:596–7.

241. Mechmann S, Pott L. Identification of Na-Ca exchange current in single cardiac myocytes. Nature 1986; 319:597–9.

242. Fedida D, Noble D, Shimoni Y, Spindler AJ. Inward currents and contraction in guinea-pig ventricular myocytes. J Physiol (Lond) 1987; 385:565–89.

243. Lipp P, Pott L. Transient inward current in guinea-pig atrial myocytes reflects a change of sodium-calcium exchange current. J Physiol (Lond) 1988; 397:601–30.

244. Campbell DL, Giles WR, Robinson K, Shibata EF. Studies of the sodium-calcium exchanger in bull-frog atrial myocytes. J Physiol (Lond) 1988; 403:317–40.

245. Egan TM, Noble D, Noble SJ, Powell T, Spindler AJ, Twist VW. Sodium-calcium exchange during the action potential in guinea-pig ventricular cells. J Physiol (Lond) 1989; 411:639–61.

246. Noble D. Sodium-calcium exchange and its role in generating electric current. In: Nathan RD, ed. Cardiac muscle: the regulation of excitation and contraction. New York: Academic Press, 1986:171–200.

247. Vassalle M. Analysis of cardiac pacemaker potential using a "voltage clamp" technique. Am J Physiol 1966; 210:1335–41.

248. Cranefield PF, Hoffman BF, Siebens AA. Anodal excitation of cardiac muscle. Am J Physiol 1957; 190(2):383–90.

249 Yanagihara K, Irisawa H. Inward current activated during hyperpolarization in the rabbit sinoatrial node cell. Pflügers Arch 1980; 385: 11–9.

250. DiFrancesco D. A new interpretation of the pace-maker current in calf Purkinje fibres. J Physiol (Lond) 1981; 314:359–76.

251. DiFrancesco D. A study of the ionic nature of the pace-maker current in calf Purkinje fibres. J Physiol (Lond) 1981; 314:377–93.

252. DiFrancesco D, Ferroni A, Mazzanti M, Tromba C. Properties of the hyperpolarizing-activated current (if) in cells isolated from the rabbit sino-atrial node. J Physiol (Lond) 1986; 377:61–88.

253. DiFrancesco D, Tromba C. Inhibition of the hyperpolarization-activated current (i_f) induced by acetylcholine in rabbit sino-atrial node myocytes. J Physiol (Lond) 1988; 405: 477 91.

254. DiFrancesco D, Tromba C. Muscarinic control of the hyperpolarization-activated current(i_f) in rabbit sino-atrial node myocytes. J Physiol (Lond) 1988; 405:493–510.

255. Endoh M, Blinks JR. Effects of endogenous neurotransmitters on calcium transients in mammalian atrial muscle. In: Fleming WW, ed. Neuronal and extraneuronal events in autonomic pharmacology. New York: Raven Press, 1984:

256. Earm YE, Shimoni Y, Spindler AJ. A pacemaker-like current in the sheep atrium and its modulation by catecholamines. J Physiol (Lond) 1983; 342:569–90.

257. Lipsius S, Vereecke E, Carmeliet E. Pacemaker current (i_f) and the inward rectifier (i_{K1}) in single right atrial myocytes from cat heart. Biophys J 1986; 49:35la.

258. Rubenstein DS, Fox LM, McNulty JA, Lipsius SL. Electrophysiology and ultrastructure of eustachian ridge from cat right atrium: a comparison with SA node. J Mol Cell Cardiol 1987; 19:965–76.

259. Colquhoun D, Neher E, Reuter H, Stevens CF. Inward current channels activated by intracellular Ca in cultured cardiac cells. Nature 1981; 294:752–4.

260. Ehara T, Noma A, Ono K. Calcium-activated non-selective cation channel in ventricular cells isolated from adult guinea-pig hearts. J Physiol (Lond) 1988; 403:117–33.

261. Wit AL, Rosen MR. Afterdepolarizations and triggered activity. In: Fozzard HA, Haber E, Jennings RB, Katz AM, Morgan HE, eds. The heart and cardiovascular system. Scientific foundations, Vol. 2 New York: Raven Press, 1986:1449–90.

262. Lederer WJ, Tsien RW. Transient inward current underlying arrhythmogenic effects of cardiotonic steroids in Purkinje fibers. J Physiol (Lond) 1976; 263:73–100.

263. Kass RS, Lederer WJ, Tsien RW, Weingart R. Role of calcium ions in transient inward

currents and aftercontractions induced by strophanthidin in cardiac Purkinje fibres. J Physiol (Lond) 1978; 281:187–208.

264. Karagueuzian HS, Katzung BG. Voltage clamp studies of transient inward current and mechanical oscillations induced by ouabain in ferret papillary muscle. J Physiol (Lond) 1982; 327:255–71.

265. Arlock P, Katzung BG. Effects of sodium substitutes on transient inward current and tension in guinea-pig and ferret papillary muscle. J Physiol (Lond) 1985; 360:105–20.

266. Noma A. ATP-regulated K^+ channels in cardiac muscle. Nature 1983; 305:147–8.

267. Trube G, Hescheler J. Inward-rectifying channels in isolated patches of heart cell membrane: ATP-dependence and comparison with cell-attached patches. Pflügers Arch 1984; 401:178–184.

268. Kakei M, Noma A, Shibasaki T. Properties of adenosine-triphosphate-regulated potassium channels in guinea-pig ventricular cells. J Physiol (Lond) 1985; 363:441–62.

269. Findlay I. ATP-sensitive K^+ channels in rat ventricular myocytes are blocked and inactivated by internal divalent cations. Pflügers Arch 1987; 410:313–20.

270. Kakei M, Noma A. Adenosine-5'-triphosphate-sensitive single potassium channel in the atrioventricular node cell of the rabbit heart. J Physiol (Lond) 1984; 352:265–84.

271. Arena JP, Kass RS. Enhancement of potassium-sensitive current in heart cells by pinacidil. Circ Res 1989; 65:436–445.

272. Belles B, Hescheler J, Trube G. Changes of membrane currents in cardiac cells induced by long whole-cell recordings and tolbutamide. Pflügers Arch 1987; 409:582–8.

273. Sanguinetti MC, Scott AL, Zingaro GL, Siegl PKS. BRL 34915 (cromakalim) activates ATP-sensitive K^+ current in cardiac muscle. Proc Natl Acad Sci USA 1988; 85:8360–4.

274. Smallwood JK, Steinberg MI. Cardiac electrophysiological effects of pinacidil and related pyridylcyanoguanidines: relationship to antihypertensive activity. J Cardiovasc Pharmacol 1988; 12:102–9.

275. Naylor RE, Hoffman BF. Methods for the study of atrial electrophysiology. In: Little RC, ed. Physiology of atrial pacemakers and conductive tissues. Mount Kisco, NY: Futura, 1980:143–69.

276. Franz MR, Bargheer K, Raffenbeul W, Haverich A, Lichtlen PR. Monophasic action

potential mapping in human subjects with normal electrocardiograms: direct evidence for the genesis of the T wave. Circulation 1987; 75:379–86.

277. Gavrilescu S, Luca C. Right atrium monophasic action potentials during atrial flutter and fibrillation in man. Am Heart J 1975; 90:199–205.

278. Olsson SB, Cotoi S, Varnauskas E. Monophasic action potential and sinus stability after conversion of atrial fibrillation. Acta Med Scand 1971; 190:381–7.

279. Gavrilescu S, Cotoi S. Monophasic action potentials of right atrium during atrial flutter and after conversion to sinus rhythm. Br Heart J 1972; 34:396–401.

280. Wu KM, Ross SM, Hoffman BF. Monophasic action potentials during reentrant atrial arrhythmias in the dog: Effects of clofilium and acetylcholine. J Cardiovasc Pharm 1989;

281. Olsson SB, Brorson L, Varnauskas E. Class 3 antiarrhythmic action in man. Observations from the monophasic action potential recordings and amiodarone treatment. Br Heart J 1973; 35:1255–9.

282. Gavrilescu S, Dragulescu SI, Luca C, Streian C, Comsulea L, Popovici V. The effects of quinidine on the monophasic action potential of the right atrium in patients with atrial fibrillation. Agressologie 1976; 17:111–8.

283. Boineau JP, Schuessler RB, Mooney CR, et al. Multicentric origin of the atrial depolarization wave: the pacemaker complex. Relation to dynamics of atrial conduction, P-wave changes and heart rate control. Circulation 1978; 58:1036–48.

284. Waldo AL, Bush HL Jr, Gelband H, Zorn GL Jr, Vitikainen KJ, Hoffman BF. Effects on the canine P wave of discrete lesions in the specialized tracts. Circ Res 1971; 29:452–67.

285. Sherf L, James TN. Functional anatomy and ultrastructure of the internodal pathways. In: Little RC, ed. Physiology of atrial pacemakers and conductive tissues. Mount Kisco, NY: Futura, 1980:67–112.

286. Sano T, Takayama N, Shimamoto T. Diectional difference of conduction velocity in the cardiac ventricular synctium studied by microelectrodes. Circ Res 1959; 7:262–7.

287. Clerc L. Directional differences of impulse spread in trabecular muscle from mammalian heart. J Physiol (Paris) 1976; 255:335–46.

288. Woodbury JW, Crill, WE. On the problem of impulse conduction in the atrium. In: Florey E, ed. Nervous inhibition. New York: Pergamon, 1961:124–35.

289. Spach MS, Dolber PC. Relating extracellular potentials and their derivatives to anisotropic propagation at the microscopic level in human cardiac muscle. Circ Res 1986; 58:356–71.

290. Randall WC, Talano J, Kaye MP, Euler DE, Jones SB, Brynjolfsson G. Cardiac pacemakers in the absence of the SA node: responses to exercise and autonomic blockade. Am J Physiol 1978; 234:H465–70.

291. Jones SB, Euler DE, Randall WC, Brynjolfsson G, Hardie EL. Atrial ectopic foci in the canine heart: hierarchy of pacemaker automaticity. Am J Physiol 1980; 238:H788–93.

292. Rozanski GJ, Lipsius SL. Electrophysiology of functional subsidiary pacemakers in canine right atrium. Am J Physiol 1985; 249:H594–603.

293. Rubenstein DS, Lipsius SL Mechanisms of automaticity in subsidiary pacemakers from cat right atrium. Circ Res 1989; 64:648–57.

294. Rozanski GJ, Jalife J. Automaticity in atrioventricular valve leaflets of rabbit heart. Am J Physiol 1986; 250:H397–406.

295. Boyden PA, Tilley LP, Albala A, Liu SK, Fenoglio JJ Jr, Wit AL Mechanisms for atrial arrhythmias associated with cardiomyopathy: a study of feline hearts with primary myocardial disease. Circ 1984; 69:1036–47.

296. Ten Eick RE, Singer DH. Electrophysiological properties of diseased human atrium. I. Low diastolic potential and altered response to potassium. Circ Res 1979; 44:545–57.

297. Cranefield PF, Aronson RS. Cardiac arrhythmias: the role of triggereed activity. Mount Kisco, NY: Futura, 1988:

298. Wit AL, Cranefield PF. Triggered activity in cardiac muscle fibers of the simian mitral valve. Circ Res 1976; 38:85–98.

299. Wit AL, Fenoglio JJ Jr, Hordof AJ, Reemtsma K. Ultrastructure and transmembrane potentials of cardiac muscle in the human anterior mitral valve leaflet. Circulation 1979; 59:1284–92.

300. Wit AL, Fenoglio JJ Jr, Wagner BM, Bassett AL. Electrophysiological properties of cardiac muscle in the anterior mitral valve leaflet and the adjacent atrium in the dog. Possible implications for the genesis of atrial arrhythmias. Circ Res 1973; 32:731–45.

301. Wit AL, Cranefield PF. Triggered activity in cardiac muscle fibers of the canine coronary artery sinus. Circ Res 1977; 41:435–45.

302. Saito T, Otoguro M, Matsubara T. Electrophysiological studies on the mechanism of electrically induced sustained rhythmic activity in the rabbit atrium. Circ Res 1978; 42:199–206.

303. Matsubara T. Electrophysiological studies on triggered activity in the rabbit right atrum. J Tokyo Med Coll 1981; 39:673–84.

304. Nilius B, Boldt W, Scheufler K. Analysis of hyperpolarizing afterpotentials in the atrial myocardium. Biomed Biochim Acta 1984; 43:101–10.

305. Nilius B, Boldt W, Scheufler K, Herrmann V. Pacing dependent properties of the transmembrane potential in plateau fibers of the mammalian atrial myocardium. Biomed Biochim Acta 1983; 42:203–13.

7

Electrophysiology of the Atrioventricular Node
Conduction, Refractoriness, and Ionic Currents

Jacques Billette

Faculty of Medicine, University of Montreal
Montreal, Quebec, Canada

Wayne R. Giles

University of Calgary Health Science Centre
Calgary, Alberta, Canada

INTRODUCTION

A large fraction of the delay (PR interval) between atrial and ventricular activation occurs at the atrioventricular (AV) node. This favors ventricular filling as a result of the atrial contraction and thereby augments the pumping function of the heart. Even more essential to the pumping function is the relatively long refractory period of the AV node. This period, besides imposing a critical minimum time that assures an effective ventricular filling, protects the ventricles against early atrial activation that could otherwise trigger life-threatening ventricular tachyarrhythmias.

Both the conduction delay and the refractory period can vary markedly from beat to beat in a wide variety of patterns. These have been the subject of numerous anatomic and functional studies (1–5). Many of these variations arise from intrinsic functional properties (2,6–8) in the AV node, but they can also be modulated by extrinsic mechanisms (5,9,10). The goal of this chapter is to briefly summarize the present state of knowledge concerning the characterization procedures for nodal function, the intrinsic regulation of conduction time and refractory period in the AV node, the corresponding electrical activation of nodal cells, and the ionic currents that underlie the resting and action potentials.

CHARACTERIZATION OF NODAL FUNCTION

The AV node can be viewed as a black box (Fig. 1A), with an input and an output representing the atrium (A) and the His bundle (H), respectively. The AH interval then specifically represents the nodal conduction time. By varying the pattern of the electrical events occurring at the entrance to the AV node with properly designed stimulation sequences, the AH interval can be varied in characteristic patterns that can be used to define the functional properties of the AV node. A technique called periodic premature stimulation of the atrium is frequently used for this purpose. This stimulation paradigm consists of periodically introducing a premature beat after a fixed number of basic beats. It thus tests conduction for a given phase of the nodal recovery cycle. By varying the interval with which the premature beat is coupled to the last beat

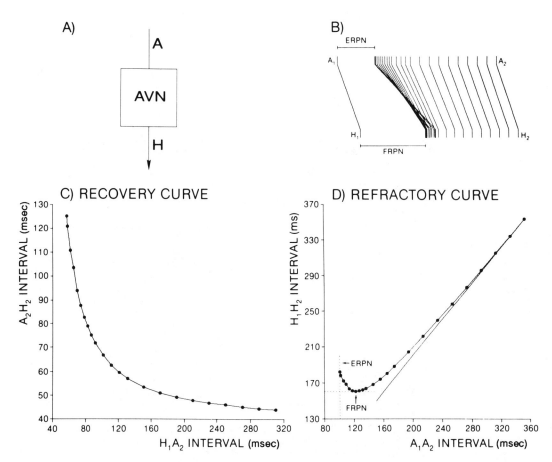

Figure 1 Methods used for the functional characterization of conduction and refractoriness in the atrioventricular node.(A) The node as a black box with an input (A, atrium) and an output (H, His bundle). (B) A superimposition, in reference to the corresponding constant basic conduction time (A_1H_1 interval), of different premature nodal conduction times (A_2H_2 intervals) obtained during a periodic premature stimulation of the atrium in an isolated rabbit heart preparation. (C) The recovery curve obtained by plotting the A_2H_2 intervals against the corresponding H_1A_2 intervals. (D) The refractory curve (H_1H_2 intervals versus A_1A_2 intervals) with the effective (ERPN) and the functional (FRPN) refractory periods.

of the basic rate, a range of premature conduction times (A_2H_2 intervals) can be obtained (Fig. 1B). As the nodal recovery time, or H_1A_2 interval (i.e., the time elapsed between last basic His bundle activation and the premature atrial activation), is shortened, the A_2H_2 interval increases progressively until conduction block within the AV node occurs. These results are used to construct a typical recovery curve (Fig. 1C), which has a characteristic form that can be fitted with either an exponential (7,11) or an hyperbolic function (12). This relationship shows that nodal conduction time increases more and more rapidly as the nodal recovery time is shortened.

Using the same data, the output (H_1H_2) intervals can be plotted against the corresponding input (A_1A_2) intervals to form a refractory curve (Fig. 1D) from which nodal refractoriness can be obtained (13). This curve can yield two parameters that are frequently determined in clinical and experimental studies on the specialized conduction system: (1) the effective refractory period (ERPN) and (2) the functional refractory period (FRPN) of the AV node. ERPN is defined as the longest A_1A_2 interval that does not result in a propagated response to the His bundle (14). When an atrial block develops before nodal block during this type of stimulation, ERPN can be approximated by the shortest atrial test interval that results in a conducted beat through the node (15). FRPN is given by the minimum H_1H_2 interval that reflects the shortest interval with which two consecutive activations can be recorded at the nodal output. This definition can be extended to the minimum interval reached between two consecutive propagated events at the nodal output during other atrial activation modes, such as those associated to incremental pacing, step pacing, or atrial fibrillation (16,17).

INTRINSIC REGULATION OF NODAL FUNCTIONAL PROPERTIES

Conduction Time

For a given homeostatic condition there is a minimal value for the nodal conduction time. This is called the basal conduction time (3,7) and can be determined from the data points on the right-hand or flat portion of the recovery curve (Fig. 1C). However, this measurement is often not possible because of the occurrence of spontaneous sinus or atrial beats that prevent the application of premature beats following long recovery times. Nodal conduction times can differ from the basal depending upon the ongoing sequence of stimulation. The most important factor governing this deviation from the basal value is the nodal recovery time. As shown by the recovery curve (Fig. 1C), the increase in nodal conduction time is more and more rapid as the nodal recovery time is shortened. Since this occurs even in presence of a slow and constant basic stimulus rate, this increase in the AV nodal conduction time depends only on the recovery time preceding the premature beat.

When the basic rate is suddenly increased, the conduction times obtained during a periodic premature stimulation are prolonged after long recovery times and are shortened after short recovery times compared to those obtained at a control slow basic rate. As demonstrated with analytic procedures (18), these changes correspond to the net effect of opposing facilitatory (facilitation) and inhibitory (fatigue) phenomena that the imposed fast rate

induces on the conduction. The combined use of computer-assisted stimulation and of specifically designed stimulation sequences has permitted selective and independent characterization of these properties (18,19). From these studies facilitation (Fig. 2) has been defined as a shorter nodal conduction time than expected from the recovery time and the prevailing level of fatigue. Facilitation, which affects only the conduction time of premature beats introduced with short recovery times, can be induced by a single short recovery time occurring at the penultimate cycle. Facilitation persists unchanged during a fast rate as long as the penultimate cycle remains short. Facilitation dissipates immediately and completely when a single long cycle equivalent to that of the sinus rhythm occurs.

The fatigue produced by a 5 min fast stimulus train induces a systematic upward shift of the recovery curve (Fig. 2), indicating that fatigue increases the nodal conduction time of all beats regardless of prematurity (19). In contrast to facilitation, fatigue develops and dissipates slowly so that it only starts to affect conduction time several beats after the beginning of a fast rate and it keeps changing for several minutes until a steady state is reached. Fatigue is more marked at faster rates. Fatigue may thus be defined as a time- and rate-dependent prolongation in nodal conduction time occurring for comparable recovery time and facilitation level. It develops and dissipates with relatively slow, almost symmetrical time courses.

The combined effects of facilitation and fatigue can also be studied with an independent protocol (Fig. 2). The resulting recovery curve is tilted increasingly to the left of the "fatigue" curve in the short recovery time range. This shows that, in conditions of interacting facilitation and fatigue, the net result on AV node conduction is determined by the sum of the effects produced by these two factors.

When applying these intrinsic functional properties to explain other rate-induced nodal responses, such as those obtained during incremental pacing, linear increases and decreases in rate, and step stimulations, one must be particularly careful about controlling

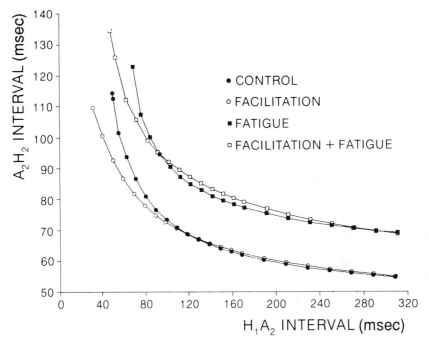

Figure 2 Changes in A_2H_2 intervals with changing H_1A_2 intervals observed during a control, a facilitation, a fatigue, and a combined facilitation and fatigue protocol in a superfused isolated rabbit heart preparation.

and/or measuring the factors that affect the dynamics of these properties. For instance, whether a new steady state was reached before measuring the effects of a given rate markedly affects the observed changes in conduction time. Since fatigue increases with time, the number of basic beats used and the rate of decrease of the coupling interval can markedly affect the fatigue influence by changing the time at which any premature beat is applied after the beginning of a fast rate. Similarly, the degree of facilitation, which changes from beat to beat when the penultimate recovery time is changing, markedly affects the characteristics of the response under conditions of changing cycle length. Another important factor that can modulate rate-induced nodal responses is the conduction time of the basic beat. This conduction time can markedly affect the recovery time preceding a premature beat and thereby change its conduction time by a process governed by the recovery curve, independently of the prevailing level of facilitation and fatigue (20). Very different and complex nodal responses can arise from these interactions.

Refractoriness

FRPN constitutes the best index reflecting the capacity of the AV node to impose a minimum ventricular cycle length. The physiologic importance of this parameter is well recognized, although its relationship to AV nodal refractoriness has been questioned because of discrepancies between changes in recovery and refractory properties (7,12). According to a recent study (16), these discrepancies can be explained by the fact that FRPN may be altered in different ways and directions by a given fast rate (Fig. 3). During the selective effects of facilitation, FRPN is systematically shortened. In contrast, under the selective effects of fatigue, FRPN is systematically prolonged. Under the combined effects of facilitation and fatigue, FRPN can be either slightly shortened or prolonged depending on the magnitude of the individual effects. These effects are cycle length dependent, reaching a maximum at the shortest cycle length tested (Fig. 3). Moreover, in conditions involving dynamic interactions between facilitation and

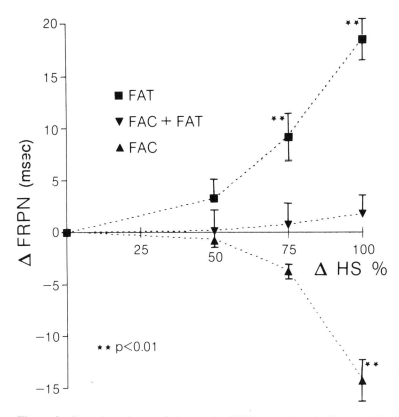

Figure 3 Rate dependence of changes in FRPN caused by facilitation (FAC), fatigue (FAT), and combined facilitation and fatigue (FAC + FAT) as studied for a 50, 75 and 100% shortening of the His stimulus interval (HS%) in six isolated rabbit heart preparations. The baseline corresponds to control. Note that both the fatigue and facilitation effects on FRPN are small for HS interval shortening below 50% and increase rapidly thereafter, but in opposite directions, to reach their maxima at the 100% shortening. Note also that, when facilitation and fatigue interact (middle curve) there are only small (not statistically significant) changes in FRPN. [Reproduced with permission from the American Heart Association (16).]

fatigue (16), the net change in FRPN can vary from a shortening to a prolongation, depending on the duration of the fast rate, which determines the level of the fatigue. These changes in FRPN are in all circumstances parallel with those seen on the recovery curve, so that rate-induced changes in nodal conduction and refractoriness are concordant.

Rate-induced variations in ERPN and FRPN usually diverge. This divergence has been interpreted as evidence that the FRPN cannot accurately reflect nodal refractoriness (7,12). However, recent evidence (21) suggests that changes in ERPN are affected by changes in recovery time due to alterations in conduction time of basic beats that cause a phase shift of the recovery cycle rather than a real

change in excitability. When rate-induced changes in ERPN are corrected for this recovery-dependent bias, changes in ERPN and FRPN also concord (16,21).

INTRANODAL ORIGIN OF NODAL FUNCTIONAL PROPERTIES

The intranodal origin of conduction and refractoriness properties of the AV node remain only partly understood, despite numerous microelectrode studies. Although the reasons for this difficulty are numerous and complex, an important one is that most studies, done mainly in isolated rabbit heart preparations (2–4,22), involved only short-lasting impalements; it was therefore difficult to correlate

BASIC PREMATURE

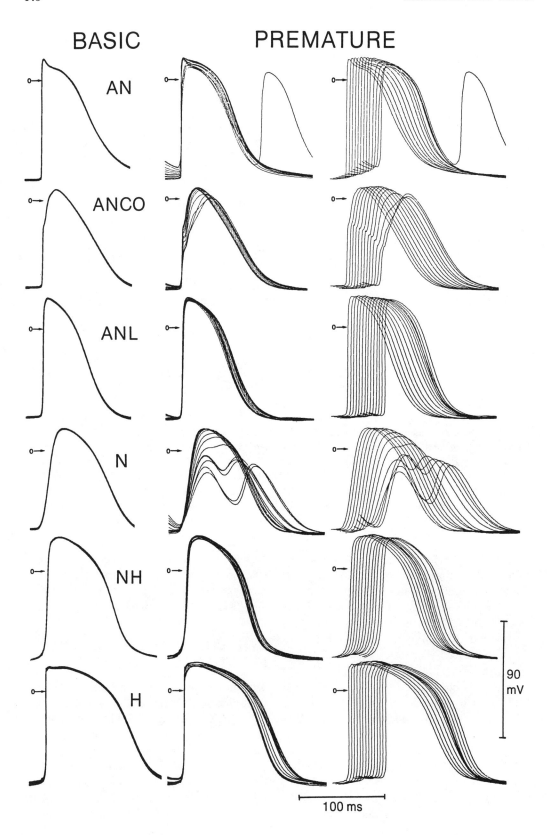

AN

ANCO

ANL

N

NH

H

90 mV

100 ms

directly the nodal functional properties with corresponding cellular activation. Recently, significant improvements were reported; stable cell impalements of sufficient duration to characterize the cell response directly during an entire periodic premature stimulation were obtained (23). This has made possible the identification of several properties of nodal recovery which are summarized here. However, the intranodal origin of facilitation and fatigue remain unknown.

Classification of Nodal Cells

The cells in the rabbit AV node can be subdivided into six groups, AN, ANCO, ANL, N, NH, and H cells, according to their responses to periodic premature stimulation (Fig. 4). AN cells have a definite phase 1 followed by a plateau and are activated at a constant time after atrial activation. ANCO cells have activation times similar to those of AN cells but have lower amplitudes and a notch on their upstrokes. ANL designates late AN cells; these have characteristics intermediate between those of AN and N cells. Comparison of N and ANL cells shows that N cells have a slower rate of rise, a more positive resting potential, a smaller amplitude, and a greater prematurity-dependent increase in duration. The N cells are also characterized by a marked reduction in amplitude and by frequent dissociations into two components with increasing prematurity. N and NH cells are distinguished mainly on the basis of the close relationship of their activation time with that of atrium and His bundle, respectively. The action potential duration characteristically increases with prematurity in N, but not in NH cells. The H cells have a characteristically long action potential and are considered AV

nodal cells despite their similarities with Purkinje fibers because they contribute significantly to the nodal properties.

Activation Time of Nodal Cells During Basic and Premature Beats

The recovery-dependent increase in conduction delay represented by the recovery curve is a complex phenomenon (Fig. 5) (23). The proximal nodal cells, including the N cells, account for 21% of the mean nodal delay (53 msec) at slow stimulation rates. The proximal node contributes similarly to all nodal delays regardless of the coupling interval, except at very short coupling intervals when its contribution increases slightly. The distal node (NH and H cells) contributes a fraction of the overall nodal delay, which is similar to that of the proximal node. However, its contribution shows a biphasic dependence on prematurity. Thus as the recovery time decreases, the distal conduction time first increases until it reaches a maximum at a recovery time near that at which FRPN occurs and then decreases to return to the same value at the shortest recovery time than it had at the longest one. The central node (N-NH cell zone) accounts for about 50% of the basal delay and for the greatest fraction of the recovery-dependent increase in this delay. Thus the nodal recovery curve represents the sum of three different patterns of changes in conduction time that occur at three different levels in the node in response to changes in recovery time.

Mechanism of N-NH Delay

No action potential upstrokes can be recorded during the mean 18 msec delay between latest N cells and earliest NH cells (23). Insight into

Figure 4 Transmembrane action potential characteristics from six typical nodal cells recorded in isolated rabbit heart preparations during basic and premature beats. For each cell the superimposed basic action potentials (left) are compared with corresponding superimposed premature action potentials (center). To illustrate their individual characteristics, the same premature potentials are also presented with a constant rightward shift of subsequent potentials (right). Note for all cells the similarity of action potentials obtained during basic beats, the marked changes in action potential characteristics induced by premature beats, and the variation in these changes with cell type. The action potential after premature potential in AN cell was caused by an atrial reentrant beat. [Reproduced with permission from the American Physiological Society (23).]

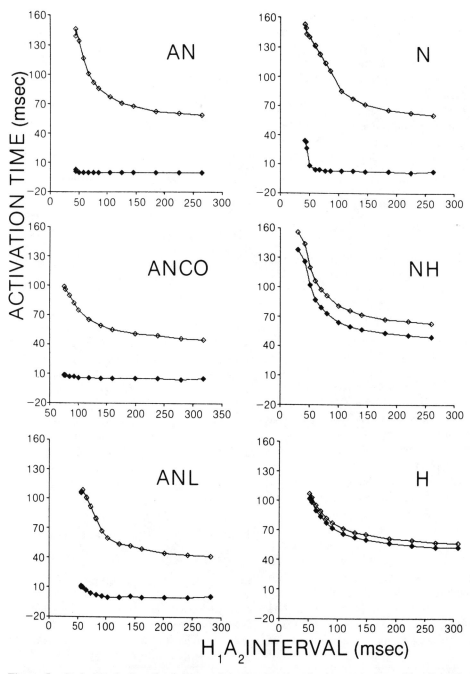

Figure 5 Cycle length-dependent changes in activation time in the same six nodal cells as in Figure 4. Cell activation times (closed symbols representing interval from low interatrial septum complex to the upstroke of the action potential) and total nodal activation times (A_2H_2 intervals, open symbols) were both plotted against corresponding preceding H_1A_2 interval (20). The shape of the resulting two curves differs markedly for AN, ANCO, ANL, and N cells, but not for NH and H cells. The largest fraction of the cycle-length-dependent increase in A_2H_2 intervals develops between N and NH cells. [Reproduced with permission from the American Physiological Society (23).]

how the electrical activation crosses this zone was obtained from transmembrane action potential recordings taken during progressively longer nodal delays induced with an accelerating train of impulses that caused a progressive dissociation of the electrical activity in these cells into two components (24). The first component started simultaneously in all cells but showed a progressive decrease in amplitude from N cells to NH cells. In NH cells, the first component was reduced to a prepotential, the beginning of which nevertheless remained closely linked to the beginning of the upstroke in the N cells. These phenomena can best be explained by an electrotonic decay of the voltage resulting from the current provided by the proximal node. In other words, the conduction through the N-NH cell zone could be largely electrotonic and thus similar to that frequently seen in the depressed zone of other myocardial tissues (25–29). The explanation is supported by the finding that, once active propagation resumes in the distal node, it produces a second electrotonic wave that is reflected back, as seen by a second component in the action potential that decays in amplitude in going from distal to proximal nodal cells. Furthermore, this second component is eliminated, while the first component is largely unchanged, when a premature beat is blocked between the N and NH cells. According to this hypothesis (1) the decrement in amplitude of the first component of the action potential represents a decaying voltage in a resistive, cable like structure; (2) the delay arises from the time taken to bring the NH cells to threshold; and (3) the earlier the NH cells are in their slow and progressive recovery of excitability, the longer this time is.

Nodal Recovery Time

The cycle length dependence of the delay in the AV node depends directly on the recovery time that the node experiences before it receives a new impulse from the atrium. However, the node consists of many cells that are activated in sequence. Hence there is no common recovery time for all nodal cells; proximal cells are activated earlier and recover earlier than distal cells. Moreover, this dispersion in recovery of excitability may be enhanced by the differences in action potential duration and/or in the time course of recovery of the different nodal cells. Therefore determination of a global or of a representative nodal recovery time is difficult and has been the center of significant controversy. When the preceding atrial interval is used to assess nodal recovery time (6,7), the latter is overestimated in the distal node in conditions in which the conduction time of the preceding beat increases. For a given atrial interval the recovery time of the distal node is shortened proportionally to the increase in the conduction time of the preceding beat. When the preceding RP or His-atrial interval is used to assess recovery time in similar circumstances (20,30), the recovery time of the proximal node is underestimated (recovery time of proximal nodal cells is longer than estimated by the RP or His-atrial interval). Nevertheless, the His-atrial interval (11,20,31,32) has been found to be a more reliable predictor of ensuing nodal conduction time than the atrial interval. The reasons for this could be that activation of the proximal node is largely cycle length independent so that the recovery time has little effect on the conduction time in this part of the node. As a result the timing of the A_2 beat reflects quite accurately the time at which the proximal node starts to provide the distal node with depolarizing current via electrotonic conduction through the N-NH zone. The most important determinant of the increment in delay is not the absolute atrial cycle length: it is the timing of the atrial input with respect to the phase of recovery in the distal node. Since the His-atrial interval is more closely linked to the recovery of the distal node than to the atrial interval, it can provide an index of nodal recovery time that is more reliable when conduction time is changing. A recent study (33) has shown that differences in rate-induced nodal responses according to the measure of recovery time used are indeed entirely due to the changes in the conduction time of basic beats. The otherwise identical results similarly reflect underlying changes in nodal function for both measures of recovery time.

Nodal Refractoriness

By comparing the minimum interval between the basic and the premature upstrokes to the duration of the ERPN and FRPN, it has been shown (23) that ERPN reflects refractoriness of the cells located at the entrance of the node while FRPN reflects refractoriness of cells located in the distal node. Moreover, no statistically significant correlation was found between corresponding ERPN and FRPN values, indicating that these variables are independent and presumably are controlled by different mechanisms. The FRPN is observed when the distal nodal cells reach a limit in their response to proximal input. That is, despite continued shortening of the coupling interval, the interval between the basic and the premature upstrokes cannot be shortened further. Conduction of the action potential may be maintained for short coupling intervals when these intervals result in sufficient delays in the proximal node; these intervals are then "converted" into longer input intervals for the distal node. FRPN corresponds to refractoriness in NH cells plus a time increment corresponding to the delay between NH and H cells. Assuming a constant level of excitability during a given steady-state condition and assuming that the electrical coupling between the proximal and the distal node is also constant, the main other factor that may affect the minimum interval between two consecutive responses is the reduction of the input current provided. The reduction in rate of rise of the upstroke and the amplitude of the action potential with increasing prematurity (see next section) may provide a substratum for such a reduced input current. However, given the numerous unknowns concerning propagation of currents in the node, it is difficult to determine with accuracy the magnitude of the reduction of the depolarizing current or to assess its impact on the response of the distal node.

CYCLE LENGTH-DEPENDENT CHANGES IN TRANSMEMBRANE ACTION POTENTIAL CHARACTERISTICS

A complete explanation of the intrinsic functional properties of the AV node requires an understanding of the various ionic currents involved and of the anatomic and geometric factors affecting the propagation within the node. A first step toward understanding these electrical events has been the definition of the changes in transmembrane action potentials observed following various degrees of prematurity (Fig. 4) (23). Although these action potentials do not provide detailed information concerning the underlying ionic currents, they are representative of the net ionic currents and intercellular interactions present. For this reason high-quality action potential data recordings are important prerequisites to the study of ionic currents. As described earlier, the morphology of the control action potentials obtained during basic beats varies markedly in different nodal cells. The responses of the cells to increasing prematurity also differ in different cells.

The most significant prematurity-induced change that may be involved in the slowing of the speed of the conduction is the reduction of the rate of rise of the upstroke that occurs in all nodal cells. (Fig. 4). This reduction is most marked in AN and H cells but more easily perceived in N cells. The reduction observed in ANL, N, and NH cells is largely independent of the takeoff potential, which does not vary significantly in these circumstances, suggesting that the reduction is due to incomplete recovery of excitability, which differs from recovery of resting potential in nodal cells (6). This reduced rate of rise affects both the ability of a cell group to activate adjacent cells and the impedance that these adjacent cells present to the propagation of the currents. Another important factor affecting the energy available is the action potential amplitude, which is systematically reduced with increasing prematurity. The action potential amplitude decreases most in ANCO and N cells and is easily appreciated from the disappearance of the overshoot (Fig. 4).

Action potential duration is also markedly affected by prematurity. In AN, ANCO, ANL, and N cells changes in action potential duration are biphasic: with increasing prematurity, duration first increases slowly and then decreases more rapidly to a value close to control. The increase is particularly marked in N cells; these action potentials dissociate progressively into two components with increasing prematurity. This dissociation is of particular significance for the interpretation of conduction, since the second component occurs at a time and a level of potential at which the membrane cannot be reactivated. Therefore, the second component appears not to represent a reactivation of the ionic current(s) responsible for the upstroke. However, as this second component diminishes markedly, but not completely, during a block (24), the participation of some active ionic current remains possible. In contrast with the pattern of action potential changes in the proximal node, the action potential in NH and H cells decreases monotonically with increasing prematurity. This reduction is most marked in H cells. However, it is uncertain to what extent these changes in action potential duration are accompanied by parallel changes in excitability, since action potential duration and excitability are clearly dissociated in nodal cells (6).

IONIC CURRENTS IN THE AV NODE

At present relatively little is known about any of the ionic currents that underlie the electrophysiologic activity of the mammalian AV node (34–36). Although voltage clamp techniques were applied to this tissue almost 10 years ago by Irisawa and his colleagues (34,37–40), the intrinsic heterogeneity of the tissue and the technical difficulty of recording either from small synthetic strips or from viable isolated cells has limited both the amount and the quality of data that are available. A number of quite recent reviews have dealt with general topics concerning the ionic current changes that underlie cardiac pacemaker activity and have summarized available informa-

tion concerning both sinoatrial and atrioventricular nodes (34–38). The purpose of this section is to summarize previous findings that may be important determinants of frequency-dependent action potential formation and/or conduction within the AV node. Virtually all this information was obtained with conventional electrophysiologic recordings or suction microelectrode voltage clamp measurements on AV nodal tissue of the rabbit or dog heart (34,38).

The Resting Potential: Time-Independent Background Ionic Currents

Microelectrode recordings confirm the AV node functions as an electrical syncytium (41–43) and that most cells from within the AV node are not quiescent; rather, viable cells pace spontaneously even if input from the SA node is interrupted (34). As a result, the concept of a resting potential is usually not appropriate. Quiescent AV node cells may have a resting potential near -50 mV. No quantitative information is available regarding which types of ionic currents generate this resting potential (or maximum diastolic potential), but it is likely that these currents resemble those in adjacent tissue, for example from the crista terminalis, atrium or SA node of the rabbit. If this is the case, the resting potential is mainly due to an ionic current that is quite selective for K^+ ions and exhibits inward rectification. However, the density of the K^+ channels underlying the whole-cell or macroscopic current appears to be much less than that in ventricle (35,44). It is even possible that some of the cells in the AV node have no inwardly rectifying background K^+ conductance, as appears to be the case in cardiac pacemaker tissue (45,46). Two consequences of having a very small background K^+ current in AV node cells are (1) the cells have a relatively high input resistance, and (2) the resting membrane potential is rather unstable. Thus, even very small applied currents can elicit relatively high voltage perturbations.

Since the quiescent AV node can exhibit a resting potential that has relatively high K^+ selectivity, and yet this membrane potential is

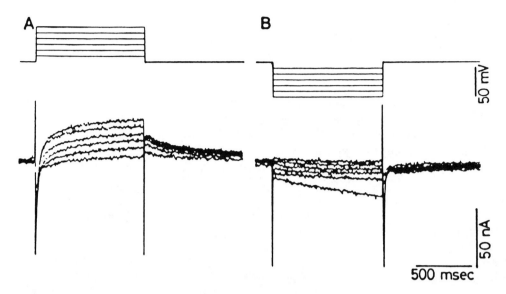

Figure 6 Ionic currents recorded from a cluster of AV node cells from rabbit heart. The preparation was approximately 50 μm wide and 100 μm long. The holding potential was -40 mV, and the voltage clamp depolarizations (-30 to 30 mV) and hyperpolarization (-90 to -50 mV) were applied in 10 mV steps. The straight lines on the current traces represent the zero level. (A) The voltage clamp depolarizations (top) elicit a transient inward current I_{Ca} followed by the time- and voltage-dependent activation of the delayed rectifier I_K. (B) The voltage clamp hyperpolarizations (top) elicit a small, slow inward current I_f. [Reproduced from Taniguchi et al. (40), with permission.]

significantly depolarized from E_K, (the electrochemical equilibrium potential for potassium), suggests that a parallel inward current mechanism is also present. Although virtually no information is available concerning the exact type of ionic permeability mechanism responsible for this, it is speculated that an inward background Na^+ current is present, as is the case in a number of other cardiac tissues.

Na^+/K^+ Pump Current

Almost 10 years ago Irisawa and his colleagues (47,48) obtained indirect evidence for the presence of an electrogenic Na^+/K^+ pump in strips of tissue from the rabbit AV node. Since that time the voltage and cation dependence of this pump mechanism has been well studied. At present, although many functionally important properties of the cardiac Na^+/K^+ pump are known (49,50), the specific ways in which it can directly or indirectly influence electrical activity within the AV node remain uncertain. Since much of the electrical activity in the AV node is characterized by depolarizing or repolarizing phases of action po-

tentials with very low dV/dt, it is possible that even rather small currents (as expected from a Na^+/K^+ pump mechanism) can significantly influence action potential duration and/or resting potential. Recently, some evidence in favor of this has been obtained from experiments in which cardiac glycosides were used to block the Na^+/K^+ pump in small strips of AV nodal tissue from rabbit heart (51), and significant changes in the height and duration of the action potentials were observed.

Sodium Current, I_{Na}

No recordings of a time- and voltage-dependent transient inward sodium current have been reported, either from small synthetic strips or from single cells obtained from AV nodal tissue. However, it has been known for some time that partial or total removal of $[Na^+]$ can markedly change the rate of rise of the action potential in this tissue (52,53). Moreover, Shigeto and Irisawa (54,55) have shown that hyperpolarization of the cat or rabbit AV node yields more rapid $[Na^+]_o$-dependent upstrokes or initial depolarization

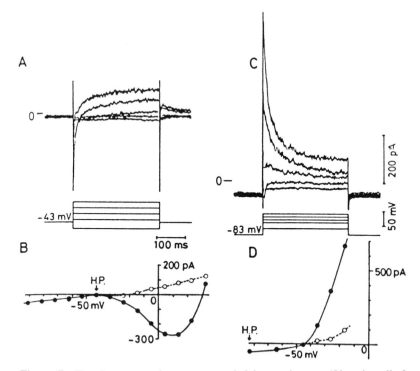

Figure 7 Transient outward current recorded in a quiescent AV node cell. In A and C, both current (upper) and the voltage traces (lower) are illustrated. (A) Depolarizing test pulses of 10, 30, 50, and 70 mV and a hyperpolarizing pulse of -20 mV from the holding potential of -43 mV activate the Ca^{2+} current and the delayed rectifier current I_K. The fast inward sodium current I_{Na} is almost entirely inactivated at this holding potential. The current I_f that can be activated by hyperpolarizations was not observed in this cell but was recorded in 4 of 11 other cells. (B) *I-V* relations corresponding to the raw data in A. The peak amplitude of the Ca^{2+} current and the initial (10 msec after the onset of the pulse) current during hyperpolarizing clamp pulses are plotted (filled circles). The current amplitudes at 300 msec are also plotted (open circle). (C) Depolarizing clamp pulses of 20, 40, 50, 60, and 70 mV from the HP of -83 mV activate the transient outward current at potentials positive to -40 mV. The peak of the current is recorded within 10 msec after the onset of the clamp pulse and becomes larger with increasing depolarization. (D) *I-V* relations corresponding to the raw data in C. The input resistances measured at -40 mV in B and D are 0.98 and 0.80 GΩ, and the specific membrane resistances are 26.0 and 21.2 kΩ/cm², respectively. The duration of the clamp pulses are 300 msec in A and C. Symbols in D are the same as in B. This cell was 24 × 40 μm in size. [Reproduced from Nakayama and Irisawa (68) with permission from the American Heart Association.]

phases of the action potential. It is possible that certain cell types or regions of the AV node have a sodium current, whereas others do not, as is the case in the sinoatrial node (38). Tetrodotoxin (TTX), a selective blocker of I_{Na}, has been demonstrated to be effective in conventional electrophysiologic recordings (56–58). Alternatively, it is also possible that reduction or removal of $[Na^+]_o$ indirectly alters the transmembrane electrochemical gradient for calcium, as a consequence of a change in Na^+/Ca^{2+} activity (59). Recent demonstrations of a TTX-insensitive but cadmium-sensitive Na^+ current in nerve (60) and in cardiac tissue (61–64) raise the question, Does a similar current exist in AV node? No relevant data are available at present.

Calcium Current, I_{Ca}

Two-microelectrode voltage clamp recordings from small synthetic strips of AV node (Fig.

6) and suction microelectrode measurements from single cells (Fig. 7) consistently identify a TTX-resistant, Ca^{2+}-dependent, slow inward current (65,66). Although this current has not been studied in detail in the AV node, it appears to be very similar to the L-type Ca^{2+} current studied in other cardiac tissues (67,68); that is, its kinetics, amplitude, and selectivity are very similar to those of the Ca^{2+} currents in atrium or in ventricle of the rabbit heart. However, additional work is needed to confirm these important points. At present no conclusive information is available concerning whether there is a T-type Ca^{2+} current in the AV node of the mammalian heart. This information is needed to answer such questions as (1) What types of Ca^{2+} currents are available in the various cell types of the AV node? (2) What is the mechanism of the action of substances like autonomic transmitters or adenosine within AV node tissue? (3) How do therapeutic agents such as verapamil exert their actions on AV nodal tissue?

During each cardiac cycle there is a substantial Ca^{2+} influx. Thus it is very likely that an electrogenic Na^+-Ca^{2+} exchange mechanism is present in mammalian AV node as in the atrium and ventricle. The Na^+-Ca^{2+} exchanger current is expected to be small relative to channel-mediated currents, but AV node tissue (cells) has both a high input resistance and, apparently, a relatively low density of Na^+ channels. As a result, under some circumstances the current generated by a Na^+-Ca^{2+} exchanger could contribute to an action potential shape change, for example, the plateau or repolarization phases (59).

Potassium Currents, I_t and I_K

Recordings from multicellular tissue (66) and those from single cells agree in demonstrating that in the rabbit AV node there is a relatively large K^+-selective time- and voltage-dependent delayed rectifier of potassium current I_K. In addition, Nakayama and Irisawa (69) have shown that in some cells a relatively large transient outward current that appears to be carried by both Na^+ and K^+ ions can be recorded. The properties of this type of transient outward current I_t have been studied in detail in the atrium, crista terminalis, and ventricle of rabbit heart (44,70).

In the absence of a significant inwardly rectifying background K^+ current, these two outward currents (I_K and I_t) are likely to be responsible for initiating and controlling repolarization. In this regard it is important to recall the different patterns of frequency-dependent changes in action potential duration (see the preceding section). In some cells within the AV node (NH cells, Fig. 4) the action potential shortens in response to an increase in stimulus frequency; this pattern of changes is expected from additional or residual activation of the delayed rectifier type of K^+ current, I_K. In contrast, in other cell types within the AV node (AN cells, Fig. 4) an increase in stimulus frequency results in an increase in action potential duration and height. This pattern of action potential shape changes is expected from the transient outward type of K^+ current, I_t, since once it has been inactivated its reactivation is both time and voltage dependent. The failure of Irisawa and his colleagues (69) to observe the transient outward K^+ current in some of their single-cell recordings presumably indicates that within the AV node there are different complements of K^+ currents in different cell types, so that I_t is not present in all cells.

At least two other K^+ currents are likely to exist within the AV node. A Ca^{2+}-activated K^+ current may be present normally and/or may develop under conditions in which the cells have abnormally high diastolic levels of calcium. For example, after treatment with ouabain a relatively large transient outward current can be recorded (51). This current is likely a mixture of the Ca^{2+}-independent transient outward current already described and a Ca^{2+}-activated K^+ current. In addition, Kakei and Noma (71), using torn-off patch recordings, have shown that under some circumstances an ATP-dependent K^+ channel can be activated. This type of K^+ conductance is activated when ATP levels within the cell are very low (approximately 1 mM). As a result it is reasonable to speculate that I_{KATP} is active only during extreme metabolic derangement.

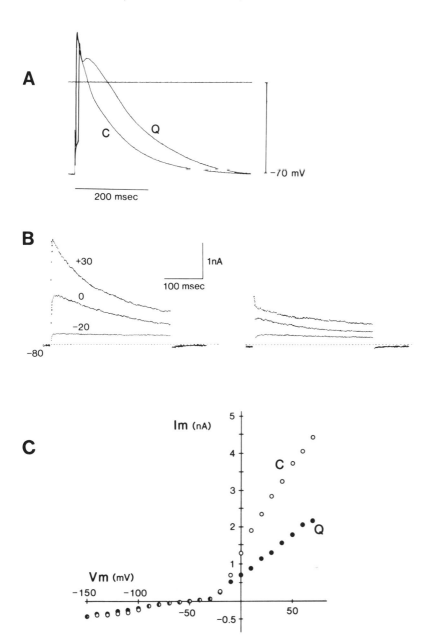

Figure 8 Effects of quinidine on the action potential and transient outward current in an atrial cell from rabbit heart. (A) Quinidine (Q) lengthens (113% at 50% repolarization) the action potential. Action potentials were elicited by 700 μsec depolarizing current pulses applied at 2 Hz. (B) Control (left) and quinidine-blocked (right) transient outward currents. In each row three current traces are superimposed. These were elicited by 300 msec depolarizations applied at 0.5 Hz to -20, 0, and 30 mV from the holding potential of -80 mV. The transient outward current was pharmacologically isolated by adding $CdCl_2$ (3.0 × 10^{-4} M) and tetrodotoxin (5 μM) to Tyrode's solution. The dotted line denotes zero current level. (C) The current-voltage (*I-V*) relationship for the transient outward current and the inward background current measured as the peak outward current or the minimum inward current in response to 300 msec pulses applied at 0.5 Hz. These data represent the averages from two experiments. I_m, membrane ionic current; V_m, membrane potential. [Reproduced from Imaizumi and Giles [76] with permission from American Physiological Society.]

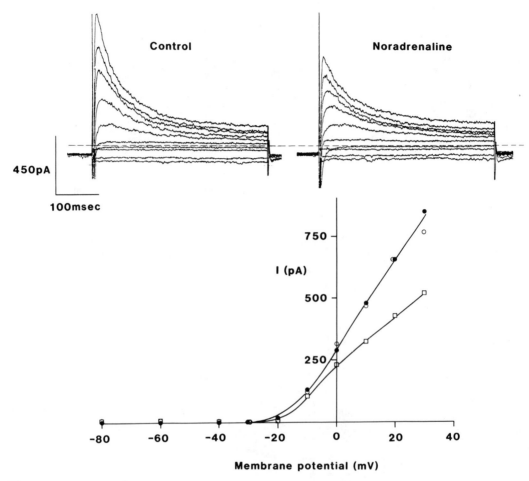

Figure 9 Effect of 10^{-5} M norepinephrine on current-voltage relation of transient outward current. Current traces were recorded during 400 msec voltage-clamp pulses from -80 mV to a range of different potentials at a frequency of 0.1 Hz. Records in the upper left panel were obtained in control conditions for pulses from -80 mV to 30, 20, 10, 0, -10, -20, -40, -60, -90, and -100 mV (top trace downward, respectively). Traces on the upper right are for identical voltages after exposure to 10^{-5} M norepinehprine for 4 min. The dotted line indicates zero current. Time-dependent current change is plotted against pulse potential in the graph at the bottom. (o) Before norepinephrine exposure; (□) during exposure; (•) after wash off of norepinephrine for 9 min. Curves through data points were fitted by eye. [Reproduced from Fedida et al. [77] with permission from the American Physiological Society.]

Other Ionic Currents

Inward Current Activated by Hyperpolarization, I_f

Recordings from both multicellular tissue and from single cells of the AV node quite consistently demonstrate the presence of a slowly activating inward current when hyperpolarizations are applied from the resting potential or the maximum diastolic potential of spontaneously active tissue (34,66). Although this current change has not been studied in detail in the AV node, it has many of the characteristics of the current I_f, which is present in pacemaker tissue from the SA node as well as in Purkinje fibers (72). In the SA node this current may contribute to the slow diastolic depolarization or pacemaker potential (38), and in Purkinje tissue it does serve this function. It will be important to study in detail the selectivity and gating characteristics of this current as well as to determine whether its channel density, for example, differs in the various cell types of the mammalian AV node.

Ca²⁺-Activated Transient Inward Current, I_{ti}

A recent study of the actions of ouabain on mammalian AV node (51) demonstrated quite clearly that under conditions of glycoside toxicity, that is, when the cells of the AV node are Ca^{2+} loaded, I_{ti} currents can be elicited. These small depolarizations occurring in cells with relatively high input resistances can interrupt rhythm and/or generate ectopic foci. The characteristics of the I_{ti} current have been studied in detail in ventricular tissue. It has recently been shown that at least part of this current is generated by calcium-activated channels which are permeable to most monovalent cations(73).

MATHEMATICAL MODELS: COMPUTER SIMULATIONS

Despite the lack of information concerning the properties of ionic currents present in mammalian AV node, a number of investigators have attempted to formulate mathematical models of conduction, refractoriness, and conduction block. This work (74,75) has been partially successful; certain well-recognized patterns of conduction block can be adequately simulated. Nevertheless, models of this type, which are based upon incomplete information concerning the ionic currents present, must be viewed as useful tools that, unfortunately, have rather limited predictive value.

SUMMARY AND FUTURE DIRECTIONS

Much additional work is needed before the ionic basis of the action potential or pacemaker potential in any of the distinct cell types within the AV node can be understood satisfactorily. This work must recognize the electrical heterogeneity of the AV node and make recordings under conditions (1) in which the nodal cells behave in a normal physiologic way, as well as (2) under conditions more amenable to quantitative biophysical analyses. It is encouraging that even with the information available at present, certain functional properties of the AV node can begin to be understood. The slow conduction through the AV node appears to result from the lack of Na^+ current in certain cell types and/or the relatively low density of sodium channels, even when I_{Na} is present. As stated previously, the presence and relative sizes of the delayed rectifier K^+ current I_K and the transient outward current I_t provide a basis for beginning to understand how it is that certain action potentials in the AV node can broaden and increase in height when the stimulus rate in increased, whereas others can show the opposite pattern of responses. Recent information (Fig. 8) on the transient outward current can perhaps be used to understand the well-known actions of quinidine in the AV node. Imaizumi and Giles (76) have shown that quinidine can inhibit the transient outward current; thus in cells of the AV node in which this current is present, quinidine is expected to broaden the action potential and thus lengthen the refractory period. Interestingly, α_1-adrenergic agonists have a rather similar effect (Fig. 9) in atrial tissue from rabbit heart (77). Finally, it is well known that the AV node in various mammalian species is exquisitely sensitive to the metabolite adenosine. It will be interesting to determine whether these actions are direct, that is, involve opening of K^+ channels through a G protein-linked mechanism, or whether they are indirect, that is, entail a suppression of the Ca^{2+} current, particularly when it has been enhanced by a β-adrenergic agonist, perhaps due to adrenergic tone in the mammalian heart, for example (78,79).

ACKNOWLEDGMENTS

The authors acknowledge research support from the Medical Research Council of Canada, the Alberta Heritage Foundation for Medical Research, and the Heart and Stroke Foundations of Alberta and Quebec. The authors also thank Ms. Lenore Doell for skilled secretarial assistance.

REFERENCES

1. Scherf D, Cohen J. The atrioventricular node and selected cardiac arrhythmias New York: Grune & Stratton, 1964:1–46.
2. Hoffman BF, Cranefield PF. Electrophysiology of the heart. New York: McGraw-Hill, 1960:132–74.
3. Childers, R. The AV node: normal and abnormal physiology. Prog Cardiovasc Dis 1977; 19:361–84.
4. Meijler FL, Janse MJ. Morphology and electrophysiology of the mammalian atrioventricular node. Physiol Rev 1988; 68:608–47.
5. Mazgalev T, Dreifus LS, Michelson EL. Electrophysiology of the sinoatrial and atrioventricular nodes. New York: Alan R Liss, 1988.
6. Merideth J, Mendez C, Mueller WJ, Moe GK. Electrical excitability of atrioventricular nodal cells. Circ Res 1968; 23:69–85.
7. Ferrier GR, Dresel PE. Relationship of the functional refractory period to conduction in the atrioventricular node. Circ Res 1974; 35:204–14.
8. Gendreau R, Billette J, Zhao J, Couture R. Intrinsic origin of atrioventricular nodal functional properties in rabbits. Can J Physiol Pharmacol 1989; 67:722–727.
9. Levy MN, Martin PJ. Neural control of the heart. In: Berne RM, Sperelakis N, Geiger SR, ed. Handbook of physiology. The cardiovascular system. Bethesda: American Physiological Society, 1979:581–620.
10. Spear JF, Moore EN. Influence of brief vagal and stellate nerve stimulation on pacemaker activity and conduction within the atrioventricular conduction system of the dog. Circ Res 1973; 32:27–41.
11. Shrier A, Dubarsky H, Rosegarten M, Guevara MR, Nattel S, Glass L. Prediction of complex atrioventricular conduction rhythms in humans using the atrioventricular conduction recovery curve. Circulation 1987; 76:1196–205.
12. Simson MB, Spear J, Moore EN. The relationship between atrioventricular nodal refractoriness and the functional refractory period in the dog. Circ Res 1979; 44:121–6.
13. Krayer O, Mandoki JJ, Mendez C. Studies on veratrum alkaloids. XVI. Action of epinephrine and veratramine on the functional refractory period of the ayriculoventricular transmission in the heart-lung preparation of the dog. J Pharmacol Exp Ther 1951; 103:412–9.
14. Denes P, Wu D, Dhingra R, Pietras RJ, Rosen KM. The effects of cycle length on cardiac refractory periods in man. Circulation 1974; 49:32–41.
15. Simson MB, Spear J, Moore EN. Electrophysiologic studies on atrioventricular nodal Wenckebach cycles. Am J Cardiol 1978; 41:244–58.
16. Billette J, Metayer R. Origin, domain and dynamics of rate-induced variations of functional refractory period in rabbit atrioventricular node. Circ Res 1989; 65:164–175.
17. Billette J, Nadeau RA, Roberge F. Relation between the minimum RR interval during atrial fibrillation and the functional refractory period of the AV junction. Cardiovasc Res 1974; 8:347–51.
18. Billette J, St.-Vincent M. Functional origin of rate-induced changes in atrioventricular nodal conduction time of premature beats in the rabbit. Can J Physiol Pharmacol 1987; 65:2329–37.
19. Billette J, Metayer R, St.-Vincent M. Selective functional characteristics of rate-induced fatigue in rabbit atrioventricular node. Circ Res 1988; 62:790–9.
20. Billette J. Preceding His-atrial interval as a determinant of atrioventricular nodal conduction time in the human and rabbit heart. Am J Cardiol 1976; 38:889–96.
21 Young ML, Wolff GS, Castellanos A, Gelband H. Application of the Rosenblueth hypothesis to assess atrioventricular nodal behavior. Am J Cardiol 1986; 57:131–4.
22. Janse MJ, van Capelle FJL, Anderson RH, Touboul P, Billette J. Electrophysiology and structure of the atrioventricular node of the isolated rabbit heart. In: Wellens HJJ, Lie KI, Janse MJ eds. The conduction system of the heart: structure, functions and clinical implications. Leiden: Stenfert Kroese, 1986:296–315.
23. Billette J. Atrioventricular nodal activation during periodic premature stimulation of the atrium. Am J Physiol 1987; 252:H163–77.
24. Billette J, Janse MJ, van Capelle FJL, Anderson RH, Touboul P, Durrer P. Cycle-length-dependent properties of AV nodal activation in rabbit hearts. Am J Physiol 1976; 231:H1129–39.
25. Wennemark JR, Ruesta VJ, Brody DA. Microelectrode study of delayed conduction in the canine right bundle branch. Circ Res 1968; 23:753–69.

26. Antzelevitch C, Moe GK. Electrotonically mediated delayed conduction and reentry in relation to slow responses in mammalian ventricular conducting tissue. Circ Res 1981; 49:1129–39.

27. Cranefield PF, Klein HO, Hoffman BF. Conduction of the cardiac impulse. 1. Delay, block, and one way block in depressed Purkinje fibers. Circ Res 1971; 28:199–219.

28. Jalife J, Moe GK. Excitation, conduction, and reflection of impulses in isolated bovine and canine Purkinje fibers. Circ Res 1981; 49:233–47.

29. Waxman MB, Downar E. Unidirectional block in Purkinje fibers. Can J Physiol Pharmacol 1980; 58:925–33.

30. Lewis T, Master AM. Observations upon conduction in the mammlian hearts. A-V conduction. Heart 1925; 12:209–69.

31. Levy MN, Martin PJ, Zieske H, Adler D. Role of positive feedback in the atrioventricular nodal Wenckebach phenomenon. Circ Res 1974; 34:697–710.

32. Billette J, Gossard JP, Lepanto L, Cartier R. Common functional origin for simple and complex responses of atrioventricular node in dogs. Am J Physiol 1986; 251:H920–5.

33. Zhao J, Billette J, Metayer R. Atrioventricular nodal functional properties and assessment of nodal recovery time in rabbit heart. Physiologist 1988; 31:A132.

34. Irisawa H, Noma A, Kokubun S, Kurachi Y. Electrogenesis of pacemaker potential as revealed by AV nodal experiments. In: Sperelakis N, ed. Physiology and pathophysiology of the heart. Boston: Kluwer Academic Publishers, 1984:97–107.

35. Giles WR, van Ginneken ACG, Shibata EF. Ionic currents underlying cardiac pacemaker activity: a summary of voltage-clamp data from single cells in cardiac muscle. In: Nathan RD, ed. The regulation of excitation and contraction. New York: Academic Press, 1986:1–27.

36. Irisawa H, Giles W. Sinus and atrioventricular cells: cellular electrophysiology. In: Zipes DP, Jalife J, eds. Cardiac electrophysiology and arrhythmias: from cell to bedside. Philadelphia: Saunders, 1990:95–103.

37. Irisawa H, Hagiwara N. Pacemaker mechanism of mammalian sinoatrial node cells. In: Mazgalev T, Dreifus LS, Michelson EL, eds. Electrophysiology of the sinoatrial and atrioventricular nodes. New York: Alan R. Liss, 1988:33–52.

38. Irisawa H, Brown H, Giles WR. Cardiac pacemaking in the sino-atrial node. Physiol Rev 1991 (in press).

39. Kokubun S, Nishimura M, Noma A, Irisawa H. The spontaneous action potential of rabbit atrioventricular node cells. Jpn J Physiol 1980; 30:529–40.

40. Taniguchi J, Kokubun S, Noma A, Irisawa H. Spontaneously active cells isolated from the sino-atrial and atrio-ventricular nodes of the rabbit heart. Jpn J Physiol 1981; 31:547–58.

41. DeMello WC. Passive electrical properties of the atrioventricular node. Pfluger Arch 1977; 371:135–9.

42. Hoffman BF, Paes de Carvalho A, DeMello WC, Cranefield PF. Electrical activity of single fibers of the atrioventricular node. Circ Res 1959; 7:11–18.

43. Paes de Carvalho A, DeAlmeida DF. Spread of activity through the atrioventricular node. Circ Res 1960; 8:801–9.

44. Giles WR, Imaizumi Y. Comparison of potassium currents in rabbit atrial and ventricular cells. J Physiol (Lond) 1988; 405:123–45.

45. Noma A, Nakayama T, Kurachi Y, Irisawa H. Resting K conductance in pacemaker and nonpacemaker heart cells of rabbit. Jpn J Physiol 1984; 34:245–54.

46. Giles WR, Shibata EF. Voltage clamp of bull-frog cardiac pace-maker cells: a quantitative analysis of potassium currents. J Physiol (Lond) 1985; 368:265–92.

47. Kurachi Y, Noma A, Irisawa H. Electrogenic sodium pump in rabbit atrio-ventricular node cell. Pfluger Arch 1981; 391:261–6.

48. Kurachi Y, Noma A, Irisawa H. Electrogenic Na pump evidenced by injecting various Na salts into the isolated A-V node cells of rabbit heart. Pfluger Arch 1981; 392:89–91.

49. Gadsby DC. The Na/K pump of cardiac cells. Annu Rev Biophys Bioeng 1984; 13:373–98.

50. DeWeer P, Gadsby DC, Rakowski RF. Voltage-dependence of the Na-K pump. Annu Rev Physiol 1988; 50:225–41.

51. Watanabe Y, Noda T, Habuchi Y. Effects of cardiac glycosides on AV nodal impulse formation and conduction. In: Mazgalev T, Dreifus LS, Michelson EL, eds. Progress in clinical and biological research, Vol. 275. New York: Alan R. Liss, 1988:111–33.

52. Ruiz-Ceretti E, Ponce Zumino A. Action potential changes under varied $[Na^+]_o$ and $[Ca^{2+}]_o$ indicating the existence of two inward currents in cells of the rabbit atrioventricular node. Circ Res 1976; 39:326–36.

53. Akiyama T, Fozzard HA. Ca and Na selectivity of the active membrane of rabbit AV nodal cells. Am J Physiol 1979; 236:C1–8.

54. Shigeto N, Irisawa H. The effect of polarization on the action potentials of the rabbit AV nodal cells. Jpn J Physiol 1974; 24:605–16.

55. Shigeto N, Irisawa H. Slow conduction in the atrioventricular node of the cat: a possible explanation. Experientia 1972; 28:1442–3.

56. Paes de Carvalho A, Hoffman BF, de Paula Carvalho M. Two components of the cardiac action potential. I. Voltage-time course and the effect of acetylcholine on atrial and nodal cells of the rabbit heart. J Gen Physiol 1969; 54:607–35.

57. Ruiz-Ceretti E, Pnce Zumino A, Parisii IM. Resolution of two components in the upstroke of the action potential in atrioventricular fibers of the rabbit heart. Can J Physiol Pharmacol 1971; 49:642-8.

58. Zipes DP, Mendez C. Action of manganese ions and tetrodotoxin on atrioventricular nodal transmembrane potentials in isolated rabbit hearts. Circ Res 1973; 32:447–54.

59. Mullins LJ. Role of Na-Ca exchange in heart. In: Sperelakis N, ed. Physiology and pathophysiology of the heart, 2nd Ed. New York: Kluwer Academic, 1989:241–51.

60. Ikeda SR, Schofield GG. Tetrodotoxin-resistant sodium current of rat nodose neurones: monovalent cation selectivity and divalent cation block. J Physiol (Lond) 1987; 389:255–70.

61. DiFrancesco D, Ferroni A, Visentin S. Cadmium block of I_{Na} in calf Purkinje fibers. J Physiol (Lond) 1984; 353:73P.

62. DiFrancesco D, Zaza A. Cadmium-induced blockade of the cardiac fast Na channels in calf Purkinje fibers. Proc Roy Soc Lond [Biol] 1985; 223:475–84.

63. Makielski JC, Sheets MF, Hanck DA, January CT, Fozzard HA. Sodium currents in voltage clamped internally perfused canine cardiac Purkinje cells. Biophys J 1987; 52:1–11.

64. Frelin C, Cognard C, Vigne P, Lazdunski M. Tetrodotoxin sensitive and tetrodotoxin resistant Na^+ channels differ in their sensitivity to Cd^{2+} and Zn^{2+}. Eur J Pharmacol 1986; 122:245–50.

65. Noma A, Irisawa H, Kokubun S, Kotake H, Nishimura M, Watanabe Y. Slow current systems in the A-V node of the rabbit heart. Nature 1980; 285:228–9.

66. Kokubun S, Nishimura M, Noma A, Irisawa H. Membrane currents in the rabbit atrioventricular node cells. Pfluger Arch 1982; 393: 15–22.

67. Hess P. Elementary properties of cardiac calcium channels: a brief review. Can J Physiol Pharmacol 1989; 66:1218–23.

68. Bean BP. Classes of calcium channels in vertebrate cells. Annu Rev Physiol 1989; 51:367–84.

69. Nakayama T, Irisawa H. Transient outward current carried by potassium and sodium in quiescent atrioventricular node cells of rabbits. Circ Res 1985; 57:65–73.

70. Clark RB, Giles WR, Imaizumi Y. Properties of the transient outward current in rabbit atrial atrial cells. J Physiol (Lond) 1988; 405:147–68.

71. Kakei M, Noma A. Adenosine 5′ - triphosphate-sensitive single potassium channel in the atrioventricular node cell of the rabbit heart. J Physiol (Lond) 1984; 352:265–84.

72. DiFrancesco D. The cardiac hyperpolarization-activated current, I_f. Origin and developments. Proc Biophys Mol Biol 1985; 46: 163–83.

73. Ehara T, Noma A, Ono K. Calcium-activated non-selective cation channel in ventricular cells isolated from guinea pig hearts. J Physiol (Lond) 1988; 403:117–33.

74. Urushibara S, Kawato M, Nakazawa K, Suzuki R. Simulation analysis of conduction of excitation in the atrioventricular node. J Theor Biol 1987; 126:275–88.

75. Nishimura M, Huan RM, Habuchi Y, Tsuji Y, Nakanishi T, Watanabe Y. Membrane actions of quinidine sulphate in the rabbit atrioventricular node studied by voltage clamp method. J Pharmacol Exp Ther 1988; 244: 780–9.

76. Imaizumi Y, Giles W. Quinidine-induced inhibition of a transient outward current in cardiac muscle. Am J Physiol 1987; 253: H704–8.

77. Fedida D, Shimoni Y, Giles WR. A novel effect of norepinephrine on cardiac cells is mediated by α_1-adrenoceptors. Am J Physiol 1989; 256:H1500–4.

78. Belardinelli L, Klockner U, Isenberg G. Modulation of potassium and calcium currents in atrial and nodal cells. In: Piper HM, Isenberg G, eds. Isolated adult myocytes. Vol. II. Electrophysiology and contractile function. Boca Raton, FL: CRC Press, 1989: 155–80.

79. Belardinelli L, Giles W, West A. Ionic mechanism of adenosine action in pacemaker cells from rabbit heart. J Physiol (Lond) 1988; 405:615–33.

8

Electrophysiology of the Purkinje Fiber

Kenneth H. Dangman

College of Physicians and Surgeons, Columbia University
New York, New York

INTRODUCTION

The Purkinje fibers of the mammalian heart are organized into a branching network called the intraventricular conduction system (1–5). The primary function of these Purkinje fibers is to provide a coordinated sequence of electrical activation in the ventricles (6). This sequence of activation leads to organized contraction. This means that efficient ventricular ejection occurs with each normal sinus beat. Thus normal physiology of the cardiac Purkinje fibers is required for proper cardiac function, and abnormal physiology of these fibers can lead to significant ventricular dysfunction.

Studies of the electrophysiology of the cardiac Purkinje fibers have passed through several phases. The development of intracellular micropipette electrodes in the late 1940s made it possible to record transmembrane action potentials (Fig. 1) from single cells in preparations of cardiac tissue (7). Pioneering experiments in the early 1950s by Weidmann et al. (8–12), Trautwein et al. (13–15), and Coraboeuf et al. (16,17) described the normal automaticity, transmembrane action potential characteristics, and basic electrical properties

of the Purkinje fiber. Then, studies through the late 1950s and 1960s further characterized these electrical properties using microelectrode and voltage clamp techniques and began to study the electropharmacology of Purkinje fibers.

Starting in the early 1970s, interest developed in models of ventricular ectopic activity in isolated tissue preparations. These models included the "digitalis-poisoned Purkinje fibers," which generates arrhythmias via enhanced automaticity as well as by triggered activity from delayed afterdepolarizations, and the "infarct zone Purkinje fiber," which generates arrhythmias by abnormal automaticity. Finally, in the late 1980s, patch clamp techniques were developed that allowed study of ionic currents and single-channel conductance in enzymatically isolated Purkinje cells.

STRUCTURE AND FUNCTION OF THE INTRAVENTRICULAR CONDUCTION SYSTEM

Functional Anatomy

The intraventricular conduction system begins proximally with the His bundle and extends distally to the subendocardial Purkinje fibers

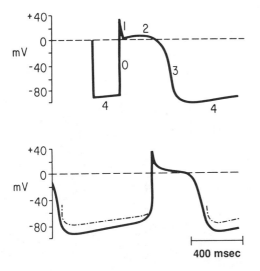

Figure 1 Diagrams of transmembrane action potentials in Purkinje fibers. Heavy lines show transmembrane potential; lighter horizontal line shows extracellular reference potential. Voltage shown at left in both panels. (Top) Electrode potential moves from zero to about -85 mV when cell is impaled. During diastole, transmembrane potential is about -90 mV. When an action potential occurs, transmembrane potential transiently spikes at $+35$ to $+40$ mV. This rapid upstroke is phase 0. Repolarization then occurs in three phases, as indicated. (Bottom) Spontaneously firing Purkinje fiber; threshold potential shown as dot-dash line above transmembrane potential. (Reprinted from Ref. 56, with permission of the publisher.)

and transitional cells on the apical surfaces of both ventricular cavities (3,4). The intraventricular conduction system is therefore also called the His-Purkinje system.

In the human heart the His bundle begins on the inferior septal surface of the right atrium, penetrates the central fibrous body, and descends via the posterior margin of the membranous septum to the muscular septum. Normally the His bundle provides the only route of propagation from the atria to the ventricles. The common His bundle consists of a series of parallel fascicles of Purkinje fibers. The fascicles are separated by fibrous septa (18,19), and the entire bundle is surrounded by a collagenous sheath. With age the fibrous septa grow thicker, and fatty infiltration may occur in the cellular tissue (19,20). The left and right bundle branches begin in the proxi-

mal muscular septum at the distal end of the His bundle. The right bundle branch typically consists of a discrete band of fibers that extends from the right margin of the common bundle, over the central right septum, toward the apex of the right ventricle, where it makes contact with the right ventricular papillary muscle. The left bundle branch fans out diffusely over the left septum; it generally separates variably into two or three indistinct fascicles. As in the His bundle, the bundle branches consist of arrays of parallel fascicles separated from the surrounding ventricular myocardium by a fibrous sheath that becomes thicker with age (20,21). These divisions run directly to the anterior and posterior papillary muscles. This arrangement has functional significance. It permits activation of the papillary muscles early in the ventricular cycle, so that the mitral and tricuspid valve leaflets are held taut during isovolumic contraction, and regurgitation of ventricular blood into the atria is avoided.

Cellular Structure

Typically cardiac Purkinje cells are larger and more elongated than ordinary ventricular muscle cells (Table 1). Purkinje cells vary in size from species to species but generally are between 15 and 70 μm in diameter and 100–200 μm in length. Contiguous Purkinje cells make end-to-end contact and are joined to each other by intercalated disks. These disks form low-resistance bridges between the cells and permit fairly large molecules (up to 40,000 daltons) to diffuse along the strand. Purkinje cells contain large amounts of glycogen and the glycogen-synthesizing enzymes glycogen synthetase and UDP glucose pyrophosphorylase (22). Glycolytic enzyme levels of Purkinje fibers and myocardial cells are similar, but the oxidative enzyme levels of the Purkinje fibers are relatively low (23). Myofibrils in Purkinje fibers are sparse and are not organized in regular arrays as in ordinary myocardial cells. Therefore Purkinje fibers contract less than ventricular or atrial muscle strands.

The Purkinje cells of the various warm-blooded animals can be classified into three groups according to their histology (24).

Table 1   Structure and Electrophysiology of Various Types of Cardiac Cells

	Sinus node cell	Atrial muscle cell	AV nodal cell	Purkinje fiber	Ventricular muscle cell
Cell diameter, μm	5–10	5–10	5–10	15–70	10–25
Cell length, μm	5–10	20	5–10	150–200	50–100
Diastolic potential, mV	-55 ± 5	-85 ± 5	-60 ± 5	-90 ± 5	-85 ± 5
Action potential amplitude, mV	60–70	110–120	70–80	120–140	110–120
dV/dt_{max}, V/sec	1–10	120–180	5–15	400–1000	100–200
Action potential duration, msec	100–300	100–200	100–300	300–500	150–300
Conduction velocity, m/sec	0.05	0.3–0.4	0.1	2–3	0.3–1.0

In one group (ungulates, whales, and birds) the Purkinje cells are large and closely packed; they are connected by extensive desmosomes and have few myofibrils. The cells are arranged in "cables," which are surrounded by well-developed connective tissue sheaths.

In the second group (dogs, rabbits, cats, and humans) the Purkinje cells are not arranged in cables as in ungulates. The cells have relatively large diameters, few myofibrils, and typically are embedded in connective tissue. In these species, therefore, the Purkinje cells can still be distinguished from ordinary working myocardial cells fairly easily. However, this is somewhat more difficult for this group that for ungulate Purkinje cells.

In the third group (rodents, such as mice, rats, and guinea pigs) the Purkinje cells contain abundant myofibrils and are difficult to distinguish from working myocardial cells by microscopy.

False Tendons

In many species of animals, including dogs, baboons, guinea pigs, rabbits, and ungulates (including sheep, cows, and goats), "free-running Purkinje fiber bundles" or "false tendons" occur. These false tendons carry the two divisions of the left bundle branch across the ventricular cavity to the left ventricular papillary muscles, and the right bundle branch across the right ventricular cavity to the free wall. The false tendons can be isolated easily and maintained in a tissue bath for many hours and so have been widely used for electrophysiologic studies. Canine and baboon false tendons are 1–3 cm long and 0.5–2 mm in diameter and are pink or reddish white in color. The "true" tendons in the ventricular cavities, the chordae tendinae, have similar dimensions. The false tendons can be distinguished from the chordae because the chordae connect the tips of the papillary muscles to the leaflets of the atrioventricular valves and have a whitish sheen.

Interspecies histologic differences may affect the electrophysiology of false tendon preparations. In ungulate (sheep) Purkinje fibers the transverse resistance to current flow is much greater than the longitudinal resistance. These directional differences in resistivity can be explained by the cable arrangement of the cell columns in the ungulate His-Purkinje system and can lead to anisotropic conduction within a false tendon (25). In contrast, the histology of the canine Purkinje fiber resembles that of the human, in that it has smaller directional differences in resistivity (26). For this reason, "the canine [false tendon] has a more favorable anatomy than the sheep [false tendon] for most physiological experiments" (26). In canine and ungulate hearts, false tendons are relatively abundant, whereas in the hearts of other species (27), such as the baboon, rabbit, and guinea pig, false tendons are more sparse. The Purkinje system of the human heart generally runs in subendocardial bundles; false tendons are relatively rare.

Although electrophysiologic studies of false tendon preparations provide much information that is relevant to clinical problems, limitations may occur because the human Purkinje bundles are surrounded by ventricular myocardium. Cells in subendocardial Purkinje bundles may be influenced electronically by action potentials occurring in the adjacent

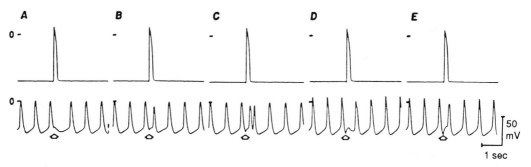

Figure 2 Effects of single extrastimuli during phase 3 on automaticity in a partially depolarized right bundle branch (RBB) preparation. Upper record in each panel shows recording from ventricular muscle cell one cell layer beneath the fibers of the right bundle. Lower record shows impalement in RBB. Impulses from RBB do not conduct to ventricular muscle. Premature impulses (arrows below RBB trace) delivered to RBB via ventricular muscle. Note subthreshold electrotonic responses (A) and suprathreshold electrotonic responses (B–E). (Reprinted from Ref. 28, by permission of the American Heart Association, Inc.)

ventricular muscle cells. Electrotonic interactions can be significant when the Purkinje fibers are partially depolarized (Fig. 2). This may contribute to ventricular ectopic rhythms (28). These interactions between Purkinje cells and muscle are difficult to mimic in simple false tendon preparations.

ELECTROPHYSIOLOGIC CHARACTERISTICS OF PURKINJE FIBER

Two types of action potentials occur in mammalian heart cells (Fig. 3). "Slow-response action potentials" occur in cells with maximum diastolic potentials of -60 or less, whereas "fast-response action potentials" occur in cells with maximum diastolic potentials of -80 mV or more. Normal Purkinje fibers show fast-response action potentials in which the current causing the rapid upstroke is carried by sodium. In partially depolarized Purkinje cells a range of maximum diastolic potentials exists (-60 to -40 mV) over which slow-response action potentials occur (Fig. 4). The inward current that generates slow-response action potentials is carried largely by calcium ions.

Conduction Velocity and Phase 0

Normal Purkinje fibers conduct impulses relatively rapidly. Conduction velocity is 1–1.5

m/sec in the His bundle and 3–3.5 m/sec in false tendons but 0.3–1.0 m/sec in ventricular muscle (6). Normal impulse conduction by Purkinje system activates the endocardial

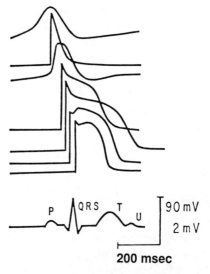

Figure 3 Diagrams of transmembrane action potentials during normal sinus rhythm. Traces show action potentials (from top) of sinus node pacemaker, atrial muscle cell, AV node cell, His bundle fiber, distal Purkinje cell, endocardial ventricular muscle cell, and epicardial ventricular muscle cell. Surface electrocardiogram (ECG), voltage, and time calibrations shown below. Voltage bar is 90 mV for action potentials, 2mV for ECG. (Reprinted from Ref. 56, with permission of the publisher.)

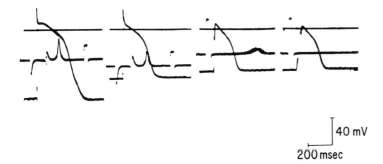

$$\Big]\, 40\,mV$$
$$\overline{\quad}\ 200\,msec$$

Figure 4 Decrease in diastolic potential in a Purkinje fiber. Each panel shows a transmembrane potential with reference potential (horizontal line) and a differentiated trace obtained during phase 0. Square wave in each differential trace is 200 V/sec calibration signal, symmetrical upward waveform in differential trace of first three panels is dV/dt of phase 0. Peak of this waveform represents dV/dt_{max}. The sharp downward and upward waveforms in differential traces (first two signals) in the two panels to the left are stimulus artifacts. First panel shows control records in normal Tyrode's solution with KCl = 2.7 mM; maximum diastolic potential (MDP) is -92 mV. Second panel, KCl approximately 10 mM, MDP is -66 mV. Third panel, MDP is -58 mV, with dV/dt_{max} of 20–26 V/sec. In fourth panel, MDP is -55 mV, and slow response action potential occurs with upstroke velocity of less than 5 V/sec. (Reprinted from Ref. 56, with permission of the publisher.)

muscle layers of the lower ventricular septum and free walls during the first 5–10 msec of the QRS complex (Fig. 5). This synchronous activation is critical for the mechanical function of the heart.

Conduction of the impulse along the Purkinje system depends on the active response of the cell membranes and the generation of a robust action potential upstroke. To elicit this upstroke a depolarizing stimulus is needed to bring the membrane potential to a critical value, at or beyond the "threshold potential" (Fig. 1). This leads to a series of changes in the permeability of the cell membrane, an influx of cations, and the generation of the upstroke of a fast-response action potential.

As shown by Draper and Weidmann nearly 40 years ago (8), the amplitude of the upstroke of the fast-response action potential is reduced linearly if the extracellular sodium concentration $[Na^+]_o$ is decreased progressively to 20–30 mM from normal values (130–140 mM). If $[Na^+]_o$ is reduced below about 20 mM (while osmotic pressure is maintained by replacing extracellular Na^+ with an impermeable cation), the cell becomes inexcitable. Therefore it was concluded that the upstroke of the normal Purkinje fiber action potential is carried by sodium ions.

The Voltage Clamp Model

The classic voltage clamp studies of Hodgkin, Huxley, and Katz in the squid axon led to a mathematical model for the inward sodium currents and outward potassium currents responsible for the nerve action potential (29,30). The inward current in the squid axon is also carried by "sodium" channels. According to the Hodgkin-Huxley theory, the current through the channel are controlled by "gating variables" called m and h. The m gates are closed, and the h gate is open, when the membrane is resting at diastolic potentials of -80 to -90 mV. If the transmembrane potential is then moved abruptly to values that are beyond the threshold potential (-75 to -60 mV), the m gates begin to open. The m gate is therefore called the activation gate. When the m gates begin to open, sodium ions flow into the cell in response to an "electrochemical concentration gradient." An electrical gradient exists because the interior of the fiber is about 90 mV negative compared to the exterior. The chemical gradient exists because the concentration of sodium ions in the extracellular fluid is 130–140 mM and, in the cytoplasm, is 10 mM or less. Thus both chemical diffusion and the orientation of the electrostatic field work to draw sodium ions into the

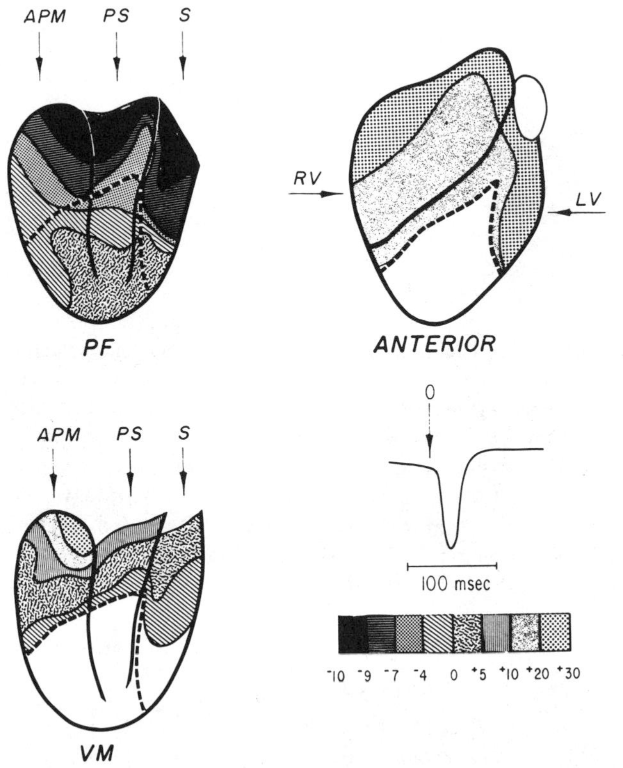

Figure 5 Activation sequence map of supraventricular beat in isolated, blood perfused canine heart 24 hr after coronary ligation. Sketch at upper left shows activation of Purkinje fibers on left ventricular endocardial surface, anterior papillary muscle (APM), paraseptum (PS), and septum (S) shown below arrows. At lower left, left ventricular subendocardial muscle activation is shown in similar sketch. Epicardial activation sequence shown at upper right. Border of anteroseptal infarct zone shown by dashed line in each sketch. Trace of atrioventricular electrogram shown at center right, with zero reference time indicated by arrow, 100 msec calibration bar below. Activation time zone codes shown by array below calibration bar. Activation of endocardial muscle closest to apex begins about 15 msec after start of Purkinje fiber activation; epicardial activation begins about 15 msec later. (Reprinted from Ref. 125, by permission of the American Heart Association, Inc.)

cell. Following a suprathreshold stimulus, the permeability of the membrane to sodium ion increases sigmoidally, reaching a maximum within 1–2 msec. The sodium current becomes the major current flowing across the cell membrane. The influx of positive charge (sodium ions) into the cytoplasm reduces the net negative potential of the cell. Transmembrane potential continues to move in the positive direction, toward the sodium equilibrium potential E_{Na}, which is about 50 mV (see Ref. 6).

As the transmembrane potential becomes depolarized, the h gates begin to close in a time-dependent manner. When the h gates close the sodium current terminates. It declines over 3–10 msec. The h gate is thus referred to as the inactivation gate.

The Hodgkin-Huxley model of the sodium current is summarized in a simple formula:

$$g_{Na} = g^{*}_{Na}\, m^3 h$$

For channel activation to occur, three m gates must move from the "closed" to the "open" position. The probability that all three gates are open is denoted in the formula as m^3. In contrast, inactivation is controlled by a single gate, and the probability that this is open is denoted by h. The values of m^3 and h vary between 0 and 1. The values are independent of each other and depend upon the membrane potential. The sodium conductance g_{Na} of the membrane is therefore determined by the maximum sodium conductance that the membrane can support if all the channels are open fully (g_{Na}^*) multiplied by the open probability (m^3) and the closed probability (h). Once the sodium channels have become inactivated, the cell must be repolarized (i.e., transmembrane voltage must be returned to resting membrane potential levels) before they can be activated again. That is, the sodium channels can exist in three states: resting, active, and inactivated. They must recover from inactivation and return to the resting state before they can be activated again. The conversion from inactivated to resting state is voltage dependent. The recovery process occurs during repolarization and proceeds as the transmembrane potential changes from about -60 to -90 mV.

The Sodium Channels

Recent studies indicate that the sodium channels are composed of several protein subunits that are embedded in the membrane (31,32). These subunits provide an aqueous pore between them. The channel subunits contain polar structures that project into the pore; the position of these polar groups within the aqueous pore can change according to the electrostatic field across the membrane. In one position the polar groups block diffusion of ions through the channel, and in a second position the polar groups allow unimpeded diffusion. Therefore the polar groups may be the equivalent of the Hodgkin-Huxley gates. Calcium and potassium ions do not move through the sodium channels as easily as the sodium ions. This has been explained by a "selectivity filter," a moiety that prevents other ions from penetrating the aqueous pore (33). Alternatively, ion selectivity of the channels has been explained by specific binding of the permeant ions with oppositely charged (polar) sites within the channel. Two factors are involved: the partition coefficient between the extracellular fluid and the channel, and the mobility

of the ion through the channel, quantified as the transition rate constant (34).

Threshold Potential and the Spike of Purkinje Fibers

The membrane potential at which the voltage-dependent activation of the sodium channels occurs varies somewhat from channel to channel. As the membrane potential becomes less and less negative, at the "foot" of the action potential, more and more sodium channels become activated as their m gates swing open. Thus as transmembrane voltage approaches the threshold potential, progressively more sodium channels open. This process is therefore called the regenerative response.

As the inside of the cell becomes positively charged in comparison to the extracellular fluid, the inward movement of more positive charge (Na^+) should be inhibited. However, the sodium current continues and results in an "overshoot" positive to zero potential of the upstroke. The overshoot, coupled with subsequent rapid repolarization (phase 1), produces the "spike" of the action potential, with its peak occurring about 30–40 mV in most Purkinje fibers.

Even though enough Na^+ enters the cell during phase 0 to change the membrane potential by at least 100 mV, this amount (approximately 10 pM/cm^2 per action potential) does not normally change either the intracellular or extracellular sodium concentration significantly. Therefore the chemical diffusion gradient remains constant throughout the upstroke. The continuation of inward current in the positive voltage range during the spike reflects the significant driving force that is generated by the chemical gradient for Na^+ alone, after the electrical gradient reverses. The peak of the spike is thus limited by E_{Na} to a maximum of about 40 mV.

Maximum Upstroke Velocity dV/dt_{max}

Some antiarrhythmic drugs work by reducing the rate and amplitude of phase 0 and thus decreasing propagation velocity or causing bidirectional conduction block in normal or pathologic tissues. These effects on the rate and amplitude of phase 0 can be studied in isolated Purkinje fiber preparations using standard microelectrode techniques. This is done by taking the first derivative of the maximum upstroke velocity (dV/dt_{max} or $\dot{V}_{max}$) during phase 0 of the transmembrane action potential. In normal Purkinje fibers the dV/dt_{max} is between 300 and 1000 V/sec, whereas in working myocardial cells it is typically between 100 and 200 V/sec (Table 1).

The dV/dt_{max} in a Purkinje fiber largely reflects the fast inward (sodium) current. However, dV/dt_{max} may be influenced by other factors, including the slow inward current, passive membrane properties of the fiber, and electrotonic interactions between the recording site and the surrounding syncytium (35–39). Therefore, for studies designed to elucidate drug effects on QRS duration or impulse propagation (topics of considerable interest in clinical cardiology), it may be better to study dV/dt_{max} or conduction times in tissue preparations than to study g_{Na} by whole-cell patch clamp. In essence, the upstroke provides the stimulus for conduction of the impulse along the Purkinje fiber. A voltage gradient occurs between the depolarized (phase 0) and resting (phase 4) areas of the fiber. This voltage gradient induces an electrotonic current, which brings the membrane in advance of the activation wavefront to threshold potential, while the dV/dt_{max} influences conduction via its effects on the availability of the fast channels. The more in advance a regenerative response occurs, the faster is the conduction velocity. Conduction velocity thus depends on a complex interaction of the active response and the core conductor properties of the tissue during rest and activity, as well as on the threshold and diastolic potential in the tissues (6,40).

Sodium Current

The magnitude of sodium currents can be measured accurately by patch clamp techniques in single isolated cells ("whole cell" or "cell-attached" patch clamp) and fairly well by two-microelectrode voltage clamp techniques in very small Purkinje fiber segments (41–47). Thus far, most studies of sodium current in isolated cardiac cells by patch

clamp techniques have been done in atrial or ventricular muscle cells; only a few studies of i_{Na} in isolated Purkinje cells have appeared (48,49). In the near future the use of cDNA clones should allow production of native and modified sodium channels. It will then be possible to study the function of these Na channels in either artificial lipid bilayers or frog (e.g., *Xenopus*) oocyte membranes (50). By studying unitary conductances of a variety of channels from mutant clones, the structure and function of the native sodium channels may be elucidated. One area of interest will be the role that different domains, or specific amino acid sequences, of the channel protein play in voltage- and time-dependent gating of ionic currents. It should also be possible to obtain insights into the basis of the ionic selectivity of the channels (51,52).

Thus, although studies of g_{Na} in collagenase-isolated Purkinje cells may not provide information that is directly applicable to clinical problems, these studies may provide essential information for the elucidation of the biochemistry of the sodium channel.

Phases 1, 2, and 3 of the Action Potential: Action Potential Duration and Refractoriness

The action potential duration of Purkinje fibers is relatively long compared to that of normal ventricular muscle (Figs. 3 and 6). Significant variations in action potential duration occur in the Purkinje fibers as they progress from the His bundle to the periphery. Action potential duration is longest in the middle of the His-Purkinje system and shorter toward the His bundle and the subendocardial Purkinje fibers (53,54). "Transitional" cells are the most peripheral fibers of the His-Purkinje system. They have action potential durations similar to those of the ventricular muscle cells in the subendocardium. This distribution of action potential durations allows the His-Purkinje system to function as a gate (53) that prevents premature beats from propagating easily throughout the heart. Thus propagation of very early premature supraventricular impulses block in the conduction sys-

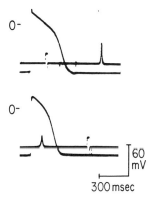

Figure 6 Transmembrane action potentials recorded from baboon left ventricular endocardium. (Top) Trace from Purkinje fiber; (bottom) trace from ventricular muscle cell impaled immediately underneath this Purkinje fiber. Note calibration bars at lower right, differential trace with 200 V/sec square-wave calibration signal in each panel, and zero reference potentials at left. (Reprinted from Ref. 27, with permission of the *British Medical Journal*.)

tem and are less likely to cause R-on-T beats and ventricular fibrillation.

The gate function of the His-Purkinje system depends on the refractoriness of the Purkinje and transitional cells of both ventricles. In either in situ or in vitro myocardial preparations, *refractoriness* describes the recovery of

excitability following an action potential, as has been reviewed in detail previously (6). It is possible to divide the recovery of excitability into four different periods (Fig. 7).

After a propagated impulse has been elicited, a period occurs during which a second propagated impulse normally cannot be evoked by a second (premature) stimulus. This is called the effective refractory period (ERP). In 1926 Drury and Love (55) defined the ERP as the recovery interval that ends when a response to a stimulus propagates throughout the myocardium. With the advent of microelectrode techniques, the phases of refractoriness of the individual Purkinje cells in a bundle could be studied. ERP was found to begin with phase 0, persist throughout phases 1 and 2, and end during phase 3. The end of ERP occurs when the transmembrane potential has repolarized to about -60 mV. At that point in time the sodium channels are beginning to recover from inactivation. That is, refractoriness is voltage dependent in Purkinje fibers (Fig. 8), rather than time dependent as it is in the AV node (56).

At the point during phase 3 at which it is again possible to elicit a premature (propagated) response, the ERP ends and the relative refractory period (RRP) begins. Typically, the

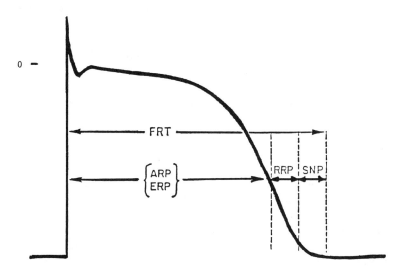

Figure 7 Purkinje fiber action potential with full recovery time (FRT), absolute or effective refractory period (ARP, ERP), relative refractory period (RRP), and supernormal period (SNP) indicated. For further discussion, see text. (Redrawn from Ref. 6.)

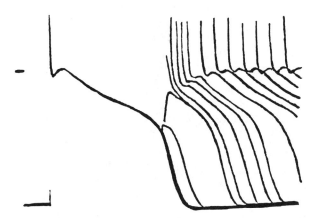

Figure 8 Voltage-dependent refractoriness in a Purkinje fiber. Premature stimuli (right) delivered at 14 different coupling intervals after the primary beat (at left). First two premature stimuli, delivered early during phase 3, elicit only local and secondary response, respectively. As fiber repolarizes after primary beat, premature impulses abruptly reach more normal amplitudes. Calibration bars at lower right represent 020 mV (vertical) and 100 msec (horizontal). (Reprinted from Ref. 56, with permission of the publisher.)

earliest premature responses are elicited by high-amplitude electrical stimuli (i.e., several times diastolic threshold voltage) and occur only after relatively long latent periods. During the latter portion of phase 3, as the transmembrane potential begins to approach full repolarization, premature responses can be elicited by progressively smaller stimuli at more and more normal latencies. The RRP can be defined as ending when the stimulus-response latency becomes equivalent to that of phase 4 (6). The end of RRP is thus defined the "full recovery time." Alternatively, the end of the relative refractory period can be defined as the instant when the stimulus threshold has declined to the value that prevails during diastole. If this definition is used the end of the RRP is not coincident with the full recovery time.

The repolarization phases of the action potential (phases 1, 2, and 3) are determined by a complex balance of outward (potassium) and inward (sodium and calcium) currents. Essentially, phase 0 depolarization occurs when the net currents across the membrane are in the inward direction; repolarization begins when the net currents across the membrane shift to the outward direction. This transition from net inward current to net outward current can re-

sult from inactivation of inward (sodium or calcium) currents, from activation of an outward (sodium-potassium or cation pump) current, or from some combination of the two. As indicated earlier, the time course of repolarization of Purkinje fiber action potentials is of interest because it controls refractoriness.

Phase 1

Phase 1 of repolarization refers to the descending limb of the action potential spike (Fig. 1). It is prominent in ungulate and dog Purkinje fibers. In these tissues the amplitude or phase 1 is about 25–40 mV. This represents one-fourth to one-third of the total amplitude of the action potential. Phase 1 is less prominent in human and baboon Purkinje fibers (27).

Changes in both inward and outward currents contribute to phase 1 of repolarization. First, the inactivation of the fast inward channels and reduction of the sodium current reduces net inward current. In addition, the onset of an outward current also contributes to phase 1. This second current has been called by several names, including the transient outward current i_{to} (57), the positive dynamic current (58), and the early outward current (59,60). Early evidence suggested that i_{to} was carried by chloride ions (58,61), but subsequent studies indicated that it is predominantly a potassium current (60).

The transient outward current is thought to consist of two components. These are a voltage-dependent component $i_{to,1}$ and a calcium-dependent component $i_{to,2}$ (62). The voltage-dependent component of i_{to} is activated at potentials of about -25 mV and is inactivated in a voltage- and time-dependent manner. It is blocked by 4-aminopyridine. In contrast, the calcium-dependent component is not affected by 4-aminopyridine but is inhibited if the amplitude of the activity-dependent intracellular calcium transient is reduced. This can be done by blocking the transmembrane calcium current, i_{Ca} or i_{SI} (57,63,64). The amplitude of $i_{to,2}$ may also be modulated by release of calcium from the sarcoplasmic reticulum (64). One recent study in isolated bovine Purkinje myocytes identified single channels that carry i_{to}; it reported that the conductance of these channels is about 18 pS (65).

Phases 2 and 3

The typical action potential of a cardiac Purkinje fiber has a plateau duration of 200–400 msec. The plateau duration is largely determined by the second phase of repolarization (phase 2), during which there are minimal changes in membrane potential. The action potential is then terminated by a phase of relatively rapid repolarization, called phase 3, that carries the transmembrane potential back to diastolic levels (Figs. 1 and 8).

Phase 0 shifts transmembrane voltage, which induces voltage- and time-dependent currents that are responsible for the plateau. Inward currents, carried by both sodium and calcium, are induced after the membrane is depolarized to -50 to -10 mV. These include a "slowly inactivating" sodium current and the slow inward current (now called the L-calcium current). The plateau voltage and duration are also influenced by outward-going potassium currents and by an outward-going current generated by the Na/K pump function of the sarcolemmal Na^+, K^+-ATPase. It is known that membrane resistance is high and transmem-

brane current is very small during phase 2 in Purkinje fibers (9). Thus the slope and duration of the plateau depends on a delicate balance of inward and outward currents.

The exact nature of the sodium current(s) that contributes to the plateau is controversial. It has been described as a unique "late" current through a population of sodium channels independent of the normal "fast" channels, as a slowly inactivating component of the fast sodium current, and as a "window current" resulting from a voltage-dependent overlap of fast sodium channel activation and inactivation (66–69). It appears that at least two components of sodium current can be identified pharmacologically; low concentrations of tetrodotoxin that do not decrease dV/dt_{max} significantly decrease the action potential duration of Purkinje fibers (66).

Two types of calcium current have been identified as contributing to the action potential of cardiac Purkinje fibers. These are $i_{Ca,T}$ and $i_{Ca,L}$ or the T- and L-calcium currents, respectively (70–72). The two currents have been distinguished on the basis of different voltage ranges and kinetics for activation and inactivation, single-channel conductance, and blockade by drugs (71,72). During depolarization, the Purkinje fiber T-current activates at a threshold of about -50 mV; the L-current activates at -10 to -20 mV (71). It has been reported that the L-current is blocked by verapamil, diltiazem, and nifedipine, whereas the T-current is blocked by 50 μM nickel (70,72,73). However, the specificity of block of the two types of channels in Purkinje cells has been questioned (71). The $i_{Ca,L}$ has a larger amplitude and slower inactivation rates than $i_{Ca,T}$; $i_{Ca,L}$ may therefore be more important than $i_{Ca,T}$ for maintaining plateau duration in Purkinje fibers (71). The time course of inactivation of $i_{Ca,L}$ is a function of both voltage and intracellular calcium activity. Increasing intracellular calcium levels accelerates inactivation of the current and decreases action potential duration.

Potassium is the major intracellular cation of cardiac cells, and outward potassium currents are important for Purkinje fiber repolarization. Several potassium currents have now been identified in cardiac cells (74–87):

1. Transient outward current i_{to}
2. Delayed rectifier current i_K
3. Inward rectifier current $i_{K,1}$
4. Acetylcholine-regulated current $i_{K,ACh}$
5. ATP-regulated current $i_{K,ATP}$
6. Sodium-regulated current $i_{K,Na}$

In particular, i_{to} and i_K are important determinants of the time course of Purkinje fiber repolarization.

The transient outward current is important for genesis of the plateau. It has been stated that in the Purkinje fiber i_{to} "governs the rapid repolarization (phase 1) which is a characteristic feature of the action potential. In turn, the rapid repolarization helps give the Purkinje fiber its long plateau by reducing the degree of voltage dependent activation of i_x [now called i_K] and inactivation of i_{si} [$i_{Ca,L}$]" (57). It was also suggested that i_{to} functions to offset the charge carried by i_{si} and "minimize the possibility of slow responses" that could "help cause cardiac arrhythmias involving either ectopic foci or re-entrant circuits" (57). Finally, i_{to} also can accumulate to contribute to rate-dependent shortening of action potential duration in Purkinje fibers (86,87).

The delayed rectifier current (i_K) was described in sheep Purkinje fibers in 1969 and "is the major outward current activated during the action potential plateau in cardiac Purkinje fibers" (88). Noble and Tsien (75) reported that the delayed rectifier current develops with time following depolarizing voltage clamp steps and has two activation components. The rapid component (initially called $i_{x,1}$) had a time constant of a few hundred milliseconds; the slower component ($i_{x,2}$) was activated over several seconds. The term X was used here because Noble and Tsien thought that the delayed rectifier current is not a pure potassium current but is carried by a mixture of ions (75). Subsequent studies in calf (78) and sheep Purkinje fibers (89,90) did not confirm this two-component X current model but suggested that a one-component K current, with superimposed effects of an in-

ward calcium current, could explain the results of Noble and Tsien (75).

The Purkinje cells in the false tendons face numerous "narrow clefts" filled with extracellular fluid. The ions in these narrow clefts do not equilibrate quickly with ions in the extracellular fluid bulk phase. In other words, there are significant diffusion barriers between the clefts and the bulk phase of the extracellular fluid. Diffusion barriers allow accumulation and depletion of potassium and other ions to occur during the voltage clamp protocols (91–93). These fluctuations in cleft ion levels complicate the analysis of the voltage clamp data obtained from multicellular preparations of Purkinje fibers. Indeed, because intracellular and extracellular potassium, sodium, and calcium concentrations can influence transmembrane conductances, it was suggested that it is almost impossible to accurately study the biophysics of ionic currents in the intact Purkinje fiber.

In the past 8–10 years techniques for acutely isolating single cardiac cells and studying them by microelectrode and patch clamp techniques have been developed. These techniques have eliminated the accumulation-depletion problem that previously confounded studies of ionic currents in Purkinje fibers. Studies of the single Purkinje cell preparations provided further insights into repolarization and ionic currents, such as i_K. Robinson et al. (94) studied the "restitution" process in isolated canine Purkinje cells. They found that following an abrupt increase in stimulation rate the action potential duration decreased to a new steady-state value with a time constant of about 60 sec (94). This time constant is similar to that for transmembrane action potentials recorded from cells in intact Purkinje tissues. On the basis of these results Robinson et al. suggest that K^+ accumulation and depletion in the clefts is not critical for shortening of action potential duration (94), contrary to earlier reports (95–97).

Studies of the delayed rectifier current in single Purkinje cells (77) indicated that it is highly selective for K^+ and activates at plateau potentials, that is, in the voltage range positive to -50 mV. Maximal activation occurs at about -10 mV. The activation and deactivation of the current are described as a sum of a fast and a slow exponential process. It was concluded that i_K in these Purkinje fibers represents a single voltage-gated conductance with one open and two closed states. Recent studies indicate that i_K is modulated by intracellular calcium and protein kinase A and C (98,99), as well as the extracellular cleft potassium and sodium concentrations (100).

Finally, the background (inward rectifier) potassium current $i_{K,1}$ has been suggested to contribute to the terminal phases of repolarization (101,102). Carmeliet (103) reported that the background potassium current in sheep Purkinje fibers does not show simple voltage-dependent gating. Rather, $i_{K,1}$ shows time-dependent activation during hyperpolarizing voltage clamp steps from plateau levels to diastolic levels of membrane potential. These time-dependent conductance changes were blocked by 0.1–3 mM Ba^{2+}. The results were explained by interaction of extracellular potassium ions with a site in the membrane. "During hyperpolarization from a low level K ions are moved to the activation site and the conductance pathway is activated in a slow time-dependent way" (103). The potassium level in the extracellular clefts, $[K^+]_c$, fluctuates during the action potential and transiently increases during the plateau in Purkinje fibers (95–97). Therefore, under physiologic conditions, activation of the delayed rectifier (i_K) begins during phase 3. This delayed rectifier current increases $[K^+]_c$, which subsequently may increase $i_{K,1}$ and accelerate the final stages of phase 3.

Measurement of Action Potential Duration

The action potential duration can be quantified in a variety of ways. A reasonable estimate of the duration of the action potential plateau can be made by measuring the interval between phase 0 and repolarization to a level of -60 mV; this is abbreviated as the action potential duration, -60 mV, or APD_{-60}. This value has the utility of also providing an estimate of the shortest possible effective refractory period of the Purkinje fiber. This is because, as discussed earlier, the sodium fast channels become inactivated during the plateau but begin to reactivate in a voltage-dependent manner as the membrane repolarizes during phase 3. Reactivation begins to occur at -55 to -60 mV. Thus in most Purkinje fibers the earliest moment during phase 3 that an upstroke can be elicited by premature stimuli is when the membrane potential reaches about -60 mV. Of course, if the Purkinje fiber has been exposed to a local anesthetic antiarrhythmic drug, the relationship between repolarization and recovery of excitability can change. That is, many antiarrhythmic drugs slow the rate at which the sodium channels recover from inactivation. These drugs tend to make the recovery of excitability more time-dependent than use dependent (56).

If APD_{-60} provides an estimate of the end of the effective refractory period, other commonly used measures of action potential duration, the $APD_{95\%}$ and $APD_{100\%}$, provide rough estimates of the end of the relative refractory period or full recovery time. These values are measured after 95% repolarization and 100% repolarization, respectively. In the typical Purkinje fiber transmembrane action potential, 95% repolarization occurs at about -85 mV and 100% repolarization occurs at maximum diastolic potential (MDP), or -90 to -95 mV. If a premature action potential is elicited between $APD_{95\%}$ and $APD_{100\%}$, the resulting dV/dt_{max} is usually equal to that of an upstroke of a "nonpremature" action potential, stimulated at the end of the normal diastolic interval during steady-state drive at the control basic cycle length.

Significance and Mechanisms of Rate-Dependent Changes in Action Potential Duration

Changes in heart rate alter the electrical and mechanical activity of the myocardium (104,105). The QT interval decreases during sinus tachycardia and increases during bradycardia. These QT changes reflect underlying changes in action potential duration in the ventricles. During bradycardia action potentials are prolonged. This allows $i_{Ca,L}$ to persist longer and thus helps to maintain sarcoplasmic calcium levels ($[Ca^{2+}]_i$) and contractility dur-

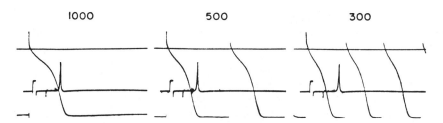

Figure 9   Rate-dependent effects on Purkinje fiber transmembrane action potentials. Format of panels as in figure 6, with zero potential shown by horizontal line. Action potentials at basic cycle lengths of 1000, 500, and 300 msec. Note decrease in action potential duration, minimal changes in dV/dt_{max}. For further discussion, see text.

ing bradycardia. This supports the increased stroke volume needed at lower heart rates. Conversely, during tachycardia the QT interval and ventricular muscle action potential duration decrease. The percentage of time that the cells are in electrical systole is increased, however, and so there is a net increase in $[Ca^{2+}]_i$ and contractility. This is shown in the "positive staircase phenomenon" (105).

Thus changes in action potential duration and $I_{Ca,L}$ (104,105) can explain the mechanisms for rate-dependent control of contractility. In general, rate-dependent changes in action potential duration of the Purkinje fiber (Fig. 9) parallel those of ventricular muscle. This is consonant with the concept of the gate function of the His-Purkinje system. During steady-state stimulation at a cycle length of 2000 msec (30 beats/min), the plateau duration of canine Purkinje fibers can be as long as 350–400 msec, whereas in ventricular muscle it is rarely more than 250 msec. At a steady-state cycle length of 300 msec Purkinje fiber plateau duration is between 230 and 260 msec, whereas that of ventricular muscle cells is between 150 and 200 msec. However, significant differences exist between Purkinje fibers and ventricular muscle cells, relative to the ways in which their action potential durations and refractory periods respond to abrupt changes in stimulation rate (106,107).

The adaptation of action potential duration of ventricular muscle to changes in rate probably depends on $[Ca^{2+}]_i$ and $i_{Ca,L}$. In contrast, the rate-dependent changes in action potential duration in Purkinje tissue may be controlled by the same currents that regulate it under normal circumstances (106); these include sev-

eral outward currents, including i_{to}, i_K, and $i_{K,1}$, as well as $i_{Ca,L}$. It is well established that after an increase in rate of stimulation in a Purkinje fiber the cells are "loaded" with sodium. This increase in $[Na^+]_i$ stimulates the sarcolemmal Na^+, K^+-ATPase (the Na/K pump) to produce a net outward current (108). This current has long been known to result in hyperpolarization of the maximum diastolic potential and overdrive suppression of automaticity (108). It also has been reported to contribute to action potential shortening after the increase in rate (109).

During rapid stimulation of Purkinje tissue there is an accumulation of potassium in the extracellular clefts (95–97). The potassium currents responsible for repolarization are affected by K^+ accumulation. As discussed earlier, action potential duration in isolated Purkinje myocytes decreases after an increase in the rate of stimulation; it has been concluded that because potassium accumulation does not occur in extracellular clefts in these single cell preparations, it cannot be critical for the rate-dependent repolarization changes (94). Moreover, in some cardiac tissues "plateau duration is insensitive to extracellular K^+ while action potentials are clearly shortened when the rate of stimulation is increased. These latter findings would indicate that K^+ accumulation is not even responsible for the shortening of the action potential as observed at high rates of stimulation" (110). Tissue differences may occur, however, and it is possible that in Purkinje fibers K^+ accumulation may make some small contribution to the time course of the rate-dependent shortening of action potential duration (111).

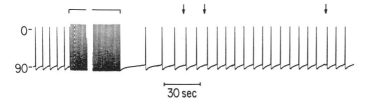

Figure 10 Automaticity in a baboon Purkinje fiber. Rapid stimulation at cycle length of 1000 msec for 5 min (bracketed zone) produces overdrive suppression of automaticity. Note voltage calibrations at left, time calibrations below. (Reprinted from Ref. 27, with permission of the *British Medical Journal*.)

Automaticity in Purkinje Fibers

Microelectrode studies in isolated cardiac tissue preparations have shown that automaticity results from slow depolarization during the "diastolic" period (6,8). This slow change in membrane potential is called phase 4 depolarization and typically occurs at 3–10 mV/sec in normal Purkinje fibers. If in any given cell or group of cells phase 4 depolarization occurs sufficiently rapidly to bring the diastolic membrane potential to the threshold value, an action potential upstroke is initiated.

In the normal heart the vast majority of the cells (i.e., the working myocardial cells) do not show phase 4 depolarization and automaticity (6). Only cells of the sinus node, atrial specialized conduction tracts, atrioventricular junctional region, and the His-Purkinje system are normally automatic. The pacemakers follow a hierarchy. Spontaneous rates of the various pacemaker sites in the heart decline as the cells become more distal from the sinus node. Thus, automaticity in the Purkinje fibers is relatively slow compared to that of the atrial or junctional pacemakers. False tendon Purkinje fiber preparations in vitro, with maximum diastolic potentials of about -90 mV, fire action potentials at 5–15 beats/min (Fig. 10). Even with maximal stimulation by catecholamines, normal Purkinje fibers rarely fire more rapidly than 40 beats/min. Nevertheless, Purkinje fiber pacemaker activity can be important biologically. During complete heart block (third-degree atrioventricular block), this pacemaker activity can produce a ventricular rate of 30–70 beats/min that is fast enough for survival.

Because automaticity is voltage dependent (112), any acute or chronic pathology that de-creases maximum diastolic potential in the Purkinje fibers will probably enhance ventricular pacemaker activity (56). The exact quantitative relationship between rate and maximum diastolic potential has not been reported for Purkinje tissues partially depolarized by pathology. In general, automaticity seems to increase progressively as maximum diastolic potential is reduced to about -70 mV from normal (-90 mV) ranges. At maximum diastolic potentials of about -65 mV, Purkinje fiber preparations typically fire at rates of 60–100 beats/min. If maximum diastolic potentials is decreased more, to as low as -45 mV, pacemaker activity may increase only slightly. Further reduction in maximum diastolic potential, beyond -45 mV, tends to decrease pacemaker activity. Purkinje fibers with transmembrane potentials of -40 mV or less are seldom automatic, or even excitable. This may be because it is difficult to elicit even the L-calcium current by depolarizing steps from these potentials.

However, one significant change in pacemaker activity occurs with depolarization beyond maximum diastolic potentials of about -60 mV (Fig. 11). Overdrive hyperpolarization and suppression of automaticity can no longer be elicited (112). This can be explained by a change in character of the upstrokes of the action potentials.

In Purkinje fibers with normal maximum diastolic potentials, the action potential upstrokes are carried by the fast sodium current. During rapid stimulation, therefore, the cells are "loaded" with sodium. Following 15 sec or more of overdrive stimulation the activity of the Na/K pump is increased. The pump current directly hyperpolarizes the cell and

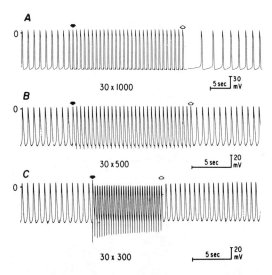

Figure 11 Effects of 30 beat trains of overdrive on normal (upper trace, 1000 msec cycle length) and abnormal automaticity (B and C, 500 and 300 msec cycle lengths, respectively). Zero potentials shown at left; voltage and time calibrations at lower right. For further discussion see text. (Reprinted from Ref. 112, with permission from the American College of Cardiology.)

suppresses phase 4 depolarization and automaticity (113,114). Pacemakers that fire from maximum diastolic potentials of -80 mV or more generally are highly susceptible to overdrive suppression. We refer to the automatic activity of these fibers as "normal automaticity" or "high-potential automaticity" (112).

Similarly, Purkinje fibers with maximum diastolic potentials of about -70 mV have ac-

tion potentials with "depressed sodium-dependent upstrokes" during overdrive stimulation. These pacemakers show some degree of overdrive hyperpolarization and suppression of automaticity. However, they are not nearly as susceptible to the effects of overdrive as are the fibers with high potential automaticity. Generally they must be driven at a rate much faster than the spontaneous rate, for periods of 3–5 min, before overdrive hyperpolarization and suppression occur (Fig. 12). We refer to the automatic activity of these fibers as "intermediate-potential automaticity" (112).

In Purkinje fibers with maximum diastolic potentials of -40 to -60 mV, the fast sodium channels are largely or completely inactivated. The upstrokes of the action potentials of these fibers are carried by the L-calcium current, not by sodium currents. Therefore overdrive of a pacemaker of this type does not result in stimulation of the Na/K pump, and overdrive hyperpolarization and suppression do not occur (Figs. 11 and 12). We refer to the automatic activity of these fibers as "abnormal automaticity" or "low-potential automaticity" (112). A convenient model of abnormal automaticity (Fig. 13) can be induced in normal Purkinje fibers by treatment with low concentrations of barium chloride (250–500 μM).

Thus normal and abnormal automaticity are two types of impulse initiation that occur in Purkinje fibers, at the high and low ends of continuum. This continuum is the physiologic

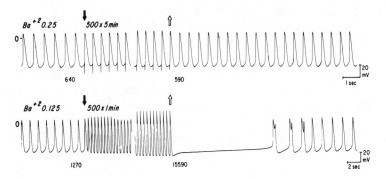

Figure 12 Effects of longer periods of overdrive on a Purkinje fiber with abnormal automaticity (top) and with automaticity from maximum diastolic potentials of about -65 mV ("intermediate potential automaticity"). Format as in Figure 11. (Reprinted from Ref. 112, with permission from the American College of Cardiology.)

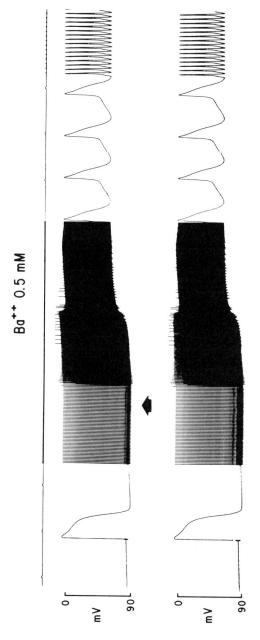

Figure 13 Effects of 500 uM barium on normal canine Purkinje fiber. Barium added to superfusate at the arrow below the first trace. Within a minute the maximum diastolic potential begins to decrease, and soon abnormal automaticity occurs (right). In a healthy Purkinje fiber this abnormal automaticity persists unchanged for hours. (Reprinted from Dangman KH, Hoffman BF. In vivo and in vitro antiarrhythmic and arrhythmogenic effects of *N*-acetyl procainamide. J Pharmacol Exp Ther 1981; 217: 851–62, with permission of the American Society for Pharmacology and Experimental Therapeutics.)

range for maximum diastolic potential. Significant voltage-dependent changes occur in the transmembrane fluxes of sodium, potassium, and calcium ions over this voltage range.

Mechanisms of Normal Automaticity

Until the early 1980s, diastolic depolarization in Purkinje fibers was explained by the time-dependent decay of an outward potassium current $i_{K,2}$, coupled with an inward current carried by sodium ions "leaking" through the sarcolemma (85,115). Since then a new model of automaticity has been developed, which turns $i_{K,2}$ "upside down" (85). Today, an inward current (i_f) is widely believed to be the primary cause of automaticity in normal Purkinje fibers (85,115–118). Voltage clamp studies indicate that i_f is activated by hyperpolarization from plateau potentials. The i_f activation curve is S-shaped in the voltage range of -50 to -100 mV. Half-maximal i_f on this curve occurs at about -80 mV. The time constant for activation is about 3 sec at -75 mV and decreases to about 175 msec at -120 mV (85). Thus the voltage ranges for the activation of i_f and for diastolic depolarization in Purkinje fibers are similar. Moreover, "the kinetics of i_f are on the same time scale as diastolic depolarization" (88).

The "reversal potential" for i_f is between -60 and -20 mV (85,88,118). This reversal potential does not coincide with that of any cation; it lies between the reversal potential for potassium (-110 mV) and that of sodium (about 50 mV). Therefore it is thought that i_f is carried by both sodium and potassium. The two ions carrying i_f "probably cross the membrane via an identical channel. The permeability of the channel for K^+ is about 10–20 times larger than for Na^+" (118).

Thus during the action potential i_f is deactivated during phase 0. It remains deactivated during the plateau. Then during phase 3, when the membrane potential moves negative to about -50 mV, i_f begins to activate. This activation is a time- and voltage-dependent process. The magnitude of i_f gradually increases during the later part of phase 3, but the long time constant for activation of i_f dictates that the current does not become maxi-

mal until well after the end of repolarization. The magnitude of i_f can continue to increase during diastole while the transmembrane potential is gradually declining toward threshold. Thus i_f is reported to be "the main current that initiates pacemaker depolarization" (115).

However, other currents also flow during diastole. One such current is $i_{K,1}$ (the "background" potassium conductance or "inward rectifier"). It is "the major potassium conductance during diastole and is the major reason why the maximum diastolic potential approaches the potassium equilibrium potential, E_K" (88,82). While i_f carries about 14 nA of inward current during diastole, $i_{K,1}$ carries about 31 nA of outward current (34).

Time-dependent decreases in the chemical activity of K^+ in the narrow intracellular clefts (aK^+_c) of the Purkinje fiber may occur during diastole (96). This decrease in aK^+_c occurs as a result of the activity of the Na/K pump. The Na/K pump transports sodium ions out of the fiber and potassium ions into the fiber in a 3:2 ratio. During repolarization potassium ions leave the cell as the outward currents i_{to}, i_K, and $i_{K,1}$ are activated. As a consequence aK^+_c rises during phase 3. Then during phase 4 the Na/K pump decreases aK^+_c. The amplitude of the variation in aK^+_c with time depends on the rate of diffusion to and from the cleft sites and the rate and degree of activation of the Na/K pump (96). Measurements using potassium ion-selective microelectrodes in Purkinje fibers in vitro indicate that the variation in aK^+_c during a single beat can be as large as 4 mEq/L (96).

The background potassium current $i_{K,1}$ shows inward-going rectification (115,119) and is extremely sensitive to K^+_o (115). When current-voltage (I-V) curves for $[K^+]_o$ at 2.7 and 5.6 mM are plotted on the same axes, a "crossover" occurs a few millivolts positive to the reversal potential for the curve obtained in 5.6 mM KCl (119). At voltages that are positive to the crossover point, more outward current is carried by $i_{K,1}$ in the higher aK^+_c than in the lower aK^+_c. Therefore, as the Na/K pump decreases aK^+_c during diastole, the I-V curve of $i_{K,1}$ shifts. This decreases $i_{K,1}$

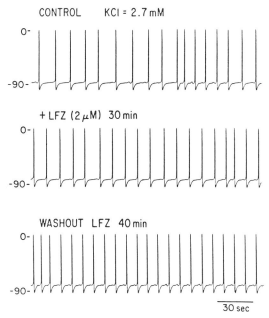

CONTROL   KCl = 2.7 mM

Figure 14. Lack of effect of lidoflazine 2 μM (LFZ) on normal automaticity in a Purkinje fiber. LFZ in these concentrations has been reported to suppress i_f. (Top) Control data; (middle) drug effects; (bottom) activity after drug washout. Note characteristic triphasic voltage changes during diastole. (Reprinted from Ref. 120, with permission of the publisher.)

with time and tends to depolarize the cell. It is therefore likely that "fluctuations [of K^+ permeability] may play an important role in Purkinje fiber automaticity" (85).

Thus both inward and outward currents influence diastolic depolarization in the normal Purkinje fiber. What is the primary mechanism of pacemaker activity in Purkinje fibers? Is it caused by increases in inward current through the f channel, by decreases in outward current through a K channel, or by some other mechanism (e.g., decline of Na/K pump current, or time- and voltage-dependent changes in a chloride current)? At this time the answer is controversial. Studies of the effects of cesium (115) suggest that i_f is critical for pacemaker activity in normal Purkinje fibers. Studies of the effects of lidoflazine on pacemaker activity (120) and i_f (121), however, suggests the opposite. Lidoflazine reduces i_f in sheep Purkinje fibers (121). When the effects

of lidoflazine at 2 and 5 μM were studied on dog and sheep Purkinje fibers with normal maximum diastolic potentials (Fig. 14), no significant decrease in diastolic depolarization or normal automaticity occurred (120).

If the i_f hypothesis is correct, and "i_f is the main current that initiates pacemaker depolarization," the f channels of each individual Purkinje cell should impose phase 4 depolarization and automaticity in the single-cell preparations. The evidence from collagenase-dispersed canine Purkinje fibers indicates that automaticity and diastolic depolarization are essentially absent in single canine Purkinje cell preparations with normal maximum diastolic potentials, -85 to -95 mV (94). The i_f hypothesis is not disproven conclusively by this, because the loss of pacemaker activity in the single cells may be caused by effects of the dispersion technique on the function of the f channels. That is, the Purkinje cells are dispersed by incubating false tendon segments in zero calcium buffer solutions with collagenase and proteolytic enzymes. Therefore, if the dispersion enzyme and zero calcium solutions damage the f channels, they could reduce or abolish diastolic depolarization and normal automaticity in the single cells.

Canine false tendons can be mounted in a stop-flow tissue bath and can be exposed to the same series of disaggregation solutions that are used to disperse single cells from false tendon segments. After this enzyme treatment the anatomy of the Purkinje fibers is clearly affected. When the enzyme-treated fiber is then superfused with normal Tyrode's solution, however, normal automaticity is restored. The cells have normal maximum diastolic potentials and fire at a rate similar to (and often faster than) that during the preenzyme period (Dangman, KH, unpublished observations). This suggests that the critical channels for pacemaker activity are not damaged by exposure to collagenase per se. This, coupled with the loss of normal automaticity in the single cells, suggests that the i_f hypothesis does not explain automaticity in the normal canine Purkinje fiber.

On the other hand, if the $i_{K,1}$ fluctuation hypothesis is correct single Purkinje cells

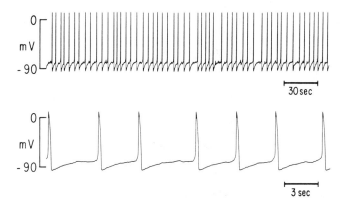

Figure 15   Normal automaticity in a "dense pack" aggregate of Purkinje cells. Format as in Figure 10.

should not be expected to generate phase 4 depolarization or automaticity. This is because the single cell is not surrounded by the cleft spaces that are critical for generating the necessary fluctuations in aK^+_c. Instead, if the $i_{K,1}$ hypothesis is correct, the minimal "element" (i.e., the smallest Purkinje cell structure) that should support normal automaticity would be an aggregate of cells. This aggregate would have to contain a sufficient number of clefts with diffusion barriers to the extracellular (bulk phase) media.

Both single Purkinje cells and small aggregates of Purkinje cells are produced by enzyme dispersion of false tendon segments. The single cells have been studied previously (94,122), but the aggregates have not been studied. Recently we began to examine the electrophysiology of the aggregates using standard single-cell techniques (Dangman KH, Boyden PA, Hoffman BF, unpublished observations). Briefly, the Purkinje cells are disaggregated (94,122), allowed to settle on a polylysine-coated coverslip on the bottom of a custom-designed 0.3 ml cell bath, and superfused at 5 ml/min (122). This cell bath is placed on the stage of an inverted microscope (Nikon diaphot), and impalements are made with standard KCl-filled microelectrodes with 30–50 MΩ tip resistances. Transmembrane action potentials are recorded using an Axoclamp-2 amplifier and are displayed on an oscilloscope and a Gould 2400 polygraph. Single Purkinje cells have stable resting potentials in the range of -80 to -90 mV and do not show diastolic depolarization. These results

are similar to those previously reported by Robinson et al. (94). If the time allowed for the diaggregation step has been kept relatively short, numerous aggregates of Purkinje cells are also encountered on the coverslip. These include preparations with only a few cells, as well as larger preparations with up to approximately 100 cells. Impalements of fibers in small aggregates (3–8 Purkinje cells) also have stable resting transmembrane potentials of about -85 mV and are quiescent.

In the larger aggregates (containing 20–100 Purkinje cells), the fibers also have maximum diastolic potentials of -85 to -95 mV. The cells in these aggregates appear as either "loose" or "dense" packs. In loose pack aggregates the Purkinje cells run end to end in strands; each aggregate consists of three or more strands with sparse connections between them. The lateral margins of the cells are not facing cleft spaces but are in direct contact with the bulk-phase superfusate. In dense pack aggregates the Purkinje cells are closely opposed side to side; therefore, restricted extracellular clefts are preserved in these preparations.

When cells in these aggregates are impaled, it is found that the dense pack Purkinje cells have diastolic depolarization and normal automaticity that closely resemble that of the intact false tendon preparations of Purkinje fibers (Fig. 15). This automaticity is stable for many hours and is similar in cells at all sites within the aggregate. This normal automaticity can be accelerated by exposure to catecholamines (Fig. 16). In contrast, the cells in the loose pack aggregates are usually quies-

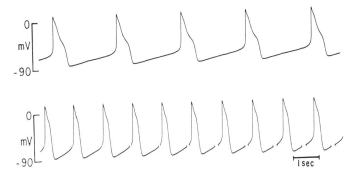

Figure 16 Acceleration of normal automaticity in a second "dense pack" aggregate of Purkinje cells by catecholamine. Control record shown at top; norepinephrine effects shown at bottom. Format as in Figure 14.

cent. No phase 4 depolarization is apparent in these cells (Fig. 17).

Thus it appears that the minimal element of a Purkinje fiber that is required for normal automaticity is the dense pack aggregate. This result is better explained by the $i_{K,1}$ fluctuation hypothesis than by the i_f hypothesis. However, it is necessary to understand that the answer may not be simple.

Phase 4 depolarization and automaticity in Purkinje fibers may not be a one-step process. In canine and primate Purkinje fibers the diastolic depolarization that leads to normal automaticity is often triphasic (Figs. 10, 14, and 18). There is an early phase of relatively rapid depolarization, during which the transmembrane potential changes by 3–10 mV over

200–1000 msec. This is followed by a plateau phase during which the transmembrane potential may change by 2–3 mV (or less) over several seconds. Finally, the diastolic period is ended in the pacemaker fiber with a final, relatively rapid phase of depolarization that blends with the "foot" of the action potential. The voltage-time course of each of these phases of diastolic depolarization, and the transitions between them, need not be controlled by only one current. That is, the three phases of diastolic depolarization may reflect as complex an interplay of currents as the three phases of action potential repolarization. It is quite possible that both outward potassium currents (120) and inward sodium currents (121,123) may be the primary currents

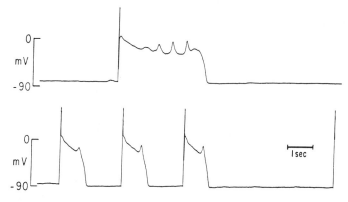

Figure 17 Lack of automaticity in a "loose pack" Purkinje cell aggregate. Note lack of phase 4 depolarization despite the long intervals between action potentials (30 sec at top; 12 sec before first action potential at bottom). At these long cycle lengths, action potentials are prolonged and have early afterdepolarizations. Action potential repolarization was normal when this preparation was stimulated at 30 beats/min or faster. Format, dispersed tissue suspension, same as in Figure 16.

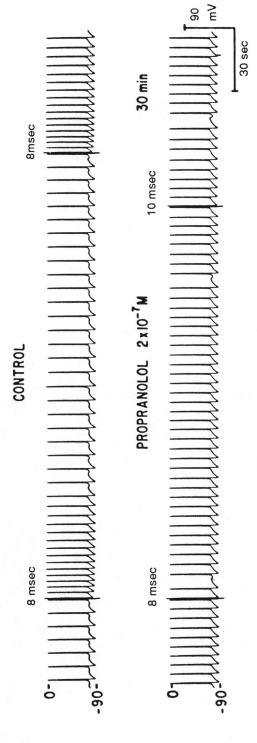

Figure 18 Effects of long-duration single stimuli on normal automaticity in canine Purkinje fiber. Control record (top) shows transient increases following each electrical stimulus. This response was abolished by 0.2 μM propranolol, indicating that it was caused by liberation of endogenous catecholamines in the false tendon. Format as in Figure 10. Note the varieties of triphasic phase 4 depolarization evident over a short time period. (Reprinted from Ref. 28, by permission of the American Heart Association, Inc.)

during different phases of phase 4 depolarization.

Mechanisms of Abnormal Automaticity

Abnormal automaticity in Purkinje fibers is an important cause of ventricular arrhythmias after myocardial infarction (124,125). Abnormal automaticity occurs in Purkinje fibers after stretch, hypoxia, or trauma (126) and during exposure to lactate (127) and amphiphiles (128,129). It occurs in Purkinje fibers and ventricular muscle from 24 hr infarct zones (130–133).

Abnormal automaticity can be induced in Purkinje fibers by artificial means (Fig. 13), including current clamp techniques (134) and by treatment with 250–500 µM barium chloride (135,136). Treatment of Purkinje fibers with high concentrations of barium, 2–5 mM, induces abnormal automaticity with peculiar early afterdepolarizations (120). Barium is thought to induce abnormal automaticity by decreasing g_K and by enhancing the L-type calcium current (137–139).

The cellular mechanism for abnormal automaticity has not been studied as intensively as have the ionic currents that produce normal automaticity in Purkinje fibers. Early on, abnormal automaticity was related to fluctuations of the delayed rectifier K^+ current (140). More recently, Escande et al. (141) suggested that the cellular mechanisms for abnormal automaticity and of delayed afterdepolarizations are similar in that both are influenced by sarcoplasmic reticulum-dependent processes. That is, delayed afterdepolarizations are caused by evoked oscillations in intracellular Ca^{2+} activity and abnormal automaticity results if the calcium transients are prolonged. Therefore small changes in the calcium transient may shift the character of impulse initiation from abnormal automaticity to triggering, or vice versa.

EFFECTS OF CATECHOLAMINES ON PURKINJE FIBERS

In the heart, both the epinephrine (adrenaline) liberated from the adrenal medulla and the norepinephrine liberated from the sympathetic nerves in the myocardium stimulate the cells by diffusing through the plasma or extracellular fluid to the sarcolemma. There, on the cell membrane, the catecholamines bind to specific membrane proteins called adrenergic receptors. Although it was long thought that the effects of catecholamines on the heart were mediated largely or entirely through stimulation of one type of receptor, termed the β-adrenergic receptor (142), it is now well established that cardiac tissues have a second class of adrenergic receptor, the α-receptor.

The β-receptor is still regarded, however, as generally more important than the α-receptor for control of cardiac function. The β-receptors are known to fit into at least two categories, called the $β_1$ and $β_2$ subtypes (143). Initially it was thought that the two subtypes were tissue specific, that is, that the heart contained $β_1$-receptors and smooth muscle cells contained $β_2$-receptors. This for a time led to hopes that $β_1$-blocking drugs could be developed that would be "cardioselective," but this goal has been abandoned (144). This is because it is now known that although the β-receptors in the myocardium are predominantly of the $β_1$ subtype, $β_2$-receptors are also present in sufficient numbers to be functionally significant (145,146). At this time the extent to which $β_2$-receptors function in Purkinje fibers is unknown.

Stimulation of β-adrenergic receptors by catecholamines or sympathomimetic drugs leads to both electrophysiologic and mechanical responses. Although mechanical responses occur in false tendon Purkinje fiber preparations, they are more physiologically significant in ventricular or atrial muscle cells. This is because the muscle cells are ultimately responsible for the "positive inotropic effects" of catecholamines in the in situ heart. In Purkinje fibers the biologically and clinically relevant actions of the catecholamines are electrophysiologic (Fig. 18).

Catecholamines elicit their cellular responses through a cascade of intracellular messengers (147,148): (1) binding of the catecholamine to the β-receptor activates a membrane guanine nucleotide regulatory protein called G_s. G_s consists of three subunits (called

α, β, and γ). Activation releases the α subunit, called α_s, into the cytoplasm. (2) The α_s subunit diffuses to the enzyme adenylylcyclase and stimulates it to begin to produce the "second messenger," $3',5'$-cyclic adenosine monophosphate (cAMP), from ATP. (3) The cAMP diffuses to protein kinase enzymes and binds to a regulatory subunit, which activates the protein kinase. (4) The protein kinase then phosphorylates and activates a variety of channels and cellular enzyme systems. The target structures for protein kinase action include the membrane channels for calcium (149), sodium (150), and potassium; phospholamban (which facilitates calcium sequestration in the sarcoplasmic reticulum) (151), and phosphorylase kinase, which breaks down glycogen stores into glucose (152). In addition, it has been reported that the G_s proteins can directly activate ion channels for calcium, sodium, or potassium independently of the cAMP cascade (153).

Catecholamines exert multiple effects on the electrophysiology of the Purkinje fibers; these effects depend upon which of the catecholamines is administered, the dose, and the condition of the fiber. Stimulation of the α- and β-adrenergic receptors leads to increases or decreases in conduction velocity and action potential duration, changes in normal and abnormal pacemaker activity, and induction of triggered activity in Purkinje fibers.

Action Potential Duration

Qualitatively, the effects of stimulation of α- and β-adrenergic receptors in Purkinje fibers by catecholamines are different. Stimulation of β-adrenergic receptors decreases action potential duration (154–159), whereas stimulation of α-adrenergic receptors increases it (154,156). Hoffman and Cranefield wrote in 1960 that "the effect of epinephrine on action potential duration in Purkinje fibers seems to be slight" (6).

Subsequent studies that quantitatively studied the effects of α- and β-adrenergic receptor stimulation on action potential duration largely confirmed this observation. β-Agonists

decrease action potential duration by only 7–12% in sheep and dog Purkinje fibers (147,148). The effects of α-stimulation on action potential duration in Purkinje fibers are similarly small. The effects in sheep Purkinje fibers, 11–13%, appear to be larger than in dog fibers, 0–2% (156,157).

In addition, Hoffman and Cranefield (6) reported that during treatment of canine Purkinje fibers with very high concentrations of epinephrine or norepinephrine, "the transmembrane action potentials recorded from a single fiber initially show one or more hump-like depolarizations during the latter part of the plateau and the initial stages of phase 3. These depolarizations appear to prolong the plateau considerably." Today, we call these hump-like depolarizations "early afterdepolarizations." The effects of α- and β-adrenergic blockers on these abnormally prolonged action potentials have not been tested.

Mechanisms of β-Receptor-Mediated Responses

Changes in action potential duration after β-receptor stimulation can result directly from decreases in i_K (155,158,160–162), decreases in i_{Na} (150), or increases in $i_{Ca,L}$ (71,162,163), or indirectly by increases in background potassium conductance. That is, β-agonists increase $[Ca^{2+}]_i$ (163–165) and this augments background potassium conductance $i_{K,1}$ (166). Finally, it has been reported that β-agonists stimulate the Na/K pump (167–168). This too could contribute to acceleration of repolarization of the action potential (170).

Mechanisms of α-Receptor-Mediated Responses

The ionic mechanism that causes the increase on action potential duration by α-adrenergic agonists has not been studied. It is possible that one or both of the reported effects of α-agonists on outward currents $i_{K,1}$ (171) or the Na/K pump current (171–173) could contribute to the action potential prolongation. The effects of α-adrenergic agonists on the delayed rectifier current i_K, on the inward calcium current, and on the sodium window current have not been studied.

Impulse Initiation

The primary effects of epinephrine and norepinephrine on normal Purkinje fibers are to increase the slope of diastolic depolarization and shift the threshold potential toward E_K (6,174). "Both these effects increase the rate of spontaneous activity in Purkinje fibers" (6). This "positive chronotropic" effect has been shown to be caused ot β-adrenergic stimulation. It has been studied repeatedly in spontaneously firing cardiac Purkinje fibers (143,154,155,157,158,175–181). In contrast, α-adrenergic agonists have been shown to produce negative chronotropic effects in Purkinje fibers (171).

β-Adrenergic Receptor Responses

The quantitative effects of β-agonists on automatic rate have been studied in isolated bovine (175) and canine (157) Purkinje fibers as well as the in situ canine heart (177). Dose-response curves for isoproterenol indicate that the threshold response of normal automaticity occurs at concentrations of about 1 nM, and near maximal increases occur at levels of about 1 μM in isolated bovine and canine Purkinje fibers (175,157). Studies of the effects of epinephrine in Purkinje preparations with normal (157) and abnormal (178) automaticity indicate that the dose-response curve was shifted an order of magnitude to the right, so that a maximal response was obtained with an epinephrine concentration of at least 10 μM.

Voltage clamp studies of Purkinje fibers designed to elucidate the ionic mechanisms responsible for the increases in normal automaticity that occur after β-adrenergic stimulation were carried out by Tsien and coworkers (179–181). Tsien interpreted the effects of epinephrine on the pacemaker current in terms of the then (1974) accepted $i_{K,2}$ model (180). He concluded that the β-agonist increased the pacemaker activity because it "speeds the deactivation of $i_{K,2}$ . . . by displacing the kinetic parameters of $i_{K,2}$ toward less negative potentials." The maximum voltage shift was about 20 mV, and it was produced by exposure to epinephrine concentra-

tions of 1 μM or more (180). Contrary to the earlier reports (6), Tsien concluded that epinephrine did not change "the threshold for i_{Na}" (180). It also appeared that epinephrine did not change "the inward leakage current" carried by sodium ions (180). The interpretations have been changed with the advent of the i_f model. The acceleration of normal automaticity by epinephrine and other β-adrenergic agonists is today interpreted as an increase in the inward pacemaker current i_f (182–184).

Tsien also concluded that the effects of epinephrine on normal automaticity in Purkinje fibers are mediated through an elevation of intracellular cyclic AMP (154,181). A later report suggests that epinephrine can increase automaticity in Purkinje fibers without elevating cAMP (176). A cAMP-independent mechanism may be explained by a direct action of a G protein of the β-receptor to modulate conductance of an ion channel or the Na/K pump (153,171).

α-Adrenergic Receptor Responses

In spontaneously firing canine Purkinje fibers, stimulation of α-adrenergic receptors often decreases automaticity (171,185–189). This decrease is reported to result from a G protein-mediated (188) activation of the Na/K pump (171,189). In contrast to the decrease in automaticity that occurs in normal Purkinje fibers, α-agonists are reported to increase impulse initiation in partially depolarized Purkinje fibers (190–192). In canine fibers these positive chronotropic responses appear to be mediated through $α_1$-receptors (190), but in sheep Purkinje tissue they can be mediated through $α_2$-receptors (192).

Anomalous Effects of Isoproterenol on Automaticity

Previous studies (155,157,174–177,186) indicate that β-adrenergic stimulation produces positive chronotropic effects in isolated Purkinje fibers. The prototypical β-adrenergic agonist, isoproterenol, induces maximal increases in normal automaticity (50–60%) at concentrations of 1 μM (186,157). The increase in automaticity is blocked by

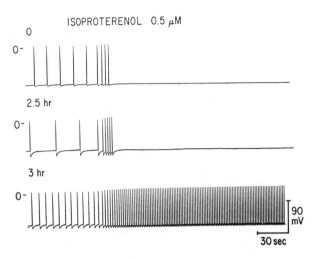

Figure 19 Induction of quiescence in a baboon Purkinje fiber by isoproterenol (upper two traces). Two periods of exposure 2.5 hr apart for 15 min each suppresses automaticity. Isoproterenol (0.5 μM) added to superfusate just after start of each trace. Third exposure at 30 min after second exposure evoked normal positive chronotropic response. Format as in Figure 10.

propranolol, indicating that it is mediated by β-receptor responses. However, lower concentrations of isoproterenol (0.1 nM) decrease normal automaticity (186,157). The decrease in automaticity could be blocked by phentolamine and therefore was attributed to an α-receptor response (157). Similar α-adrenergic responses were induced by other adrenergic agonists, including phenylephrine, norepinephrine, and epinephrine (157).

Anomalous effects of isoproterenol on normal automaticity occur in baboon and canine Purkinje fibers (Dangman, unpublished results). In the baboon Purkinje fibers normal automaticity consistently arrested within 1–2

min after the start of exposure to isoproterenol 0.5–1 μM. The quiescent period lasted for periods of 5 min to more than 30 min (Fig. 19). The preparations were stimulated for 15–30 sec intervals before exposure to isoproterenol, during the quiescent period, and during recovery from the catecholamine effects (Fig. 20). Action potential duration for the action potentials elicited during the quiescent period was decreased greatly, such that the plateau duration was reduced by more than 80% at a cycle length of 1000 msec. During the recovery period, beat-to-beat variations in action potential duration could occur (Fig. 20, bottom). This observation could be repeated if the prepara-

Table 2 Effects of Isoproterenol on Transmembrane Potentials Recorded from Baboon Purkinje Fibers[a]

	Cycle length (msec)	APA (mV)	MDP (mV)	dV/dt_{max} (V/sec)	$APD_{50\%}$ (msec)	$APD_{100\%}$ (msec)
Control	1000	123 ± 2	-90 ± 1	383 ± 101	275 ± 8	423 ± 9
	500	125 ± 1	-90 ± 2	367 ± 98	228 ± 2	360 ± 6
	300	121 ± 2	-89 ± 3	330 ± 85	163 ± 9	267 ± 7
ISO	1000	114 ± 1[b]	-92 ± 7	303 ± 55	44 ± 3[b]	170 ± 15[b]
	500	118 ± 1[b]	-92 ± 7	303 ± 61	48 ± 4[b]	173 ± 15[b]
	300	121 ± 1	-94 ± 7	300 ± 57	58 ± 8[b]	180 ± 15[b]

[a]All drug treatment values after 5–7 min in isoproterenol-Tyrode's solution, $N = 3$: APA, action potential amplitude; MDP, maximum diastolic potential; dV/dt_{max}, maximum rate of depolarization; $APD_{50\%}$ action potential duration to repolarization to 50% level; and $APD_{100\%}$, total action potential duration.
[b]$p < 0.05$ compared to control values.

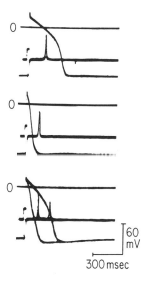

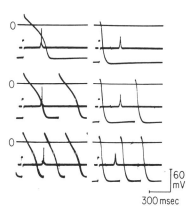

Figure 20 Action potential changes evoked by isoproterenol (ISO) during quiescent periods. (Top) Transmembrane action at basic cycle length (BCL) of 1000 msec before exposure to ISO. (Middle) Action potential during first period of quiescence (Fig. 19); preparation was driven at BCL 1000 msec just after end of top trace of Figure 19. (Bottom) Transmembrane action potentials during drive at BCL 1000 msec, 5 minutes after washout of isoproterenol was begun. Some action potentials have relatively normal repolarization, but most action potentials were still short. For further discussion, see text.

Figure 21 Cycle length-dependent action potential changes before and during second exposure to isoproterenol (ISO). Same preparation as in Figures 19 and 20. The preparation was driven at basic cycle lengths (BCLs) of 1000 (top), 500 (middle), and 300 msec (bottom) before and after exposure to ISO (Fig. 19, second trace). Control recordings (panels in left-hand column) were obtained about 3 min before ISO; the Purkinje fibers showed normal rate-dependent decreases in action potential duration. Then, about 5 min after ISO, the stimulation protocol was repeated (panels in right-hand column); action potential duration was radically shortened and the rate-dependent changes were abolished. Panel format as in Figure 20.

tions were again exposed to isoproterenol after a wait of 2–3 hr (Fig. 19, middle, and Fig. 21). For action potentials elicited during the quiescent periods the usual cycle length dependence of action potential duration was lost (Fig. 21, right column, and Table 2). These responses to isoproterenol showed tachyphylaxis; the more normal positive chronotropic effect of isoproterenol occurred if the interval between drug infusions was too short (Fig. 19, bottom). When action potentials were elicited at cycle lengths of 1000–300 msec during these isoproterenol-induced normal (acceleration) responses, they were not shortened greatly (Fig. 22). Treatment of canine or baboon Purkinje fibers with comparable concentrations of epinephrine and norepinephrine did not produce this anomalous response of quiescence with acceleration or repolarization.

In canine Purkinje fibers a similar phenomenon occurs in about 40% of the preparations.

After treatment of the canine preparations (n = 11) with 1 µM isoproterenol for about 1 min, the period of arrest averaged 4.9 ± 1.8 min. Diastolic membrane potential increased by 2.5 ± 0.5 mV during this arrest. The quiescent period was terminated by a period of accelerated automaticity, during which the rate was 50–100% faster than control. This arrest of automaticity was completely blocked by 0.5 µM propranolol (Fig. 23), indicating that it is caused by β-adrenergic responses. Action potential duration in the canine Purkinje fibers was markedly decreased 2 min after the start of the quiescent period (Fig. 24). Control studies indicated that 1 µM isoproterenol did not significantly decrease action potential duration in canine ventricular muscle cells recorded from the left or right ventricular endocardium.

The mechanisms by which β-adrenergic receptor stimulation by isoproterenol can

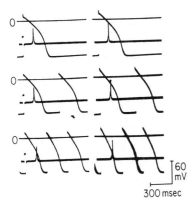

Figure 22 Cycle length-dependent action potential changes before and during third exposure to isoproterenol (ISO). Same preparation as in Figures 19 through 21. Format and stimulation protocol the same as in Figure 22. After third exposure to ISO a "normal" increase in automaticity occurs. During this period, about 5 minutes after the start of ISO, driven action potentials show normal durations and cycle length-dependent changes.

suppress automaticity and radically shorten action potential duration in Purkinje fibers are unknown. It is possible that these effects result from increases in i_K, $i_{K,1}$, or the Na/K pump current induced by isoproterenol. These effects

clearly cannot be explained by an increase in i_f induced by the catecholamine. Although we can only speculate about the ionic mechanism for the anomalous effect on repolarization, it is clear that the phenomenon itself could be of clinical significance. The results suggest that rapid injection of isoproterenol during attempts to increase cardiac contractility or resuscitate a patient could increase dispersion of refractoriness in the ventricles. This could promote reentrant activation and ventricular fibrillation.

Delayed Afterdepolarizations

Delayed afterdepolarizations (also called transient depolarizations and oscillatory afterpotentials) are oscillations in membrane potential that occur shortly after full repolarization (192–195). If the amplitude of a delayed afterdepolarization is large enough, it attains threshold and causes a triggered impulse. Catecholamines can induce delayed afterdepolarizations and increase triggered activity in isolated Purkinje fibers (192,196–200). The amplitude of catecholamine-induced delayed afterdepolarizations in Purkinje fibers is deter-

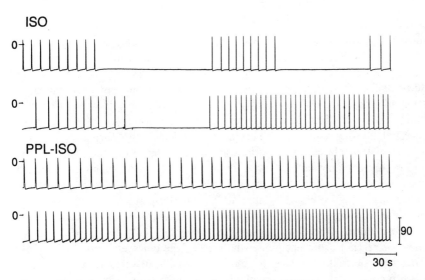

Figure 23 Induction of quiescence by isoproterenol (ISO) in two canine Purkinje fibers (top). ISO (1 μM) arrived in the tissue bath near start of each trace. The period of quiescence was generally shorter in canine Purkinje fibers than in baboon fibers. In the canine fibers, rapid automaticity occurred after the quiescent period. The quiescent period was eliminated by treating the fibers with propranolol (PPL), 0.5 μM (lower panel).

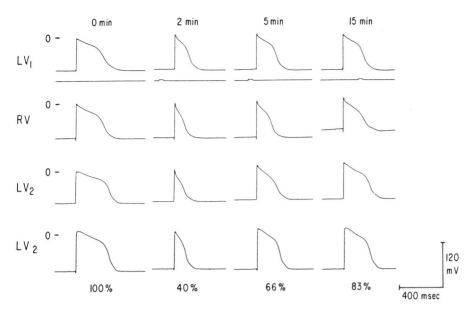

Figure 24 Decrease in action potential duration by isoproterenol in canine Purkinje fibers. Three preparations from one dog heart (two false tendons from the left ventricle and one from the right) were studied, with four simultaneous impalements. Zero reference potential at left of each row of panels; time and voltage calibration at lower right. The preparation was allowed to fire spontaneously and was periodically driven at a cycle length of 1000 msec for 10–15 beats. Polygraph traces were taken at 100 mm/sec on a Gould 2400 recorder during these stimulation periods; the last action potential of each drive train is displayed here and represents a quasi–steady-state configuration. Control records are displayed in the "0 min" column, and the effects of ISO after 2, 5, and 15 min are displayed in the next three columns. Overall, action potential duration was reduced to about 40% of control at 2 min but had recovered to 83% of control by 15 min.

mined by both the cycle length (Fig. 25) and the number of the action potentials in the train (Fig. 26) used to induce them (56).

As mentioned earlier, catecholamines augment L-calcium currents in Purkinje fibers. This tends to increase cytoplasmic calcium levels. Simultaneously, catecholamines activate phospholamban via the cAMP-protein kinase A cascade. Activated phospholamban stimulates the Ca^{2+}-ATPase of the sarcoplasmic recticulum (SR) and accelerates the rate of sequestration of cytoplasmic calcium in the

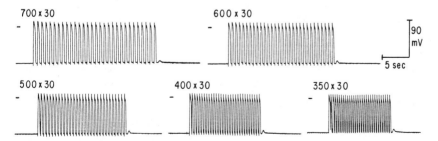

Figure 25 Delayed afterdepolarizations induced in a goat Purkinje fiber by 1 µM isoproterenol. Each panel shows the effects of a stimulus train of 30 beats at cycle lengths between 700 and 350 msec. As the cycle length decreases, the amplitude of the delayed afterdepolarizations increases, and the coupling interval decreases. Voltage and time calibrations are shown at the upper right; zero reference potential shown by horizontal mark to left of each panel.

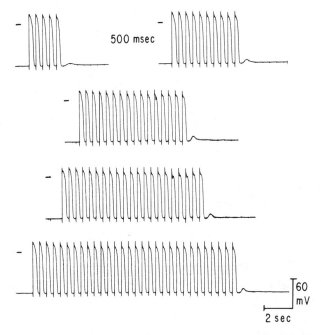

500 msec

60 mV

2 sec

Figure 26 Delayed afterdepolarizations in a goat Purkinje fiber induced by 1 μM isoproterenol. The preparation was stimulated at a cycle length of 500 msec for trains of 5–30 beats. Note that the amplitude of the delayed afterdepolarizations increases between 5 and 15–20 beats; minimal increases occur with longer stimulus trains. Same preparation as Figure 25. Reference potential marked to left of each panel; time and voltage calibrations at lower right.

SR. If stimulation by catecholamine is excessive, it may lead to "overloading" of the SR with calcium. Overloading can lead to oscillatory releases of calcium from the SR after the action potentials and in turn produces aftercontractions and delayed afterdepolarizations (201–203). The delayed afterdepolarizations result from a transient inward current (i_{TI}), which is thought to be evoked by the oscillatory calcium release. The transient inward current may reflect inward currents through either a calcium-activated nonspecific ion channel or an electrogenic Na^+-for-Ca^{2+} exchange current, or both (115,204–207).

CONCLUSION

Even though it is true that "the purpose of heart muscle is to develop tension and shorten, not to generate electrical signals" (208), over the past 40 years studies of Purkinje fiber action potentials have greatly increased our understanding of the physiology and pathology of the heart. These 40 years were the era of the microelectrode and the iso-

lated tissue preparation. Today we appear to be entering a new era, a time of membrane patch recordings, biochemical responses to receptor stimulation, cloned mutant channels, and electrical activity of reconstituted membranes. Studies of the Purkinje fiber may well be deemphasized in the future, as most of the new techniques will probably be more easily carried out in isolated ventricular myocytes or amphibian oocytes. The insights provided by these new techniques will still have to be integrated into our understanding of the physiology and pathology of the Purkinje fiber, however. This is because the cells of the His-Purkinje system play a central role in the function of the heart.

ACKNOWLEDGMENTS

The preparation of this chapter was supported by Grant HL-24354 from the NHLBI. Dr. B. F. Hoffman reviewed a preliminary version of this manuscript; his comments and suggestions are gratefully acknowledged.

REFERENCES

1. Tarawa S. Da Reizleitungssystem des Saugetierherzens. Jena: Gustav-Fischer Verlay, 1906.
2. Lewis T. The mechanism and graphic registration of the heart beat. London: Shaw, 1925.
3. Baird J A, Robb J S. Study, reconstruction, and gross dissection of the atrioventricular conducting system of the dog heart. Anat Rec 1950; 108:747–64.
4. Kugler J H, Parkin J B. Continuity of Purkinje fibres with cardiac muscle. Anat Rec 1956; 126:335–41.
5. Purkinje J G. Mikroscopisch-neurologische Beobachtungen. Arch Anat Physiol Wissensch Med 1845; 281–95.
6. Hoffman B F, Cranefield P F. Electrophysiology of the heart. New York: McGraw-Hill, 1960.
7. Ling G N, Gerard R W. The normal membrane potential of frog sartorius fibers. J Cell Comp Physiol 1949; 34:383–96.8.
8. Draper M H, Weidmann S. Cardiac resting and action potentials recorde with an intracellular electrode. J Physiol (Lond) 1951; 115:74–94.
9. Weidmann S. Effect of current flow on the membrane potential of cardiac muscle. J Physiol (Lond) 1951; 115:227–36.
10. Weidmann S. The electrical constants of Purkinje fibers. J Physiol (Lond) 1952; 118:348–60.
11. Coraboeuf E, Weidmann S. Temperature effects on the electrical activity of Purkinje fibers. Helv Physiol Pharmacol Acta 1954; 12:32–41.
12. Weidmann S. The effect of cardiac membrane potential on the rapid availability of the sodium-carrying system. J Physiol (Lond) 1955; 127:213–24.
13. Trautwein W, Gottstein U, Federschmidt K. Der Einfluss der Temperatur auf den Aktionstrom des excidierten Purkinje-Fadens, gemessen mit einer intracellularen Elektrode. Pflugers Arch Ges Physiol 1953; 258:243–60.
14. Trautwein W, Dudel J. Aktionspotential und Mechanogramm des Warmbluterherzmuskels als Funktion der Schlagfrequenz. Pflugers Arch Ges Physiol 1954; 260:24–39.
15. Dudel J, Trautwein W. Das Aktionpotential und Mechanogramm des Herzmuskels unter dem Einfluss der Dehnung. Cardiologia 1954; 25:344–62.
16. Coraboeuf E, Boistel J. L'Action des taux eleves de gaz carbonique sur le tissu cardiaque, etudiee a l'aide de microelectrodes intracellulaires. C R Soc Biol (Paris) 1953; 147:654–8.
17. Coraboeuf E, Zacouto F, Boistel J. L'Entrainment electrique du tissu cardiaque. Effets favorables sur les fibres de Purkinje. C R Soc Biol (Paris) 1954; 148:68–71.
18. Titus J L. Normal anatomy of the human cardiac conduction system. Mayo Clin Proc 1973; 48:24–30.
19. Anderson R H, Becker A E, Brechenmacher C. The human atrioventricular junctional area: a morphological study of the AV node and bundle. Eur J Cardiol 1975; 3:11–25.
20. Erickson E E, Lev M. Aging changes in the human atrioventricular node, bundle and bundle branches. J Gerontol 1952; 1:1–12.
21. Davies M J, Anderson R H, Becker A E. The conduction system of the heart. London: Butterworths, 1983; 9–94.
22. Henry C G, Lowry O H. Enzymes and metabolites of glycogen metabolism in canine cardiac Purkinje fibers. Am J Physiol 1985; 248:H599–605.
23. Henry C G, Lowry O H. Quantitative histochemistry of canine cardiac Purkinje fibres. Am J Physiol 1983; 245:H824–9.
24. Thornell L E, Eriksson A. Filament systems in the Purkinje fibers of the heart. Am J Physiol 1981; 241:H291–305.
25. Pressler M L. Cable analysis in quiescent and active sheep Purkinje fibres. J Physiol (Lond) 1984; 352:739–57.
26. Eisenberg B R, Cohn I S. The ultrastructure of the cardiac Purkinje strand in the dog. A morphometric analysis. Proc R Soc Lond [Biol] 1983; 217:191–213.
27. Dangman K H, Dresdner K P, Michler R E. Transmembrane action potentials and intracellular K+ activity of baboon cardiac tissues. Cardiovascu Res 1988; 22:204–12.
28. Dangman K H, Hoffman B F. Effects of single premature stimuli on automatic and triggered rhythms in isolated canine Purkinje fibers. Circulation 1985; 71:813–22.
29. Hodgkin A L, Huxley A F, Katz B. Measurement of current voltage relations in the membrane of the giant axon of Loligo. J Physiol (Lond) 1952; 116:424–48.
30. Hodgkin A L, Huxley A F. A quantitative description of membrane currents and its application to conduction and excitation in nerve. J Physiol (Lond) 1952; 117:500–44.

31. Noda M, Shimizu S, Tanabe T, et al. Primary structure of electrophorus electricus sodium channel deduced from cDNA sequence. Nature 1984; 312:121–7.

32. Catterall W A. Structure and function of voltage sensitive ion channels. Science 1988; 242:50–61.

33. Hille B. Gating in sodium channels of nerve. Annu Rev Physiol 1976; 38:139–52.

34. Barry P H, McLachlan E M. Electrochemistry of membranes and excitable cells. In: Eckert GM, Gutmann F, Keyzer H, eds. Electropharmacology. Boca Raton, Fl: CRC Press, 1990:107–38.

35. Mary-Rabine L, Hoffman B F, Rosen M R. Participation of the slow inward current in the Purkinje fiber action potential overshoot. Am J Physiol 1979; 237:H201–12.

36. Strichartz G, Cohen I. $\dot{V}_{max}$ as a measure of G_{Na} in nerve and cardiac membranes. Biophys J 1978; 23:153–6.

37. Cohen I, Attwell D, Strichartz G. The dependence of the maximum rate of rise of the action potential upstroke on membrane properties. Proc R Soc Lond [Biol] 1981; 214:85–98.

38. Cohen C J, Bean B P, Tsien R W. Maximal upstroke velocity ($\dot{V}_{max}$) as an index of available sodium conductance. Comparison of $\dot{V}_{max}$ and voltage clamp measurements of I_{Na} in rabbit Purkinje fibers. Circ Res 1984; 54:636–51.

39. Hondeghem L. Letter to the editor. Circ Res 1985; 57:192–3.

40. Peon J, Ferrier G R, Moe G K. The relationship of excitability to conduction velocity in canine Purkinje tissue. Circ Res 1978; 43:125–35.

41. Colatsky T J. Voltage clamp measurements of sodium channel properties in rabbit cardiac Purkinje fibers. J Physiol (Lond) 1980; 305:215–34.

42. Kass R S, Siegelbaum S A, Tsien R W. Three microelectrode voltage clamp experiments in calf cardiac Purkinje fibers. Is slow inward current adequately measured? J Physiol (Lond) 1979; 290:201–25.

43. Lee K S, Weeks T A, Kao R L, Akaike N, Brown B M. Sodium current in single heart muscle cells. Nature 1979; 278:269–71.

44. Brown B M, Lee K S, Powell T. Sodium current in single rat heart muscle cells. J Physiol (Lond) 1981; 318:479–500.

45. Colquhoun D, Neher E, Reuter H, Stevens C F. Inward current channels activated by intracellular Ca in cultured cardiac cells. Nature 1981; 294:752–4.

46. Nilius B, Hess P, Lansman J B, Tsien R W. A novel type of cardiac calcium channel in ventricular cells. Nature 1985; 316:443–6.

47. Lansman J B, Hess P, Tsien R W. Blockade of currents through single calcium channels by Cd^{2+}, Mg^{2+}, and Ca^{2+}. Voltage and concentration dependence of calcium entry into the pore. J Gen Physiol 1986; 88:321–47.

48. Makielski J C, Sheets M F, Hanck D A. Sodium current in voltage clamped internally perfused canine cardiac Purkinje fibers. Biophys J 1987; 52:1–11.

49. Sheets M F, Hanck D A, Fozzard H A. Nonlinear relation between $\dot{V}_{max}$ and I_{Na} in canine cardiac Purkinje cells. Circ Res 1988; 63:386–98.

50. Sutton F, Davidson N, Lester H A. Tetrodotoxin sensitive voltage-dependent Na currents recorded from *Xenopus* oocytes injected with mammalian cardiac muscle RNA. Mol Brain Res 1988; 3:187–92.

51. Vassivlev P M, Scheuer T, Catterall W A. Identification of an intracellular peptide segment involved in sodium channel inactivation. Science 1989; 241:1658–61.

52. Stuhmer W, Conti F., Suzuki H. Structural parts involved in activation and inactivation of the sodium channel. Nature 1989; 339:597–603.

53. Myerburg R J, Gelband H, Hoffman B F. Functional characteristics of the gating mechanism in the canine A-V conducting system. Circ Res 1971; 28:136–47.

54. Lazzara R, El-Sherif N, Befeler B, Scherlag B J. Regional refractoriness within the ventricular conduction system. An evaluation of the "gate" hypothesis. Circ Res 1976; 39:254–62.

55. Drury A N, Love W S. The supposed lengthening of the absolute refractory period of frog's ventricular muscle by veratrine. Heart 1926; 13:77–84.

56. Dangman K H, Boyden P A. Cellular mechanisms of cardiac arrhythmias. In: Fox PR, ed. Canine and feline cardiology. New York: Churchill Livingstone, 1988:269–87.

57. Siegelbaum S A, Tsien R W. Calcium-activated transient outward current in calf Purkinje fibers. J Physiol (Lond) 1980; 299:485–506.

58. Fozzard H A, Hiraoka M. The positive dynamic current and its inactivation properties

in cardiac Purkinje fibers. J Physiol (Lond) 1973; 239:211–40.

59. Kenyon J L, Gibbons W R. 4-Aminopyridine and the early outward current of sheep cardiac Purkinje fibers. J Gen Physiol 1979; 73:139–57.

60. Kenyon J L, Gibbons W R. Influence of chloride, potassium, and tetraethylammonium on the early outward current of sheep cardiac Purkinje fibers. J Gen Physiol 1979; 73:117–38.

61. Dudel J, Peper K, Rudel R, Trautwein W. The dynamic chloride current in Purkinje fibers. Pfugers Arch 1967; 295:197–212.

62. Coraboeuf E, Carmeliet E. Existence of two transient outward currents in sheep cardiac Purkinje fibers. Pflugers Arch 1982; 392:352–9.

63. Berger F, Borchard U, Hafner D. Effects of the calcium entry blocker bepridil on repolarizing and pacemaker currents in sheep cardiac Purkinje fibers. Naunyn Schmiedebergs Arch Pharmacol 1989; 339:638–46.

64. Siegelbaum S A, Tsien R W, Kass R S. Role of intracellular calcium in the transient outward current of calf Purkinje fibers. Nature 1977; 269:611–3.

65. Callewaert G, Vereecke J, Carmeliet E. Existence of a calcium-dependent potassium channel in the membrane of cow cardiac Purkinje cells. Pflugers Arch 1986; 406:424–6.

66. Coraboeuf E, Deroubaix E, Coulombe A. Effect of tetrodotoxin on action potentials of the conducting system in the dog heart. Am J Physiol 1979; 236:H561–7.

67. Gintant G A, Daytner N, Cohen I S. Slow inactivation of a tetrodotoxin sensitive current in canine cardiac Purkinje fibers. Biophys J 1984; 45:509–12.

68. Carmeliet E. Voltage dependent block by tetrodotoxin of the sodium channel in rabbit cardiac Purkinje fibers. Biophys J 1987; 51:109–14.

69. Attwell D, Cohen I S, Eisner D, Ohba M, Ojeda C. The steady state TTX-sensitive (window) sodium current in cardiac Purkinje fibers. Pflugers Arch 1979; 379:137–41.

70. Tsien R W, Hess P, McCleskey E W, et al. Calcium channels: mechanisms of selectivity, permeation, and block. Annu Rev Biophys Chem 1987; 16:265–90.

71. Tseng G N, Boyden P A. Multiple types of Ca currents in single canine Purkinje cells. Circ Res 1989; 65:1735–50.

72. Hirano Y, Fozzard H A, January C T. Characteristics of L- and T-type Ca^{++} currents in canine cardiac Purkinje cells. Am J Physiol 1989; 256:H1476–92.

73. Hagiwara N, Irisawa H, Kameyama M. Contribution of two types of calcium currents to the pacemaker potentials of rabbit sino-atrial node cells. J Physiol (Lond) 1986; 395:233–53.

74. McAllister R E, Noble D. The time and voltage dependence of the slow outward current in cardiac Purkinje fibres. J Physiol (Lond) 1966; 186:632–62.

75. Noble D, Tsien R W. Outward membrane currents activated in the plateau range of potentials in cardiac Purkinje fibres. J Physiol (Lond) 1969; 200:205–31.

76. Kass R S. Delayed rectification in the cardiac Purkinje fiber is not activated by intracellular calcium. Biophys J 1984; 45:837–9.

77. Gintant G A, Datyner N B, Cohen I S. Gating of delayed rectification in acutely isolated canine cardiac Purkinje myocytes. Evidence of a single voltage gated conductance. Biophys J 1985; 48:1059–64.

78. Bennett P B, McKinney L C, Kass R S, Begenisich T. Delayed rectification in the calf cardiac Purkinje fiber. Evidence for multiple state kinetics. Biophys J 1985; 48:553–67.

79. Bennett P, McKinney L, Begenisich T, Kass R S. Adrenergic modulation of the delayed rectifier potassium channel in calf cardiac Purkinje fibers. Biophys J 1986; 49:839–48.

80. Kenyon J L. Sutko J L. Calcium- and voltage activated plateau currents of cardiac Purkinje fibers. J Gen Physiol 1987; 89:921–58.

81. Carmeliet E, Biermans G, Callewaert G, Vereeke J. Potassium currents in cardiac cells. Experientia 1987; 43:1175–84.

82. Shah A K, Cohen I S, Datyner N B. Background K current in isolated canine cardiac Purkinje myocytes. Biophys J 1987; 52:519–25.

83. Cohen I S, DiFrancesco D, Mulrine N K, Pennefeather P. Internal and external K^{+} help gate the inward rectifier. Biophys J 1989; 55:197–202.

84. Bennett P B, Kass R, Begenisich T. Nonstationary fluctuation analysis of the delayed rectifier K channel in cardiac Purkinje fibers. Actions of norepinephrine on single channel current. Biophys J 1989; 55:731–8.

85. DiFrancesco D, Noble D. A model of cardiac electrical activity incorporating ionic

pumps and concentration changes. Philos Trans R Soc Lond [Biol] 1985; 307:335–98.

86. Boyett M R. A study of the effect of the rate of stimulation on the transient outward current in sheep cardiac Purkinje fibres. J Physiol (Lond) 1981; 319:1–22.

87. Boyett M R. Effects of rate-dependent changes in the transient outward current on the action potential of sheep Purkinje fibers. J Physiol (Lond) 1981; 319:23–41.

88. Gintant G A, Cohen I S. Advances in cardiac cellular electrophysiology: implications for automaticity and therapeutics. Annu Rev Pharmacol Toxicol 1988; 28:61–81.

89. Jaeger J M, Gibbons W R. A re-examination of the late outward plateau currents of cardiac Purkinje fibers. Am J Physiol 1985; 249:H108–21.

90. Jaeger J M, Gibbons W R. Slow inward current may produce many results attributed to $i_{x,1}$ in cardiac Purkinje fibers. Am J Physiol 1985; 249:H122–32.

91. Baumgarten M C, Isenberg G, McDonald T, Ten Eick R E. Depletion and accumulation of potassium in the extracellular clefts of cardiac Purkinje fibers during voltage clamp hyperpolarization and depolarization. J Gen Physiol 1977; 70:149–69.

92. Cohen I S, Kline P R. K fluctuations in the extracellular space of cardiac muscle: evidence from voltage clamp and extracellular K selective microelectrodes. Circ Res 1982; 50:1–16.

93. Levis R A, Mathias R T, Eisenberg R S. Electrical properties of sheep Purkinje strands. Electrical and chemical potentials in the clefts. Biophys J 1983; 44:225–48.

94. Robinson R B, Boyden P A, Hoffman B F, Hewett KW. Electrical restitution process in dispersed canine cardiac Purkinje and ventricular cells. Am J Physiol 1987; 253:H1018–25.

95. Kline R P, Cohen I S, Falk R, Kupersmith J. Activity dependent extracellular K fluctuations in canine Purkinje fibers. Nature 1980; 286:68–71.

96. Kline R P, Kupersmith J. Effects of extracellular potassium accumulation and sodium pump activation on automatic canine Purkinje fibers. J Physiol (Lond) 1982; 324:507–33.

97. Kline R P, Morad M. Potassium efflux in heart muscle during activity. Extracellular accumulation and its implications. J Physiol (Lond) 1978; 280:537–58.

98. Tohse N, Kemeyama M, Irisawa H. Intracellular Ca^{++} and protein kinase C modulate K^+ current in guinea pig heart cells. Am J Physiol 1987; 253:H1321–4.

99. Walsh K B, Kass R S. Regulation of a heart potassium channel by protein kinase A and C. Science 1988; 242:67–9.

100. Scamps F, Carmeliet E. Delayed K current and external K in single cardiac Purkinje cells. Am J Physiol 1989; 257:C1086–92.

101. Hall A, Hutter O, Noble D. Current-voltage relations of Purkinje fibres in sodium deficient solutions. J Physiol (Lond) 1963; 166:225–40.

102. Giles W, Imaizumi Y. Comparison of potassium currents in rabbit atrial and ventricular cells. J Physiol (Lond) 1988; 405:123–45.

103. Carmeliet E. Induction and removal of inward-going rectification in sheep cardiac Purkinje fibers. J Physiol (Lond) 1982; 327:285–308.

104. Beeler G W, Reuter H. Reconstruction of the action potential of ventricular myocardial fibres. J Physiol (Lond) 1977; 268:177–210.

105. Koch-Weser J, Blinks J R. The influence of the interval between beats on myocardial contractility. Pharmacol Rev 1963; 15:601–52.

106. Saitoh H, Bailey J C, Surawicz B. Action potential duration alternans in dog Purkinje and ventricular muscle fibers. Further evidence in support of two mechanisms. Circulation 1989; 80:1421–31.

107. Tchou P J, Lehmenn M H, Dongas J, Mahmud R, Denker S T, Aktar M. Effect of sudden rate acceleration on the human His-Purkinje system: adaptation of refractoriness in a dampened oscillatory pattern. Circulation 1986; 73:920–9.

108. Vassalle M. Cardiac automaticity and its control. Am J Physiol 1977; 233:H625–34.

109. Gadsby D C, Cranefield P F. Effects of electrogenic sodium extrusion on the membrane potential of cardiac Purkinje fibers. In: Normal and abnormal conduction in the heart. Paes de Carvalho A, Hoffman B, Lieberman M, eds. Mt. Kisco, NY: Futura, 1982: 225–46.

110. Weidmann S. Heart: electrophysiology. Annu Rev Physiol 1974; 155–69.

111. Attwell D, Cohn I, Eisner D A. The effects of heart rate on the action potential of guinea pig and human ventricular muscle. J Physiol (Lond) 1981; 313:439–61.

112. Dangman K H, Hoffman B F. Studies on overdrive stimulation of canine cardiac Purkinje fibers: maximal diastolic potential as a determinant of the response. J Am Coll Cardiol 1983; 2:1183–90.

113. Browning D J, Strauss H C. Effects of stimulation frequency on potassium activity and cell volume in cardiac tissue. Am J Physiol 1981; 240:C39–55.

114. Vassalle M. Electrogenic suppression of automaticity in sheep and dog Purkinje fibers. Circ Res 1970; 27:361–77.

115. Noble D. The surprising heart: a review of recent progress in cardiac electrophysiology. J Physiol (Lond) 1984; 353:1–50.

116. DeFrancesco D. A new interpretation of the pace-maker current in calf Purkinje fibres. A study of the ionic nature of the pace-maker current in calf Purkinje fibers. J Physiol (Lond) 1981; 314:359–93.

117. DeFrancesco D. Characterization of the pace-maker current kinetics in calf Purkinje fibres. J Physiol (Lond) 1984; 348:341–67.

118. Glitsch H G, Pusch H, Verdonck F. The contribution of Na and K ions to the pacemaker current in sheep cardiac Purkinje fibres. Pflugers Arch 1986; 406:464–71.

119. Coulombe A, Coraboeuf E. Simulation of potassium accumulation in clefts of Purkinje fibers: effect on membrane electrical activity. J Theor Biol 1983; 104:211–29.

120. Dangman K H, Miura D S. Does i_f control normal automatic rate in canine cardiac Purkinje fibers? Studies on the negative chronotropic effects of lidoflazine. J Cardiovasc Pharmacol 1987; 10:332–40.

121. Hart G, Dukes I D. An analysis of the rate-dependent action of lidoflazine in mammalian sinoatrial node and Purkije fibers. J Mol Cell Cardiol 1984; 16:33–42.

122. Boyden P A, Dresdner K P. Electrogenic Na^+-K^+ pump in Purkinje myocytes isolated from control noninfarcted and infarcted hearts. Am J Physiol 1990; 258:H766–72.

123. Dangman K H, Hoffman B F. Antiarrhythmic effects of ethmozin in cardiac Purkinje fibers: suppression of automaticity and abolition of triggering. J Pharmacol Exp Ther 1983; 227:578–86.

124. LeMarec H, Dangman K H, Danilo P, Rosen M R. An evaluation of automaticity and triggered activity in the canine heart 1 to 4 days after myocardial infarction. Circulation 1985; 71:1224–36.

125. Dangman K H, Dresdner K P, Zaim S. Automatic and triggered impulse initiation in canine subepicardial ventricular muscle cells from border zones of 24 hr transmural infarcts. New mechanisms for malignant cardiac arrhythmias? Circulation 1988; 78:1020–30.

126. Singer D H, Lazzara R, Hoffman B F. Interrelationships between automaticity and conduction in Purkinje fibers. Circ Res 1967; 21:537–53.

127. Wissner S B. The effects of excess lactate on the excitability of sheep Purkinje fibers. J Electrocardiol 1974; 7:17–26.

128. Arnsdorf M F, Sawicki G J. The effects of lysophosphatidylcholine, a toxic metabolite of ischemia, on the components of cardiac excitability in sheep Purkinje fibers. Circ Res 1981; 49:16–30.

129. Corr P B, Snyder D W, Caine M E, Crafford W A, Gross R W, Sobel B E. Electrophysiological effects of amphiphiles on canine Purkinje fibers. Circ Res 1981; 49:354–63.

130. Lazzara R, El Sherif N, Scherlag B J. Electrophysiological properties of canine Purkinje cells in one-day-old myocardial infarction. Circ Res 1973; 33:722–34.

131. Friedman P L, Stewart J R, Wit A L. Spontaneous and induced cardiac arrhythmias in subendocardial Purkinje fibers surviving extensive myocardial infarction. Circ Res 1973; 33:612–26.

132. Allen J D, Wit A L. Some observations on abnormal pacemaker activity in endocardial Purkinje fibers surviving myocardial infarction. J Physiol (Lond) 1976; 263:248–9P.

133. Allen J D, Brennan F J, Wit A L. Actions of lidocaine on transmembrane potentials of subendocardial Purkinje fibers surviving in infarcted canine hearts. Circ Res 1978; 43:470–81.

134. El Harrar V, Zipes D P. Voltage modulation of automaticity in cardiac Purkinje fibers. In: Zipes D P, Bailey J C, El Harrar V, eds., The slow inward current and cardiac arrhythmias. 1980:357–73.

135. Dangman K H, Hoffman B F. The effects of EN-313 on abnormal automaticity in canine cardiac Purkinje fibers. Circulation 1978; 58:II–104.

136. Dangman K H, Hoffman B F. The effects of nifedipine on abnormal automaticity in canine cardiac Purkinje fibers. Circulation 1979; 60:II–209.

137. Hiraoka M, Ikeda K, Sano T. The mechanism of Ba-induced automaticity in ventricular muscle fibers. J Mol Cell Cardiol 1978; 10:I–35.

138. Hermsmeyer K, Sperelakis N. Decrease in K^+ conductance and depolarization in frog cardiac mucle produced by Ba^{++}, Am J Physiol 1970; 219:1108–14.

139. Ehara T, Inazawa M. Calcium dependent slow action potentials in potassium depolarized guinea pig ventricular myocardium enhanced by barium ions. Naunyn Schmeidebergs Arch Pharmacol 1980; 315:47–54.

140. Hauswirth O, Noble D, Tsien R W. The mechanism of oscillatory activity at low membrane potentials in cardiac Purkinje fibers. J Physiol (Lond) 1969; 200:255–65.

141. Escande D, Coraboeuf E, Planche C. Abnormal pacemaking is modulated by sarcoplasmic reticulum in partially depolarized myocardium from dilated right atria in humans. J Mol Cell Cardiol 1987; 19: 231–41.

142. Innes I R, Nickerson M. Drugs acting on postganglionic adrenergic nerve endings and structures innervated by them (sympathomimetic drugs). In: Goodman LS, Gilman A, eds. The Pharmacological basis of therapeutics, 4th ed. New York: Macmillan, 1970:478–523.

143. Kaumann A J. Is there a thrid heart β-adrenoceptor? Trends Pharmacol Sci (TIPS) 1989; 10:316–20.

144. Prichard B N C. Beta adrenoceptor blocking drugs. In: Hombach V, Hilger HH, Kennedy HL, eds. Electrocardiography and cardiac drug therapy. Kluwer, Dordrecht: 1989:298–322.

145. Liang B T, Frame L H, Molinoff P B. $β_2$-Adrenergic receptors contribute to catecholamine stimulated shortening of action potential duration in dog atria. Proc Natl Acad Sci USA 1985; 82:4521–5.

146. Brodde OE. The functional importance of $β_1$ and $β_2$-adrenoceptors in the human heart. Am J Cardiol 1988; 62:24C–9C.

147. Gilman A G.. G proteins and regulation of adenyl cyclase. JAMA 1989; 262:1819–25.

148. Cohen P. Protein phosphorylation and hormone action. Proc R Soc Lond 1988; 234:115–44.

149. Yatani A, Brown A M. Rapid β-adrenergic modulation of calcium currents by a fast G protein pathway. Science 1989; 245:71–4.

150. Schubert B, VanDongen A, Kirsch E, et al. β-Adrenergic inhibition of cardiac sodium channels by dual G-protein pathways. Science 1989; 245:516–9.

151. Lindemann J, Jones L, Hathaway D, et al. Beta-adrenergic stimulation of phospholamban phosphorylation and Ca^{+2} ATPase activity in guinea pig ventricles. J Biol Chem 1983; 258:464–71.

152. Insel P A, Rasnas L A. G proteins and cardiovascular disease. Circulation 1988; 78:1511–3.

153. Brown A M, Birnbaumer L. Direct G protein gating of ion channels. Am J Physiol 1988; 254:H401–10.

154. Tsien R W. Adrenaline-like effects of intracellular iontophoresis of cyclic AMP in cardiac Purkinje fibers. Nature New Biol 1973; 245:120–2.

155. Tsien R W, Giles W, Greengard P. Cyclic AMP mediates the effects of adrenaline on cardiac Purkinje fibers. Nature New Biol 1972; 240:181–3.

156. Giotti A, Ledda F, Mannaioni P F. Effects of noradrenaline and isoprenaline, in combination with α- and β-receptor blocking substances, on the action potential of cardiac Purkinje fibers. J Physiol (Lond) 1973; 220:99–113.

157. Rosen M, Hordof A, Ilvecto J P, Danilo P. Effects of adrenergic amines on electrophysiological properties and automaticity of neonatal and adult cardiac Purkinje fibers. Circ Res 1977; 40:390–400.

158. Kass R S, Wiegers S E. The ionic basis of concentration related effects of noradrenaline on the action potential of calf cardiac Purkinje fibres. J Physiol (Lond) 1982; 322:541–58.

159. Rosen M, Weiss R M, Danilo P. Effect of alpha adrenergic agonists and blockers on Purkinje fiber transmembrane potentials and automaticity in the dog. J Pharmacol Exp Ther 1984; 231:566–71.

160. Bennett P, McKinney L, Begenisich T, Kass R S. Adrenergic modulation of the delayed rectifier potassium channel in calf cardiac Purkinje fibers. Biophys J 1986; 49:839–48.

161. Bennett P, Begenisich T. Catecholamines modulate the delayed rectifying potassium current in guinea pig ventricular myocytes. Pflugers Arch 1987; 410:217–9.

162. Walsh K. Begenisich T, Kass R S. Beta adrenergic modulation of cardiac ion channels. J Gen Physiol 1989; 93:841–54.

163. Reuter H. Calcium channel modulation by neurotransmitters, enzymes, and drugs. Nature 1983; 301:569–74.

164. Kameyama M, Hofmann F, Trautwein W. On the mechanism of β-adrenergic regulation of the Ca channel in the guinea pig heart. Pflugers Arch 1985; 405:285–93.

165. Trautwein W, Hescheler J. Regulation of cardiac L-type calcium current by phosphorylation and G proteins. Annu Rev Physiol 1990; 52:257–74.

166. Isenberg G. Cardiac Purkinje fibres. [Ca^{++}], controls the potassium permeability via the conductance components g_{k1} and g_{k2} Pflugers Arch 1977; 371:77–85.

167. Desilets M, Baumgarten C M. Isoproterenol directly stimulates the Na^+-K^+ pump in isolated cardiac myocytes. Am J Physiol 1986; 251:H218–25.

168. Lee C O, Vasalle M. Modulation of intracellular Na^+ activity and cardiac force by norepinephrine and Ca^{++}. Am J Physiol 1983; 244:C110–4.

169. Wasserstrom J A, Schwartz D, Fozzard H A. Catecholamine effects on intracellular sodium activity and tension in dog heart. Am J Physiol 1982; 243:H670–5.

170. Gadsby D C. Influence of the sodium pump current on electrical activity of cardiac cells. In: Blaustein M P, Lieberman M, eds. Electrogenic transport: fundamental principles and physiological implications. New York: Raven Press, 1984:215–38.

171. Shah A, Cohen I S, Rosen M R. Stimulation of cardiac alpha receptors increases Na/K pump current and decreases g_K via a pertussis toxin-sensitive pathway. Biophys J 1988; 54:219–25.

172. Vassalle M, Barnabei O. Norepinephrine and potassium fluxes in cardiac Purkinje fibers. Pflugers Arch 1971; 322:287–303.

173. Posner P, Vassalle M. The inhibitory action of norepinephrine on potassium uptake in cardiac Purkinje fibers. Life Sci 1971; 1:67–78.

174. Otsuka M. Die Wirkung von Adrenalin auf Purkinje-Fasern von Saugetierherzen. Pflugers Arch 1958; 266:512–7 (with a correction in Pflugers Arch 1958; 267:312).

175. Grabowski W, Luttgau H C, Schulze J J. The effects of isoprenaline and a new β-sympathomimetic amine upon spontaneous activity, diastolic depolarization, and plateau height in cardiac Purkinje fibres. Br J Pharmacol 1978; 63:427–34.

176. Danilo P, Vulliemoz Y, Verosky M, Rosen M R. Epinephrine induced automaticity of canine cardiac Purkinje fibers and its relationship to the adenylate cyclase adenosine 3',5'-monophosphate system. J Pharmacol Exp Ther 1978; 205:175–82.

177. Hordof A J, Rose E, Danilo P, Rosen M. Alpha- and beta-adrenergic effects of epinephrine on ventricular pacemakers in dogs. Am J Physiol 1982; 242:H677–82.

178. Han J, Cameron J S. Effects of epinephrine on automaticity of Purkinje fibers from infarcted ventricles. In: Zipes D, Jalife J, eds. Cardiac electrophysiology and arrhythmias. New York: Grune & Stratton, 1985: 331–5.

179. Hauswirth O, Noble D, Tsien R W. Adrenaline: mechanism of action on the pacemaker potential in cardiac Purkinje fibers. Science 1968; 162:916–7.

180. Tsien R W. Effects of epinephrine on the pacemaker potassium current of cardiac Purkinje fibers. J Gen Physiol 1974; 64:293–319.

181. Tsien R W. Mode of action of chronotropic agents in cardiac Purkinje fibers. Does epinephrine act by directly modifying the external surface charge? J Gen Physiol 1974; 64:320–42.

182. Glitsch H G, Rasch R. An effect of noradrenaline on resting potential and Na activity in sheep cardiac Purkinje fibres. Pflugers Arch 1986; 406:144–50.

183. Terris S, Wasserstrom J A, Fozzard H A. Depolarizing effects of catecholamines in quiescent sheep cardiac Purkinje fibres. Am J Physiol 1986; 251:H1056–61.

184. Chang F, Gao J, Tromba C, Cohen I, DeFrancesco D. Acetylcholine reverses effects of β-agonists on pacemaker current in canine cardiac Purkinje fibers but has no direct action. Circ Res 1990; 66:633–6.

185. Posner P, Farrar E L, Lambert C R. Inhibitory effects of catecholamines in canine cardiac Purkinje fibers. Am J Physiol 1976; 231:1415–20.

186. Rosen M R, Mary-Rabine L, Danilo P, Hordof A J. Alpha and beta-adrenergic effects on cardiac arrhythmias due to automaticity. In: Braunwald E, ed., Beta-adrenergic blockade, a new era in cardiovascular medicine. Amsterdam: Princeton Exerpta Medica, 1978: 179–89.

187. Reder R F, Danilo P, Rosen M R. Developmental changes in alpha adrenergic effects

on canine Purkinje fiber automaticity. Dev Pharmacol Ther 1984; 7:94–108.

188. Rosen M R, Steinberg S, Chow Y K, Bilezikian J P, Danilo P. Role of a pertussis toxin sensitive protein in the modulation of canine Purkinje fiber automaticity. Circ Res 1988; 62:315–23.

189. Zaza A, Kline R P, Rosen M R. Effects of alpha adrenergic stimulation on intracellular sodium activity and automaticity in canine Purkinje fibers. Circ Res 1990; 66:416–26.

190. Hamra M, Rosen M R. Alpha adrenergic receptor stimulation during simulated ischemia and reperfusion in canine cardiac Purkinje fibers. Circulation 1988; 78:1495–502.

191. Amerini S, Piazzesi G, Giotti A, Mugelli A. Alpha adrenoceptor stimulation enhances automaticity in barium-treated cardiac Purkinje fibers. Arch Int Pharmacodyn Ther 1984; 270:97–105.

192. Mugelli A, Amerini S, Piazzesi G, Cerbai E, Giotti A. Enhancement by norepinephrine of automaticity in sheep cardiac Purkinje fibers exposed to hypoxic glucose-free Tyrode's solution: a role for alpha adrenoceptors? Circulation 1986; 73:180–8.

193. Ferrier G R, Moe G K. Effect of calcium on acetylstrophanthidin-induced transient depolarizations in canine Purkinje tissue. Circ Res 1973; 33:508–15.

194. Ferrier G R, Saunders J H, Mendez C. A cellular mechanism for the generation of ventricular arrhythmias by strophanthidin. Circ Res 1973; 32:600–9.

195. Cranefield P F. Action potentials, afterpotentials and arrhythmias. Circ Res 1977; 41:415–23.

196. Dangman K H, Danilo P, Hordof A J, Mary-Rabine L, Reder R F, Rosen M R. Electrophysiologic characteristics of human ventricular and Purkinje fibers. Circulation 1982; 65:362–8.

197. Valenzuela F, Vassalle M. Interaction between overdrive excitation and overdrive suppression in canine Purkinje fibers. Cardiovasc Res 1983; 10:608–19.

198. Coetzee W A, Dennis S C, Opie L H, Muller C A. Calcium channel blockers and early ischemia arrhythmias. Electrophysiological versus anti-ischemic effects. J Mol Cell Cardiol 1987; 19(Suppl. II):77–97.

199. Adamantidis M M, Caron J F, Dupuis B A. Triggered activity induced by combined mild hypoxia and acidosis in guinea pig Purkinje fibers. J Mol Cell Cardiol 1986; 18:1287–99.

200. Hewett K, Rosen M R. β-Adrenergic modulation of digitalis induced delayed afterdolarizations and triggered activity. Am J Cardiol 1982; 49:913–8.

201. Fabiato A, Fabiato F. Contractions induced by a calcium triggered release from the sarcoplasmic reticulum of single skinned cardiac cells. J Physiol (Lond) 1975; 249:469–95.

202. Allen D G, Eisner D A, Orchard C H. Oscillations of intracellular [Ca^{++}] in resting ferret cardiac muscle. J Physiol (Lond) 1983; 345:23P.

203. Hiraoka M, Kawano S. Regulation of delayed afterdepolarizations and aftercontractions in dog ventricular muscle fibres. J Mol Cell Cardiol 1984; 16:285–9.

204. Vassalle M, Mugelli A. An oscillatory current in sheep cardiac Purkinje fibers. Circ Res 1981; 48:618–31.

205. Eisner D A. The role of intracellular Ca ions in the therapeutic and toxic effects of cardiac glycosides and catecholamines. J Cardiovasc Pharmacol 1986; 8(Suppl.3):S2–9.

206. Lederer W J, Tsien R W. Transient inward current underlying arrhythmogenic effects of cardiotonic steroids in Purkinje fibers. J Physiol (Lond) 1976; 263:73–100.

207. Tsien R W, Kass R S, Weingart R. Cellular and subcellular mechanisms of cardiac pacemaker oscillations. J Exp Biol 1979; 81:205–15.

208. Fozzard H A, Gibbons W R. Action potential and contraction of heart muscle. Am J Cardiol 1973; 31:182–92.

9

Electrophysiology of Mammalian Ventricular Muscle

J. Andrew Wasserstrom and Robert E. Ten Eick

Northwestern University
Chicago, Illinois

INTRODUCTION

Channel Function and the ECG

Normally the cardiac impulse is initiated by specialized pacemaker cells of the sinoatrial node (SAN). It spreads from the SAN to excite the atrial myocardium, propagates to the atrioventricular node (AVN), conducts slowly through this structure, and then enters the His bundle, the bundle branches, and Purkinje fibers to spread rapidly to and activate the ventricular myocardium. The various cells in the heart also repolarize sequentially and are then ready for another activation sequence. The electrocardiogram (ECG) is a voltage signal generated by the heart that is detected at the body surface. It reflects the vector strength and direction of the electrical field generated by the integrated cellular currents underlying the conducted electrical excitatory event associated with the propagation of cellular action potentials throughout the heart. The most prominent feature of the ECG is the R wave, the next most prominent feature being the T wave. Both reflect the mean integrated electrophysiologic activity of ventricular cells, with the R wave reflecting depolarization and

the T wave reflecting repolarization (see Fig. 1). It follows that the QT interval reflects the mean integrated duration of action potentials elicited by the cells of the ventricle. We now know that the depolarization is mediated by membrane current governed by Na and/or Ca channels, that repolarization is governed by a mix of K channels, and that the action potential duration is derived from an interplay between the several aforementioned channels (and perhaps even still other channels). In the final analysis, clearly, it is the membrane ion channels that define the waveform of the electrocardiogram and govern the electrical activity of the ventricles as well as the whole heart.

Heart Disease and Cardiac Drugs Alter Cellular Electrophysiology by Altering Ion Channel Function

If the cardiologist arrhythmologist, cardiac electrophysiologist (either clinical or research), or student attempting to fathom the heart is to understand the electrophysiology of the ventricle at a level beyond this very simple analysis, he or she must understand the electrophysiology of ventricular cells; this understanding should even extend beyond the level of the sarcolemmal membrane per se to that of the ion channels regulating the transmembrane ion fluxes that underlie cellular action potentials and transmembrane currents. This is particularly true if one hopes to understand the effects of disease that make "sick" hearts more prone to rhythm disturbances than "normal, healthy" hearts and the effects of pharmacologic agents used clinically to suppress the risk of sudden death often associated with these rhythm disturbances.

DESCRIPTION OF THE VENTRICULAR RESTING AND ACTION POTENTIALS

Resting Potential and Its Origin

The resting potential of most normal, healthy cardiac ventricular cells ranges from -80 to -95 mV. During the diastolic or resting period, termed phase 4, cardiac fibers sustain a transmembrane resting potential because the membrane is selectively permeable to K ions and because an active transport mechanism maintains the concentration gradients for Na^+ and K^+ such that intracellular potassium concentration $[K^+]_i$ is higher than the extracellular value $[K^+]_o$ and the intracellular sodium concentration $[Na^+]_i$ is lower than the extracellular concentration $[Na^+]_o$. In the resting state the transmembrane potential is determined largely by the ratio of $[K^+]_i$ to $[K^+]_o$ and by the permeability of the membrane to K^+ relative to the permeabilities for other important ions, such as Na^+, Ca^{2+}, and Cl^-. Resting potential approaches but usually does not quite equal the potassium equilibrium potential E_K, defined by the Nernst equation (i.e., $E_K = RT/F$ ln $([K^+]_o/[K^+]_i)$; or at 37°C, $E_K = 61$ log $([K^+]_o/[K^+]_i)$. A better prediction of resting potential can be derived using an equation based on the now classic Goldman-Hodgkin-Katz (GHK) formulation

where V_{rest} is resting potential; P_K, P_{Na}, P_{Ca}, and so on, are the permeability coefficients for the subscripted ion species; and $[K^+]_i$ and $[K^+]_o$, etc. are the intra- and extracellular activities for each of the ion species identified by subscript (the activity of ion A = the concentration of A × its activity coefficient).

The GHK equation is based on the assumption of steady state and therefore probably applies to the membrane voltage only at the end of fairly long but otherwise normal diastolic intervals. When the K permeability decreases or the Na or Ca permeabilities increase, cardiac cells depolarize from their normal resting potentials to levels that may be as low as -40 to -50 mV. Such depolarization is not uncommon in diseased myocardium exhibiting dysrhythmia and probably occurs primarily because P_K to P_{Na} or P_{Ca} ratios are decreased in cells found in diseased heart.

To predict the resting potential during non-steady-state conditions, especially during beating at or above usual physiologic rates, a Hodgkin-Huxley-like formulation defining the time and voltage dependencies of the several components of the transmembrane current is needed. Using this approach, V_{rest} occurs when the net transmembrane current is zero. That is, the sum of I_{Na}, I_{Ca}, I_{to}, I_{K1}, I_K, I_{KATP}, I_{leak}, I_{Napump}, $I_{Na-Caexchange}$, and so on (i.e., the net sum of all components of the total membrane current capable of flowing at V_{rest}) is zero at V_{rest}. The solution of this equation requires the simultaneous solution of the several equations defining the steady-state and kinetic time and voltage dependencies of each of the several components of the composite transmembrane current I_m. Using a fairly powerful personal computer and commercially available enabling software, solutions to this rather formidable set of equations can be obtained in several seconds to minutes. Solution by hand, however, is out of the question for all but the most compulsive diehards, so for the sake of simplicity steady state is usually assumed and V_{rest} is calculated from the GHK equation. As long as it is recognized that the GHK equation

$$V_{rest} = 61 \log \frac{([K^+]_o + P_{Na}/P_K[Na^+]_o + P_{Ca}/P_K[Ca^{++}]_o + \ldots + P_x/P_K[X^-])}{([K^+]_i + P_{Na}/P_K[Na^+]_i + P_{Ca}/P_K[Ca^{++}]_i + \ldots + P_x/P_K[X^-])}$$

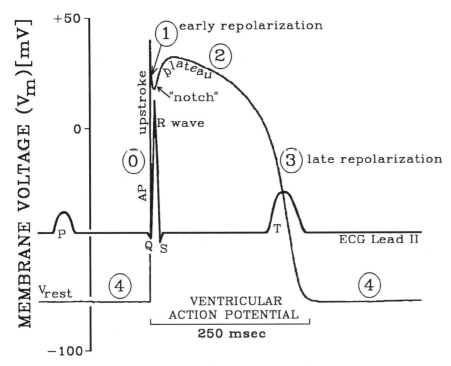

Figure 1 An action potential (AP) recorded from an freshly isolated feline ventricular myocyte using a conventional patch pipette technique while stimulated at 0.5 Hz (37°C). A depiction of an ECG lead II is shown in superimposition with the AP to dramatize the relationship between the upstroke and repolarization of the AP and the R and T waves of the ECG. The five operational phases of the AP are indicated by the circled numbers 0–4 placed near the appropriate position along the time course of the AP. The voltage scale on the left pertains to the transmembrane voltage of the AP. Notice that the plateau voltage is about 10 mV positive to levels typically recorded from ventricular strips or papillary muscles (i.e., 35–40 versus 20–25 mV). No voltage scale is given for the ECG (see text for more detail).

is valid only for the steady state and its use is predicated accordingly, this approach is reasonable and acceptably accurate.

The Ventricular Action Potential and Its Ionic Basis

As is the case for other excitable cells, the transmembrane potential of a cardiac fiber changes because the conductance (conductance equals resistance^{-1}) of ion channels in the sarcolemmal membrane can change, permitting ions to move across the cell membrane in a direction and at a rate governed by the transmembrane concentration and voltage gradients. Current, in the form of ion fluxes, carries charge across the sarcolemma and changes the amount of charge "separated" by the 100Å thick membrane and thus effects a change in the transmembrane potential (voltage V_m). The ionic currents flowing during the depolarization and repolarization of normal generic action potentials should be understood before the membrane bases of arrhythmias, the actions of antiarrhythmic drugs, or the effects of cardiac disease are considered at the level of the ion channels.

The Normal Cellular Action Potential

During phase 4 in the absence of excitation, ventricular cells maintain a stable resting potential. Normally in response to an excitatory stimulus, a transmembrane action potential with a voltage-time course (shape of the voltage versus time projection) characteristic for cardiac cells is inscribed (Fig. 1). The cardiac action potential traditionally has been considered to be composed of five distinctly definable temporal phases termed phases 0, 1, 2, 3, and 4 (see Fig. 1). The initial event of an action potential typically is a depolarization (phase 0) during which V_m changes very rapidly from V_{rest} to $\sim$ 35 or 40 mV. The depolarization rate for ventricular cells is typically 150–250 V/sec and rarely can be as much as 400–500 V/sec. This is followed by repolarization, which occurs with a multiphasic time course that has been divided into three periods (phases 1, 2, and 3). In some ventricular cells (usually epicardially located myocardial cells), phase 1 carries the membrane potential to a level that is slightly negative to the level seen during the early portion of the action potential plateau (phase 2). This results in the inscription of a "notch" between phases 1 and 2. The plateau of a typical ventricular action potential has a "hump and shoulder" appearance, with a gradual transition from phase 2 to the more rapidly repolarizing period of phase 3. Repolarization during phase 3 can, but usually does not, carry membrane potential to a value slightly more negative than the resting potential (termed maximum diastolic potential, MDP), and then, slowly, resting potential is restored to its steady-state level during early phase 4.

Ventricular action potentials can be distinguished from Purkinje fiber action potentials by the longer plateau duration and fairly sharp inflection between phases 2 and 3 that are typical of Purkinje fibers. Purkinje fibers also exhibit the property of automaticity and as a result can spontaneously depolarize during phase 4, whereas ventricular cells do not ordinarily exhibit this ability. The action potentials exhibited by ventricular cells can also be distinguished from those of atrial myocardial cells by the shorter, more rapidly repolarizing phase 2 blending into phase 3 typical of atrial action potentials. The most prominent distinctions between sinoatrial nodal and atrioventricular nodal potentials and ventricular potentials are the much less polarized levels of V_{rest} (i.e., -60 to -70 versus -80 to -95 mV) and much slower depolarization rates during phase 0 (i.e., 5–20 V/sec versus 150–250 V/sec) for both types of nodal cells. These latter differences contribute to the much faster conduction velocity of impulses in the ventricles compared to that through the AV node.

The Ionic Basis of the Ventricular Action Potential

The fairly complex time course of ventricular action potentials is the result of a complex coordinated sequence of changes in the conductances regulating the flow of transmembrane ionic current that involves at least five and possibly more ion channels (DiFrancesco and Noble, 1985). For the discussions in this chapter, the notation I refers to current produced by a cell or a tissue, and the notation i refers to the current passed by single ion channels. The action potential upstroke (phase 0) is generated whenever the membrane potential is reduced from resting potential to threshold potential (TP). This occurs because depolarization to TP causes the fast sodium channels to activate (i.e., open rapidly) and sodium ions to rush into the cell carrying positive charge across the cell membrane. The result of the inrush of positive charge is depolarization of the cell from V_{rest} to 30 $\pm$ 10 mV (see Fig. 2). The sodium channels subsequently undergo voltage-dependent inactivation, and most but not quite all close within a very few milliseconds (i.e., < 10 msec; Fig. 2, lower panel). Sodium current I_{Na} is greatly reduced but not totally eliminated during phase 1 and the early portion of phase 2 (the plateau phase).

The shutdown of the sodium influx and a concomitant surge of effluxing K^+ carried by the transient outward current I_{to} allows the cell to undergo the early phase of repolarization (phase 1). Cells eliciting a robust I_{to} exhibit a notch between phases 1 and 2; those with a weak or absent I_{to} may not exhibit the notch. Inscription of a notch is presumptive evidence that the cell in question can elicit I_{to}. The transient nature of I_{to} causes it subsequently to turn off rather quickly (typically within 4–10 msec) when the membrane potential returns to the vicinity of 0 $\pm$ 10 mV and the repolarization process is temporarily arrested by the plateau phase, with V_m often undergoing a secondary depolarization to the ultimate plateau voltage of 20 $\pm$ 10 mV.

A. ACTION POTENTIAL

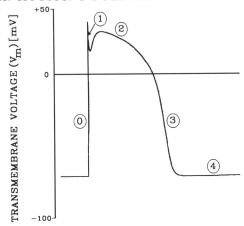

B. WHOLE CELL CONDUCTANCES

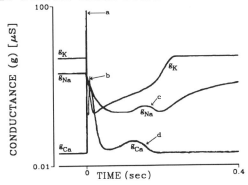

Figure 2 (A) The same action potential (AP) as that in Figure 1. (B) The time courses of the conductances g for the Na, Ca, and K currents (g_{Na}, g_{Ca}, and g_K, respectively) that flow during the AP (in A) on the same time scale as used for the AP. The arrow a depicts the peak g_{Na} observed during the AP upstroke; b depicts the outward spike of g_K associated with the transient outward current flow during phase 1; c and d represent the increases in g_{Na} and g_{Ca}, respectively, associated with the Na and Ca "window currents." Notice the sequential changes in each conductance component and the corresponding effect on the AP. The time courses of the conductance changes depicted here are approximate, having been calculated by a DEC 11/73 running a version of OXSOFT HEART (license 1.015) compiled for cat ventricular myocytes.

In heart, complete repolarization does not occur immediately following the action potential upstroke (phase 0) as it does in neurons because phase 2, the plateau phase, interrupts

the process. Three factors underlie the plateau. First, a very small fraction of the Na channels remain open during early phase 2. Second, the initial depolarization produced by the Na current causes Ca channels to open, allowing Ca^{2+} and perhaps some Na^+ to enter the cell though Ca channels during the plateau. The entry of positive charge through the Ca channels, termed Ca current I_{Ca}, keeps membrane potential near zero mV during phase 2 even though the depolarized membrane begins to open delayed outwardly rectifying potassium channels I_K (the third factor) to augment the sustained but weak repolarizing K currents carried by the inwardly rectifying K current I_{K1} and possibly by other K channels conducting repolarizing K current when V_m is in the plateau range (e.g., I_{Kp}). The resulting K^+ efflux begins to carry some of the excess positive charge out of the cell, thus tipping the balance between inward and outward movements of charge in favor of repolarization. Toward the end of phase 2, the Ca current gradually shuts down as result of both voltage-dependent deactivation and inactivation so that calcium ions no longer enter to oppose the repolarizing action of the now strengthening K^+ current effluxing from the cells. During phase 3 the now well-developed flow of K^+ from the cell through a slowly increasing number of open K channels rapidly carries charge across the membrane and repolarization proceeds to completion. As phase 4 begins, K channel conductance again slowly returns to the resting condition at which it is the most prominent resting conductance, setting V_{rest} at or near the level predicted by the GHK equation.

To recapitulate, the action potential arises primarily because of a specific sequence of ion movements that are controlled by the sequential opening and closing of Na, Ca, and K channels and whose function is to carry charge first into and then out of the cell. Such a simplistic and qualitative description of the ionic basis of the ventricular action potential, however, can only be used as an embarkation point for even a semi-quantitative understanding of how ion channel activity underlies the cellular action potential. The time course of ventricular action potentials changes radically in response to interventions as innocuous as increasing the beat rate or increasing or decreasing the $[K^+]$ of the interstitial fluid by 1 or 2 mM. The action potential can change even more drastically if interstitial pH is allowed to drop by only 0.1–0.3 pH units below normal, if the resting potential decreases or if the heart becomes ischemic, even if only transiently. Exposure to sympathomimetic and parasympathomimetic drugs (e.g., norepinephrine and acetylcholine), to many antiarrhythmic agents, or to cardiac glycosides can also alter the action potential in quite obvious ways. The alterations in the action potential associated with each of these interventions can be quite different, implying that each can modify one or more of the individual components of the membrane current governing the shape of the action potential in a specific, perhaps unique way. An apparently seldom recognized corollary to this notion is that specific current(s) and channels modified by an intervention cannot be deduced definitively from examination of the intervention-induced change in the time course of the action potential. To illustrate, a decrease in plateau voltage and/or duration could be the result of either decreasing the inwardly flowing I_{Ca} or increasing an outwardly flowing component of the K current, or both. If one wishes to explain the effect of an intervention on the ventricular action potential or on the electrocardiogram at the level of the ion channels, the most powerful approach currently available is to address each of the several possibilities in a straightforward manner using voltage clamp techniques.

In keeping with the notion just discussed, explanations for the decrease in action potential duration associated with increased interstitial $[K^+]$, depolarization of V_{rest}, and increased stimulus rate are derived from considerations of the voltage and time dependencies of the steady-state and kinetic parameters governing the components of the membrane current flowing at V_m relevant to the plateau and late repolarization phases (i.e., phases 2 and 3). Explanations for the decreases in the amplitude and depolarization rate of the up-

stroke associated with depolarization of V_{rest} and with increased beat rate are also derived from similar considerations involving I_{Na} and I_{Ca}. When pertinent data are available, the effects on action potentials of pH, intracellular "second messenger" systems, and such ions as Ca^{2+} and Na^+, said to modulate several components of the membrane current, are correlated with their effects on membrane current to further demonstrate that it is the electrophysiologic behavior of the ion channels that mainly governs the electrical activity of the myocardium.

Role of Electrogenic Ion Pumps and Exchangers

In addition to the major conductances just mentioned, a few minor players contribute a small amount of current to the resting and action potentials. These are the currents generated by the ATPase-dependent Na/K pump, usually termed the Na pump, and by the sarcolemmal Na-Ca exchanger (see Fig. 3). Their effects on the level of the resting potential and on the time course of the normal ventricular action potential are usually considered minor, amounting to no more than 1–4 mV of the resting potential and probably even less of the plateau voltage, yet the plateau duration of normal cells exhibiting a membrane resistance in the normal range can be shortened by as much as 10% by a strongly activated Na pump current. The extent to which current generated by Na pumping or Na-Ca exchange can influence V_{rest} and plateau voltage and duration depends on the resistance of the sarcolemmal membrane r_m to current flow through ion conductance channels. For example, when resting (i.e., steady-state) r_m is higher than normal, the hyperpolarization of V_{rest} that occurs in response to a 100 pA current generated by Na pumping is greater than if r_m is normal. This is because less of the current generated by Na pumping is short-circuited through the sarcolemma by the higher r_m. Currents arising from electrogenic pumps and exchangers should be regarded differently from the currents carried by ions passively flowing down their electrochemical gradients through ion channels because they do not contribute to r_m. Exchange

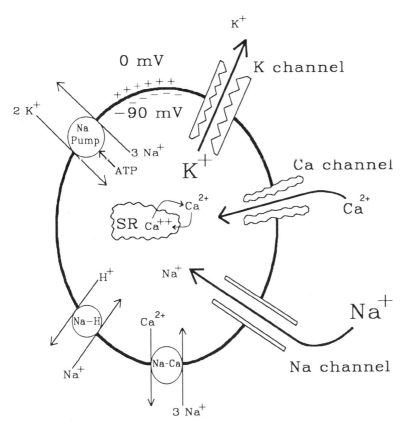

Figure 3 A cartoon model of an idealized isolated ventricular cell. The cell contains channel proteins for the Na, Ca, and K conductances to provide routes for the passive voltage- and time-dependent fluxes of these ions; it also contains an ATP-dependent Na/K pump (Na pump), a Na-proton exchanger (Na-H), a Na-Ca exchanger (Na-Ca), and a representation of the sarcoplasmic reticulum (SR) Ca^{2+} handling mechanism. The cartoon depicts with arrows how the several ions cycle into, around, and out of the cell via the channels, pumps, and exchangers (see text for detailed discussion).

and pump currents operate as current generators to transfer charge from one side of the membrane capacity c_m to the other rather than by regulating the flow of (ionic) current from one side to the other through a resistance (i.e., r_m) in parallel with c_m.

The Na Pump

The role of the Na pump is to maintain the level of $[K^+]_i$ high (i.e., ≥ 120–130 mM) and that for $[Na^+]_i$ low (i.e., ≤ 10 mM). These intracellular levels of K^+ and Na^+ provide the electrochemical ion gradients needed to drive the Na and K currents directly and indirectly to drive the Ca current (because the Na^+ gradient drives the Na-Ca exchange; see next section and refer to Fig. 3). There is an enormous literature concerning the Na pump; we have

not attempted even a cursory review of it in this chapter. The interested reader should consult a comprehensive review of the Na pump literature (e.g., Chapman, 1984; Gadsby, 1984; DeWeer, 1984) because only very key points are mentioned here. The exchange of intracellularly located Na^+ for extracellularly located K^+ requires energy in the form of ATP and is accomplished electrogenically because for each cycle of the pump mechanism three Na^+ are moved out of the cell but only two K^+ are recovered. This yields an efflux of one net charge per pump cycle, which becomes an outward hyperpolarizing current (Isenberg and Trautwein, 1974). The cycling rate of the pump, and therefore the size of the Na pump current, is governed by the levels of $[Na^+]_i$ and $[K^+]_o$. However, with the level of

$[K^+]_o$ for half-maximal activation $\sim$1–2 mM (Gadsby, 1984) and the typical interstitial $[K^+]$ 4–5 mM, the rate of Na pumping is predominantly governed by $[Na^+]_i$. The level of $[Na^+]_i$ producing half-maximal stimulation has been estimated as anywhere between approximately 10 mM (Sejersted et al., 1988) and $\geq$20 mM (Mogul et al., 1990). As result of the usually prevalent levels of $[Na^+]_i$ and $[K^+]_o$, minor changes in either can increase or decrease the level of Na pump current depending on the direction of change in $[K^+]_o$ or $[Na^+]_i$.

A principal source of intracellular Na^+ that the Na pump must extrude arises from the operation of the Na-proton exchange, which performs a major role in the regulation of the intracellular pH (Lazdunski et al., 1985). This exchange is electroneutral (see Fig. 3), transferring Na^+ into cells in exchange for protons out in equimolar amounts, but any accumulation of Na^+ intracellularly when exchanging Na^+ for protons is expected to increase the rate of Na pumping and generate more outward current (Rasmussen et al., 1989).

The Na-Ca Exchange

The Na-Ca exchange process was discovered first in heart by Reuter and Seitz (1968) nearly a quarter of a century ago and is now generally recognized as common to nearly all living cells. Like the Na pump, the Na-Ca exchange can generate current. However, the generation of current does not involve energy derived from ATP. Instead the potential energy stored in the transmembrane electrochemical gradients of Na^+ and Ca^{2+} drives the exchange process. The current arises because for each Ca^{2+} translocated, at least three, possibly four, Na^+ move in the opposite direction, generating a net charge transfer of at least one for each cycle of the exchanger. Whereas the Na pump only produces outward current when membrane potential is within even the most extreme range of physiologically possible levels, the Na-Ca exchange can generate either inward or outward current depending on the whether V_m is negative or positive (respectively) to the conjoint equilibrium potential for the Na^+ and Ca^{2+} concentration gradients

($E_{Na\text{-}Ca}$). From thermodynamic considerations, $E_{Na\text{-}Ca}$ for normal physiologic conditions is expected to be about -40 mV, with inward current generated at V_m negative to that level and outward current generated at V_m positive to it. The consequences of $E_{Na\text{-}Ca}$ normally being approximately -40 mV are (1) that the current generated by Na-Ca exchange exerts a depolarizing influence when V_m is at or near V_{rest} and a repolarizing influence when V_m is in the plateau voltage range, and (2) that the Na-Ca exchange can translocate Ca^{2+} into cardiac cells during the action potential plateau and out of them during phase 4. This last effect is believed to contribute importantly to both the phasic changes in $[Ca^{2+}]_i$ occurring during action potentials and to the steady-state levels of Ca^{2+} in both the cytosol and the sarcoplasmic reticulum (SR) (see Eisner and Lederer, 1985).

Perhaps the most important role of the Na-Ca exchanger is to prevent the development of an intracellular Ca^{2+} overload and the consequences of such an overloaded condition, for example, serious disruption of many cellular processes and even cell "death." Conditions that cause $[Ca^{2+}]_i$ to increase cause $E_{Na\text{-}Ca}$ to shift to a less polarized level. This in turn serves to augment the inward flux of Na^+ and outward flux of Ca^{2+} and establishes a new, at least somewhat elevated, steady-state level for $[Ca^{2+}]_i$ that persists for as long as the Na^+ gradient can be maintained at its new steady-state level (by the Na pump or other mechanisms). Conversely, when exposed to a Na^+-free external environment or to one in which the $[Na^+]_i$ is "forced" to increase, cardiac cells experience an increase in their $[Ca^{2+}]_i$ (Reuter and Seitz, 1968). The consequence of an increase in $[Ca^{2+}]_i$ when V_m is at or near V_{rest} is that the exchanger can then generate a stronger than normal inward (depolarizing) current. The augmented exchange current can reduce (depolarize) the level of V_{rest} and increase the intrinsic automaticity of the involved cells. From this discussion it follows that conditions leading to an instability in the ability of the SR to sequester Ca^{2+} should contribute to the development of oscillations in the strength of the Na-Ca exchange current and possibly to oscillations in V_m during phase

4. There has been speculation that the Na-Ca exchange may have a role in the generation of the transient inward current said to underlie at least some early (EAD) and/or delayed after-depolarizations (DAD), but the evidence to date has not been completely convincing either for or against this notion.

From this discussion the nature of the intimate intertwining of the roles in the homeostasis of intracellular cation activities played by the Na pump, the Na-proton exchanger, and the Na-Ca exchanger should begin to be appreciated, and it should be clear why any intervention leading to an elevation of $[Na^+]_i$ may cause $[Ca^{2+}]_i$ to rise also. Therefore it is difficult to isolate the electrophysiologic effect of an intervention intended to modify any one of the ion translocation processes specifically to the particular process of interest because of the involvement of Na^+_i in the regulation of all three. There are substances said to inhibit Na-Ca exchange (e.g., Mn^{2+}, amiloride, and dibenzamil), but none are sufficiently selective to warrant their use as an experimental tool, even for the purpose of definitively identifying the Na-Ca exchange process. Currently, the only feasible approach available to enable a detailed electrophysiologic study of the exchange current is the whole-cell patch, voltage clamp technique using dialyzed or internally perfused myocytes. However, despite the substantial difficulties obscuring the interpretations of the results of experiments intended to elucidate the details of the Na-Ca exchanger, its existence has been amply demonstrated by its physiologic behavior and accepted as fact for more than two decades.

THE COMPONENTS OF MEMBRANE CURRENT: KINETIC DESCRIPTIONS AND MODULATION

We have already qualitatively described the ionic basis of the ventricular action potential. From those discussions it is apparent that a number of specific ionic currents are responsible for the changes in V_m that result in the inscription of an action potential. Each component of the membrane current is regulated by the conductance properties of the specific ion channel governing that particular component. Each channel has its own unique ionic selectivity and kinetic properties governing the opening and closing events of the ion channels specific for each particular current. In this section we describe the kinetic properties of the major components of the cardiac transmembrane ionic currents thought to have a role in generating action potentials in mammalian ventricular cells. We also discuss factors believed to modulate these currents.

Sodium Current I_{Na}

The current responsible for the rapid phase of cardiac cell depolarization is carried by Na^+. In many ways it is similar to the I_{Na} described for nerves (Hodgkin and Huxley, 1952). A family of I_{Na} recorded from an isolated feline ventricular myocyte recorded using the whole-cell patch voltage clamp technique is shown in Figure 4 along with its current-voltage (I-V) relationship. I_{Na} is very large, flows very briefly, and appears to result from the opening of several hundred to several thousand channels per square micrometer of surface area. I_{Na} activates when transmembrane potential depolarizes into the range in which channel openings can occur (the activation threshold), that is, around -70 mV. The opening of these Na^+-selective channels allows an inward flow of Na^+, causing additional depolarization, which in turn causes additional channels to open. This regenerative process ensures that stimulation produced by either a voltage clamp pulse or a conducted action potential activates all the available Na channels that it can and produces as large a I_{Na} possible for the conditions in effect at that particular moment. In the case of a conducted action potential in vivo, a large depolarizing wavefront normally ensures that conduction velocity is fast enough to cause a nearly simultaneous activation of the entire ventricular muscle mass. I_{Na}, because it is a principal determinant of the upstroke velocity (i.e., the depolarization rate) of the action potential, is an important determinant of the success or failure of cardiac conduction.

In addition to a dependence on voltage, cardiac Na^+ channel activation is also time

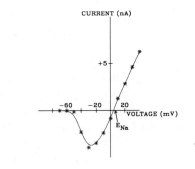

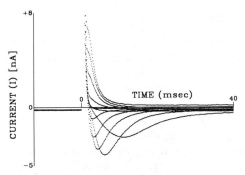

Figure 4 [Sodium current] I_{Na} in a cat ventricular myocyte. (Top) The peak I_{Na} versus voltage relationship of the family of whole-cell patch current recordings shown in the bottom panel. The measured reversal potential was within 3 mV of the calculated E_{rev}. The holding potential was -120 mV, and voltage was stepped to different test potentials for 75 msec at a frequency of 0.2 Hz. The voltage threshold occurred at about -60 mV, and the peak current occurred at -30 mV. Notice (lower panel) that the outward flowing I_{Na} elicited at V_m positive to E_{Na} exhibit activation and inactivation phases, as do the more familiar inward-flowing I_{Na}. The data were obtained with $[Na^+]_i = 10$ mM and $[Na^+]_o = 15$ mM at a temperature of 14°C so that the I_{Na} elicited would be less than 4 nA and reasonable quality voltage clamp would be possible. (Data kindly provided and processed by E. Schackow.)

dependent in that it does not instantaneously achieve its maximal amplitude. Ordinarily, the activation time constant is very brief (probably within 0.1–0.2 msec at physiologic temperatures). The time to the peak current, however, is less than the time to reach full activation because, at the same instant the Na channels begin to activate, a second process

causing Na channels to close and preventing their reopening, termed inactivation, is also set in motion by depolarization. Inactivation occurs with a short delay following the onset of the depolarization, contributes to the rate of channel closure, and may limit the peak current that can flow during channel opening. Recent evidence also indicates that inactivation may occur even in the absence of previous channel opening (Follmer et al., 1987) or after extremely brief open times (Grant, 1990; Grant et al., 1989), thus reducing the peak current to less than that expected based on the number of available channels.

The rate of recovery from the inactivation developed during a previous excitation determines the fractional amount of the maximal I_{Na} available for the next excitatory event. The process of recovery from inactivation therefore governs the rate at which a series of impulses can be repetitively conducted throughout the ventricle; recovery has been shown to occur as the result of at least two separate processes (Follmer et al., 1987), one with a time constant of roughly 3–5 msec and the other with a time constant of about 10–40 msec. Usually both are brief enough to allow nearly complete recovery of I_{Na} during diastole when heart rate is in the physiologic range (i.e., 40–200 beats/min). However, since the rate of recovery from inactivation is time dependent, being slower at depolarized potentials than at well-polarized potentials (i.e., exhibits voltage dependence), an early extrasystole would find fewer Na^+ channels available for opening and thus would be expected to conduct more slowly than the regular beat. This slowing of conduction also could contribute significantly to a delay in ventricular activation. Still, the major cause of refractoriness is the slow recovery from inactivation that occurs during the repolarization of the action potential.

In addition to the roles of activation and inactivation in governing I_{Na}, a third process, deactivation, is also involved in determining the behavior of cardiac I_{Na}. Deactivation is believed to be responsible for Na^+ channel closure upon repolarization following depolarizations too brief (1–2 msec) to allow significant inactivation to occur. Deactivation is said to result from closure of the activation gate rather than channel occlusion by the inactivation gate. The distinction lies in the fact that inactivation occurs *during* depolarization whereas deactivation occurs *following* repolarization of membrane potential. Although it is unlikely that deactivation is very important physiologically, deactivation probably accounts for some of the shutdown of I_{Na} that occurs when action potentials exhibiting very short durations repolarize, the resulting reduction of I_{Na} both being caused by and contributing to the rapid repolarization.

Although most I_{Na} inactivates within a few milliseconds after depolarization, a small fraction of I_{Na} inactivates with a rather prolonged time course in ventricular cells in some species (Wasserstrom and Salata, 1988). This slowly inactivating I_{Na} takes several hundred milliseconds to several seconds to inactivate fully and is similar to that described for Purkinje fibers (Gintant et al., 1984; Carmeliet, 1987). In addition, in hearts of some species there is very small fraction of I_{Na} that does not appear to inactivate (Attwell et al., 1979). This steady-state current component of I_{Na} may result from the crossover of the curves describing the voltage dependencies for I_{Na} activation and inactivation in the voltage range of approximately -55 ± 10 mV. The analogous current found in sheep and canine Purkinje fibers has been named the Na "window" current (Attwell et al., 1979). Since both the slowly inactivating and steady-state components of I_{Na} are blocked by the specific Na channel blocker tetrodotoxin (TTX), the often dramatic decrease in action potential duration associated with exposure to TTX (10–30 μM) is taken to indicate that these two components of I_{Na} can importantly contribute inward current during both phases 2 and 3 of the action potential. Slowly inactivating I_{Na} also recovers from inactivation much more slowly than the rapidly inactivating component of I_{Na}, and as with the fast inactivating current, it is also voltage dependent, being slower the more depolarized the recovery potential. Although a slowly inactivating or noninactivating component of I_{Na} has not yet been identified in human heart, channels in the slowly inacti-

vated state are thought to be an important site of action of a variety of type I antiarrhythmic agents (Hondeghem and Katzung, 1977; Starmer et al., 1984).

The properties of Na^+ current are closely mimicked by single Na^+ channel activity, which has been extensively studied in recent years (for review, see Grant, 1990). Single-channel conductance in heart is about 10 picosiemens (pS). The threshold voltage for brief channel openings is about -70 mV. Openings occur after a very brief latency, usually within 1 msec after a depolarizing voltage pulse. Channel opening is responsible for current activation, whereas inactivation causes a rapid decline in open probability within several milliseconds (Cachelin et al., 1983).

Some characteristics of single-channel activity have shown important deviations from the channel behavior predicted from Hodgkin-Huxley (HH) formulations derived from nerve data: (1) Na^+ channels can enter either of at least two inactivated states directly from the available state without first having to undergo an open transition. (2) In an apparent contrast with certain neurally derived cells (Aldrich et al., 1983), the rate of inactivation in heart appears to be voltage dependent (Grant et al., 1989; Yue et al., 1989). However, the kinetic behavior of long openings and bursts of openings is not consistent with a simple HH kinetic scheme; the long openings could represent a transient shift to a completely distinct alternative mode of gating (Hess et al., 1984). This channel behavior could be responsible for the TTX-sensitive, slowly inactivating Na^+ current reported in myocardium (Patlack and Ortiz, 1986). (3) Cardiac Na channels also appear to exhibit subconductance states, suggestive of multiple channel types (Scanley and Fozzard, 1987; Grant et al., 1989). Continued examination of single-channel activity will without doubt reveal much new information about how the behavior of single channels and the several putative channel subtypes contribute to the macroscopic I_{Na} current component of the action potential.

Cardiac I_{Na} can be sensitive to change in either of the intracellular or extracellular environments. It is well known that increasing Ca^{2+}_o decreases both the maximum rate of depolarization of the upstroke (Weidmann, 1955) and I_{Na} (Sheets et al., 1987). This has been ascribed to a ''shielding'' or ''screening'' effect of divalent cations that serves to neutralize negative surface charge residing on either the inner or outer surfaces of the sarcolemma (Frankenhauser and Hodgkin, 1957). Ca^{2+} also exerts a direct blocking action on I_{Na} in sheep Purkinje cells (Sheets et al., 1987). In a similar fashion, lowering external pH by as little as 0.2–0.4 pH units reduces I_{Na}, also possibly due to an effect on surface charge acting in addition to a direct effect on Na channels (Hille et al., 1975; Hille, 1984; Hisatome et al., 1989). The direct blocking action of protons has not been examined in single-channel experiments, so it is not yet known what site(s) on the Na^+ channel is affected by H^+ ions. The effects of ischemia include a reduction in external pH by as much as 1–1.4 units, which is expected to reduce I_{Na} markedly. These results suggest that ischemia and the resulting metabolic acidosis are expected to reduce I_{Na} directly. It has recently been reported that when cardiac Na^+ channels are phosphorylated, their conductance decreases (Schubert et al., 1989). This effect, plus an ischemia-induced depolarization of V_{rest} causing the fractional amount I_{Na} in the inactivated state to increase, could combine to decrease I_{Na}. Any or all of these effects of ischemia would reduce the likelihood of evoking a I_{Na}-dependent action potential with a slowly rising upstroke that, when conducting slowly, would provoke impulse reentry. However, it is also possible that reduced channel availability is compensated for by the increase in I_{Na} that results from channel dephosphorylation. This would minimize the effects of ischemia on the amplitude of I_{Na} and ensure the fastest conduction velocity possible under these proarrhythmic conditions that predispose the heart to reentry.

Transient Outward Current(s) I_{to}

The earliest phase of repolarization of the action potential is the result of activation of the transient outward current, a current carried by an outward movement of K^+. The homology of the gene(s) regulating the cellular expression of the membrane protein responsible for governing this current is remarkably similar across a wide range of excitable cell types and species. I_{to} has been identified in human atrial cells (Escande et al., 1987; Shibata et al., 1989). Although not yet identified in human ventricular cells, there is no reason to believe that it is not a feature of their membrane current. Recent observations in dog heart suggest epicardial cells have a much more pronounced I_{to} than endocardial cells (Litovsky and Antzelevitch, 1988), thus providing an explanation for the shorter action potential duration and earlier repolarization in epicardium than in endocardium that is said to determine the polarity of the T wave of the electrocardiogram. Although putative differences between the I_{to} elicited by endo- and epicardial cell types have not yet been investigated using voltage clamp analysis, Tseng and Hoffman (1989) showed that dog ventricular cells can be segregated into two distinct cell populations distinguished by the amplitude of the notch associated with phase 1 of the action potential (see Fig. 1). Differences in properties of I_{to} in different regions of the ventricle may be important in determining how physiologic and pharmacologic interventions affect the ventricle.

A typical family of I_{to} recorded from a feline ventricular myocyte using the whole-cell patch voltage clamp technique is shown in Figure 5 along with its I-V curve. I_{to} can be activated in cat myocytes by depolarizing from V_m negative to -30 mV to V_m positive to -10 mV. This behavior permits the current to be evoked in response to depolarizations from most physiologically relevant levels of V_{rest} by an action potential upstroke induced by I_{Na} activation and thus provide repolarizing current to effect phase 1. I_{to} rapidly rises within 2–5 msec to a peak outward level (see Fig. 5) and then decays as the result of inactivation. The onset of the decay begins within 2–5 msec of activation. I_{to} amplitude falls back nearly to baseline with a time constant of 10–15 msec (in cat) and often leaves a steady-state out-

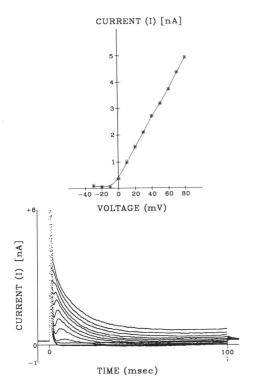

Figure 5 Transient outward current I_{to} in a cat ventricular myocyte. (Top) A graph of the peak I_{to} versus voltage relationship derived from the family of currents recorded using the whole-cell patch mode voltage clamp shown in the bottom panel. The holding potential was -40 mV; V_m was stepped for 100 msec to test potentials ranging from -30 to 60 mV in 10 mV increments at a frequency of 0.2 Hz. The peak outward current occurred within 2–5 msec after the pulse onset, and then the current declined to a steady-state level above zero. $[K^+]_o$ = 5.4 mM and temperature = 37°C. (Data kindly provided and processed by E. Schackow.)

tricular cells (Hiraoka and Kawano, 1989); the first is blocked by aminopyridine derivatives (in millimolar concentrations) and the second seems to be sensitive to intracellular Ca^{2+} The 4-aminopyridine-sensitive component represents about three-fourths of the current identified as I_{to}. The Ca^{2+}-sensitive component accounts for the remaining portion of I_{to} and is reduced by exposure to ryanodine or caffeine, which prevents Ca^{2+} release from the sarcoplasmic reticulum. This effect may contribute to the increase in action potential duration seen in the presence of ryanodine (Kenyon and Sutko, 1987). The implication is that tissues that release more Ca^{2+} from SR during contractions would have a greater Ca^{2+}-sensitive component of I_{to}. In addition, physiologic and pharmacologic interventions that increase Ca^{2+}_i and therefore SR Ca^{2+} release may cause action potential abbreviation as a result of activation of the Ca^{2+}-sensitive component of I_{to} under certain conditions.

It is unclear whether both components are generally present in ventricles of mammalian species, including humans, or whether tissues from different areas of the same heart can exhibit both components. Neither is it clear what role either or both components of I_{to} may play in arrhythmogenesis and in the efficacy of antiarrhythmic drugs. However, it is not absurd to suggest that I_{to} is importantly involved in arrhythmia associated with at least one kind of cardiac pathology. For instance, hypertrophic hearts are more prone to malignant rhythm disturbances and to the arrhythmic effects of concurrent ischemia (Cameron et al. 1987). The only striking changes in the cellular electrophysiology of cells from hypertrophied cat right ventricle (resulting from right ventricular pressure overload) are an increased mean amplitude of I_{to} and an increased fraction of cells in the right ventricle that exhibit I_{to} (Ten Eick, unpublished data).

I_{to} was first thought to be a Cl^- current (Dudel et al., 1967; Hiraoka and Fozzard, 1973). Although this notion was ultimately determined to be incorrect, recent evidence suggests that an outward Cl^- current can be superimposed on I_{to} (Harvey and Hume, 1989a). This Cl^- current is rapidly activating,

ward current component that probably has little to do with I_{to} because it is not sensitive to agents that can inhibit the phasic component of I_{to}. However, I_{to} appears to have a steady-state "window" component (voltage range around -20 mV) that may also contribute to repolarization during early phase 3.

Although much is known about the kinetics and significance of I_{to}, the precise mechanisms of current flow in ventricular cells have not been fully clarified. Two components of I_{to} have been identified in human atrium (Escande et al., 1987) and in isolated rabbit ven-

noninactivating, voltage dependent, and enhanced by β-agonists (Nakayama and Fozzard, 1988; Harvey et al., 1990). The kinetics of this current suggest that it probably contributes to the acceleration of repolarization observed in the presence of catecholamines.

Calcium Current I_{Ca}

I_{Ca} was initially thought to be a mixed cationic current but has more recently been identified in cardiac myocytes as a "pure" Ca^{2+} current composed of either one or two components (for review, see Bean, 1989). All cardiac myocytes exhibit the so-called L-type I_{Ca}, but only some cardiac tissues, notably dog Purkinje cells (Tseng and Boyden, 1989) and atrium (Bean, 1985) and guinea pig ventricle (Mitra and Morad, 1986), exhibit the T type of I_{Ca}. These two components can be distinguished by the differences between their voltage dependencies and kinetics and by the differences in the behavior of the single-channel currents that underlie them. T current activates rapidly in the voltage range between about -80 and -50 mV. It also inactivates rapidly and virtually completely. It received the designation "T current" to denote the transient nature of the whole-cell macroscopic current and the briefly opening, small (tiny) conductance channels (~7 pS) that underlie T current. Single-channel recordings reveal channels exhibiting short opening latencies and short open dwell times, with closing typically occurring within only a few milliseconds after opening (Nilius et al., 1985). T current is blocked by Ni^{2+} but only somewhat selectively (Mitra and Morad, 1986). It seems to be absent in most ventricular preparations (e.g., dog and cat), although a number of exceptions will no doubt be identified with time. The physiologic function of T channels and their current remains to be clarified. Based on considerations about the properties of the T current, two roles have been suggested. Because of the range of its activation voltage dependence (i.e., approximately -80 mV to around -60 mV), it may influence Purkinje fiber automaticity, and because it appears to provide a small but necessarily rapid surge of

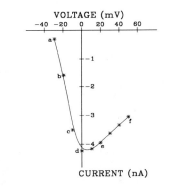

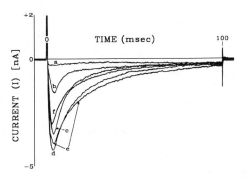

Figure 6 Whole-cell calcium current I_{Ca} recorded from patch-clamped cat ventricular myocytes. (Top) A graphic representation of peak I_{Ca} versus voltage relationship derived from the family of Cd^{2+}-sensitive currents shown in the bottom panel. The holding potential was -40 mV, and the voltage was stepped to different test potentials for 100 msec at a frequency of 0.2 Hz. The extrapolated reversal potential in this experiment is very positive because 1 mM EGTA was in the pipette, so $Ca^{2+}{}_i$ was set to a very low level. Cd^{2+} (0.5 mM) was added to the external solution to extract I_{Ca} from the membrane current, which is often a composite of I_{Ca} plus I_{to}. Some feline cells do not exhibit I_{to}, and currents from these cells have been used to verify that the Cd^{2+}-sensitive current reflects I_{Ca}. Temperature = 37°C. (Data kindly provided and processed by E. Schackow.)

Ca^{2+} influx it may be a (or, possibly, the) source of "trigger" Ca^{2+} for initiating contraction (Marban and Wier, 1985).

A typical family of L-type, Cd^{2+}-sensitive I_{Ca} are shown in Figure 6 along with its corresponding *I-V* curve. From these recordings it is evident that L-type I_{Ca} also activates rapidly but inactivates much more slowly than T current. Like the T current, the L current derives its name from its electrophysiologic behavior, being characterized by long-duration openings. The L channel conductance is 18 pS when the charge is Ba^{2+}, 7 pS when Ca^{2+}. It is the binding site for dihydropyridines, including such agonists as Bay K 8644 and antagonists like nifedipine and nitrendipine. L-type I_{Ca} is blocked by Cd^{2+} and several other divalent alkaline-earth ions; it is activated by rapid depolarizations into the voltage range positive to -40 mV. Inactivation of L-type channels is Ca^{2+} sensitive, inactivation being enhanced by increased Ca^{2+}_i and suppressed when Ba^{2+} (rather than Ca^{2+}) is the charge carrier of the L current. L-type current exhibits a "window" or steady-state current in the voltage range in which the voltage dependencies of activation and inactivation overlap (approximately -20 ± 10 mV) (Josephson et al., 1984).

In addition to producing a steady-state or "window" component, a small fraction of the total L-type current may not fully inactivate. An explanation for this finding can be derived from data obtained from single-channel recordings. In the presence of the dihydropyridine L-type Ca channel agonist Bay K 8644, during sustained depolarizations from around -40 mV to 0 ± 10 mV, L channels can exhibit a persistent activation (characterized by very long open dwell times) that does not appear to undergo any significant degree of inactivation. During long trains of repetitive depolarizations this behavior tends to occur in groups and is the predominant pattern. Occasionally the channels briefly revert to the pattern of short open dwell times occurring in bursts that is typical in the absence of Bay K 8644. This noninactivating channel behavior has been interpreted as an alternative, entirely different mode of channel gating rather than simply the result of an alteration of the normal gating kinetics (Hess et al, 1984). The importance of this finding is not restricted to when Bay K 8644 is present because it has been observed in the absence of the agonist, albeit the frequency of appearance was very much less, suggesting that this mode of channel gating may have physiologic importance. It may underlie the noninactivating component exhibited by the family of L-type I_{Ca} shown in Figure 6. A similar shift in gating mode has also been identified in cardiac Na^+ channels (Patlack and Ortiz, 1986).

Hess et al. (1984) suggest that there are, in fact, three modes of Ca^{2+} channel gating that can occur during a series of repetitive depolarizations. Mode 0 occurs when channels are unavailable to open (possibly when channels become dephosphorylated). This mode accounts for when no opening events are seen during a depolarization. The normal, most commonly observed type of L channel activity is designated mode 1 gating. Channel activity of this variety can be greatly enhanced by the development of an increase in the frequency of bursting behavior when in the presence of β-agonists (Tsien et al., 1986). Mode 2 shows the behavior described at length for the effect of Bay K 8644 during depolarizing steps. From an operational point of view the principal difference between modes 1 and 2 is the following. During mode 1 operation, channels are predominantly in the closed state and go to the open state in bursts of openings that can be sustained for many milliseconds, whereas during mode 2 channels are predominantly open and close occasionally, sometimes in bursts of closings. Finally, the role of switching between modes in the normal function of ventricular cells remains to be determined. In principle, mode switching could be a source of arrhythmogenic inward current (January et al., 1988).

Several important intracellularly based regulatory mechanisms influence I_{Ca}. The most prominent of these is mediated via activation of β-adrenoceptors and increased intracellular cAMP. The resulting phosphorylation of Ca^{2+} channels is associated with an increased open probability that favors an increased number of channels being open at any time (Tsien et al., 1986). This effect can fully explain the increase in I_{Ca} amplitude that occurs in response to β-agonists. I_{Ca} is markedly reduced by low pH (Irisawa and Sato, 1986), probably as the result of effects that both reduce single-channel conductance directly (Pietrobon et al., 1988) and alter membrane surface charge in a fashion similar to that described for

I_{Na}. Elevation of $[Ca^{2+}]_i$ can accelerate the decay of I_{Ca} by enhancing the rate of inactivation. As result the action potential duration is expected to shorten under conditions of increased cytoplasmic Ca^{2+} (such as during Ca^{2+} overload or during the Ca^{2+} paradox resulting from reexposure to Ca^{2+} following Ca^{2+} removal) and possibly during exposure to positive inotropic interventions.

The modulation of I_{Ca} by cellular factors probably also plays an important role during ischemia when cellular K^+ "leaks" into the myocardial interstitium and locally elevates K^+_o. This results in the levels of V_m of cells in the immediate vicinity becoming partially depolarized, and in turn their I_{Na} can become inactivated. Under such conditions action potentials can still be generated as the result of activating I_{Ca} and producing "slow upstroke action potentials," the slow conduction of which can establish conditions for reentrant excitation and arrhythmias (Wit and Rosen, 1986). Low local pH tends to suppress such activity, whereas high regional and circulating catecholamines tend to increase the amplitude and duration of the slow action potentials. The net effect of these opposing factors determines the actual activity level of Ca^{2+} channels and the proarrhythmic potential of this type of Ca^{2+}-dependent activity.

I_{Ca} serves several important functions in the heart. First, it serves as the trigger for cardiac contraction. It is the primary source of Ca^{2+} influx that causes Ca^{2+}-induced Ca^{2+} release from the SR (Marban and Wier, 1985). In addition, although the Ca^{2+} entering the cell through I_{Ca} appears not to directly activate contractile proteins in mammalian heart (Fabiato, 1983), "trigger" Ca^{2+} appears to load the SR stores for subsequent contractions; therefore I_{Ca} contributes to the modulation of contractile force. Finally, because L-type I_{Ca} inactivates slowly and can even exhibit a small component that does not appear to inactivate, it can provide a small but sustained inward current during step depolarizations and action potentials. Such a sustained I_{Ca} would contribute to the inward current needed to maintain the action potential at plateau voltage levels, thus influencing both plateau voltage and action potential duration, both of which influence twitch force as well as the electrophysiologic activity of ventricular myocardium.

Inward Rectifying K Current

The inwardly rectifying K current I_{K1}, as it is known in cardiac cells, is found ubiquitously in polarized cells throughout the plant and animal kingdoms (Hagiwara, 1983). Its similarity from species to species is striking, and the principal difference in its character between species or between tissues from the same species seems to be only in channel density. That is, the specific conductance for the inward rectifier may vary but its basic electrophysiologic nature is qualitatively uniform across most life-forms. This holds even when considering differences between atrial and ventricular cells from cat heart, I_{K1} of atrial cells normalized to cell membrane area usually being a quarter to a tenth of that found in ventricular cells (Hume and Uehara, 1985; Harvey and Ten Eick, unpublished observation). The single-channel conductance is said to be around 27 pS with normal $[K^+]_i$ and $[K^+]_o$ (Hume, 1989).

Figure 7 shows a typical family of I_{K1} currents elicited from isolated feline (left panels) and guinea pig (right panels) ventricular myocytes along with their respective I-V curves. I_{K1} can be elicited by hyperpolarizing voltage clamp pulses from holding potentials V_{hold} at least 20 mV positive to E_K. Typically -40 mV is used because the conductance is maximally deactivated at or positive to this V_m (refer to Harvey and Ten Eick, 1988 for a comprehensive description of I_{K1} in feline ventricular myocytes). During pulses to V_m positive to E_K, I_{K1} is outward and negative to E_K it is inward. The reversal potential tracks E_K very closely regardless of the level of $[K^+]_o$, indicating that I_{K1} is a "pure" K current. The peak current versus voltage curve indicates the current rectifies inwardly, making the conductance of outwardly flowing I_{K1} very much less than that for inwardly flowing current (Sakmann and Trube, 1984a). When hyperpolarizing from -40 mV to V_m positive to -120 mV, I_{K1} is

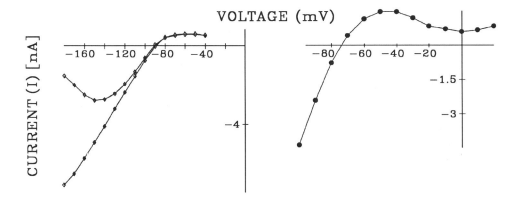

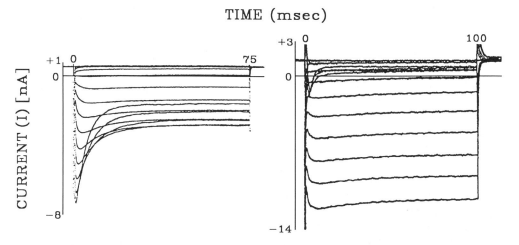

Figure 7   Inward rectifier potassium current I_{K1} in a cat ventricular myocyte (left panels) and a guinea pig ventricular myocyte (right panels). Both families of whole-cell recordings were initiated from a holding potential of -40 mV, and steps were made to test potentials ranging from -50 to -100 mV (guinea pig) or to -180 mV (cat). In both examples each negative voltage step rapidly activates an inward current. At potentials negative to -120 mV in cat, a prominent inactivation phase follows the peak inward current (identical results can be obtain in guinea pig but are not shown here). Cat myocyte shows a very flat response (i.e., voltage insensitive) to changes in voltage between -40 and -80 mV, indicating high membrane resistance and strong inward rectification in the plateau voltage range. Current in the guinea pig myocyte shows not only inward rectification with depolarization but also a region of negative slope conductance, giving an *n* shape to the current-voltage relationship. [Cat data modified from Harvey and Ten Eick; unpublished guinea pig data provided by S. Eager; figure prepared by E. Schackow.]

a rapidly activating ($\tau \leq$ 1–4 msec) current (Kurachi, 1985). When elicited at V_m negative to approximately -120 mV, the shape of the time course of the current changes from essen-

tially rectangular (i.e., it does not exhibit any evidence of an inactivation process) to one displaying a peak within 1–3 msec after the onset of the clamp pulse and then decays with a half-time of about 10 msec to a steady-state level that can be substantially less (i.e., 40–50%) than the peak current. This decay of I_{K1} that follows inscription of the peak behaves as though a sizable fraction of the peak current undergoes an inactivation process (Sakmann and Trube, 1984b). This "inactivation" process involves the extracellular presence of Na^+ and saturates at a $[Na^+]_o$ of around 60 mM (Harvey and Ten Eick, 1989a). Na^+-dependent inactivation appears to involve a monovalent cation binding site having a role in ion permeation (Harvey and Ten Eick, 1989a). Extracellular divalent cations also influences inactivation (Biermanns et al., 1987), although it is not known if their effect is mediated by the monovalent cation binding site.

Removing Na^+ from the external solution, in addition to reducing the extent of I_{K1} inactivation, can also decrease the conductance governing I_{K1}. This effect appears to be the result of the intracellular acidification caused by the reduction in Na-proton exchange brought about by decreasing $[Na^+]_o$ (Harvey and Ten Eick, 1989b). It is well known that the conductance for the inward rectifier is very sensitive to rather minor decreases (i.e., 0.1–0.3 pH units) in the intracellular pH (Hagiwara et al., 1978). This effect of pH alters the current-voltage relationship (I-V curve) by decreasing the conductance at V_m negative to E_K, decreasing inward rectification and linearizing the peak I-V curve. Removing Mg^{2+} from the intracellular solution can also abolish inward rectification. However, in this instance, in contrast to the effect of removing extracellular Na^+, the linearization of the I-V curve results from an increase in the conductance at V_m positive to E_K (Horie and Irisawa, 1987).

The I-V curves shown in Figure 7 are for ventricular myocytes derived from cat (left panel) and guinea pig (right panel) hearts. The slope between -70 and -30 mV (or even less negative) is virtually flat (i.e., zero slope) in cat ventricular myocytes. This finding may be unique to cat insofar as the slope of the I_{K1} I-V curve for dog and guinea pig ventricular cells and for dog Purkinje fibers exhibits a region of negative slope in this range of V_m with the I-V curve having an n-shaped appearance (see right upper panel, Fig. 7). There are several possible consequences of an n-shaped I_{K1}-V curve. One is that as repolarization proceeds during phase 3, outward I_{K1} is recruited in the range of V_m between -30 and -60 mV. This aids the repolarization to get through the voltage region that is most prone to initiate early afterdepolarizations. The effect is construed as beneficial for normal cardiac electrical activity. Another effect, which may not be beneficial, is that, should an n-shaped I-V curve move downward in the I-V domain, as can occur in the presence of a Na pump inhibitor (Isenberg and Trautwein, 1974), it may cross the zero current level three times, causing the cell to have two stable levels of V_{rest} rather than the customary one. This situation can cause the repolarization process to "hang" at the less polarized of the two stable levels until such time that additional outward current is somehow generated. An I_{K1}-V curve resembling that for the cat ventricle does not produce such an event. This difference in the I_{K1}-V curves of different species may explain some of the diversity in the effects that have been reported for interventions said to operate through an action on this current. Whether I_{K1} in human ventricle is more like that of dog or that of cat remains to be determined.

The inward rectifying K current seems to serve several electrophysiologic roles. The first is to "set" V_{rest} at or near E_K and make V_{rest} quite sensitive to $[K^+]_o$ (typically $\geq$ 55–60 mV per 10-fold change in $[K^+]_o$). It also contributes to the repolarizing currents flowing during phase 3, particularly during the later portion when the other K^+-based currents have undergone substantial voltage-dependent deactivation. Although the belief is not universally shared, I_{K1} appears to contribute a major portion of the repolarizing current that flows during phase 3. This notion arises largely because alternative sources of significant repolarizing current have not been demonstrated. Finally, that the current is inwardly rectifying with such a striking increase in conductance at V_m negative to E_K suggests that its principal purpose is to prevent V_{rest} from ever becoming significantly negative to E_K in the event that the Na pump became strongly activated. In essence, the inward rectification serves to short-circuit the current generated by the Na pump when V_m is near or exceeds E_K. Were V_{rest} to exceed E_K, excitation and conduction could become tenuous and impulse conduction could fail as a result of a need for much larger than normal depolarizing currents to achieve excitation. The changes in V_{rest} associated with intracellular acidosis, chronic disease states (Ten Eick and Singer, 1979), and exposure to lysophosphatidylcholine, a metabolite of the phosphatidylcholine found as a constituent component of the myocyte sarcolemma produced during ischemia, may result from a decrease in the conductance for I_{K1} (Clarkson and Ten Eick, 1983). All these changes are accompanied by an increase in steady-state membrane resistance and, incidentally, in the ability of an activated Na pump current to hyperpolarize V_{rest} to levels well negative to E_K (Rasmussen et al., 1986).

Delayed Outward Rectifying K Current I_K

Although a prominent voltage- and time-dependent delayed outward rectifying K current, termed I_K (or I_X in Noble's original notation for Purkinje fibers; Hauswirth et al., 1972), has been described in multicellular preparations of guinea pig and cat papillary muscles using the single-sucrose gap voltage clamp technique by many investigators (Ten Eick et al., 1983; Clarkson and Ten Eick, 1983; Nawrath et al., 1977; McDonald and Trautwein, 1978), the evidence from isolated cat ventricular myocytes indicates that it is not much more than a very minor component of the outward current when elicited by depolarizing pulses from V_{hold} negative to -40 mV to V_m in the plateau range. Even when strongly depolarizing pulses are applied (e.g., $V_m \geq 40$ mV), the delayed outward K current is rather small (i.e., typically only 100–200 pA) and it develops with a very slow time constant, which can be up to several seconds. It is an enigma why the delayed outward current recorded from cat papillary muscle by McDonald and Trautwein (1978) using the sucrose gap voltage clamp method was so robust and

so rapidly developing (time constants were typically ≤300–500 msec) in comparison to the analogous I_K-like current recorded from isolated cat ventricular myocytes (Ten Eick, Harvey, and Barrington, unpublished data). The differences may not be real, possibly having arisen from artifacts generated with the sucrose gap approach (e.g., interstitial K^+ accumulation), or they could reflect a fundamental difference between the I_K of papillary muscles and that of cells isolated from the ventricular wall.

A larger, more rapidly developing I_K has been elicited from dissociated canine Purkinje fibers (Cohen et al., 1986) and from guinea pig ventricular myocytes (Matsuura et al., 1987). However, even in these types of cells, the current cannot be regarded as robust because only rarely is it larger than 0.5 nA even when fully developed after a 10 sec pulse to 60 mV. In guinea pig ventricular myocytes I_K appears to be modulated by the autonomic nervous system. The amplitude of the current is enhanced during exposure to β-adrenergic agonists, an effect that can be antagonized by concomitant exposure to cholinergic agonists and that involves a G protein-based regulatory mechanism (Harvey and Hume, 1989b). However, even when fully enhanced with 1 μM isoproterenol the whole-cell currents flowing during 5 sec voltage clamp pulses to V_m relevant to the action potential plateau are only 100–200 pA. In addition, I_K appears to "run down" in a manner similar to I_{Ca} over a period of 5–15 min after gaining intracellular access with a patch pipette. This rundown can be prevented by dialyzing the cell with an internal solution containing nonhydrolyzable GTP analogs, a finding that again implicates a G protein as a modulator of I_K even when it is not stimulated by β-agonists (Harvey and Hume, 1989b).

To what extent failure to find a robust I_K in cat ventricular cells is related to rundown is uncertain. Curiously, in our hands, isoproterenol in concentrations that clearly increase I_{Ca} (1–10 μM) does not detectably enhance the tiny I_K seen in cat myocytes (Schackow and Ten Eick, unpublished data). This suggests that I_K in cat and guinea pig ventricular myocytes are qualitatively different. Which, if either, is the relevant model for human ventricle remains to be clarified. The several uncertainties concerning I_K are amplified by the fact that convincing recordings of single-channel currents with a behavior appropriate to support the whole-cell I_K have apparently not yet been reported for ventricular cells from any species.

Based on the behavior of I_K in papillary muscle, McDonald and Trautwein (1978) concluded that I_K was a major contributor of the late repolarizing current when action potential duration was more than 200–300 msec long, as they are when the heart rate (or the stimulus rate) is low (<0.5 Hz). This view no longer seems tenable because whole-cell I_K is so small and slow to activate. However, if the voltage dependencies of activation and deactivation allow I_K to activate at plateau voltages faster than it deactivates during diastole, I_K could "accumulate" during a long series of beats at a rapid rate. The gradually increasing (accumulating) I_K is expected to cause a gradual shortening of the action potential duration after an abrupt increase in the beat rate. Therefore it is not unreasonable to speculate that I_K may modulate repolarization during phase 3. The ability of some selective blockers of I_K to inhibit rate-dependent changes in action potential duration supports this notion (Hume, 1989). However, I_K cannot be regarded as a major source of late repolarizing current, a least not in cat ventricular myocytes and probably not even in guinea pig ventricular myocytes, despite the fact that it is a larger current in the latter than in the former. There must surely be a source of outward current whose role is to effect the repolarization of the action potential elicited by cultured cells, but it apparently is not provided by either I_{to} or I_K. Much earlier in this chapter we indicated that a strongly activated Na pump current could abbreviate the action potential duration by as much as 10% but when $[Na^+]_i$ is normal (e.g., ~10 mM) this too appears unable to account for but a small fraction of the current needed for repolarization during phase 3. Can (must) I_{K1} by itself provide most of the needed

current, or are there other sources of repolarizing current?

"Instantaneous" Outward "Plateau" K Current I_{Kp}

Yue and Marban (1988) described "a novel K channel." It was Ba^{2+} sensitive, Ca^{2+} and TEA insensitive, "ohmic" in nature, very rapidly activating (<1–2 msec), noninactivating, and exhibited a Boltzmann-like relationship between V_m and open probability (P_o), with a P_o of zero when V_m is negative to around -60 mV and maximal ($P_o = 0.3$–0.4) when V_m is about 50 mV. The single-channel conductance when internal and external $[K^+]$ were "normal" was 14 pS. Yue and Marban (1988) proposed that the channel's current be named "i_{Kp}," because it would be expected to support K current during an action potential plateau and contribute to repolarization. The channel was quite selective for K^+, but unlike I_{K1}, at least when V_m is negative to E_K, the conductance was insensitive to change in $[K^+]_o$. It is pertinent to mention that these properties are similar to those of I_K in cat papillary muscle when examined using the sucrose gap voltage clamp method (McDonald and Trautwein, 1978). Also pertinent is the finding that the inwardly rectifying K current described by Harvey and Ten Eick (1988) as I_{K1} was also insensitive to changing extracellular $[K^+]$ at V_m positive to E_K by at least 10 mV. Despite these two curious parallels, a contribution by the "novel" channel to either the papillary muscle I_K or the cat myocyte I_{K1} seems unlikely because of its lack of either outward or inward rectification and because the single-channel conductances for these currents are different from one another. They also argued that i_{Kp} can be distinguished from $i_{K(ATP)}$ by the difference in their single-channel conductances (14 versus 80 pS).

The channel may underlie the rather small (i.e., <0.5 nA) steady-state outward current remaining in cat right ventricular myocytes during strong depolarizing pulses after all time-dependent components are accounted for. However, the sole source of convincing evidence that an I_{Kp} current exists has been derived from single-channel recordings. At the time of this writing there has been no evidence reported from whole-cell patch currents that can support the existence of this current. Solid support may be difficult to achieve because the pharmacology of the i_{Kp} channel is not yet sufficiently explored to know whether this particular K current can be selectively, if not specifically, blocked, or if blockers of the other channel types that one would use to isolate I_{Kp} pharmacologically for study will also in some way alter, if not inhibit, I_{Kp}. To further complicate matters, there is still insufficient information at the single-channel level to predict with reasonable assurance how large the whole-cell current should be and the nature of its kinetics. It is conceivable that the number of channels for i_{Kp} are so few that they produce an insignificant contribution to the whole-cell current. However, it must be recognized that there is a component of the whole-cell current that we do not acknowledge by assigning it a formal name. It is called the "linear leak" current simply because we do not know what else to call it. Interestingly enough, however, the leak current is inhibited by <0.5–1.0 mM concentrations of Ba^{2+}. Is the leak current, or at least part of it, I_{Kp}? This is an interesting possibility, but too little is known to do more than idly speculate at this time.

ATP-Sensitive K Current $I_{K(ATP)}$

Another K current has recently been identified under conditions in which intracellular ATP is reduced to rather low levels (<200 μM). The single-channel conductance is larger than either i_{K1} or i_K channels, approximately 80 pS (Noma, 1983). Since this channel is detectable only under conditions that exist during extreme metabolic duress, $I_{K(ATP)}$ is assumed to activate during ischemic or hypoxic conditions. Activation of $I_{K(ATP)}$ may partially explain the remarkable shortening of the action potential duration that occurs under such conditions. In addition, channel activation may provide some outward current to hyperpolarize the V_{rest} of partially depolarized, ischemic

cells to a level closer to E_K than would otherwise be possible. Both effects would protect cells against the damaging effects of Ca overload during ischemia. Action potential shortening would reduce ion fluxes (Na^+ influx and K^+ efflux) whose homeostatic mechanisms require energy derived from an already depleted intracellular pool of ATP. A foreshortened action potential duration would also limit Ca^{2+} influx via I_{Ca}, thus reducing ATP requirements for the SR Ca^{2+}-ATPase. In addition, cell hyperpolarization would improve the chances of conduction through ischemic regions by at least partially maintaining I_{Na} availability.

The ATP sensitivity of the channels has been found to decrease into the millimolar range within several minutes after obtaining intracellular access with large-bore patch electrodes (Kirsch et al., 1990); also, the sensitivity of $I_{K(ATP)}$ has been reported to decrease relative to normal in myocytes derived from hypertrophied ventricle (Cameron et al., 1988). These findings suggest that this channel may occasionally come into play even at normal levels of ATP. Much research effort has recently been directed toward the development of antiarrhythmic drugs targeted to the ATP-sensitive K channels and the whole-cell current they serve. However, the precise role and physiology of these channels remains to be fully characterized.

Na-Sensitive K Current $I_{K(Na)}$

Still another K^+ current system operating under conditions of elevated Na^+_i has recently been identified. $I_{K(Na)}$ channels have a very large conductance (~210 pS) and can open when Na^+_i is about 25 mM or higher (Kameyama et al., 1984). The role of $I_{K(Na)}$ has not yet been defined but an increased outward current would be expected to shorten action potential duration and possibly hyperpolarize V_{rest}. Elevation of Na^+_i could occur when normal Na^+_i extrusion mechanisms are inadequate to balance Na^+ influx, for example during Na, K-ATPase inhibition, ATP depletion, and/or massive Na^+ influx, among other conditions. The effects of turning on this current would be protective and similar to those already described for $I_{K(ATP)}$ including abbreviation of the action potential to reduce Na^+ and Ca^{2+} influx and ATP utilization and to hyperpolarize V_{rest} so that impulse conduction is at least partially normalized. However, since elevation of Na^+_i (and Ca^{2+}_i via Na-Ca exchange) to a level high enough to activate this current is usually toxic if not lethal, we surmise that $I_{K(Na)}$ would only be operative under extreme physiologic conditions and does not have any role in normal cell function.

Transient Inward Current I_{ti}

The transient inward current was identified as a principal source of inward current underlying delayed afterdepolarizations (DAD; see Fig. 8 for an example) and subthreshold voltage oscillations that can occur in cardiac tissues under conditions of Ca^{2+}_i overload (for reviews, see Ferrier, 1977; Wit and Rosen, 1986; January and Fozzard, 1988). Its importance lies in the fact that the generation of many triggered ventricular tachyarrhythmias, particularly those associated with Ca^{2+}_i overload (including digitalis intoxication and the Ca^{2+} paradox), most likely arise as result of DAD and the attendant oscillations in V_m. I_{ti} is activated by elevated Ca^{2+}_i, as evidenced by its enhancement following an iontophoretic injection of Ca^{2+} and abolition by EGTA (Matsuda et al., 1982). There are two main notions concerning the ionic basis of I_{ti}. The first was offered by Kass and coworkers (1978) after they found an apparent reversal potential for I_{ti} of around -4 mV. They concluded that I_{ti} is a mix of inward and outward cationic current. This idea received support from the discovery in heart of a discrete nonspecific cation channel, activated by Ca^{2+}_i (Colquhoun et al., 1981) that could serve as the conductance pathway for I_{ti}.

In contrast, the dependence of I_{ti} on an elevation of Ca^{2+}_i was the basis for the suggestion that I_{ti} actually represents an oscillating current generated by electrogenic Na-Ca exchange (Arlock and Katzung, 1985; Noble, 1985; Lin et al., 1986; Lipp and Pott, 1988). A

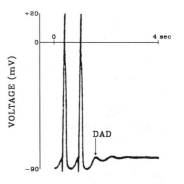

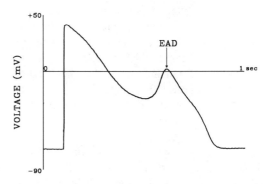

Figure 8 Abnormal automaticity in ventricular tissues. (Top) Example of a delayed afterdepolarization (DAD) in a sheep Purkinje fiber exposed to acetylstrophanthidin. The last two beats of a 20 beat train (600 msec basic cycle length) were followed by a pause during which three DAD occurred before a stable resting potential was achieved. This behavior is virtually identical to that seen in atrial and ventricular muscle. (J. A. Wasserstrom, unpublished observation.) (Bottom) Example of an early afterdepolarization (EAD) occurring spontaneously in cat ventricular myocyte that had been kept in a conventional primary culture environment for several days. The internal and external solutions were entirely conventional and contained no drugs. Temperature = 37°C. (E. Schackow and R. E. Ten Eick, unpublished data.)

transient elevation of Ca^{2+}_i favors a transient increase in the inward current generated electrogenically during the associated increase in the rate of Na-Ca exchange. This suggestion has found support from data failing to identify either a clear reversal potential for I_{ti} or an increase in membrane conductance during I_{ti}. In addition, the responses of I_{ti} to changes in either the Ca^{2+}_i load or $[Na^+]_o$ and $[Ca^{2+}]_o$ are similar to those predicted for a mechanism involving electrogenic Na-Ca exchange. The lack of a selective blocker for either I_{Na-Ca} or I_{ti} precludes distinguishing between these possibilities with any reasonable certainty.

Since myocytes exhibit this current only under conditions that are toxic and are associated with disturbances in cardiac electrical activity, it is assumed to be more of an arrhythmogenic influence than a contributor to current normally underlying the action potential. Since delayed afterdepolarizations are maximal in amplitude when V_m is approximately -70mV (Ferrier, 1977; Wasserstrom and Ferrier, 1981), it is likely that depolarization from the normal level of V_{rest} (e.g., about -90 mV) promotes the abnormal ventricular automaticity that is induced by this mechanism. Conversely, hyperpolarization by pharmacologic or physiologic means would tend to decrease DAD amplitude and therefore reduce their potential to initiate arrhythmias. Thus the level of regional interstitial K^+_o, particularly when it varies from locale to locale during regional ischemia, may have significant effects on the arrhythmogenic influences of I_{ti}. In addition, any intervention that would increase Ca^{2+}_i (e.g., increasing the rate of beating; Wit and Rosen, 1986) would be expected to increase the likelihood of I_{ti} and enhance their amplitude, thereby increasing the likelihood of DAD-induced triggered arrhythmias. The role of this type of activity in vivo remains to be clarified fully.

Stretch-Activated Channels i_{SAC}

Stretch-activated channels are membrane-bound channels that function as mechanoreceptors (Sachs, 1986). These channels respond to deformation of the cell membrane by opening a nonspecific conductance that exhibits an open probability proportional to the pressure (positive or negative) applied to deform the surrounding membrane (Guhary and Sachs, 1984). The conductance of the stretch-activated channels in neonatal rat ventricular cells has been reported to be 120 ± 45 pS; i_{SAC} reversed at -31 ± 13 mV positive to V_{rest} be 5.4 mM $[K^+]_o$ (this probably translates to be about -20 to -10 mV), suggesting that i_{SAC} is a

mixed current (Craelius et al., 1988). Stretch-activated channels in cardiac cell membranes are expected to open in response to osmotically induced cell swelling or shrinking or in response to stretch resulting from the contraction of neighboring cells, diastolic filling of the ventricular chambers, or the effects of hypertrophy, heart failure, development of akinetic ischemic regions (e.g., in the ventricular free wall), or other wall motion (contraction) abnormalities. It is not inconceivable that inward current flowing through stretch-activated channels contributes inward current to fuel the spontaneous depolarization associated with either normal or abnormal automaticity. However attractive any speculations concerning the role(s) of cardiac stretch-activated channels may seem, at present they are merely speculations. All we can say at this time is that they appear to be present in ventricular myocytes, but the details about their behavior remain to be clarified. These channels apparently respond only to deformation of the surrounding membrane, so they apparently are devoid of a pharmacology. It will therefore be exceedingly difficult to determine unequivocally the nature of any effects they may have on the electrophysiologic activity of cardiac ventricular cells.

IMPULSE FORMATION AND ABNORMAL AUTOMATICITY IN VENTRICULAR CELLS

Many cardiac cells, under appropriate conditions, can generate action potentials in the absence of external stimuli. This capacity to beat spontaneously is known as "*automaticity*" and in many cardiac cells is a completely intrinsic characteristic (Hoffman and Cranefield, 1960). In automatic cells, after repolarization (phase 3) has been completed and phase 4 has been initiated, the transmembrane potential decreases slowly from the maximal level of diastolic potential until it reaches threshold potential and initiates a new action potential. Automaticity is not ordinarily a property of ventricular cells exposed to extracellular conditions approximating those believed to exist normally. However, even ventricular cells can, under unusual but nonetheless physiologic conditions, exhibit what has been termed by Hoffman and Cranefield (1964) *"abnormal"* automaticity, and initiate ectopic beating.

Automaticity in Purkinje fibers undergoing slow spontaneous depolarization during phase 4 (termed diastolic depolarization) results from (1) the development of an inward component of current termed the *"funny"* or pacemaker current I_f which is carried mostly by Na^+ and activated with rather slow kinetics by (re)polarization of V_m into the range of -60 to -90 mV; and (2) the decay of the outward K currents activated during the plateau and phase 3. The conjoint effect of these several currents is to tip the balance from net outward (or zero) current to net inward current and a slowly developing depolarization from the MDP results. Spontaneous beating that is abolished by 1–2 mM Cs^+ is generally presumed to be supported by I_f or an I_f-like current; slowly developing inward current evoked by hyperpolarizing voltage clamps from -40 mV to around -100 mV, which is inhibited by Cs^+, is presumed to be I_f. By these criteria I_f has not been demonstrated in isolated ventricular myocytes. Curiously, however, neither has the I_f that is so prominent in intact sheep and canine Purkinje fibers been evoked from single, enzymatically isolated Purkinje cells. This could mean that the involved channels may be inactivated (or destroyed, removed, inactivated, or otherwise altered) by enzyme treatment, but other interpretations are possible. For example, just because we do not expect to find i_f channels in ventricular cells and in fact we do not, can we justifiably conclude they are not present when they also cannot be found in isolated single Purkinje cells? Clearly this is an area needing further experimental work.

Although the best information at the present time indicates that ventricular cells do not exhibit automaticity supported by I_f or an I_f-like current, it is clear that ventricular cells can be induced to beat spontaneously and that, when they do, it must result from the production of net inward current that develops following the completion of the repolarization process. There could be several sources of the inward current underlying spontaneous beating in ventricular cells. One of the most likely sources is that arising from I_{ti}. Another is that arising from oscillations in the current generated by the Na-Ca exchanger in response to fluctuations in intracellular Ca^{2+} activity. Inward current having such origins could give rise to DAD, but EAD would be unlikely. These notions were discussed in detail in the previous section devoted to the transient inward current.

When impulse initiation occurs only after previous stimulation, it is considered to represent *triggered* rather than truly spontaneous activity (Cranefield, 1977). In general, any depolarizing influence promotes triggered beating (Surawicz, 1980) whereas hyperpolarization reduces the likelihood of a DAD reaching threshold. However, there is one exception to this generalization. It is unlikely that a localized accumulation of K^+ would have similar actions because, in addition to depolarizing V_m, increased $[K^+]_o$ also decreases membrane resistance, making it more difficult for a I_{ti}-induced DAD to achieve the voltage threshold for I_{Na} activation. On the other hand, electrotonic influences from adjoining depolarized myocardial regions could reduce membrane potential sufficiently to permit a coincident DAD to depolarize V_m to the activation voltage threshold for I_{Na}. For a DAD to successfully induce an extra beat, two conditions must be met: (1) the rate of depolarization during the DAD must be sufficiently rapid to achieve the voltage threshold for an upstroke without producing additional inactivation (accommodation); (2) V_{rest} must be fairly negative (-70 mV or more) to have an adequate number of Na^+ channels available for activation. Activation may result if the membrane resistance is high because large voltage changes can be produced with relatively small I_{ti}. This probably excludes conditions that favor $I_{K(Na)}$ or $I_{K(ATP)}$ since resting membrane conductance is markedly elevated by these currents. Higher than normal intercellular resistance also favors activation of triggered beats when I_{ti} is small.

Abnormal automaticity generated by early afterdepolarizations (see Fig. 8 for an example) is also considered triggered because of the necessity to have an initiating action potential that triggers the production of an EAD (Damiano and Rosen, 1984). Recent reports suggest that EADs may play a role in the generation of arrhythmias in vivo, such as during antiarrhythmic therapy with agents that prolong the action potential, such as quinidine and sotalol (Roden and Hoffman, 1985) and in patients with drug-induced torsade des points (multiform ventricular tachycardia) (Brachmann et al., 1983). EAD have also been reported to produce spontaneous beating in isolated cardiac cells under a variety of conditions. A recent study of EAD suggests that they are not governed by the same mechanisms responsible for DAD (January et al., 1988). Instead, EAD are promoted by altering the net balance of current during the plateau. These conditions are favored by decreasing the outward, repolarizing current or increasing the inward current. Agents that block outward currents, including Ba^{2+}, Cs^+, and amantadine, prolong action potential duration and favor EAD production. Agents that increase inward current can produce virtually identical effects. Maintained I_{Ca} activation with Bay K 8644, reduced K conductance caused by reduced $[K^+]_o$, or any other intervention that slows repolarization can increase the incidence of EAD (January and Riddle, 1989). The data suggest that if repolarization is slow enough for I_{Ca} to recover sufficiently and to reactivate before full repolarization occurs, then EAD can occur and abnormal automaticity may be initiated. In contrast, any intervention that abbreviates the action potential, including blocking I_{Na} with tetrodotoxin or I_{Ca} with dihydropyridines or increasing $[K^+]_o$, can antagonize EAD.

Theoretically, for an EAD to occur net inward current must develop at some time during the period at least 10 msec or more after the onset of depolarizing clamp pulses to voltages in the range relevant to the plateau voltage. This situation can arise when the inactivation kinetics and current densities of I_{Ca} and I_{to} are just different enough that I_{to} can briefly carry net membrane current to zero or net outward but then decays so fast that a more slowly decaying i_{Ca} can reestablish a short period of net inward current before I_{Ca} inactivates during the remainder of the depolarizing pulse (Hauswirth et al., 1969). Such behavior has been recorded from patch-clamped feline right ventricular (RV) cells isolated from cats with RV hypertrophy induced by RV pressure overload (Harvey and Ten Eick, unpublished data). Whether this interplay between I_{Ca} and I_{to} underlies the EAD that are more frequent in this particular preparation than in "normal" cells is not certain, but the possibility is interesting. Spontaneous beating due to this mechanism is expected to be inhibited by blockers of either I_{Ca} or I_{to}. A role for this mechanism in clinical rhythm disturbances has not been recognized, but it has never been systematically investigated, either.

CABLE PROPERTIES, INTERCELLULAR RESISTANCE, AND IMPULSE CONDUCTION

Cable Properties and Their Analysis in Cardiac Tissue

Impulse propagation in cardiac tissue is the product of an interplay between the so-called active and passive properties of the sarcolemma of the cells comprising the tissue. Together they are termed the *membrane properties*. Active properties include the voltage- and time-dependent behavior of the different ion channels in the sarcolemma. The preceding sections were primarily concerned with the active properties. Ionic current regulated by the active properties serves two purposes. One is to serve as the source for the transmembrane current to generate the locally occurring membrane action potential. The other is to provide the voltage difference that causes excitatory current to flow from excited cells to unexcited cells located distally along the conduction pathway (see Fig. 9, top). It is this excitatory current that depolarizes the V_m of

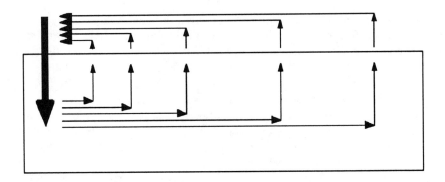

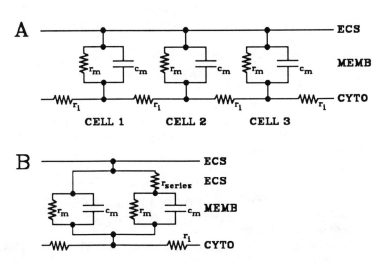

Figure 9 (Top) Local circuit currents during conduction of an action potential. The large thick arrow can represent either a point source of current injected into the cell or the depolarizing leading edge of an action potential upstroke as it moves from left to right. The internally located positive charge brought in by the upstroke or the injected current is electrostatically (electrotonically) repelled forward, ahead of the depolarizing wavefront, and discharges the negatively charged membrane capacitance. The combination of increasing positivity just inside the membrane and the relative negativity on the extracellular surface of the membrane in the depolarized region draws external positive charges away from the inactive region and toward the active region, thus completing the circuit. The thin arrows represent the electrotonically driven local circuit currents. The decreasing current density with distance ahead of the depolarizing current source is depicted by the distance between the thin arrows.

(Bottom, A) A schematic diagram of the equivalent circuit for a cell membrane showing three successive membrane elements (cells) from left to right. If current is "injected" into the cytoplasmic (cyto) side of cell 1, the current flows to cells 2 and 3, producing the pattern of current flow shown in the upper panel. (B) The unitary equivalent circuit with more detail (i.e., the series resistance of the T tubules is represented).

the distal unexcited cells to the voltage threshold for I_{Na} (or I_{Ca}) and thereby initiates an action potential at the distal site. This process of an action potential in a proximal cell serving as the source of current to excite a distal cell is repeated element by element, again and again, to effect impulse propagation along the length of a cardiac fiber (Rushton, 1937). The passive membrane properties regulate the current flowing between cells that exhibit differences in the levels of their V_m. The passive properties therefore describe the electrical properties of the sarcolemma that regulate the cell-to-cell charge flow required for impulse conduction (Weidmann, 1951; Jack et al., 1975). Passive properties of the sarcolemma are often ignored because they seem difficult to understand and of little consequence in arrhythmogenesis and drug actions. However, recently their possible importance to our understanding of antiarrhythmic drug actions and the pathophysiology of cardiac disease has received a deserved increased level of attention (Arnsdorf and Wasserstrom, 1986).

The passive membrane properties are the direct result of the structure and physical and chemical properties of the cardiac cell membrane interacting with the intra- and extracellular milieu. The sarcolemma is composed of a lipid bilayer, with each half of the bilayer consisting of polar head groups attached to a hydrophobic tail. Monolayers are oriented by hydrophobic interactions of the tail groups, leaving the charged hydrophilic heads directed toward the aqueous extracellular and intracellular milieus. The amphipathic properties of the membrane lipid are largely responsible for the orientation and interactions of lipids within the membrane. It is the dielectric property of the hydrophobic tails of the lipid bilayer that allows the membrane to separate charge across a rather small distance (around 100 Å) at quite high field strength. As result the bilayer can be polarized, allowing the membrane to store charge as though it were a capacitor. The membrane is highly resistant to transmembrane current flow, except through the channel proteins inserted into the membrane. Their voltage sensitivity and ionic selectivity permit them to serve as aqueous

conduits for transmembrane current in the form of ion fluxes. These structural features endow the sarcolemma with the electrical properties of both resistance and capacitance (Fozzard and Arnsdorf, 1986), and most models of membrane electrical function place these elements oriented in parallel across the membrane (see Fig. 9, bottom).

Much of the work on the cable properties of cardiac tissue has been performed in discrete bundles of Purkinje fibers because they approximate the behavior of an infinite cable with regard to how current spreads (Weidmann, 1952; Schoenberg and Fozzard, 1979). Assuming an infinite cable, a coaxial conductor model simplifies the analysis of nonconducted current spread in appropriate cardiac tissues. The component cells in cardiac tissues are connected by low-resistance pathways called gap junctions that can allow both movement of small molecules and spread of ionic current between cells (Weingart et al., 1975). Gap junctions are located mostly at the ends of Purkinje cells, favoring current flow along the length of the fiber while restricting transverse current spread, whereas in ventricular cells junctions are also present along the sides, allowing for both longitudinal and transverse (anisotropic) conduction (Clerc, 1976). The location of gap junctions therefore appropriately influences impulse spread in both tissues so that Purkinje fibers can conduct the impulse from the AVN to the distal ventricular muscle mass as rapidly as possible and ensure nearly simultaneous activation of the entire ventricular mass to obtain an efficient ventricular contraction and ejection of blood.

Early experiments examining the passive behavior of cardiac cell membranes used intracellular current injection through an intracellular microelectrode to examine the spread of current along a fiber bundle (Weidmann, 1960). An intracellular injection of current results in a time-dependent change in V_m along the entire length of the fiber; the time constant τ describing the rate of this voltage change is expressed by

$$\tau_m = r_m c_m \tag{1}$$

where r_m is membrane resistance (g_m^{-1}) and c_m is membrane capacitance. The voltage decline with distance is described by

$$V_x = V_0 \, e^{-x/m} \tag{2}$$

where V_x is the transmembrane potential at any given distance x from the current source, V_0 is the voltage at the point of current injection (i.e., $x = 0$), and λ_m is the length constant of the membrane. The length constant is defined as the distance over which V_m falls by a factor of e^{-1} (i.e., to approximately 37% of V_0). The experimentally defined profile for the decay of V_m with distance from the injection site along the length of a thin fiber appears well fit to an exponential. Fitting the data to these equations allows λ_m and r_m to be calculated and then used to determine r_i, the internal (or axial) resistance of the cable, from

$$\lambda_m = \left(\frac{r_m}{r_i + r_o} \right)^{1/2} \tag{3}$$

External resistance r_o is usually regarded as negligible and therefore is neglected, but when dealing with long, narrow interstitial spaces this may not be a justified assumption.

The input resistance R_{in} describes the relationship between current input I_0 and the voltage response V_0 at $x = 0$ where

$$R_{in} = \frac{V_0}{I_0} = (r_m r_i)^{1/2} \tag{4}$$

The relation between passive and active membrane properties can be best understood through the application of the concept of liminal length. This concept was used in nerve (Rushton, 1937) and, more recently, in heart (Schoenberg and Fozzard, 1979) to describe the minimum length of a fiber that must be depolarized at least to its threshold voltage to activate enough inward depolarizing current to exceed the outward repolarizing current flowing into the depolarized region from the fully polarized region beyond and achieve excitation.

$$\text{Liminal length} = \frac{0.855 Q_{th}}{2\pi^{3/2} a C_m \lambda_m V_{th}} \tag{5}$$

where Q_{th} is charge threshold, a is the radius of the tissue, and V_{th} is threshold voltage. Defining the liminal length helps to relate electrotonic current spread to the regenerative depolarization necessary to sustain impulse conduction. Although its utility to precisely calculate the effects of arrhythmogenic and antiarrhythmic interventions is limited, it is a useful means of mathematically relating passive membrane properties to the generation and propagation of action potentials.

This brief treatment of cable properties provides a cursory quantitative description of passive current spread in cardiac cells. A detailed treatment of cable analysis and the theory of current flow in excitable cells can be found in definitive sources, such as the now classic treatment by Jack et al. (1975).

Factors Influencing Intercellular Current Flow and Impulse Conduction

Conduction in the heart depends upon current flowing from one cell to the next. A number of factors affect the resistance to current flow (the so-called *intercellular coupling*) between adjacent cells mediated by action involving the resistance characteristics of gap junctions. The healing process after tissue injury (De Mello, 1972) or the mechanical or enzymatic separation of cells is effected by "closing" the gap junctions. This process allows polarized "healthy" cells to electrically disconnect (uncouple) themselves from injured depolarized cells so that the former are not depolarized by the electrotonic flow of injury current from the latter. Uncoupling also prevents the diffusion of the products of cell damage, such as proteases and Ca^{2+}_i, from injured cells to normal cells. Both decreasing pH_i and increasing pCa_i promotes uncoupling (Weingart, 1982; Dahl and Isenberg, 1980), apparently as the result of a direct effect of these ions to close gap junction channels. In addition, because of the interaction of H^+ and Ca^{2+} for common intracellular binding sites (Bers and Ellis, 1982), an increase in either of these ions results in a higher cytosolic concentration of the other, an effect that magnifies an action to close gap junctional channels. Reduced metabolic function can limit the ATP available for various membrane ion extrusion mechanisms, such as the sarcolemmal Na, K-ATPase and the Ca^{2+}-ATPase in the sarcolemma and mitochondria, and allow Na^+, protons, and Ca^{2+} to accumulate intracellularly and thereby induce gap junctional closure.

Positive inotropic agents that increase free cytosolic $Ca^{2+}{}_i$, such as digitalis, can increase intercellular resistance, thereby impairing conduction. Conversely, agents that produce their positive inotropic actions via cAMP, including phosphodiesterase inhibitors and β-adrenergic agonists, can reduce free cytoplasmic $[Ca^{2+}]$ and are expected to improve conduction. Toxic metabolites that accumulate during ischemia, such as lysophosphatidylcholine (LPC), can alter cable properties (Arnsdorf and Sawicki, 1981) and increase V_0, R_{in}, and λ_m, among other actions. It is possible that the effects of LPC and several related cellular metabolites on cell-to-cell coupling can at least partially explain their effects on impulse conduction. The importance of the findings with LPC is derived from the fact that myocardial ischemia appears to promote the accumulation of LPC in ischemic cardiac tissue. However, whether LPC has a role in the cardiac rhythm disturbances associated with ischemia remains to be proven.

INTERACTIONS BETWEEN PASSIVE AND ACTIVE MEMBRANE PROPERTIES: IMPLICATIONS FOR ANTIARRHYTHMIC DRUG EFFICACY AND FOR ARRHYTHMOGENESIS

An interaction between electrotonically flowing current and membrane current may be involved in the genesis of certain cardiac arrhythmias (Janse, 1986). It has been thought for many years that alterations in both passive and active membrane properties in one limb of a bifurcated conduction pathway may lead to reentrant excitation (Wit et al., 1972a, b; Jalife and Moe, 1976). These interactions have been studied in some detail in vitro through the use of a "gap of limited excitability" imposed along the length of a Purkinje fiber (Antzelevitch et al., 1980). The results clearly demonstrate that the electrotonic spread of current across this gap has important influences on the electrical activity of the tissue distal to the gap, including pacemaker entrainment and the generation of coupled rhythms (Jalife, 1984). Impulse "reflection" can also occur as result of electrotonic current, with subsequent reentry of the reflected beat through the gap and reinvading the tissue proximal to the gap (Antzelevitch et al., 1980). In addition, electrotonus is capable of bringing the previously quiescent distal segment to threshold and generating action potentials purely via passive processes, giving the appearance that conducted impulses can "jump" across inexcitable areas of membrane. It is therefore clear that the mechanisms responsible for the generation of arrhythmias probably include a combination of alterations in the passive as well as the active membrane properties.

One implication of this important interplay between the active and passive properties of cardiac cells and tissues is that the efficacy of many antiarrhythmic agents may be derived not only from their effects on ion channels but also from their ability to alter the passive membrane cable properties, thereby altering excitability and conduction. One means by which passive current spread can be altered by antiarrhythmic drugs is via their ability to influence the intracellular concentrations of ions that modulate intercellular coupling. All antiarrhythmic agents that reduce Na^+ and/or Ca^{2+} influx through their respective channels, including most clinically useful class I–IV drugs, should improve intracellular coupling by limiting the extent to which the resistance of the gap junctions increases. The result is to improve conduction by a mechanism that is conceptually independent of any direct membrane effects of the drugs either to improve or inhibit conduction.

Several recent reports have described the effects of some antiarrhythmic drugs on passive membrane properties. For instance, lidocaine can decrease V_0, τ_m, and λ_m and some other passive properties in Purkinje fibers, whereas procainamide has opposite effects (Sawicki and Arnsdorf, 1985). These effects on the passive properties are particularly prominent in cases in which the cellular pathology includes elevated Na^+_i and/or Ca^{2+}_i, such as during reperfusion following ischemia and digitalis toxicity. The contribution of these changes in the passive properties of cardiac tissue to the antiarrhythmic efficacy of these agents remains to be determined, but they may in fact be quite substantial. In addition, it is also possible that agents that increase r_m or λ_m increase the contribution of electrotonic currents to the excitatory process and tissue conductivity and thereby enhance the effectiveness of extrasystoles to spread and activate the heart or to promote slow conduction.

To take into account the multiplicity of drug actions on these passive membrane properties as well as their potent blocking effects on ionic currents, an integrated, multifactorial approach to the analysis of antiarrhythmic efficacy was put forth (Arnsdorf, 1990; Arnsdorf and Wasserstrom, 1986). This matrix approach takes into consideration not only the voltage, time, state, and use dependence of the drug-channel interaction but also considers potential drug actions directly on the substrate or electrophysiologic basis of the underlying arrhythmia, including the effects on electrotonic current spread.

SUMMARY, CONCLUSIONS, AND CONNECTIONS

Our purpose in this chapter was to explore the notion that the electrical activity of a patient's heart is the result of biologically derived currents whose purposes are to depolarize and then repolarize the cells of the myocardium and to flow from cell to cell to propagate the excitatory event around the heart. We have indicated that the current source is derived from the transmembrane flow of charge in the form of ions and that this flow is not willy-nilly in

nature. Rather, it is highly regulated by specific, specialized proteins that have been inserted into the sarcolemma to serve as conductance channels, which confer the voltage- and time-dependent characteristics special to each component of the membrane current. Membrane channels are gene products, and therefore channel behavior is ultimately controlled by the nuclear genes. The challenge of the next decade is to understand *how* genes regulate channel expression. If our original postulate that heart disease and cardiac drugs alter the cellular electrophysiology of the heart by altering ion channel function is correct, understanding the regulation of channel function at the level of the gene may provide the handle needed to better understand how drugs act and how acute and chronic heart disease alters channel function.

ACKNOWLEDGMENTS

The authors thank Eric Schackow for allowing us to steal his time to create the nine computer-generated text figures and for allowing us to use some of his thesis data as examples. We also thank, most deeply, our wives for their support and understanding and for not divorcing us while we allowed the writing of this chapter to take over our lives.

We apologize to our colleagues if we did not cite their very important contributions to the field. There are so many of you, and we were allowed only so many pages, and ran over anyway.

Portions of work not yet published by the authors in journal form were supported by grants from the United States Public Health Service, National Institutes of Health to Wasserstrom (HL30724) and to Ten Eick (HL27026 and HL38041).

REFERENCES

1. Aldrich RW, Corey DP, Stevens CF. A reinterpretation of mammalian sodium channel gating based on single channel recording. Nature 1983; 306:436–41.
2. Antzelevitch C, Jalife J, Moe GK. Characteristics of reflection as a mechanism of re-

entrant arrhythmias and its relationship to parasystole. Circulation 1980; 61:182–91.

3. Arlock P, Katzung BG. Effects of sodium substitutes on transient inward current and tension in guinea-pig and ferret papillary muscle. J Physiol (Lond) 1985; 360:105–20.

4. Arnsdorf MF. Arnsdorf's paradox. J Cardiovasc Electrophysiol 1990; 1:42–52.

5. Arnsdorf MF, Sawicki GJ. The effects of lysophosphatidylcholine, a toxic metabolite of ischemia, on the components of cardiac excitability in sheep Purkinje fibers. Circ Res 1981; 49:16–30.

6. Arnsdorf MF, Sawicki GJ. Effects of quinidine sulfate on the balance among active and passive cellular properties that comprise the electrophysiological matrix and determine excitability in sheep Purkinje fibers. Circ Res 1987; 61:244–55.

7. Arnsdorf MF, Wasserstrom JA. Mechanisms of action of antiarrhythmic drugs: a matrical approach. In: Fozzard HA et al., eds. The heart and cardiovascular system. New York: Raven Press, 1986; 1259–316.

8. Attwell D, Cohen I, Eisner D, Ohba M, Ojeda C. The steady state TTX-sensitive ("window") sodium current in cardiac Purkinje fibers. Pfluegers Arch 1979; 379:137–42.

9. Bean BP. Multiple types of calcium channels in heart muscle and neurons. In: Wray D, Norman RJ, Hess P, eds. Calcium channels: structure and function. New York: NY Acad Sci, 1989.

10. Bean BP. Two kinds of calcium channels in canine atrial cells. Differences in kinetics, selectivity and pharmacology. J Gen Physiol 1985; 86:1–30.

11. Beeler GW, Reuter H. Reconstruction of the action potential of ventricular myocardial fibers. J Physiol (Lond) 1977; 268:177–210.

12. Bers DM, Ellis D. Intracellular calcium and sodium activity in sheep heart Purkinje fibres. Pfluegers Arch 1982; 393:171–8.

13. Biermanns G, Vereecke J, Carmeliet E. The mechanism of the inactivation of the inward-rectifying K current during hyperpolarizing steps in guinea pig ventricular myocytes. Pfluegers Arch 1987; 410:604–13.

14. Brachmann J, Scherlag BJ, Rosenshtraukh LV, Lazzara R. Bradychardia-induced triggered activity: relevance to drug-induced multiform ventricular tachycardia. Circulation 1983; 68:846–56.

15. Cachelin AF, DePeyer JE, Kokubun S, Reuter H. Sodium channels in cultured cardiac cells. J Physiol (Lond) 1983; 340:389–401.

16. Cameron JS, Bassett AL, Gaide MS, Wong SS, Lodge NJ, Kozlovskis PL, Myerburg RJ. Cellular electrophysiological effects of coronary artery ligation in chronically pressure overloaded cat hearts. Int J Cardiol 1987; 14:155–68.

17. Cameron JS, Kimura S, Jackson-Burns DA, Smith DB, Bassett AL. ATP-sensitive K⁺ channels are altered in hypertrophied ventricular myocytes. Am J Physiol 1988; 255: H1254–8.

18. Carmeliet E. Slow inactivation of sodium current in rabbit cardiac Purkinje fibers. Pfluegers Arch 1987; 408:18–26.

19. Chapman JB. Thermodynamics and kinetics of electrogenic pumps. In: Blaustein MP, Lieberman M, eds. Electrogenic transport: fundamental principles and physiological implications. New York: Raven Press, 1984: 17–32.

20. Clarkson CW, Ten Eick RE. On the mechanism of lysophosphatidylcholine induced depolarization of cat ventricular myocardium. Circ Res 1983; 52:543–56.

21. Clerc L. Directional differences of impulse spread in trabecular muscle from mammalian heart. J Physiol (Lond) 1976; 255:335–46.

22. Cohen IS, Daytner NB, Gintant GA, Kline RP. Time-dependent outward currents in the heart. In: Fozzard HA et al., eds. The heart and cardiovascular system. New York: Raven Press, 1986:637–70.

23. Colquhoun D, Neher E, Reuter H, Stevens CF. Inward current channels activated by intracellular Ca in cultured cardiac cells. Nature 1981; 294:752–4.

24. Craelius W, Chen V, El-Sherif N. Stretch activated ion channels in ventricular myocytes. Biosci Rep 1988; 8:407–14.

25. Cranefield PF. Action potentials afterpotentials and arrhythmia. Circ Res 1977; 41: 415–23.

26. Dahl G, Isenberg G. Decoupling of heart muscle cells: correlation with increased cytoplasmic calcium activity and with changes in nexal ultrastructure. J Membr Biol 1980; 53:63–75.

27. Damiano BP, Rosen MR. Effect of pacing on triggered activity induced by early afterdepolarizations. Circulation 1984; 69:1013–25.

28. DeMello WC. The healing over process in cardiac and other muscle fibers. In: DeMello

WC, ed. In: Electrical phenomena in the heart. New York: Academic Press, 323–51.

29. De Weer P. Electrogenic pumps: theoretical and practical considerations. In: Blaustein MP, Lieberman M, eds. Electrogenic transport: fundamental principles and physiological implications. New York: Raven Press, NY, 1984:1–15.

30. DiFrancesco D, Noble D. A model of cardiac electrical activity incorporating ionic pumps and concentration changes. Philos Trans R Soc Lond [Biol] 1985; 307:353–98.

31. Dudel J, Peper K, Rudel R, Trautwein W. The dynamic chloride component of membrane current in Purkinje Fibers. Pfluegers Arch 1967; 295:197–212.

32. Eisner DA, Lederer WJ. Na-Ca exchange: stoichiometry and electrogenicity. Am J Physiol 1985; 248:C189–202.

33. Escande D, Coulombe A, Faives J, Deroubaix E, Coraboeuf E. Two types of transient outward currents in adult human atrial cells. Am J Physiol 1987; 252:H142–8.

34. Fabiato A. Calcium-induced release of calcium from the cardiac sarcoplasmic reticulum. Am J Physiol 1983; 245:C1–14.

35. Ferrier GR. Effects of transmembrane potential on oscillatory afterpotentials induced by acetylstrophanthidin in canine ventricular tissues. J Pharmacol Exp Ther 1977; 215:332–41.

36. Ferrier GR. Digitalis arrhythmias, role of oscillatory afterpotentials. Prog Cardiovasc Dis 1977; 19:459–74.

37. Follmer CH, Ten Eick RE, Yeh JZ. Sodium current kinetics in cat atrial myocytes. J Physiol (Lond) 1987; 384:169–97.

38. Fozzard HA, Arnsdorf MF. Cardiac electrophysiology. In: Fozzard HA et al., eds. The heart and cardiovascular system. New York: Raven Press, 1986:1–30.

39. Frankenhauser G, Hodgkin AL. The action of calcium on the electrical properties of squid axons. J Physiol (Lond) 1957; 137:218–44.

40. Gadsby DC. The Na/K pump of cardiac cells. Ann Rev Biophys Bioeng 1984; 13:373–98.

41. Gintant GA, Datyner NB, Cohen IS. Slow inactivation of tetrodotoxin-sensitive current in canine cardiac Purkinje fibers. Biophys J 1984; 45:509–12.

42. Grant AO. Evolving concepts of cardiac sodium channel function. J Cardiovasc Electrophysiol 1990; 1:53–67.

43. Grant AO, Dietz MA, Gilliam FR III, Starmer CF. Blockade of cardiac sodium channels by lidocaine: Single channel analysis. Circ Res 1989; 65:723–60.

44. Guhary F, Sachs F. Stretch-activated single ion channel currents in tissue cultured embryonic chick skeletal muscle. J Physiol (Lond) 1984; 352:685–701.

45. Hagiwara S, Miyazaki S, Moody W, Patlak J. Blocking effects of barium and hydrogen ions on the potassium current during anomalous rectification in the starfish egg. J Physiol (Lond) 1978; 279:167–85.

46. Hagiwara S. K Channels. In: Membrane potential-dependent ion channels in cell membranes. Phylogenetic and developmental approaches. New York: Raven Press, 1983:61–86.

47. Harvey RD, Clark CD, Hume JR. A chloride current in mammalian cardiac myocytes: novel mechanism for autonomic regulation of action potential duration and resting membrane potential. J Gen Physiol 1990: 1077–1102.

48. Harvey RD, Hume JR. Autonomic regulation of delayed rectifier K^+ current in mammalian heart involves G proteins. Am J Physiol 1989; 257:H818–23.

49. Harvey RD, Hume JR. Autonomic regulation of a chloride current in heart. Science 1989; 244:983–5.

50. Harvey RD, Hume JR. Autonomic regulation of a chloride current in heart. Science 1989; 244:983–5.

51. Harvey RD, Ten Eick RE. Characterization of an inward rectifying potassium current in cat ventricular myocytes. J Gen Physiol 1988; 91:593–615.

52. Harvey RD, Ten Eick RE. On the role of sodium ions in the regulation of the inward rectifying potassium conductance in cat ventricular myocytes. J Gen Physiol 1989a; 94:329–48.

53. Harvey RD, Ten Eick RE. Voltage-dependent block of inward rectifying K^+ current by monovalent cations in cat ventricular myocytes. J. Gen Physiol 1989b; 94:349–61.

54. Hauswirth O, Noble D, Tsien RW. The mechanism of oscillatory activity at low membrane potentials in cardiac Purkinje fibers. J Physiol (Lond) 1972; 200:255–65.

55. Hauswirth O, Noble D, Tsien RW. The dependence of plateau currents in cardiac

Purkinje fibers on the interval between action potentials. J Physiol (Lond) 1972; 222:27–49.

56. Hess P, Lansman JB, Tsien RW. Different modes of Ca channel gating behavior favoured by dihydropyridine Ca agonists and antagonists. Nature 1984; 311:538–44.

57. Hille BA, Woodhull M, Shapiro BI. Negative surface charge near sodium channels of nerve: divalent ions, monovalent ions, and pH. Philos Trans R Lond [Biol] Soc 1975; 270:301–18.

58. Hille B. Ionic channels of excitable membranes. Sunderland, MA: Sinauer Associates, 1984.

59. Hiraoka M, Fozzard HA. The positive dynamic current and its inactivation properties in cardiac Purkinje fibres. J Physiol (Lond) 1973; 234:569–86.

60. Hiraoka M, Kawano S. Calcium-sensitive and insensitive transient outward current in rabbit ventricular myocytes. J Physiol (Lond) 1989; 410:187–212.

61. Hisatome I, Sato R, Singer DH. Direct proton block of sodium current in guinea pig ventricular myocytes. Biophys J 1989; 55:288a.

62. Hodgkin AL, Huxley AF. A quantitative description of membrane current and its application to conduction and excitation in nerve. J Physiol (Lond) 1952; 117:500–44.

63. Hoffman BF, Cranefield PF. Physiological basis of cardiac arrhythmias. Am J Med 1964; 37:670–89.

64. Hoffman BF, Cranefield PF. Electrophysiology of the heart. McGraw-Hill, New York, 1960.

65. Hondeghem LM, Katzung BG. Time- and voltage-dependent interactions of antiarrhythmic drugs with cardiac sodium channels. Biochim Biophys Acta 1977; 472: 373–98.

66. Horie M, Irisawa H. Rectification of muscarinic K^+ current by magnesium ion in guinea pig atrial cells. Am J Physiol 1987; 253:H210–4.

67. Hume J. Properties of myocardial K^+ channels and their pharmacological modulation. In: Hondeghem L, ed. Molecular and cellular Mechanisms of antiarrhythmic agents. Mount Kisco, NY: Futura, 1989:113–31.

68. Hume JR, Uehara A. Ionic basis of the different action potential configurations of single guinea-pig atrial and ventricular myocytes. J Physiol (Lond) 1985; 368:525–44.

69. Irisawa H, Sato R. Intra- and extracellular actions of protons on the calcium current of isolated guinea pig ventricular cells. Circ Res 1986; 59:348–55.

70. Isenberg G, Trautwein W. The effect of dihydro-ouabain and lithium-ions on the outward current in cardiac Purkinje fibers. Pfluegers Arch 1974; 350:41–54.

71. Jack JJB, Noble D, Tsien RW. Electric current flow in excitable cells. Oxford: Clarendon Press, 1975.

72. Jalife J. Mutual entrainment and electrical coupling as mechanisms for synchronous firing of rabbit sino-atrial pacemaker cells. J Physiol (Lond) 1984; 356:221–43.

73. Jalife J, Moe GK. Effect of electrotonic potentials on pacemaker activity of the isolated sinus node of the cat. Circ Res 1976; 39:801–8.

74. Janse MJ. Reentry rhythms. In: Fozzard HA et al., eds. The heart and cardiovascular system. New York: Raven Press, 1986:1203–8.

75. January CT, Fozzard HA. Delayed afterdepolarizations in heart muscle: mechanisms and relevance. Pharmacol Rev 1988; 40: 219–27.

76. January CT, Riddle JM, Salata JJ. A model for early afterdepolarization: Induction with the Ca^{2+} channel agonist Bay K 8644. Circ Res 1988; 62:563–71.

77. January CT, Riddle JM. Early afterdepolarization: mechanism for induction and block. Circ Res 1989; 64:977–90.

78. Josephson IR, Sanchez-Chapula J, Brown AM. A comparison of calcium currents in rat and guinea-pig single ventricular cells. Circ Res 1984; 54:144–56.

79. Kameyama M, Kakei M, Sato R, Shibasaki T, Matsuda H, Irisawa H. Intracellular Na^+ activates a K^+ channel in mammalian cardiac cells. Nature 1984; 309:354–6.

80. Kass RS, Tsien RW, Weingart R. Ionic basis of transient inward current induced by strophanthidin in cardiac Purkinje fibres. J Physiol (Lond) 1978; 281:209–26.

81. Kenyon J, Sutko J. Calcium- and voltage-activated plateau currents of cardiac Purkinje fibers. J Gen Physiol 1987; 89:921–58.

82. Kirsch GE, Kodina J, Birnbaumer L, Brown AM. Direct G-protein effects on ATP-sensitive channels in rat ventricular myocytes. Biophys J 1990; 57:290a.

83. Kurachi Y. Voltage-dependent activation of the inward-rectifying potassium channel in

the ventricular cell membrane of guinea-pig heart. J Physiol (Lond) 1985; 366:365–85.

84. Lazdunski M, Frelin C, Vigne P. The sodium/hydrogen exchange system in cardiac cells: its biochemical and pharmacological properties and its role in regulating internal concentrations of sodium and internal pH. J Mol Cell Cardiol 1985; 17:1029–42.

85. Lin C-I, Katake H, Vassalle M. On the mechanism underlying the oscillatory current in cardiac Purkinje fibers. J Cardiovasc Pharmacol 1986; 8:906–14.

86. Lipp P, Pott L. Transient inward current in guinea pig atrial myocytes reflects a change of sodium-calcium exchange current. J Physiol (Lond) 1988; 397:601–30.

87. Litovsky SH, Antzelevitch C. Transient outward current prominent in canine ventricular epicardium but not endocardium. Circ Res 1988; 62:116–27.

88. Marban E, Wier WG. Ryanodine as a tool to determine the contributions of calcium entry and calcium release to the calcium transient and contraction of cardiac Purkinje fibers. Circ Res 1985; 56:133–8.

89. Matsuda H, Noma A, Kurachi Y, Irisawa H. Transient depolarization and spontaneous fluctuations in isolated single cells from guinea pig ventricles. Calcium-mediated membrane potential fluctuations. Circ Res 1982; 51:142–51.

90. Matsuura H, Ehara T, Imoto Y. An analysis of the delayed outward current in single ventricular cells of the guinea-pig. Pfluegers Arch 1987; 410:596–603.

91. McAllister RE, Noble D, Tsien RW. Reconstruction of the electrical activity of cardiac Purkinje fibers. J Physiol (Lond) 1975; 251:1–59.

92. McDonald TF, Trautwein W. The potassium current underlying delayed rectification in cat ventricular muscle. J Physiol (Lond) 1978; 274:217–46.

93. Mitra R, Morad M. Two types of calcium channels in guinea-pig ventricular myocytes. Proc Natl Acad Sci USA 1986; 83:5340–4.

94. Nakayama T, Fozzard HA. Adrenergic modulation of the transient outward current in isolated canine Purkinje cells. Circ Res 1988; 62:162–72.

95. Nilius B, Hess P, Lansman JB, Tsien RW. A novel type of cardiac calcium channel in ventricular cells. Nature 1985; 316:443–6.

96. Noble D. The surprising heart: a review of recent progress in cardiac electrophysiology. J Physiol (Lond) 1985; 353:1–50.

97. Noble D, Tsien RW. The kinetics and rectifier properties of the slow potassium current in cardiac Purkinje fibers. J Physiol (Lond) 1968; 195:185–214.

98. Nawrath H, Ten Eick RE, McDonald TF, Trautwein W. On the mechanism underlying the action of D-600 on slow inward current and tension in mammalian myocardium. Circ Res 1977; 40:408–14.

99. Noma A. ATP-regulated K^+ channels in cardiac muscle. Nature 1983; 305:147–8.

100. Patlack J, Ortiz M. Two modes of gating during late Na^+ channel currents in frog sartorius muscle. J Gen Physiol 1986; 87:305–26.

101. Pietrobon D, Prud'hom B, Hess P. Conformational changes associated with ion permeation of L-type calcium channels. Nature 1988; 333:373–6.

102. Rasmussen HH, Singer DH, Ten Eick RE. Characterization of an electrogenic Na pump induced hyperpolarization in human atrial myocardium. Am J Physiol 1986; 20:H331–9.

103. Rasmussen HH, Cragoe EH, Ten Eick RE. Na^+-dependent activation of Na^+, K^+ pump in human myocardium during recovery from acidosis. Am J Physiol 1989; 256(Heart Circ Physiol 25):H256–64.

104. Reber WR, Weingart R. Ungulate cardiac Purkinje fibres: the influence of intracellular pH on the electrical cell-to-cell coupling. J Physiol (Lond) 1982; 328:87–104.

105. Reuter H, Seitz N. The dependence of calcium efflux from cardiac muscle on temperature and external ion composition. J Physiol (Lond) 1968; 195:451–70/

106. Roden DM, Hoffman BF. Action potential prolongation and induction of abnormal automaticity by low quinidine concentrations in canine Purkinje fibers, Relationship to potassium and cycle length. Circ Res 1985; 56:857–67.

107. Rushton WA. Initiation of the propagated disturbance. Proc R Soc Lond [Biol] 1937; 124:210–43.

108. Sachs F. Biophysics of mechanoreception. Membr Biochem 1986; 6:173–95.

109. Sakmann B, Trube G. Voltage-dependent inactivation of inward-rectifying single-channel currents in the guinea-pig heart cell membrane. J Physiol (Lond) 1984; 347:659–83.

110. Sawicki GJ, Arnsdorf MF. Electrophysiological actions and interactions between lysophophatidylcholine and lidocaine in the

nonsteady state: the match between multiphasic arrhythmogenic mechanisms and multiple drug effects in cardiac Purkinje fibers. J Pharmacol Exp Ther 1985; 235: 829–38.

111. Scanley BE, Fozzard HA. Low conductance sodium channels in canine cardiac Purkinje cells. Biophys J 1987; 52:487–95.

112. Schoenberg M, Fozzard HA. The influence of intercellular clefts on the electrical properties of sheep cardiac Purkinje fibers. Biophys J 1979; 25:217–34.

113. Schubert B, Van Dangen AMJ, Kirsch GE, Brown AM. β-Adrenergic inhibition of cardiac sodium channels by dual G-protein pathways. Science 1989; 245:516–9.

114. Sejersted OM, Wasserstrom JA, Fozzard HA. Na, K pump stimulation by intracellular Na in isolated, intact sheep cardiac Purkinje fibers. J Gen Physiol 1988; 91:445–66.

115. Sheets MF, Scanley BE, Hanck DA, Makielski JC, Fozzard HA. Open sodium channel properties of single canine cardiac Purkinje cells. J Gen Physiol 1987; 52:13–22.

116. Shibata EF, Drury T, Refsum H, Aldrete V, Giles W. Contributions of a transient outward current to repolarization in human atrium. Am J Physiol 1989; 257:H1773–81.

117. Starmer CF, Grant AO, Strauss HC. Mechanisms of use-dependent block of sodium channels in excitable membranes by local anesthetics. Biophys J 1984; 46:15–27.

118. Surawicz B. Depolarization-induced automaticity in atrial and ventricular myocardial fibers. In: Zipes DP, Bailey JC, Elharrar V, eds. The slow inward current and cardiac arrhythmias. The Hague: Martinus Nijhoff, 1980:375–96.

119. Ten Eick RE, Singer DH. Electrophysiological properties of diseased human atrium (I): low resting potential and altered sensitivity to potassium. Circ Res 1979; 44:545–7.

120. Tseng G-N, Boyden PA. Multiple types of Ca^{2+} currents in single canine Purkinje cells. Circ Res (1989); 65:1735–50.

121. Tseng G-N, Hoffman BF. Two components of transient outward current in canine ventricular myocytes. Circ Res 1989; 64:633–47.

122. Tsien RW, Bean BP, Hess P, Lansman JB, Nilius B, Nowycky MC. Mechanisms of calcium channel modulation by β-adrenergic agents and dihydropyridine calcium agonists. J Mol Cell Cardiol 1986; 18:691–710.

123. Trautwein W, Pelzer D. Gating of single calcium channels in the membrane of enzymatically isolated ventricular myocytes from adult mammalian hearts. In: Zipes D, Jalife J, eds. Cardiac electrophysiology and arrhythmias. Orlando, FL: Grune and Stratton, 1985:31–42.

124. Wasserstrom JA, Salata JJ. Basis for tetrodotoxin and lidocaine effects on action potentials in dog ventricular myocytes. Am J Physiol 1988; 254:H1157–66.

125. Wasserstrom JA, Ferrier GR. Voltage dependence of digitalis afterpotentials, aftercontractions and inotropy. Am J Physiol 1981; 241:H646–53.

126. Weidmann S. Effect of current flow in the membrane potential of cardiac muscle. J Physiol (Lond) 1951; 115:227–36.

127. Weidmann S. The electrical constants of Purkinje fibres. J Physiol (Lond) 1952; 118:348–60.

128. Weidmann S. Effects of calcium ions and local anaesthetics on electrical properties of Purkinje fibers. J Physiol (Lond) 1955; 129:568–82.

129. Weingart R, Imanaga I, Weidmann S. Low resistance pathways between myocardial cells. In: Fleckenstein A, Dhalla NS, eds. Basic functions of cations in myocardial activity. Baltimore: University Park Press, 1975:227–32.

130. Wit AL, Hoffman BF, Cranefield PF. Slow conduction and reentry in the ventricular conducting system. I Return extrasystole in canine Purkinje fibers. Circ Res 1972; 30:1–10.

131. Wit AL, Cranefield PF, Hoffman BF. Slow conduction and reentry in the ventricular conducting system. II. Single and sustained circus movement in networks of canine and bovine Purkinje fibers. Circ Res 1972; 30:11–22.

132. Wit AL, Rosen MR. Afterdepolarizations and triggered activity. In: Fozzard HA, et al., eds. The Heart and Cardiovascular System New York: Raven Press, 1986:1449–90.

133. Yue DT, Lawrence JH, Marban E. Two molecular transitions influence cardiac sodium channel gating. Science 1989; 244:349–52.

134. Yue DT, Marban E. A novel cardiac potassium channel that is active and conductive at depolarized potentials. Pfluegers Arch 1988; 413:127–33.

III
MODELS AND MECHANISMS OF CARDIAC ARRHYTHMIAS

This section is concerned with models and mechanisms of cardiac arrhythmias, and it consists of nine chapters. Arrhythmias may result from abnormalities of impulse propagation or impulse initiation. Abnormalities of propagation can lead to conduction blocks or reentrant excitation. Abnormalities of impulse initiation can lead to ectopic pacemaker activity. Ectopic activity at the cellular level can be caused by enhanced normal automaticity, abnormal automaticity, or triggered activity caused by either early or delayed afterdepolarizations. The first two chapters discuss circus movement or reentrant activation in atrial and ventricular myocardium. The next chapter discusses the mechanisms of arrhythmias caused by digitalis toxicity. This is followed by three chapters that discuss arrhythmias that occur following myocardial ischemia. The seventh chapter in this section discusses mechanisms of arrhythmias caused by antiarrhythmic drug toxicity, and the eighth chapter discusses arrhythmias caused by cardiac hypertrophy and cardiomyopathy. The final chapter in this section concerns naturally occurring arrhythmias in dogs and cats. Cardiovascular scientists and clinicians rarely consider this topic, although most of the relevant models of cardiac arrhythmias and sudden death require the use of dog or cat heart preparations. Information about spontaneous arrhythmias in experimental animals may therefore prove to be useful to evaluate these models.

The chapters in this section largely deal with data obtained by physiologic techniques. That is, methods that have proved useful for study of certain arrhythmias necessarily involve either whole-animal or isolated tissue models, not single-cell biophysical studies. For the foreseeable future this will certainly remain the case. For instance, it is impossible to study reentrant arrhythmias in single-cell models. This is because, as explained in the following chapters, reentry requires zones of tissue with at least two pathways and a one-way conduction block.

Cellular mechanisms of arrhythmias caused by enhanced impulse initiation are of great interest, and these have been studied for many years using in vitro tissue preparations. Bozler, using extracellular recording techniques, in the late 1930s described oscillatory afterpotentials that occurred in electrical diastole. The development of microelectrode techniques allowed Rosen, Ferrier, Moe, and others to de-scribe these oscillatory phenomena in more detail in digitalis-intoxicated Purkinje fibers. These are currently called delayed afterdepo-larizations or oscillatory afterpotentials; they are known to cause "triggered activity." Like-wise, although the concept of ectopic automa-ticity originated in the late 1800s, one of the goals of Weidmann's first microelectrode stud-ies in the mid-1950s was to describe automa-ticity in sheep and dog Purkinje fibers. Current investigators continue this research using whole-cell or membrane patch clamp techniques in single cells, which may be use-ful for elucidating the biophysical mechanisms of ectopic impulse initiation. As discussed in the previous sections, however, it is difficult to know whether impulse initiation occurring in a single myocyte or Purkinje cell is truly comparable to the impulse initiation that oc-curs within tissue preparations. This is be-cause much of spontaneous activity that routinely occurs in single-cell models may dis-appear if the cell is integrated (coupled) into the syncytial mass of a tissue segment. Cells that are part of a syncytium generally are sub-jected to significant electrotonic influence from the surrounding cells. Current flow from the surrounding cells that have relatively shorter action potential durations or more negative resting potentials could suppress afterdepolarizations or abnormal phase 4 de-polarization in any given focus of partially depolarized cells under study.

The significance and size of the electronic influences themselves is becoming an impor-tant subject of study. Obviously, single-cell preparations cannot be utilized for these stud-ies; electrotonic interaction requires communi-cations of two or more (coupled) cells. Moreover, studies of tissue preparation have provided the basis for our understanding the physiology of the arrhythmogenic focus. For quantifying abnormal pacemaker activity or for studying cardiotonic drug effects on auto-matic or triggered arrhythmic mechanisms, the "classic" tissue (e.g., 24 hr infarct zone or digitalis-intoxicated Purkinje fibers) models are still useful for study. This is because the cells in an "arrhythmogenic focus" of an ap-

propriate tissue preparation probably provide a more physiologic model of ectopic activity in the intact heart than does impulse initiation, which occurs in single cells.

One must recognize that the clinical need for improved therapy of malignant cardiac ar-rhythmias is the primary driving force behind much of our scientific investigation. The jus-tification for use of animal models of cardiac arrhythmias in vitro or in vivo is to gain de-tailed knowledge of arrhythmic mechanisms. Through study of these models the basic sci-entist can contribute to clinical progress, help rationalize therapy, and may improve the out-come for patients with cardiac disease.

Before the 1970s it was generally taught that there are two possible mechanisms for tachyarrhythmias: enhanced ectopic automatic-ity and reentry. Reentrant arrhythmias of atria, atrio-ventricular node, or ventricles were those that started and stopped abruptly. These were "paroxysmal" tachycardias, which can sud-denly interrupt normal sinus rhythm. Reen-trant arrhythmias were most easily observed as "coupled" extrasystoles. These coupled ex-tra beats, in either the atria or ventricles, were "unifocal" premature complexes that occur at one ("constant") coupling interval. The cou-pling interval is the time between the begin-ning of the QRS complex of the last sinus beat and the beginning of the QRS complex of the premature beat.

Automatic arrhythmias, which occur in ei-ther the atria or ventricles, could gradually ac-celerate and then subside. As such, these tachycardias were called nonparoxysmal. Au-tomaticity was also thought to produce "para-systolic" beats. These extrasystoles may occur at any time during electrical diastole. These beats can be seen to follow a pattern: the intervals between complexes represent multiples of an underlying basic cycle length. That is, a "protected" automatic focus could exist, which would not be affected by normal sinus impulses. It was assumed that there was "entry block" into this automatic focus. That is, the pacemaker in this focus was not sup-pressed by sinus impulses because they cannot conduct into the focal site and "reset" the rhythm. In addition to entrance block, variable exit block can occur from the focus. That is, ectopic activity initiated from the parasystolic pacemaker could occasionally escape from the focal site from time to time and lead to the observed premature complex.

Today we know that reentry is not the only possible cause of paroxysmal tachycardias. These arrhythmias can be caused by triggered activity from delayed afterdepolarizations or early afterdepolarizations. Automatic foci can also show abrupt changes in rate. This can happen if there is a sudden increase in sympathetic tone in or around the focus, or if the diastolic potential of the cells of the focus suddenly depolarizes by 2–10 mV. In addition, triggered impulses can also lead to "coupled" extrasystoles. Under some circumstances triggered activity can complicate diagnosis. For example, if sinus rate accelerates transiently this could make delayed afterdepolarizations (DAD) in a potential triggered focus grow in amplitude. If these DAD reach threshold potential they could lead either to single extrasystoles or a burst of tachycardia. DAD can generate impulses over a "warm-up period" in which there is a gradual decrease in the cycle length of the premature beats. Then, after maximum rate is achieved, a gradual hyperpolarization of maximum diastolic potential be-

gins. This hyperpolarization resembles the progressive increase in diastolic potential that occurs during overdrive stimulation, as described by Vassalle in 1970. The gradual hyperpolarization carries diastolic potential further and further from threshold potential and thus slows the discharge rate of the focus. Triggered activity can therefore show gradual rate acceleration and deceleration and thus lead to nonparoxysmal arrhythmias. Finally, as shown at the Masonic Research Laboratory some years ago, coupled extrasystoles can also result from parasystolic (automatic) foci that are influenced by electrotonic inputs across an inexcitable gap.

In view of these complicated issues the current basis for therapy of cardiac arrhythmias (whether by pharmacologic or electrical means) is largely empirical. Ultimately these empirical therapies should be replaced by approaches based on identification of the cellular mechanism that has caused the specific arrhythmia. At this time techniques to routinely identify these mechanisms in the in situ heart do not exist. It is possible that development of new techniques will provide the basis for a rapid clinical diagnosis and therapeutic intervention.

10

Reentrant Excitation in the Atrium

Penelope A. Boyden

College of Physicians and Surgeons, Columbia University
New York, New York

INTRODUCTION

Circus movement or reflection of a cardiac impulse could result in a single or multiple beats of reentrant excitation. In this chapter we address the major points underlying our existing knowledge of the various subtypes of circus movement that occur in the atrium leading to single or multiple reentrant beats. These subtypes include reentrant excitation around an anatomic or inexcitable barrier, reentrant excitation around a functional barrier, or, last, a combination of these.

The historical experiments of Mayer (1), Mines (2), and Garrey (3) provide us with the early models of the "entrapped circuit wave" (4) that we now refer to as circus movement. Several points made when using these early models are still valid today, particularly when discussing the particular subtype of circus movement in the atrium, reentry around an inexcitable barrier. In brief, Mayer found that only when he made a single ring out of the disk portion of a jellyfish could he momentarily stimulate it to produce a rapid regular pulsation of the tissue (1).

Further investigations into the conditions necessary for the initiation of the circulating impulse led Mines in 1913 to clearly outline that for reentry to occur: (1) there must be blockade of the initiating impulse at some site within the potential pathway, (2) there must be slowed conduction in an alternate pathway, (3) there must be slowed or delayed activation in the pathway beyond the area of block, and (4) there must be reexcitation of the tissue proximal to the site of block (2). Finally he reported:

> once started in this way it (the impulse) will continue unless interfered with by some external stimulus arriving during the part of the cycle when the portion of the muscle that is stimulated is neither in the excited state nor in the condition of depressed excitability which outlasts it.

This last criterion must be thoroughly satisfied if one wishes to ascribe reentrant excitation as the mechanism of any tachycardia. These conditions have been carefully

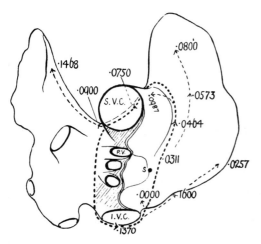

Figure 1 A two-dimensional representation of the dog right and left atrial chambers showing readings (in seconds) from a probe type of electrode during a period of sustained flutter in the dog. All times are in reference to an arbitrary zero time (at a site near the IVC). The broken lines indicate the proposed path of impulse propagation during this one "beat" of atrial flutter. [From Lewis et al. (6).]

analyzed, and subsequent studies by Schmidt and Erlanger (5) provided the first direct evidence of unidirectional block and circus movement in the ventricle as early as 1928. On the contrary, experimental demonstration of conditions that conclusively defined a circus pathway in the intact atrium during tachycardia was almost lacking until recently. In early studies most investigators relied heavily on surmised evidence in their explanations of the mechanism of atrial arrhythmias.

ATRIAL REENTRY AROUND AN ANATOMIC OR INEXCITABLE BARRIER

Intensive observations by Lewis and his colleagues (6) from 1918 to 1921 of one episode of atrial flutter inducible in a canine heart were best explained by circus movement of the impulse along a pathway that circumscribed the caval openings in the right atrium (Fig. 1). In another episode the pattern of activation was assumed to be consistent with circus movement of the impulse in the atrial tissue that surrounds the mitral valve orifice. In both

cases an anatomic obstacle provided an inexcitable barrier around which the impulse circulated.

The involvement of an anatomic (and now surgically induced) inexcitable barrier in reentry was further emphasized by the studies of Rosenblueth and Garcia Ramos (7). In their model of atrial flutter the size of the anatomic barrier was increased by actually crushing the atrial tissue between the two vena cavae. This decreased the rate of the inducible flutter. In their original report (7), as well as in the supplementary data supplied by others using this model (8–10), studies of activation sequences using probe mapping techniques during this regular tachyarrhythmia allowed these authors to conclude that the sustained flutter was due to circus movement of the impulse around an inexcitable barrier; that is, the path of the impulse was around the intercaval lesion and involved tissue of both the right and left atria.

In more recent studies using a modification of the experimental model originally used by Rosenblueth and Garcia Ramos, Frame et al. (11) further defined the characteristics of this subtype of atrial reentry. In their model, in addition to the incision made in the right atrium in the intercaval region, they made an incision from this region that ran parallel to the atrioventricular groove extending to the base of the right atrial appendage. In this atrium, now with a Y-shaped lesion, a sustained rapid regular atrial tachycardia resembling atrial flutter was easily inducible with appropriate electrical stimulation. Based upon the knowledge and extrapolation from the conclusions of previous studies, Frame et al. (11) hypothesized that after creating this Y-shaped lesion, the reentering impulse should follow a path coursing around the inexcitable barrier of the large Y-shaped lesion. However, in a follow-up study, detailed sequences of endocardial atrial activation during the inducible flutter clearly demonstrated that reentry occurred in atrial tissues not surrounding the Y-shaped lesion but those surrounding the tricuspid valve orifice (Fig. 2)(12).

In discussing the role of the Y-shaped lesion in stabilizing the inducible arrhythmias, a more general concept of the extent and nature

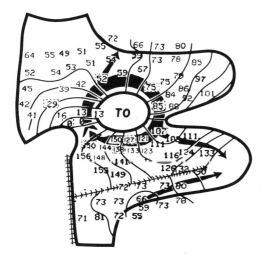

Figure 2 Map of clockwise right atrial endocardial activation sequence around the tricuspid orifice (TO) during one beat of atrial flutter. The cycle length of the tachycardia was 158 msec, and there was a sequential activation of sites that encircle the TO (wide arrow). The position of the Y-shaped lesion in the right atrial free wall is depicted by the hatched lines. Isochrones are drawn at 10 msec intervals. Individual activation times are indicated. [From Frame et al. (12).]

of the boundaries required for circus movement of the impulse to occur was presented. This discussion has particular applicability to reentry as it occurs in the atria, since unlike the large ventricular surface, the intact atrial chambers are not two-dimensional sheets of tissue or simple linear cables. Rather, they are irregularly shaped spheres with several types of surfaces and naturally occurring orifices (e.g., orifices of the caval veins, the orifices of the pulmonary veins, and the orifices of the mitral and tricuspid valves).

The pathway of a reentering impulse must be protected by adequate boundaries. An adequate boundary is one that protects the reentrant pathway from becoming invaded by other wavefronts that would in one way or another "short-circuit" the reentrant circuit. In an atrial chamber in which impulse conduction can occur over excitable tissue that is contiguous but surrounds a central cavity, only two boundaries seem necessary for reentrant excitation. In these chambers short-circuiting cannot occur via impulse propagation "through" the cavity or via the "outside" surface. There-

fore, any theoretical pathway must have two edges on the atrial surface and it must be bounded along its entire length for circus movement to occur.

We now know that boundaries for reentrant pathways in atria can be of two general types. Circus movement can take place around the first type of boundary, an inexcitable barrier or scar. The second type of boundary can be functional in nature. For instance, the boundary or barrier is temporarily inexcitable (refractory) during the reentry but not during sinus rhythm, or the "boundary" can be in the form of an alternate pathway of perfectly excitable tissue that is either longer or has conduction properties different from those of the reentrant path. This alternate pathway is "functional" in that any impulse that might leave the reentrant path and follow this alternate path is able to reconnect with the reentrant path. However, if conduction time over this path is longer (because of the path length or the conduction properties of the tissue in the path) than the time it takes to proceed along the reentrant path, then the impulse would arrive too late to short-circuit the reentrant path.

In the case of the atrial flutter induced in the atrium with the Y-shaped lesion (12), maps of the activation sequence during a single beat of the rapid rhythm clearly illustrate the two boundaries that protect and are necessary for this type of reentry (Fig. 2). In this example one boundary is the tricuspid valve orifice (TO). The other boundary consists of the inexcitable region produced by the Y-shaped lesion and the bulge of the right atrial appendage. For this latter component, conduction time over any alternate path the impulse might take is longer than conduction time via the path the impulse would follow around a part of the tricuspid orifice.

CHARACTERISTICS OF SUSTAINED CIRCUS MOVEMENT AROUND AN INEXCITABLE OR ANATOMIC BARRIER

From the experiments of Mines (2) conditions of circus movement around an inexcitable barrier or anatomic barrier were discussed. If the length of the path is large, if the conduction velocity of the circulating impulse is low, or if the refractory period is short, then reentrant excitation can occur via a defined pathway in this subtype of reentry. Importantly, the length of the path of the circulating impulse is fixed by its barriers and is determined by the perimeter of the anatomic barrier. Given that the path length taken is constant, then in the ideal case the rate of the reentrant arrhythmia would equal the conduction velocity of the impulse (cm/sec)/path length (cm), or the cycle length of the tachycardia (sec) would equal the path length (cm)/conduction velocity (cm/sec).

Another characteristic of circus movement around an anatomic or inexcitable barrier is the existence of an excitable gap. If the path around an inexcitable barrier is fixed and longer than the wavelength of the circulating impulse (conduction velocity × refractory period), then atrial fibers just in front of the head of the wavefront have completely restored their excitability. If these fibers have completely restored their excitability, then a stimulus or a depolarizing impulse arriving at the circuit via an alternate path could interrupt and depolarize this tissue and alter the reentrant excitation. An excitable gap thus exists in the circuit. A fully excitable gap during a reentrant tachycardia may only exist in tachycardias in which paths are very long (e.g., in hearts with an accessory atrioventricular pathway).

As early as 1920 Lewis et al. (6) observed and commented that in experimental canine atrial flutter the calculated conduction velocity of the atrial impulse was about one-half to one-third of impulse velocity determined in fully recovered or fully excitable atrial tissue. This has been interpreted to mean that in flutter the wavefront must be propagating through partially recovered or relatively refractory atrial tissue. The existence of a partially excitable gap in reentry involving an inexcitable barrier has now been quantified (12, 13).

In these latter studies the degree of recovery of refractoriness of tissue along the reentrant path after each impulse of the rhythm

was determined by observing the response to single premature stimuli delivered at various times during the reentrant cycle. By determining the duration of the period during which premature stimuli advanced the following tachycardia beat, the duration of the excitable gap during the arrhythmia was determined. The duration varied from 50 to 95 msec, representing an average gap that was 47% of the flutter cycle length. Furthermore, because every premature stimulus that reset the arrhythmia conducted *more* slowly around the circuit than the circulating impulse, it was concluded that there was incomplete recovery of tissue excitability during the excitable gap (12). This implies that in this model of reentry around an inexcitable barrier recovery of tissue excitability is incomplete by the end of the excitable gap. Consequently, the normal reentrant impulse propagates through partially refractory tissue at all sites within the reentrant path. Monophasic potential recordings from atrial fibers during the tachycardia in this model also support this notion (Fig. 3)(14).

The presence of an excitable gap in some types of human atrial flutter has been demonstrated using similar stimulation protocols (15, 16). In one study, the duration of the excitable gap was approximately 20% of the flutter cycle length (15). Furthermore, as for the experimental models of flutter, monophasic recordings of human atrial fibers during atrial tachycardias suggest a partially excitable gap (Fig. 4)(17–20).

ATRIAL REENTRY AROUND A FUNCTIONAL BARRIER

Reentrant excitation not around an anatomic barrier but around a functional barrier was first addressed theoretically by Garrey, who suggested that perhaps naturally occurring rings were not always essential, for circus movement (3). Lewis, in his 1925 treatise dealing with arrhythmias (21), described the important electrophysiologic properties of an impulse circulating in a sheet of excitable tissue. In his discussion of this type of circus movement he emphasized that a change in

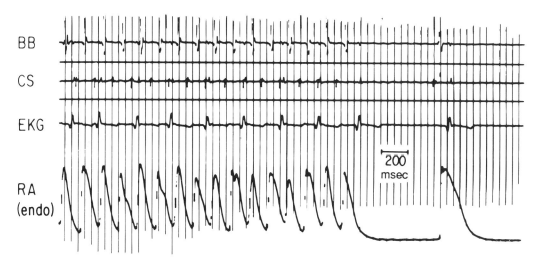

Figure 3 Monophasic action potentials recorded from the right atrial (RA) endocardium during atrial flutter induced in dogs with the Y-shaped lesion. Also shown are electrograms recorded from sites on Bachmann's bundle (BB) and coronary sinus (CS). The ECG is also shown. Note that the monophasic potentials obtained during flutter clearly showed incomplete repolarization between upstrokes. [From Wu et al. (14).]

conduction or a change in the refractoriness of the muscle would alter the pathway of the circulating impulse. In the illustration accompanying these speculations, Lewis included a central inexcitable barrier in his drawing but concluded that it may not be essential for sustaining the circus movement. However, the possible nature of the central barrier in this type of reentrant excitation was never discussed.

The possibility that refractoriness of cardiac tissue could serve as a functional barrier was demonstrated in an early mathematical (computer) model of an arrhythmia by Moe et al. (22). In this model of an atrial tachyarrhyth-

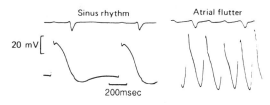

Figure 4 Surface ECG (upper traces) recorded simultaneously with in vivo endocardial monophasic action potentials (lower traces) during sinus rhythm and atrial flutter (atrial rate 320 beats/min) in a 54-year-old patient. [From Lauribe et al. (20).]

mia, a functional type of reentry could occur in a sheet of similar normal elements only if there existed a "functional abnormality", that is, a nonuniform distribution of refractoriness. No large anatomic obstacles were needed. Several studies have also suggested that "functional longitudinal dissociation" can exist in normal atrioventricular (AV) nodal tissue and underlie reentrant tachycardias involving this tissue (see later).

The phenomenon of circus movement in the atria in the absence of an anatomic obstacle is now well documented. Several studies have shown that properly timed electrical stimuli can induce nondriven rhythmic activity in small isolated sections of rabbit atrial muscle (23–25). Presumably these latter preparations lacked specific anatomic barriers. However, by accurately determining the sequence of activation in this small atrial section, Allessie et al. (23) clearly described constant circuits without a demonstrable obstacle. During these tachycardias the circulating impulse coursed around a barrier of refractory tissue and a small zone of inactive tissue (Fig. 5). The region of block did not recover sufficient excitability during the reentry because it was continually being invaded by colliding centripetal wavelets (24,

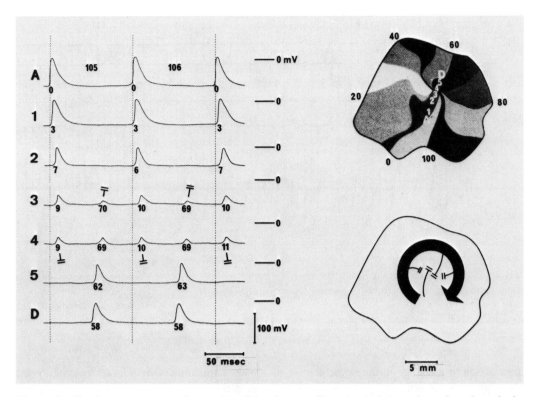

Figure 5 Simultaneous transmembrane potentials of seven fibers located at various sites through the center of the reentrant circuit observed in a section of rabbit atrium. The location of electrodes A, 1–5, and D are depicted on the activation map seen in the upper right-hand corner. Note the double responses in the most central area of the circuit (electrodes 3 and 4). Both responses were unable to propagate beyond the center, thus preventing a short circuiting of the circuit. A schematic of this type of reentry around a functional line of block is depicted in the lower right-hand corner. [From Allessie et al. (25).]

25). The central barrier in these tachycardias was therefore "functional". These studies led directly to the description of the *leading circle* type of reentrant excitation (25).

In leading circle reentrant excitation the impulse travels along the shortest pathway around the functional barrier. As a consequence the rate of this type of arrhythmia is completely determined by the electrophysiologic properties of the tissue in the pathway.

Second, because of these important properties the path the reentrant impulse takes need not be fixed but can be variable. Importantly for this type of reentrant excitation as it occurs in the intact atrium, even though the pathway is not fixed, for such an arrhythmia to be sustained in the atrial chamber two boundaries must remain to protect the pathway during the reentry. For instance, one boundary can be the

central functional barrier and the other could be anatomic or functional in nature.

In the original description of the leading circle, it was illustrated and assumed that the isolated atrial tissue was isotropic. Under this special condition the length of the circuit is variable, but since the impulse conducts uniformly around the circuit, the head and the tail always meet and therefore there would be no gap of full excitability. In this ideal condition the path of the impulse around the barrier would equal the wavelength of the impulse ($CV \times RP$).

A number of animal models of rapid atrial tachycardias have now been described in which the sustained rhythm is not due to circus movement around an anatomic obstacle but due to circus movement around a functional barrier. Whether these arrhythmias are exam-

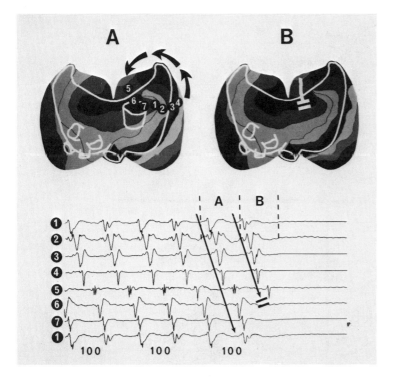

Figure 6 Maps of spontaneous termination of an episode of acetylcholine-induced atrial flutter in the right atrium of an isolated dog heart. Endocardial maps of the last two cycles of the flutter. Seven electrograms recorded simultaneously during this episode are shown at the bottom. The sites of these electrode recordings are shown on the maps. The flutter was due to circus movement of the impulse around an area of block located on the superior aspect of the right atrial appendage (A). Termination occurred when the impulse blocked in a narrow part of the circuit (B). [From Allessie et al. (26).]

ples of the classic leading circle type of arrhythmia in vivo is controversial.

In normal isolated and perfused canine hearts, Allessie et al. (26) determined the pattern of atrial endocardial activation during atrial flutter induced by a low dose of acetylcholine and rapid pacing. In all six cases of flutter mapped, the rhythm was due to circus movement of the impulse in the atrial myocardium; however, there was marked variation in both the rate of the flutter and the location of the circuits (Fig. 6). The estimated size of the circuits varied between 5 and 10 cm (conduction velocity ranged from 0.6 to 0.8 m/sec). In all cases a specific anatomic barrier was not central to the circus movement, since endocardial activation maps during sinus rhythm showed a normal spread of the impulse conduction.

In another model it was suggested that the atrial flutter inducible in dogs after the production of pericardiotomy pericarditis results from reentry in the absence of discrete atrial lesions (27). These flutters are similar to those occurring in patients after open heart surgery (28, 29). Complete details of the activation sequence of the atria during these arrhythmias are lacking, but preliminary reports (30) suggest that an anatomic obstacle is not required for the reentry. Furthermore, the nature of the functional barrier in these diseased and inflamed atria is not known. Perhaps alternations in cellular electrophysiology resulting from the pericarditis process predispose certain areas of the right atrium to conduction abnormalities.

An animal model developed to mimic the pathophysiologic circumstances that lead to

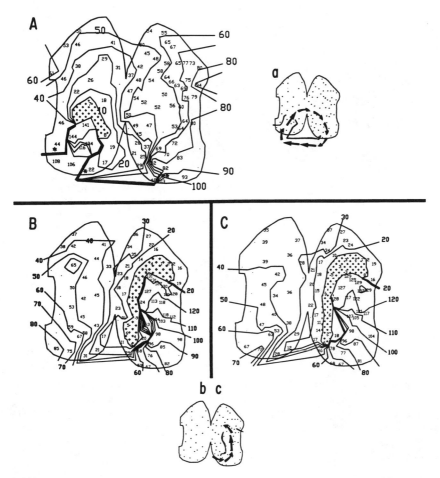

Figure 7 Detailed maps of the right atrial endocardial activation in two different episodes of sustained flutter induced in the same TI/PS dog heart. (A) An episode of a clockwise pattern of activation during the flutter with an area in the intraatrial septum providing the location of two functional types of block. (a) The major path of the impulse during a single beat. (B, C) Maps illustrating two successive beats of a flutter also induced in this heart. Isochrones at 10 msec are depicted. Zero time is different for each map, yet the zero time of C is exactly 132 msec (the flutter cycle length) after the zero time in B. The path of the impulse is again depicted in bc. Note the location of the arc of functional block. [From Boyden (33).]

atrial flutter in humans is the model of flutter in dogs with surgically induced tricuspid insufficiency and pulmonary artery stenosis (TI/PS dogs)(31). In these dogs the change in susceptibility to atrial flutter (31), as well as the existence of chronic atrial fibrillation in markedly enlarged left atria of dogs with naturally occurring mitral valvular disease (32), occurs in atrial tissues with reasonably normal transmembrane action potentials. Analysis of the patterns of sustained flutters inducible in the TI/PS dogs showed that one of the boundaries needed for the circular pathway in the enlarged right atrium was an area of functional block (Fig. 7). This area of block was functional since during examination of conduction during normal sinus rhythm no areas of total inexcitability or slowed conduction were found (33). Importantly, conduction velocity of the impulse along the circuit was not uniform and seemed to depend on the direction of the wavefront. Although the underlying nature of this functional block was not the objective of this study, it was hypothesized that this type of block was related to the anisotropic nature of the enlarged atrial myocardium.

The structural complexities and resultant geometric anisotropic nature of the normal atrial tissue have been described by many, and its role in initiating atrial reentrant impulses has been examined. Functional dissociation of Bachmann's bundle (34) and the crista terminalis bundle (35) into several pathways for impulse conduction makes them likely structures where functional block can easily occur in the atrial myocardium.

CHARACTERISTICS

For all the development of models of reentrant arrhythmias around functional barriers, much of our characterization of the electrophysiology of such circuits still relies on the in vitro studies on isolated rabbit atrium by Allessie et al. (23–25).

In addition to the concept that the path of the impulse is variable, some data have been presented that suggest that in the reentry inducible in isolated rabbit atrium there is a tight fit between the crest and tail of the reentering impulse. Therefore, no excitable gap exists in the circuit. In fact, transmembrane potential recordings from sites around the circuit during the induction of this rhythm suggest that fibers do not complete repolarization before the return of the reentrant impulse (24). Furthermore, the ability to alter this type of reentrant circuit with premature stimuli was difficult, and the timing of the stimuli had to be precise to perturb the circuit. In only a 15 msec window could the arrhythmia be perturbed, suggesting that the gap of partial excitability was not large.

Extrapolation of these findings to the functional circuits defined in the several animal models is difficult. First, unlike the "ideal" leading circle circuit described for the isolated rabbit atrial tissue, functional reentrant circuits in the enlarged right atria (31) or in atria with pericarditis (30) are somewhat different. The single largest difference is in the nonuniform conduction of the impulse as it courses through atrial tissue around the area of functional block (see Fig. 7). In both examples there is always at least one area in the circuit in which isochrones are bunched together. A bunching of isochrones suggests an area of slowed conduction. Obviously, then, as conduction slows tissue distal to this area has more time to recover excitability.

At best, in these functional circuits the duration of the excitable gap is not the same at all sites within the circuit. Specific stimulation studies designed to determine the size and nature of an excitable gap in these types of circuits remain to be done.

CIRCUS MOVEMENT INVOLVING THE TISSUES OF THE ATRIOVENTRICULAR NODES

As mentioned, perhaps a special case of the type of reentrant excitation around a functional barrier is reentrant excitation that involves the cells of the AV node. Reentry seems to occur in this region of the heart because functional differences exist between the different groups of cells that make up the AV node (36–39). The presence of this functional dissociation was demonstrated in isolated rabbit atrial and nodal tissue (37). From this experimental work it was hypothesized that two pathways with different electrical properties in terms of refractoriness and conduction velocity exist at the atrial interface of nodal tissues. These pathways then merge within the nodal tissue to form a final common pathway that then proceeds distally toward the His bundle. In 1971 a map of the impulse during the initiation and perpetuation of tachycardia involving the tissues of the AV node provided the most direct evidence for AV nodal reentrant excitation (Fig. 8)(36). Whether the functional barriers existing in the node during the tachycardia have an anatomic basis was a matter of speculation at that time. Subsequent studies that attempted to associate specific anatomic pathways with these electrophysiologic observations have not as yet decided this issue. What has been found is that the AV node has two atrial inputs, and they may be the functional pathways (40). However, definite proof is lacking. More likely, as has been hypothesized for functional reentry in sheets of atrial and ventricular myocardium, the anisotropic nature of AV nodal tissue could provide the substrate for AV nodal reentrant arrhythmias.

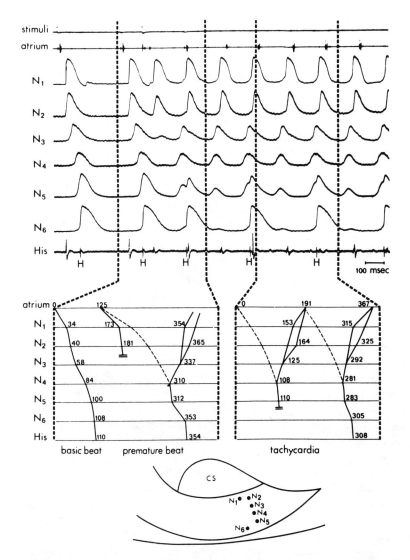

Figure 8 Simultaneous transmembrane action potentials of six AV nodal cells during initiation of a supraventricular tachycardia with a single atrial premature stimulus in isolated rabbit atrium. The middle diagram shows the activation pattern (time in mseconds) during the basic beat, during the premature beat, and during the tachycardia. The bottom diagram illustrates the position of cells N_1–N_6. CS is the coronary sinus. Note that the premature stimulus in N_1 propagates to N_2 but then blocks at N_3. N_4 is then activated, however, presumably by the impulse from N_2 following another pathway (dotted line). N_3, N_2, and N_1 are then activated in a retrograde fashion. This pattern of activation is maintained during the tachycardia. [From Janse et al. (36).]

REFERENCES

1. Mayer AG. Rhythmical pulsation in scyphomedusae. II. Papers from Tortugas Laboratory of the Carnegie Institution of Washington, Publication No. 2, 1908; I:115–31.

2. Mines GR. On dynamic equilibrium in the heart. J Physiol (Lond) 1913; 46:349–83.

3. Garrey WE. The nature of fibrillary contraction of the heart. Its relation to tissue mass and form. Am J Physiol 1914; 33:397–414.

4. Rytand DA. The circus movement (entrapped circuit wave) hypothesis and atrial flutter. Ann Intern Med 1966; 65:125–59.

5. Schmidt FO, Erlanger J. Directional differences in the conduction of the impulse

through heart muscle and their possible relation to extrasystolic and fibrillary contractions. Am J Physiol 1928; 87:326–47.

6. Lewis T, Feil HS, Stroud WD. Observations upon flutter and fibrillation. Part II. The nature of auricular flutter. Heart 1920; 7:191–245.

7. Rosenblueth A, Garcia Ramos J. Studies on flutter and fibrillation. II. The influence of artificial obstacles on experimental auricular flutter. Am Heart J 1946; 677–84.

8. Lanari A, Lambertini A, Ravin A. Mechanism of experimental atrial flutter. Circ Res 1956; 4:282–6.

9. Hayden WG, Hurley EJ, Rytand DA. The mechanism of canine atrial flutter. Circ Res 1967; 20:496–505.

10. Kimura E, Kato K, Murao S, Ajisaka H, Koyama S, Omiya Z. Experimental studies on the mechanism of the auricular flutter. Tohoku J Exp Med 1954; 60(2):197–207.

11. Frame LH, Page RL, Hoffman BF. Atrial reentry around an anatomic barrier with a partially excitable gap. A canine model of flutter. Circ Res 1986; 58:495–511.

12. Frame LH, Boyden PA, Page RL, Fenoglio JJ Jr, Hoffman BF. Circus movement in the canine atrium around the tricuspid ring during experimental atrial flutter and during reentry in vitro. Circulation 1987; 76:1155–75.

13. Spinelli W, Hoffman BF. Mechanisms of termination of reentrant atrial arrhythmias by class I and class III antiarrhythmic agents. Circ Res 1989; 65:1565–79.

14. Wu KM, Ross SM, Hoffman BF. Monophasic action potentials during reentrant atrial arrhythmias in the dog: effects of clofilium and acetylcholine. J Cardiovasc Pharmacol 1989; 13:908–14.

15. Inoue H, Matsuo H, Takayanagi K, Murao S. Clinical and experimental studies of the effects of atrial extrastimulation and rapid pacing on atrial flutter cycle. Evidence of macroreentry with an excitable gap. Am J Cardiol 1981; 48:623–31.

16. Disertori M, Inama G, Vergara G, Guarnerio M, Del Favero A, Furlanello F. Evidence of a reentry circuit in the common type of atrial flutter in man. Circulation 1983;67:434–40.

17. Gavrilescu S, Cotoi S. Monophasic action potentials of right atrium during atrial flutter and after conversion to sinus rhythm. Br Heart J 1972; 34:396–401.

18. Olsson SB, Cotoi S, Varnauskas E. Monophasic action potential and sinus stability after conversion of atrial fibrillation. Acta Med Scand 1971; 190:381–7.

19. Gavrilescu S, Luca C. Right atrium monophasic action potentials during atrial flutter and fibrillation in man. Am Heart J 1975; 90:199–205.

20. Lauribe P, Escande D, Nottin R, Coraboeuf E. Electrical activity of human atrial fibers at frequencies corresponding to atrial flutter. Cardiovasc Res 1989; 23:159–68.

21. Lewis T. The mechanism and graphic registration of the heart beat. London: Shaw and Sons, 1925.

22. Moe GK, Rheinboldt WC, Abildskov JA. A computer model of atrial fibrillation. Am Heart J 1964; 67:200–20.

23. Allessie MA, Bonke FIM, Schopman FJG. Circus movement in rabbit atrial muscle as a mechanism of tachycardia. Circ Res 1973; 36:54–62.

24. Allessie MA, Bonke FIM, Schopman FJG. Circus movement in rabbit atrial muscle as a mechanism of tachycardia. II. The role of nonuniform recovery of excitability in the occurrence of unidirectional block, as studied with multiple microelectrodes. Circ Res 1976; 39:168–77.

25. Allessie MA, Bonke FIM, Schopman FJG. Circus movement in rabbit atrial muscle as a mechanism of tachycardia. III. The "leading circle" concept: a new model of circus movement in cardiac tissue without the involvement of an anatomical obstacle. Circ Res 1977; 41:9–18.

26. Allessie MA, Lammers, WJEP, Bonke IM, Hollen J. Intra-atrial reentry as a mechanism for atrial flutter induced by acetylcholine and rapid pacing in the dog. Circulation 1984; 70(1):123–35.

27. Page' PL, Plumb VJ, Okumura K, Waldo AL. A new animal model of atrial flutter. J Am Coll Cardiol 1986; 8:872–9.

28. Wells JL, MacLean WAH, James TN, Waldo AL. Characterization of atrial flutter: studies in man after open heart surgery using fixed electrodes. Circulation 1979; 60:665–71.

29. Waldo AL, MacLean WAH, Karp RB, Kouchoukos NT, James TN. Entrainment and interruption of atrial flutter with atrial pacing. Studies in man following open heart surgery. Circulation 1977; 56:737–45.

30. Okumura K, Waldo AL, Plumb VJ. Leading circle type of reentry as a mechanism of rapid atrial flutter in a canine model. Circulation 1984; 70 (Suppl. II):223.

31. Boyden PA, Hoffman BF. The effects on atrial electrophysiology and structure of surgically induced right atrial enlargement in dogs. Circ Res 1981; 49:1319–31.

32. Boyden PA, Tilley LP, Pham TD, Liu SK, Fenoglio J Jr, Wit AL. Effects of left atrial enlargement on atrial transmembrane potentials and structure in dogs with mitral valve fibrosis. Am J Cardiol 1982; 49:1896–908.

33. Boyden PA. Activation sequence during atrial flutter in dogs with surgically induced right atrial enlargement. I. Observations during sustained rhythms. Circ Res 1988; 62:596–608.

34. Ogawa S, Dreifus LS, Osmick MJ. Longitudinal dissociation of Bachmann's bundle as a mechanism of paroxysmal supraventricular tachycardia. Am J Cardiol 1977; 40:915–22.

35. Spach MS, Miller WT III, Dolber PC, Kootsey JM, Sommer JR, Mosher CE Jr. The functional role of structural complexities in the propagation of depolarization in the atrium of the dog. Cardiac conduction disturbances due to discontinuities of effective axial resistivity. Circ Res 1982; 50:175–91.

36. Janse MJ, van Capelle FJL, Freud GE, Durrer D. Circus movement within the A-V node as a basis for supraventricular tachycardia as shown by multiple microelectrode recordings in the isolated rabbit heart. Circ Res 1971; 28:403–14.

37. Mendez C, Moe GK. Demonstration of a dual A-V nodal conduction system in the isolated rabbit heart. Circ Res 1966; 19:378–93.

38. Watanabe Y, Dreifus LS. Inhomogeneous conduction in the AV node. A model for reentry. Am Heart J 1965; 70:505–14.

39. Wit AL, Goldreyer BN, Damato AN. An in vitro model of paroxysmal supraventricular tachycardia. Circulation 1971; 43:862–75.

40. Janse MJ, van Capelle FJL, Anderson RH, Touboul P, Billette J. Electrophysiology and structure of the atrioventricular node of the isolated rabbit heart. In: Wellens HJJ, Lie KI, Janse MJ, eds. The conduction system of the heart. The Hague: Martinus Nijhoff, 1976: 298–315.

11

Reflection and Circus Movement Reentry in Isolated Atrial and Ventricular Tissues

Charles Antzelevitch and Anton Lukas

Masonic Medical Research Laboratory
Utica, New York

INTRODUCTION

The mechanisms responsible for cardiac arrhythmias have generally been categorized under two major headings: enhanced or abnormal impulse formation and reentry. Reentry, simply defined, is a phenomenon that occurs when a propagating impulse fails to die out after normal activation of the heart but persists to reexcite the heart after expiration of the refractory period. The evidence implicating reentry as a mechanism of cardiac arrhythmias originates at the turn of the century (1–5), and a number of excellent reviews are available that describe the evolution of concepts that have contributed to our present understanding of reentrant mechanisms (6–17).

Circus movement was long thought to be the sole mechanism responsible for reentrant reexcitation in the heart. More recent studies have provided evidence in support of a second subclass of reentry, termed reflection (Fig. 1). Recent findings have also led to the subdivision of circus movement reentry into three mechanistic models. In this chapter our aim is to provide an overview of these different models with a focus on experimental data derived

from in vitro studies devoted to the demonstration and characterization of reentrant phenomena in isolated atrial and ventricular tissues.

CIRCUS MOVEMENT REENTRY

A circus movement, broadly defined, is the circuitous propagation of an impulse around an anatomic or functional obstacle leading to reexcitation of the heart. Three basic models of circus movement reentry have been described: (1) the ring model; (2) the leading circle model; and (3) the figure eight model. The ring model of reentry differs fundamentally from the other two in that an anatomic obstacle is required. The leading circle and figure eight models of reentry require only a functional obstacle around which the reentrant wavefront circulates.

The Ring Model

The first experimental demonstration of circus movement reentry was in a ring model consisting of the subumbrella tissue of a jellyfish *(Sychomedusa cassiopea)* (1,2). Upon isolating this muscular tissue, Mayer noted that the disk

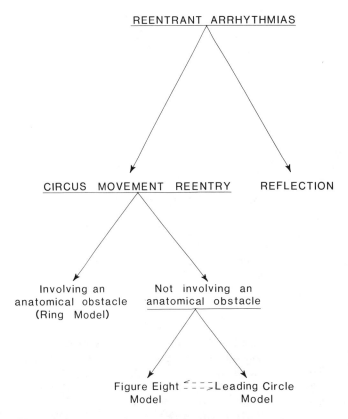

Figure 1 Classification of reentrant arrhythmias.

did not contract unless ringlike cuts were made and a stimulus applied. The disk then "springs into rapid rhythmical pulsation so regular and sustained as to recall the movement of clockwork" (1). Although Mayer also demonstrated circus movement excitation in strips cut from the ventricles of turtle hearts, he did not consider this a likely mechanism for the development of cardiac arrhythmias, since he believed the intact heart to be constructed in such a way as to make reentrant reexcitation impossible. Mayer's experiments identified two conditions essential for the initiation and maintenance of circus movement excitation: (1) the impulse initiating the circulating wave must travel in one direction only, and (2) for the circus movement to continue, the circuit must be long enough to allow each site in the circuit to recover before the return of the circulating wave.

The concept of circus movement reentry as a cause for cardiac arrhythmias was first developed by Mines (3,4). Using ringlike preparations from the atria and ventricles of canine hearts and atrioventricular rings from turtle hearts in which the chambers were electrically connected (Fig. 2A), Mines confirmed Mayer's observations and suggested that "a circulating mechanism of this type may be responsible for some cases of paroxysmal tachycardia observed clinically"(3). He reaffirmed this conviction (4) upon reading of the discovery by Kent of an extra accessory pathway connecting the atrium and ventricle of a human heart (18). The criteria developed by Mines for the identification of circus movement reentry, in use today, can be summarized as follows: (1) an area of unidirectional block must be demonstrated; (2) the movement of the excitatory wave should be observed to progress along a distinct pathway, to return to its point of origin and then follow the same path; and (3) interruption of the reentrant circuit at any point along its path should terminate the circus movement. Although amenable for testing in isolated tissues, the use of

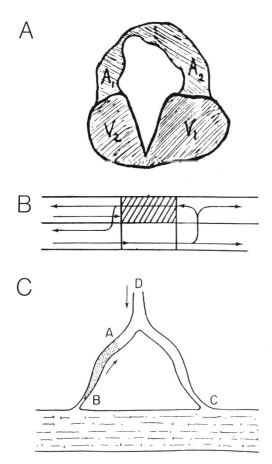

Figure 2 Ring models of reentry. (A) Mines diagram of a ring preparation comprised of the auricles and ventricles of a tortoise heart in which he observed reciprocating rhythm. Both connections between auricle and ventricle could transmit an excitation wave. During reciprocating rhythm, the four portions of the ring marked V_1, V_2, A_1, and A_2 contracted in that order [From Mines (3) with permission.] (B) Diagramatic representation of circus movement reentry in a linear bundle of tissue as proposed by Schmitt and Erlanger (19). The upper pathway contains a depressed zone (shaded) that serves as a site of unidirectional block and slow conduction. Anterograde conduction of the impulse is blocked in the upper pathway but succeeds along the lower pathway. Once beyond the zone of depression the impulse crosses over through lateral connections and reenters through the upper pathway. (C) A mechanism for reentry in a Purkinje-muscle loop as proposed by Schmitt and Erlanger (19). The diagram shows a Purkinje fiber bundle (D) that divides into two branches, both connected distally to ventricular muscle. Circus movement was considered possible if the stippled segment,

Mines' criteria for the identification of reentrant arrhythmias in the in situ heart has proven to be difficult, if not impossible, in all but a few instances.

In 1928, Schmitt and Erlanger (19) reported another important study aimed at characterization of reentry in isolated ventricular tissues. Using strips of turtle ventricle mounted in a multicompartment tissue bath divided by rubber curtains, they created segmental depression of the preparation by perfusing one of the chambers with a high-K^+ solution. They evaluated conduction by monitoring contraction along the various segments of the preparation. When the distal end of the preparation was depressed with high K^+, stimulation of the proximal end induced a contraction wave that propagated slowly in the anterograde direction, often giving rise to a contraction wave at the distal site that propagated in the retrograde direction, causing recurrent activation of the proximal end. To explain this observation, the authors proposed that the high-K^+ environment had created longitudinal dissociation in the muscle such that anterograde conduction of the impulse would be blocked through one pathway but succeed through an adjacent parallel pathway. Once beyond the major zone of depression, the impulse would cross over through lateral connections to the pathway in which it was initially blocked, which would then serve as a conduit for the retrograde passage of the impulse back to its point of origin (Fig. 2B).

Based on their observations of reentrant activity in muscle strips, Schmitt and Erlanger hypothesized that coupled ventricular extrasystoles in mammalian hearts could also arise as a consequence of circus movement reentry within loops composed of terminal Purkinje

---

$A \rightarrow B$, showed unidirectional block. An impulse advancing from D would be blocked at A but would reach and stimulate the ventricular muscle at C by way of the other terminal branch. The wavefront would then reenter the Purkinje system at B, traversing the depressed region slowly to arrive at A following expiration of refractoriness. [B and C from Schmitt and Erlanger (19) with permission.]

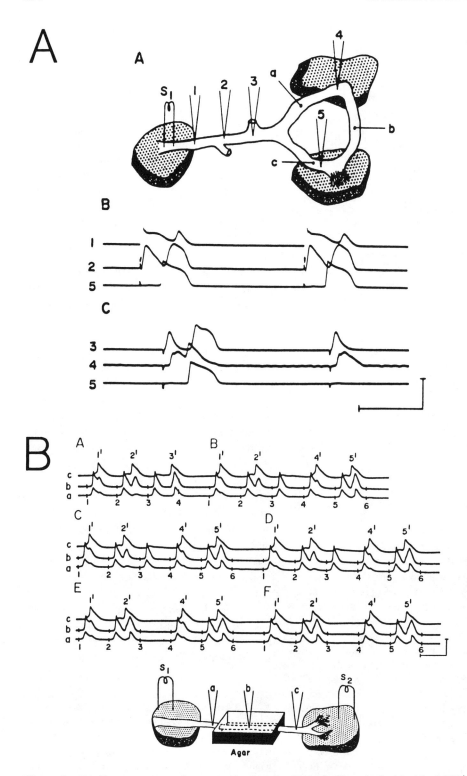

Figure 3 (A) Circus movement in a network of canine Purkinje fibers bathed in 15 mM K$^+$ and 5 × 10^{-6} M epinephrine. Panel A diagrams the preparation from which the records in panels B and C were obtained. The preparation was stimulated through electrodes at S$_1$. The records in B show reentrant excita-

fibers and ventricular muscle. Using a theoretical model consisting of a Purkinje bundle that divides into two branches that insert distally into ventricular muscle (Fig. 2C), they suggested that a region of depression within one of the terminal Purkinje branches could provide unidirectional block and conduction slow enough to permit successful reexcitation within a loop of limited size (i.e., 10–30 mm).

The early investigators realized that one of the conditions required for successful reentry was that the impulse be sufficiently delayed in an alternate pathway to allow expiration of the refractory period in the tissue proximal to the site of unidirectional block. Initially the theoretical minimum path length required for development of reentry was quite long. Not until the early 1970s was microreentry within narrowly circumscribed loops shown to be within the realm of possibility.

In 1971 Cranefield and Hoffman and coworkers (20,21) demonstrated that segments of canine Purkinje fibers that normally display impulse conduction velocities of 2–4 m/sec can conduct impulses with apparent velocities of 0.01–0.1 m/sec when encased in high-K^+ agar. This finding, coupled with the demonstration by Sasyniuk and Mendez (22) of a marked abbreviation of action potential duration and refractoriness in terminal Purkinje fibers just proximal to the site of block, greatly reduced the theoretical limit of the path length required for the development of reentry. Indeed, Sasyniuk and Mendez were able to induce single reentrant responses in isolated canine Purkinje fiber-papillary muscle preparations using critically timed premature stimuli (22).

In 1972 Wit and coworkers (23) demonstrated single and repetitive reentry in small loops of canine and bovine conducting tissues bathed in a high-K^+ solution containing catecholamines. In some of their experiments simultaneous microelectrode recordings from several sites clearly suggested that the impulse traveled around the loop in one direction, thereby causing reexcitation via a circus movement mechanism (Fig. 3A). In other experiments conducted in linear unbranched bundles of Purkinje tissue, they demonstrated a phenomenon similar to that observed by Schmitt and Erlanger in which slow anterograde conduction of the impulse was at times followed by a retrograde wavefront that produced a "return extrasystole" (Fig. 3B) (24). They proposed that the nonstimulated impulse was caused by a circus movement reentry at the level of the syncytial interconnections made possible by longitudinal dissociation of the bundle, as in the model proposed by Schmitt and Erlanger. The authors, however, considered another possibility (24,25). They noted that in many of their experiments "the rapid upstroke within the depressed segment arises after the rapid upstroke of the normal fiber" and that "this raises the possibility that the reflected impulse that travels slowly backward through the depressed segment is evoked by retrograde depolarization of the cells within the depressed segment by the rapid upstrokes of the cells beyond" (25). Thus arose the suggestion that reexcitation could occur in a single fiber through a mechanism other than circus movement, namely reflection. Although both explanations appeared plausible, proof for either was lacking at the time. Reflection

---

tion at sites 1 and 2, apparently caused by excitation that traveled around the loop to reenter the bundle. The first set of records in C shows the same phenomenon recorded at different sites; the second set shows that when block occurs at site 4, reentry does not occur. Vertical calibration, 100 mV; horizontal, 500 msec. [From Wit et al. (23); with permission.] (B) Reentry across a depressed segment in a linear bundle of Purkinje fibers. The central fiber segment was encased in agar containing high K^+ and epinephrine (see diagram below). The numbers 1, 2, and so on identify stimuli, and the numbers 1′, 2′, and so on identify delayed impulses in the forward direction. Responses elicited by stimulation at S_1 (trace a) propagate relatively promptly to site b but are either blocked or delayed in reaching site c. A delayed impulse that appears at site c may or may not return in a retrograde direction to b and a. The entire figure is a continuous tracing. The horizontal calibration represents 500 msec for all records; the vertical, 100 mV for traces a and c and 50 mV for trace b. [From Wit et al (24) with permission.]

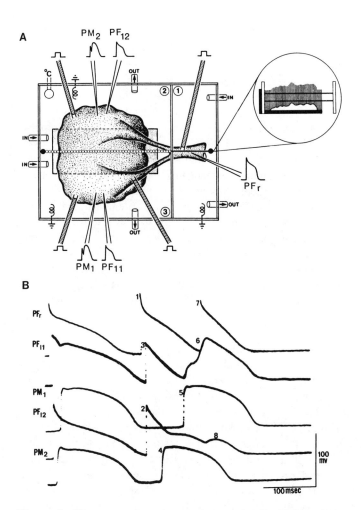

Figure 4 Circus movement reentry in a canine Purkinje-papillary muscle preparation. (A) Schematic diagram of the preparation. The inset shows a side view of the partition separating chambers 2 and 3 (consisting of adjustable slats of fiber optic tubing) and the foam pad on which the preparation rested. The free-running portion of the Purkinje fiber was threaded through a hole preformed in the rubber partition separating the left and right chambers. Chambers 1 and 2 were superfused with normal Tyrode's solution, and chamber 3 was superfused with Tyrode's containing elevated KCl and heptanol. Bipolar stimuli were delivered to the Purkinje fiber in chamber 1. Transmembrane recordings were obtained from Purkinje cells and from papillary muscle cells near the Purkinje-muscle junction (notched action potentials). (B) Transmembrane recordings obtained during a typical reentry cycle. Recordings were obtained from a Purkinje cell in chamber 1 (PF_r), Purkinje and junctional cells in chamber 2 (PF_{12} and PM_2, respectively), and Purkinje and junctional cells in chamber 3 (PF_{11} and PM_1, respectively) following the last stimulus of a train of stimuli (BCL = 300 msec) and a premature stimulus (S_1-S_2 = 166 msec). The sequence of activation following the premature stimulus is indicated by numbers 1–8. [From Gilmour, (26) with permission.]

as a mechanism of reentrant activity is discussed in greater detail in the third section.

Since the classic studies of the early 1970s, the development of in vitro ring models of reentry has been rather limited. The most recent addition to the field is that developed by Gilmour (26). In this model isolated canine ventricular Purkinje fiber-papillary muscle preparations containing two distinct Purkinje-muscle (P-M) junctions were mounted in a three-compartment chamber such that the free-running end of the Purkinje fiber and each of the two P-M junctions could be superfused independently (Fig. 4A). Conduction across one P-M junction was then depressed by superfusion with Tyrode's solution containing 6–10 mM KCl and 0.5mM heptanol. Under these conditions single stable cycles of circus movement reentry could be induced by the application of premature stimuli (Fig. 4B). These data provide a direct demonstration of the theoretical model conceived by Schmitt and Erlanger (see Fig. 2C)(19). Gilmour also showed that the delivery of subthreshold current pulses to the depressed P-M junction can accelerate, delay, or suppress the reentrant beat, depending on the polarity of the current pulse and the phase of the cycle at which the pulse is introduced.

The Arc of Block and the Leading Circle Model

A major advance in our understanding of mechanisms of reentry stemmed from the demonstration by Allessie and coworkers (27–29) of circus movement reentry in the absence of an anatomic obstacle. Garrey in 1924 was the first to suggest that reentry could be initiated without the involvement of anatomic obstacles and that "natural rings are not essential for the maintenance of circus contractions" (30). He reasoned that local differences in refractoriness could give rise to regions in which the conduction of a premature impulse is blocked and around which the reentrant wavefront may circulate. Allessie and coworkers first provided evidence in support of this hypothesis in experiments in which they induced a tachycardia in isolated preparations of rabbit left atria by applying properly timed premature extrastimuli (28). Using multiple extracellular electrodes, they carefully mapped out the activation sequence and refractory periods throughout the preparation before and during the tachycardia. They showed that although the basic beats elicited by stimuli applied near the center of the tissue spread radially throughout the preparation, premature impulses propagated only in the direction of shorter refractory periods and blocked upon approaching the region that displayed longer refractory periods. An arc of block thus developed around which the impulse was able to circulate and reexcite the tissue.

In another series of experiments, Allessie and coworkers employed microelectrode techniques to record transmembrane activity from the center of a reentrant circuit. In the example illustrated in Figure 5, they exposed the isolated rabbit left atrial preparation to carbachol to facilitate reentry. The circus movement revolved in a clockwise direction around a central zone that showed only subthreshold responses (sites 3 and 4) representing the decrement of impulses attempting to propagate into the region from opposite ends of the preparation. Thus arose the concept of the leading circle (29). In this model, circus movement reentry can occur in structurally uniform tissue; no anatomic obstacle is necessary. The functionally refractory region that develops at the vortex of the circulating wavefront prevents the centripetal waves from short-circuiting the circus movement and thus serves to maintain the reentry. Since the head of the ciculating wavefront usually travels on relatively refractory tissue, a fully excitable gap of tissue may not be present; unlike other forms of reentry, the leading circle model may not be readily influenced by extraneous impulses initiated in areas outside the reentrant circuit. The length of the circuit (pathlength) in the leading circle model is therefore essentially defined by the product of the conduction velocity and the refractory period.

Our understanding of the leading circle mechanism of reentry depends in part on our ability to explain the functionally inexcitable zone at the vortex of the circulating wavefront. Although postrepolarization refractoriness (i.e., a phenomenon in which the refractory period outlasts the action potential duration) is observed in tissues that display this type of activity, a long enduring refractoriness of the type illustrated in Figure 5 cannot be explained on the basis of conventional mechanisms, since refractoriness is generally thought of as a period that follows a

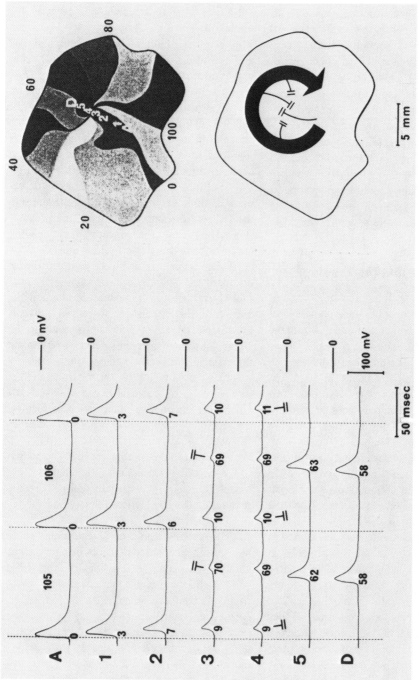

Figure 5 Activation maps during steady-state tachycardia induced by a premature stimulus in an isolated rabbit atrium (upper right). On the left are transmembrane potentials recorded from seven fibers located on a straight line through the center of the circus movement. Note that the central area is activated by centripetal wavelets and that the fibers in the central area show double responses of subnormal amplitude. Both responses are unable to propagate beyond the center, thus preventing the impulse from short-circuiting the circuit. The activation pattern (lower right) is schematically represented, showing the leading circuit and the converging centripetal wavelets. Block is indicated by double bars. [From Allessie et al. (29) with permission.]

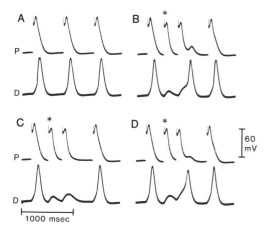

Figure 6 Electrotonic inhibition and summation in an ischemic gap preparation of calf crista terminalis. (A) Conduction of 1:1 across the gap at a BCL of 600 msec. (B) Interpolation of a premature stimulus (denoted by the asterisk; S_1-S_2 = 320 msec) elicited a premature proximal response that failed to propagate to the distal site but markedly delayed the conduction of the next stimulated beat. (C) A premature stimulus interpolated slightly later in diastole (S_1-S_2 = 330 msec) caused conduction failure of the next basic beat. (D) Summation of two subthreshold responses (S_1-S_2 = 350 msec) lead to an active response in the distal segment. [From Lukas and Antzelevitch (32) with permission.]

regenerative activation of cardiac tissue. The zone of functional block in Figure 5 shows only subthreshold responses (sites 3 and 4), which probably represent electrotonic images of activity in tissues adjacent to these zones (since they appear at the same instant in time). Refractoriness could be perpetuated under these conditions if the subthreshold or electrotonic event is capable of resetting the excitability of the tissue in the vortex region and thus resetting its refractory period. This phenomenon has been described in atrial and ventricular tissues and has been termed electrotonic inhibition (31, 32).

An example of electrotonic inhibition in atrial tissue is illustrated in Figure 6. The two transmembrane traces were recorded from the proximal and distal segments of a calf crista terminalis preparation whose central segment was depressed by exposure to an "ischemic"

solution. In Figure 6A, conduction across the depressed zone is 1:1 during stimulation of the proximal segment at a BCL of 600 msec. Introduction of an extrastimulus at an S_1-S_2 interval of 320 msec (Fig. 6B) elicits a premature response in the proximal segment that fails to propagate to the distal site but nevertheless causes a prominent delay in the conduction of the next basic beat. When the extra beat is interpolated slightly later in the cycle (S_1-S_2 = 330 msec), it again fails to propagate, but in this instance leads to conduction failure of the next basic beat (Fig. 6C). Finally, interpolation of the extra beat even later in the cycle (S_1-S_2 = 350 msec) results in summation of the two subthreshold responses, giving rise to an active response at the distal site (Fig. 6D). A single subthreshold event has been shown to be capable of prolonging refractoriness by hundreds of milliseconds (31, 32). The mechanism underlying electrotonic inhibition has been shown to be due to the ability of the subthreshold response (electrotonic image of the blocked beat) to reset the excitability of the sink (distal tissue)(31). Postrepolarization refractoriness, normally present under these conditions (Fig. 6B), is thus further prolonged by the subthreshold event. As a consequence, complete functional block can be achieved at rapid rates of stimulation in preparations that conduct in a 1:1 manner at slower rates (Fig. 7).

The leading circle mechanism has also recently been proposed to mediate tachycardia induced in isolated ventricular tissues. Kamiyama and coworkers (33) used microelectrode techniques to map thinly sliced sheets of canine ventricular epicardium. Sustained tachycardia could be readily induced in these preparations with a single premature stimulus. The reentrant wavefront was calculated based on measurements of the refractory period and construction of the depolarizing and repolarizing wavefronts obtained from action potential measurements during normal pacing. Based on these calculations the authors concluded that the wavefront revolved around an arc of functional block and that a leading circle with a diameter of 8–10 mm was involved. In a preliminary report Allessie and coworkers (34)

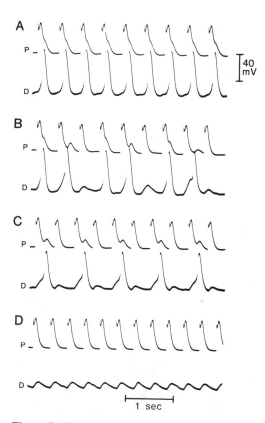

Figure 7 Rate dependence of conduction in a segmentally depressed atrial preparation. The two transmembrane traces in each panel were recorded from the proximal (P) and distal (D) segments of an ischemic gap preparation of calf crista terminalis. (A) Conduction of 1:1 across the gap at a BCL of 450 msec. (B) A 3:2 conduction ratio at a BCL of 440 msec. (C) A 2:1 block at a BCL of 400 msec. (D) At a BCL of 350 msec, conduction across the depressed zone was completely blocked and only subthreshold (electrotonic) responses were recorded at the distal site. [From Lukas and Antzelevitch (32) with permission.]

recently described the development of circus movement reentry without the involvement of an anatomic obstacle in a two-dimensional model of ventricular epicardium created by freezing the endocardial layers of a Langendorff perfused rabbit heart. A sustained ventricular tachycardia with a cycle length of 130 msec and an excitable gap of 30 msec was induced with rapid stimulation. High-resolution mapping of the surviving epicardial layer revealed that the tachycardia was due to circulation of the wavefront around a line of functional block oriented parallel to the long axis of the myocardial fibers. Microelectrode recordings from the center of the ellipsoid circuit showed markedly prolonged action potentials with 2:1 or 3:1 activation patterns.

The development of functional arcs or lines of block in epicardium leading to circus movement reentry without the involvement of anatomic obstacles has been well established in in vivo models of canine infarction in which a thin surviving epicardial rim overlies the infarcted ventricle (10, 35–40). In most cases the lines of block observed during tachycardia have been found to be oriented parallel to the direction of the myocardial fibers, suggesting that anisotropic conduction properties (due to differences in the end-to-end versus side-to-side electrical coupling of cells) (41–43) in addition to differences in local refractoriness, play an important role in defining this zone. The lines of block observed during the initiation of the tachycardia, however, are often transverse to the direction of the fibers.

It is not as yet clear whether the long lines of functional block that sustain large reentrant circuits and the small vortices of functional block described by Allessie and coworkers represent different mechanisms or different manifestations of the same electrophysiologic phenomenon. In a recent study Dillon and coworkers (40) presented evidence to suggest that the long lines of functional block that sustain reentry in the epicardial rim overlying canine infarction may in fact represent zones of very slow conduction (Fig. 8). Slow conduction of the wavefront across the lines of apparent block occurred in a direction transverse to the long axis of the myocardial fibers, suggesting that this phenomenon may be due in part to the anisotropic properties of the tissue. According to this interpretation, although long lines of block may appear to be present on gross examination of data obtained from mapping studies, the dimensions of the area of functional block may in fact be relatively small and may even approach those of the vortex of functional block described by Allessie and coworkers.

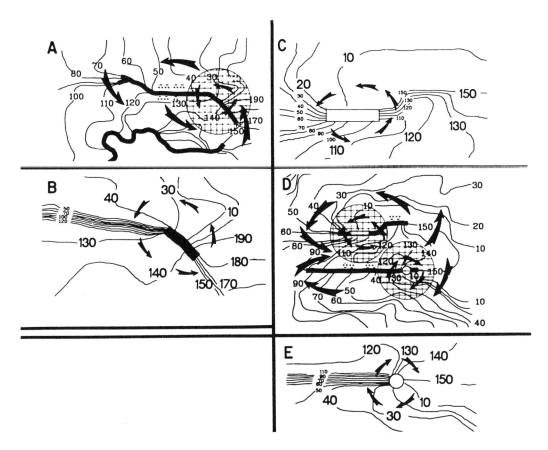

Figure 8 The possible effects of anisotropy on reentrant circuits. (A–D) Isochrones from reentrant circuits recorded during sustained tachycardia in the epicardial border zone of subacute canine infarcts. In A, the large black arrows point out a sequence of excitation that appears to be progressing around the long line of apparent block, indicated by the horizontal thick black line. An analysis of electrogram characteristics and isochrones adjacent to this line suggests that there is slow activation across it, and thus the center of the circuit is smaller as indicated by the smaller black arrows within the shaded circle. This region is enlarged in B, where the thick black line of apparent block has been resolved into closely bunched isochrones, indicating slow activation in the part of the circuit transverse to the fiber orientation. In D, the large black arrows point out a sequence of excitation that appears to be progressing around two long lines of apparent block, indicated by the horizontal thick black lines. The smaller arrows in D within the shaded circles are shown enlarged in C (upper circuit) and E (lower circuit). The activation maps suggest that there is rapid activation in the parts of the circuit where activation occurs parallel to the long axis of the fibers and slow activation in the parts where activation occurs transversely. [From Dillon et al. (40) with permission.]

The Figure Eight Model

Although the figure eight model has not been described in isolated tissues, a brief discussion seems appropriate. The figure eight model (pretzel configuration) of reentry was first described by El-Sherif and coworkers in their mapping studies of the surviving epicardial layer overlying infarction produced by occlusion of the left anterior descending artery in canine hearts (15,35–37,44). In this model the reentrant premature beat produces a wavefront that circulates in both directions around a long line of functional conduction block (Fig. 9; see also Fig. 8D). The wavefront proceeds to rejoin on the distal side of the block and then breaks through the arc of block to reexcite the tissue proximal to the block. The single arc of block is thus divided into two, and the reentrant activation continues as two

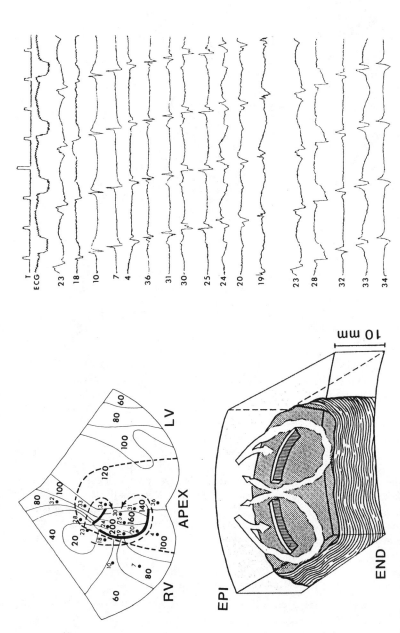

Figure 9 Figure eight model of reentry. Isochronal activation map during monomorphic reentrant ventricular tachycardia occurring in the surviving epicardial layer overlying an infarct. Recordings were obtained from the epicardial surface of a canine heart 4 days after ligation of the left anterior descending coronary artery. Activation isochrones are drawn at 20 msec intervals (upper left). The reentrant circuit has a characteristic figure eight pattern. Two circulating wavefronts advance in clockwise and counterclockwise directions, respectively, around two zones (arcs) of conduction block (represented by heavy solid lines). The epicardial surface is depicted as if the ventricles were unfolded following a cut from the crux to the apex. The right panel shows selected simultaneous electrograms recorded along the two arcs of functional conduction block and the common reentrant wavefront. A three-dimensional diagrammatic illustration of the ventricular activation pattern during the reentrant tachycardia is shown at the lower left corner. RV = right ventricle, LV = left ventricle, EPI = epicardium, END = endocardium, T = time lines at 100 msec intervals. [From El-Sherif (15) with permission.]

circulating wavefronts that travel in clockwise and counterclockwise directions around the two arcs. The diameter of the reentrant circuit in the ventricle may be as small as a few millimeters or as large as several centimeters. El-Sherif et al. (45) have suggested that figure eight reentry could occur in the epicardial, intramural, or subendocardial regions of the heart, depending on the distribution of pathologic features in the myocardium. These authors (15,44) have also suggested that the leading circle model described by Allessie and coworkers may be a special modification of the figure eight model, the former being more likely to occur in isolated tissues of limited size.

REFLECTION

Reflection is a term used since the turn of the century to describe a variety of phenomena characterized by the to-and-fro propagation of an impulse over the same pathway, leading to recurrent activation of the tissue at a proximal site (19,24,25,46–49). The term "pseudo-reflection" has been applied occasionally to describe phenomena in which a single beat elicited by stimulation of a proximal site is observed at some distal site to be followed by a closely coupled response that develops spontaneously and travels retrogradely to reexcite the proximal tissue (12,25,47). This phenomena results in a coupled response at both the proximal and distal sites and is generally thought to be due to triggered activity. In "true" reflection, a coupled response occurs at the proximal site but only a single response is seen at the distal site.

The concept of reflection as we know it today was first suggested by Cranefield and Wit and coworkers based on their studies of the propagation characteristics of slow responses in K^+-depolarized Purkinje fibers (20,21, 23–25). Using linear unbranched bundles of Purkinje tissue, Wit and coworkers demonstrated a phenomenon similar to that observed by Schmitt and Erlanger in which slow antegrade conduction of the impulse was at times followed by a retrograde wavefront that produced a "return extrasystole" (24). They pro-

posed that the nonstimulated impulse was caused by circuitous reentry at the level of the syncytial interconnections, made possible by longitudinal dissociation of the bundle, as the most likely explanation for the phenomenon but also suggested the possibility of reflection.

The demonstration and characterization of electrotonically mediated conduction and return extrasystoles across inexcitable gaps created in linear bundles of Purkinje tissue by Antzelevitch and coworkers provided the first direct line of evidence in support of reflection as a mechanism of arrhythmogenesis (48,49). Several models of reflected reentry have been developed (48–51). The first of these consisted of a preparation in which an "ion-free" solution of isotonic sucrose was used to create a narrow (1.5–2 mm) central inexcitable zone (gap) in unbranched Purkinje fibers mounted in a three-chamber tissue bath (48).

The characteristics of conduction in such a preparation are illustrated in Figure 10. Stimulation of the proximal (P) segment elicits an action potential that propagates to the proximal border of the sucrose gap. Although active propagation across the gap is not possible because of the ion-depleted extracellular milieu, local circuit current continues to flow through the intercellular low-resistance pathways (a Ag/AgCl extracellular shunt pathway is provided). This electrotonic current, much diminished upon emerging from the gap, slowly discharges the capacity of the distal (D) tissue. The resulting depolarizations manifest as either subthreshold responses (last distal response) or as foot potentials that bring the distal excitable element to its threshold potential. Active impulse propagation therefore stops and then resumes after a delay that may be as long as several hundred milliseconds. When anterograde (P → D) transmission time is sufficient to permit recovery of refractoriness at the proximal end, electrotonic transmission of the impulse in the retrograde direction reexcites the proximal tissue, thus generating a closely coupled reflected reentry. Reflection therefore results from the to-and-fro electrotonically mediated transmission of the impulse across the same blocked segment; neither longitudinal dissociation nor cir-

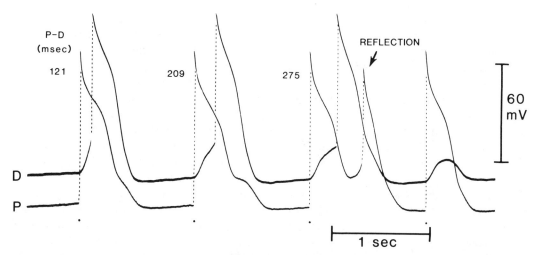

Figure 10 Delayed transmission and reflection across an inexcitable gap created by superfusion of the central segment of a Purkinje fiber with an "ion-free" isotonic sucrose solution. The two traces were recorded from proximal (P) and distal (D) active segments. P-D conduction time (indicated in the upper portion of the figure, in msec) increased progressively with a 4:3 Wenckebach periodicity. The third simulated proximal response was followed by a reflection [From Antzelevitch (56) with permission.]

cus movement need be invoked to explain the phenomenon.

A second model more consistent with the conditions likely to impair conduction in a diseased heart was subsequently developed (49). A narrow zone of depression was created by superfusion of a central segment of a Purkinje bundle with a solution designed to mimic the extracellular milieu at a site of ischemia. With a K^+ concentration of between 15 and 20 mM, the "ischemic" solution induced delays in conduction as long as 500 msec across the 1.5 mm wide gap. Under these conditions the gap segment was shown, with the aid of such pharmacologic tools as verapamil and tetrodotoxin (blockers of the inward currents), to be largely comprised of an inexcitable cable across which conduction of impulses was electrotonically mediated (Fig. 11). The long delays for conduction of the impulse across the ischemic gap permitted the manifestation of reflection (Fig. 12A). When propagation across the gap was mediated by "slow responses," transmission was relatively prompt and reflection did not occur (49).

Under similar conditions reflected reentry has also been demonstrated in isolated ventricular tissues (51,52). In all cases step delays attended by subthreshold foot potentials at the

distal site were apparent, and an inexcitable zone was a prerequisite (Fig. 12B). More recently, Lukas and Antzelevitch (32) demonstrated delayed conduction and reflection in segmentally depressed canine and calf atrial preparations (Fig. 12C).

Reflection has also been demonstrated in Purkinje tissues in which a functionally inexcitable zone was created by focal depolarization of the preparation with long-duration constant current pulses (53). Reflected reentry can also be observed in homogeneously depressed isolated canine Purkinje fibers as well as in branched preparations of "normal" Purkinje fibers (Figs. 13 and 14). In these preparations as in the models already described, a distinct discontinuity (step delay) in conduction is observed with careful mapping of the preparation using microelectrodes.

Although the presence of phase 4 depolarization (pacemaker activity) in the tissue distal to the site of conduction impairment facilitates reflection by making possible longer delays for the transmission of the impulse across the depressed zone, phase 4 depolarization is not a prerequisite for the manifestation of reflected reentry (see Figs. 12B and 13B).

Reflection depends critically on the magnitude of conduction delays in both directions

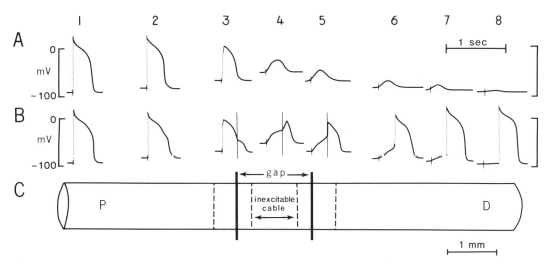

Figure 11 Schematic representation of an ischemic gap preparation depicting transmembrane activity characteristic of the various sites along the preparation. The model consists of a Purkinje fiber whose central segment (gap) is exposed to an "ischemic" solution. Because part of the gap tissue is rendered inexcitable, an impulse initiated by stimulation of the proximal (P) segment propagates normally up to the border of the block and stops there. Local circuit current continues to flow axially along the inexcitable cable, generating an electrotonically mediated depolarization, which may (B) or may not (A) bring the distal (D) membrane to threshold. When transmission is successful, propagation of the active impulse resumes at the distal site, but after a delay. Transmembrane potentials recorded near the distal border of the gap (B-5) display foot potentials representative of the electrotonic image of the proximal responses (A-5). [From Antzelevitch (14) with permission.]

across the functionally inexcitable zone. These transit delays depend on several factors, including the width of the blocked segment, the intracellular and extracellular impedance to the flow of local circuit current across the inexcitable zone, and the excitability of the distal active site. Because excitability of cardiac tissues continues to recover for hundreds of milliseconds after an action potential, transmission of impulses across an inexcitable gap is a sensitive function of frequency (31,48, 54,55). Not surprisingly, the incidence and patterns of manifest ectopic activity encountered in models of reflection are highly frequency dependent (50–52, 54, 56–58).

Figure 15 illustrates an example of frequency-dependent alterations in impulse transmission across an inexcitable gap and the resultant changes in arrhythmic patterns obtained in a model in which an in vitro sucrose gap-Purkinje fiber preparation was allowed to interact with the activity of an intact canine heart (50). In this model of reentry (representative of both circus movement and reflec-

tion), a ventricular electrogram (middle trace) recorded from the right ventricle (in vivo) triggers the delivery of a stimulus to the proximal segment of the sucrose gap-Purkinje fiber preparation. The activity thus elicited, when successful in propagating across the inexcitable zone, leads to an active response at the distal site (top trace) whose upstroke triggers the delivery of a stimulus back to the right ventricle of the intact heart.

Similar rate-dependent changes in extrasystolic activity have been reported in patients with frequent premature ventricular responses evaluated with Holter recordings (59) and in patients evaluated by atrial pacing (Fig. 16) (56,60).

The frequency dependence of reflection depends critically on the level of electrotonic communication across the functionally inexcitable zone. When communication is weak, major delays in conduction and reflection occur at slow rates of stimulation. When the level of electrotonic interaction is relatively high, delayed conduction and reflected reentry are

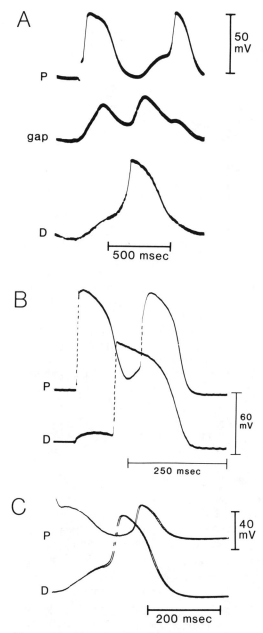

only observed following a premature beat or at rapid stimulation rates.

Although much of the data relative to the frequency-dependent behavior of premature beat manifestation stems from models of reflection, there is little reason to believe that a circus movement mechanism should behave differently. Microreentry with either mechanism depends on delayed conduction, and it is the frequency dependence of delayed conduction that is in large part responsible for the rate dependence of microreentry.

The reciprocal interactions that generate reflected reentry can, under the right conditions, generate a self-sustained tachycardia. The capability of a reflection model to reciprocate in the generation of two consecutive reflected responses has been demonstrated (57). The conditions necessary for initiating sustained runs, although difficult to achieve in the in vitro preparation, may be readily attained in the coupled in vitro-in vivo preparation in which anterograde and retrograde conduction can be independently controlled. The ability to initiate and terminate ventricular tachycardia by using programmed electrical stimulation, long considered evidence of an underlying mechanism of circus movement (61), is shared in this model of reentrant tachycardia in which an inexcitable zone provides the necessary conduction delay.

Because reflection can occur within areas of tissue as small as 1–2 mm^2, its identification as a mechanism of arrhythmia requires very high spatial resolution mapping of the electrical activity of discrete sites. Extracellular mapping studies conducted to date have generally fallen far short of the requirements necessary to define reflected reentry or the

Figure 12 Examples of reflected reentry in segmentally depressed Purkinje, ventricular muscle, and atrial preparations. (A) Reflection in an "ischemic" (high K$^+$, low pH, and hypoxia) gap preparation of calf Purkinje fiber. The three traces were recorded from the proximal (P), gap, and distal (D) segments of the preparation. Stimulation of the proximal segment elicits a response that fails to activate the central segment but is nevertheless transmitted to the distal site with a step delay of 340 msec. Electrotonic transmission of the distal response in the retrograde direction gives rise to a reflected reentrant beat (coupling interval = 650 msec). (B) Reflection in a high-K$^+$ gap preparation of feline papillary muscle. BCL = 1000 msec, 1 mm gap, with 30 mM KCl. [From Rozanski et al. (51) with permission.] (C) Reflected reentry in an ischemic gap preparation of calf crista terminalis. [From Lukas and Antzelevitch (32) with permission.]

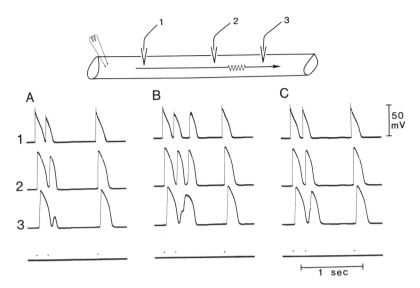

Figure 13 Disparity of local refractoriness contributes to conduction delay and reflection in a canine Purkinje fiber bathed in 20 mM K$^+$ and 0.3μM epinephrine. The diagram at the top shows the arrangement of stimulating and recording electrodes. In the lower panels, the upper three traces are transmembrane recordings from sites 1–3 and the lower trace is the stimulus marker. (A) Application of an extrastimulus at an S_1-S_2 = 180 msec elicits a premature impulse that propagates to site 2 but is blocked between sites 2 and 3. (B) An extrastimulus applied at an S_1-S_2 interval of 190 msec conducts successfully between sites 2 and 3 with a step delay of 120 msec, which is long enough to permit reflection of the impulse. (C) An extrastimulus applied at a longer S_1-S_2 interval (210 msec) conducts between sites 2 and 3 with a delay too short to permit reflection.

mechanism of very slow or delayed conduction that has been suggested to occur at lines of apparent conduction block (40). Activation patterns in these regions can be quite complex as judged by the polyphasic extracellular waveforms recorded from such sites; high-resolution recording with very fine tipped unipolar electrodes (50 μm) may be helpful in this regard (62). The precise delineation of impulse conduction mechanisms at discrete sites of marked conduction impairment, however, will most likely require the use of intracellular microelectrode techniques in conjunction with high-resolution extracellular mapping techniques. These limitations considered, reflection has been suggested as the mechanism underlying reentrant extrasystolic activity in ventricular tissues excised from 1-day-old infarcted canine heart (63) and in a clinical case of incessant ventricular bigeminy in a young patient with no evidence of organic heart disease (64).

SLOW AND DELAYED CONDUCTION

Slow or delayed impulse conduction can greatly facilitate circus movement involving large reentrant circuits (macroreentry) and is a prerequisite for reflection and circus movement microreentry. A number of factors determine the velocity at which an action potential propagates through cardiac tissue. Among these is the intensity of the fast inward sodium current that flows during the upstroke of the action potential. This current is gated by channels whose activation, inactivation, and reactivation properties are finely regulated by the voltage across the cellular membrane. Changes in the rate of rise of the action potential upstroke (dV/dt_{max} or $\dot{V}_{max}$) are generally used as a measure of the changes in the magnitude of the sodium current with the recognition that there may not be a linear relationship between the two parameters (65,66). Depolar-

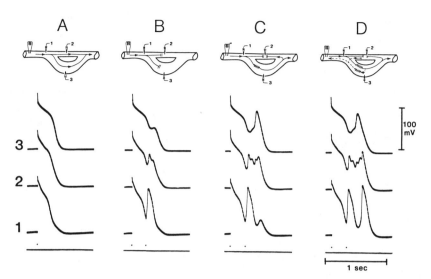

Figure 14 Contribution of geometry to delayed conduction, block, and reentry of premature beats in an isolated canine Purkinje preparation. The schematic drawing of the preparation at the top of each panel shows the location of stimulating and recording electrodes and the proposed pathways of impulse propagation. In the lower part of each panel the top three traces are transmembrane recordings from sites 1–3 and the bottom trace is the stimulus marker. (A) Basic beats at a BCL of 1000 msec. (B) Application of an extrastimulus at an S_1-S_2 = 230 msec elicits a premature response that conducts to site 1 but is blocked near the branch point before reaching sites 2 and 3. (C) A slight increase in the S_1-S_2 interval to 245 msec elicits a premature beat that once again blocks at site 2 but succeeds in activating site 3 after a 125 msec delay. (D) A premature beat elicited at an S_1-S_2 = 240 msec also blocks before reaching site 2 but activates site 3 after a longer delay (145 msec). The delay is sufficient to permit reentrant excitation of the proximal site (site 1).

ization of the resting membrane potential by whatever means can lead to steady-state inactivation of sodium channels, thereby reducing the number of channels available to carry this current during the action potential upstroke (67). In depolarized states, as well as in the presence of some drugs, the availability of sodium channels may also be diminished because of insufficient time for recovery of the channels from inactivation (incomplete reactivation) or from the blocking effect of the drug (67–70). The intensity of the sodium current accompanying a closely coupled premature beat can be greatly diminished as a result of a more positive takeoff potential (if the response occurs during the repolarization phase of the previous beat), as well as to incomplete reactivation of the sodium channels.

The sodium channels are totally inactivated when the membrane potential is depolarized to voltages positive to -55 mV. Under these conditions the action potential upstroke is maintained by a more slowly activating inward current carried largely by calcium ions. In many cases enhancement of the calcium current with catecholamines is needed to evoke an action potential at these depolarized levels (71,72). Responses solely dependent on the activation of the calcium current (slow inward current) have been referred to as "slow" responses. Because of their apparently slow conduction they have been suggested to underlie the occurrence of reentrant arrhythmias (25). Recent studies have questioned the role of the slow response in arrhythmogenesis, noting that major conduction delays recorded in depressed or diseased tissues are often accompanied by apparently normal or slightly depolarized (depressed fast response) responses (49,63,73–75). Apparently slow conduction seen in slow response preparations appears to be due to the development of discontinuities in conduction (discussed later) created under the conditions used to elicit these responses, not to the homogeneous slow conduction of the slow response (49).

Discontinuities in conduction can give rise to apparently very slow conduction and reentry in cardiac tissues by allowing the development of prominent step delays in the transmission of impulses at discrete sites. Any agent or agency capable of suppressing the active generator properties of cardiac tissues may diminish excitability to the point of rendering a localized region functionally inexcitable and thus creating a discontinuity in the propagation of the advancing wavefront. Examples include an ion-free, ischemic, or high-K^+ environment (31,48,49,51,54), as discussed earlier, as well as electrical blocking current (53,76,77), localized pressure (31, 78), and localized cooling (78). Inhibition of the inward currents using sodium and/or calcium blockers can also create discontinuities in conduction when applied to localized segments (49).

Very slow conduction under these conditions has been shown to be due to the development of major step delays caused by electrotonically mediated (saltatory) transmission of impulses across a functionally inexcitable zone (i.e., across a large cumulative axial resistance imposed between two excitable regions) rather than to a uniform or homogeneous slowing of impulse propagation. The functionally inexcitable zone effectively serves to diminish the electrical coupling between the excitable regions participating in the conduction of the impulse. The decay of the wavefront as it courses the inexcitable or refractory zone leads to slow activation of the tissue beyond and thus to a step delay in the conduction of the impulse.

The resistive barriers created secondary to the evolution of inexcitable regions fundamentally are not very different from those observed in anisotropy (42,43). With either condition small changes in the effective impedance to the flow of local circuit current from one excitable element to the next can give rise to major delays in conduction. Conduction delays of the order of tens or hundreds of milliseconds occur when the electrotonic communication between the region already

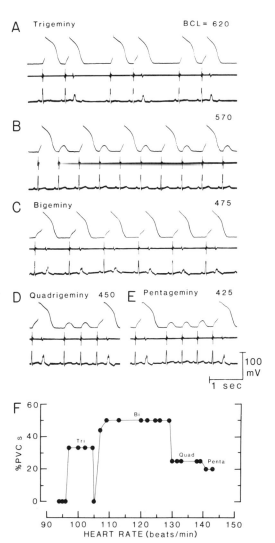

Figure 15 Frequency dependence of reentry recorded in a model consisiting of a sucrose gap preparation coupled to the intact heart of an open-chest dog. (A–E) Transmembrane potentials from the distal segment of the sucrose gap preparation; right ventricular electrogram and lead II electrocardiogram from the in vivo preparation. Right atrial drive was applied at the indicated basic cycle length (BCL). Right ventricular activation triggered the delivery of a stimulus to the proximal segment of the sucrose gap preparation. When an active response ensued at the distal site across the inexcitable gap, the transmembrane action potential recorded from that tissue effected stimulation of the right ventricle after a fixed delay of 80 msec. (F) Summary of a complete scan of stimulation frequencies. The incidence of reentrant beats (% PVC) is plotted as a function of heart rate [From Antzelevitch et al. (50) with permission.]

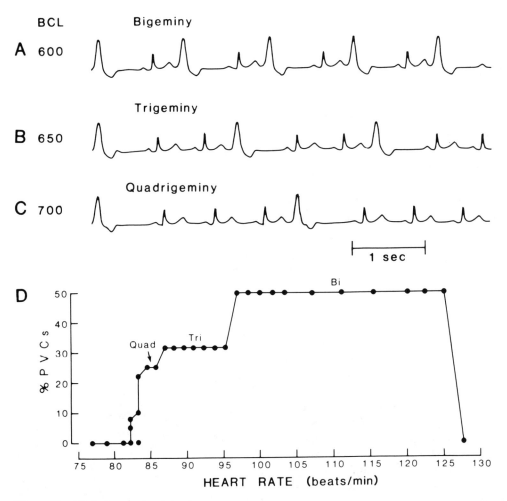

Figure 16 Clinical example of the frequency dependence of extrasystolic manifestation recorded during a routine electrophysiologic study. Right atrial drive was accelerated in 10 msec steps. (A–C) Examples of electrocardiographic activity (lead II) recorded at the indicated cycle lengths. (D) The incidence of premature ventricular responses (% PVC) is plotted as a function of heart rate. BCL = basic cycle length. Records were provided by Dr. Douglas Zipes. [From Antzelevitch (56) with permission.]

activated (source) and the region awaiting activation (sink) is weak. With progressive uncoupling between source and sink, conduction characteristics also become progressively more sensitive to changes in the active and passive membrane properties of both the source and sink (55). Although the importance of the intensity of the source current, as reflected by the action potential amplitude, duration, or maximum rate of rise, $(dV/dt)_{max}$, is well appreciated (55,75,79–82), recent studies suggest that under a variety of conditions the threshold current requirement of the sink (i.e., changes in excitability) (31,55,82) may be a

more critical determinant of conduction delay (or block).

Step delays of impulse transmission attended by electrotonic prepotentials have been observed in intracellular recordings obtained from human and animal infarcted myocardium (11,63,73,74). Extracellular mapping experiments have also uncovered step delays in the propagation of impulses in canine hearts subjected to acute regional myocardial ischemia (83). These studies lend support to an electrotonic interaction across a high impedance barrier as a mechanism responsible for apparently slow conduction.

Nonuniform recovery of refractoriness and geometric factors also play an important role in determining impulse conduction velocity as well as the success or failure of conduction. Disparity in the recovery of refractoriness has already been discussed as the basis for unidirectional block or the lines of block that develop in response to premature beats. Disparity of local refractoriness can also contribute to a major slowing of impulse propagation and thus to reentry, as illustrated in Figure 13. The three transmembrane traces shown were recorded along the length of a thin canine Purkinje fiber preparation bathed in Tyrode's solution containing 20 mM K^+ and 0.3 μM epinephrine. The resting potentials were -53, -55, and -54 mV for cells 1, 2 and 3, respectively. The action potential duration (APD_{90}) increased from a value of 155 msec at cell 1 to 190 msec at cell 3. With stimulation applied near cell 1 at a basic cycle length of 1000 msec (first and last responses), propagation is relatively prompt and unencumbered. A premature impulse elicited with an extrastimulus applied at an S_1-S_2 interval of 180 msec propagates relatively promptly to cell 2 but is blocked between sites 2 and 3 where action potential duration is longest (Fig. 13A). With an S_1-S_2 of 190 msec conduction between sites 2 and 3 succeeds, but with a step delay of 120 msec, long enough to permit reflection of the impulse and the generation of an extrasystole (Fig. 13B). With an S_1-S_2 of 210 msec conduction between cells 2 and 3 also occurred with a step delay, but one too short to permit reflected reentry (Fig. 13C). The discontinuity in conduction occurred at the site where refractoriness would be expected to be longest. These results suggest that local differences in refractoriness contribute not only to the development of directional block in the conduction of the impulse but also to the development of prominent step delays in conduction, thus setting the stage for circus movement and reflected reentry.

The influence of geometry on impulse conduction has long been appreciated. Regions in which the cross-sectional area of interconnected cells increases abruptly are known to be potential sites for the development of unidirectional block or delayed conduction. Slowing or block of conduction generally occurs when the impulse propagates in the direction of increasing diameter because the local circuit current provided by the advancing wavefront is insufficient or barely sufficient to charge the capacity of the larger volume of tissue ahead and thus bring the larger mass to its threshold potential. The Purkinje-muscle junction is one example of a site at which unidirectional block and conduction delays are commonly observed (26,84–86). The preexcitation (Wolff-Parkinson-White) syndrome is another example, where a thin bundle to tissue (Kent bundle) inserts into a large ventricular mass.

Figure 14 illustrates an example in which the geometry of the preparation contributes to delayed conduction, block, and reentry of premature beats in a normal isolated Purkinje fiber preparation. The preparation, shown schematically at the top of the figure, was excised from the right ventricle of a canine heart. With stimulation at a BCL of 1000 msec, conduction of the basic beat (first beat in each panel) was unimpeded and the action potential durations at sites 1, 2, and 3 were 300, 330, and 340 msec, respectively (Fig. 14A). A premature beat elicited with an extrastimulus applied at an S_1-S_2 interval of 230 msec conducted to site 1 but was blocked near the branch point before reaching sites 2 and 3 (Fig. 14B). When the S_1-S_2 interval was increased by 15 msec (245 msec), the premature wavefront was once again blocked at site 2 but succeeded in activating site 3 after a delay of 125 msec (Fig. 14C). With a slight (5 msec) abbreviation of the S_1-S_2 interval to 240 msec (Fig 14D), the premature wavefront blocked before reaching site 2 and the activation of site 3 was further delayed (145 msec). The delay was then long enough to permit reentrant reexcitation of the proximal site. The records suggest that retrograde conduction of the impulse (dotted line) may have occurred along the same path as anterograde conduction, thus giving rise to a reflected reentry. An alternative interpretation is that the impulse traveled around the preparation in a counterclockwise direction, returning through site 2 and thus causing reentry through a circus movement mechanism. Regardless of the mechanism involved, it seems clear that the geometry of the preparation (branching leading to a near doubling or the total cross-sectional area), as well as the gradient of action potential duration, contributed to the unidirectional block and the major step delay in conduction of the impulse, both of which were required for reentry to occur.

CONCLUSION

Although it is difficult to extrapolate findings from in vitro models of reentry directly to cardiac arrhythmias in the human or even to arrhythmias observed in in vivo animal models, such findings, some stemming back to the turn of the century, have greatly advanced our understanding of the mechanisms by which reentrant arrhythmias occur. Studies of isolated tissue models have been especially helpful in furthering our understanding of the complex factors influencing conduction in the cardiac syncytium, especially in pathophysiologic states. Many questions remain to be answered, and many answers will undoubtedly be questioned in the years ahead as we approach yet another level of understanding of the intricate mechanisms contributing to the genesis and maintenance of reentrant cardiac arrhythmias.

REFERENCES

1. Mayer AG. Rhythmical pulsations in Scyphomedusae. Publication 47 of the Carnegie Institute, Washington, D.C., 1906:1–62.
2. Mayer AG. Rhythmical pulsations in Scyphomedusae. II. Publication 102 of the Carnegie Institute, Washington, D.C., 1908: 115–31.
3. Mines GR. On dynamic equilibrium in the heart. J Physiol (Lond) 1913; 46:349–82.
4. Mines GR. On circulating excitation in heart muscle and their possible relation to tachycardia and fibrillation. Trans R Soc Can 1914; 8:43–52.
5. Lewis T. The mechanism and graphic registration of the heart beat, 3rd ed. London: Shaw and Sons, 1925.
6. Cranefield, PF, Wit AL, Hoffman BF. Genesis of cardiac arrhythmias. Circulation 1973; 47:190–204.
7. Moe GK. Evidence for reentry as a mechanism for cardiac arrhythmias. Rev Physiol Biochem Pharmacol 1975; 72:56–66.
8. Kulbertus HE, ed. In: Reentrant arrhythmias, mechanisms and treatment. Baltimore: University Park Press, 1977.
9. Wit AL, Cranefield PF. Re-entrant excitation as a cause of cardiac arrhythmias. Am J Physiol 1978; 235:H1–17.
10. Wit AL, Allessie MA, Fenoglio JJ Jr, Bonke FIM, Lammers W, Smeets J. Significance of the endocardial and epicardial border zones in the genesis of myocardial infarction arrhythmias. In: Harrison D, ed. Cardiac arrhythmias: a decade of progress. Boston: GK Hall, 1982:39–68.
11. Spear JF, Moore EN. Mechanisms of cardiac arrhythmias. Ann Rev Physiol 1982; 44:485–97.
12. Janse MJ. Reentry rhythms. In: Fozzard HA, Haber E, Jennings RB, Katz AM, Morgan HE, eds. The heart and cardiovascular system. New York: Raven Press, 1986:1203–38.
13. Hoffman BF, Dangman KH. Mechanisms for cardiac arrhythmias. Experientia 1987; 43: 1049–56.
14. Antzelevitch C. Reflection as a mechanism of reentrant cardiac arrhythmias. Prog Cardiol 1988; 1(1):3–16.
15. El-Sherif N. Reentry revisited. PACE 1988; 11:1358–68.
16. Lazzara R, Scherlag BJ. Generation of arrhythmias in myocardial ischemia and infarction. Am J Cardiol 1988; 161:20A–26A.
17. Rosen MR. The links between basic and clinical cardiac electrophysiology. Circulation 1988; 77:251–63.
18. Kent AFS. Observations on the auriculoventricular junction of the mammalian heart. Q J Exp Physiol 1913; 7:193–7.
19. Schmitt FO, Erlanger J. Directional differences in the conduction of the impulse through heart muscle and their possible relation to extrasystolic and fibrillary contractions. Am J Physiol 1928; 87:326–47.
20. Cranefield PF, Hoffman BF. Conduction of the cardiac impulse. II. Summation and inhibition. Circ Res 1971; 28:220–33.
21. Cranefield PF, Klein HO, Hoffman BF. Conduction of the cardiac impulse. I. Delay, block and one-way block in depressed Purkinje fibers. Circ Res 1971; 28:199–219.

22. Sasyniuk BI, Mendez C. A mechanism for reentry in canine ventricular tissue. Circ Res 1971; 28:3–15.

23. Wit AL, Cranefield PF, Hoffman BF. Slow conduction and reentry in the ventricular conducting system. II. Single and sustained circus movement in networks of canine and bovine Purkinje fibers. Circ Res 1972; 30:11–22.

24. Wit AL, Hoffman BF, Cranefield PF. Slow conduction and reentry in the ventricular conducting system. I. Return extrasoles in canine Purkinje fibers. Circ Res 1972; 30:1–10.

25. Cranefield PF. In: The conduction of the cardiac impulse. Mount Kisco, NY: Futura, 1975:153–97.

26. Gilmour RF Jr. Phase resetting of circus movement reentry in cardiac tissue. In: Zipes DP, Jalife J, eds. Cardiac electrophysiology, from cell to bedside. New York: W. B. Sanders, 1990: 396–402.

27. Allessie MA, Bonke FIM, Schopman FJG. Circus movement in rabbit atrial muscle as a mechanism of tachycardia. Circ Res 1973; 33:54–62.

28. Allessie MA, Bonke FIM, Schopman FJG. Circus movement in rabbit atrial muscle as a mechanism of tachycardia. II. The role of non-uniform recovery of excitability in the occurrence of unidirectional block as studied with multiple microelectrodes. Circ Res 1976; 39:168–77.

29. Allessie MA, Bonke FIM, Schopman FJG. Circus movement in rabbit atrial muscle as a mechanism of tachycardia. III. The "leading circle" concept: a new model of circus movement in cardiac tissue without the involvement of an anatomical obstacle. Circ Res 1977; 41:9–18.

30. Garrey WE. Auricular fibrillation. Physiol Rev 1924; 4:215–50.

31. Antzelevitch C, Moe GK. Electrotonic inhibition and summation of impulse conduction in mammalian Purkinje fibers. Am J Physiol 1983; 245:H42–53.

32. Lukas A, Antzelevitch C. Reflected reentry, delayed conduction and electrotonic inhibition in segmentally depressed atrial tissues. Can J Physiol Pharmacol 1989; 67:757–64.

33. Kamiyama A, Eguchi K, Shibayama R. Circus movement tachycardia induced by a single premature stimulus on the ventricular sheet. Jpn Circ J 1986; 50:65–73.

34. Allessie MA, Schaly MJ, Huybers MSP, Boersma LVA. Ventricular anisotropy causes an excitable gap in reentry without an anatomic obstacle (abstract). Circulation 1988; 78:II–612.

35. El-Sherif N, Smith RA, Evans K. Canine ventricular arrhythmias in the late myocardial infarction period. 8. Epicardial mapping of reentrant circuits. Circ Res 1981; 49:255–65.

36. El-Sherif N, Mehra R, Gough WB, Zeiler RH. Ventricular activation pattern of spontaneous and induced ventricular rhythms in canine one-day-old myocardial infarction. Evidence for focal and reentrant mechanisms. Circ Res 1982; 51:152–66.

37. Mehra R, Zeiler RH, Gough WB, El-Sherif N. Reentrant ventricular arrhythmias in the late myocardial infarction period. 9. Electrophysiologic-anatomic correlation of reentrant circuits. Circulation 1983; 67:11–24.

38. El-Sherif N, Mehra R, Gough WB, Zeiler RH. Reentrant ventricular arrhythmias in the late myocardial infarction period. Interruption of reentrant circuits by cyrothermal techniques. Circulation 1983; 68:644–56.

39. Wit AL, Allessie MA, Bonke FIM, Lammers W, Smeets J, Fenoglio JJ Jr. Electrophysiologic mapping to determine the mechanism of experimental ventricular tachycardia initiated by premature impulses. Am J Cardiol 1982; 49:166–85.

40. Dillon SM, Allessie MA, Ursell PC, Wit AL. Influences of anisotropic tissue structure on reentrant circuits in the epicardial border zone of subacute canine infarcts. Circ Res 1988; 63:182–206.

41. Clerc L. Directional differences of impulse spread in trabecular muscle from mammalian heart. J Physiol (Lond) 1976; 255:335–46.

42. Spach MS, Miller WT, Geselowitz DB, Barr RC, Kootsey JM, Johnson EA. The discontinuous nature of propagation in normal canine cardiac muscle. Evidence for recurrent discontinuities of intracellular resistance that affect the membrane currents. Circ Res 1981; 48:39–54.

43. Spach MS, Kootsey JM, Sloan JD. Active modulation of electrical coupling between cardiac cells of the dog. A mechanism for transient and steady state variations in conduction velocity. Circ Res 1982; 51:347–62.

44. El-Sherif N. The figure 8 model of reentrant excitation in the canine post-infarction heart. In: Zipes DP, Jalife J, eds. Cardiac electrophysiology and arrhythmias. New York: Grune and Stratton, 1985:363–78.

45. El-Sherif N, Gough WB, Zeiler RH, Hariman R. Reentrant ventricular arrhythmias in the late myocardial infarction period. 12. Spontaneous versus induced reentry and intramural versus epicardial circuits. J Am Coll Cardiol 1985; 6:124–32.

46. Bethe A. In: Allgemeine anatomie und physiologie des nervensystems. Leipzig: George Thieme, 1903:427–32.

47. Scherf D, Cohen J. In: The atrioventricular node and selected cardiac arrhythmias. New York: Grune and Stratton, 1964:230–59.

48. Antzelevitch C, Jalife J, Moe GK. Characteristics of reflection as a mechanism of reentrant arrhythmias and its relationship to parasystole. Circulation 1980; 61:182–91.

49. Antzelevitch C, Moe GK. Electrotonically mediated delayed conduction and reentry in relation to "slow responses" in mammalian ventricular conducting tissue. Circ Res 1981; 49:1129–39.

50. Antzelevitch C, Bernstein MJ, Feldman HN, Moe GK. Parasystole, reentry and tachycardia: a canine preparation of cardiac arrhythmias occurring across inexcitable segments of tissue. Circulation 1983; 68:1101–15.

51. Rozanski GJ, Jalife J, Moe GK. Reflected reentry in nonhomogeneous ventricular muscle as a mechanism of cardiac arrhythmias. Circulation 1984; 69:163–73.

52. Davidenko J, Antzelevitch C. The effects of milrinone on action potential characteristics, conduction, automaticity, and reflected reentry in isolated myocardial fibers. J Cardiovasc Pharmacol 1985; 7:341–9.

53. Rosenthal JE, Ferrier GR. Contribution of variable entrance and exit block in protected foci to arrhythmogenesis in isolated ventricular tissues. Circulation 1983; 67:1–8.

54. Jalife J, Moe GK. Excitation, conduction, and reflection of impulses in isolated bovine and canine cardiac Purkinje fibers. Circ Res 1981; 49:233–47.

55. Davidenko JM, Antzelevitch C. Electrophysiological mechanisms underlying rate-dependent changes of refractoriness in normal and segmentally depressed canine Purkinje fibers. The characteristics of post-repolarization refractoriness. Circ Res 1986; 58: 257–68.

56. Antzelevitch C. Clinical applications of new concepts of parasystole, reflection and tachycardia. Cardiol Clin 1983; 1:39–50.

57. Antzelevitch C, Davidenko JM, Shen XT, Moe GK. Reflected reentry: electrophysiol-ogy and pharmacology. In: Zipes DP, Jalife J, eds. Cardiac electrophysiology and arrhythmias. New York: Grune and Stratton, 1985:253–64.

58. Davidenko JM, Antzelevitch C. The effects of milrinone on conduction, reflection and automaticity in canine Purkinje fibers. Circulation 1984; 69:1026–35.

59. Winkle RA. The relationship between ventricular ectopic beat frequency and heart rate. Circulation 1982; 66:439–46.

60. Nau GJ, Aldariz AE, Acunzo RS, Elizari MV, Rosenbaum MB. Clinical studies on the mechanism of ventricular arrhythmias. In: Rosenbaum MB, Elizari MV, eds. Frontier of cardiac electrophysiology. Amsterdam: Martinus Nijhoff, 1983:239–73.

61. Zipes DP. The contribution of artificial pacemaking to understanding the pathogenesis of arrhythmias. Am J Cardiol 1971; 28:211–22.

62. Spach MS, Dolber PC. Relating extracellular potentials and their derivatives to anisotropic propagation at a microscopic level in human cardiac muscle. Evidence for uncoupling of side-to-side fiber connections with increasing age. Circ Res 1986; 58:356–71.

63. Rosenthal JE. Reflected reentry in depolarized foci with variable conduction impairment in 1 day old infarcted canine cardiac tissue. J Am Coll Cardiol 1988; 12:404–11.

64. Van Hemel NM, Swenne CA, De Bakker JMT, Defauw JJAM, Guiraudon GM. Epicardial reflection as a cause of incessant ventricular bigeminy. PACE 1988; 11:1036–44.

65. Walton M, Fozzard HA. The relation of V_{max} to I_{Na}, G_{Na} and h_{∞} in a model of the cardiac Purkinje fiber. Biophys J 1979; 25:407–20.

66. Cohen I, Attwell D, Stricharz G. The dependence of the maximum rate of rise of the action potential upstroke on membrane properties. Proc R Soc Lond [Biol] 1981; 214: 85–98.

67. Weidmann S. The effect of the cardiac membrane potential on the rapid availability of the sodium carrying system. J Physiol (Lond) 1955; 127:213–24.

68. Gettes LS, Reuter H. Slow recovery from inactivation of inward currents in mammalian myocardial fibers. J Physiol (Lond) 1974; 240:703–24.

69. Hondeghem LM, Katzung BG. Time- and voltage-dependent interactions of antiarrhythmic drugs with cardiac sodium channels. Biochim Biophys Acta 1977; 472:373–98.

70. Kunze DL, Lacerda AE, Wilson DL, Brown AM. Cardiac Na currents and the inactivating, reopening, and waiting properties of single cardiac Na channels. J Gen Physiol 1985; 86:691–719.

71. Carmeliet E, Vereecke J. Adrenaline and the plateau phase of the cardiac action potential. Pfluegers Arch 1969; 379:300–15.

72. Tsien RW. Calcium channels in excitable cell membranes. Ann Rev Physiol 1983; 45:341–58.

73. Gilmour RF Jr, Heger JJ, Prystowsky EN, Zipes DP. Cellular electrophysiologic abnormalities of diseased human ventricular myocardium. Am J Cardiol 1983; 51:137–44.

74. Gilmour RF Jr, Zipes DP. Cellular basis for cardiac arrhythmias. Cardiol Clin 1983; 1:3–11.

75. Lazzara R, El-Sherif N, Scherlag BJ. Electrophysiological properties of canine Purkinje cells in one-day-old myocardial infarction. Circ Res 1973; 33:722–34.

76. Ferrier GR, Rosenthal JE. Automaticity and entrance block induced by focal depolarization of mammalian ventricular tissues. Circ Res 1980; 47:238–48.

77. Wennemark JR, Ruesta VJ, Brody DA. Microelectrode study of delayed conduction in the canine right bundle branch. Circ Res 1968; 23:753–69.

78. Downar E, Waxman MB. Depressed conduction and unidirectional block in Purkinje fibers. In: Wellens HJJ, Lie KI, Janse MJ, eds. The conduction system of the heart. Philadelphia: Lea and Febiger, 1976:393–409.

79. Antzelevitch C, Jalife J, Moe GK. Frequency-dependent alterations of conduction in Purkinje fibers. A model of phase-4 facilitation and block. In: Rosenbuam MB, Elizari MV,

eds. Frontiers of cardiac electrophysiology. Amsterdam: Martinus Nijhoff, 1983:397–415.

80. Jalife J, Antzelevitch C, Lamanna V, Moe GK. Rate-dependent changes in excitability of depressed cardiac Purkinje fibers as a mechanism of intermittent bundle branch block. Circulation 1983; 67:912–22.

81. Janse MJ, Kleber AG, Capucci A, Coronel R, Wilms-Schopman F. Electrophysiological basis for arrhythmias caused by acute ischemia. Role of the subendocardium. J Mol Cell Cardiol 1986; 18:339–55.

82. Gilmour RF Jr, Salata JJ, Zipes DP. Rate-related suppression and facilitation of conduction in isolated canine cardiac Purkinje fibers. Circ Res 1985; 57:35–45.

83. Janse MJ, van Capelle FJL. Electrotonic interactions across an inexcitable region as a cause of ectopic activity in acute regional myocardial ischemia. A study in intact porcine and canine hearts and computer models. Circ Res 1982; 50:527–37.

84. Matsuda K, Kamiyama A, Hoshi T. Configuration of the transmembrane potential of the Purkinje-ventricular fiber junction and its analysis. In: Sano T, Mizuhira J, Matsuda K, eds. Electrophysiology and ultrastructure of the heart. New York: Grune and Stratton, 1967:177–88.

85. Mendez C, Mueller WJ, Urguiaga X. Propagation of impulses across the Purkinje fiber-muscle junctions in the dog heart. Circ Res 1970; 26:135–50.

86. Overholt ED, Joyner RW, Veenstra RD, Rawling D, Wiedmann R. Unidirectional block between Purkinje and ventricular layers of papillary muscles. Am J Physiol 1984; 247:H584–95.

12

Digitalis Toxicity

Gregory R. Ferrier

Dalhousie University
Halifax, Nova Scotia, Canada

INTRODUCTION: DIGITALIS ARRHYTHMIAS

Cardiac glycosides and aglycones can elicit a wide variety of toxic manifestations in many organs and systems. The most serious of these are cardiac arrhythmias. When William Withering published his famous treatise, *An Account of the Foxglove, and Some of Its Medical Uses: With Practical Remarks on Dropsy and Other Diseases* (1), he did not attribute the therapeutic benefits of digitalis to its actions on the heart. Yet, Withering was well aware of the profound decrease in heart rate that the drug could induce and its potential to cause syncope and death. Subsequently we have recognized that digitalis causes a wide variety of cardiac arrhythmias ranging from sinus arrhythmias and atrioventicular (AV) block to ventricular premature beats, tachycardia, and fibrillation (2–5). The effects of digitalis on the sinoatrial (SA) and AV nodes are largely mediated by autonomic effects, whereas ventricular and atrial ectopy, although influenced by the autonomic nervous system, primarily reflect direct actions of digitalis on cardiac tissues. Discussion of the toxic cardiac actions of digitalis falls naturally into these two categories.

BRADYCARDIAS

Effects of Cardiac Glycosides on SA Node

Decreased heart rate is frequently observed at therapeutic levels of digoxin in patients with congestive heart failure and is usually attributed to the autonomic consequences of improved cardiac performance (4,5). In animal studies slowing of heart rate involves both cholinomimetic and antisympathetic actions (6). The cholinergic component is believed to be mediated by a combination of hypersensitization of the carotid sinus baroreceptors (7), stimulation of the central vagal nucleus and nodose ganglia (7), increased excitability of the vagus nerve (8), and potentiation of the effects of acetylcholine on the sinus node (9). Evidence for the antisympathetic actions of cardiac glycosides comes from several studies (6,10,11).

Studies in isolated sinus node tissues and patients with transplanted hearts failed to demonstrate a direct slowing of pacemaker activity by cardiac glycosides (9,12). In contrast to animals, patients with innervated hearts and normal ventricular function also show little change or even an increase in rate in response to cardiac glycosides (4). Patients with sinus dysfunction, however, frequently exhibit increased sinoatrial conduction block (13).

At toxic levels of digitalis, acceleration of sinus pacemaker activity has been reported and attributed to adrenergic stimulation (9,11, 14,15). However, speeding of pacemaker activity also occurs in denervated preparations and in isolated sinus nodes (10,16,17). Increase in sinus rate can be accompanied by SA conduction block. These apparently opposing effects depend on electrotonic interactions of SA nodal cells. SA node function depends on mutual entrainment of multiple pacemaker cells (18). At toxic levels cardiac glycosides decrease electrical coupling between cardiac cells, probably by increasing intracellular calcium (19,20). Both acceleration of sinus rate and SA conduction block can be explained by progressive decreases in entrainment of neighboring cells (17).

Toxic levels of digitalis in humans primarily induce sinoatrial conduction block or sinus arrest (21). However, paroxysmal atrial tachycardia with block, a common manifestation of digitalis intoxication, has been suggested to represent sinus acceleration analogous to that seen in animals (16,22).

Effects of Cardiac Glycosides on AV Nodal Conduction and Refractoriness

Therapeutic and toxic levels of digitalis slow conduction and prolong the refractory period in AV node in animals and humans (4). At therapeutic levels these effects can be attributed to autonomic actions (23,24). Although a major component can be attributed to parasympathetic actions, antisympathetic actions have also been reported (25,26). Studies in transplant patients indicate that the effects of therapeutic concentrations on AV conduction and refractoriness in humans are mediated primarily by autonomic actions, possibly with a small direct component (27,28).

Toxic concentrations of cardiac glycosides clearly depress the AV node directly (23,29). Ouabain decreases maximum diastolic potential, action potential amplitude, and maximum upstroke velocity and conduction of action potentials in isolated rabbit AV nodes.

ATRIAL AND VENTRICULAR ARRHYTHMIAS: PREMATURE BEATS AND TACHYCARDIAS

Digitalis can induce a wide range of arrhythmias in animals and humans (4,15,30–32). Digitalis-induced atrial arrhythmias in the human include atrial premature beats and atrial tachycardia with or without AV block, flutter, and fibrillation (31). However, ouabain can also cause a paradoxical decrease in atrial vulnerability to induction of fibrillation by programmed stimulation (33). Digitalis-induced atrial arrhythmias may be caused by depolarization and depression of atrial cells or induction of afterpotentials (29,34).

Ventricular arrhythmias attributed to digitalis intoxication include ventricular premature beats (especially bigeminy and trigeminy), AV junctional tachycardia, multifocal rhythms originating in the specialized conducting system, tachycardia, bidirectional tachycardia, and ventricular flutter and fibrillation (4,32). None of these arrhythmias are clearly pathognomonic for digitalis intoxication; however, AV junctional rhythm is frequent (4).

Induction of ventricular arrhythmias by digitalis likely involves both automaticity and reentry, and both mechanisms ultimately may depend on inhibition of the sarcolemmal ATPase associated with active Na and K exchange (35). With progressive digitalis intoxication the excitability of ventricular tissues, assessed by epicardial stimulation, shows an initial increase followed by depression (36). Premature ventricular beats first appear during enhanced excitability but become more numerous as excitability becomes depressed. Conduction velocity is unchanged or even accelerated when extrasystoles first appear. Conduction then slows to approximately 50% of control values immediately before the

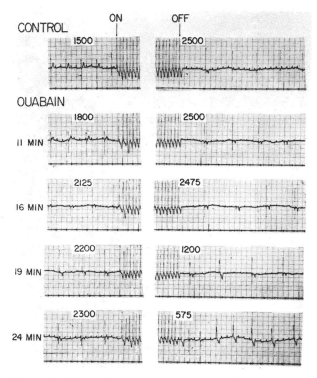

Figure 1 Effect of ouabain on idioventricular automaticity and its response to pacing in an anesthetized dog with AV block. Ouabain caused progressive prolongation of prepacing cycle length (indicated in msec above left panels). However the escape interval following pacing showed progressive abbreviation, indicating development of postpacing acceleration (indicated above right panels). On and off refer to the beginning and end of ventricular pacing in each panel. [Reproduced by permission of the American Heart Association, Inc., from *Circulation Research* (43).]

onset of ventricular fibrillation. This study suggests that reentry may be involved in late arrhythmias when conduction is depressed, but some other mechanism must be involved earlier when excitability, and frequently conduction, are enhanced. The participation of automaticity is supported by the ability of vagal stimulation to unmask enhanced ventricular ectopic activity before toxicity becomes overt (30).

CELLULAR BASIS FOR DIGITALIS-INDUCED ATRIAL AND VENTRICULAR ARRHYTHMIAS

Afterpotentials and Triggered Activity

Historical Development
Elucidation of the cellular bases for digitalis arrhythmias has occurred gradually. Vassalle

et al. (37) characterized the effects of a toxic concentration of ouabain on transmembrane electrical characteristics of canine muscle and Purkinje tissues. Ouabain decreased the membrane potential, action potential amplitude, and action potential duration in both, but the effects were greater and earlier in Purkinje tissue. Enhancement of diastolic depolarization and automaticity was also noted in Purkinje tissue. However, studies in isolated tissues and intact dogs identified other ectopic activity that required an initiating beat for induction, a characteristic identified with reentry (15,37).

In dogs, automaticity was first depressed and only later enhanced (15). Depression of idioventricular rate has been reported in many studies, including one in humans during interruption of artificial pacing (14,15,30,38,39).

Eventually it became apparent that the distinction between enhanced automaticity and reentry was not clear. Lown et al. (40) demonstrated that digitalis promoted the induction of coupled activity by direct stimulation of the ventricles. This phenomenon, which he called the repetitive ventricular response (RVR), could be elicited in animals or humans before overt electrical toxicity. Increases in heart rate promoted the appearance of the RVR and decreased its coupling interval (41). Observations that the RVR occurred at a relatively long coupling interval that was not necessarily fixed led these authors to question the supposed reentrant basis. In the same year Wittenberg et al. (42) published evidence that cardiac glycosides modified the response of automatic foci to preceding pacing. Following exposure to ouabain, dog hearts exhibited postpacing acceleration instead of normal postpacing depression. Rapid pacing shortened the escape interval seen upon termination of pacing (43). Infusion of ouabain caused progressive depression of idioventricular automaticity (Fig. 1). However, even though automaticity slowed, ventricular pacing induced greater and greater postpacing acceleration until the escape beat was indistinguishable from the RVR. Transmembrane recordings from isolated tissues also suggested that toxic levels of ouabain induced postpacing acceleration of phase 4 depolarization (44,45).

The marked changes induced by digitalis in the characteristics of automaticity suggest that these agents either greatly modify the cellular basis for pacemaker activity or that they induce a different mechanism of automaticity that supplants "normal" phase 4 depolarization. Overwhelming evidence supports the latter alternative. Experiments by Ferrier et al. (46) on isolated canine Purkinje tissue demonstrated that the aglycone acetylstrophanthidin suppressed phase 4 depolarization and actually increased postpacing depression of this mechanism of automaticity. At the same time acetylstrophanthidin induced oscillations in the transmembrane potential that were coupled to the preceding action potentials. These oscillatory afterpotentials (OAP) could reach threshold and induce premature beats (Fig. 2). Also, OAP and resultant premature beats demonstrated the postpacing acceleration necessary

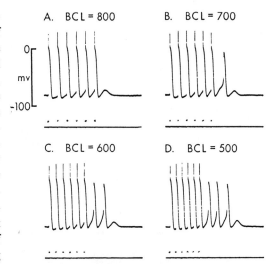

Figure 2 Induction of OAP in isolated canine Purkinje fibers by acetylstrophanthidin. (A) A subthreshold OAP can be seen following the last driven action potential. Abbreviation of the cycle length of stimulation (BCL) from 800 to 700 msec (B) caused the OAP to reach threshold. Further abbreviation of BCL (C and D) caused multiple responses. [Reproduced by permission of the American Heart Association, Inc., from *Circulation Research* (46).]

to explain the RVR and similar phenomena in whole-animal experiments. Premature beats initiated by OAP were also followed by OAP. This novel mechanism of automaticity, which required an initiating beat, could therefore become self-perpetuating and result in tachycardias (Fig. 3) (46). The dependence of the coupling interval of OAP on the preceding cycle length also caused repetitive patterns of driven and spontaneous beats. Thus with continuous pacing at physiologic heart rates, OAP frequently generated bigeminal and trigeminal rhythms (Fig. 3). OAP were also shown to occur in canine Purkinje tissue exposed to ouabain (47). Rosen et al. (47) suggested that OAP may transiently increase the excitability of the membrane. Modulation of excitability by OAP has since been confirmed. However, the effect appears to be biphasic. Early in intoxication OAP reduce the strength of stimuli needed to initiate action potentials (48). Later, the peaks of OAP are associated with depressed excitability and conduction block of

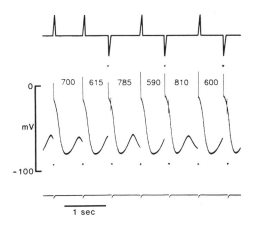

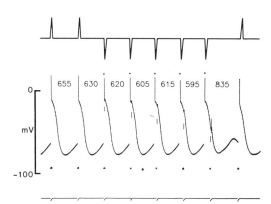

Figure 3 Induction of bigeminy (top) and runs of extrasystoles (bottom) by acetylstrophanthidin-induced OAP in isolated canine Purkinje tissue. In each panel the top trace is a schematic indicating driven beats as upward deflections and OAP-induced beats as downward deflections; the second trace is an intracellular microelectrode recording; and the bottom trace is a record of stimulation. The numbers between action potentials are measured cycle lengths. (Previously unpublished records.)

beats initiated at a distant site (49). Thus OAP provide a mechanism for both automaticity exhibiting postpacing acceleration and conduction block that could participate in reentry.

In isolated canine Purkinje tissues superfused in an external circuit by blood from a anesthetized animal to which ouabain was administered, the first ectopic activity in the ECG of the whole animal corresponded in

time with the appearance of OAP in the isolated tissues (50).

Nomenclature

The most common terms used to describe cardiac afterpotentials are based on two overlapping systems. One system places afterpotentials in categories based on the transmembrane currents leading to their generation. Afterpotentials caused by the transient inward current I_{ti} are referred to as oscillatory afterpotentials (51). This term was first used by Bozler (52) in reference to afterpotentials induced by high Ca-low Na solutions. This system of nomenclature differentiates OAP from afterpotentials caused by aborted phase 4 depolarization (dependent on I_f) or automaticity generated by the slow inward (calcium) current in depolarized tissues (53). Automaticity caused by the latter mechanism is referred to as depolarization-induced automaticity (DIA) (54,55). The functional significance of this differentiation is underscored by the observation that toxic concentrations of digitalis that induce OAP depress phase 4 depolarization (46) and abolish DIA (55,56). However, the membrane potentials over which the different mechanisms operate overlap. Thus, some afterpotentials may be generated by a combination of ionic mechanisms (57).

The other common system of nomenclature is based on the phase of repolarization of the preceding action potential at which the afterpotential occurs (58,59). The afterpotential is referred to as an early afterdepolarization (EAD) when it occurs before full repolarization of the cell (Fig. 4A). EAD represent failure of normal repolarization and can lead to repetitive firing without attainment of resting potential (Fig. 4A, dotted line). Repetitive activity of this type corresponds to DIA in the other system of nomenclature. When the membrane potential following an action potential hyperpolarizes with respect to the resting potential, the voltage excursion is called an early afterhyperpolarization (EAH) (Fig. 4B). Depolarization occurring after the resting membrane potential has been attained or exceeded is referred to as a delayed afterdepolarization (DAD). The total excursion (EAH

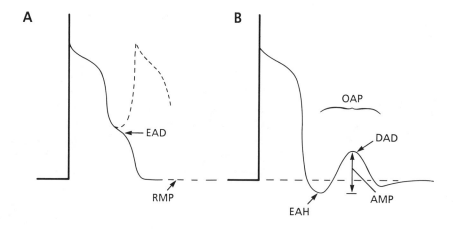

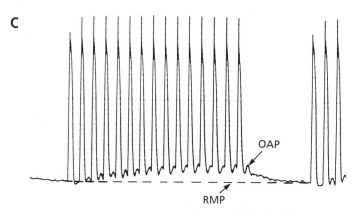

Figure 4 Nomenclature of afterpotentials. (A, B) Early after depolarization (EAD), early afterhyperpolarization (EAH), delayed afterdepolarization (DAD), and an oscillatory afterpotential (OAP). The resting membrane potential is indicated by RMP, and the amplitude of the OAP is indicated as AMP. (C) An intracellular recording from a canine Purkinje fiber exposed to acetylstrophanthidin. In this example digitalis-induced OAP occur before the resting membrane potential of the fiber is achieved, both following termination of stimulation and in the diastolic intervals during stimulation, after the first two driven beats.

plus DAD) is called an oscillatory afterpotential (OAP) (58).

The latter system avoids difficulties associated with overlapping ionic mechanisms since it is based on morphology rather than mechanism. However, it is subject to other difficulties. For example, digitalis afterpotentials are usually referred to as DAD, but with advancing digitalis intoxication Purkinje tissue often exhibits beat-by-beat decreases in maximum diastolic potential (Fig. 4C). When this happens OAP occur before the resting potential has been reached and therefore fit the defini-

tion of EAD rather than DAD, even though the ionic mechanism has not changed.

The amplitudes of OAP are measured from the maximum polarization immediately preceding the afterpotential to the peak depolarization (Fig. 4B) (46). This total excursion has a functional significance since it is the total excursion that is the potential stimulus to the cell. To avoid ambiguity, and because the term has functional significance and belongs to both systems of nomenclature, the term "oscillatory afterpotential" (OAP) is used throughout this discussion. OAP is used to

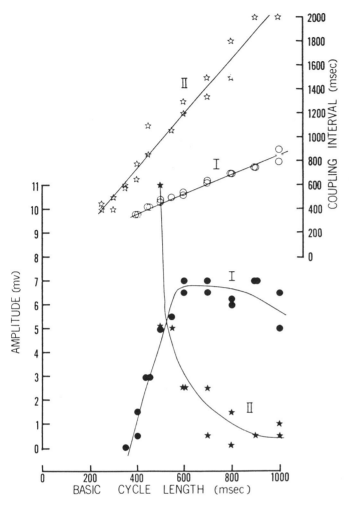

Figure 5 Effect of basic cycle length of pacing on the coupling intervals and amplitudes of the first two OAP coupled to driven beats. Data for the first and second OAP are indicated by I and II. Amplitude was measured as shown in Figure 4. The coupling interval was measured from the upstroke of the last of a train of 10 driven action potentials to the peak depolarization of the OAP. [Reproduced by permission of the American Heart Association, Inc., from *Circulation Research* (46).]

designate the total depolarizing excursions whether or not resting potential is achieved but is restricted to those afterpotentials believed to be generated by the transient inward current and that typically occur at membrane potentials between -60 and -90 mV.

Characteristics of OAP

Digitalis-induced OAP have characteristics that determine the properties of OAP-generated ectopic activity (46,51,61). Action potentials may be followed by two or more sequential OAP. The amplitude of the first OAP

is maximal when the preceding BCL is approximately 700 msec, whereas the amplitude of the second OAP becomes maximal only with very short preceding basic cycle length (BCL, ≤300 msec, Fig. 5) (46). Thus the probability of the first OAP reaching threshold is increased at moderately high heart rates but decreases again at higher rates.

The peak of the first OAP occurs at an interval of approximately 80% of the preceding basic cycle length. The second OAP occurs at about twice this interval. Thus, during regular rhythm at normal or slightly elevated heart rates, ectopic beats are most likely to appear as late premature beats. An example of this eventuality is shown in Figure 3.

The timing and amplitudes of OAP are influenced primarily by the immediately preceding cycle during continuous pacing. However, the cumulative effects of the preceding 8–10 beats can readily be demonstrated when interruptions of stimulation are brief ($\leq$3 sec) (46). Cumulative effects on OAP amplitude lasting hundreds of beats can be demonstrated following interruption of pacing for 30–60 sec. Thus, either elevation of average heart rate or single short cycles can exacerbate OAP-induced ectopy (46,61). These characteristics result in premature beats and arrhythmias that are "triggered" by the preceding activity (58).

Attainment of threshold by OAP often results in accelerating spontaneous rhythms (Fig. 3). Acceleration is expected because the peak of each OAP in sequence occurs at an interval shorter than the preceding cycle length. Such rhythms usually terminate abruptly or stabilize at cycle lengths of approximately 400–500 msec. Further acceleration is likely prevented by the diminishing amplitude of OAP at short BCL. Thus OAP seldom generate tachycardias with rates faster than 150 per min.

The second of the two OAP commonly coupled to action potentials may also contribute to arrhythmogenesis. Clearly, an afterpotential that occurs at approximately twice the preceding cycle length cannot maintain a continuous rhythm. The second OAP normally reaches threshold following very early interpolated beats (at which time the first OAP is very small). For example, during a regular rhythm at a BCL of 800 msec, a test beat at an interval of 300 msec may trigger an OAP-induced beat at 600 msec. The spontaneous beat would be followed by a first OAP with near-maximal amplitude at an interval slightly shorter than 600 msec. If this OAP reaches threshold a sustained rhythm may result. Thus the spontaneous beat initiated by a second OAP can trigger a sustained tachycardia maintained by the sequential first OAP. This interplay of first and second OAP can regularly be demonstrated in canine Purkinje tissues (46).

Tachycardias induced by OAP can be terminated abruptly by interpolation of single premature stimuli (46). The interpolated beat is usually followed by one final ectopic beat. Termination of arrhythmias by a single interpolated beat was previously considered diagnostic of reentry (60). Bursts of rapid stimulation may either accelerate or terminate the tachycardia. Termination may be abrupt or occur after 1–10 terminal triggered beats (61). Suppression appears not to occur by the postpacing depression characteristic of normal phase 4 depolarization. Once the rhythm is interrupted it will not resume unless it is again triggered. Tachycardias initiated by rapid pacing may terminate spontaneously. When this occurs, the cycle length first shows gradual prolongation (46).

Relationship of OAP to Digitalis Arrhythmias in the Whole Animal and in Humans

If OAP represent an important mechanism of digitalis arrhythmias, digitalis arrhythmias in animals and humans should have characteristics similar to those of OAP-induced ectopic activity in isolated tissues. Observations on digitalis arrhythmias in anesthetized dogs were published by Vassalle and colleagues (15) 10 years before the description of digitalis-induced OAP. However, the characteristics of the arrhythmias clearly parallel those of OAP. Ventricular automaticity showed gradual depression before ectopic activity was enhanced. Ventricular ectopic activity exhibited triggering by sinus beats. Although the activity was triggered the coupling intervals were not always fixed. When runs of activity terminated spontaneously, the rhythm did not recur unless it was triggered again.

Bigeminal rhythms corresponding to those seen in isolated tissues can also be recorded from whole animals administered toxic concentrations of cardiac glycosides (15). An example is illustrated in Figure 6. As predicted by observations in isolated tissues (see Fig. 3), the bigeminal rhythm occurred at moderately elevated heart rate and the ectopic beats occurred as late premature beats.

Zipes et al. (62) demonstrated that both the RVR and the escape interval of digitalis-

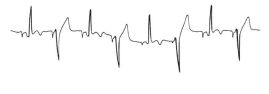

Figure 6 Bigeminal rhythm induced by digoxin in an anesthetized dog. The top trace is the lead II ECG, and the bottom trace shows a record of stimulation delivered to the right atrium. The SA node was destroyed by crushing. Driven beats generated upward deflects, whereas premature beats were downward. Stimulus artifacts are apparent in the ECG. The coupled beats occur as late premature beats similar to those shown in Figure 3 (top). (Unpublished record from a study by T. Lawley, G. R. Ferrier, and P. E. Dresel.)

induced ectopic activity seen following the interruption of pacing showed a dependence on preceding cycle length that closely resembled the relationship described for OAP. A similar relationship between the rate of programmed stimulation and the first poststimulation interval has been demonstrated in dogs with ventricular tachycardia induced by digoxin (63).

OAP can be induced by ouabain in human cardiac tissue (64). Since the "rules" governing the response of OAP to heart rate and interpolated beats are defined, there have been attempts to demonstrate similar responses in clinical arrhythmias. It is important to note that as OAP become greater in amplitude, threshold is achieved earlier on the ascending limb. Thus extrasystoles can occur earlier than 80% of the preceding cycle length. Rosen et al. (65) analyzed electrocardiograms of patients exhibiting accelerated junctional escape. Escape intervals varied with dominant R-R interval as predicted by OAP. However, no distinction could be made between patients receiving digitalis and those not. Many patients not receiving digitalis had ischemic heart disease or myocardial infarcts. OAP can be induced by catecholamines in human tissues (64) and have been reported in experimental 24 hr infarcts in dogs (66). Thus the

occurrence of OAP in response to a wide variety of conditions may hinder the definitive association of digitalis toxicity with arrhythmias with OAP-like characteristics. Also, it is not possible to exclude other mechanisms simply on the basis of the responses of a given rhythm to overdrive or programmed stimulation (67–69).

Cellular Mechanism of OAP

Although there is controversy concerning the role of Na pump inhibition in the inotropic actions of digitalis, it is generally accepted that the toxic effects occur in the presence of substantial inhibition of the Na pump (4,35). Inhibition of the Na pump may promote the occurrence of ventricular arrhythmias by induction of OAP, reduction of transmembrane potential, and elevation of intercellular resistance. Induction of OAP by digitalis is strongly promoted by elevation of extracellular Ca^{2+} and inhibited by lowering extracellular Ca^{2+} levels or by inhibiting the slow inward (Ca^{2+}) current by Mn^{2+} (70). Voltage clamp studies have identified a transmembrane current responsible for OAP, the I_{ti} (71). The reversal potential of the I_{ti} was not altered by changes in extracellular Ca^{2+} concentration. Thus it was clear that, although the current was very sensitive to Ca^{2+}, the charge carrier of this current was not Ca^{2+} (72,73).

Evidence that an oscillatory rise in intracellular free Ca^{2+} induces the I_{ti}, and therefore OAP, comes from several sources. Toxic levels of glycosides induce aftercontractions that likely represent direct activation of the myofilaments by internally released Ca^{2+} (74,75). The coupling intervals and amplitudes of aftercontractions and OAP change in parallel (75), and the contractile event appropriately lags behind the I_{ti} by 40–140 msec (Fig. 7) (72). Oscillatory Ca^{2+} transients can be detected by intracellular injection of the Ca^{2+}-sensitive fluorescent agent, aequorin (76,77). Augmentation of intracellular Ca^{2+} load by the calcium agonist Bay K 8644 (78) or by intracellular injection of Ca^{2+} (79) induces OAP or I_{ti}, whereas intracellular injection of EGTA inhibits OAP or I_{ti} induced by digitalis

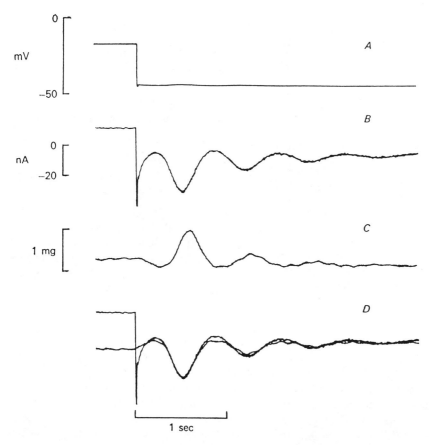

Figure 7 Induction of the transient inward current I_{ti} and aftercontraction by strophanthidin in a calf Purkinje fiber under voltage clamp conditions. (A) A voltage clamp repolarizing step to -44 mV from -17 mV. The repolarizing step induced oscillations in inward current (B) associated with aftercontractions (C). (D) The current and force traces are superimposed by inverting the force record and advancing to 80 msec. [Reproduced by permission of the *Journal of Physiology (London)* (72).]

(79). In addition, inhibition of Ca^{2+} release from the sarcoplasmic reticulum by ryanodine inhibits OAP (77,80) as well as Ca^{2+} transients detected by aequorin light emission (81). Caffeine, which inhibits the reuptake of Ca^{2+} by the sarcoplasmic reticulum, inhibits the I_{ti}, OAP, and triggered activity induced by digitalis (80,82). However, at low concentrations caffeine can transiently stimulate or even induce the I_{ti}, presumably through enhancing the manifestations of calcium overload (83,84).

Induction of OAP is believed to be a consequence of inhibition of the sarcolemmal Na^+,K^+-ATPase (Fig. 8) (72). Inhibition of the Na pump causes an increase in intracellular Na^+ activity (85,86). Because Na^+ can

exchange for Ca^{2+} across the sarcolemma by means of a specific Na^+-Ca^{2+} exchanger, a secondary rise in intracellular Ca^{2+} occurs (87). Much of this Ca^{2+} is taken up by the sarcoplasmic reticulum and can be released upon excitation. Normally the release of Ca^{2+} from the sarcoplasmic reticulum is believed to occur in response to elevation of intracellular Ca^{2+} activity (calcium-induced Ca^{2+} release) (88). In the presence of Ca^{2+} overload consequent to Na^+ pump inhibition, spontaneous release of Ca^{2+} from the sarcoplasmic reticulum may occur even in quiescent preparations (89,90). The resulting spontaneous fluctuations in Ca^{2+} can cause corresponding fluctuations in transmembrane ionic conductances and tension (91). Spectral analysis of these

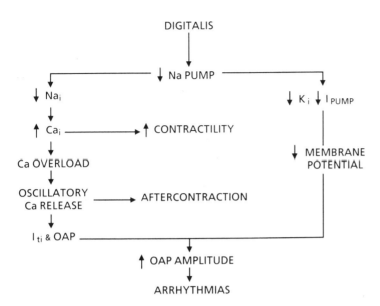

Figure 8 Mechanisms of induction and potentiation of OAP-induced arrhythmias by digitalis and the relationship to induction of mechanical effects. See text for explanation.

fluctuations demonstrated the same frequency distribution as seen in the larger I_{ti} evoked by hyperpolarizing voltage clamp steps. This observation led these authors to propose that the natural resonance frequency of the spontaneous fluctuations represents the cytoplasmic clock that determines the periodicity of the I_{ti} and OAP. The voltage clamp step, or action potential, could act by synchronizing independent oscillatory units by resetting their phase and thereby generating a large summated response, the I_{ti} (91,92). If the I_{ti} represents synchronization of a spontaneous event, one would predict that the mechanism for generation of the I_{ti} is an inherent property of cardiac cells that can be unmasked or augmented by a variety of conditions. In support of this hypothesis Vassalle and Mugelli (93) have demonstrated the spontaneous occurrence of the I_{ti} (I_{os}) in sheep Purkinje fibers in the absence of inhibition of the Na$^+$ pump and at physiologic concentrations of K$^+$ and Ca^{2+}.

The identity of the charge-carrying mechanism of the I_{ti} is not clear (94–96). Two different mechanisms have been suggested by Kass et al. (73). The first is a relatively nonspecific cation membrane channel that is activated by a rise in intracellular Ca^{2+} activity. The I_{ti} had a reversal potential close to -5 mV.

The reversal potential was sensitive to changes in extracellular Na$^+$ concentration but was too negative for the current to be carried by Na$^+$ alone. Therefore, a K$^+$ permeability approximately equal to that for Na$^+$ was also proposed. In addition, it was also necessary to propose a Ca^{2+} permeability to account for the reversal potential measured in the absence of Na$^+$. The channel was impermeant to anions, such as chloride.

Nonspecific cation channels that are activated by Ca^{2+} have been identified by single-channel recording techniques (95,97,98). The reversal potential of a channel documented in adult guinea pig myocytes was close to that of the I_{ti} (95). This channel was activated by Ca^{2+} in the micromolar range similar to that which activates the I_{ti}.

The other charge-carrying mechanism proposed for the I_{ti} is the Na^2-Ca^{2+} exchange mechanism. Normally this exchange system transports Ca^{2+} out of the cell and Na$^+$ into the cell. However, approximately three Na$^+$ are exchanged for one Ca^{2+}, and the exchange is electrogenic (99,100). Kass et al. (73) suggested that the oscillatory release of Ca^{2+} from the sarcolemmal stores may transiently stimulate electrogenic Na$^+$-Ca^{2+} exchange and result in the I_{ti}.

Several experimental studies favor Na^+-Ca^{2+} exchange as the mechanism for the I_{ti} largely because of the lack of a clear reversal potential (101–104). In addition, OAP induced in coronary sinus and I_{ti} in sinus node rapidly disappear when Li^+ is substituted for Na^+ (102,104). Inhibition of OAP would not be expected if OAP are caused by nonselective cation channels, because these channels are permeable to Li^+ (95). Amiloride, an inhibitor of Na^+-Ca^{2+} exchange, suppresses the inotropic and arrhythmogenic effects of digitalis (105). However, these observations may reflect a reversal of Ca^{2+} overload rather than specific inhibition of the I_{ti}.

Experiments favoring Na^+-Ca^{2+} exchange as the mechanism for the I_{ti} were conducted in muscle or sinoatrial node, whereas studies favoring a nonspecific cation channel were mostly done in Purkinje tissue. Indeed, Cannell and Lederer (106) showed that the I_{ti} persists in Purkinje tissue equilibrated with Tyrode's solution in which Na^+ was replaced with isotonic $CaCl_2$ to remove the Na^+-Ca^{2+} exchanger as a possible current carrier. It has also been possible to separate Na^+-Ca^{2+} exchange from the I_{ti} in isolated rabbit myocytes (107). Taken together these studies suggest that the I_{ti} can be generated by either mechanism, and the predominant mechanism may vary from one tissue or species to another.

Effects of Electrolyte Imbalances on Digitalis Arrhythmias and OAP

Patients with hypokalemia are more likely to develop digitalis arrhythmias (4). The mechanisms are complex. Animal studies indicate that potassium depletion promotes the myocardial uptake of cardiac glycosides, whereas hyperkalemia reduces uptake (108). In addition, elevation of potassium concentration interferes with digitalis binding and inhibition of the Na^+,K^+-ATPase. In isolated Purkinje tissues, reduction of potassium concentration increases the amplitudes of OAP and promotes triggered activity (70). However, varying extracellular potassium concentration has no immediate effect on the peak I_{ti} or its reversal potential (73). Therefore, the effect of potassium may reflect changes in the binding of

digitalis to the Na^+, K^+-ATPase or changes in potassium conductance that would attentuate the OAP. Very low concentrations of potassium would be expected to facilitate induction of the I_{ti} because the activity of the Na^+, K^+-ATPase is decreased, and indeed low or zero potassium can induce OAP in the absence of digitalis (109).

Elevation of Ca^{2+} concentration increases and reduction of Ca^{2+} concentration decreases the amplitudes of OAP (70). Very high concentrations of Ca^{2+} induce OAP in the absence of digitalis (70). Parallel changes in peak I_{ti} have been reported (72,73). Elevation of Ca^{2+} increases the intracellular levels of Ca^{2+} and oscillatory release of calcium as detected by aequorin light emission (110). These effects are primarily mediated by Na^+-Ca^{2+} exchange. The same exchange system results in changes in intracellular Ca^{2+} levels in response to changes in extracellular Na^+ concentration (110). Thus the elevation of extracellular Na^+ levels suppresses triggered activity induced by digoxin (111). However, very rapid changes in Na^+ concentration may have the opposite effect because Na^+ is also a charge carrier for the I_{ti} (104).

Hypomagnesemia enhances sensitivity to digitalis (112). In isolated tissue experiments, Mg^{2+} depletion has been shown to increase OAP amplitude and incidence of triggered activity, whereas elevation of Mg^{2+} concentration suppresses OAP and triggered activity (113,114). Parallel effects are seen on the I_{ti} (72). Hypomagnesemia may promote digitalis toxicity by decreasing the activity of the sarcolemmal Na^+, K^+-ATPase (115) or by increasing sympathetic nerve discharge (116). Parenteral magnesium has been found to be effective in managing massive digoxin intoxication (117).

Effects of Pathophysiologic Conditions

Sensitivity to the toxic effects of digitalis is greatly increased by cardiac ischemia or congestive heart failure. Conversely, digitalis may increase the infarct size and incidence of arrhythmias following coronary artery ligation (118). Evidence for an increased mortality associated with digitalis therapy following in-

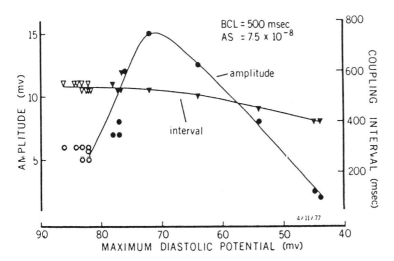

Figure 9 Effects of membrane potential on the amplitudes and coupling intervals of OAP induced by acetylstrophanthidin in isolated canine Purkinje tissue. Membrane potential was changed by extracellular application of electric current. The amplitudes of OAP were maximal when the maximum diastolic potential was close to -70 mV. Coupling intervals were essentially unaffected by changes in membrane potential. Open symbols represent data collected without current application. BCL = basic cycle length; AS = acetylstrophanthidin. [Reproduced by permission of the American Society for Pharmacology and Experimental Therapeutics, from the *Journal of Pharmacology and Experimental Therapeutics* (55).]

farction is accumulating from clinical (119) and experimental studies (120). This synergistic effect may stem from the common ability of both toxic levels of digitalis and ischemic heart disease to induce OAP (66,121). Also, conditions of ischemia followed by reperfusion induce OAP and triggered activity in isolated canine tissues (122,123), and induction of both electrical abnormalities is potentiated by subtoxic concentrations of digitalis (124).

Factors associated with ischemia or reperfusion may sensitize the heart to digitalis. Partial depolarization of cardiac tissues occurs in ischemia. The amplitudes of digitalis OAP and the incidence of triggered activity increase greatly as the membrane potential decreases (Fig. 9) (55,125). In addition, lysophosphatidylcholine, which accumulates in ischemic myocardium, can induce OAP (126). Also, digitalis stimulates the release of cardiac prostaglandins that promote digitalis toxicity and sensitize ischemic hearts to the arrhythmogenic actions of digitalis (127–129). Endogenous prostaglandins may also be involved in the potentiation of reperfusion arrhythmias by subtoxic concentrations of digitalis (124,130). Synergistic arrhythmogenic action

between ischemia and digitalis may also involve sympathetic nerve discharge. In addition, one cannot exclude the possible involvement of endogenous digitalis-like substances that have been shown to have electrical toxic effects virtually identical to those induced by ouabain (131).

Specific components of ischemia may also modulate the effects of digitalis. Clearly hyperkalemia exerts an inhibitory effect on digitalis toxicity (70). Hypoxia, substrate deprivation, acidosis, and lactate, in combination but in the absence of hyperkalemia, also abolish digitalis OAP (124). OAP induced by norepinephrine in rabbit papillary muscles are enhanced by moderate decrease in pH (7.0) but inhibited by further acidification of superfusate (pH 6.0–6.7) (132). Lactate also abolished OAP at physiologic pH, but not in the presence of acidosis (pH = 6.8) (133). Hypoxia by itself inhibits digitalis OAP in muscle but much less, or not at all, in Purkinje tissue (134). In fact, Chilson and Davis (135) reported that hypoxia promoted arrhythmic activity in Purkinje tissues pretreated with subtoxic levels of ouabain. In isolated myocytes metabolic inhibition suppresses OAP by inhibiting the I_{ti}, possibly by inhibiting Ca^{2+} uptake by the sarcoplasmic reticulum or by elevating potassium conductance (136).

These observations suggest that OAP are more likely an important mechanism of arrhythmia in reperfusion than in ischemia and conflict with the observation that digitalis toxicity is promoted by ischemic heart disease. This interaction may still be possible if the ischemic area experiences transient periods of reperfusion or if OAP occurring in the border zone of ischemic areas are subjected to a net stimulatory effect (e.g., norepinephrine release, moderate acidosis, stimulatory autacoids, etc.) rather than inhibition. Indeed, Purkinje fibers removed from the endocardial surface of canine infarcts are hypersensitive to ouabain (137).

Other disease conditions also alter sensitivity to digitalis. Ventricular muscle from streptozotocin-diabetic rats are more prone than normal myocardium to develop OAP and triggered activity in response to ouabain (138). This interaction may be mediated by opposing effects of insulin and digitalis on the Na^+, K^+-ATPase (139).

Ouabain-induced arrhythmias are significantly enhanced in rats with renal hypertensive hypertrophy (140). Potentiation of digitalis toxicity in hypertrophy, or in failure, may in part reflect the effect of increasing fiber tension or length to enhance digitalis OAP and triggered activity (75). Dystrophic mice are also hypersensitive to digitalis toxicity (141). Here enhanced sensitivity may be related to a significantly longer action potential duration and Ca^{2+} loading, in addition to the possible effects of stretch.

Disease-related hypersensitivity to digitalis may be complicated by age-related increases in sensitivity to the toxic effects of digitalis (4). Neonatal dogs are relatively insensitive to digoxin compared to adults (142). This difference persists at the cellular level (143,144). One can demonstrate a progressive increase in sensitivity in hearts from old as opposed to young adult rats and guinea pigs (145, 146). Old hearts demonstrate a decrease in Na^+,K^+-ATPase activity; however, greater Na^+ leak may also be involved (145).

Effects of Autonomic Mediators on Digitalis Arrhythmias and OAP

The sympathetic nervous system plays an important role in digitalis arrhythmias. Surgical or pharmacologic sympathectomy increases the lethal dose of digitalis. Also, the terminal event becomes cardiac standstill rather than tachyarrhythmia (38). Toxic concentrations of digitalis increase neural activity to the heart, at least partly through a central action (147, 148). Isoproterenol can induce OAP in isolated ventricular myocardium (149), and stimulation of the left stellate ganglion can elicit OAP in vivo as detected by monophasic action potential recording (150). Not surprisingly, β-adrenergic agonists potentiate the amplitudes of OAP induced by ouabain (Fig. 10) (151). However, other studies have failed to show potentiation of digitalis toxicity by β-adrenergic stimulation in conscious dogs (152). In anesthetized guinea pigs, α_1-adrenergic agonists increase and α_2-adrenergic agonists decrease sensitivity to ouabain toxicity (153). α_1-adrenergic agonists have no effect or even inhibit digitalis-induced OAP or I_{ti} in Purkinje tissues, however (151,154,155), whereas α-adrenergic agonists potentiated OAP or I_{ti} induced by high concentrations of Ca^{2+} (154–156).

Actions and Effects of Antiarrhythmic Drugs on OAP and I_{ti}

Digitalis OAP are sensitive to agents that alter intracellular Ca^{2+} and/or Na^+. The possibility that the I_{ti} may be blocked by local anesthetics was addressed by Kass et al. (73). They concluded that tetrodotoxin did not inhibit the I_{ti} directly but acted by decreasing the intracellular Na^+ concentration by blocking the fast inward current. Sheu and Lederer (157) concluded that lidocaine had a similar action but also decreased Ca^{2+} influx by shortening action potential duration (Fig. 11). Triggered activity was also terminated by depression of excitability. Local anesthetics that have been shown to suppress OAP include lidocaine, quinidine, procainamide, disopyramide, aprindine, ethmozine, mexiletine, and phenytoin (158–165). In humans, quinidine increases plasma levels of digoxin and may promote arrhythmias

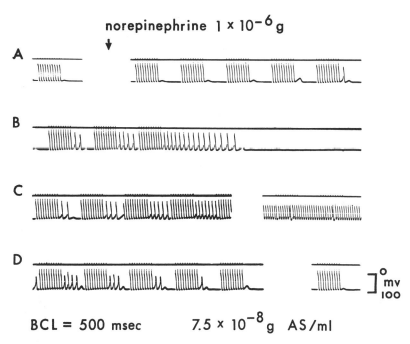

Figure 10 Effects of norepinephrine on OAP and triggered activity induced by acetylstrophanthidin in isolated canine Purkinje tissue. In each panel the top trace is a record of stimulation and the bottom record is an intracellular microelectrode recording. Acetylstrophanthidin alone induced subthreshold OAP (A, left). At the arrow, 1 μg norepinephrine was added directly to the Tyrode's solution flowing through the tissue bath. The amplitudes of OAP progressively increased (A, right) and induced triggered activity (B). The cycle length of triggered activity progressively shortened, and eventually spontaneous activity became continuous except for occasional driven beats (C). The effects of norepinephrine reversed as the catecholamine washed from the bath (D). (Panels show previously unpublished records.)

and is less effective in reversing digitalis toxicity than lidocaine or phenytoin (4).

Digitalis-induced OAP and I_{ti} are inhibited by blockade of the slow inward (calcium) current, presumably by decreasing Ca^{2+} overload (70,72). Similarly, verapamil decreases the amplitudes of OAP and inhibits triggered activity (160). Although verapamil increases plasma levels of digitalis in animals and humans, the antiarrhythmic effects predominate (166). The inhibitory effects of several calcium channel blockers on OAP have been compared (167). Verapamil and nifedipine were more effective than diltiazem. Nicardipine and nitrendipine were not effective at similar concentrations.

Other agents also antagonize digitalis toxicity. Halothane suppresses ouabain-induced ectopy, thereby leaving subthreshold OAP (illustrated but not described) in isolated ca-

nine Purkinje fibers (168). Several phenothiazines have been shown to suppress OAP in isolated myocytes, possibly by an action on calmodulin (169). Doxorubicin appears to be highly specific for suppressing OAP-dependent rhythms and may be a useful experimental tool for identifying mechanisms (170). For massive overdoses of digitalis, antibodies (digoxin-specific Fab fragments) have proven useful in reversing toxicity (4,171).

Reentry in Digitalis Arrhythmias

Moe and Mendez (36) noted that intraventricular conduction, although slightly improved initially, became depressed with advanced intoxication with digitalis. It seems likely that disturbances in conduction and reentry may be involved in the late stages of intoxication, including transition to fibrillation. More recently it has been shown in muscle and

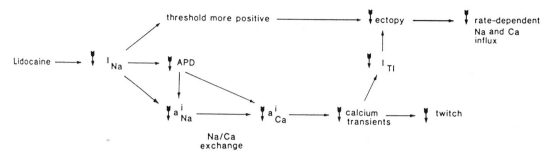

Figure 11 Schematic showing how lidocaine may antagonize digitalis-induced OAP and triggered activity. Therapeutic actions may include the effects of lidocaine to decrease excitability, shorten action potential duration, and decrease Na^+ influx. The last two effects would exert antiarrhythmic effect by decreasing intracellular Ca^{2+} activity and, thus, the magnitude of the I_{ti} and amplitudes of OAP. The effect on excitability threshold would further decrease the probability of OAP reaching threshold. [Reproduced by permission of the American Heart Association, Inc., from *Circulation Research* (157).]

Purkinje tissues that digitalis causes slowing of conduction by increasing intercellular resistance (20,172). The increase in resistance probably represents the effects of elevated intracellular Ca^{2+} on gap junctions (19). In addition, in advanced intoxication OAP may cause conduction block (49).

REFERENCES

1. Withering W. An account of the foxglove, and some of its medical uses: with practical remarks on dropsy, and other diseases. In: Willus, FA, Keys, TE, eds. *(Cardiac classics)*. St. Louis: C. V. Mosby, 1941: 231–52.
2. Pick A, Igarashi M. Mechanisms, differential diagnosis and clinical significance of digitalis-induced arrhythmias. In: Fisch C, Surawicz B, eds. Digitalis. New York: Grune & Stratton, 1969:148–173.
3. Bigger JT, Strauss HC. Digitalis toxicity: drug interactions promoting toxicity and the management of toxicity. Semin Drug Treat 1972; 2:147–77.
4. Smith TW, Antman EM, Friedman PL, Blatt CM, Marsh JD. Digitalis glycosides: mechanisms and manifestations of toxicity. Prog Cardiovasc Dis 1984; Part I, 26:413–58; Part II, 26:495–540; Part III, 27:21–56.
5. Antman EM, Smith TW. Digitalis toxicity. Annu Rev Med 1985; 36:357–67.
6. Ten Eick RE, Hoffman BF. Chronotropic effect of cardiac glycosides in cats, dogs and rabbits. Circ Res 1969; 25:365–78.
7. Chai CY, Wang HH, Hoffman BF, Wang SC. Mechanisms of bradycardia induced by digitalis substances. Am J Physiol 1967; 212:26–34.
8. Ten Eick RE, Hoffman BF. The effect of digitalis on the excitability of autonomic nerves. J Pharmacol Exp Ther 1969; 169: 95–108.
9. Toda N, West TC. The influence of ouabain on cholinergic responses in the sinoatrial node. J Pharmacol Exp Ther 1966; 153: 104–13.
10. Mendez C, Aceves J, Mendez R. Inhibition of adrenergic cardiac acceleration by cardiac glycosides. J Pharmacol Exp Ther 1961; 131:191–8.
11. James TN, Nadeau RA. The chronotropic effect of digitalis studied by direct perfusion of the sinus node. J Pharmacol Exp Ther 1963; 139:42–52.
12. Goodman DJ, Rossen RM, Ingham R, Rider AK, Harrison DC. Sinus node function in the denervated human heart. Effect of digitalis. Br Heart J 1975; 37:612–8.
13. Reiffel JA, Bigger JT, Cramer M. Effects of digoxin on sinus nodal function before and after vagal blockade in patients with sinus nodal dysfunction. Am J Cardiol 1979; 43:983–9.
14. Sherlag BJ, Abelleira JL, Narula OS, et al. The differential effects of ouabain on sinus, A-V nodal, His bundle, and idioventricular rhythms. Am Heart J 1971; 81:227–35.
15. Vassalle M, Greenspan K, Hoffman BF. Analysis of arrhythmias induced by ouabain in intact dogs. Circ Res 1963; 13:132–48.

16. Steinbeck G, Bonke FIM, Allessie MA, Lammers WJEP. The effects of ouabain on the isolated sinus node preparation of the rabbit studied with microelectrodes. Circ Res 1980; 46:406–14.
17. Takayanagi K, Jalife J. Effects of digitalis intoxication on pacemaker rhythm and synchronization in rabbit sinus node. Am J Physiol 1986; 250:H567–78.
18. Jalife J. Mutual entrainment and electrical coupling as mechanisms for synchronous firing of rabbit sino-atrial pace-maker cells. J Physiol (Lond) 1984; 356:221–43.
19. De Mello WC. Effects of intracellular injection of calcium and strontium on cell communication in heart. J Physiol (Lond) 1975; 231:231–45.
20. Weingart R. The actions of ouabain on intercellular coupling and conduction velocity in mammalian ventricular muscle. J Physiol (Lond) 1977; 264:341–65.
21. Friedberg CK, Donoso E. Arrhythmias and conduction disturbances due to digitalis. Prog Cardiovasc Dis 1960; 2:408–31.
22. Geer MR, Wagner GS, Waxman M, Wallace AG. Chronotropic effect of acetylstrophanthidin infusion into the canine sinus nodal artery. Am J Cardiol 1977; 39:684–9.
23. Toda N, West TC. The action of ouabain on the function of the atrioventricular node in rabbits. J Pharmacol Exp Ther 1969; 169:287–97.
24. Amlie JP, Storstein L. Effects of autonomic blockade on the inotropic and electrophysiologic response to digitoxin in the intact dog. J Cardiovasc Pharmacol 1980; 2:55–66.
25. Carleton RA, Miller PH, Graettinger JS. Effects of ouabain, atropine, and ouabain and atropine on A-V nodal conduction in man. Circ Res 1967; 20:283–8.
26. Mendez C, Aceves J, Mendez R. The antiadrenergic action of digitalis on the refractory period of the A-V transmission system. J Pharmacol Exp Ther 1961; 131:199–204.
27. Goodman DG, Rossen RM, Cannom DS, et al. Effect of digoxin on atrioventricular conduction. Studies in patients with and without cardiac autonomic innervation. Circulation 1975; 51:251–6.
28. Ricci DR, Orlick AE, Reitz BA, et al. Depressant effect of digoxin on atrioventricular conduction in man. Circulation 1978; 57:898–903.
29. Hoffman BF, Singer DH. Effects of digitalis on electrical activity of cardiac fibers. Prog Cardiovasc Dis 1964; 7:226–60.
30. Rotherberger CJ, Winterberg H. Uber den einfluss von strophantin auf die reizbildungsfahigkeit der automatishen zentren des herzens. Pflugers Arch 1913; 150:217–61.
31. Church G, Schamroth L, Schwartz NL, Marriott HJL. Deliberate digitalis intoxication. Ann Intern Med 1962; 57:946–56.
32. Fisch C, Knoebel SB. Digitalis cardiotoxicity. J Am Coll Cardiol 1985; 5:91A–98A.
33. Engel TR, Gonzalez, AC. Effects of digitalis on atrial vulnerability. Am J Cardiol 1978; 42:570–6.
34. Hashimoto K, Moe GK. Transient depolarizations induced by acetylstrophanthidin in specialized tissue of dog atrium and ventricle. Circ Res 1973; 32:618–24.
35. Schwartz A, Lindenmayer GE, Allen JC. The sodium-potassium adenosine triphosphatase: Pharmacological, physiological and biochemical aspects. Pharmacol Rev 1975; 27:3–134.
36. Moe GK, Mendez R. The action of several cardiac glycosides on conduction velocity and ventricular excitability in the dog heart. Circulation 1951; 4:729–34.
37. Vassalle M, Karis J, Hoffman BF. Toxic effects of ouabain on Purkinje fibers and ventricular muscle fibers. Am J Physiol 1962; 203:433–9.
38. Erlij D, Mendez R. The modification of digitalis intoxication by excluding adrenergic influences on the heart. J Pharmacol Exp Ther 1964; 144:97–103.
39. Edhag O, Rosén A. A study on the effect of lanatoside C on ventricular automaticity in man. Scand J Clin Lab Invest 1967; 23:43–7.
40. Lown B, Cannon RL III, Rossi MA. Electrical stimulation and digitalis drugs: repetitive response in diastole. Proc Soc Exp Biol Med 1967; 126:698–701.
41. Hagemeijer F, Lown B. Effect of heart rate on electrically induced repetitive ventricular responses in the digitalized dog. Circ Res 1970; 27:333–44.
42. Wittenberg SM, Streuli F, Klocke FJ. Acceleration of ventricular pacemakers by transient increases in heart rate in dogs during ouabain administration. Circ Res 1970; 26:705–16.
43. Wittenberg SM, Gandel P, Hogan PM, et al. Relationship of heart rate to ventricular

automaticity in dogs during ouabain administration. Circ Res 1972; 30:167–76.

44. Hogan PM, Wittenberg SM, Klocke FJ. Relationship of stimulation frequency to automaticity in the canine Purkinje fiber during ouabain administration. Circ Res 1973; 32:377–84.

45. Davis LD. Effect of changes in cycle length on diastolic depolarization produced by ouabain in canine Purkinje fibers. Circ Res 1973; 32:206–14.

46. Ferrier GR, Saunders JH, Mendez C. A cellular mechanism for the generation of ventricular arrhythmias by acetylstrophanthidin. Circ Res 1973; 32:600–9.

47. Rosen MR, Gelband H, Merker C, Hoffman BF. Mechanisms of digitalis toxicity: effects of ouabain on phase four of canine Purkinje fiber transmembrane potentials. Circulation 1973; 47:681–9.

48. Peon J, Ferrier GR, Moe GK. Speeding of conduction associated with depression of action potential upstroke velocity in Purkinje tissue. Circ Res 1978; 43:125–35.

49. Saunders JH, Ferrier, GR, Moe GK. Conduction block associated with transient depolarizations induced by acetylstrophanthidin in isolated Purkinje fibers. Circ Res 1973; 32:610–7.

50. Rosen MR, Gelband H, Hoffman BF. Correlation between effects of ouabain on the canine electrocardiogram and transmembrane potentials of isolated Purkinje fibers. Circulation 1973; 47:65–72.

51. Ferrier GR. Digitalis arrhythmias: role of oscillatory afterpotentials. Prog Cardiovasc Dis 1977; 19:459–74.

52. Bozler E. The initiation of impulses in cardiac muscle. Am J Physiol 1943; 138:273–82.

53. Hauswirth O, Noble D, Tsien RW. The mechanism of oscillatory activity at low membrane potentials in cardiac Purkinje fibres. J Physiol (Lond) 1969; 220:225–65.

54. Katzung BG, Morgenstern JA. Effects of extracellular potassium on ventricular automaticity and evidence for a pacemaker current in mammalian ventricular myocardium. Circ Res 1977; 40:105–11.

55. Ferrier GR. Effects of transmembrane potential on oscillatory afterpotentials induced by acetylstrophanthidin in canine ventricular tissues. J Pharmacol Exp Ther 1980; 215:332–41.

56. Karagueuzian H, Katzung BG. Biphasic effects of acetylstrophanthidin on automaticity in guinea pig ventricular muscle. Eur J Pharmacol 1982; 79:175–83.

57. Aronson RS, Cranefield PF. The effect of resting potential on the electrical activity of canine cardiac Purkinje fibers exposed to Na-free solution or to ouabain. Pfluegers Arch 1974; 347:101–16.

58. Cranefield PF. The conduction of the cardiac impulse: The slow response and cardiac arrhythmias. Mount Kisco, NY: Futura, 1975.

59. Cranefield PF. Action potentials, afterpotentials, and arrhythmias. Circ Res 1977; 41:414–23.

60. Moe GK. Evidence for reentry as a mechanism of cardiac arrhythmias. Rev Physiol Biochem Pharmacol 1975; 72:56–81.

61. Moak JP, Rosen MR. Induction and termination of triggered activity by pacing in isolated canine Purkinje fibers. Circulation 1984; 69:149–62.

62. Zipes DP, Arbel E, Knope RF, Moe GK. Accelerated cardiac escape rhythms caused by ouabain intoxication. Am J Cardiol 1974; 33:248–53.

63. Gorgels AP, De-Wit B, Beekman HD, Dassen WR, Wellens HJ. Triggered activity induced by pacing during digitalis intoxication: observations during programmed electrical stimulation in the conscious dog with chronic complete atrioventricular block. Pace 1987; 10:1309–21.

64. Dangman KH, Danilo P, Hordof AJ, Mary-Rabine L, Reder RF, Rosen MR. Electrophysiologic characteristics of human ventricular and Purkinje fibers. Circulation 1982; 65:362–8.

65. Rosen MR, Fisch C, Hoffman BF, Danilo P, Lovelace DE, Knoebel SB. Can accelerated atrioventricular junctional escape rhythms be explained by delayed afterdepolarizations? Am J Cardiol 1980; 45:1272–84.

66. El-Sherif N, Gough WB, Zeiler RH, Mehra R. Triggered ventricular rhythms in 1-day-old myocardial infarction in the dog. Circ Res 1983; 52:566–79.

67. Rosen MR, Reder RF. Does triggered activity have a role in the genesis of cardiac arrhythmias? Ann Intern Med 1981; 94:794–801.

68. Wellens HJJ, Brugada P. The role of triggered activity in clinical arrhythmias. In: Rosenbaum MB, Elizari MV, eds. Frontiers

of Cardiac Electrophysiology. The Hague: Martinus Nijhoff, 1983:195–216.

69. Fisch C, Knoebel SB. Accelerated junctional escape: a clinical manifestation of "triggered" automaticity? In: Zipes DP, Jalife J, eds. Cardiac electrophysiology and arrhythmias. Orlando, FL: Grune and Stratton, 1985:469–73.

70. Ferrier GR, Moe GK. Effect of calcium on acetylstrophanthidin-induced transient depolarizations in canine Purkinje tissue. Circ Res 1973; 33:508–15.

71. Lederer WJ, Tsien RW. Transient inward current underlying arrhythmogenic effects of cardiotonic steroids in Purkinje fibers. J Physiol (Lond) 1976; 263:73–100.

72. Kass RS, Lederer WJ, Tsien RW, Weingart R. Role of calcium ions in transient inward currents and aftercontractions induced by strophanthidin in cardiac Purkinje fibres. J Physiol (Lond) 1978; 281:187–208.

73. Kass RS, Tsien RW, Weingart R. Ionic basis of transient inward current induced by strophanthidin in cardiac Purkinje fibres. J Physiol (Lond) 1978; 281:209–26.

74. Reiter M. Die entstehung von "nachkontraktionen" im herzmuskel unter einwirkung von calcium und von digitalisglykosiden in abhangigkeit von der reizfrequenz. Naunyn-Schmiedebergs Arch Pharmakol 1962; 242:497–507.

75. Ferrier GR. The effects of tension on acetylstrophanthidin-induced transient depolarizations and aftercontractions in canine myocardial and Purkinje tissues. Circ Res 1976; 38:156–62.

76. Wier WG, Hess P. Excitation-contraction coupling in cardiac Purkinje fibers. Effects of cardiotonic steroids on intracellular $[Ca^{2+}]$ transient, membrane potential, and contraction. J Gen Physiol 1984; 83:395–415.

77. Marban E, Robinson SW, Wier WG. Mechanisms of arrhythmogenic delayed and early afterdepolarizations in ferret ventricular muscle. J Clin Invest 1986; 78:1185–92.

78. Nilius B. Stimulation of Ca-dependent action potentials in mammalian ventricular myocardium by a novel dihydropyridine. Biomed Biochim Acta 1984; 43:1385–97.

79. Matsuda H. Cellular and subcellular mechanism of transient depolarization. Jpn Circ J 1987; 51:172–5.

80. Chan TL, Chau TC, Bose D. Role of sarcoplasmic reticulum in digitalis-induced electrical and mechanical oscillations in the heart. Can J Cardiol 1987; 3:197–204.

81. Valdeolmillos M, Eisner DA. The effects of ryanodine on calcium-overloaded sheep cardiac Purkinje fibers. Circ Res 1985; 56: 452–6.

82. Vassalle M, Di-Gennaro M. Caffeine actions on currents induced by calcium overload in Purkinje fibers. Eur J Pharmacol 1984; 106:121 31.

83. Hasegawa J, Satoh H, Vassalle M. Induction of the oscillatory current by low concentrations of caffeine in sheep cardiac Purkinje fibres. Naunyn Schmiedebergs Arch Pharmacol 1987; 335:310–20.

84. Hiraoka M, Kawano S, Kinoshita H. Contribution of Ca^{2+}-influx to generation of the transient inward current in guinea pig ventricular muscles. Jpn J Physiol 1987; 37:479–96.

85. Deitmer JW, Ellis D. The intracellular sodium activity of cardiac Purkinje fibres during inhibition and re-activation of the Na-K pump. J Physiol (Lond) 1978; 284:241–59.

86. Wasserstrom JA, Schwartz DJ, Fozzard HA. Relation between intracellular sodium and twitch tension in sheep cardiac Purkinje strands exposed to cardiac glycosides. Circ Res 1983; 52:697–705.

87. Glitsch HG, Reuter H, Scholtz H. The effect of the internal sodium concentration on calcium fluxes in isolated guinea-pig auricles. J Physiol (Lond) 1970; 209:25–43.

88. Fabiato A. Time and calcium dependence of activation and inactivation of calcium-induced release of calcium from the sarcoplasmic reticulum of a skinned canine cardiac Purkinje cell. J Gen Physiol 1985; 85:247–89.

89. Eisner DA, Valdeolmillos M. A study of intracellular calcium oscillations in sheep cardiac Purkinje fibres measured at the single cell level. J Physiol (Lond) 1986; 372:539–56.

90. Weir WG, Kort AA, Stern MD, Lakatta EG, Marban E. Cellular calcium fluctuations in mammalian heart. Direct evidence from noise analysis of aequorin signals in Purkinje fibers. Proc Natl Acad Sci USA 1983; 80:7367–71.

91. Kass RS, Tsien RW. Fluctuations in membrane current driven by intracellular calcium in cardiac Purkinje fibers. Biophys J 1982; 38:259–69.

92. Capogrossi MC, Houser SR, Bahinski A, Lakatta EG. Synchronous occurrence of spontaneous localized calcium release from the sarcoplasmic reticulum generates action potentials in rat cardiac ventricular myocytes at normal resting membrane potential. Cir Res 1987; 61:498–503.

93. Vassalle M, Mugelli A. An oscillatory current in sheep cardiac Purkinje fibers. Circ Res 1981; 48:618–31.

94. Eisner DA, Lederer WJ. Na-Ca exchange: stoichiometry and electrogenicity. Am J Physiol 1985; 248:C189–202.

95. Ehara T, Noma A, Ono K. Calcium-activated non-selective cation channel in ventricular cells isolated from adult guinea-pig hearts. J Physiol (Lond) 1988; 403: 117–33.

96. January CT, Fozzard HA. Delayed afterdepolarizations in heart muscle: mechanisms and relevance. Pharmacol Rev 1988; 40: 219–27.

97. Colquhoun D, Neher E, Reuter H, Stevens CF. Inward current channels activated by intercellular Ca in cultured cardiac cells. Nature (Lond) 1981; 294:752–4.

98. Hill JA Jr, Coronado R, Strauss HC. Reconstitution and characterization of a calcium-activated channel from heart. Circ Res 1988; 62:411–5.

99. Horackova M, Vassort G. Sodium-calcium exchange in regulation of cardiac contractility. Evidence for an electrogenic, voltage-dependent mechanism. J Gen Physiol 1979; 73:403–24.

100. Kimura J, Shunich M, Noma A. Identification of sodium-calcium exchange current in single ventricular cells of guinea-pig. J Physiol (Lond) 1987; 384:199–222.

101. Arlock P, Katzung BG. Effects of sodium substitutes on transient inward current and tension in guinea-pig and ferret papillary muscle. J Physiol (Lond) 1985; 360:105–20.

102. Brown HF, Noble D, Noble SJ, Taupignon AI. Relationship between the transient inward current and slow inward currents in the sino-atrial node of the rabbit. J Physiol (Lond) 1986; 370:299–315.

103. Fedida D, Noble D, Rankin AC, Spindler AJ. The arrhythmogenic transient inward current I_{ti} and related contraction in isolated guinea-pig ventricular myocytes. J Physiol (Lond) 1987; 392:523–42.

104. Tseng G, Wit AL. Effect of reducing $[Na^+]_o$ on catecholamine-induced delayed afterdepo-

larizations in atrial cells. Am J Physiol 1987; 253:H115–25.

105. Kennedy RH, Akera T, Brody T. Suppression of positive inotropic and toxic effects of cardiac glycosides by amiloride. Eur J Pharmacol 1985; 115:199–210.

106. Cannell MB, Lederer WJ. The arrhythmogenic current I_{ti} in the absence of electrogenic sodium-calcium exchange in sheep cardiac Purkinje fibres. J Physiol (Lond) 1986; 374:201–19.

107. Shimoni Y, Giles W. Separation of Na-Ca exchange and transient inward currents in heart cells. Am J Physiol 1987; 253:H1330–3.

108. Farah AE. The effects of the ionic milieu on the response of cardiac muscle to cardiac glycosides. In: Fisch C, Surawicz B, eds. Digitalis. New York: Grune and Stratton, 1969:55–64.

109. Eisner DA, Lederer WJ. Inotropic and arrhythmogenic effects of potassium-depleted solutions on mammalian cardiac muscle. J Physiol (Lond) 1979; 294:255–77.

110. Allen DG, Eisner DA, Orchard CH. Factors influencing free intracellular calcium concentration in quiescent ferret ventricular muscle. J Physiol (Lond) 1984; 350:615–30.

111. Adamantidis MM, Duriez PR, Rouet RH. High extracellular sodium and digoxin-induced arrhythmias in guinea-pig ventricular myocardium. J Mol Cell Cardiol 1983; 15:207–11.

112. Berkelhammer C, Bear RA. A clinical approach to common electrolyte problems. 4. Hypomagnesemia. Can Med Assoc J 1985; 132:360–8.

113. Moe BH. On the therapeutic mechanism of Mg^{2+} in digitoxic arrhythmias and the role of cardiac glycosides in Mg depletion. Magnesium 1984; 3:8–20.

114. Saikawa T, Arita M, Ito S. Effects of magnesium on transient depolarizations and triggered activity induced by ouabain in guinea pig ventricular muscle. Magnesium 1987; 6:169–79.

115. Fischer PW, Giroux A. Effects of dietary magnesium on sodium-potassium pump action in the hearts of rats. J Nutr 1987; 117:2091–5.

116. Tackett RL. Enhanced sympathetic activity as a mechanism for cardiac glycoside toxicity in hypomagnesemia. Pharmacology 1986; 32:141–6.

117. Iseri LT. Magnesium and cardiac arrhythmias. Magnesium 1986; 5:111–26.

118. Lynch JJ, Lucchesi BR. Effect of digoxin on the extent of injury and the severity of arrhythmias during acute myocardial ischemia and infarction in the dog. J Cardiovasc Pharmacol 1988; 11:193–203.

119. Bigger JT Jr, Fleiss JL, Rolinitzky LM, Merab JP, Ferrick KJ. Effect of digitalis treatment on survival after acute myocardial infarction. Am J Cardiol 1985; 55:623–30.

120. Lynch JJ, Montgomery DG, Lucchesi BR. Facilitation of lethal ventricular arrhythmias by therapeutic digoxin in conscious post infarction dogs. Am Heart J 1986; 111:883–90.

121. Dangman KH, Dresdner KP, Zaim S. Automatic and triggered impulse initiation in canine subepicardial ventricular muscle cells from border zones of 24-hour transmural infarcts. New mechanisms for malignant cardiac arrhythmias? Circulation 1988; 78: 1020–30.

122. Ferrier GR, Moffat MP, Lukas A. Possible mechanisms of ventricular arrhythmias elicited by ischemia followed by reperfusion. Studies on isolated canine ventricular tissues. Circ Res 1985; 56:184–94.

123. Ferrier GR, Moffat MP, Lukas A, Mohabir R. A model of ischemia and reperfusion: effect of potassium concentration on electrical and contractile responses of canine Purkinje tissue. In: Zipes DP, Jalife J, eds. Cardiac electrophysiology and arrhythmias. Orlando FL: Grune and Stratton, 1985: 325–30.

124. Lukas A, Ferrier GR. Interaction of ischemia and reperfusion with subtoxic concentrations of acetylstrophanthidin in isolated cardiac ventricular tissues: effects on mechanisms of arrhythmia. J Mol Cell Cardiol 1986; 18:1143–56.

125. Wasserstrom JA, Ferrier GR. Voltage dependence of digitalis afterpotentials, aftercontractions, and inotropy. Am J Physiol 1981; 241:H646–53.

126. Pogwizd SM, Onufer JR, Kramer JB, Sobel BE, Corr PB. Induction of delayed afterdepolarizations and triggered activity in canine Purkinje fibers by lysophosphoglycerides. Circ Res 1986; 59:416–26.

127. Moffat MP, Karmazyn M, Ferrier GR. Prostaglandin involvement in hypersensitivity of ischemic hearts to arrhythmogenic influence of ouabain. Am J Physiol 1985; 249:H57–63.

128. Moffat MP, Ferrier GR, Karmazyn M. A possible role for endogenous prostaglandins in the electrophysiological effects of acetylstrophanthidin on isolated canine ventricular tissues. Circ Res 1986; 58:486–94.

129. Moffat MP, Karmazyn M, Ferrier GR. Role of prostaglandins in the arrhythmogenic effects of ouabain on isolated guinea pig hearts. Eur J Pharmacol 1987; 141:383–93.

130. Moffat MP, Ferrier GR, Karmazyn M. A direct role of endogenous prostaglandins in reperfusion-induced cardiac arrhythmias. Can J Physiol Pharmacol 1989; 67:772–9.

131. Kieval RS, Butler VP Jr, Derguini F, Bruening RC, Rosen MR. Cellular electrophysiologic effects of vertebrate digitalis-like substances. J Am Coll Cardiol 1988; 11: 637–43.

132. Kano T, Nishi K. External pH dependency of delayed afterdepolarization in rabbit myocardium. Am J Physiol 1986; 251:H324–30.

133. Coetzee WA, Opie LH. Effects of components of ischemia and metabolic inhibition on delayed afterdepolarizations in guinea pig papillary muscle. Circ Res 1987; 61:157–65.

134. Di Gennaro M, Vassalle M, Iacono G, Pahor M, Bernabei R, Carbonin PU. On the mechanisms by which hypoxia eliminates digitalis-induced tachyarrhythmias. Eur Heart H 1986; 7:341–52.

135. Chilson RA, Davis LD. Combined effects of ouabain and hypoxia on the transmembrane potential of canine cardiac Purkinje fibers. J Cardiovasc Pharmacol 1985; 7:368–76.

136. Coetzee WA, Biermans G, Callewaert G, Vereecke J, Opie LH, Carmeliet E. The effect of inhibition of mitochondrial energy metabolism on the transient inward current of isolated guinea-pig ventricular myocytes. J Mol Cell Cardiol 1988; 20:181–5.

137. Hariman RJ, Zeiler RH, Gough WB, El-Sherif N. Enhancement of triggered activity in ischemic Purkinje fibers by ouabain: a mechanism of increased susceptibility to digitalis toxicity in myocardial infarction. J Am Coll Cardiol 1985; 5:672–9.

138. Nordin C, Gilat E, Aronson RS. Delayed afterdepolarizations and triggered activity in ventricular muscle from rats with streptozotocin-induced diabetes. Circ Res 1985; 57:28–34.

139. LaManna VR, Ferrier GR. Electrophysiological effects of insulin on normal and depressed cardiac tissues. Am J Physiol 1981; 240:H636–44.

140. Capasso JM, Tepper D, Reichman P, Sonnenblick EH. Renal hypertensive hypertrophy

in the rat: a substrate for arrhythmogenicity. Basic Res Cardiol 1986; 81: 10–9.

141. Saito K, Ohkura H, Kashima T, Tanaka H. Enhanced sensitivity to digoxin in dystrophic mice. Jpn Heart J 1984; 25:765–72.

142. Murphy AM, Gaum WE, Lathrop DA, Hussain AS, Ritschel WA, Kaplan S. Age-related digoxin effects in an intact canine model. Am Heart J 1987; 114:583–8.

143. Rosen MR, Hordof AJ, Hodess AB, Verosky M, Vulliemoz Y. Ouabain-induced changes in electrophysiologic properties of neonatal, young and adult canine cardiac Purkinje fibers. J Pharmacol Exp Ther 1975; 194: 255–63.

144. Gaum WE, Lathrop DA, Kaplan S. Age-related changes in electrophysiologic properties of canine Purkinje fibers: effect of ouabain. Dev Pharmacol Ther 1983; 6: 145–56.

145. Katano Y, Akera T, Temma K, Kennedy RH. Enhanced ouabain sensitivity of the heart and myocardial sodium pump in aged rats. Eur J Pharmacol 1984; 105:95–103.

146. Khatter JC. Mechanisms of age-related differences in the cardiotoxic action of digitalis. J Cardiovasc Pharmacol 1985; 7:258–61.

147. Somberg JC, Smith TW. Localization of the neurally mediated arrhythmogenic properties of digitalis. Science 1979; 204:321–3.

148. Plunkett LM, Tackett RL. Increases in CSF norepinephrine associated with the onset of digoxin-induced arrhythmias. Eur J Pharmacol 1987; 136:119–22.

149. Nathan D, Beeler GW. Electrophysiologic correlates of the inotropic effects of isoproterenol in canine myocardium. J Mol Cell Cardiol 1975; 7:1–15.

150. Priori SG, Mantica M, Schwartz PJ. Delayed afterdepolarizations elicited in vivo by left stellate ganglion stimulation. Circulation 1988; 78:178–85.

151. Hewett KW, Rosen MR. Alpha and Beta adrenergic interactions with ouabain-induced delayed afterdepolarizations. J Pharmacol Exp Ther 1984; 229:188–92.

152. Haass M, Sponer G, Abshagen U. Arrhythmogenic dose of acetylstrophanthidin unchanged by beta-sympathomimetics in conscious dogs. Basic Res Cardiol 1984; 79:679–89.

153. Thomas GP, Tripathi RM. Effects of α-adrenoceptor agonists and antagonists on ouabain-induced arrhythmias and cardiac arrest in guinea-pig. Br J Pharmacol 1986; 89:385–8.

154. Ferrier GR, Carmeliet E. Effects of alpha-adrenergic agents on the transient inward current in isolated rabbit Purkinje fibers. Circulation 1987; 76:IV–62.

155. Han X, Ferrier GR. Effects of alpha-adrenergic agents on generation of oscillatory afterpotentials in rabbit Purkinje fibers. J Mol Cell Cardiol 1989; 21 (Suppl. II):S67.

156. Kimura S, Cameron JS, Kozlovskis PL, Bassett AL, Myerburg RJ. Delayed afterdepolarizations and triggered activity induced in feline Purkinje fibers by α-adrenergic stimulation in the presence of elevated calcium levels. Circulation 1984; 70:1074–82.

157. Sheu SS, Lederer WJ. Lidocaine's negative inotropic and antiarrhythmic actions. Dependence on shortening of action potential duration and reduction of intracellular sodium activity. Circ Res 1985, 57:578–90.

158. Rosen MR, Danilo P, Alonso MB, Pippenger CE. Effects of therapeutic concentrations of diphenylhydantoin on transmembrane potentials of normal and depressed Purkinje fibers. J Pharmacol Exp Ther 1976; 187: 594–604.

159. Elharrar V, Bailey JC, Lathrop DA, Zipes DP. Effects of aprindine on slow channel action potentials and transient depolarizations in canine Purkinje fibers. J Pharmacol Exp Ther 1978; 205:410–7.

160. Rosen MR, Danilo P. Effects of tetrodotoxin, lidocaine, verapamil, and AHR-2666 on ouabain-induced delayed afterdepolarizations in canine Purkinje fibers. Circ Res 1980; 46:117–24.

161. Wasserstrom JA, Ferrier GR. Effects of phenytoin and quinidine on digitalis-induced oscillatory afterpotentials, aftercontractions, and inotropy in canine ventricular tissues. J Mol Cell Cardiol 1982; 14:725–36.

162. Boyden PA, Wit AL. Pharmacology of the antiarrhythmic drugs. In: Rosen MR, Hoffman BF, eds. Cardiac therapy. Boston: Martinus Nijhoff, 1983:171–234.

163. Amerini S, Carbonin P, Cerbai E, Giotti A, Mugelli A, Pahor M. Electrophysiological mechanisms for the antiarrhythmic action of mexiletine on digitalis-, reperfusion- and reoxygenation-induced arrhythmias. Br J Pharmacol 1985; 86:805–15.

164. Endou K, Yammomoto H, Sato T, Nakata F. Effects of CM7857, a derivative of disopyra-

mide, on electrophysiologic properties of canine Purkinje fibers and inotropic properties of canine ventricular muscle. J Cardiovasc Pharmacol 1986; 8:507–13.

165. Dangman KH. Effects of procainamide on automatic and triggered impulse initiation in isolated preparations of canine cardiac Purkinje fibers. J Cardiovasc Pharmacol 1988; 12:78–87.

166. Khatter JC, Navaratnam S, Hoeschen RJ. Protective effect of verapamil upon ouabain-induced cardiac arrhythmias. Pharmacology 1988; 36:380–9.

167. Endou K, Yamamoto H, Sato T. Comparison of the effects of calcium channel blockers and antiarrhythmic drugs on digitalis-induced oscillatory afterpotentials on canine Purkinje fiber. Jpn Heart J 1987; 28:719–35.

168. Reynolds AK, Chiz JF, Pasquet AF. Halothane and methoxyflurane—a comparison of their effects on cardiac pacemaker fibers. Anesthesiology 1970; 33:602–10.

169. Kremers MS, Kenyon JL, Ito K, Sutko JL. Phenothiazine suppression of transient depolarizations in rabbit ventricular cells. Am J Physiol 1985; 248:H291–6.

170. le Marec H, Spinelli W, Rosen MR. The effects of doxorubicin on ventricular tachycardia. Circulation 1986; 74:881–9.

171. Smith TW, Butler VP Jr, Haber E, Fozzard H, Marcus FI, Bremner WF, Schulman IC, Phillips A. Treatment of life-threatening digitalis intoxication with digoxin-specific Fab antibody fragments. Experience in 26 cases. N Engl J Med 1982; 307:1357–62.

172. Jalife J, Sicouri S, Delmar M, Michaels DC. Electrical uncoupling and impulse propagation in isolated sheep Purkinje fibers. Am J Physiol 1989; 257:H179–89.

13

Arrhythmias in the Canine Heart Two to Twenty-Four Hours After Myocardial Infarction

Eugene Patterson, Benjamin J. Scherlag, and Ralph Lazzara

University of Oklahoma Health Sciences Center and Veterans Administration Medical Center
Oklahoma City, Oklahoma

DELAYED DEVELOPMENT OF VENTRICULAR ECTOPIC RHYTHMS FOLLOWING EXPERIMENTAL CORONARY ARTERY OCCLUSION IN THE DOG: EARLY STUDIES

The abrupt occlusion of a major coronary artery in the dog elicits a high incidence of ventricular tachycardia and fibrillation. Lethal ventricular arrhythmias are primarily limited to the first 30 min following coronary ligation (1,2) and are critically dependent upon the site of coronary artery occlusion. The incidence of ventricular fibrillation may exceed 50% even when left anterior descending coronary artery ligation occurs 1.5–2.0 cm distal to its origin and can prevent the systematic observation of the later phases of ventricular arrhythmia. A two-stage ligation of the coronary artery (a stenosis formed by ligating against, then removing a 20 gauge hypodermic needle followed 30 min later by complete ligation of the vessel) prevents or suppresses the initial lethal ventricular arrhythmias observed following abrupt coronary artery occlusion but fails to prevent the subsequent delayed phases of

ventricular ectopia (3,4). To circumvent the high mortality experienced with a single-stage coronary artery ligation, most experimental studies examining ventricular arrhythmia mechanisms during the 2–24 hr period have been performed using the canine two-stage left anterior descending ligation model as described by Harris (3,4).

The three periods of ventricular arrhythmia following coronary artery occlusion in the dog have been characterized by their time of evolution. The first phase, with its high attendant danger for ventricular tachycardia and ventricular fibrillation, develops within 2–5 min following coronary artery ligation. In the absence of lethal ventricular arrhythmia, ventricular ectopy resolves within 30 min. The early phase of ventricular arrhythmia development is not examined in this chapter. The second phase begins with the decline of the initial paroxysm of ventricular ectopy to an incidence of 0–5 beats/min and lasts for 4–8 hr. Ventricular ectopic beats are infrequent until the quiescent phase is interrupted by the evolution of the late phase, or delayed ventricular arrhythmias (Figures 1 and 2). During the 8–48 hr period following canine coronary artery

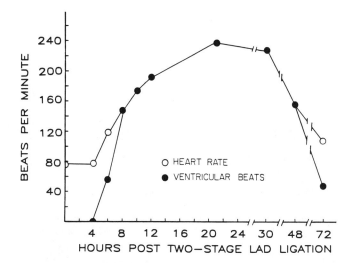

Figure 1 The temporal development of ventricular ectopic beats after left anterior descending coronary artery occlusion. The total ventricular rate (open circles) and the incidence of ventricular ectopic beats (closed circles) are shown at intervals from 4 to 72 hr after coronary artery ligation. (The data are excerpted from A. S. Harris, *Circulation* 1950; 1:1318–28, with permission from the American Heart Association.)

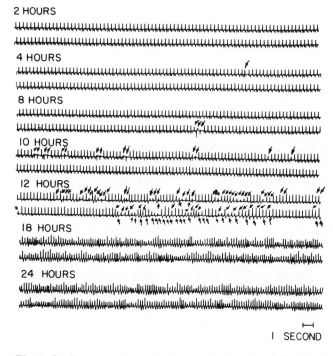

Figure 2 Spontaneous ventricular arrhythmias after left anterior descending coronary artery occlusion in the dog. A surface electrocardiogram is shown at various intervals after left anterior descending coronary artery occlusion in the dog. Ventricular ectopic beats in the 2–12 hr periods are marked with arrows. The electrocardiograms at 18 and 24 hr consisted entirely of ectopic beats of ventricular origin.

ligation, the majority of ventricular beats are ectopic and originate within ventricular tissue (Figures 1 and 2). The duration of the delayed arrhythmia phase varies, with a partial resolution usually apparent by 72–96 hr. Although sinus rhythm predominates after 3–4 days, intermittent ventricular ectopic beats can be recorded as late as 7 days after coronary artery ligation.

Harris and colleagues (4) examined the role of the sympathetic nervous system in the genesis of delayed ventricular arrhythmias. The bilateral excision of the stellate ganglia and the sympathetic chain ganglion from T1 to T5 failed to prevent or alter the time course for the inexorable development of the delayed ventricular arrhythmias; however, bilateral sympathectomy reduced both the rate and duration of the delayed ventricular arrhythmias. The maximum rate of ventricular ectopy during the delayed phase of arrhythmia development failed to exceed 210 beats/min in all 12 dogs undergoing bilateral cardiac sympathectomy before coronary artery ligation. The observation contrasts with the frequent presence of ventricular ectopia exceeding 250 beats/min in dogs with coronary artery ligation and an intact sympathetic nervous system. In 11 of the 12 animals undergoing bilateral cardiac sympathectomy, the delayed arrhythmia phase ceased between 44 and 57 hr after occlusion. When the sympathetic nervous system remained intact, ventricular ectopic activity lasted until 72–120 hr after coronary artery occlusion.

SPONTANEOUS DEVELOPMENT OF LETHAL VENTRICULAR ARRHYTHMIA IN THE 2–24 HR PERIOD AFTER LEFT ANTERIOR DESCENDING ARTERY LIGATION IN THE DOG

Although the two-stage occlusion of the left anterior descending coronary artery in the dog markedly reduces the incidence of ventricular fibrillation observed within the initial minutes following coronary artery ligation (3,5), the two-stage ligation fails to prevent sudden

death occurring during the subsequent 2–24 hr period. The initial studies by Harris in 1950 (3) described a 33% mortality (5 of 15 animals) in dogs surviving the initial, early phase of ventricular arrhythmia. Later studies examining the electrophysiologic bases for sudden death after two-stage coronary artery ligation in the dog (6–8) described a similar mortality of 25–35% in the 2–24 hr period.

The following data were obtained from 100 consecutive left anterior descending coronary artery occlusions performed in mongrel dogs over a 24 month period (Patterson, Scherlag, and Lazzara, unpublished results). Continuous surface electrocardiograms were obtained throughout the 2–24 hr period after coronary artery occlusion. Sudden death was observed in 33 animals, at a mean of 13.3 ± 0.8 hr ($\overline{X} \pm$ standard error of the mean, SEM) after coronary artery ligation (Figure 3). Sudden death resulted from rapid (>300 beats/min), sustained monomorphic ventricular tachycardia degenerating to ventricular fibrillation (Figure 4). In 30 of 33 recorded episodes the duration of monomorphic ventricular tachycardia exceeded 15 sec ($X \pm$ SEM = 66 ± 7 sec) before ultimately deteriorating into ventricular fibrillation. A total of 48 episodes of spontaneous, sustained monomorphic ventricular tachycardia with rates greater than 300 beats/min (385 ± 15 beats/min) and lasting in excess of 30 sec were observed in the 2–24 hr period after canine coronary artery ligation (Figure 5).

The absence of rapid, spontaneous sustained monomorphic ventricular tachycardia in the 24 hr survivors of coronary artery ligation was not dependent solely upon the inability of ischemically injured myocardium to sustain the tachyarrhythmia. Previous studies by Scherlag et al. (6) and El-Sherif et al. (7) have demonstrated that sustained monomorphic ventricular tachycardia can be induced by ventricular pacing in the majority of infarcted hearts studied 24 hr after coronary artery occlusion. Two separate and distinct events appear to be necessary for the initiation and maintenance of spontaneous sustained monomorphic ventricular tachycardia in the 2–24 hr period after coronary artery occlusion in the

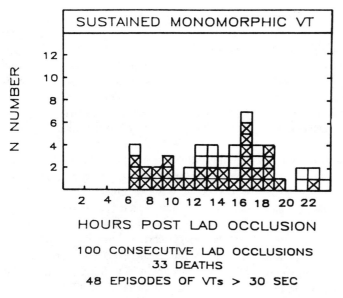

Figure 3 Spontaneous sustained monomorphic ventricular tachycardia during the first 24 hr after left anterior descending coronary artery occlusion. The incidence of spontaneous sustained monomorphic ventricular tachycardia is shown for 100 consecutive left anterior descending coronary artery occlusions in the dog. No sustained monomorphic ventricular tachycardia was observed before 6 hr. A total of 48 spontaneous episodes of sustained monomorphic ventricular tachycardia lasting more than 30 sec were observed; 33 animals died during the 6–24 hr period. (Lethal events marked by X.)

dog (8–10). The first exigency is an underlying substrate capable of sustaining rapid, monomorphic ventricular tachycardia. Provocative ventricular pacing produces sustained monomorphic ventricular tachycardia in 25% of animals at 6 hr (11) and in 50–88% of animals at 24 hr (8–10). The tachycardia is rapid (>350 beats/min) and can be induced only with provocative ventricular pacing at rates exceeding 330 beats/min (Table 1). The sustained monomorphic ventricular tachycardia induced with ventricular pacing in the surviving animals at 24 hr is similar in both rate and form to spontaneous rhythms observed in animals dying suddenly during the 6–24 hr period (Table 1). A second event, however, appears to be necessary to initiate sustained monomorphic ventricular tachycardia in the

Table 1 Spontaneous and Pacing-Induced Ventricular Tachycardias in the 2–24 Hr Period After Coronary Artery Ligation in the Dog

	Spontaneous sustained Monomorphic Ventricular Tachycardia ($N = 37$)	Paced Sustained Monomorphic Ventricular Tachycardia ($N = 67$)
Ventricular tachycardia rate, beats/min	385 ± 15	356 ± 18
Paced Rate to Induce Ventricular Tachycardia, beats/min	—	369 ± 13
Maximum rate of spontaneous triplets in 2–24 hr period, beats/min	360 ± 11	313 ± 19[a]
Infarct Mass, % LV	28 ± 3	29 ± 2

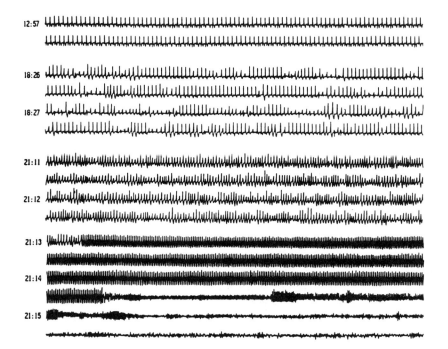

Figure 4 Ventricular fibrillation in the 2–24 hr period after anterior descending coronary artery occlusion in the dog. Surface electrocardiograms are shown at 12 hr 57 min, 18 hr 26–27 min, and 21 hr 11–15 min after left anterior descending coronary artery occlusion in the dog. At 21 hr 13 min 2 sec, rapid monomorphic ventricular tachycardia is initiated. The tachycardia is sustained for 122 sec before disintegrating into ventricular fibrillation. A close examination of the electrocardiogram reveals the presence of rapid ventricular triplets during the 21 hr 11–13 min recordings.

presence of the underlying substrate. Sustained monomorphic ventricular tachycardia fails to develop spontaneously in all animals capable of sustaining rapid, monomorphic ventricular tachycardia at 24 hr. The spontaneous rhythm is not observed in the absence of rapid, ventricular triplets, exceeding 330 beats/min, during the 6–24 hr period (Tables 1 and 2). The rate of the rapid triplets observed in animals developing spontaneous sustained ventricular tachycardia is not different from the rapid ventricular pacing rates needed to initiate ventricular tachycardia in the surviving animals at 24 hr (Table 1).

The electrophysiologic mechanism responsible for the genesis of the rapid ventricular triplets is unknown. The rate of the triplets, 300–390 beats/min is inconsistent with abnormal automaticity or the triggering of delayed afterdepolarizations as a basic mechanism and is more consistent with localized myocardial

reentry. Based upon the limited information available using two electrocardiographic leads, the morphology of the ventricular triplets may or may not have the same morphology as the subsequent sustained tachycardia. The rate and the frequency of both rapid ventricular couplets and triplets develops slowly and reaches a maximum at 14–18 hr after ligation (Figure 6). β-Adrenergic receptor blockade with d,l-nadolol (8) and left stellate ganglionectomy (but not right stellate ganglionectomy) (12)

Table 2 Incidence of Sustained Monomorphic Ventricular Tachycardia (Spontaneous + Paced) and Rapid Ventricular Triplets

		Sustained Ventricular +	Monomorphic Tachycardia −
Rapid			
Ventricular	+	37	4
Triplets	−	42	17

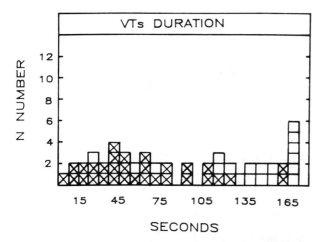

Figure 5 Duration of spontaneous sustained monomorphic ventricular tachycardia during the 2–24 hr period after left anterior descending coronary artery occlusion in the dog. The data were obtained from 100 consecutive dogs undergoing left anterior descending coronary artery occlusion. The duration of sustained monomorphic ventricular tachycardia before ventricular fibrillation (closed boxes) or spontaneous termination and the resumption of a slower ventricular ectopic rhythm (open boxes) is shown. Only three episodes of rapid sustained ventricular tachycardia lasted for less than 15 sec before spontaneous termination.

reduce the maximal rate (8,12) and/or the incidence (8) of rapid ventricular tachycardia and sudden death during the 6–24 hr period. The reduced incidence of sudden death occurs without the suppression of pacing-induced sustained monomorphic ventricular tachycardia in the survivors at 24 hr (Figures 7–9).

Experiments performed by Scherlag and colleagues over a 3 year period (10) examined the incidence of spontaneous sustained monomorphic ventricular tachycardia and pacing-induced ventricular tachycardia during the 6–24 hr period after left anterior descending coronary artery occlusion in 184 dogs. Spon-

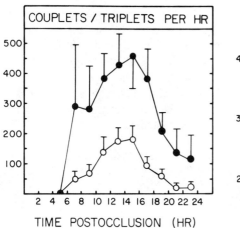

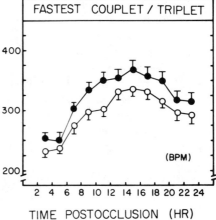

Figure 6 Incidence of rapid ventricular couplets (●) and triplets (○) after left anterior descending coronary artery occlusion in the dog. The incidence of rapid ventricular couplets and triplets (>240 beats/min) and the rate of the fastest couplets and triplets during the 2–24 hr period are shown for 27 consecutive left anterior descending coronary artery occlusions.

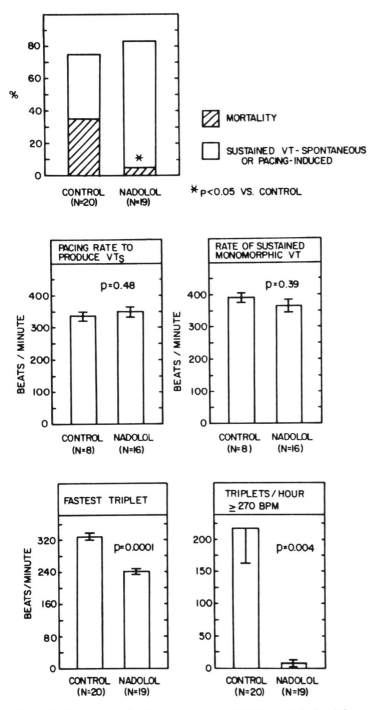

Figure 7 Prevention of sudden death in the 6–24 hr period after left anterior descending coronary artery occlusion in the dog. Saline and nadolol (1 mg/kg IV) were administered randomly to dogs 6 hr after left anterior descending coronary artery occlusion. Provocative ventricular pacing was performed in the surviving animals at 24 hr. Nadolol administration reduced the incidence of sudden death in the 6–24 hr period with a corresponding decrease in the incidence of spontaneous sustained monomorphic ventricular tachycardia. Nadolol treatment failed to alter the pacing rate necessary to induce ventricular tachycardia, the rate of tachycardia, or the incidence of pacing-induced sustained monomorphic ventricular tachycardia in surviving animals at 24 hr. Nadolol significantly reduced the rate and the number of rapid ventricular triplets in the 6–24 hr period.

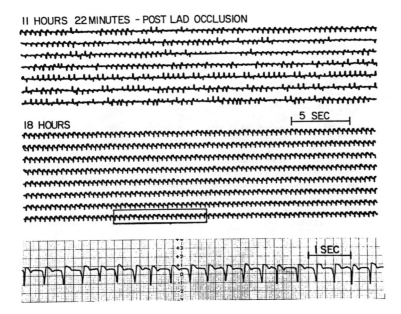

II HOURS 22 MINUTES - POST LAD OCCLUSION

18 HOURS

5 SEC

I SEC

Figure 8   Ventricular arrhythmias in the 6–24 hr period after coronary artery occlusion in the dog: nadolol administration. A surface electrocardiogram is shown at 11 hr 22 min and 18 hr after left anterior descending coronary artery occlusion. Note the slow ventricular rate and the absence of rapid ventricular couplets and triplets with nadolol administration. (Reproduced from Patterson et al. *J Am Coll Cardiol* 1986; 8:1369, with permission from Elsevier Science Publishing Co., New York).

taneous sustained monomorphic ventriculartachycardia followed by ventricular fibrillation was observed in 46 dogs (25%). Provocative ventricular pacing produced sustained monomorphic ventricular tachycardia in 60 of the 138 survivors (43%). The overall incidence of sudden death and sustained monomorphic ventricular tachycardia roughly approximate that observed by previous investigators (3,8,10) but varied according to the time of year the study was performed. The highest incidence of sudden death and pacing-induced ventricular tachycardia occurred during November–February, with an eight fold lower incidence in July-August (Figure 10). Seasonal differences in infarct mass, left ventricular mass, or the pacing rate needed to induce ventricular tachycardia were not observed (Figure 11). A higher incidence of nontransmural infarction was observed in the May–August period (Figure 11) and may reflect a different pattern or myocardial injury with a lower intrinsic ability to sustain spontaneous or pacing-induced monomorphic ventricular tachycardia (10).

SPONTANEOUS NON-LETHAL VENTRICULAR ARRHYTHMIAS 24 HR AFTER CORONARY ARTERY OCCLUSION

A number of dissimilar electrophysiologic mechanisms have been proposed to contribute to the spontaneous ventricular ectopy present 24 hr after coronary artery ligation in the dog. Some of the proposed electrophysiologic mechanisms and their salient characteristics are briefly described in Table 3. The wide variety of elecrophysiologic changes produced by myocardial ischemic injury in muscle and Purkinje tissue and the enormous complexity provided by attempts to determine electrophysiologic mechanisms in vivo, as well as the artificial environment imposed by in vitro studies of ischemically injured myocardial tissues combine to make the identification of exact roles and contributions of individual mechanisms problematic. Some mechanisms may contribute little to the overall ventricular ectopy in vivo despite the clear ability to

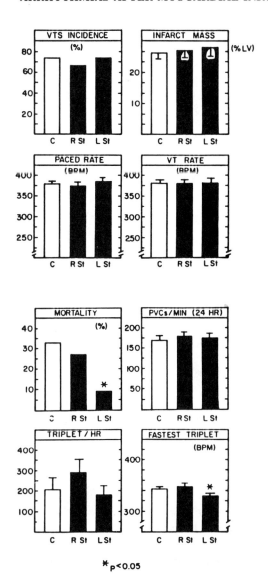

Figure 9 Prevention of lethal ventricular arrhythmia during the 2–24 hr period after coronary artery occlusion in the dog by left stellate ganglionectomy. Dogs were randomly assigned to control (C), left stellate ganglionectomy (L ST), and right stellate ganglionectomy (R ST) groups 15 min before left anterior descending coronary artery occlusion. Left stellate ganglionectomy (but not right stellate ganglionectomy) reduced mortality in the 2–24 hr period. The beneficial actions of left stellate ganglionectomy were observed in the absence of alterations in the incidence or rate of ventricular tachycardia induced by provocative ventricular pacing in the surviving animals at 24 hr. Neither left nor right stellate ganglionectomy altered infarct mass (expressed as a percentage of total LV mass),

become manifest in ischemically injured tissues preparations in vitro.

A representative electrocardiogram taken 24 hr after left anterior descending coronary artery occlusion is shown in Figure 2. The most common spontaneous rhythm present at 24 hr is an irregular ventricular ectopic rate of 160–220 beats/min with a multiform morphology. If the ectopic ventricular activity is masked by sinus tachycardia, the underlying rhythm can be uncovered by vagally induced sinus arrest. The ectopic ventricular beats occur predominantly but not exclusively in association with an early activation of ischemically injured subendocardial Purkinje tissue underlying the infarct zone (6,7,12–16). The activation of subendocardial Purkinje fibers underlying the infarct zone precedes left bundle and His bundle activation. The early activity of Purkinje fibers on the endocardial surface is characterized by rapid low-voltage deflections of 0.2–1.0 mV that precede low-voltage, slow deflections coincident with the surface QRS complex (distant ventricular activation). During sinus rhythm, the rapid deflection, low-voltage potentials presumed to represent local Purkinje fiber activation are observed within the 5–20 msec period immediately preceding the surface QRS complex (Figure 12 and 13). Electrical pacing at the site of earliest endocardial activation roughly reproduces the surface electrocardiogram and pattern of ventricular activation observed with the premature ventricular beat (Figure 14) (14). The spontaneous rhythm is only mildly suppressed by prolonged rapid ventricular pacing. Single premature ventricular beats neither interrupt nor accelerate the ventricular ectopic rhythm (17).

the number of rapid ventricular triplets present in the 2–24 hr period, or the ectopic ventricular rate present at 24 hr. The decreased incidence of sudden arrhythmic death observed with left stellate ganglionectomy was associated with a decrease in the maximal rate of rapid ventricular triplets observed in the 2–24 hr period.

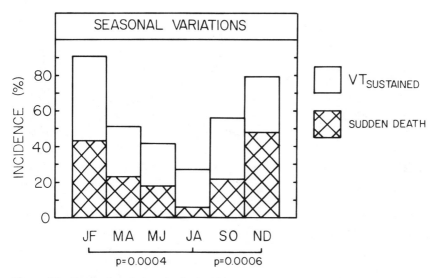

Figure 10 Seasonal variations in the incidence of lethal and paced ventricular arrhythmia during the first 24 hr after left anterior descending coronary artery ligation in the dog. The incidence of sudden death and pacing-induced sustained ventricular tachycardia at 24 hr is shown for 184 animals subjected to left anterior descending coronary artery ligation over a 36 month period. The incidence of both pacing-induced and spontaneous ventricular tachycardia was greater in the winter versus the summer months. JF = January–February, MA = March–April, MJ = May–June, JA = July–August, SO = September–October, ND = November–December.

Some of the individual mechanisms that have been proposed as bases for the spontaneous ectopic rhythms present at 24 hr are now discussed in greater detail. Despite extensive characterization of spontaneous ventricular rhythms in the intact canine heart, the cellular electrophysiologic mechanisms responsible for the spontaneous rhythms can be revealed at present only with in vitro studies using isolated, superfused tissue preparations from in-

farcted canine hearts. These studies and proposed mechanisms are described in the following sections.

Enhanced Normal Automaticity

Specialized conducting fibers in the normal canine ventricle have the intrinsic ability to develop spontaneous electrical activity. Free-running cardiac Purkinje fibers from canine

Table 3 Mechanisms for Ventricular Arrhythmia Formation 24 Hr After Coronary Artery Occlusion in the Dog

Proposed Mechanism	Rate (beats/min)	Involved Tissue	Mode of Induction	Mode of Termination	References
Abnormal Automaticity	60–250	Subendocardial Purkinje Fibers	None	None	3,4,6,7,12–22
	60–130	Epicardium	None	None	16
Triggered Rhythms	90–150	Subendocardial Purkinje Fibers	Rapid Pacing, Premature Beat	Rapid Pacing, Premature Beat	17–19,29
	90–150	Epicardium	Rapid Pacing, Premature Beat	Rapid Pacing, Premature Beat	16
Reentry	300–400	Subendocardial Purkinje fibers	Premature beat	Premature beat	20,30,40–43
	300–400	Epicardium	Rapid Pacing	Rapid Pacing	6–11

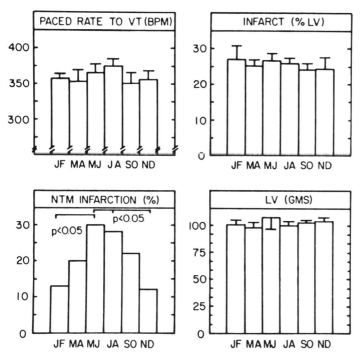

Figure 11 Seasonal variations in the incidence of lethal and paced ventricular arrhythmia during the first 24 hr after left anterior descending coronary artery ligation in the dog. The paced rate necessary to induce sustained monomorphic ventricular tachycardia in surviving animals at 24 hr after coronary artery occlusion, infarct mass (expressed as a percentage of total LV mass), left ventricular mass (LV mass), and the incidence of electrocardiographic nontransmural infarction (NTM) are shown over a 36 month period. The incidence of nontransmural infarction was higher in the summer versus the winter months.

left ventricle demonstrate slow spontaneous depolarization during diastole (phase 4 of the action potential) and have automatic rates ranging from 1 to 10 beats/min (18). An augmentation of automaticity or the sensitization of excitable cells within ischemically injured myocardium by sympathoadrenal excitation, histamine liberation, or proteins or peptides released from damaged myocardium were initially suggested by Harris et al. (3) as potential factors contributing to the generation of ectopic foci. Later experiments performed in the intact dog (12–17) or in isolated cardiac tissue (19–22) preparations have identified many fundamental differences in the basic electrophysiologic properties of enhanced automaticity in normal canine Purkinje fibers and ''abnormal'' automaticity in ischemically injured subendocardial Purkinje fibers surviving myocardial infarction. Normal automaticity is markedly suppressed by rapid pacing and

cesium chloride (an inhibitor of I_f current), interventions failing to alter spontaneous ventricular rhythm formation after myocardial infarction in the dog (23). No strong evidence currently exists suggesting a marked enhancement of normal automatic mechanisms in Purkinje or ventricular muscle after coronary artery ligation in the dog. Experiments examining rhythm formation in normally automatic tissues (His bundle and bundle branches) distant from the site of infarction have noted a paradoxical depression rather than an augmentation of spontaneous rhythm formation within the specialized tissue (18,24).

Abnormal Automaticity

When the surviving subendocardial tissue underlying infarcted myocardium is removed and superfused with normal Tyrode's solution, spontaneous depolarization and conducted

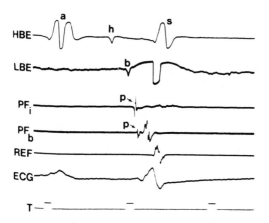

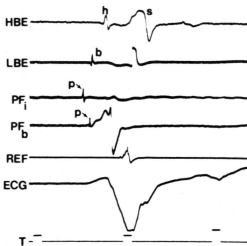

Figure 12 Depolarization of ventricular specialized conduction system (VCS) and electrocardiogram during normal sinus rhythm. The first record is the His bundle electrogram (HBE) recorded by a catheter electrode. In the HBE, a = atrial septal activation, h = His bundle depolarization, and s = ventricular septal activation. The seconds record is the left bundle electrogram (LBE) recorded with a multiple-lead electrode in the left bundle branch. The ventricular and atrial electrograms in the HBE and LBE are electronically clipped. Note that left bundle activation (b) follows h. The third and fourth electrograms were recorded from the left ventricular endocardium and show Purkinje fiber depolarization within the area of the infarct (PFi) and in the border (periinfarction) zone (PFb). These follow b. The fifth record recorded in noninfarcted myocardium is the reference electrogram (REF) used in the mapping protocol of each experiment. The last record is the lead II electrocardiogram (ECG). The timing signal indicates 100 msec intervals. (Reproduced from Horowitz et al., *Circulation* 1976; 53:59, with permission from the American Heart Association.)

Figure 13 Depolarization of the ventricular specialized conduction system (VSCS) and electrogram during a ventricular ectopic depolarization. The records from top to bottom are the His bundle electrogram recorded through a catheter electrode (HBE), left bundle electrogram (LEB), infarct zone Purkinje fiber (PFi), border zone Purkinje fiber (PFb), reference electrogram (REF), and lead II electrocardiogram (ECG). The timing signal (T) indicates 100 msec intervals. Labeling is identical to that in Figure 12. Note that the activation of PFi precedes both b and h, which are activated in the retrograde direction, and PFb, REF, and ECG, representing the distal VSCS and ventricular myocardium, which are activated in the antegrade direction. (Reproduced from Horowitz et al., *Circulation* 1976; 53:59, with permission from the American Heart Association.)

beats originate from within the ischemically injured Purkinje tissue (13,18–23). The majority of the studies describing the electrophysiologic mechanisms responsible for spontaneous arrhythmia formation have been performed in vitro utilizing small (2–10 cm^2) superfused tissue samples removed from ischemically injured canine subendocardium (1–3 mm thick).

Spontaneous ectopy in ischemically injured canine left ventricular Purkinje fibers studied 24 hr after coronary artery ligation is observed in depolarized fibers with reduced maximum diastolic potentials (-50 to -70 mV)

and depressed amplitudes (40–120 mV) (Figure 15) (25). As a consequence of an increased rate of phase 4 depolarization, continuous impulse formation in the isolated tissue preparation is observed at rates of 40–90 beats/min. Multiple sites of spontaneous impulse formation can be observed in larger tissue preparations. With an increased duration of superfusion with normal Tyrode's solution, the maximal diastolic potential and the action potential amplitude are slowly increased. The rate of spontaneous impulse formation then decreases (Table 4). With a prolonged period

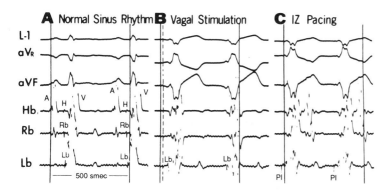

Figure 14 Localization of the site of origin of accelerated ventricular rhythm in an infarcted heart. The recordings represent the standard limb leads I (L-1), aVR, and aVF and electrograms recorded from the His bundle (H), proximal right bundle branch (Rb), and proximal left bundle branch (Lb). The recordings are shown for normal sinus rhythm (A), an underlying idioventricular rhythm during vagus nerve stimulation (B), and during ventricular pacing from the site of earliest activation during the ventricular ectopic beats (C). Note the close similarity between the QRS complexes in B and C. (Reproduced from Hope et al., *Circ Res* 1976; 885, with permission from the American Heart Association.)

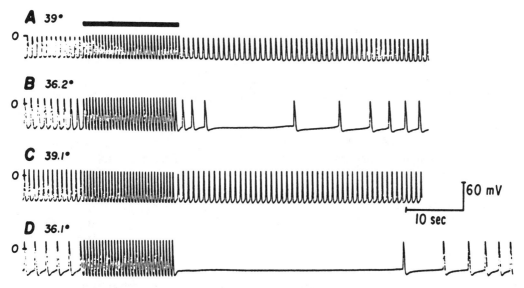

Figure 15 Effects of bath temperature on rhythms of two isolated infarcts. (A) A preparation at 39°C. The rhythm appeared to be automatic, and pacing (black bar) induced no change in it. (B) Same preparation at 36.2°C. The preparation hyperpolarized and pacing-induced further hyperpolarization was followed by a delayed afterdepolarization and three beats that appeared to be triggered. After quiescence there was warm-up of an apparently automatic rhythm. (C) Another preparation showing sustained rhythmic activity at 39.1°C. Pacing had no effect. (D) At 36.1°C, pacing-induced hyperpolarization and quiescence. There again was a gradual warm-up of an apparently automatic rhythm. (Reproduced from Le Marec et al., *Circulation* 1985; 71:1235, with permission from the American Heart Association.)

Table 4 Changes in Transmembrane Potential Characteristics with time $(N = 6)^a$

	MDP (MV)	AV (MV)	OS (MV)	SRA CL (Msec)
Control	-64.5 ± 1.3	-51.6 ± 2.6	11.3 ± 2.8	737 ± 96
4 hr later	-75.8 ± 1.2[b]	-65.6 ± 4.7[c]	28.7 ± 4.7[c]	972 ± 44[d]

[a]MDP = Maximum diastolic potential; AV = Activation Voltage; OS = Overshoot; SRA CL = Cycle length of sustained rhythmic activity. Statistical comparisons (versus control).
[b]$p < 0.001$.
[c]$p < 0.01$.
[d]$p < 0.02$.
Source: From Reference 17, with permission.

(>10 hr) of superfusion with normal Tyrode's solution, the rate of phase 4 depolarization and the spontaneous heart rate slow to become indistinguishable in normal and ischemically injured Purkinje tissue (25). As we discuss later, even though spontaneous automaticity diminishes with a partial recovery of maximum diastolic potential and action potential amplitude, the ischemically injured subendocardial tissue remains capable of initiating and sustaining rapid ventricular rhythms.

Few experiments have been performed to identify the ionic currents involved with phase 4 automaticity in the ischemically injured heart. The nature of the experimental preparation at 24 hr (a thin sheet of interconnected surviving subendocardial Purkinje fibers and ventricular muscle underlying infarcted myocardium) and the continued normalization of the electrophysiologic properties of the fibers observed with prolonged superfusion preclude accurate determination of membrane currents under voltage clamp conditions. Only recently have studies elucidating basic electrophysiologic alterations in the tissue been performed using intracellular microelectrode recordings with ion-specific microelectrodes. Intracellular potassium ion concentrations determined as intracellular potassium ion activity are moderately to severely reduced in ischemically injured canine subendocardial Purkinje fibers 24 hr after coronary artery ligation (Table 5). The potassium equilibrium potential in the ischemically injured tissue is reduced from -97 ± 5 to -81 ± 7 mV (25). With prolonged superfusion (3–6 hr) the equilibrium potential in ischemically injured tissue is returned toward normal (-94 ± 6 mV). Only a portion of the

maximum diastolic potential changes can be attributed to a change in potassium equilibrium potential. A similar determination of intracellular sodium ion concentrations has demonstrated increased internal sodium ion activity at 24 hr, with a significant recovery after 3–6 hr of superfusion with normal Tyrode's solution (Table 5) (25). The small accumulation of intracellular sodium is less than expected with the observed decreases in intracellular potassium ion activity. The electrophysiologic abnormalities and/or spontaneous automaticity observed in subendocardial Purkinje fibers at 24 hr may be dependent upon additional derangements, such as intracellular acidosis, altered sensitivity or specificity of ion-selective channels, or altered sodium-potassium/sodium-calcium exchange pumps in the sarcolemma (25).

Spontaneous impulse formation present in ischemically injured subendocardial canine Purkinje fibers after myocardial infarction has many characteristics in common with automaticity induced in normal Purkinje fibers by barium administration (26,27) or local current injection (28,29). With barium-or-depolarization-induced automaticity, it is proposed that a loss of membrane potential enhances or unmasks background I_f current, leading to spontaneous phase 4 depolarization. Antagonists of sodium channel-mediated window current, such as tetrodotoxin (26), and calcium antagonists, such as nifedipine (27), suppress abnormal automaticity resulting from barium administration. Neither antagonist produces a consistent depression of ventricular rhythms present 24 hr after canine myocardial infarction (27,28).

Table 5 Temporal Changes in MDP, a_K^i, and MDP-E_K in Subendocardial Purkinje Cells of Apical Infarct[a]

	Purkinje fibers in infarcts—hr after start of superfusion						Control
	0–1	1–2	2–3	3–4	4–5	5–6	
MDP, mV	-50.1 ± 13.7[b]	-60.3 ± 12.1[b]	-64.3 ± 8.5[b]	-71.7 ± 7.4[b]	-72.7 ± 11.0[b]	-78.9 ± 8.7[c]	-85.0 ± 4.5
a_K^i mM	61.6 ± 16.1[b]	73.1 ± 15.1[b]	90.8 ± 18.5[c]	87.2 ± 36.2[c]	95.4 ± 15.8[d]	98.6 ± 21.9[e]	112 ± 19.8
E_K mV	-81.2 ± 6.9[b]	-85.8 ± 5.5[b]	-91.6 ± 5.4[c]	-90.5 ± 10.8[c]	-92.9 ± 4.4[e]	-93.8 ± 5.9[e]	-97.2 ± 4.7
MDP-E_K, mV	31.1	25.5	27.3	18.8	20.2	14.9	12.2
n	32	26	31	16	25	30	56

[a]Data are means ± SD; MDP is maximum diastolic potential, a_K^i is intracellular potassium ion activity. E_K is the transmembrane potassium equilibrium potential, and n is the number of cell impalements with potassium ion-selective electrode.
[b]$p < 0.0005$ compared to control
[c]$p < 0.05$ compared to control
[d]$p > 0.05$ compared to control
[e]$p > 0.20$ compared to control.
Source: From Reference 25 with permission from the American Heart Association.

316 PATTERSON ET AL.

The spontaneous rhythms present 24 hr after coronary artery occlusion in the intact canine heart and in surviving subendocardial tissue preparations are (1) increased in rate with β-adrenergic receptor agonists and sympathetic nervous system stimulation (18,30–32), and (2) modestly reduced in rate but only incompletely suppressed with β-adrenergic receptor blockade or sympathetic nervous system denervation (4,8,17,31,32). The increased rate of phase 4 depolarization (and increased rate of ectopic impulse formation) occurs in the presence of an increased maximum diastolic potential (30). The stimulation of α-receptors in surviving ischemically injured tissue with phenylephrine (30,31) or blockade by phentolamine (31) fails to significantly alter the rate or pattern of spontaneous rhythm formation.

Delayed Afterdepolarizations and Triggered Rhythms

After prolonged periods of superfusion with normal, oxygenated Tyrode's solution, the depolarized subendocardial Purkinje fibers (-50 to -70 mV) underlying infarcted myocardium slowly regain normal membrane potential with a corresponding decrease in spontaneous automaticity to normal in vitro rates (Table 4). Despite the absence of spontaneous rhythm and a recovery of resting membrane potential, the subendocardial tissue preparations demonstrate marked electrophysiologic abnormalities, most notably the formation of delayed afterdepolarizations and triggered ventricular rhythms. Ventricular rhythms at rates of 50–120 beats/min can be initiated by ventricular pacing at cycle lengths less than 1000 msec or by the introduction of single premature ventricular beats (17,18,27,33). The initiation of repetitive ventricular rhythms is associated with an increase in delayed afterdepolarization amplitude initiated by a reduction in the cycle length of stimulation using a closely coupled single premature ventricular beat and using an increased duration of rapid pacing (17,18). Rapid pacing and/or premature stimuli were also capable of terminating the sustained rhythms, termination being characterized by a delayed after depolarization failing to reach

threshold voltage. Examples of the repetitive rhythms that can be initiated at 24 hr are shown in Figures 16 through 18. Unlike the automatic rhythms present 24 hr after infarction in the canine subendocardium, the ability to initiate and terminate sustained ventricular rhythms in ischemically injured subendocardial Purkinje fibers did not subside with periods of superfusion lasting to 8 hr (19).

The amplitude of delayed afterdepolarizations and the ability to initiate sustained rhythms in ischemically injured subendocardium are facilitated by epinephrine (10-6 M) (19) and by elevated extracellular calcium ion concentrations (2.7–8.1 mM) (19,33). The calcium entry blockers verapamil (10-6 M) (19), nifedipine (200 μg/L) (27), and diltiazem (1 mg/L) (33), attenuate the increase in afterdepolarization amplitude observed with elevated extracellular calcium ion concentrations and can prevent the induction of sustained ventricular rhythms with rapid pacing (19,33). The anticancer antibiotic doxorubicin (50 mM) does not significantly alter fast- or slow-response action potentials but suppresses the formation of delayed afterdepolarizations and pacing-induced repetitive rhythms in ischemically injured subendocardial tissue (34).

The relative contributions of triggered ventricular rhythms and abnormal automaticity to the spontaneous rhythms present 24 hr after coronary artery occlusion in the dog remain controversial. It is somewhat difficult to directly extrapolate the electrophysiologic mechanisms observed in vitro to the intact dog heart in vivo. The extracellular milieu provided in vivo by lysophosphatides, high concentrations of catecholamines, activated leukocytes, and inhomogeneous extracellular potassium ion concentrations is difficult to duplicate with in vitro superfusion. Even relatively small changes in temperature during superfusion (a reduction of temperature from 39° to 36°C)suppresses abnormal automaticity and facilitates delayed after depolarization formation (Figure 15) (17). Most of our knowledge concerning the comparison of spontaneous ventricular arrhythmia formation in vivo versus in vitro has been indirect, through the use of relatively nonspecific phar-

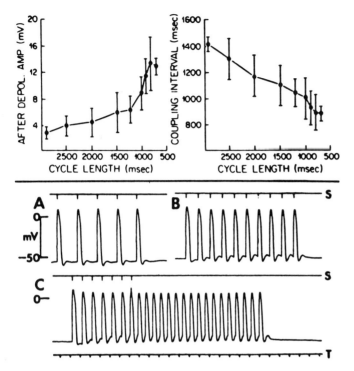

Figure 16 The effect of decreasing the cycle length of stimulation on the amplitude and coupling interval of the delayed afterdepolarization. (Top) The results from 18 preparations presented as mean ± standard deviation (SD). In each preparation the mean of at least two impalements was used for analysis. The shortest cycle length shown is the shortest cycle length at which triggered activity did not occur. Reduction of the cycle length of stimulation was associated with an increase of the amplitude of the delayed afterdepolarization and a decrease in its coupling interval. (Bottom) Transmembrane recordings from a Purkinje cell in the ischemic zone of one of the preparations. The preparation was stimulated at cycle lengths of 2000, 1200, and 1000 msec. Reduction in the cycle length of stimulation resulted in an increase in the amplitude of the afterdepolarization, which reached threshold and initiated a triggered rhythm in lower recordings. S denotes the timing of stimulation. The time scale (T) represents 1 sec intervals. (Reproduced from El-Sherif et al., *Circ Res* 1983; 52:568, with permission from the American Heart Association.)

macologic probes (28,33–36) or through the changes in spontaneous rhythm observed with the introduction of premature ventricular beats (17,19,34). The results of these studies are summarized in Table 6. The majority of the studies are consistent with the predominance of abnormal automaticity rather than triggered rhythms in ischemically injured subendocardium at 24 hr.

Spontaneous Ventricular Ectopic Beats Originating in Surviving Ventricular Epicardium

In a paper published in 1974, Scherlag and colleagues described a small subset of sponta-neous ventricular ectopic beats originating from ischemically injured canine subepicar-dium 24 hr after coronary artery occlusion (13). More recent studies have described two possible electrophysiologic mechanisms re-sponsible for the epicardial origin of ventricu-lar ectopic beats (16,37).

Dangman and coworkers have recently described automaticity and delayed afterdepo-larizations in superfused epicardial muscle preparations 24 hr after canine coronary ar-tery occlusion (16). Spontaneous impulse for-mation over a prolonged period was described in three depolarized epicardial tissue prep-arations with a maximum diastolic potential of -64 ± 6 mV. In the presence of catechola-

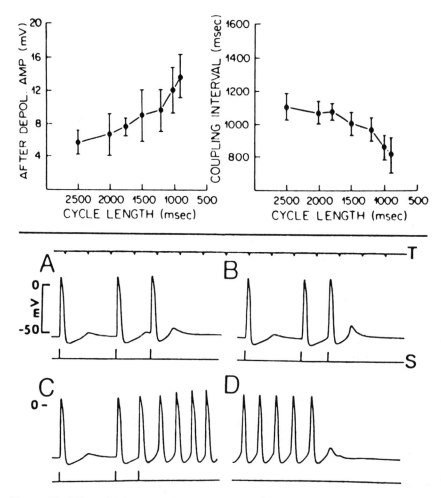

Figure 17 Effect of premature stimulation on the amplitude and coupling interval of the delayed afterdepolarization. (Top) The results from five preparations presented as mean ± SD. The shortest cycle length shown is the shortest cycle length at which triggered activity did not occur. As the coupling interval of the premature impulse was decreased, the amplitude of the delayed afterdepolarizations increased and its coupling interval decreased. (Bottom) Transmembrane recordings from a Purkinje cell in the ischemic zone of one of the preparations. The coupling interval of the premature stimulus was shortened from 1500 msec in A to 1200 msec in B and 1000 msec in C. This resulted in an increase in the amplitude of the afterdepolarization that reached threshold and initiated a triggered rhythm in C. The rhythm terminated following a subthreshold afterdepolarization in D. S designates the time of stimulation. The time scale (T) represents 1 sec intervals. (Reproduced from El-Sherif et al., *Circ Res* 1983;52:5698, with permission from the American Heart Association.)

mines, delayed afterdepolarizations and triggered rhythms could be initiated in an additional nine preparations with rapid pacing and/or single premature stimuli. The amplitude of the delayed afterdepolarizations and the incidence of triggered repetitive beats were increased with more rapid pacing rates (Figures 19 and 20). Rapid pacing also terminated the

triggered rhythms. The maximal diastolic potential in tissue preparations demonstrating delayed afterdepolarizations and triggered rhythms in the absence of spontaneous rhythm (-78 ± 1 mV) is greater than the maximal diastolic potential observed in Purkinje cells demonstrating abnormal automaticity. Both the electrophysiologic changes and arrhythmia

Table 6   Comparison of Arrhythmia Mechanisms

	Abnormal Automaticity	Triggered Rhythms	Spontaneous Rhythms at 24 hr
Single premature beats	Resetting of first recovery beat	Initiation, termination, or acceleration	Resetting of first recovery beat
Rapid pacing	Resetting of first recovery beat	Initiation, termination, or acceleration	Resetting of first recovery beat
Ethmozin	Suppression	Suppression	Suppression
Doxorubicin	No Effect	Suppression	No Effect
Lidocaine	No Effect	Suppression	Mild Suppression
β-Adrenergic Agonist	Increased Rate	Enhancement or increased rate	Increased rate

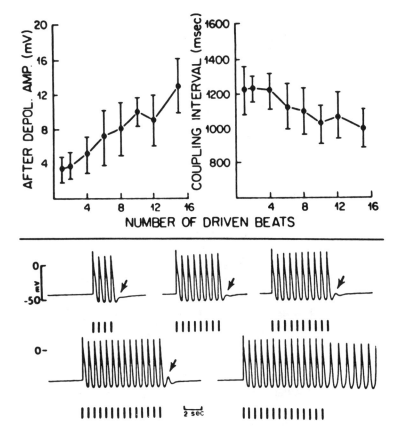

Figure 18   Effect of the number of driven beats on the amplitude and coupling interval of the delayed afterdepolarization. (Top) The results from eight preparations presented as mean ± SD, with the last plotted point in the longest driven train giving an afterdepolarization but no triggered activity. The increase in the number of driven beats was associated with an increase in the amplitude of the delayed afterdepolarization and a decrease in its coupling interval. (Bottom) Transmembrane recordings from a Purkinje cell in the ischemic zone of one of the preparations. The amplitude of the delayed afterdepolarizations (marked by arrows) showed a gradual increase as the number of stimulated impulses was increased. The afterpotential reached threshold and initiated a triggered rhythm in the lower right panel. The timing of stimulation is indicated at the bottom of each panel by heavy vertical bars. (Reproduced from El-Sherif et al., *Circ Res* 1983; 52:569, with permission from the American Heart Association.)

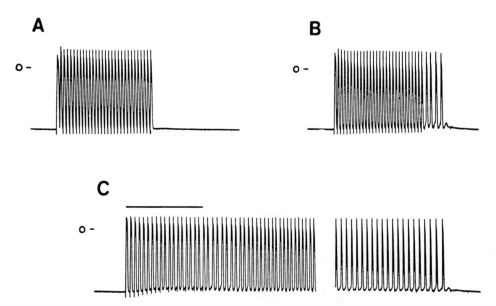

Figure 19 Tracings of induction of delayed afterdepolarizations (DAD) and triggered activity in 24 hr infarct zone supepicardial muscle by isoproterenol. (A) The 30 beat, 300 msec train does not induce DAD. (B,C) Effects of 1 μM isoproterenol after stimulus trains at 300 and 400 msec, respectively. The horizontal bar above trace C shows period of stimulation; voltage and time calibration bar (60 mV and 4 sec, respectively). (Reproduced from Dangman et al., *Circulation* 1988; 78:1022, with permission from the American Heart Association.)

mechanisms described for superfused ventricular muscle (epicardium) preparations are similar to the changes described for superfused subendocardium (Purkinje fibers) at 24 hr.

Patterson and colleagues (37) described spontaneous ventricular beats originating in epicardium overlying infarcted myocardium at 24 hr following canine coronary artery occlusion. The premature ventricular beats had the following characteristics: (1) early epicardial activation in ischemically injured left ventricular epicardium, clearly preceding His bundle and Purkinje activation; (2) a constant coupling interval with the preceding ventricular beat; (3) a left bundle branch block ECG pattern; and (4) Δ-wave formation on the anterior ECG leads corresponding with the early epicardial activation (Figure 21). The Δ-wave preceding endocardial activation and corresponding with early epicardial activation in the composite electrogram or with a handheld bipolar electrode can be clearly observed in Figure 22. Using closely spaced bipolar recordings from ischemically injured left ventricular subendocardium, ventricular beats

were observed with both early subendocardial and early epicardial activation (Figure 23). Premature beats originating on the epicardium with coupling intervals of 391 ± 17 msec represented from 36 to 100% (58 ± 13%) of total ventricular beats in the 12 animals studied. The epicardial origin of the beats is also suggested by the ability to reversibly ablate the ventricular beats of subepicardial origin by placing lidocaine-soaked pledgets on the site of earliest epicardial activation or irreversibly by injecting latex into the coronary artery at the site of occlusion (Figure 24). Neither intervention interfered with ventricular rhythms originating from ischemically injured subendocardium. The electrophysiologic basis for the subepicardial beats is unknown. The beats are moderately suppressed by systemic lidocaine administration and enhanced by systemic epinephrine administration but are also enhanced with the intravenous administration of D-600, a calcium entry blocker. The results of systemic drug administration are only partially consistent with the expected response of delayed afterdepolarization formation and triggering.

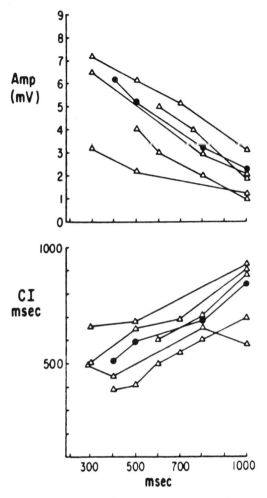

The interaction of multiple pacemaker sites and the entrance and exit block present at individual sites may help to explain the polymorphic nature of the spontaneous rhythms present at 24 hr. Examples of the following types of pacemaker interactions are clearly demonstrable in ischemically injured subendocardium: (1) variable entrance block, (2) variables exit block, (3) modulation and entrainment of ectopic (automatic) foci, and (4) type I and type II reflected reentry. The possible roles and individual contributions of the previously mentioned pacemaker interactions in the intact canine heart 24 hr after coronary artery occlusion are unclear. An in-depth discussion of the pacemaker interactions is provided in another chapter in the present book.

VENTRICULAR RHYTHMS INITIATED AND TERMINATED WITH VENTRICULAR PACING 24 HR AFTER CORONARY ARTERY OCCLUSION IN THE DOG

Experimental Results in the Intact Dog Heart

Provocative ventricular pacing can initiate rapid, sustained ventricular tachycardias in the intact dog heart 24 hr after coronary artery occlusion (6–10). The incidence of pacing-induced sustained monomorphic ventricular tachycardia at 24 hr is 60–90% in animals with electrocardiographically defined transmural myocardial infarction (6,8–10). The ventricular tachycardias induced by ventricular pacing can be clearly distinguished from spontaneous ventricular rhythms based upon rate, form, site of origin, and mode of initiation or termination (Table 7). A direct comparison of the spontaneous rhythm and a pacing-induced sustained monomorphic ventricular tachycardia is shown in Figure 25. The composite electrogram during the interectopic interval of the pacing-induced sustained monomorphic ventricular tachycardia is closely reproducible on a beat-to-beat basis during the tachycardia. The continuous diastolic electrical activity appears only in ischemically injured ventricular

Figure 20 Plots of amplitude (top) and coupling interval (bottom) of delayed afterdepolarizations induced by isoproterenol. The horizontal axis shows the cycle length of stimulation in msec; vertical axes show amplitude in V and coupling intervals in msec. Circles show the results of 30 beat trains; triangles show results of 10 beat trains. (Reproduced from Dangman et al., *Circulation* 1988; 78:1023, with permission from the American Heart Association.)

Reflected Reentry and Variable Impaired Conduction as Modulators of Spontaneous Rhythms 24 hr After Canine Myocardial Infarction

Variable entrance and exit block of pacemaker potentials has long been demonstrated in ischemically injured canine subendocardium after coronary artery occlusion (21,22,38,39).

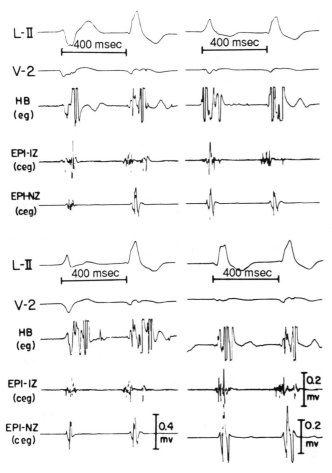

Figure 21 Ectopic ventricular beats demonstrating early epicardial activation. Four premature ventricular beats with a constant coupling interval are shown from a representative experiment 24 hr after myocardial infarction. The recordings represent a lead II electrocardiogram (L-II), anterior chest lead (V-2), a His bundle electrogram (HB), an epicardial composite electrogram recorded from ischemically injured left ventricular epicardium (EPI-IZ), and a composite electrogram from normal myocardium (EPI-NZ). The electrocardiographic morphology of the premature beats and the coupling interval were consistent throughout the experiment. Early epicardial activation was present in ischemically injured left ventricular epicardium.

epicardium and is not observed in composite electrograms from normal myocardial tissue. The continuous diastolic electrical activity ceases with the termination of the ventricular tachycardia. Sustained monomorphic ventricular tachycardias induced by provocative ventricular pacing at 24 hr are very rapid and produce marked hypotension. If not terminated by rapid pacing or electrical countershock, the rhythm degenerates to ventricular fibrillation (6–10). The pacing-induced sus-

Table 7 Comparison of Spontaneous and Pacing-Induced Rhythms 24 hr After Canine Coronary Artery Occlusion

	Spontaneous	Pacing-Induced
Rate, beats/min	150–200	300–400
Morphology	Multiform	Uniform
Regularity	Irregular	Regular
Initiation	Spontaneous	Pacing-Induced
Effect of Rapid		Initiation and
Ventricular Pacing	Resetting	Termination

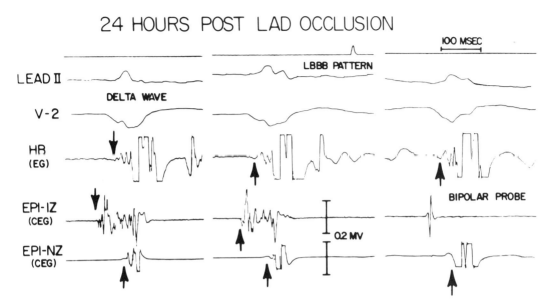

Figure 22 Ectopic ventricular beats present 24 hr after left anterior descending coronary artery occlusion in the dog. Three examples of ventricular ectopic beats demonstrating early activation in ischemically injured left ventricular epicardium. The ectopic beats were characterized by (1) a left bundle branch morphology, (2) a δ-wave in the V-2 electrocardiogram, and (3) early activation on the epicardial surface in the infarct zone. The two left-hand panels demonstrate early epicardial activation in the composite electrogram preceding His activation. The right-hand panel demonstrates early epicardial activity in a closely spaced bipolar electrode on the epicardial surface of the heart.

tained monomorphic ventricular tachycardias observed at 24 hr are similar in rate and morphology to those occurring spontaneously in animals developing sudden death during the 6–24 hr period after coronary artery occlusion. The spontaneous development of sustained monomorphic ventricular tachycardia is discussed in an earlier section of this chapter.

The sustained monomorphic ventricular tachycardias observed with provocative ventricular pacing are believed to result from localized reentry within the thin surviving epicardial layer overlying infarcted myocardium. The site of origin can be localized to the epicardial surface using continuous diastolic electrical activity recorded from composite electrodes as a marker (6,8–10) or by using multielectrode mapping of the putative reentrant circuit (7). The mapping of a reentrant circuit, as well as the rapid rate and mode of initiation or termination of the tachycardia, is suggestive of localized myocardial reentry.

Pacing-Induced Repetitive Rhythms in Ischemically Injured Subendocardium, 24 Hr After Canine Myocardial Infarction

Early experiments examining the electrophysiologic alterations present in surviving subendocardial tissue preparations 24 hr after myocardial infarction demonstrated repetitive beat formation with the introduciton of properly timed premature stimuli (21,22,40–43). The rhythms induced by the premature stimuli are faster than the rhythms observed to result from abnormal automaticity and delayed afterdepolarizations in their rate (>300 beats/min), timing in the cardiac cycle (the next beat occurs before full repolarization), failure to terminate in a delayed afterdepolarization, and dependence upon the development of a critical conduction delay (21,22,24,40–43). The electrophysiologic basis for the repetitive rhythms induced by the single premature beats is

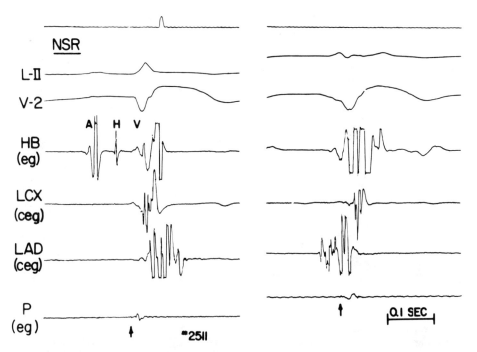

Figure 23 Ectopic ventricular beats recorded in the dog 24 hr after anterior descending coronary artery occlusion. The recordings are as given in Figure 21. A subendocardial recording representing Purkinje activation (P) is also shown. In the left-hand panel during sinus rhythm, Purkinje activation in injured subendocardium follows His bundle activation and precedes ventricular activation. During an ectopic beat with early epicardial activation, subendocardial Purkinje fiber activation follows epicardial activation.

believed to be localized myocardial reentry. This hypothesis is supported by the following data. (1) Repetitive rhythms are observed only with early premature stimuli and the development of activation delays sufficient to exceed localized refractoriness (Figure 26). (2) Antiarrhythmic agents that slow conduction (increased activation delays) and fail to produce local conduction block exacerbate arrhythmia formation (Figure 27). (3) Antiarrhythmic agents that increase local refractoriness and reduce the development of delayed activation prevent the development of repetitive ventricular beats. (4) The repetitive ventricular beats can occur in the absence of delayed afterdepolarizations and/or spontaneous automaticity. The repetitive rhythms induced by single premature stimuli in infarcted subendocardial Purkinje fibers may or may not be present in the intact heart at 24 hr after coronary artery occlusion. A reentrant mechanism in ischemically injured subendocardium underlying the infarct may potentially explain some of the closely coupled ventricular ectopic beats or ventricular triplets present 24 hr after coronary artery occlusion in the intact canine heart. There are, however, no data available at present to directly support this hypothesis.

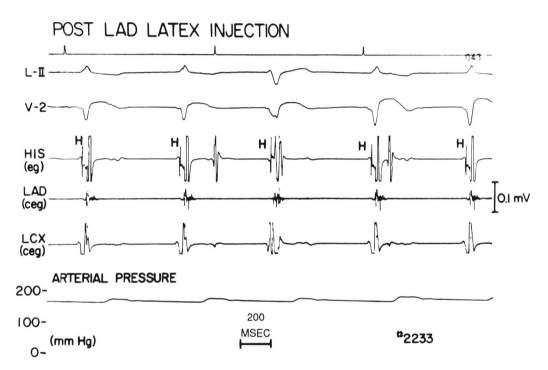

Figure 24 Ectopic ventricular beats recorded in the dog 24 hr after coronary artery occlusion, a continuation of the experiment shown in Figure 23. Latex, 0.2 ml, was injected into the occluded LAD artery distal to the occlusion site. The latex injection reduced the amplitude of the infarct zone electrogram. After latex injection no beats with early epicardial activation were observed, and all ventricular ectopic beats were accompanied by early His bundle activation and Purkinje fiber activation.

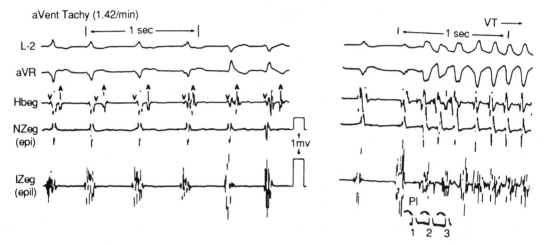

Figure 25 Ventricular rhythms observed in the anesthetized dog 24 hr after left anterior descending coronary artery occlusion. (Left) Recordings of a spontaneous rhythm present 24 hr after left anterior descending coronary artery occlusion. The recordings from top to bottom are a lead II electrocardiogram (L-2), aVR surface lead, a His bundle electrogram (HB eg), a normal zone composite electrogram (NZeg) from epicardium, and a ischemically injured zone epicardial composite electrogram (IZeg). Ventricular activation occurs first on the endocardial surface. Although there is some delay and fractionation in the IZ composite electrogram, the delayed activity remains localized to the QRS interval. (Right) Three premature ventricular beats are introduced, resulting in increased epicardial activation delays with each successive premature beat. The delayed electrical activity observed with the third premature beat spans diastole and initiates a sustained monomorphic ventricular tachycardia with a repetitive pattern of continuous electrical activity spanning the diastolic interval between ventricular beats. (Reproduced from Scherlag et al., *Am J Cardiol* 1983; 51:208–9, with permission from York Medical Publications.)

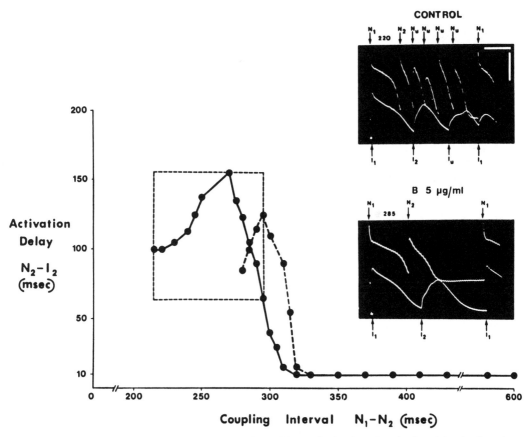

Figure 26 Prevention of Reexcitation by bretylium without elimination of activation delay in the subendocardial Purkinje fiber network of an anterior papillary muscle preparation 24 hr after coronary occlusion. Increased conduction delays between the normal and ischemic zone action potential recordings are shown on the ordinate with increasing prematurity of stimulated beats. The break in the control curve from 250 to 270 msec indicates that during this period the impulse initiated in the normal region failed to propagate to the recording site in the infarcted region. Responses initiated earlier than 250 msec reached the infarcted region again but with slightly less delay, suggesting that perhaps the pattern of activation of the infarcted zone was altered. The panels above and to the right of the graph indicate the responses obtained under control conditions (top) and after equilibration with bretylium (bottom) when the N_1–N_2 coupling intervals were 5 msec greater than the local refractory period in each case. In both cases the activation delays to the recording site within the infarcted region were similar. In the absence of bretylium the premature response was followed by four unstimulated responses in the normal region and one unstimulated response in the infarcted region. In the presence of bretylium no unstimulated responses followed the premature response. (Reproduced from Cardinal and Sasyniuk, *J Pharmacol Exp Ther* 1978; 204:169, with permission from the Williams and Wilkins Co.)

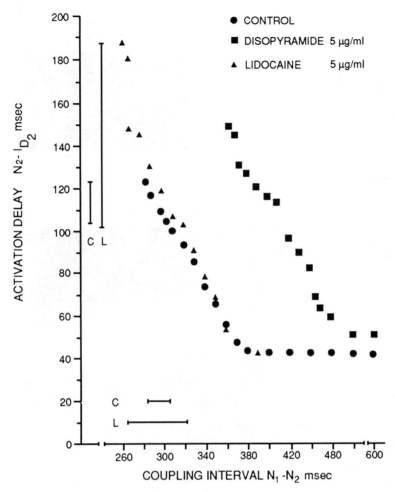

Figure 27 Comparison of the effects of lidocaine, 5 μg/ml, and disopyramide, 5 μg/ml, on the relationship between the coupling interval of the premature response initiated in the normal region (N_1–N_2) and its conduction to the recording site in the distal infarcted region (N_2–ID_2). Horizontal bars indicate the unstimulated response (Nu) zone under control conditions (C) and after exposure to lidocaine (L). No Nu occurred in the presence of disopyramide. The vertical bars indicate the range of delays associated with Nu. (Reproduced from Sasyniuk and McQuillan, Mechanisms by which antiarrhythmic drugs influence induction of reentrant responses. In: Zipes and Jalife, eds. Cardiac Electrophysiology. With permission from Grune and Stratton, Inc., New York.)

REFERENCES

1. Harris AS, Guevara Rojas A. The initiation of ventricular fibrillation due to coronary occlusion. Exp Med Surg 1943; 1:105–21.
2. Harris AS. Terminal electrocardiographic patterns in experimental anoxia, coronary occlusion, and hemorrhagic shock. Am Heart J 1948; 35:895–909.
3. Harris AS. Delayed development of ventricular ectopic rhythms following experimental coronary occlusion. Circulation 1950; 1318–28.
4. Harris AS, Estandia A, Tillotson RF. Ventricular ectopic rhythms and ventricular fibrillation following cardiac sympathectomy and coronary occlusion. Am J Physiol 1951; 165:505–12.
5. Kabell G, Scherlag BJ, Hope RR, Lazzara R. Regional myocardial blood flow and ventricular arrhythmias following one-stage and two-stage coronary artery occlusion in anesthetized dogs. Am Heart J 1982; 104:537–44.
6. Scherlag BJ, Kabell G, Brachmann J, Harrison L, Lazzara R. Mechanisms of spontaneous and induced ventricular arrhythmias in the 24 hour infarcted dog heart. Am J Cardiol 1983; 51:207–13.
7. El-Sherif N, Mehra R, Gough WB, Zeiler RH. Ventricular activation patterns of spontaneous and induced rhythms in canine one-day-old myocardial infarction. Circ Res 1982; 51:152–66.
8. Patterson E, Scherlag BJ, Lazarra R. Mechanism of prevention of sudden death by nadolol: differential actions on arrhythmia triggers and substrate after myocardial infarction. J Am Coll Cardiol 1986; 1365–72.
9. Scherlag BJ, Patterson E, Berbari EJ, Lazzara R. Experimental simulation of sudden coronary death in man: electrophysiological mechanisms and role of adrenergic influences. In: Schomig AS, Brachmann J, eds. Adrenergic system and ventricular arrhythmia in myocardial infarction. New York: Springer-Verlag, 1989:299–312.
10. Scherlag BJ, Patterson E, Lazzara R. Seasonal variation in sudden cardiac death after experimental myocardial infarction. J Electrocardiol 1990; 23:223–230.
11. Patterson E, Scherlag BJ, Szabo B, Lazzara R. Different reentrant substrates induced by permanent versus transient ischemia. Clin Res 1989; 37:284A.
12. Friedman PL, Stewart JR, Fenoglio JJ, Wit AL. Survival of subendocardial Purkinje fibers after extensive myocardial infarction in dogs. Circ Res 1973; 33:597–611.
13. Scherlag BJ, El-Sherif N, Hope R, Lazzara R. Characterization and localization of ventricular arrhythmias resulting from myocardial ischemia and infarction. Circ Res 1974; 35:372–83.
14. Horowitz LN, Spear JF, Moore EN. Subendocardial origin of ventricular arrhythmias in 24-hour-old experimental myocardial infarction. Circulation 1976; 35:56–63.
15. Dangman KH, Wang HI, Wit AL. Effects of intracoronary potassium chloride on electrograms of canine Purkinje fibers in six-hour- to four-week-old myocardial infarcts. Circ Res 1979; 44:392–405.
16. Dangman KH, Dresdner KP, Zaim S. Automatic and triggered initiation in canine subepicardial ventricular muscle cell from border zones of 24 hour transmural infarcts. Circulation 1988; 78:1020–30.
17. Le Marec H, Dangman KH, Danilo P, Rosen MR. An evaluation of automaticity and triggered activity in the canine heart one to four days after myocardial infarction. Circulation 1985; 71:1224–36.
18. Hope RR, Scherlag BJ, El-Sherif N, Lazzara R. Hierarchy of ventricular pacemakers. Circ Res 1976; 39:883–8.
19. El-Sherif N, Gough WB, Zeiler RH, Mehra R. Triggered ventricular rhythms in 1-day-old myocardial infarctions in the dog. Circ Res 1983; 52:566–79.
20. Dangman KH, Hoffman BF. The effects of single premature stimuli on automatic and triggered rhythms in isolated canine Purkinje fibers. Circulation 1985; 71:813–22.
21. Friedman PL, Stewart JR, Wit AL. Spontaneous and induced cardiac arrhythmias in subendocardial Purkinje fibers surviving extensive myocardial infarctions in dogs. Circ Res 1973; 33:612–26.
22. Lazzara R, El-Sherif N, Scherlag BJ. Electrophysiologic properties of canine Purkinje cells in one-day-old myocardial infarction. Circ Res 1973; 33:722–34.
23. Rosenshtraukh LV, Brachmann J, Scherlag BJ, Harrison L, Lazarra R. Mechanisms of ventricular automaticity in the normal and infarcted dog heart. Clin Res 1981; 29:212A.
24. Patterson E, Scherlag BJ, Lazzara R. Depression of left bundle automaticity after coronary

artery occlusion and reperfusion. J Am Coll Cardiol 1986; 7:85A.

25. Dresdner KP, Kline RP, Wit AL. Intracellular K^+ activity, intracellular Na^+ activity and maximum diastolic potential of canine subendocardial Purkinje cells from one-day-old infarcts. Circ Res 1987; 60:122–32.

26. Dangman KH. Effects of procainamide on automatic and triggered impulse initiation in isolated preparations of canine cardiac Purkinje fibers. J Cardiovasc Pharmacol 1988;12:78–87.

27. Dangman KH, Hoffman BF. Effects of nifedipine on electrical activity of cardiac cells. Am J Cardiol 1980; 46:1059–67.

28. Katzung BG. Electrically-induced automaticity in ventricular myocardium. Life Sci 1974;14:1133–40.

29. Katzung BG. Effects of extracellular calcium and sodium on depolarization-induced automaticity in guinea pig papillary muscle. Circ Res 1975; 37:118–27.

30. Cameron JS, Han J. Effects of epinephrine on automaticity and the incidence of arrhythmias in Purkinje fibers surviving myocardial infarction. J Pharmacol Exp Ther 1982; 223:573–9.

31. Martins JB. Autonomic control of ventricular tachycardia: sympathetic neural influence on spontaneous tachycardia 24 hours after coronary occlusion. Circulation 1985; 72:933–42.

32. Constantin L, Martins JB. Autonomic control of ventricular tachycardia: direct effects of beta-adrenergic blockade in 24 hour old canine myocardial infarction. J Am Coll Cardiol 1987; 9:366–73.

33. Gough WB, Zeiler RH, El-Sherif N. Effects of diltiazem on triggered activity in canine 1 day old infarction. Cardiovasc Res 1984; 18:339–43.

34. Le Marec H, Spinelli W, Rosen MR. The effects of doxorubicin on ventricular tachycardia. Circulation 1986; 74:881–6.

35. Hashimoto K, Satoh H, Shibuya T, Imai S. Canine-effective plasma concentrations of antiarrhythmic drugs on the two-stage coronary ligation arrhythmia. J Pharmacol Exp Ther 1982; 223:801–10.

36. Dangman KH, Hoffman BF. Antiarrhythmic effects of ethmozin in cardiac Purkinje fibers: suppression of automaticity and abolition of triggering. J Pharmacol Exp Ther 1983; 227: 578–86.

37. Patterson E, Scherlag BJ, Lazzara R. Subepicardial origin of spontaneous ectopic beats in the infarcted dog heart. J Am Coll Cardiol 1986; 7:98A.

38. Rosenthal JE. Reflected reentry in depolarized foci with variable conduction impairment in one day old infarcted canine cardiac tissue. J Am Coll Cardiol 1988; 12:404–11.

39. Rosenthal JE. Contribution of depolarized foci with variable conduction impairment to arrhythmogenesis in one day old infarcted canine cardiac tissue: an in vitro study. J Am Coll Cardiol 1986; 8:648–56.

40. Cardinal R, Sasyniuk BI. Electrophysiologic effects of bretylium tosylate on subendocardial Purkinje fibers from infarcted canine hearts. J Pharmacol Exp Ther 1978; 204:159–74.

41. Sasyniuk BI. In vitro preparation of infarcted myocardium. Environ Health Perspect 1978; 26:233–42.

42. Sasyniuk BI, McQuillan J. Mechanism by which antiarrhythmic drugs influence induction of reentrant responses in the subendocardial Purkinje network of 1-day-old infarcted canine ventricle. In: Zipes DP, Jalife J, eds. Cardiac electrophysiology and arrhythmias. New York: Grune and Stratton, 1985:389–96.

43. Dersham GH, Han J. Actions of verapamil on Purkinje fibers from normal and infarcted heart tissues. J Pharmacol Exp Ther 1981; 216:261–64.

14

Reentrant Ventricular Rhythms in the Three- to Five-Day-Old Canine Postinfarction Heart

Nabil El-Sherif, Mark Restivo, and William B. Gough

State University of New York Health Sciences Center and the Veterans Administration Medical Center
Brooklyn, New York

INTRODUCTION

Reentrant excitation is an important mechanism of ventricular arrhythmias associated with myocardial ischemia and infarction. In 1977 El-Sherif and associates made the observation that in dogs that survived the initial stage of myocardial infarction arrhythmias and that were studied 3–5 days postinfarction, reentrant ventricular rhythms occurred spontaneously but were more commonly induced by programmed electrical stimulation (1–3). The anatomic and electrophysiologic substrates for the reentrant rhythms were later characterized in a series of reports (4–12). These studies showed that reentrant excitation occurred around zones (arcs) of functional conduction block. The arcs were attributed to ischemia-induced spatially nonhomogeneous lengthening of refractoriness. Sustained reentrant tachycardia was found to have a figure eight activation pattern whereby a clockwise and counterclockwise wavefront oriented around two separate arcs of functional conduction block. The two circulating wavefronts coalesced into a common wavefront that conducted slowly between the two arcs of block.

Using reversible cooling reentrant excitation could be successfully terminated only from localized areas along the common reentrant wavefront (7). In this chapter we describe in more detail the electrophysiologic characteristics of reentrant excitation in the canine postinfarction heart.

ANATOMIC AND ELECTROPHYSIOLOGIC SUBSTRATES OF REENTRANT EXCITATION

After left anterior descending coronary artery ligation in dogs, blood flow is reduced more in the subendocardium, and resistance to flow in the infarcted tissue causes a redistribution of flow in the epicardial layers. Combined with the enlargement of collateral vessels, this results in sufficient flow to the epicardium that it usually survives (13). Although the geometry of the infarction varies in different experiments, pathologic studies consistently reveal a layer of surviving epicardial tissue overlying the core of necrotic myocardium (Figure 1). The epicardial layer varies in

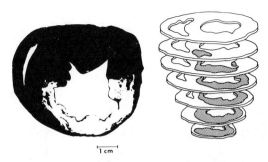

Figure 1 Anatomic characteristics of the infarction 4 days postligation of the left anterior descending coronary artery in the dog. (Right) A composite of sections stained with nitroblue tetrazolium. The shaded area represents necrotic tissue. The infarction is localized to the anteroseptal region and extends to the endocardial surface. A layer of surviving epicardium of varying thickness is present in all the sections. (Left) The fourth section from the top. The dark-stained zone represents normal myocardium; the necrotic areas are unstained.

thickness from a few cells to a few millimeters (up to 200 cell layers), as verified histologically. The surviving epicardial layer is generally wedge shaped, with more depth at the border than at the central portion of the infarction. Although the surviving epicardial layer looks intact on microscopic examination, this layer has a reduced myocardial blood flow (13).

Intracellular recordings from the surviving "ischemic" epicardial layer show cells with variable degrees of partial depolarization, reduced action potential amplitude, and decreased upstroke velocity (14–16). Full recovery of responsiveness frequently outlasts the action potential duration, reflecting the presence of postrepolarization refractoriness (14,15). In these cells premature stimuli could elicit graded responses over a wide range of coupling intervals. Slowed conduction, Wenckebach periodicity, and 2:1 or higher degrees of conduction block could easily be induced by fast pacing or premature stimulation (Figure 2). Isochronal mapping studies have shown that both the arcs of functional conduction block and their slow activation wavefronts of the reentrant circuit develop in the surviving electrophysiologically abnormal epicardial layer overlying the infarction.

The ionic changes induced by ischemia that explain abnormal transmembrane action potentials of ischemic myocardial cells have not been fully explored. Some studies suggest that ischemic transmembrane action potentials may be generated by a depressed fast Na^+ channel. This was based on experiments that showed that ischemic cells are sensitive to the depressant effect of the fast channel blocker tetrodotoxin but not to the slow channel blocker methoxyverapamil (D600); (Figure 3) (14,15). The fast channel may be depressed in ischemia for various reasons. This can only be partly explained by cellular depolarization because the depression is usually out of proportion to the degree of depolarization of the resting potential (14). The Na^+/K^+ pump may be depressed in surviving ischemic myocardial cells, leading to intracellular Na^+ loading (17). This can diminish the electrochemical driving force for the inward Na^+ current. Ultrastructural changes in the sarcolemmal membrane, as well as the effects of products released by ischemia, including lysophosphoglycerides (18), have also been implicated.

Abnormal membrane properties of ischemic myocardial cells may not be the only cause for slowed conduction and block in the surviving ischemic epicardial layer. Electrical uncoupling and increase in extracellular resistance after ischemia have also been suggested (19). Ischemia-induced increase in intracellular Ca^{2+} and low pH may increase the resistance of the gap junctions of the intercalated disk (20).

Another factor considered by some authors is the anisotropic structure of the surviving epicardial layer (21,22). The epicardial muscle fibers are closely packed together and arranged parallel to each other in a direction generally perpendicular to the left anterior descending artery. Conduction in the direction along the long axis of myocardial fibers is more rapid than in the transverse direction (23–26). The slower conduction in the transverse direction is due to higher axial resistivity, which may be partly explained by fewer and shorter intercalated disks in a side-to-side direction (24). The normal uniform anisotropic conduction properties of the epicardial

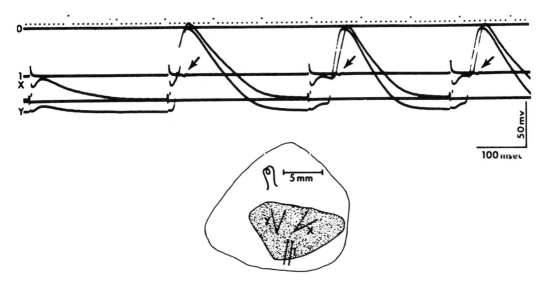

Figure 2 Recordings from a dog with a 3-day-old infarction illustrating action potential characteristics in ischemic epicardium. The sketch shows two intracellular recordings (X and Y) and a close bipolar recording (1) from the infarction zone (hatched area). Ischemic cells had decreased upstroke velocity, reduced action potential amplitude, and a variable degree of partial depolarization. The two cells were recorded 5 mm apart in the infarction zone but showed a significant difference in their resting potentials. The resting potential of the Y cell was only slightly reduced (-80 mV), but it still had a poor action potential. The preparation was stimulated at a cycle length of 290 msec, which resulted in a Wenckebach-like conduction pattern. Note that the pacing cycle length exceeded the action potential duration of the two cells, suggesting that refractoriness extended beyond the completion of the action potential, that is, postrepolarization refractoriness. (Reprinted with permission from N. El-Sherif and R. Lazzara, *Circulation* 1979; 6:605–15.)

layer may be further altered following ischemia. It was suggested that the site of conduction block of premature stimuli in the ischemic epicardial layer may be determined by its anisotropic properties, that is, premature stimuli block along the long axis of epicardial muscle fibers (21). We have shown that functional conduction block of premature stimuli in the ischemic epicardial layer is due to an abrupt and discrete change in refractoriness. The spatially nonuniform refractory distribution occurs both along and across fiber direction, as are the arcs of conduction block (27).

EPICARDIAL ACTIVATION PATTERNS OF REENTRANT EXCITATION INDUCED BY PREMATURE STIMULATION

Reentrant rhythms could be induced 1–5 days postinfarction in the canine heart by the introduction of one or more premature stimuli (S₂S₃) during regular cardiac pacing (S₁) at relatively long cycle lengths (Figure 4). Isochronal activation maps during S₁ usually show relatively fast conduction over the epicardial surface of the infarction. In a few dogs, however, areas of conduction block and slow conduction could be seen during S₁. In some of these areas myocardial necrosis was seen to extend to the epicardial surface or within a few cell layers from the surface. The introduction of S₂ results in the development of an arc of unidirectional conduction block, forcing the activation wavefront to travel around the two ends of the arc. The arc of conduction block is functional in nature and does not exist during S₁ stimulation.

The length of the arc of conduction block and the degree of slow conduction distal to the arc are crucial factors for the creation of a reentrant circuit. A premature beat that success-

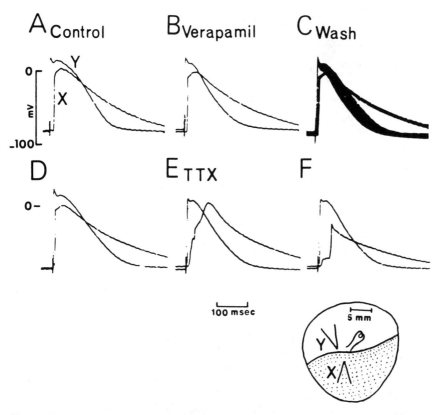

Figure 3 Action potential recordings of ischemic (X) and normal (Y) myocardial cells from an epicardial preparation from a 3-day-old canine infarction comparing the effects of tetrodotoxin (TTX) and verapamil. The resting potential of the ischemic cell was similar to that of the normal cell at -82 mV. However, the ischemic cell had a reduced action potential amplitude, decreased upstroke velocity, and a prolonged action potential duration. Verapamil (1×10^{-6} g/ml) had no significant effect on the ischemic cell but resulted in acceleration of the early repolarization phase of the normal cell. On the other hand, TTX (1×10^{-6} g/ml) resulted in marked depression of the ischemic action potential with fractionation of the upstroke and, later, abbreviation of the action potential due to loss of the large-amplitude hump on the plateau. This was associated with evidence of conduction delay and block in the ischemic zone.

fully initiates reentry results in a longer arc of conduction block and/or slower conduction compared to one that fails to induce reentry. When a single premature stimulus (S_2) fails to initiate reentry, the introduction of a second premature stimulus (S_3) may be necessary. S_3 usually results in a longer arc of conduction block and/or slower conduction around the arc. The slower activation wavefronts travels around a longer, more circuitous route, thus providing more time for refractoriness to expire along the proximal side of the arc of unidirectional block. Reexcitation of this site initiates reentry. The beat that initiates the first reentrant cycle, whether it is an S_2 or an S_3, results in a continuous arc of conduction

block. The activation front circulates around both ends of the arc of block and rejoins on the distal side of the arc of block before breaking through the arc to reactivate an area proximal to the block. This results in splitting of the initial single arc of block into two separate arcs. Subsequent reentrant activation continues with a figure eight activation pattern whereby two circulating wavefronts advance in clockwise and counterclockwise directions, respectively, around two arcs of conduction block. During a monomorphic reentrant tachycardia the two arcs of block and the two circulating wavefronts remain fairly stable. The two arcs of functional conduction block are usually oriented parallel to the long axis of the epicar-

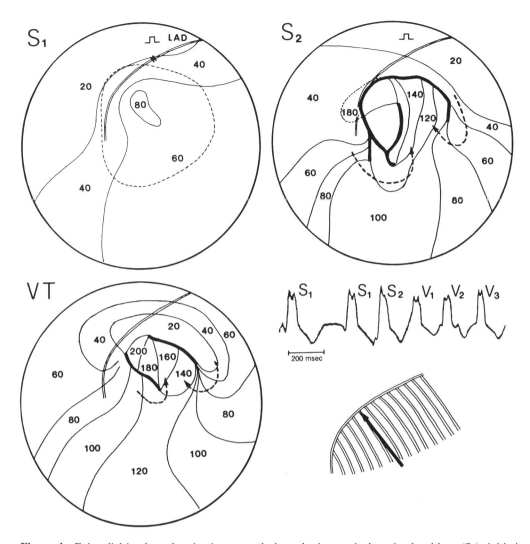

Figure 4 Epicardial isochronal activation maps during a basic ventricular stimulated beat (S₁), initiation of reentry by a single premature stimulus (S₂), and sustained monomorphic reentrant ventricular tachycardia (VT). A representative electrocardiogram is shown in the lower right. The recordings were obtained from a dog 4 days postligation of the left anterior descending artery (LAD). The site of ligation is represented by a double bar. In this and subsequent maps epicardial activation is displayed as if the heart is viewed from the apex located at the center of the circular map. The perimeter of the circle represents the AV junction. The outline of the epicardial ischemic zone is represented by the dotted line. Activation isochrones are drawn at 20 msec intervals. Arcs of functional conduction block are represented by heavy solid lines and are depicted to separate contiguous areas that are activated at least 40 msec apart. During S₁, the epicardial surface was activated within 80 msec, with the latest isochrone located in the center of the ischemic zone. S₂ resulted in a long continuous arc of conduction block within the border of the ischemic zone. The activation wavefront circulated around both ends of the arc of block and coalesced at the 100 msec isochrone. The common wavefront advanced within the arc of block before reactivating an area on the other side of the arc at the 180 msec isochrone to initiate the first reentrant cycle. During sustained VT, the reentrant circuit had a figure eight activation pattern in the form of clockwise and counterclockwise wavefronts around two separate arcs of functional conduction block. The two wavefronts joined into a common wavefront that conducted between the two arcs of block. The sites of the two arcs of block during sustained VT were different to a varying degree from the site of the arc of block during the initiation of reentry by S₂ stimulation. (Lower right) The orientation of myocardial fibers in the surviving ischemic epicardial layer perpendicular to the direction of the LAD. The arrow represents the longitudinal axis of propagation of the slow common reentrant wavefront during sustained figure eight activation pattern, which is oriented parallel to fiber orientation and perpendicular to the nearby LAD segment.

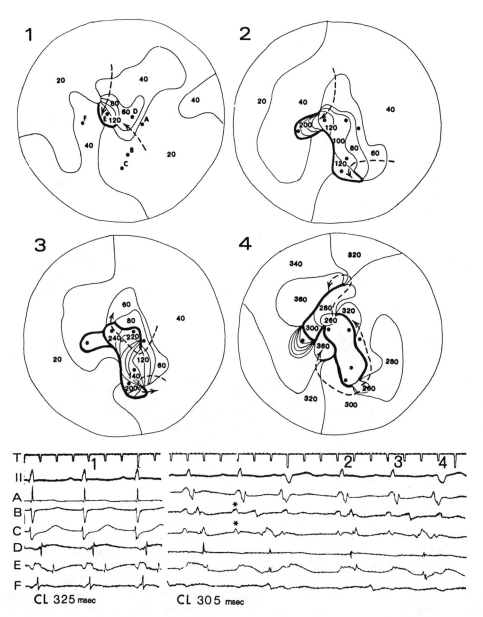

Figure 5 Isochronal maps of a reentrant trigeminal rhythm: epicardial activation maps as well as selected electrographic recordings from a dog 4 days postinfarction in which a reentrant trigeminal rhythm developed during sinus tachycardia. During sinus rhythm at a cycle length of 325 msec there was a consistent small arc of functional conduction block near the apical region of the infarct and relatively slow activation of nearby myocardial zones (map 1). The activation pattern, however, was constant in successive beats, reflecting a 1:1 conduction pattern. Spontaneous shortening of the sinus cycle length to 305 msec resulted in the development of a single reentrant beat following every second sinus beat. During the reentrant trigeminal rhythm the epicardial activation map of the first sinus beat showed the development of a longer arc of functional conduction block compared to that during sinus rhythm at a cycle length of 325 msec (map 2). The activation front circulated around both ends of the arc of block but was not sufficiently delayed on the distal side of the arc of block. On the other hand, the activation map of the second sinus beat showed more lengthening of the arc of block at one end but, more characteristically, a much slower conduction of the two activation fronts circulating around both ends of the arc of block (map 3). The

dial muscle fibers (22,28). On the other hand, during a pleomorphic reentrant rhythm both arcs of block and the circulating wavefronts can change their geometric configurations while maintaining their synchrony. Reentrant activation spontaneously terminates when the leading edge of both reentrant wavefronts encounters refractory tissue and fails to conduct. This results in coalescence of the two arcs of block into a single arc and termination of reentrant activation (6).

The majority of reentrant circuits in the canine postinfarction model develop in the surviving epicardial layer and could be viewed as having an essentially two-dimensional configuration. However, some reentrant circuits were identified in intramyocardial (9) or subendocardial locations (5). The latter location is of special interest because it may be comparable to reentrant circuits described in the surviving subendocardial muscle layer in the heart of patients with chronic myocardial infarction (29,30). This underscores the fact that, depending on the particular anatomic features of the infarction and the geometric configuration of ischemic surviving myocardium, reentrant circuits could be located in epicardial, subendocardial, or intramyocardial zones (31).

"SPONTANEOUS" REENTRANT EXCITATION VERSUS REENTRANT EXCITATION INDUCED BY PREMATURE STIMULATION (9)

Conduction delay and conduction block in ischemic myocardium are characteristically tachycardia dependent, meaning that conduction worsens at higher, but not necessarily high rates and improves at relatively slow rates (1,2). In dogs 1–5 days postinfarction, reentrant excitation commonly develops following a premature beat that interrupts an otherwise regular cardiac rhythm with a critically short cycle length. The regular rhythm can be either a sinus rhythm or paced atrial or ventricular rhythms (2). For reentry to occur during regular cardiac rhythm, the heart rate should be within the relatively narrow critical range of rates during which conduction in a potentially reentrant pathway shows a Wenckebach-like pattern (1). During a Wenckebach-like conduction cycle, a beat-to-beat increment in the length of the arc of conduction block and/or the degree of conduction delay occurs until the activation wavefront is sufficiently delayed for certain parts of the myocardium proximal to the arc of block to recover excitability and become reexcited by the delayed activation front. A Wenckebach-like conduction sequence may be the initiating mechanism for repetitive reentrant excitation, for example a reentrant tachycardia, or may result in a single reentrant cycle in a repetitive pattern giving rise to a reentrant extrasystolic rhythm (Figure 5).

INTERRUPTION OF A FIGURE EIGHT REENTRANT CIRCUIT

The criteria for proving the presence of circulating excitation as established by Mines (32,33) are (1) an area of unidirectional block must be demonstrated; (2) the movement of

degree of conduction delay was sufficient for refractoriness to expire at two separate sites on the proximal side of the arc, resulting in two simultaneous breakthroughs close to the ends of the arc and thus initiating reentrant excitation. The leading edge of the two reentrant wavefronts coalesced but failed to conduct to the central part of the epicardial surface of the infarct, that is, to areas that showed slow conduction during the preceding cycle. This limited the reentrant process to a single cycle (map4). It also resulted in recovery of those myocardial zones in the central part of the infarct, allowing the next sinus beat to conduct with a lesser degree of conduction delay, thus perpetuating the reentrant trigeminal rhythm. Analysis of the two electrograms recorded from each of the two reentrant pathways (B and C and D and E, respectively) shows a characteristic 3:2 Wenckebach-like conduction pattern. The complexity of conduction patterns in ischemic myocardium and the presence of a zone of dissociated conduction are shown, represented by site F, which showed a 2:1 conduction pattern during the 3:2 Wenckebach cycle and the reentrant trigeminal rhythm already described. (Reprinted with permission from N. El-Sherif et al., *J Am Coll Cardiol* 1985; 6:124–32.)

the excitatory wave should be observed to progress through the pathway, to return to its point of origin, and then to again follow the same pathway; and (3) "the best test for circulating excitation is to cut through the ring at one point. If impulses continue to arise in the cut ring, circus movement as a cause can be ruled out." We used reversible cooling and/or cryoablation of a localized area of the epicardial surface of the reentrant circuit to fulfill the Mines criteria for proving the presence of circulating excitation and to identify the critical site along the reentrant pathway at which interruption of reentrant activation could be successfully accomplished (7). These studies demonstrated that a figure eight reentrant activation could be successfully interrupted when cooling or cryoablation was applied to the part of the common reentrant pathway immediately proximal to the zone of earliest reactivation (Figure 6). At this site the common reentrant wavefront is usually narrow and is surrounded on each side by an arc of functional conduction block. On the other hand, localized cooling to the site of earliest reactivation commonly failed to interrupt reentry. The common reentrant wavefront usually broke through the arc of functional conduction block and reactivated other sites close to the original reactivation site without necessarily changing the overall reentrant activation pattern.

ROLE OF SPATIAL NONHOMOGENEOUS LENGTHENING OF REFRACTORINESS IN THE INITIATION OF REENTRY

In the surviving ischemic epicardial layer refractoriness was found to be prolonged in a spatially nonuniform manner (10). The pattern of refractoriness resembled concentric rings of isorefractoriness that increased in a monotonic fashion from the normal zone toward the center of the ischemic zone (Figure 7). The disparity of refractoriness per unit distance was more marked along the septal border of the ischemic zone, resulting in a more crowded refractory isochrones. The arc of functional conduction block induced by premature stimu-

lation was found to occur along the steep gradient of refractoriness. The length and location of the arc depended on the degree of prematurity of the extrastimulus (S_1S_2 interval).

When a single extrastimulus (S_2) failed to induce reentry there were fewer adjacent sites with disparate refractoriness and hence a shorter arc of conduction block. The circulating wavefront reached the distal side of the arc of block before refractoriness expired proximal to the arc. The introduction of a second extrastimulus (S_3) could further shorten refractoriness in normal and ischemic zones by 10–40 msec. If shortening of refractoriness at some border zones occurred differentially, that is, more in normal than in ischemic zones, this could result in lengthening of the arc of block. The longer arc of block would force the circulating wave to travel a longer pathway, reaching the distal side of the arc after expiration of refractoriness in areas proximal to the arc. These areas could then be reexcited to initiate reentry. When reentrant excitation was confined to a single beat, this was again explained by failure of refractoriness to shorten further in the central zone of the ischemic layer, resulting in conduction block in this zone and termination of reentry. Differential shortening of refractoriness in successive short cardiac cycles could thus modify the initial changes of refractoriness due to ischemia and explain both the induction of reentry by multiple premature stimuli and the spontaneous termination of reentrant excitation.

The correlation of activation and refractory isochronal maps shown in Figure 7 was obtained from epicardial sites that were spaced 5–10 mm apart. Because of the relatively lower density of measurements of activation and refractoriness several isochrones may have to be interpolated. From these studies a refractory gradient of 20 msec/cm was suggested as a threshold for the occurrence of functional conduction block. However, a higher resolution of both activation and refractory measurements would be necessary to discern: (1) whether functional conduction block occurs abruptly or is preceded by decremental conduction, (2) whether the spatially disparate

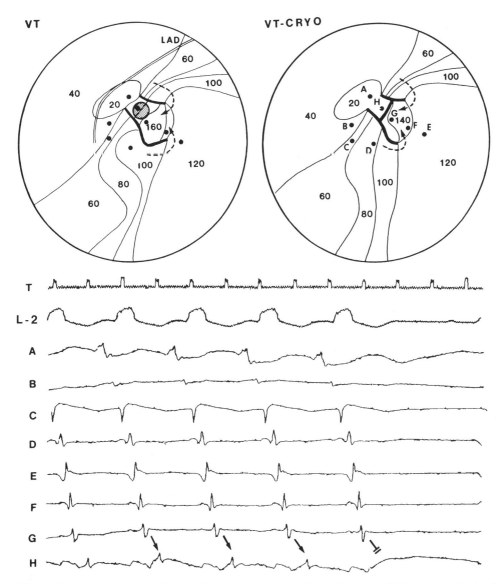

Figure 6 Interruption of a figure eight reentrant tachycardia in the epicardial layer overlying 4-day-old canine infarction by cryothermal techniques. The control activation map is shown on the left (VT), and the map of the last reentrant beat before termination on the right (VT-Cryo). Selected epicardial electrograms are shown on the bottom. The position of the cryoprobe is represented by the shaded circle. The reentrant circuit was interrupted by reversible cooling of the distal part of the common reentrant wavefront (site H). During control, the conduction time between the proximal electrode site G and the more distal site H was 33 msec. Before termination of the tachycardia an incremental beat-to-beat increase in the conduction time between sites G and H occurred, associated with equal increases in the tachycardia cycle length. When conduction block developed between the two sites, the reentrant circuit was terminated and electrogram H and electrotonic potential recorded but no local activation potential. This is represented on the isochronal map by an arc of conduction block (heavy solid line) that joins the two separate arcs of conduction block into one.

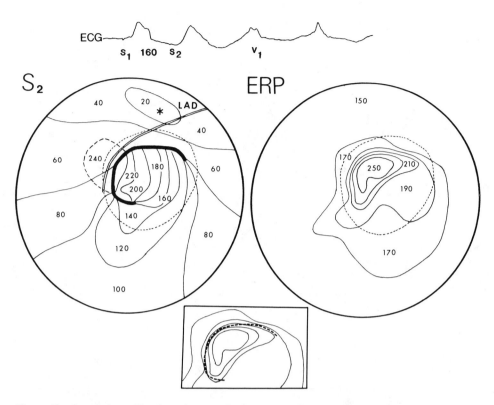

Figure 7 Correlation of isochronal maps of reentrant activation and refractory distribution in the epicardial surface from a 4-day-old infarction in the dog. (Top) The electrocardiogram shows that a single premature stimulus S_2 at a coupling interval of 160 msec initiated a reentrant rhythm. (Left) The epicardial activation map of S_2 and (right) the refractory map of S_1 as encountered by S_2 is labeled ERP. Both maps were drawn at 20 msec isochrones. The border of the ischemic zone is outlined on both maps by the dotted line. The refractory map shows a nonuniform refractory distribution with effective refractory periods (ERP) of 150–170 msec located in the normal right and left ventricular epicardium; the longer ERP of 250 msec is located in the center of the ischemic region. The dispersion of refractoriness is 100 msec, with concentric isochrones of refractoriness producing a graded increase in ERP from the border zone toward the center of the ischemic zone. The steepest dispersion of refractoriness is inside the septal and basal borders of the infarction. The arc of functional conduction block encountered by S_2 developed between adjacent sites of short and long refractoriness, with the sites of longer refractoriness distal to the arc of block. This is shown in the inset at the bottom of the figure in which the arc of block (represented by a heavy dotted line) is superimposed on the refractory isochronal map. Note that both disparate refractoriness and the functional arc of conduction block occur both parallel and perpendicular to the long axis of epicardial muscle fibers.

refractory gradient is due to gradual (albeit steep) increase in refractoriness or to abrupt and discontinuous jumps of refractoriness, and (3) whether the line of functional conduction block correlates with the abrupt change in refractoriness at the high resolution level. Figure 8 was obtained from an experiment in which a high-density electrode plaque (1 mm interelectrode distance) was utilized to obtain activation and refractory measurements

at sites of functional conduction block during premature stimulation. Functional conduction block was found to occur abruptly (within 1 mm distance), and the activation wavefront before block did not show decremental conduction. The site of conduction block correlated with an aburpt increase in refractoriness of 10–85 msec over a 1 mm distance. Electrograms obtained 1 mm distal to the site of conduction block usually revealed an electrotonic

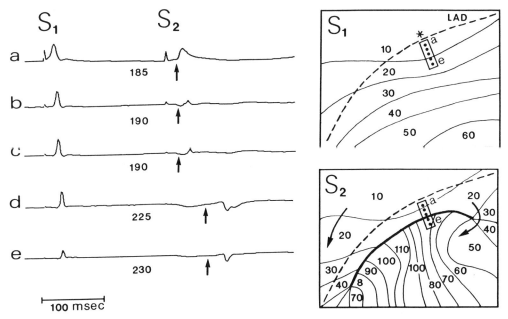

Figure 8 High-resolution determination of spatial refractory gradients and their relationship to the arc of functional conduction block from a 4-day-old canine infarction. A high-density bipolar electrode plaque with 1 mm interelectrode spacing was positioned on the epicardial surface at the site of the arc of block induced by premature stimulation (S_2) as determined from an earlier low-resolution sock electrode array. The plaque was oriented with the electrode rows perpendicular to the arc. Five bipolar electrograms were recorded successively at a 1 mm distance (a through e). The values in msec of the effective refractory period at each site are shown. The arrows indicate the end of the effective refractory period relative to S_1 activation at each site. (Right) The S_1 and S_2 activation maps. The asterick on the S_1 map denotes the site of stimulation. During S_1 sites a–e were activated sequentially within a 12 msec interval (conduction velocity of 42 cm/sec). During S_2 conduction between sites a and c was relatively slow compared to S_1. Conduction block developed abruptly between sites c and d. Sites d and e were activated 65 msec later by the wavefront that circulated in a clockwise direction around one end of the arc of block. The site of conduction block coincided with a 35 msec abrupt increase in the effective refractory period between sites c and d. Note that the arc of block was parallel to the left anterior descending artery (LAD) represented by the dashed line.

deflection synchronous with the activation potential proximal to block. It was sometimes possible to demonstrate that the amplitude of the electrotonic deflection diminished with distance from the site of block (Figure 9).

The role of differential refractoriness and fiber orientantion in the formation of the arc of functional conduction block was examined utilizing high-resolution activation and refractory maps generated at 1 mm intervals in the area of the arc functional block (27). An abrupt increase in refractoriness was found both along the fiber axis (27 ± 9 msec/mm) and across the fiber axis (14 ± msec/mm). Although the difference along the fiber axis was

greater, the arc of functional conduction block occurred in both orientations where there was an abrupt change in refractoriness. The study suggests that in the ischemic ventricle an arc of functional block occurs as a consequence of differentially graded refractoriness and can be independent of fiber orientation.

EFFECTS OF MODIFICATION OF THE SPATIAL PATTERN OF RECOVERY TIME ON THE INITIATION OF REENTRY

Further evidence of the role of the spatially nonhomogeneous distribution of refractoriness

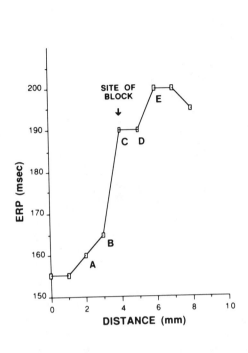

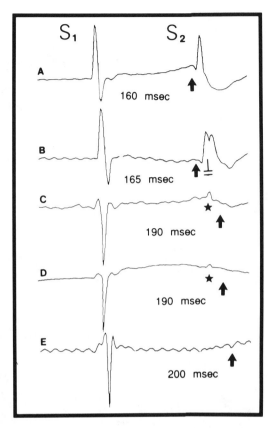

Figure 9 Five successive bipolar electrograms (A–E) recorded at a 1 mm distance across an arc of functional conduction block induced by S_2 stimulation (right). The layout of the high-density plaque was similar to that shown in Figure 5, but the recordings were obtained from a different experiment. The effective refractory period (ERP) at each site is shown, and the arrows indicate the end of the ERP relative to S_1 activation. Abrupt conduction block occurred during S_2 stimulation between sites B and C and coincided with an abrupt increase in ERP of 25 msec. The asterisks indicate the electrotonic deflection recorded in electrograms C and D distal to block. The amplitude of the electrotonic deflection diminished with distance from the site of block. (Left) Graph of the distribution of ERP across an 8 mm distance.

in the formation of the arc of functional conduction block was obtained from experiments in which the initiation of reentry could be prevented by changing the activation pattern of the basic stimulated beat (S_1) (12). The spatial patterning of recovery time depended on the activation pattern of the basic beat, in addition to the spatially nonhomogeneous refractory distribution induced by ischemia. The dispersion of recovery time could be modified by stimulation at two ventricular sites during the basic beat. The arc of conduction block could be modified or abolished entirely by appropriate selection of the secondary stimulation site in the ischemic zone and the temporal sequencing of the paired stimuli (Figure 10).

Asynchronous dual stimulation, with preexcitation of an appropriate site in the ischemic zone, was frequently successful in preventing the initiation of reentry by a fixed coupled premature stimulus. In all instances that resulted in the prevention of reentry, the secondary site was distal to the arc of block that formed following the control S_2 stimulation. The secondary site should be in an area of long refractoriness that activated late during the basic beat. Properly applied dual stimulation differentially peels back refractoriness in the ischemic zone. Successful dual stimulation depended on the reduction of two factors: the spatial gradient of recovery time and the dispersion of recovery time across the arc. The

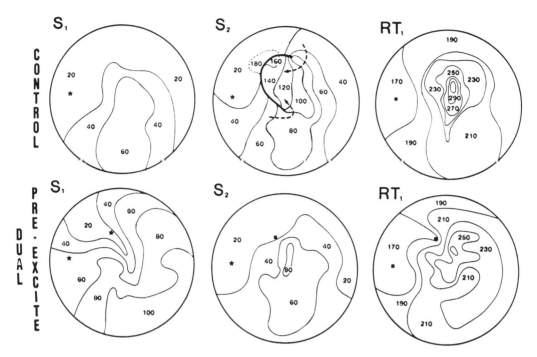

Figure 10 Abolition of the arc of functional conduction block by dual S_1 stimulation. (Top) Control, S_1 activation occurred within 60 msec. A gradient of recovery time between the 190 and 230 msec isochrones supported the formation of an arc of block during (Bottom) dual asynchronous stimulation. The two sites of stimulation, one from the right ventricle (as in control) and one from the ischemic zone distal to the arc of block, are represented by stars. When the dual ischemic site was preexcited by 40 msec, no two adjacent sites differed in recovery time by more than 20 msec. A zone of graded recovery time that could support functional conduction block was not present. An arc of conduction block did not form. In this experiment the recovery time was computed by the sum of the activation time (stimulus artifact to response during S_1) plus the effective refractory period at each site.

former determines the extent and location of the continuous arc of conduction block. The latter determines whether areas distal to block are recovered during the premature stimulation. Reducing the difference in activation time across the arc of block to a value less than the effective refractory period of the premature stimulus (ERP_2) proximal to the arc is the mechanism by which dual S_1 stimulation can prevent the initiation of reentry.

SUSTAINED REENTRY ORIENTS AROUND CONTINUOUS ARCS OF FUNCTIONAL CONDUCTION BLOCK

We and others (22,28) have shown that during sustained figure eight monomorphic reentrant tachycardia the two arcs of functional conduction block around which the reentrant wave-

fronts circulate are usually oriented in parallel with the long axis of the epicardial muscle fibers. Some authors have suggested that these areas represent apparent or pseudoblock and are in fact due to very slow and possibly discontinuous conduction across the myocardial fibers (22). In this case reentrant activation may be oriented around a small central region of functional block rather than a long line of block. Electrograms recorded from these sites had a long duration and were fractionated, a characteristic that was shown to result from activation transverse to the myocardial fiber long axis (34). These conclusions, however, were based on relatively low-resolution recordings (3.5 mm interelectrode distance) (22). We have analyzed close bipolar electrograms obtained at high resolution (1 mm interelectrode distance) from sites of the arcs of block during sustained stable reentry (Figure

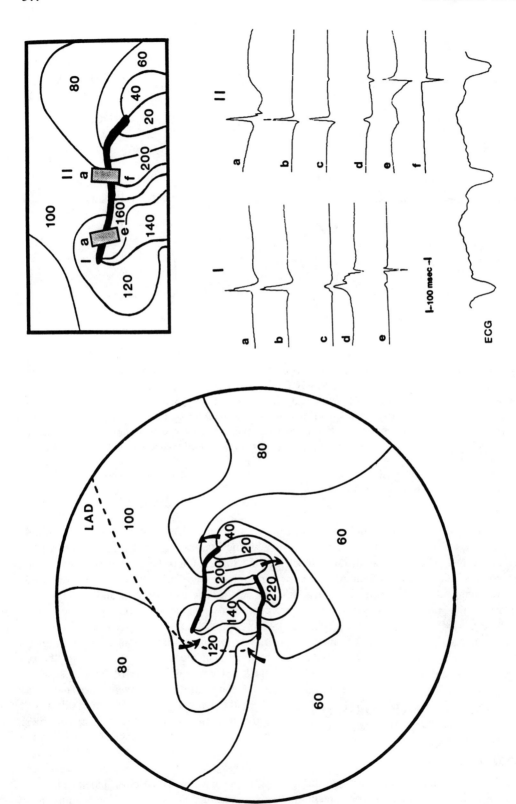

Figure 11

11). Electrograms recorded at each side of theline of block showed two distinct deflections: one represented local activation and the second an electrotonus corresponding to activation recorded 1 mm away. Both deflections were separated by a variable isoelectric period that correlated with the isochronal differences across the arc. In recordings obtained from the center of the arc local activation and electrotonus were separated by 90–110 msec. This interval successively decreased toward both ends of the arc. These observations provide evidence that circus movement reentry was sustained around a continuous arc of abrupt functional conduction block (7–25 mm long), not very slow conduction across fibers. Although refractoriness could not be measured during sustained reentry, the electrogram configurations reflecting conduction block were similar to those obtained during functional conduction block induced by premature stimulation across refractory gradient (Figures 7 and 8). This suggests that disparate refractoriness along the line of block rather than anisotropic properties of the epicardial layer may be responsible for sustained reentrant excitation.

ENTRAINMENT, TERMINATION, OR ACCELERATION OF FIGURE EIGHT REENTRANT TACHYCARDIA BY PROGRAMMED STIMULATION

In the figure eight reentrant circuit the two arcs of conduction block and the slow common reentrant wavefront are functionally determined and cycle length dependent (Figures 12 and 13) (11). A tight fit exists at certain locations during the reentrant tachycardia, with the circulating wavefront closely following the refractory tail of the previous revolution. This is particularly significant in the zone of the slow common reentrant wavefront. The reentrant circuit conduction time is determined by the area with the longest refractoriness in the zone of the slow common reentrant wavefront. It is safe to assume that during reentrant tachycardia the duration of refractoriness in the zone with the longest refractoriness probably cannot shorten further. This is not the case, however, with the rest of the reentrant pathway. A stimulated wavefront at a cycle length shorter than the tachycardia cycle

Figure 11 High-resolution recordings of activation across one of the two arcs of functional conduction block around which sustained figure eight reentrant activation occurred. (Left) The epicardial activation pattern during a figure eight reentrant tachycardia as obtained from a sock electrode array with 5–10 mm interelectrode distance. A high-density electrode plaque (1 mm interelectrode distance) was positioned at two locations across the upper arc of block. (Upper right) An expanded map of the counterclockwise circuit around the upper arc of block and the electrograms along one row of bipolar electrodes at each location. Plaque location II is situated near the center of the arc of block. Conduction between sites a and c during the left-to-right wavefront on the upper side of the arc was fast. Conduction block probably occurred between sites c and d. Similarly, conduction between sites f and e during the returning wavefront on the distal side of the arc was fast and conduction block probably occurred between sites e and d. The two deflections recorded at site d are separated by an isoelectric interval of 85 msec, which corresponds to the isochronal activation difference across the site of 81–100 msec. Both deflections most probably represent electrotonic potentials. It is possible, however, that one of the deflections, but not both, represents an activation potential. Both electrograms c and e show small deflections synchronous with the two potentials in electrogram d. These may reflect gradual diminution of the amplitude of the electrotonus with distance from the site of block at d. Plaque location I was obtained close to the septal end of the arc of block. The exact site of conduction block during the right-to-left wavefront on the upper side of the arc of block was not clear but probably occurred between sites b and c, with the first deflection in electrograms c, d, and e representing electrotonic potentials. On the other hand, conduction block occurred between sites d and c during the returning wavefront on the lower side of the arc. An electrotonic potential corresponding to the activation potential at site d was not clearly visible at site c. The two potentials at site d are separated by 30 msec and correspond to the difference in isochronal activation at this site of 21–40 msec.

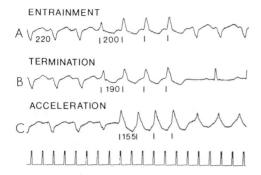

Figure 12 Electrocardiographic recording showing that a train of four stimulated beats (marked by vertical bars) resulted in entrainment, termination, or acceleration of a monomorphic reentrant tachycardia depending on the cycle length of stimulation. Recordings were obtained from 4-day-old canine infarction. The numbers are in msec. The times lines represent 100 msec.

length can still conduct in these zones. In other words, these zones have a gap of excitability. For stimulated termination of reentrant tachycardia the stimulated wavefront must arrive at the area with the longest refractoriness in the zone of the slow common reentrant wavefront before refractoriness expires, thus resulting in conduction block. If this area is stragetically located between the two arcs of functional conduction block, reentrant excitation is terminated. The three factors that determine whether the stimulated wavefront can reach this zone in time for conduction block are (1) the cycle length of stimulation, (2) the number of stimulated beats, and (3) the site of stimulation. The most optimal situation for stimulated termination of reentry is to apply a critically coupled single stimulus to the proxi-

mal side of the slow common reentrant wavefront that conducts prematurely to the strategic zone for conduction block. The stimulus can only result in local capture and does not have to conduct to the rest of the ventricles (i.e., concealed conduction). When a single stimulated wavefront fails to terminate reentry, one or more subsequent wavefronts may succeed. However, the stimulated train must be terminated following the beat that interrupts reentry. Otherwise, a subsequent stimulated beat could reinitiate the same reentrant circuit or induce a different circuit. The new circuit could have a shorter revolution time, resulting in tachycardia acceleration, and occasionally degeneration into ventricular fibrillation. Overdrive termination of reentry requires both a critical cycle length of stimulation and a critical number of beats in a stimulated train. Otherwise the stimulated train can establish a new balance of refractoriness and conduction velocity in the reentrant pathway. This may perpetuate the reentrant process at the shorter cycle length of the stimulated train, resulting in entrainment, and spontaneous reentry resumes on termination of the train. Studies of the effects of programmed stimulation on figure eight reentrant tachycardia illustrate the significance of the site of stimulation and emphasize the need for more precise localization of the slow zone of reentry and the direction of the activation front in this zone in the clinical setting.

ACKNOWLEDGMENTS

Supported by National Institutes of Health Grants HL36680 and HL31341 and Veterans Administration Medical Research Funds.

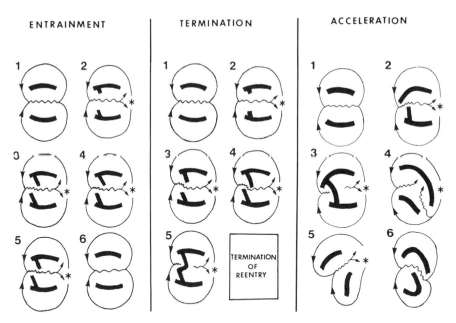

Figure 13 The mechanisms of entrainment, termination, and acceleration of reentrant ventricular tachycardia by overdrive stimulation as shown in Figure 12. The control reentrant circuit is labeled 1 and the four beats of the stimulated train are labeled 2–5. The control circuit has a figure eight configuration, and conduction in the slow zone of reentry proceeds from left to right. The heavy solid lines represent arcs of functional conduction block. Stimulation was applied at the distal side of the slow zone, as shown by the astericks. During entrainment the stimulated wavefront collides with the emerging slow reentrant wavefront. It then circulates and arrives earlier at the proximal part of the slow zone of reentry. This is consistently associated with a change in the conduction pattern in the slow zone with the development of new functional arcs of block and much slower conduction in parts of this zone. However, a new equilibrium quickly develops in which successive stimulated beats, represented by cycles 3, 4, and 5, maintain the same new conduction pattern at the shorter cycle length of stimulation, thus entraining the tachycardia. On cessation of stimulation reentry resumes as shown in cycle 6. For termination of reentry, on the other hand (middle), successive stimulated beats, now applied at a relatively shorter cycle compared to the entraining train, result in gradually more conduction delay. Eventually conduction block develops at the proximal part of the slow zone of reentry, as shown in cycle 5. (Left) The same four-beat stimulated train is applied at an even shorter cycle length. In this case and because of the short cycle length of stimulation, the second stimulated beat represented by cycle 3 has already blocked in the proximal part of the slow zone of reentry. If stimulation is stopped at this point the reentrant tachycardia terminates. If stimulation is continued, however, the third and fourth stimulated beats represented by cycles 4 and 5 initiate new arcs of block and different reentrant pathways so that on termination of the stimulated train a new and possibly faster reentrant circuit occurs.

REFERENCES

1. El-Sherif N, Scherlag BJ, Lazzara R. Reentrant ventricular arrhythmias in the late myocardial infarction period. 1. Conduction characteristics in the infarction zone. Circulation 1977; 55:686-701.

2. El-Sherif N, Scherlag BJ, Lazzara R. Reentrant ventricular arrhythmias in the late myocardial infarction period. 2. Patterns of initiation and termination of re-entry. Circulation 1977; 55:702-19.

3. El-Sherif N, Lazzara R, Hope RR, Scherlag BJ. Reentrant ventricular arrhythmias in the late myocardial infarction period. 3. Manifest and concealed extrasystolic grouping. Circulation 1977; 56:225-34.

4. El-Sherif N, Smith RA, Evans K. Canine ventricular arrhythmias in the late myocardial infarction period. 8. Epicardial mapping of reentrant circuits. Circ Res 1981; 49:255-65.

5. El-Sherif N, Mehra R, Gough WB, Zeiler RH. Ventricular activation pattern of spontaneous and induced ventricular rhythms in canine one-day-old myocardial infarction. Evidence for focal and reentrant mechanisms. Circ Res 1982; 51:152-66.

6. Mehra R, Zeiler RH, Gough WB, El-Sherif N. Reentrant ventricular arrhythmias in the late myocardial infarction period 9. Electrophysiologic-anatomic correlation of reentrant circuits. Circulation 1983; 67:11-24.

7. El-Sherif N, Mehra R, Gough WB, Zeiler RH. Reentrant ventricular arrhythmias in the late myocardial infarction period. Interruption of reentrant circuits by cyrothermal techniques. Circulation 1983; 8:644-56.

8. El-Sherif N, Mehra R, Gough WB, Zeiler RH. Reentrant ventricular arrhythmias in the late myocardial infarction period. 11. Burst pacing versus multiple premature stimulation in the induction of reentry. J Am Coll Cardiol 1984; 4:295-304.

9. El-Sherif, Gough WB, Zeiler RH, Hariman R. Reentrant ventricular arrhythmias in the late myocardial infarction period. 12. Spontaneous versus induced reentry and intramural versus epicardial circuit. J Am Coll Cardiol 1985; 6:124-32.

10. Gough WB, Mehra R, Restivo M, Zeiler RH, El-Sherif N. Reentrant ventricular arrhythmia in the late myocardial infarction period in the dog. 13. Correlation of activation and refractory maps. Circ Res 1985; 57:432-42.

11. El-Sherif N, Gough WB, Restivo M. Reentrant ventricular arrhythmias in the late myocardial infarction period. 14. Mechanisms of resetting, entrainment, acceleration, or termination of reentrant tachycardia by programmed electrical stimulation. Pace 1987; 10:341-71.

12. Restivo M, Gough WB, El-Sherif N. Reentrant ventricular rhythms in the late myocardial infarction period: prevention of reentry by dual stimulation during basic rhythm. Circulation 1988; 77:429-44.

13. Hirzel HO, Nelson GR, Sonnenblick EH, Kirk ES. Redistribution of collateral blood flow from necrotic to surviving myocardium following coronary occlusion in the dog. Circ Res 1976; 39:214-22.

14. El-Sherif N, Lazzara R. Reentrant ventricular arrhythmias in the late myocardial infarction period. 7. Effects of verapamil and D-600 and role of the "slow channel." Circulation 1979; 60:605-15.

15. Lazzara R, Scherlag BJ. The role of the slow current in the generation of arrhythmias in ischemic myocardium. In: Zipes DP, Bailey JC, Elharrar V, eds. The slow inward current and cardiac arrhythmias. The Hague: Martinus Nijhoff 1980:399-416.

16. Ursell, PC, Gardner PI, Albala A, Fenoglio JJ Jr, Wit AL. Structural and electrophysiological changes in the epicardial border zone of canine myocardial infarcts during infarct healing. Circ Res 1985; 56:436-51.

17. Schwartz A, Wood JM, Allen JC, Bornet E, Entman ML, Goldstein MA, Sordahl LZ, Suzuki M, Lewis RM. Biochemical and morphologic correlates of cardiac ischemia. I. Membrane system. Am J Cardiol 1973; 32:46-61.

18. Sobel BE, Corr PB, Robinson AK, Golstein RA, Witkowski FX, Klein MS. Accumulation of lysophosphoglycerides with arrhythmogenic properties in ischemic myocardium. J Clin Invest 1978; 62:546-53.

19. Spear JF, Michelson EL, Moore EN. Reduced space constant in slowly conducting regions of chronically infarcted canine myocardium. Circ Res 1983; 52:176-85.

20. Page E, Shibata Y. Permeable junctions between cardiac cells. Annu Rev Physiol 1981; 43:431-41.

21. Wit AL, Dillon S, Ursell PC. Influences of anisotropic tissue structure a reentrant ventricular tachycardia. In: Brugada P, Wellens HJJ, eds. Cardiac arrhythmias. Where to go from here? Mount Kisco, NY: Futura 1987:27-50.

22. Dillon S, Allessie MA, Ursell PC, Wit AL. Influences of anisotropic tissue structure on reentrant circuits in the epicardial border zone of subacute canine infarcts. Circ Res 1988; 63:182–206.

23. Clerc L. Directional differences of impulse spread in trabecular muscle from mammalian heart. J Physiol (Lond) 1976; 255:335–46.

24. Spach M, Miller WT, Geselowitz DB, Barr RC, Kootsey IM, Johnson FA. The discontinuous nature of propagation in normal canine cardiac muscle: evidence for recurrent discontinuities of intracellular resistance that affect the membrane currents. Circ Res 1981; 48:39–54.

25. Spach MS, Miller WT, Dolber PC, Kootsey JM, Summer JR, Moscher CE. The functional role of structural complexities in the propagation of depolarization in the atrium of the dog: cardiac conduction disturbances due to discontinuities of effective axial resistivity. Circ Res 1982; 50:175–91.

26. Spach MS, Kootsey JM. The nature of electrical propagation in cardiac muscle. Am J Physiol 1983; 13:H3–22.

27. Restivo M, Gough WB, Wu K-M, Williams C, El-Sherif N. Role of abrupt changes in refractoriness and fiber orientation in the formation of functional conduction block (abstract). Circulation 1987; 76:IV–241.

28. Cardinal R, Vermeulen M, Shenasa M, Roberge F, Page P, Helie F, Savard P. Anisotropic conduction and functional dissociation of ischemic tissue during reentrant ventricular tachycardia in canine myocardial infarction. Circulation 1988; 77:1162–76.

29. Fenoglio JJ Jr, Pham TD, Harken AH, Horowitz LN, Josephson ME, Wit AL. Recurrent sustained ventricular tachycardia: structure and ultrastructure of subendocardial regions, where tachycardia originates. Circulation 1983; 68:518–33.

30. Harris L, Downar E, Mickelborough L, Shaikh N, Parsons I, Chen T, Gray G. Activation sequence of ventricular tachycardia: endocardial and epicardial mapping studies in the human ventricle. J Am Coll Cardiol 1987; 10:1040–7.

31. El-Sherif N. The figure 8 model of reentrant excitation in the canine postinfarction heart. In: Zipes DP, Jalife J, eds. Cardiac electrophysiology and arrhythmias. Orlando, FL: Grune & Stratton 1985:365–78.

32. Mines GR. On dynamic equilibrium in the heart. J Physiol (Lond) 1913; 46:350–83.

33. Mines GR. On circulating excitations in heart muscles and their possible relation to tachycardia and fibrillation. Trans R Soc Can (ser 3, sect IV) 1914; 8:43–52.

34. Spach MS, Dolber PC. Relating extracellular potentials and their derivatives to anisotropic propagation at a microscopic level in human cardiac muscle: evidence for uncoupling of side to side fiber connections with increasing age. Circ Res 1986; 56:356–71.

15

Arrhythmias in the Cat Heart with Chronic Myocardial Infarction

Shinichi Kimura, Arthur L. Bassett, and Robert J. Myerburg

University of Miami School of Medicine
Miami, Florida

INTRODUCTION

Ventricular arrhythmias are common in patients with myocardial ischemia or infarction. These arrhythmias may be caused by abnormal electrophysiologic properties of cardiac cells in the ischemic or infarcted regions of the ventricle. A rationale approach to the therapy of ischemic arrhythmias is provided by a better understanding of the electrophysiologic mechanisms of ventricular arrhythmias occurring in ischemic and infarcted hearts. Since the early 1970s extensive experimental studies have been carried out in canine models of acute and subacute myocardial infarction, and these studies have provided important new insights into the electrophysiology of the early phase of myocardial infarction.

Increasing attention has recently been focused on chronic electrophysiologic changes in the late postmyocardial infarction period, which corresponds to chronic ischemic heart disease in the human. It has been emphasized, based on clinical and epidemiologic studies, that a preexisting healed myocardial infarction is a major factor contributing to risk for potential lethal ventricular arrythmias. Approximately three-fourths of patients who died

suddenly as a result of coronary artery disease had a previous myocardial infarction, many of which were unrecognized before death (1). It is thus important to understand the electrophysiologic abnormalities associated with chronic or healed myocardial infarction and their interactions with other contributing factors, such as neural activity, metabolic changes, and transient acute ischemia, to define the tran sition from an abnormal but stable myocardium to an electrically unstable muscle mass. Experimental preparations that have a previous myocardial infarction more closely mimic the clinical circumstances, and several canine and feline models have been developed. In this chapter we present some of our observations on electrophysiologic abnormalities in chronic myocardial infarction and discuss possible pathophysiologic mechanisms responsible for the development of chronic ventricular arrhythmias.

EXPERIMENTAL MODELS OF HEALED MYOCARDIAL INFARCTION

In the mid-1970s Friedman et al. (2–4) studied electrophysiologic and structural abnormalities in canine hearts 24 hr to 7 weeks after ligation of the left anterior descending coronary artery using the technique described by Harris. In their studies ventricular arrhythmias disappeared by 3 days after coronary artery occlusion, and the rapid, repetive spontaneous activity recorded in vitro from subendocardial Purkinje fibers to 24 hr infarcts was not observed at later stages of infarction. Lazzara et al. (5) also studied electrophysiologic abnormalities 10 days to 3 months after ligation of the left anterior descending coronary artery in dogs. They found no arrhythmias and no enhanced automaticity in surviving Purkinje fibers in the infarct zone, and they could not record transmembrane action potentials from the ventricular muscle cells overlying the region of the infarction. Pathologic studies by Friedman et al. (4) showed that coronary artery ligation by the Harris method produced massive destruction of muscle, little subendocardial ventricular muscle survived the acute events, and the surviving subendocardial Purkinje fibers appeared structurally normal after a period of healing. In humans, however, pathologic data suggest that both Purkinje fibers and ventricular muscle cells may survive in the endocardium overlying the infarction, and clinical and epidemiologic evidence suggests persistence of electrophysiologic instability for variable periods after healing of an acute myocardial infarction (1).

Different techniques and different species have been used in attempts to develop experimental models characterized by the persistence of electrophysiologic abnormalities and spontaneous or induced ventricular arrhythmias. Garan et al. (6,7) ligated the left anterior descending artery and all visible epicardial branches in the left ventricular apical area originating from the left circumflex or posterior descending arteries. This results in large and easily identifiable transmural infarction. Michelson et al. (8,9) have used a model in which myocardial infarction is produced by 2 hr of occlusion of the left anterior descending coronary artery followed by reperfusion. This procedure results in a region of infarction that is transmural but mottled in appearance with close interspersing of normal and abnormal tissues. Klein et al. (10) ligated one or more diagonal or obtuse marginal arteries to produce a parietal wall infarction of the left ventricle. In such canine models of myocardial infarction ventricular tachycardia can be induced by programmed electrical stimulation after healing, although few data are available on the incidence of spontaneous ventricular arrhythmias.

In our laboratory we developed a feline model of chronic myocardial infarction (11–14). In this model myocardial infarction is created by a closed circle of multiple overlapping sutures through the anterior wall of the left ventricle near the apex. This procedure produces a transmural infarction involving the base of the anterior papillary muscle and surrounding free wall, sometimes extending onto areas of the apex, and of the apical free wall and lower septum. Anatomically the infarction is characterized by dense scar tissue with an overlying layer of endocardium, three to ten cell layers deep, and an overlying layer of epicardium of similar thickness. Interdigitation between surviving muscle cells and scar tissue is often observed at the periphery of the scar 2 months after coronary artery ligation. The surviving bands of subendocardial fibers overlying the infarction scar appear histologically normal. Detailed studies of the incidence of spontaneous ventricular arrhythmias or the inducibility of ventricular tachycardia or fibrillation have not been done in this model. However, when spontaneous arrhythmias were monitored for 60 min in 61 anesthetized cats with 2- to 4-month-old myocardial infarction, ventricular tachycardia was recorded in 4 of the 61 cats (7%), complex premature ventricular contractions in 6 (10%), and unifocal premature ventricular contractions in 13 (21%). In total, 19 of the 61 cats (31%) had some form of ventricular arrhythmia, either premature ventricular contractions or more complex ventricular arrhythmias. During studies of isolated tissue preparations, sustained ventricular activity, perhaps equivalent to ventricular tachycardia in vivo, could be induced by premature stimulation in 20 of 61 (33%) left ventricular preparations with 2- to 4-month-old infarcts. In this model cellular electrophysiologic abnormalities persist after healing of myocardial infarction, which are described later.

Other investigators have also used cats as a model of chronic myocardial infarction. Wetstein et al. (15) studied the inducibility of arrhythmias and ventricular fibrillation threshold 2 weeks after coronary artery occlusion in cats. In their studies myocardial infarction was created by occlusion of the left anterior descending artery just distal to the circumflex coronary artery, which produced extensive, transmural homogeneous infarcts of approximately 30% of the anterior wall of the left ventricle. The infarcted regions were thinned, approximately one-third to one-half of the normal ventricular wall thickness. There were no surviving islands of myocardial tissue within the infarcted area, but continuous intact endocardial and epicardial rims of viable myocardial fibers were observed. In this model ventricular fibrillation was more frequently induced by programmed electrical stimulation compared to normal cat hearts, but sustained monomorphic ventricular tachycardia was rarely induced. Data on spontaneous arrhythmias are not available from their studies.

Each of the models in both dogs and cats vary from one another in anatomic substrates and in the nature of chronic arrhythmias induced. Nevertheless, we believe that the data obtained from studies using different models of chronic infarction can be integrated and are very useful for understanding the mechanisms of electrophysiologic abnormalities and arrhythmias occurring at chronic stages of myocardial infarction.

CELLULAR ELECTROPHYSIOLOGY IN HEALED MYOCARDIAL INFARCTION

Action Potential Abnormalities

Since it is technically difficult to record electrical activity continuously for a long time after coronary artery occlusion and to record transmembrane potentials from vigorously beating in situ hearts, cellular electrophysiologic changes that occur in ventricular muscle cells and Purkinje fibers as time progresses after infarction have been determined by recording membrane potentials from the endocardial or epicardial surface of isolated ventricular tissues removed from the infarcted left ventricle and superfused with Tyrode's solution. Thus it is likely that the same phenomenon observed in studies in vitro may not always occur in vivo. Nevertheless, data obtained from these in vitro studies have provided important information on the cellular mechanisms of electrophysiologic abnormalities and arrhythmias caused by ischemia and infarction.

The membrane potentials of ventricular muscle cells in the ischemic region is affected dramatically within a few minutes after coronary artery ligation and the onset of ischemia. Resting potential, action potential amplitude, upstroke velocity, and action potential duration are reduced, and conduction velocity is slowed during acute ischemia. Figure 1A illustrates the recordings of transmembrane action potentials from the endocardial surface of the isolated left ventricle of the cat heart 90 min after coronary artery occlusion. The middle two transmembrane potentials in row C and the middle three transmembrane potentials in row D in Figure 1A were recorded from the ischemic zone; the other recordings were obtained from the surrounding normal zone. The action potential duration at 90% repolarization (APD_{90}) recorded from the cells in the ischemic zone was markedly shorter than that of normal cells. The resting potential and action potential amplitude were also reduced. In contrast, when transmembrane action potentials were recorded in the same way from the isolated left ventricle with healed myocardial infarction (2 months), the action potential duration of the cells overlying the infarct scar was significantly longer than that of the normal zone cells, as shown in Figure 1B. In Figure 1B the first transmembrane potential in row B and the first two transmembrane potentials in rows C and D were recorded from surviving cells overlying the infarct zone. Careful mapping of action potentials from the normal, border, and infarct zones in hearts with healed myocardial infarction have demonstrated that transmembrane action potentials are characterized by long action potential duration in the

PANEL **A**

90 MINUTE ACUTE MYOCARDIAL INFARCTION

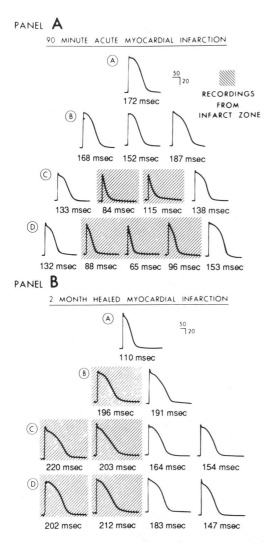

Figure 1 Transmembrane action potentials recorded from sites on the endocardium of the cat left ventricle 90 min (A) and 2 months (B) after coronary artery ligation. Transmembrane action potential duration at 90% repolarization (APD_{90}) is indicated below each recording. The hatched recordings were from cells overlying the infarct area, and the remaining recordings were from normal areas extending from the base of the heart (row A) toward the apex (row D). The cells in the acute infarct zone (A) have shorter APD_{90} values than do normal cells, and the cells in healed infarct zone (B) have longer APD_{90} values than do normal cells. [From Myerburg et al. (12), by permission of the *American Journal of Cardiology*.]

infarct zone cells and by short action potential duration and low resting membrane potential

in the border zone cells. Figure 2 illustrates representative action potentials recorded at 12 sites within a sample grid (12 mm^2) straddling areas of infarct and surrounding normal tissues from a left ventricular preparation 3 months after infarction. Action potentials having a normal configuration were recorded at the normal zone of the infarcted heart (sites A1, A3, A4, B1, and C1). Prolonged action potentials were recorded in the central infarct zone (sites C2, C3, and C4) of the same preparation. However, resting potential, action potential amplitude, and upstroke velocity were similar in cells of the normal and central infarct zones. As the electrode was moved away from the central infarct area into the border zone (sites A2, B2, B3, and B4), action potential duration shortened dramatically. In addition, action potentials recorded from the border zone cells had reduced resting potential, action potential amplitude, and upstroke velocity. Various action potential abnormalities were observed even within the border or infarct zone.

Causes for the Changes in Action Potentials

Changes in transmembrane potentials in ischemic myocardium may be caused by alteration of ionic environment and/or electrotonic interaction. Since ion-sensitive electrodes were introduced, a number of studies have focused on ionic mechanisms underlying action potential abnormalities in ischemic myocardium. The measurement of extracellular potassium concentration with potassium-sensitive electrodes has demonstrated an increase of up to 12–15 mM within 10 min after the occlusion of the coronary artery in the intact porcine heart (16,17). More recently, intracellular potassium concentration has been measured with ion-sensitive microelectrodes and has been shown to decrease during the early phase of ischemia or simulated ischemia (18,19). These changes in extracellular and intracellular potassium concentration could account for the change in resting potential in large part during acute ischemia. However, in chronic stages of infarction it is unlikely that a high potassium

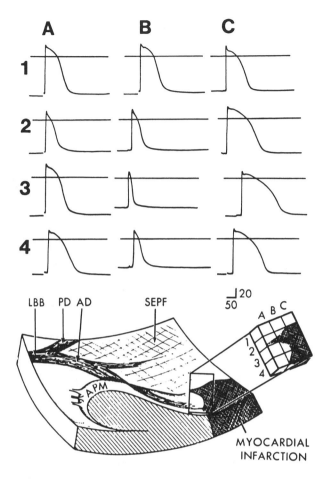

Figure 2 Transmembrane action potentials recorded from the normal, border, and infarct zones of the cat left ventricle with 3-month-old infarction. The surface of the infarct is indicated by the shaded area. The grid overlaps the border between infarct zone and surrounding normal areas. The interelectrode distance between impalements is 1.0 mm in both directions (i.e., A–C and 1–4). The cells in the border zone (A2, B2, B3, and B4) have a short action potential duration, a lower resting potential, and reduced upstroke velocity. Recordings from the infarct zone (C2, C3, and C4) show a prolongation of action potential duration compared to those recorded in normal zone cells (A1, A3, A4, B1 and C1). [From Wong et al. (13), by permission of the American Heart Association, Inc.]

concentration in the extracellular spaces is the major determinant of the loss of resting potential. When the myocardial tissues isolated from the infarcted ventricle are superfused with Tyrode's solution with a normal potassium concentration, reduced resting potentials are still recorded. Dresdner et al. (20) have shown that canine subendocardial Purkinje fibers surviving 1 day after myocardial infarction have a high intracellular sodium activity and a low potassium activity. In the feline model of chronic infarction (2–4 months) in-

tracellular sodium activity was slightly elevated and intracellular potassium activity was reduced in the border zone cells, where resting potential was reduced (21). Table 1 summarizes intracellular sodium and potassium activity measured by ion-sensitive microelectrodes in the normal, border, and infarct zone cells. The border zone cells had a higher sodium activity and a lower potassium activity, but the infarct zone cells had normal sodium and potassium activities. These findings indicate that the decrease in intracellular potassium

Table 1 Membrane Potential, Intracellular Sodium and Potassium Activity, and Calculated E_K in Normal, Border, and Infarct Zone Cells of Cat Hearts with Healed Myocardial Infarction[a]

	V_m(-mV)	$a_{Na}i$	$a_K i$	E_K (-mV)	Vm^{11}-E_K (mV)
Normal	79 ± 1	11 ± 2	90 ± 12	90 ± 4	11 ± 4
Border	68 ± 1	19 ± 6[b]	71 ± 5[b]	85 ± 2[b]	16 ± 2[b]
Infarct	79 ± 1	11 ± 3	91 ± 15	91 ± 5	12 ± 5

[a]Data are presented as mean ± standard deviation (SD). V_m = membrane potential; $a_{Na}i$ = intracellular sodium activity; $a_K i$ = intracellular potassium activity; E_K = calculated potassium equilibrium potential.
[b]Significant differences from the values in normal and infarct zone cells (P <0.01).

concentration with reduction of the potassium equilibrium potential may account for the depolarization in ischemic or border zone cells at later stages of infarction. However, the relationship between the membrane potential (V_m) and the potassium equilibrium potential (E_K) was also altered in the depolarized cells in the border zone. As shown in Table 1, the membrane potential was more positive to the potassium equilibrium potential in the border zone cells than in the normal zone cells, suggesting that a decreased potassium conductance, an increase in sodium conductance, or both is also involved in the depolarization. This hypothesis is supported by additional experiments. Figure 3 shows the relationship between membrane potential and extracellular potassium concentration in the normal zone cells and the border zone cells (depolarized cells) of the left ventricles obtained from the cat hearts with healed myocardial infarction (2–4 months). The membrane potential in border zone cells was less sensitive to the change in the extracellular potassium concentration than that in normal zone cells in the range between 2 and 10 mM [K+]. The finding that the border zone cells did not function well as a potassium electrode suggests that decreased potassium conductance and/or increased sodium conductance, in addition to decreased intracellular potassium concentration, is involved in depolarization in the border zone cells of the healed infarct hearts.

The ionic mechanisms of alterations in action potential duration in the border and infarct zone cells after healing of myocardial infarction are uncertain. The plateau of the ac-

tion potential represents a balance between inward and outward currents, and thus changes in the inward or the outward current cause alterations in action potential duration. Intracellular sodium concentration was increased in depolarized cells in the border zone, and this may lead to intracellular calcium accumulation via sodium-calcium exchange. If this is the case, increased intracellular calcium may reduce inward calcium current during the plateau phase and activate outward potassium current during repolarization, resulting in action potential shortening (22–24). If hypoxic state or irreversible metabolic changes persist in the border zone long after ischemic insults, the action potential duration may remain shortened, since hypoxia and a fall in the [ATP]$_i$ enhance the outward potassium currents (25,26). In the cells overlying the infarct with prolonged action potential duration intracellular sodium and potassium concentrations are not altered, and thus the action potential prolongation may result from electrotonic influences of surviving Purkinje fibers in the infarct zone and by electrical uncoupling from the surrounding and deeper layer cells. Further studies are required to test these hypotheses for the mechanisms underlying action potential abnormalities in the border and infarct zone cells of the heart with healed myocardial infarction.

AUTOMATICITY

Spontaneous phase 4 depolarization is enhanced in ischemic Purkinje fibers, resulting

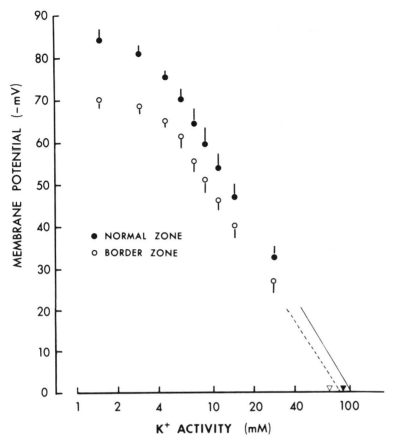

Figure 3   The relation of the membrane potential (ordinate) to the K^+ activity of the superfusate (log arithmic scale on abscissa) for the normal zone cells (filled circles) and the border zone cells (unfilled circles) of cat left ventricles with healed myocardial infarction (2–4 months). K^+ activity = K^+ coefficient (0.74) × K^+ concentration. The membrane potential in border zone cells was less sensitive to the change in the K^+ activity of the superfusate in the range between 1.5 and 7.3 mM (2 and 10 mM [K^+], respectively). [From Kimura et al. (21), by permission of the American Heart Association, Inc.]

in increased firing rates. This enhanced automaticity is not observed during the early phase of ischemia but is prominent during the first day after coronary artery occlusion in dogs. Abnormal automaticity subsides gradually over several days, and no enhanced automaticity has been observed in surviving Purkinje fibers months after coronary artery occlusion in either canine and feline models. Table 2 summarizes the action potential characteristics and automatic firing rates in Purkinje fibers in the infarct zone of the cat left ventricle with 2-to 4-month-old myocardial infarction. Action potential characteristics recorded from Purkinje fibers in the infarct zone were not statistically different from those of

Purkinje fibers in the noninfarct zone or of Purkinje fibers from normal cat hearts. Automatic firing rates were not different among Purkinje fibers from infarct or noninfarct zones or from normal cat hearts. Furthermore, automaticity in Purkinje fibers from infarct-zones was more suppressed by rapid pacing. Figure 4 illustrates the recovery cycle lengths after 15 sec of pacing at different drive rates in Purkinje fibers from infarct and noninfarct zones and from normal cat hearts. Overdrive at drive cycle lengths of less than 500 msec markedly prolonged the recovery cycle length and suppressed automaticity in Purkinje fibers from the infarct zone. These observations suggest that abnormal automaticity, if any, is a

Table 2 Action Potential Characteristics of Purkinje Fibers from the Infarct and Noninfarct Zones of Cat Hearts with Healed Myocardial Infarction and from Normal Cat Hearts[a]

	MDP (-mV)	APA (mV)	APD$_{50}$ (msec)	APD$_{90}$ (msec)	V_{max} (V/sec)	SR (b cats/min)
Normal	85 ± 1	119 ± 2	169 ± 5	237 ± 4	310 ± 17	42 ± 9
Infarct	83 ± 1	113 ± 1	156 ± 4	248 ± 7	281 ± 17	38 ± 8
Noninfarct	85 ± 1	115 ± 2	166 ± 7	231 ± 5	325 ± 18	40 ± 7

[a]Data are expressed as mean ± SEM. Normal = Purkinje fibers from normal cat hearts. Infarct = Purkinje fibers from the infarct zone of cat hearts with healed myocardial infarction. Noninfarct = Purkinje fibers from the noninfarct zone of cat hearts with head myocardial infarction. MDP = maximum diastolic potential. APA = action potential amplitude. APD$_{50}$ and APD$_{90}$ = action potential duration at 50 and 90% repolarization, respectively. V_{max} = maximum upstroke velocity of phase O of action potential. SR = spontaneous firing rate. None of the comparisons between the three groups showed statistically significant differences.

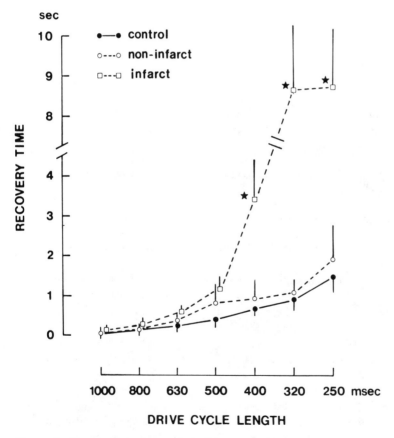

Figure 4 Corrected recovery cycle lengths in Purkinje fibers from the infarct (open squares) and noninfarct (open circles) zones of cat hearts with healed myocardial infarction (2–4 months) and from normal cat hearts (filled circles). Recovery cycle lengths were measured after 15 sec of pacing at cycle lengths from 1000 to 250 msec. The corrected recovery cycle length was longer in Purkinje fibers from the infarct zones than in Purkinje fibers from the noninfarct zones and from normal hearts at drive cycle lengths of 400 msec or less. [From Kimura et al. (27), by permission of the American Heart Association, Inc.]

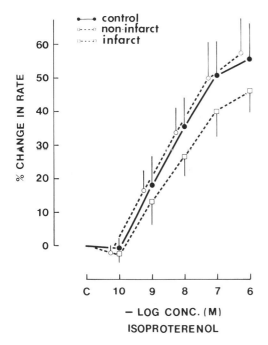

Figure 5 Concentration-response curves showing the effect of isoproterenol on automatic rates of Purkinje fibers from the infarct (open squares) and noninfarct (open circles) zones of cat hearts with healed myocardial infarction and from normal cat hearts. The response to isoproterenol was not different among the three groups. [From Kimura et al. (27), by permission of the American Heart Association, Inc.]

less likely mechanism for the arrhythmias that occur in the chronic stages of myocardial infarction.

Stimulation of β-adrenergic receptors enhances automaticity in cardiac Purkinje fibers. Such effects are exaggerated in acute myocardial infarction. Cameron and Han (28) have demonstrated that epinephrine increases the automatic rate to a greater degree in infarcted Purkinje fibers than in noninfarcted fibers 24 hr after myocardial infarction in dogs, suggesting the role of catecholamines in enhancement of arrhythmias at this stage of infarction. This enhanced response to β-adrenergic stimulation is not observed in the feline model of healed myocardial infarction. Figure 5 shows the concentration-response curves for the effect of isoproterenol (β-adrenergic stimulation) on automatic rates of Purkinje fibers in the in-

farct zone of cat left ventricles with 2- to 4-month-old myocardial infarction. Responses to isoproterenol in Purkinje fibers in the non-infarct zone and Purkinje fibers obtained from normal cat hearts are also shown in Figure 5. Isoproterenol increased the automatic rate in a concentration-dependent manner. The difference in response to isoproterenol among the three groups was not statistically significant. The response of Purkinje fibers in the infarct zone to isoproterenol rather tended to be smaller than those of Purkinje fibers from the noninfarct zone and from normal hearts, further supporting the concept that enhancement of automaticity is unlikely as a genesis of arrhythmias at chronic states of infarction.

In contrast, the response to α-adrenergic stimulation appears to be augmented in Purkinje fibers in the infarct zone. α-Adrenergic stimulation usually reduced automatic rates in Purkinje fibers of most adult mammalian hearts, and our experiments showed that this effect was enhanced in Purkinje fibers in the infarct zone. Figure 6 illustrates the changes in the spontaneous firing rate of Purkinje fibers from infarct and noninfarct zones and from normal cat hearts during superfusion with phenylephrine in the presence of propranolol (α-adrenergic stimulation). Phenylephrine at a concentration of 10^{-5} M markedly reduced the automatic rate in Purkinje fibers from the infarct zone. Corr et al. (29) have demonstrated an increase in the number of α-adrenergic receptors in acutely ischemic cat myocardium. It is conceivable that the properties of α-adrenergic receptors may be modified in Purkinje fibers from the infarct zone, but no data are available on the number or affinity of α-adrenergic receptors in hearts with healed myocardial infarction. The arrhythmogenesis associated with the enhanced α-adrenergic responses in Purkinje fibers from the infarct zone is uncertain.

TRIGGERED ACTIVITY

Triggered activity is initiated by either early or delayed afterdepolarizations. Triggered activity due to early afterdepolarizations may be initiated by high concentrations of catechola-

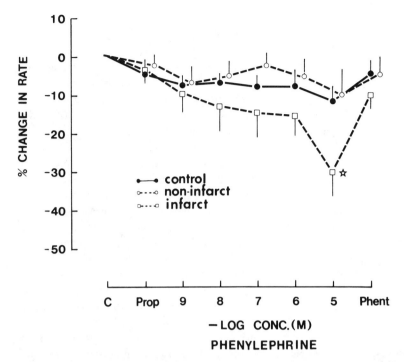

Figure 6 Concentration-response curves showing the effect of phenylephrine in the presence of 5×10^{-7} M propranolol on automatic rates of Purkinje fibers from the infarct zone (open squares) and noninfarct (open circles) zones of cat hearts with healed myocardial infarction and from normal cat hearts (filled circles). Automaticity was more suppressed by phenylephrine in Purkinje fibers from the infarct zone. C = before exposure to the drugs. Prop = propranolol (5×10^{-7} M). Phent = phentolamine (10^{-6} M).

mine, some antiarrhythmic drugs (e.g., sotalol and *N*-acetylprocainamide), and cesium (30). Delayed afterdepolarizations and triggered activity have been well demonstrated in digitalis-toxic canine Purkinje fibers, in the fibers from simian mitral valve and canine coronary sinus in the presence of catecholamines, and in diseased human atrial fibers (30). Triggered activity arising from delayed afterdepolarizations has been also observed in the 24 hr infarct, and its frequency has been reported to increase with hyperpolarization of the membrane that occurs at 48–96 hr after infarction in dogs (31,32). Delayed afterdepolarizations and triggered activity in chronic stages of myocardial infarction have also been demonstrated in the feline model (28). Figure 7 shows spontaneously developed triggered activity due to delayed afterdepolarizations in Purkinje fibers in the infarct zone isolated from the cat heart with a 3-month-old infarction. The amplitude of the delayed afterdepolarizations increased progressively as the rate

of intrinsic automaticity increased. Finally, the delayed afterdepolarizations reached threshold and induced triggered activity (indicated by stars), which persisted for several seconds to a few minutes and then stopped spontaneously. A subthreshold delayed afterdepolarization was recorded after the last action potential of the triggered activity (indicated by arrows), and then the intrinsic automaticity resumed. As the rate of intrinsic automaticity increased to a critical level, triggered activity resulting from delayed afterdepolarizations developed again. The nature of the delayed afterdepolarizations observed in Purkinje fibers from infarct zones is similar to those noted in digitalis-toxic canine Purkinje fibers. The amplitude of delayed afterdepolarizations increased and their coupling intervals decreased as the stimulation frequency or number of preceding driven beats was increased, and they were dependent on the extracellular calcium concentration. Delayed afterdepolarizations and triggered activity were recorded

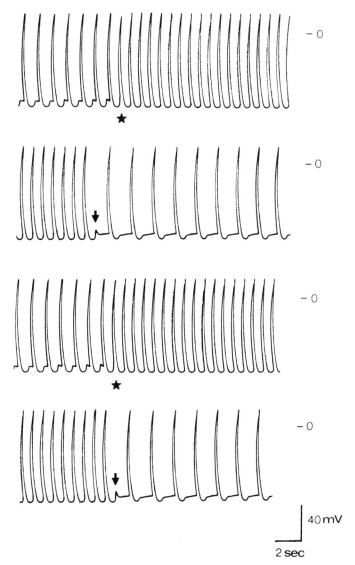

Figure 7 Delayed afterdepolarizations and triggered activity recorded from a Purkinje fiber in the infarct zone of the left ventricle isolated from cat heart with healed myocardial infarction. The amplitude of delayed afterdepolarizations increased as the intrinsic automatic rate increased. Finally, the delayed afterdepolarizations reached threshold and induced triggered activity (shown by a star in the top panel). The triggered activity stopped spontaneously after periods of several seconds to a few minutes. A subthreshold delayed afterdepolarization was recorded after the last action potential of the triggered activity (shown by an arrow in the second panel). At this point intrinsic automaticity resumed after a 1.8 sec pause, and the automatic rate gradually increased. As the rate of intrinsic automaticity increased to a critical level (third panel), triggered activity resumed. The automatic rhythm due to spontaneous depolarization appeared after cessation of triggered activity and then reinduced triggered activity as the increasing automatic rate produced afterpotentials that reached threshold. [From Kimua et al. (27), by permission of the American Heart Association, Inc.]

in 10 of 29 (34%) preparations with healed myocardial infarction. Delayed afterdepolarizations occur under conditions that cause intracellular calcium overload directly or indirectly. Cardiac glycosides increase intracellular sodium concentration inhibiting the sodium/potassium pump and thereby may increase intracellular calcium concentration via

Table 3 Functional Refractory Periods at Normal, Border, and Infarct Zones of the Cat Left Ventricles with Healed Myocardial Infarction[a]

Cycle length (msec)	Normal zone (msec)	Border zone (msec)	Infarct zone (msec)
500	156 ± 10	161 ± 14	187 ± 12[*]
630	168 ± 8	174 ± 9	190 ± 11[*]
800	167 ± 14	164 ± 16	205 ± 19[*]

[a]Data are expressed as mean ± SEM.
[*]$p < 0.05$ infarct zone versus normal and border zones.

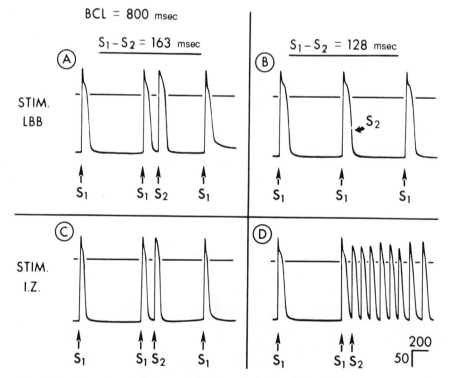

Figure 8 Induced sustained ventricular activity in an isolated left ventricular preparation with healed myocardial infarction. The action potential was recorded from a ventricular muscle cell on the endocardial surface of the infarct zone. (A, B) The recordings were made during stimulation of the left bundle branch. At an S_1-S_2 interval of 163 msec the response to the premature stimulus (S_2) is propagated to the recording electrode and initiates a single response to the premature stimulus. At a coupling interval of 128 msec (B) S_2 is blocked, presumably in the specialized conducting tissue, and no response occurs at the site of the recording electrode overlying the infarct. (C, D) The stimulus is delivered to the infarct zone, and at a coupling interval of 163 msec (C) a single response to the premature stimulus again occurs. (D) The premature stimulus delivered 128 msec after the drive stimulus initiates a run of sustained ventricular activity. Calibrations: vertical, 50 mV; horizontal, 200 msec. [From Myerburg et al. (12), by permission of the *American Journal of Cardiology*.]

sodium-calcium exchange. It is unknown at this time whether Purkinje fibers in the infarct zone that developed delayed afterdepolarizations have increased intracellular calcium or sodium concentration. Triggered activity arising from early afterdepolarizations has not been demonstrated in ischemic myocardium. Triggered activity may contribute to the genesis of some clinical ventricular tachyarrhythmias in humans, but clinical electrophysiologic methods have not yet been developed to clearly differentiate triggered activity from reentrant arrhythmias.

REENTRY

Experimental Observations

The dispersion of refractoriness and conduction abnormalities, which facilitate reentrant arrhythmias, have been demonstrated in ischemic myocardium. Refractory periods are generally determined by action potential duration in normal cardiac cells. During the early phase of acute ischemia, refractory periods shorten in parallel with action potential shortening, creating a dispersion of refractoriness between normal and ischemic regions. When the ischemia is prolonged, refractory periods commonly exceed the duration of the action potentials (postrepolarization refractoriness), producing further complex inhomogeneities of refractoriness. In healed myocardial infarction the refractory periods may be variable, depending on the degree of persistent electrophysiologic abnormalities in an area of the heart. Table 3 provides data on local functional refractory periods measured by the extrastimulus method in the normal, border, and central infarct zones of the cat left ventricles with 2- to 7-month-old infarcts. The functional refractory period of cells in the infarct zone was significantly longer than that recorded from cells in the normal and border zones, since action potential duration in the infarct zone cells was longer than that in the normal and border zone cells. The refractory period of the border zone cells was similar to that of the normal zone cells, despite the shorter action potential duration in the border

zone cells, because of postrepolarization refractoriness. However, the refractory periods may be variable even within the border and infarct zones in each heart because of variations in action potential duration and inexcitability (different degree of postrepolarization refractoriness), further facilitating the condition to induce reentrant arrhythmias. When premature stimulation was applied in these preparations sustained ventricular activity (equivalent to ventricular tachycardia) was often initiated. Figure 8 shows such repetive responses induced by a premature beat. Transmembrane action potentials were simultaneously recorded from cells in the normal, border, and infarct zones. When a premature stimulus with a coupling interval of 128 msec was delivered to the infarct zone sustained ventricular activity was initiated. During sustained activity in another preparation (Figure 9) the cells in the normal and infarct zones were activated but conduction into the border zone was blocked. When the coupling interval of the premature beat was sufficiently long the cells in the border zone were activated with significant delay. However, the premature beat with a short coupling interval did not activate the cells in the border zone, and the cells in the infarct zone were activated with delay (Figure 9). In this experiment, as the coupling interval of the basic and premature stimuli was reduced, premature activation of the recording site within the border zone occurred progressively later until, finally, it failed to respond. The border zone between the infarct and surrounding normal zones with impaired excitability and conduction may be a possible site of unidirectional block and may contribute to reentry, although reentry is not directly demonstrated in this preparation. Impaired conduction into the border zone may be related to the low resting potential and the reduced upstroke velocity or as a result of decreased coupling between cells caused by their separation by connective tissue and a reduced space constant (33,34).

The correlation between dispersion of refractoriness and arrhythmic activity in healed myocardial preparations was further suggested by experiments with procainamide. Figure 10 shows the effect of procainamide on the trans-

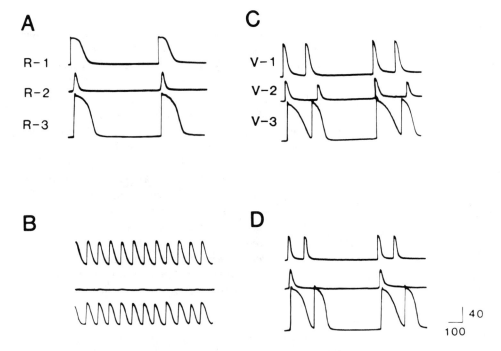

Figure 9 Effect of stimulation rate on the electrical activity of normal, border, and infarct zones of an isolated left ventricular preparation with healed myocardial infarction. (A) Simultaneous transmembrane action potentials recorded from cells in the normal (R-1), border (R-2), and infarct (R-3) zones. Drive stimuli (S_1) and premature stimuli (S_2) were delivered to a site overlying the healed infarction to induce sustained ventricular activity. (B) During sustained ventricular activity the cells from normal and infarct zones were activated, but conduction into the border zone cell was blocked. (C) V-1, V-2, and V-3 indicate action potential recordings from the cells in the normal, border, and infarct zones. At a coupling interval (S_1-S_2) of 159 msec, the cell in the border zone was activated with delay. (D) The premature beat with a shorter coupling interval (111 msec) did not activate the border zone cell but did activate the infarct zone cell with delay. Basic cycle length = 630 msec. Calibration: vertical, 40 mV; horizontal, 100 msec. [From Wong et al. (13), by permission of the American Heart Association, Inc.]

membrane action potentials recorded from the normal and infarct zones of the left ventricle with 2-month-old myocardial infarction when the preparation was superfused with Tyrode's solution containing 40 mg/L procainamide. A 45 min superfusion with the drug increased the action potential duration measured at 90% repolarization (APD_{90}) from 148 to 184 msec (+24%) in the normal zone cell and from 203 to 213 msec (+5%) in the infarct zone cell. As previously mentioned, action potential duration is longer in the infarct zone cells than in the normal zone cells. Since procainamide increased APD_{90} to a greater degree in normal zone cells than in infarct zone cells, the difference in APD_{90} between the two zone cells was reduced. As a result of such differential effects

of procainamide on action potential duration, the dispersion of local refractory periods was reduced from 28 ± 12 to 11 ± 7 msec. Accompanying these electrophysiologic effects of procainamide, sustained ventricular activity, which was reproducibly induced by premature stimulation, was no longer inducible in the presence of procainamide, as shown in Figure 11. Reduced dispersion of refractoriness by procainamide may decrease the maximum reentry frequency. Procainamide could also modify conduction properties in the reentrant circuit, with transition from unidirectional block to bidirectional block.

No mapping studies using a feline model of chronic infarction demonstrate reentrant circuits. However, the electrophysiologic proper-

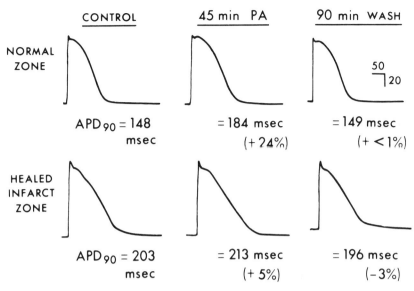

Figure 10 Effects of procainamide on transmembrane action potentials recorded from cells in the normal and infarct zones of an isolated left ventricular preparation with healed myocardial infarction. The action potential duration measured at 90% repolarization (APD_{90}) is shown under each action potential recording. Superfusion with 40 mg/L of procainamide (PA) prolonged APD_{90} to a greater extent in the normal zone cell than in the infarct zone cell. Calibration: vertical, 20 mV; horizontal 50 msec. [Modified from Myerburg et al. (14).]

ties of cat hearts with chronic, healed myocardial infarction already described can facilitate reentrant arrhythmias, such as heterogeneities in action potentials, refractory periods, and conduction. Also, sustained ventricular activity in isolated left ventricles with healed myocardial infarction can be induced by premature beats and is prevented by procainamide, which reduces heterogeneities in action potential duration and refractory periods. All these findings suggest reentry as a mechanism of such induced sustained ventricular activity.

In canine models the first experimental studies of the mechanism of chronic ventricular tachycardia were carried out 3–7 days after coronary artery ligation by El-Sherif et al. (35,36). In these studies, multiple spikes and continuous electrical activity during the entire diastolic interval were often recorded from the surviving epicardial muscle, and they were associated with the appearance of ventricular premature beats and tachycardia, suggesting the reentrant mechanism. Further evidence of

reentry as a mechanism of ventricular tachycardia in this canine model was provided by mapping activation of the epicardial muscle during tachycardia by recording up to several hundred electrograms simultaneously (37,38). In addition, Gessman et al. (39) and El-Sherif et al. (40) have demonstrated that cooling of epicardial regions over the infarcts blocks conduction in the reentrant circuit and terminates or prevents tachycardia. In more chronic stages of canine myocardial infarction ventricular tachycardia can be induced by programmed stimulation when the myocardial infarction is created by ligation of the left coronary artery and its branches (6–10). Further studies with activation mapping provide evidence of reentry as a mechanism of the induced tachycardia in the canine model of infarction of several weeks duration (6).

Clinical Observations

A large body of clinical data on the electrophysiology of chronic ventricular tachycardia

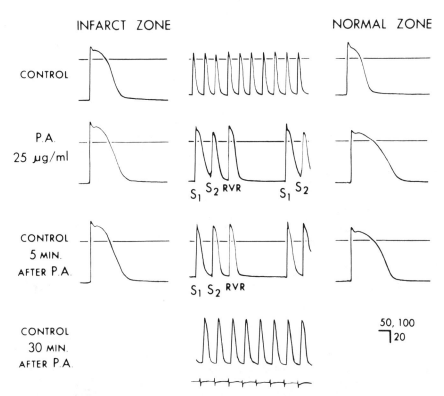

Figure 11 Effects of procainamide on transmembrane action potentials and response to premature stimulation in an isolated left ventricular preparation with healed myocardial infarction. (Left) The response of cells in the infarct zone to procainamide (PA), 25 mg/L; (right) the effects on a cell in the normal zone. (Center) The response to premature stimulation close to the refractory period before, during, and after superfusion with procainamide. Procainamide prolonged the action potential duration to a greater extent in the normal zone cell than in the infarct zone cell, and the ability to induce sustained ventricular activity disappeared during superfusion with procainamide and reappeared after washout. [From Myerburg et al. (14), by permission of the American Heart Association, Inc.]

in patients with ischemic heart disease has provided some indication about the mechanism. Ventricular tachycardia can be commonly initiated and terminated by programmed electrical stimulation or rapid pacing of the heart in patients with chronic ischemic heart disease and previous myocardial infarction who have a history of spontaneous episodes of sustained arrhythmias (41,42) Tachycardia is initiated by critically timed premature beats. When tachycardia is initiated by rapid ventricular pacing, only specific pacing cycle lengths are effective to induce the arrhythmia. Tachycardia can often be terminated by overdrive or premature stimulation. These observations provide evidence that the chronic ventricular tachycardias are caused by reentry.

However, these findings are not definitive proof of reentry. Triggered activity can also be initiated and terminated by rapid or premature stimulation (43). A direct demonstration of reentrant excitation and the reentrant circuits has been sought with mapping of the activation sequence during ventricular tachycardia. These studies have shown the site of origin of the arrhythmias, the region of earliest activation, probably where the impulse exits from the reentrant circuit, and the site of fractionated or continuous electrical activity (slow conduction) (44). Surgical resection of this region often abolishes tachycardias (45), supporting the concept that this is where arrhythmia originates. From these considerations most of chronic ventricular tachycardia may be caused by reentry.

ACUTE ISCHEMIA AND HEALED MYOCARDIAL INFARCTION

The majority of survivors of cardiac arrest have extensive coronary artery disease, usually with previous myocardial infarction (1,46,47). The high incidence of recurrent ventricular fibrillation and sudden cardiac death in this group suggests that transient ischemic events in the presence of preexisting healed myocardial infarction enhance the risk of the occurrence of fatal arrhythmias. Experimentally, the incidence of spontaneous ventricular tachycardia and fibrillation is higher when acute ischemia is superimposed on previous myocardial infarction than with acute ischemia alone in both the canine and feline models (12,48,49). Garan et al. (49) have shown that spontaneous ventricular fibrillation during transient occlusion of the marginal branch of the left circumflex coronary artery increase from 13% without infarction to 54% 2 weeks after permanent ligation of the left anterior descending coronary artery. In the feline model, spontaneous arrhythmias insitu and induced sustained ventricular activity in isolated tissues were more often observed in the preparations with acute ischemia (90 min of ligation of the coronary arteries 5–10 mm proximal to the site of the previous ligations) superimposed on healed myocardial infarction (>2 months) compared to preparations with acute ischemia or healed myocardial infarction alone (12). Enhanced arrhythmogenesis in hearts with acute ischemia and preexisting infarction may result from a greater disparity of electrophysiologic characteristics and from increased infarct size. In the studies by Kabel et al. (50) in a canine model of infarction, coronary artery stenosis markedly reduced blood flow to the collateral-dependent periinfarction zone in the epicardium; blood blow to the normal myocardium was little affected. In addition, the epicardial periinfarction zone is very sensitive to the coronary flow reduction and the site of the most severe electrophysiologic disturbances. Garan et al. (49) demonstrated that decreased myocardial blood flow in the lateral infarct border and lateral periinfarction zones during superimposed acute ischemia

was significantly lower in dogs that developed spontaneous ventricular fibrillation than in dogs that did not, indicating that the reduction in coronary blood flow to the infarct border and periinfarct zones and subsequently their electrophysiologic derangement play a role in arrhythmogenesis. These findings suggest that the surviving infarct border zones which are dependent on collateral coronary perfusion, could be the sites of origin of the arrhythmias that develop during transient occlusion in hearts with preexisting infarction.

The electrophysiologic mechanisms of enhanced arrhythmogenesis by superimposition of acute ischemia on chronic, healed myocardial infarction are complex and are not yet well understood. The concept is that the subsequent acute ischemia increases electrophysiologic heterogeneities that are already present in infarcted hearts. Figure 12 shows the disparity of the local refractory periods measured in the cat left ventricular preparations isolated from normal hearts, hearts with acute ischemia (90–120 min after coronary artery ligation), hearts with healed myocardial infarction (2–4 months), and hearts with acute ischemia superimposed on healed myocardial infarction. The range of refractory periods, from shortest to longest, was greatest in the preparations with acute ischemia superimposed on healed myocardial infarction, indicating a greater dispersion of recovery of excitability in this condition.

The dynamic cellular electrophysiologic effects of transient acute ischemia (30 min) superimposed on chronic, healed myocardial infarction were recently studied in the feline model (51). These studies were carried out in the isolated perfused coronary left ventricles with healed myocardial infarction with recordings of transmembrane action potentials from normal and infarct zone cells. Figure 13 shows action potential changes in normal and infarct zone cells when coronary perfusion was discontinued. Action potentials were markedly deteriorated in the normal zone cells during 30 min of ischemia, but they were less affected in the infarct zone cells. Local refractory periods in the normal zone shortened in parallel with the shortening of action potential

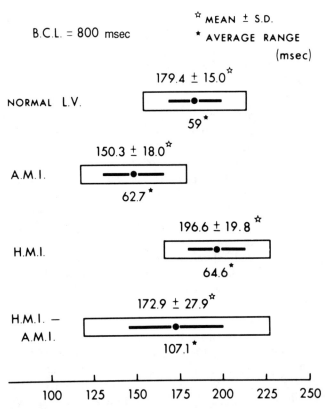

Figure 12 The range of local refractory periods for each of the four experimental conditions: normal cat left ventricle (normal L.V.), acute myocardial infarction (A.M.I.), healed myocardial infarction (H.H.I.), and acute myocardial infarction superimposed on healed myocardial infarction (H.M.I-A.M.I.). The mean refractory periods were shortest in preparations with acute infarction, longest in those with healed infarction, and intermediate and nearly equal in normal preparations and those with acute infarction superimposed on healed infarction. However, these last preparations have the greatest dispersion of refractoriness, with an average range of 107.1 msec compared to 59.0, 62.7, and 64.6 msec for normal preparations and preparations with acute and healed infarction, respectively. B.C.L. = basic cycle length. [From Myerburg et al. (12), by permission of the American Heart Association, Inc.]

duration during ischemia, but they did not change in the infarct zone. As shown in Figure 14, there were significant differences in action potential characteristics between the normal and infarct zone cells during acute ischemia. More complex electrophysiologic heterogeneities are expected between normal and acutely ischemic tissues as well as acutely ischemic and chronically infarcted tissues in hearts in situ.

CONCLUSION

An expanding body of clinical, epidemiologic, and experimental data highlight the complex-

ity of pathophysiologic mechanisms responsible for the initiation of lethal arrhythmias in chronic myocardial infarction. Although pre-existing myocardial infarction enhances the propensity to arrhythmias, the superimposition of acute ischemia and reperfusion and neurophysiologic and metabolic factors all interact in the transition from an abnormal but stable myocardium to an electrically unstable muscle mass. More studies are needed to clarify the ionic, subcellular, and molecular bases underlying electrophysiologic abnormalities in acutely and chronically ischemic myocardium to achieve a better understanding of the precise mechanisms of ischemic arrhythmias.

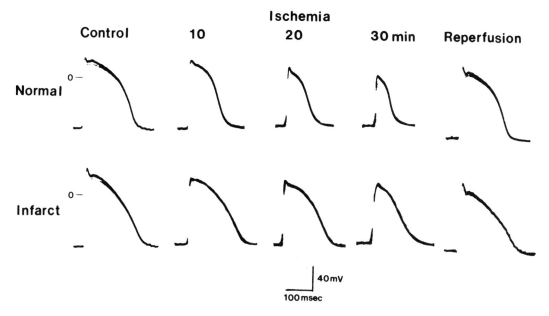

Figure 13 Effects of transient acute ischemia on transmembrane action potentials recorded from cells in the normal and infarct zones of an isolated cat left ventricular preparation with healed myocardial infarction. The preparation was perfused through the coronary arteries with oxygenated Tyrode's solution, and ischemia was produced by stopping coronary perfusion. The action potential in the normal zone cell was markedly deteriorated during 30 min of ischemia; that in the infarct zone cell was less affected. [From Kimura et al. (50), by permission of the American Heart Association, Inc.]

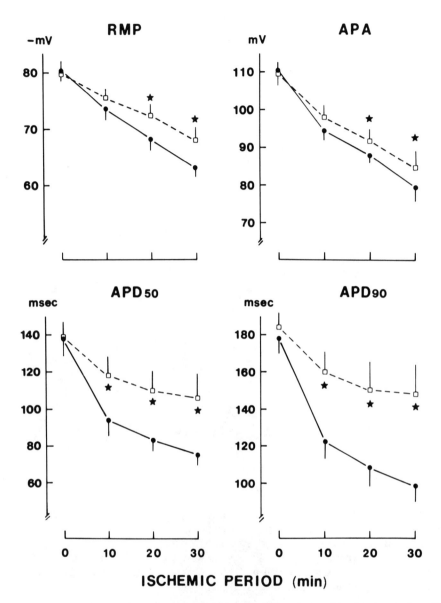

Figure 14 Changes in action potential characteristics during 30 of ischemia in cells of normal (filled circles) and infarct (open squares) zones of isolated cat left ventricular preparations with healed myocardial infarction. The preparations were perfused through the coronary arteries with oxygenated Tyrode's solution, and ischemia was produced by stopping coronary perfusion. Resting membrane potential (RMP), action potential amplitude (APA), and action potential duration at 50 and 90% repolarization (APD$_{50}$ and APD$_{90}$, respectively) were reduced to a lesser degree in cells of the infarct zone than in cells of the normal zone. [From Kimura et al. (50), by permission of the American Heart Association, Inc.]

REFERENCES

1. Myerburg R J, Castellanos A. Cardiac arrest and sudden cardiac death. In: Braunwald E ed. Heart disease: textbook of cardiovascular medicine. Philadelphia, W. B. Saunders, 1988: pp 742–7.

2. Friedman P L, Stewart J R, Fenoglio J J, Wit A L. Survival of subendocardial Purkinje fibers after extensive myocardial infaction in dogs. Circ Res 1973; 33:597–611.

3. Friedman P L, Stewart J R, Wit A L. Spontaneous and induced cardiac arrhythmias in subendocardial Purkinje fibers surviving extensive myocardial infarction in dogs. Circ Res 1973; 33:612–26.

4. Friedman P L, Stewart J R, Wit A L. Time course for reversal of electrophysiological and ultrastructural abnormalities in subendocardial Purkinje fibers surviving extensive myocardial infarction in dogs. Circ Res 1975; 36:127–44.

5. Lazzara R, El-Sherif N, Scherlag B J. Early and late effects of coronary artery occlusion on canine Purkinje fibers. Circ Res 1974; 35:391–9.

6. Garan H, Fallon J R, Ruskin J N. Sustained ventricular tachycardia in a recent canine myocardial infarction. Circulation 1980; 62: 980–7.

7. Garan H, Ruskin J N. Localized reentry: mechanism of induced sustained ventricular tachycardia in canine model of recent myocardial infarction. J. Clin Invest 1984; 74: 377–92.

8. Michelson E L, Spear J F, Moore E N. Electrophysiologic and anatomic correlates of sustained ventricular tachyarrhythmias in a model of chronic myocardial infarction. Am J Cardiol 1980; 45:583–90.

9. Michelson E L, Spear J F, Moore E N. Initiation of sustained ventricular tachyarrhythmias in a canine model of chronic myocardial infarction. Importance of the site of stimulation. Circulation 1981; 63:776–84.

10. Klein G J, Ideker R E, Smith W M, Harrison L A, Kasell J, Wallace A G, Gallangher J J. Epicardial mapping of the onset of ventricular tachycardia initiated by programmed stimulation in the canine heart with chronic infarction. Circulation 1979; 60:1375–84.

11. Myerburg R J, Gelband H, Nilsson K, Sung R J, Thurer R J, Morales A R, Bassett A L. Long-term electrophysiological abnormalities resulting from experimental myocardial infarction in cats. Circ Res 1977; 41:73–84.

12. Myerburg R J, Epstein K, Gaide M S, Wong S S,Castellanos A, Gelband H, Bassett A L. Electrophysiologic consequences of experimental acute ischemia superimposed on healed myocardial infarction in cats. Am J Cardiol 1982; 49:323–30.

13. Wong S S, Bassett A L, Cameron J S, Epstein K, Koslovskis P L, Myerburg R J. Dissimilarities in the electrophysiological abnormalities of lateral border and central infarct zone cells after healing of myocardial infarction in cats. Circ Res 1982; 51:486–93.

14. Myerburg R J, Bassett A L, Epstein K, Gaide M S, Kozlovskis P, Wong S S, Castellanos A, Gelband H. Electrophysiological effects of procainamide in acute and healed experimental ischemic injury of cat myocardium. Circ Res 1982; 50:386–93.

15. Wetstein L, Mark R, Kelliher G J, Friehling T, O'Connor K M, Kowey P R. Arrhythmia inducibility and ventricular vulnerability in a chronic feline infarction model. Am Heart J 1985; 110:955–60.

16. Hirche H J, Franz C, Bos L, Bissig R, Schramm M. Myocardial extracellular K^+ and H^+ increase and noradrenaline release as possible cause of early arrhythmias following acute coronary artery occlusion in pigs. J Mol Cell Cardiol 1980; 12:579–93.

17. Hill J L, Gettes L S. Effect of acute coronary artery occlusion on local myocardial extracellular K^+ activity in swine. Circulation 1980; 61:768–78.

18. Kleber A G. Resting membrane potential, extracellular potassium activity, and intracellular sodium activity during acute global ischemia in isolated perfused guinea pig hearts. Circ Res 1983; 52:442–450.

19. Nakaya H, Kimura S, Kanno M. Intracellular K^+ and Na^+ activities under hypoxia, acidosis and no glucose in dog hearts. Am J. Physiol 1985; 249:H1078–85.

20. Dresdner K, Kline R P, Wit A L. Intracellular K^+ activity, intracellular Na^+ activity and maximum diastolic potential of canine subendocardial Purkinje cells from one-day-old infarcts. Circ Res 1987; 60:122–32.

21. Kimura S, Bassett A L, Gaide M S, Kozlovskis P L, Myerburg R J. Regional changes in intracellular potassium and sodium activity after healing of experimental myocardial infarction in cats. Circ Res 1986; 58:202–8.

22. Tsien R W. Calcium channels in excitable cell membranes. Annu Rev Physiol 1983; 45: 341–58.

23. Isenberg G. Cardiac Purkinje fibers. $[Ca^{2+}]^i$ controls steady state potassium conductance. Pflugers Arch 1977; 371:71–6.

24. Isenberg G. Cardiac Purkinje fibers. $[Ca^{2+}]i$ controls the potassium permeability via the conductance components gK_1 and gK_2. Pflugers Arch 1977; 371:77–85.

25. Vleugels A, Vereecke J, Carmeliet E. Ionic currents during hypoxia in voltage-clamped cat ventricular muscle. Circ Res 1980; 47:501–8.

26. Noma A. ATP-regulated K^+ channels in cardiac muscle. Nature 1983; 305:147–8.

27. Kimura S, Bassett A L, Kohya T, Kozlovskis P L, Myerburg R J. Automaticity, triggered activity, and responses to adrenergic stimulation in cat subendocardial Purkinje fibers after healing of myocardial infarction. Circulation 1987; 75:651–60.

28. Cameron J S, Han J. Effects of epinephrine on automaticity and the incidence of arrhythmias in Purkinje fibers surviving myocardial infarction. J Pharmacol Exp Ther 1982; 223:573–9.

29. Corr P B, Shayman J A, Dramer J B, Kipnis R J. Increased α-adrenergic receptors in ischemic cat myocardium: a potential mediator of electrophysiological derangments. J Clin Invest 1981; 67:1232–6.

30. Zipes D P. Genesis of cardiac arrhythmias: electrophysiological considerations. In Braunwald E, ed. Heart disease: textbook of cardiovascular medicine. Philadelphia: W. B. Saunders, 1988: 581–620.

31. El-Sherif N, Gough W B, Zeiler R H, Mehra R. Triggered ventricular rhythm in one-day-old myocardial infarction in the dog. Circ Res 1983; 52:566–79.

32. Marec H L, Dangman K H, Danilo P, Rosen M R. An evaluation of automaticity and triggered activity in the canine heart one to four days after myocardial infarction. Circulation 1985; 71:1224–36.

33. Ursell P C, Gardner P I, Albala A, Fenoglio J J, Wit A L. Structural and electrophysiological changes in the epicardial border zone of canine myocardial infarcts during infarct healing. Circ Res 1985; 56:436–451.

34. Spear J F, Michelson E L, Moore E N. Reduced space constant in slowly conducting regions of chronically infarcted canine myocardium. Circ res 1983; 53:176–85.

35. El-Sherif N, Hope R R, Scherlag B J, Lazzara R. Reentrant ventricular arrhythmias in the late myocardial infarction period. 1. Conduction characteristics in the infarction zone. 1977; 55:686–702.

36. El-Sherif N. Hope R R, Scherlag B J, Lazzara R. Reentrant ventricular arrhythmias in the late myocardial infarction period. 2. Pattern of initiation and termination of reenty. Circulation 1977; 55:702–19.

37. Wit A L, Allessie M A, Bonke FIM, Lammers W, Smeets J, Fenoglio J J. Electrophysiological mapping to determine the mechanism of experimental ventricular tachycardia initiated by premature impulses. Experimental approach and initial results demonstrating reentrant excitation. Am J Cardiol 1982; 49:166–85.

38. El-Sherif N, Sith A, Evans K. Canine ventricular arrhythmias in the late myocardial infarction period. 8. Epicardial mapping of reentrant circuits. Circ Res 1981; 49:255–65.

39. Gessman L J, Agarwal J B, Endo T, Helfant R H. Localization and mechanism of ventricular tachycardia by ice mapping 1 week after the onset of myocardial infarction in dogs. Circulation 1983; 68:657–66.

40. El-Sherif N, Mehra R, Gough W B, Zeiles R H. Reentrant ventricular arrhythmias in the late myocardial infarction period: interruption of reentrant circuits by cryothermal techniques. Circulation 1983; 68:644–56.

41. Wellens H J J, Duren D R, Lie K L. Observations on mechanisms of ventricular tachycardia in man. Circulation 1976; 54:237–44.

42. Josephson M E, Horowitz L N, Farshidi A, Kastor J A. Recurrent sustained ventricular tachycardia. 1. Mechanisms. Circulation 1978; 57:431–40.

43. Wit A L, Wiggins J R, Cranefield P F. The effects of electrical stimulation on impulse initiation in cardiac fibers; its relevance for the determination of the mechanisms of clinical cardia arrhythmias. In: by Wellens H J J, Lie K I, Janse M J, eds. The conduction system of the heart; structure, function and clinical implications. Leiden: Stenfert Kroese, 1976:

44. Josephson M E, Horowitz L N, Farshidi A, Spear J F, Kastor J A, Moore E N. Recurrent sustained ventricular tachycardia. 2. Endocardial mapping. Circulation 1978; 57:440–7.

45. Josephson M E, Harken A H, Horowitz L N. Endocardial excision: a new surgical technique for treatment of recurrent ventricular tachycardia. Circulation 1979; 60:1430–9.

46. Ruskin J N, DiMarco J P, Garan H. Out-of-hospital cardiac arrest: electrophysiologic observations and selection of long-term antiarrhythmic therapy. N Engl J Med 1980; 303:607–13.

47. Josephson M E, Horowitz L N, Spielman S R, Greenspan A M. Electrophysiologic and hemodynamic studies in patients resuscitated from cardiac arrest. Am J Cardiol 1980; 46:948 55.

48. Patterson E, Holland K, ELler B T, Lucchesi B R. Ventricular fibrillation resulting from ischemia at a site remote from previous myocardial infarction. Am J Cardiol 1982; 50:1414–23.

49. Garan H, McComb J M, Ruskin J N. Sponta-neous and electrically induced ventricular arrhythmias during acute ischemia superimposed on two week-old canine myocardial infarction. J Am Coll Cardiol 1988; 11:603–11.

50. Kabel G, Brachmann J, Scherlag B J, Harrison L, Lazzara R. Mechanisms of ventricular arrhythmias in multivessel coronary disease: the effects of collateral zone ischemia. Am Heart J 1984; 108:447–54.

51. Kimura S, Bassett A L, Cameron J S, Huikuri H, Koslovskis P L, Myerburg R J. Cellular electrophysiological changes during ischemia in isolated, coronary-perfused cat ventricle with healed myocardial infarction. Circulation 1988; 78:401–6.

16

Proarrhythmic Effects of Antiarrhythmic Drugs

Kenneth H. Dangman

College of Physicians and Surgeons, Columbia University
New York, New York

Dennis S. Miura

Albert Einstein College of Medicine
Bronx, New York

INTRODUCTION

Drug-induced arrhythmias have been recognized as an important clinical problem in recent years. In fact, proarrhythmic toxicity has dominated the headlines with respect to clinical testing of antiarrhythmic drugs. Established concepts in pharmacokinetic modeling of drug plasma concentrations include "minimum effective concentration" and "threshold for toxicity." The goal of antiarrhythmic drug management is to attain drug concentrations in the therapeutic range, between ineffective (low) and toxic (high) plasma levels. Plasma levels above the therapeutic range can result from use of an inappropriately large dose, changes in drug clearance, or drug interactions (1).

However, in some patients antiarrhythmic drug toxicity can occur even if the plasma concentrations are in the therapeutic range. For antiarrhythmic drugs these toxic effects can involve not only the cardiovascular system but the central nervous system and peripheral organs (Table 1). This chapter focuses on the "proarrhythmic" effects of these agents (Table 2).

Antiarrhythmic drug toxicity may result in the development of new types of arrhythmias or in intensification of preexisting arrhythmias (2, 3). Depending on the drug and the patient population, proarrhythmic effects have been reported to occur in 5–20% of patients (4). In fact, data from the Cardiac Arrhythmia Suppression Trial (CAST) suggest that these iatrogenic arrhythmias may contribute to about 5% of out-of-hospital cardiac arrests (5).

Abnormalities of impulse initiation and/or conduction, alone or in combination, can cause a variety of cardiac arrhythmias in patients with heart disease (Table 3).

In addition to providing the anatomic and physiologic substrates for spontaneous cardiac arrhythmias, heart disease predisposes patients to the development of proarrhythmic side effects (2,3). The networks of cells that generate arrhythmias are commonly referred to as "arrhythmogenic zones." These zones typically are created by ischemia, stretch, or drug toxicity. Studies of drug toxicity in cardiac tissues from animals provide insights into the electrophysiology of arrhythmic zones. These studies suggest that the causes of arrhythmias include both abnormal impulse initiation and abnormal impulse conduction.

Table 1   Side Effects of Antiarrhythmic Drugs

Drug	Typical toxic threshold plasma level (μg/ml)	Toxic effects
Quinidine	> 6	Cardiovascular collapse and severe hypotension (quinidine syncope after IV administration)
		Conduction block (AV node, ventricles)
		Negative inotropic effects
		Ventricular arrhythmias
		Mild cinchonism: tinnitus, loss of hearing, blurring of vision
		Severe cinchonism: headache, vertigo, diplopia, photophobia, confusion, delirium, psychosis
		Gastrointestinal upset (nausea, vomiting, and diarrhea) forces discontinuation quinidine in about one-third of patients
		Hypersensitivity: fever, anaphylaxis, thrombocytopenia, asthmalike respiratory symptoms
Procainamide	> 10	Severe myocardial depression and hypotension (after rapid IV injection)
		Arrhythmias (ventricular ectopic beats, tachycardia, and fibrillation)
		Gastrointestinal effects: nausea, vomiting, anorexia occasionally occur
		CNS effects: giddiness, psychosis, hallucinations, and mental depression
		Hypersensitivity: fever, granulocytopenia, lupuslike syndrome with arthritis, arthralgia, and pleuritis
Disopyramide	> 4	Myocardial depression and arterial constriction lead to reduced cardiac output; arrhythmias and conduction disturbances possible
		Gastrointestinal symptoms: nausea, vomiting, diarrhea, abdominal pain
		Anticholinergic effects produce a significant incidence of dry mouth, blurred vision, constipation, and urinary hesitancy or retention
Lidocaine	> 5	Minimal cardiovascular toxicity but may produce adverse effects in patients with severely compromised ventricular function
		CNS effects: mild drowsiness, agitation, paresthesias leading to disorientation, hearing loss, muscle twitching, convulsion and respiratory arrest
Phenytoin	> 20	CNS effects: drowsiness, vertigo, nystagmus, ataxia, and nausea
		Cardiovascular effects (can develop if phenytoin is injected rapidly IV) include cardiac arrhythmias with or without hypotension
Propranolol	0.1–3	Sinus bradycardia or arrest, AV block, ventricular failure and hypotension; rapid withdrawal can exacerbate angina pectoris and ventricular arrhythmias or lead to myocardial infarction
		Exacerbation of asthma

Table 1 Continued

Drug	Typical toxic threshold plasma level (μg/ml)	Toxic effects
Amiodarone	—	Gastrointestinal effects include nausea, diarrhea, gastric pain, constipation CNS effects include hallucinations and insomnia Sinus bradycardia, AV block, ventricular tachycardias, and hypotension Corneal microdeposits Photodermatitis with blue-gray discoloration of the skin Thyroid dysfunction Pulmonary toxicity; pneumonitis, severe dyspnea, and pulmonary fibrosis (can be fatal)
Verapamil	> 2	Decreased cardiac contractility and hypotension (following rapid IV injection); sinus bradycardia, AV block, and ventricular asystole can occur in patients with preexisting disease of the sinus or AV node Gastrointestinal effects include constipation and nausea CNS effects include vertigo and dizziness

Some types of toxicity may reflect exaggeration of clinically useful therapeutic drug effects. This is most easily seen in those arrhythmias caused by overdoses of class I or IV antiarrhythmic drugs. Their therapeutic effect is in part to decrease action potential upstroke velocity and slow conduction in the ventricular conduction system or atrioventricular node. Toxic arrhythmias may therefore be caused by excessive reduction of depolarization velocity, which leads to conduction block or reentrant activation in the atrioventricular node or myocardium.

Toxic effects of antiarrhythmic drugs must therefore be understood in the context of their therapeutic actions. A classification system for antiarrhythmic drugs has been proposed by Vaughan-Williams that divides these agents into four categories according to therapeutic actions (6,7). These actions are (1) local anesthetic effect, that is, reduction of rapid sodium influx and the maximum upstroke velocity (dV/dt_{max}) during phase 0 of the action potential; (2) β-adrenergic receptor blockade; (3) prolongation of action potential duration and refractoriness; and (4) reduction

Table 2 Proarrhythmic Effects of Antiarrhythmic Agents

Bradycardia
  Sinus bradycardia, arrest, or sinoatrial exit block
  AV block
Tachycardia
  Supraventricular tachycardia
  Ventricular tachyarrhythmias
    Increased VPD frequency
    Uniform ventricular tachycardias
    Polymorphic ventricular tachycardias
    Torsades-de-pointes tachycardia with or without prolonged QT interval
    Ventricular fibrillation

Table 3 Electrophysiologic Mechanisms of Ventricular Arrhythmias

Arrhythmias caused by abnormal impulse conduction
   Conduction blocks
   Reentrant activation
      Macroreentry
         Fixed pathway/anatomic barrier
         Variable pathway/"leading circle"
      Microreentry
         Functional longitudinal dissociation
         Reflection
Arrhythmias caused by enhanced impulse initiation in ectopic foci
   Automatic rhythms
      Normal Purkinje fiber automaticity (MDP > -80 mV)
      Catecholamine-enhanced automaticity in normal Purkinje fibers
      Abnormal automaticity (MDP < -60 mV) in Purkinje fibers and ventricular muscle cells
   Triggered rhythms
      Early afterdepolarizations
      Delayed afterdepolarizations
Arrhythmias caused by simultaneous derangements of impulse initiation and impulse conduction
   Parasystole
   Complex arrhythmias

of transmembrane calcium influx via the "slow inward current." The class I drugs are subdivided further into several groups based on different effects on QT interval and/or on the time constants of "use-dependent effects" of the drugs on dV/dt_{max} or inward sodium current (6,7).

To produce therapeutic effects antiarrhythmic drugs exert selective actions on the arrhythmogenic zones of the heart in vivo. Most antiarrhythmic drugs are clinically useful simply because they make arrhythmogenic zones electrically silent. They also do not affect undamaged segments of the heart but allow them to continue to function normally, both electrically and mechanically. Antiarrhythmic drugs may exert these effects "directly" by blocking ionic channels in the sarcolemma, or possibly "indirectly" by altering autonomic nerve activity to the heart (8). The arrhythmogenic effects of these drugs may also result from these direct and indirect actions. Unlike therapeutic effects, toxic effects may be produced by drug actions on either the undamaged segments of the heart or on the arrhythmogenic zone.

CONDUCTION BLOCK

Antiarrhythmic drugs can cause conduction blocks and bradycardias (9,10). Patients with preexisting disease of the sinoatrial or atrioventricular nodal regions are particularly susceptible to development of conduction blocks.

Consider a patient with abnormally high vagal tone to the heart, with or without underlying disease of the junctional region. This is most commonly seen in acute inferior wall myocardial infarctions. Complete heart block may occur if antiarrhythmic drugs are given. This is caused by additive depression of atrioventricular node impulse conduction. Suppression of atrioventricular node conduction often presents as third-degree atrioventricular block or junctional rhythm. This rhythm is caused by ventricular (e.g., His bundle) automaticity. In the normal heart this automaticity results from the normal physiologic function of Purkinje cells. That is, after the effects of overdrive suppression, from faster pacemaker sites above the atrioventricular node, on the Purkinje cells have dissipated, a junctional pacemaker in the His bundle or bundle branches emerges. This pacemaker is under the influence of appropri-

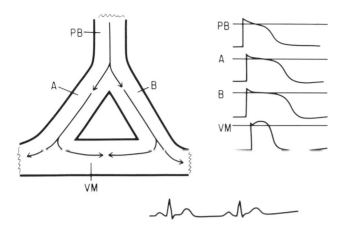

Figure 1 Normal conduction through a branch of the His-Purkinje system. Schmitt-Erlanger diagram at the left shows one of the branches of the Purkinje network. PB, proximal bundle; A and B, two distal branches; and VM, ventricular muscle. Action potential duration and refractory periods are longest in distal Purkinje fibers of A and B. The impulses normally conduct through A and B and activate ventricular muscle. The wavefronts of activation then collide in ventricular wall and terminate. Action potentials at right are from point indicated in drawing at left. Action potentials show activation sequence in the ventricle, producing normal ECG as shown below. (Republished from Dangman KH, Boyden PA. Cellular mechanisms of cardiac arrhythmias, in: Fox PR, ed. Canine and feline Cardiology. New York: Churchill Livingstone, 1988: with permission of the publisher.)

ate β-adrenergic stimulation. Treatment with β-adrenergic blockers or some antiarrhythmic drugs, such as lidocaine (11), may make the junctional rate too low to sustain an adequate cardiac output for perfusion of critical organs. If treatment with these drugs stops normal automaticity in the junctional and ventricular pacemakers in a patient with complete heart block, death can occur.

The suppression of Purkinje fiber automaticity by class I drugs illustrates why antiarrhythmic agents must be regarded as "two-edged swords." One would normally consider ventricular pacemaker activity as a cause of arrhythmias, such as parasystolic or premature beats. Under some circumstances these ventricular beats can lead to R-on-T phenomena and ventricular fibrillation. However, suppression of ventricular automaticity can also be a fatal effect if it causes ventricular asystole. In addition, even individuals being treated for other diseases may experience conduction disturbances as a result of antiarrhythmic drug interactions. Treating hypertension with a class IV drug (e.g., verapamil) in addition to therapy with a class II drug (e.g., propranolol) can precipitate complete heart block.

Complete heart block as a side effect of antiarrhythmic drug therapy is a particular danger in the setting of digitalis toxicity. This is because digitalis increases vagal tone and decreases atrioventricular node conduction velocity. Therefore antiarrhythmic drugs that can further decrease atrioventricular node conduction and suppress automaticity should be avoided whenever possible during digitalis-induced tachycardias.

Reentrant Activation

A structurally normal heart generally does not provide a good substrate for reentrant arrhythmias. This can change if toxic antiarrhythmic drug effects are superimposed on the tissues of the heart. If the electrophysiologic substrate is altered, reentry may occur by one or more mechanisms. These mechanisms include (1) classic "circus movement" arrhythmias in a defined anatomic pathway, (2) "leading circle" arrhythmias, and (3) microreentry caused by functional longitudinal dissociation in a small segment of myocardium.

A three-step process is required for reentry to occur. Conduction of the antegrade (sinus)

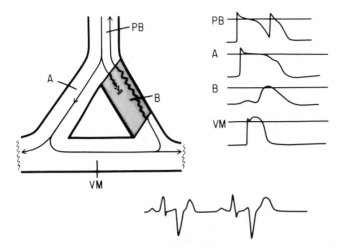

Figure 2 Reentry depicted in the Schmitt-Erlanger diagram. Same format as in Figure 1. Antegrade impulse conducts normally through proximal bundle (PB) and distal bundle A but slowly and decrementally through B (wavy line) and blocks in the damaged zone. The impulse conducts through the ventricle from insertion sites of branch A and enters the damage zone from the distal margin. It conducts slowly in the retrograde direction through B and reenters the proximal bundle. This can cause premature coupled ventricular depolarizations as depicted by action potentials at right and ECG below. (Republished from Dangman KH, Boyden PA. Cellular mechanisms of cardiac arrhythmias, in: Fox PR, ed. Canine and feline cardiology. New York: Churchill Livingstone, 1988: with permission of the publisher.)

impulse (Fig. 1) must block in the arrhythmogenic zone (Fig. 2) and must also spread to a distal margin of the arrhythmogenic zone (Fig. 2). The impulse must then conduct through a "protected" pathway in the arrhythmogenic zone. This takes the wavefront of activation in the retrograde direction, toward and then through the site of antegrade block. Finally, the retrograde impulse must propagate through the normal tissues proximal to the site of block and reactivate the rest of the heart. If the propagation velocity is too fast through the arrhythmogenic zone, the retrograde impulse arrives at a critical site in the tissue loop (i.e., at or proximal to the site of antegrade block) before these sites have recovered excitability. This produces bidirectional conduction block and prevents reentry. Thus reentry occurs only in the presence of unidirectional conduction block and slow conduction.

Antiarrhythmic drugs can produce conduction blocks and reentry in either a fixed anatomic circuit or in a variable (leading circle arrhythmia) circuit. Clinically, reentrant arrhythmias are most commonly seen in chronic myocardial infarctions in which the anatomic

substrates for reentry in fixed circuits are likely to occur. Reentry in fixed circuits depends on the occurrence of unidirectional block in a very specific site. In contrast, reentry in a variable circuit depends on functional block at shifting sites within a more generalized arrhythmogenic zone. Functional blocks occur in partially depolarized atrial and ventricular tissues (12–14).

Antiarrhythmic drugs could produce reentry by several mechanisms at the cellular level.

Reduction of Maximum Rate of Depolarization During Phase 0

Class I antiarrhythmic drugs are believed to work, in part, by eliminating reentrant activity. They appear to have selective effects on the sodium current-dependent upstrokes of partially depolarized cells in the arrhythmogenic zone. These effects can convert one-way block to bidirectional block and thus abolish reentrant activity (Fig. 3).

Class I agents may generate arrhythmias by exaggeration of these same effects (15). Figure 4 depicts such toxic effects. Under

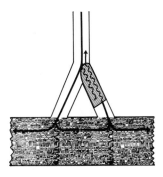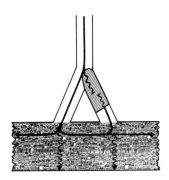

Figure 3 Abolition of reentrant activity by antiarrhythmic drug. Reentry pattern shown in Schmitt-Erlanger diagram at left, similar to Figure 2. After effects of antiarrhythmic drug (right), conduction in damaged zone is selectively depressed and unidirectional block is converted to bidirectional block.

normal conditions the supraventricular impulse propagates through both limbs of the system, although in the damaged segment the conduction velocity is subnormal. After exposure to the drug the antegrade impulse no longer propagates through the damaged limb. Next, the retrograde impulse conducts slowly through the damaged (arrhythmogenic) zone and reenters the proximal segment. In this model reentry could be abolished by either decreasing drug levels and allowing bidirectional conduction or increasing drug levels and establishing bidirectional block.

Effects on Action Potential Duration

Drugs that prolong action potential duration in Purkinje fibers may induce reentry (15,16). Such drugs include those in class IA and III. The relative refractory period occurs during phase 3 of the action potential, after the end of the absolute refractory period (Fig. 5). The

relative refractory period begins when the transmembrane potential becomes slightly negative to -60 mV as the voltage-dependent inactivation of the sodium channels begins to reverse. The threshold of excitability is increased during this time (16), and premature impulses propagate more slowly than after full recovery of excitability. The relative refractory period ends when the sodium channels are fully reactivated. In different cells this occurs at -80 to -95 mV. In some cells a "supernormal period" occurs late in phase 3, when the difference between membrane potential and threshold potential is minimal.

In normal ventricular tissues terminal repolarization is rapid, such that the duration of the relative refractory period is very brief. Antiarrhythmic drugs can prolong terminal repolarization in Purkinje fibers and myocardial cells. The relative refractory period is longer than normal in these cells. An early premature

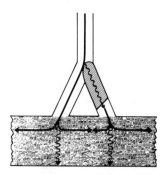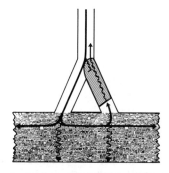

Figure 4 Genesis of arrhythmias as toxic drug effects. Damaged segment supports slow antegrade conduction before drug is given (left). After drug (right) conduction is further compromised, and unidirectional conduction block, slow retrograde conduction, and reentrant activity can occur.

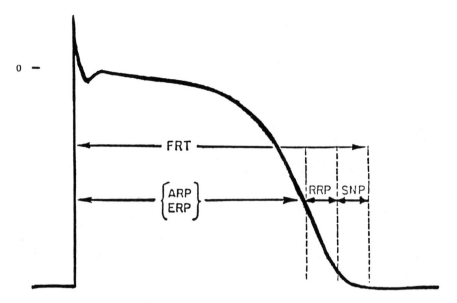

0 —

Figure 5 Recovery of excitability in a Purkinje fiber action potential. Full recovery time (FRT), absolute refractory period (ARP), effective refractory period (ERP), relative refractory period (RRP), and supernormal period (SNP) depicted diagrammatically. For discussion, see text. (Figure adapted from Hoffman BF, Cranefield PF. Electrophysiology of the heart. New York: McGraw-Hill, 1960.)

impulse occurring during the relative refractory period, or "vulnerable period," may conduct slowly through some segments of the heart and block at others. Thus antiarrhythmic drugs that prolong this vulnerable period can also promote reentry. This is thought to be one of the mechanisms for the proarrhythmic effects of these drugs (16). Clinically this can be seen as an increase in R-on-T phenomena.

Decreases in Action Potential Duration

In a similar manner it is possible that reentry can be promoted by antiarrhythmic drugs that shorten action potential duration and refractoriness (16). Class IB drugs, such as lidocaine, can decrease action potential duration and absolute refractory period in Purkinje fibers in "therapeutic" concentrations. Suppose that, before drug treatment, the absolute refractory period is 300 msec in the fibers proximal to the damaged zone (Fig. 4A), but after drug treatment it is decreased to 275 msec (Fig. 4B). After lidocaine causes one-way block, either continuously or intermittantly, reentry occurs as described earlier. Since lidocaine reduces the absolute refractory period in the proximal segment, however, the coupling interval of the earliest possible reentrant impulse

is reduced by 25 msec to 275 msec. This means that more rapid tachycardias may result (218 versus 200 beats/min).

Differential Effects on Refractoriness in Ventricular Tissues: Breakdown of the Purkinje Fiber "Gate"

Class IC drugs have variable effects on repolarization in the ventricles. For example, flecainide and encainide decrease action potential duration of Purkinje fibers but increase action potential duration of subendocardial ventricular muscle cells. The ventricular tachycardias caused by class IC agents may be related to these cellular effects (3,16).

Studies in animal models with other investigational agents have provided data that may explain the proarrhythmic effects of the class IC drugs (17, 18). These drugs prolong QT interval and promote rapid ventricular tachycardias and fibrillation in the canine heart (Fig. 6). They also decrease action potential duration of Purkinje fibers while increasing action potential duration of ventricular muscle, similar to the IC agents. This led to the hypothesis that these agents produce arrhythmias by shifting the site of the gate region and

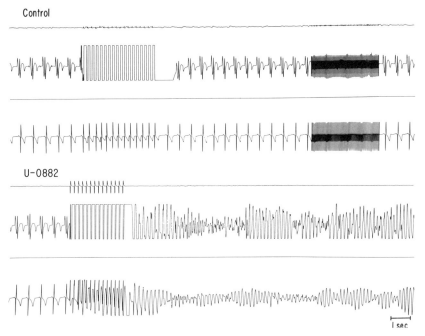

Figure 6 Effects of atrial stimulation on a canine heart before and after treatment with a class IC-type agent, U-0882. Each panel shows three traces: (top) stimulus artifact of atrial electrode (note increased amplification in lower panel); (middle) atrioventricular electrogram recorded between right atrial and right ventricular plaque electrodes; (bottom) reflects surface electrocardiogram. Control (top) shows effects of rapid atrial stimulation (200 msec) on the rate and rhythm before treatment with U-0882, 10 mg/kg IV. No arrhythmias result. QT interval is longer 10 min after drug injection (bottom), and atrial stimulation results in a rapid tachycardia that soon degenerates into ventricular fibrillation.

altering conduction. The gate region is the zone in the ventricular conduction system with the longest refractory period (19). Thus the gate is the site that determines whether early premature (supraventricular) impulses will be blocked before activating ventricular muscle. Premature impulses in the canine heart normally block in the distal regions of the bundle branches (Fig. 7A). Treatment with agents that produce "class IC-like" effects shifts the gate region distally, so that premature impulses can propagate to endocardial ventricular muscle and block occurs there (Fig. 7B).

These effects may be critical for generation of reentrant arrhythmias. Before treatment, block of premature impulses occurs in a few discrete sites in the His-Purkinje system (Fig. 8). After drug treatment, early premature impulses (S_2) may traverse the terminal branches of the His-Purkinje system, only to be blocked in the subendocardial ventricular muscle layers.

During normal sinus beats the impulse travels from the Purkinje system to ventricular muscle via transitional cells on the apical third of the left and right ventricular endocardial surfaces. Once the impulse activates these apical muscle cells, it spreads toward the epicardial and basal portions of the ventricles. This means that, during normal sinus beats, a broad band of subendocardial muscle cells in many regions of the right and left ventricles is activated simultaneously. Action potential duration and refractoriness vary greatly from site to site in these subendocardial cells (e.g., right versus left ventricle and apex versus base). Depending on the timing of the S_2 impulse (Fig. 9), conduction may be blocked at some sites in the endocardium but not at others. If the impulse blocks in most places in the ventricular apex but conducts slowly at one site, reentry may be able to occur. This happens if the impulse conducts retrogradely, back across the site of block and into the

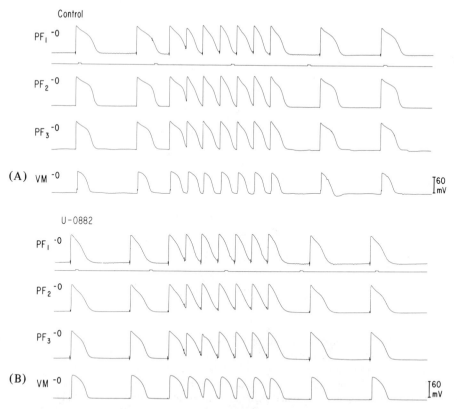

Figure 7 (A) Repolarization during superfusion with standard Tyrode's solution. Transmembrane action potentials shown are from four simultaneous impalements in a 2 × 4 cm segment of canine left ventricular endocardium. Impalements obtained from three distal (gate region) Purkinje fibers (PF$_1$, PF$_2$, and PF$_3$), and attached (distal) myocardium (VM). Basic cycle length at left and right of panel, 1000 msec. After abrupt change in stimulation rate (action potentials 4–9) at maximum 1:1 following frequency, upstrokes of Purkinje fibers are from phase 3 of preceding impulse but VM still shows full repolarization and diastolic segment. (B) Repolarization after treatment with a toxic drug (U-0882, 10 mg/L, 10 min). Same preparation, format, and impalement locations as in A. Note lack of diastolic segment in VM and (B) distal shift of gate region. For further discussion, see text.

His-Purkinje system. A single ventricular beat or a salvo of premature beats may result. The outcome varies according to the conduction velocity and dispersion of refractoriness in the ventricles, which determine how a good substrate for reentry exists.

AUTOMATICITY AND TRIGGERED ACTIVITY

Antiarrhythmic drug toxicity can increase ventricular ectopic activity. The arrhythmogenic mechanisms include increases in automaticity and triggered activity in Purkinje

fibers or ventricular muscle, as well as reentrant activity.

Automaticity

Controversy exists in the literature about whether class IA antiarrhythmic drugs cause arrhythmias by inducing automaticity (15,20). Class I drugs usually are thought to decrease pacemaker activity (21). Some class III agents (e.g., *N*-acetylprocainamide) and class IV agents (e.g., nifedipine, lidoflazine, diltiazem, and bepridil) do not decrease normal automaticity in isolated Purkinje fibers (22–

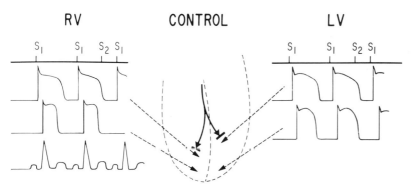

Figure 8 Block of premature junctional impulse in normal ventricular conduction system. Stimulus pattern shown by event marker lines above action potentials. Action potentials from Purkinje fiber (top trace) and ventricular muscle (bottom trace) of apices of right and left ventricles as indicated. Impulse blocks at site proximal to Purkinje impalements. ECG shown at lower left (see Fig. 9). For further discussion, see text.

26). Rather, nifedipine and *N*-acetylprocainamide (NAPA) can increase normal automaticity (22,23). The causes of this type of increase in pacemaker activity are not clear. NAPA can increase action potential duration by blocking the "delayed rectifier" potassium current. NAPA-enhanced automaticity could be explained if the drug also decreases diastolic potassium conductance in some Purkinje fibers. This may reduce maximum diastolic potential and promote enhanced automaticity.

Class IV antiarrhythmic drugs exert their effects by blocking inward currents through the "L-calcium channels." The class IV drugs suppress abnormal automaticity and triggered activity in cells with maximum diastolic potentials positive to -60 mV. These types of automaticity and triggered activity cause ventricular tachycardias in dogs 24 hr after occlusion of the left anterior descending coronary artery (21). Therefore, class IV drugs would be predicted to be very effective against these arrhythmias. However, nifedipine (10–200 μg/kg IV) is usually not effective against tachycardias in dogs with 24 hr infarcts (Dangman, unpublished observations). Occasionally, however, the arrhythmias subside completely (Fig. 10). These results can be explained by the two effects that nifedipine exerts on the heart. Nifedipine can slow or abolish

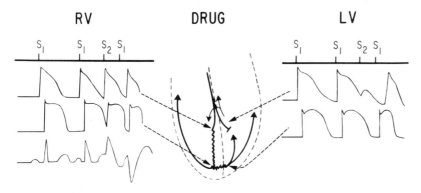

Figure 9 Reentry induced by shift of gate region from Purkinje fibers (PF) to ventricular muscle (VM) or transitional cells. Format as in Figure 8. Here the drug shortens APD and refractoriness in the PF gate region and prolongs APD and refractoriness in VM. Premature impulse may not then block in right side but will in left endocardial VM. Slow conduction through right ventricular muscle cells, reentry, and R-on-T beat may result. For further discussion, see text.

DANGMAN AND MIURA

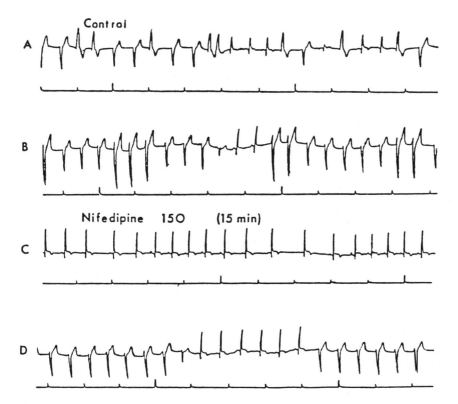

Figure 10 Effects of nifedipine on multiform ventricular tachycardias in a 24 hr infarcted canine heart. (A) Control data (lead II surface ECG above, 1 sec time marks below). Effects of nifedipine shown in B and C (cumulative doses of 100 and 150 μg/kg, IV, respectively). After the higher dose there was a gradual decrease in ventricular ectopic activity over 12–18 min. Animal was then in normal sinus rhythm, with R-R intervals up to 1100 msec. The effects of the last dose then decreased, and there was a gradual increase in the percentage of ventricular premature beats over the next 30–50 min (D).

abnormal automaticity or triggered activity in ectopic pacemakers by blocking calcium currents in myocardial cells. This represents a "direct" antiarrhythmic effect. Nifedipine also blocks calcium channels in vascular smooth muscle, however. This reduces blood pressure, which leads to increased sympathetic tone to the heart, which can accelerate ectopic activity. Nifedipine thus has both direct (antiarrhythmic) and indirect (sympathomimetic-arrhythmogenic) effects on the heart. Because the indirect effects usually overwhelm the direct effects of the drug, nifedipine does not usually change ventricular tachycardias significantly.

These results with nifedipine are of interest because many class I antiarrhythmic drugs can also reduce blood pressure or decrease cardiac contractility (27,28). These side effects can

induce reflex increases in sympathetic tone (29). Increased sympathetic tone may reverse the direct antiarrhythmic effects of the drug, exacerbate existing arrhythmias, or induce new types of ectopic activity. Thus a complete consideration of the toxicity of antiarrhythmic drugs must include evaluation of both direct and indirect effects.

Triggered Activity

Triggered impulses result when an afterdepolarization occurs, which achieves a suprathreshold voltage for an inward current. The upstroke of the triggered impulse is then carried by either the fast inward (sodium) current or a slow inward (T- or L-calcium) current. Triggered impulses do not occur de novo, which distinguishes them from automatic

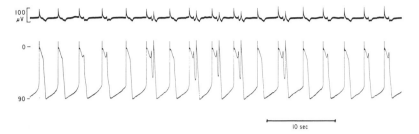

Figure 11 Extracellular and intracellular recordings of early afterdepolarizations induced by NAPA (*N*-acetylprocainamide), 80 mg/kg for 30 min, in a canine Purkinje fiber preparation. Transmembrane (bottom) trace shows action potentials with or without early afterdepolarization-triggered impulses. These triggered impulses have variable amplitudes; this is reflected in the extracellular recording (top trace) Voltage calibrations at left; time calibrations at lower right. (Republished from Dangman KH, Hoffman BF. In vivo and in vitro anti-arrhythmic and arrhythmogenic effects of *N*-acetyl procainamide. J Pharmacol Exp Ther 1981; 217:851–62, with permission of the American Society for Pharmacology and Experimental Therapeutics.)

impulses. By definition (30), triggered impulses occur only after one or more action potentials elicit an appropriate afterdepolarization. Afterdepolarizations occurring after maximum diastolic potential (MDP) are called delayed afterdepolarizations (DADs), transient depolarizations, or oscillatory afterpotentials. Afterdepolarizations that precede maximum diastolic potential, that is, occur during phase 2 or 3 of the action potential, are called early afterdepolarizations.

Triggered impulses from DAD typically occur in Purkinje fibers or ventricular muscle exposed to toxic doses of digitalis, catecholamines, or other agents that increase intracellular calcium concentrations. DAD-induced triggering is not generally associated with toxicity from any of the four classes of antiarrhythmic drugs (6,7). In contrast, several antiarrhythmic drugs may cause arrhythmias via triggered activity from early afterdepolarizations. These early afterdepolarization-triggered impulses can occur as coupled single beats or as salvos of extra beats. In Purkinje fibers triggered beats from early afterdepolarizations occur after treatment with NAPA (Fig. 11) or class I antiarrhythmic drugs, such as quinidine, pirmenol, and cibenzoline (Fig. 12).

Early afterdepolarizations typically occur in preparations in which the primary pacemaker is firing at slow rates, and once they occur they can then be suppressed by stimulation at rapid rates (23). They can also be

suppressed by drugs, such as lidocaine, that decrease action potential durations. Although it has been stated that "prolongation of repolarization appears crucial to the development of [early] afterdepolarizations" (15), they also occur frequently after treatment with cibenzoline in concentrations that significantly decrease action potential duration (31). It is therefore probably more correct to conclude that drugs that lead to early afterdepolarizations either decrease outward current (i_K or $i_{K,1}$), or increase inward currents (i_{SI} or i_{Na}), during phase 3 of repolarization. Thus early afterdepolarizations can develop following (1) a decrease in outward currents, as may occur after treatment with NAPA, quinidine, or cesium, or (2) an increase in inward current during the plateau, as may explain the effects of catecholamines (32) or cibenzoline (33).

Many investigators have observed triggered activity from early afterdepolarizations in isolated cardiac tissues exposed to toxic agents. These observations are of interest here because there is evidence that these triggered impulses can result in arrhythmias in the in situ heart. In the dog with chronic heart block (34) the ventricular rate is controlled by a junctional pacemaker. This pacemaker typically fires at 30–40 beats/min. Treatment of these dogs with NAPA, 50–150 mg/kg, typically induces coupled VPD and then salvos of VPD (Fig. 13). These arrhythmias are bradycardia dependent. If the ventricles are

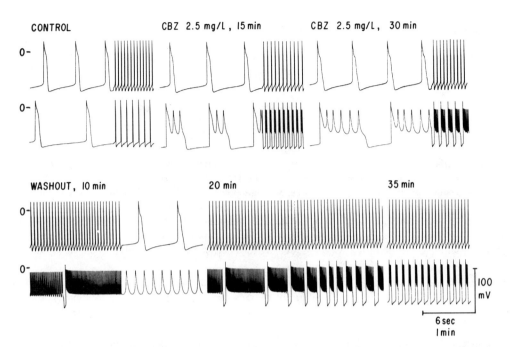

Figure 12 Effects of cibenzoline (CBZ) on automaticity in Purkinje fibers. First column shows control records; second and third columns show effects of 2.5 and 5 mg/L of CBZ, respectively. Data from three separate preparations from one heart are shown, with data from each fiber in each row of panels. Zero reference potential is the horizontal line in each panel. Time and voltage calibrations are shown at lower right. (Republished from Dangman KH. Cardiac effects of cibenzoline. J Cardiovasc Pharmacol 1984; 6:300–11, with permission of the publisher.)

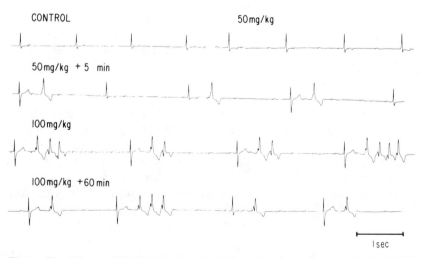

Figure 13 Effects of NAPA on rate and rhythm of a canine heart with chronic His bundle transection. Control ECG and rhythm after 50 and 100 mg/kg. Time calibration appears below. (Republished from Dangman KH, Hoffman BF. In vivo and in vitro anti-arrhythmic and arrhythmogenic effects of N-acetyl procainamide. J Pharmacol Exp Ther 1981; 217:851–62, with permission of the American Society for Pharmacology and Experimental Therapeutics.)

50 mg/kg

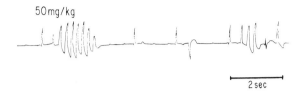

2 sec

Figure 14 Severe ventricular arrhythmias induced in a canine heart by *N*-acetylprocainamide, 50 mg/kg IV. (Republished from Dangman KH, Hoffman BF. In vivo and in vitro anti-arrhythmic and arrhythmogenic effects of *N*-acetyl procainamide. J Pharmacol Exp Ther 1981; 217:851–62, with permission of the American Society for Pharmacology and Experimental Therapeutics.)

stimulated at a rate faster than 55–60 beats/min, extrasystoles do not occur (23).

Sudden death can occur in animals with these bradycardia-dependent arrhythmias. This presumably is caused by rapid tachycardias (Fig. 14) degenerating into ventricular fibrillation. Thus there is a strong association between NAPA-induced early afterdepolarizations and bradycardia-dependent triggered arrhythmias in the in situ canine heart.

However, cibenzoline rarely produces triggered extrasystoles in the dog with chronic heart block (33). Nevertheless, it is probable that the hypothesis that these tachycardias are caused by EAD-triggered impulses is valid. These tachycardias occur in patients with QT prolongation and drug toxicity and in many cases are associated with the R-on-T phenomenon (35). It may be that the first beat of the tachycardia is initiated by an early afterdepolarization-generated impulse but that the subsequent beats are caused by reentrant activation. Data from the cesium-toxic dog (36,37) support this concept. However, the cesium ion can induce very complex ventricular arrhythmias in the dog that are not easily explained as resulting from early afterdepolarization-triggered impulses (Dangman and Hoffman, unpublished data).

Early afterdepolarizations and triggered activity often occur in isolated Purkinje fiber preparations during "washout" of local anesthetic drugs. The typical setting is in a preparation that has been treated with one or more concentrations of the drug for several hours. The highest concentration is above the therapeutic range. At the end of the drug exposure periods the preparation is "washed" with drug-free Tyrode's solution to determine whether the putative drug effects that have

occurred are reversible. With some drugs early afterdepolarizations and triggered activity develop for the first time during such a washout period. Local anesthetic drugs can decrease intracellular sodium ion activity $[Na^+]_i$, and this could lead to (1) decreased electrogenic pump current (sarcolemmal Na^+, $-K^+$-ATPase activity) and (2) decreased sodium-calcium exchange and intracellular calcium ion activity. These effects could decrease repolarization rate because the "delayed rectifier" potassium current that leads to phase 3 of repolarization is enhanced by increases in sarcoplasmic calcium activity. Also, sodium pump current accelerates repolarization.

Therefore washout of a local anesthetic drug may lead to early afterdepolarizations and triggering if the following effects occur. (1) Blockade of the sodium channels is rapidly reversed by washout of the drug. This could enhance sodium window current and increase the magnitude of the inward currents flowing at plateau voltages. (2) Reduction of potassium conductance by the drug is not rapidly reversed during drug washout. This is possible because this effect of the drug may depend, in whole or in part, on the effects of the drug on intracellular Ca^{2+}. Restoration of Ca^{2+} levels may not occur quickly.

The concept that arrhythmias may be caused by drug washout could be important clinically. During oral administration of an antiarrhythmic agent plasma drug concentrations typically vary with time depending on drug absorption and elimination. As the drug is absorbed "peak" levels occur; plasma concentration then declines toward a "trough" level until the patient takes another dose of the drug and absorption of that dose begins to increase

Table 4 Percentage of Patients with Proarrhythmic Responses
to Various Antiarrhythmic Drugs

Drug	Incidence with noninvasive testing (%)	Incidence with invasive testing (%)
Quinidine	15	20
Procainamide	9	21
Disopyramide	6	5
Mexiletine	7	20
Tocainide	8	5
Encainide	15	37
Ethmozine	11	14
Flecainide	12	NA
Indecainide	19	NA
Lorcainide	8	24
Propafenone	8	15

NA = not available.
Source: All data abstracted from Podrid et al.(42).

plasma level again. Arrhythmias may disappear at peak plasma levels but return when
levels fall below the "minimum effective concentration." Thus an increase in the incidence
of extrasystoles that occurs during trough levels of a drug may reflect either (1) the recurrence of arrhythmias from the original source,
or (2) new types of arrhythmias caused by
early afterdepolarization-triggered impulses,
which result from variable persistence of the
drug's effects during washout.

DRUG-INDUCED TACHYCARDIAS: CLINICAL CONSIDERATIONS

Tachycardias resulting from antiarrhythmic
drug effects have become a topic of increasing
interest in the past few years. It has been reported that iatrogenic tachycardias are common in patients being treated for malignant
ventricular arrhythmias (38,39). The overall
incidence of the proarrhythmic effects of antiarrhythmic drugs in patients has been
estimated as 11% by Holter monitoring (40)
and as 18% by programmed extrastimulus
(PES) techniques (41). Different antiarrhythmic drugs vary in their tendency to cause
proarrhythmic effects. Also, as summarized by
Podrid et al. (42), the incidence of proarrhythmic effects for class I drugs tends to be higher
when they are studied by invasive techniques
(Table 4). The appearance of symptomatic

new rhythm disturbances in patients with significant heart disease with preexisting ectopic
activity requiring drug treatment is a major
clinical problem. In this section a review of
the more malignant forms of arrhythmia that
have been attributed to antiarrhythmic drug
toxicity is presented.

Monomorphic Ventricular Ectopic Activity

All antiarrhythmic drugs may, in some patients, increase the frequency of ventricular
ectopic beats or even to convert nonsustained
ventricular tachycardia to sustained tachycardia. The mechanism by which arrhythmias can
be initiated by a drug can be suggested by the
known effects of that drug on reentrant circuits. Reentrant arrhythmias are initiated and
maintained by specific balance between refractoriness, unidirectional block, and slow conduction in the arrhythmogenic zone. Most
antiarrhythmic drugs can change refractoriness
and the velocity of slow conduction in the reentrant circuit. Thus they can change the relationship between them to promote or prolong
reentrant rhythms. Increasing the plasma concentration of an antiarrhythmic drug may either abolish or exacerbate this ectopic activity.

In addition, some drugs may cause ventricular ectopic beats or ventricular tachycardia
via enhanced impulse initiation. Quinidine

toxicity may increase ventricular automaticity, and class III agents may cause triggered activity from early afterdepolarizations.

"Incessant" Ventricular Tachycardias

Class IC drugs, including flecainide, encainide, propafenone, and ethmozine, can cause "incessant tachycardias" (2). These arrhythmias occur soon after starting or increasing the dose of IC agents. They are common in patients with left ventricular ejection fraction < 30% and a history of spontaneous, sustained ventricular tachycardia. The incessant arrhythmia is characterized by wide ventricular beats, as should occur during marked slowing of intraventricular conduction caused by toxic levels of IC drugs. The configuration of incessant tachycardia may be "sinusoidal"; that is, it is characterized by very broad, undulating complexes that resemble a sine wave. The configuration of the ventricular beats is quite different from those that occurred before drug toxicity, and the rate of the incessant tachycardia is usually slower than the spontaneous tachycardias (2). These drug-induced tachycardias are extremely difficult to terminate, however, and sudden death is common, even in hospitalized patients (43). Incessant tachycardias may be the cause of the increased mortality in patients treated with encainide or flecainide following myocardial infarction (5). The high incidence of sudden death in these patients suggests that the selection of patients for therapy with class IC drugs should be done with extreme care (43).

Torsades-de-Pointes

Treatment with a variety of antiarrhythmic drugs, as well as antidepressant and antipsychotic agents, has been associated with development of torsades-de-pointes arrhythmias (Table 5). Torsades-de-pointes is a paroxysmal ventricular tachycardia, with rates typically greater than 200 beats/min. The term "torsades-de-pointes," or "twisting of points," describes the progressive variation or undulation of the QRS around the baseline. That is, the amplitudes of the successive QRS complexes change gradually from beat to beat,

Table 5 Drugs Reported to Cause Torsades-de-Pointes Tachycardias

Antiarrhythmics	
Class I	Quinidine
	Procainamide
	Disopyramide
	Flecainide
	Encainide
	Ajmaline
	Aprindine
Class II	Propranolol
Class III	Amiodarone
	N-acetylprocainamide
	Sotalol
Class IV	Bepridil
	Lidoflazine
	Nifedipine
Antidepressants	Amitriptyline
	Imipramine
Antipsychotics	Thioridazine
	Trifluoperazine

Source: Modified from Raehl et al. (35) and Bhandari and Scheinman (67).

such that the main vector varies from upright to inverted in a regular sequence. It is associated with a prolonged QT interval or a prominent U wave (44,45) and a "long-short initiating sequence" (46). The sequence begins with a ventricular premature beat; this, after a compensatory pause, is followed by a sinus beat. A second ventricular beat then occurs on the T wave of this sinus beat. This "R-on-T" beat then precipitates the episode of torsades-de-pointes. Paroxysms of torsades-de-pointes are typically brief, lasting 5–20 beats (47,48), but they can lead to ventricular fibrillation (49). Episodes of torsades-de-pointes typically occur after a period of increased ventricular ectopic activity (47,50, 51). Although hypokalemia and hypomagnesemia have been associated with increased risk of developing torsades-de-pointes (52,53), determining plasma concentrations of the initiating antiarrhythmic drug may not be helpful. In most cases the drug levels are found to be in the therapeutic range (46). The risk that a given patient will develop drug-induced torsades-de-pointes is probably best followed by simple monitoring of QT interval. It has been suggested that if uncorrected QT intervals are more than 0.50 or 0.60 sec, torsades-de-pointes may occur (54,55).

Torsades-de-pointes may be caused by enhanced ventricular impulse initiation. Specifically, this arrhythmia may result from two ventricular ectopic foci firing slightly out of phase (56–58). Rapid impulse initiation from a single focus in the ventricles could also produce torsades-de-pointes, if the cycle length of the rhythm is shorter than the effective refractory period of part of the surrounding myocardium. This would allow successive wavefronts to conduct differently and produce epicardial breakthrough at different sites (57).

The impulses may be initiated by either automaticity (56) or triggering from early afterdepolarizations (43). Toxicity from quinidine (59,60) and NAPA (23) can cause both early afterdepolarizations and torsades-de-pointes arrhythmias. Early afterdepolarizations are cycle length dependent. They tend to appear during slow heart rates or after relatively long R-R intervals that may be caused by conduction blocks or transient slowing of sinus rate. Thus, during the long-short initiation sequence for torsades-de-pointes a sinus impulse occurs after a long R-R interval. Early afterdepolarizations may then occur and trigger the R-on-T beat that leads to the paroxysm of tachycardia.

However, this hypothesis cannot explain all forms of torsade-de-pointes (61). Early afterdepolarizations induced by class IA and III antiarrhythmic drugs typically occur in Purkinje fibers at sites with the longest action potential durations. They do not tend to occur in peripheral Purkinje fibers or ventricular muscle cells, which have shorter action potentials (23). Therefore, triggered impulses from these early afterdepolarizations generally occur after repolarization has been completed in ventricular muscle, and therefore after the T wave. Thus the triggered impulses give rise to early diastolic beats, not R-on-T beats. In addition, some drugs (the investigational class IV drugs, bepridil and lidoflazine) cause torsades-de-pointes (62–64) but do not elicit early afterdepolarizations (24,25).

Torsades-de-pointes may be caused by reentrant activation (65,66), which results from increased dispersion of refractoriness in the ventricles. For example, lidoflazine and bepridil prolong QT interval and cause torsades-de-pointes tachycardias. These drugs prolong ventricular muscle action potential duration but shorten plateau duration in Purkinje fibers. Thus these drugs may alter the function of the Purkinje fiber gate. Reentry is facilitated if the gate region is shifted far enough to the periphery, to the level of the endocardial ventricular muscle.

Toxicity from these drugs may prolong action potential duration and refractoriness in ventricular muscle while shortening action potential duration and refractoriness in the His bundle and both the left and right bundle branches. If, in addition, refractoriness in the left ventricular endocardial muscle is longer during this toxic effect than is refractoriness in the right ventricular endocardial muscle, reentry becomes possible. If the impulse timing is correct antegrade supraventricular impulses tend to block in the left ventricular endocardium but not in the right ventricular endocardium. The antegrade impulse may then conduct slowly across the septum and proceed back through the site of block in the left ventricular endocardium and to the left bundle branch. A single R-on-T beat, an R-on-T beat leading to a stable reentrant rhythm (e.g., in a fixed circuit consisting of the left bundle branch, the His Bundle, the right bundle branch, and the ventricular muscle in the apical septum), or an R-on-T beat leading to a chaotic reentrant rhythm and ventricular fibrillation could result. As mentioned, a reentrant rhythm in a fixed circuit may lead to a "uniform" ventricular tachycardia or to an arrhythmia morphologically similar to torsades-de-pointes if variable exit points or conduction patterns away from the circuit occur.

Finally, torsades-de-pointes tachycardias may involve both enhanced ventricular automaticity and reentry, "especially in the presence of a marked and uneven delay in myocardial repolarization" (35).

In conclusion, antiarrhythmic drug toxicity can probably cause arrhythmias via induction of reentrant activity, enhanced automaticity, or triggered activity. It is of interest to know

whether the cellular mechanisms of drug toxicity found in studies in vitro are present and
cause arrhythmias in vivo. Ventricular tachyarrhythmias that occur when plasma drug concentrations have risen above the therapeutic
range, such as incessant tachycardias caused
by class IC agents, appear to occur frequently
and to be very predictable. These arrhythmias
by their very predictability can be assumed to
result from consistent effects of excessive drug
effects on either normal or abnormal cardiac
tissues. In contrast, drug-induced torsades-
de-pointes tachycardias "are named for their
morphology rather than their etiology" (66).
They typically occur as an idiosyncratic
reaction, and usually no other indication of
drug toxicity is present (67). It is difficult to
be certain that an animal model for torsades-
de-pointes, or other idiosyncratic and unpredictable arrhythmias, is truly relevant to a
parallel clinical phenomenon. This is because
similar morphologic forms can be produced by
several different etiologies.

ACKNOWLEDGMENTS

Original studies described in this paper were
supported by Grant HL 24354 from the National Heart, Lung and Blood Institute.

REFERENCES

1. Woosley R L, Roden D M. Pharmacologic causes of arrhythmogenic actions of antiarrhythmic drugs. Am J Cardiol 1987; 59:19E–24E.
2. Bigger J T, Sahar D I. Clinical types of proarrhythmic response to antiarrhythmic drugs. Am J Cardiol 1987; 59:2E–9E.
3. Zipes D P. Proarrhythmic effects of antiarrhythmic drugs. Am J Cardiol 1987; 59:26E–30E.
4. Stanton M S, Prystowsky E N, Fineberg N S, et al. Arrhythmogenic effects of antiarrhythmic drugs: a study of 506 patients treated for ventricular tachycardia or fibrillation. J Am Coll Cardiol 1985; 14:209–15.
5. Cardiac Arrhythmia Suppression Trial Investigators. Preliminary report: effect of encainide and flecainide on mortality in a randomized

trial of arrhythmia suppression after myocardial infarction. N Engl J Med 1989; 321:406–11.
6. Vaughan-Williams E M. Classification of anti-arrhythmic drugs. In: Sandoe E, Flenstadt-Jensen E, Olesen K H, eds. Symposium on cardiac arrhythmias. Sweden: Sodertalje, 1970.
7. Vaughan-Williams E M. A classification of antiarrhythmic actions reassessed after a decade of new drugs. J Clin Pharmacol 1984; 24:129–47.
8. Dangman K H, Wang H H, Reynolds R D. Studies on bethanidine and meobentine: direct and indirect effects of antifibrillatory drugs. J Cardiovasc Pharmacol 1986; 8:1185–94.
9. Dobmeyer D, Muir W W, Schaal S F. Antiarrhythmic effects of flecainide against canine ventricular arrhythmias induced by two-stage coronary ligation and halothane-epinephrine. J Cardiovasc Pharmacol 1985; 7:238–44.
10. Ikeda N, Singh B N, Davis L D, Hauswirth O. Effects of flecainide on the electrophysiologic properties of isolated canine and rabbit myocardial fibers. J Am Coll Cardiol 1985; 5:303–10.
11. Dangman K H. Effects of procainamide on automatic and triggered impulse initiation in isolated preparations of canine cardiac Purkinje fibers. J Cardiovasc Pharmacol 1988; 12:78–87.
12. Allessie M A, Bonke F I M, Schopman F J G. Circus movement in rabbit atrial muscle as a mechanism of tachycardia. III. The "leading circle" concept: a new model of circus movement in cardiac tissue without the involvement of an anatomic obstacle. Circ Res 1977; 41:9–18.
13. Kamiyama A, Eguchi K, Shibayama R. Circus movement tachycardia induced by a single premature stimulus on the ventricular sheet—evaluation of the leading circle hypothesis in the canine ventricular muscle. Jpn Circ J 1986; 50:65–73.
14. El Sherif N, Smith A, Evans K. Canine ventricular arrhythmia in the late myocardial infarction period: epicardial mapping of reentrant circuits. Circ Res 1981; 49:255–64.
15. Rosen M R, Wit A L. Arrhythmogenic actions of antiarrhythmic drugs. Am J Cardiol 1987; 59:10E–7E.
16. Surawicz B. Contributions of cellular electrophysiology to the understanding of the electrocardiogram. Experientia 1987; 43:1061–8.

17. Moore J I, Swain H H. Sensitization to ventricular fibrillation. I. Sensitization by amarine and congeners of U-0882. J Pharmacol Exp Ther 1960; 128:243–58.

18. Dangman K H, Hoffman B F. Is reduction of Purkinje fiber ''gate'' function a primary mechanism for drug-induced ventricular tachycardias? Circulation 1987; 76 (Suppl. IV):112.

19. Myerburg R J, Gelband H, Hoffman B F. Functional characteristics of the gating mechanism in the canine A-V conducting system. Circ Res 1971; 28:136–47.

20. Bellet S. Clinical disorders of the heart beat. Philadelphia: Lea & Febiger, 1971.

21. LeMarec H, Dangman K H, Danilo P, Rosen M R. An evaluation of automaticity and triggered activity in the canine heart one to four days after myocardial infarction. Circulation 1985; 71:1224–36.

22. Dangman K H, Hoffman B F. Effects of nifedipine on electrical activity of cardiac cells. Am J Cardiol 1980; 46:1059–67.

23. Dangman K H, Hoffman B F. In vivo and in vitro anti-arrhythmic and arrhythmogenic effects of N-acetyl procainamide. J Pharmacol Exp Ther 1981; 217:851–62.

24. Dangman K H. Effects of bepridil on transmembrane action potentials recorded from canine cardiac Purkinje fibers and ventricular muscle cells; insights into antiarrhythmic mechanisms. Naunyn Schmied ebergo Arch Pharmacol 1985; 329:326–32.

25. Dangman K H, Miura D S. Does i_f control normal automatic rate in canine cardiac Purkinje fibers? Studies on the negative chronotropic effects of lidoflazine. J Cardiovasc Pharmacol 1987; 10:332–40.

26. Dangman K H, Zaim S, Miura D S. Local anesthetic and negative chronotropic effects of diltiazem on canine cardiac Purkinje fibers. Am Heart J 1989; 117:1271–7.

27. Hoffmeister H M, Hepp A, Seipel L. Negative inotropic effect of class I antiarrhythmic drugs: comparison of flecainide with disopyramide and quinidine. Eur Heart J 1987; 8:1126–32.

28. Honerjager P, Loibl E, Steidl I, Schonsteiner G, Ulm K. Negative inotropic effects of tetrodotoxin and seven class I antiarrhythmic drugs in relation to sodium channel blockade. Naunyn Schmiedebergs Arch Pharmacol 1986; 332:184–95.

29. Gulamhusein S, Ko P, Carruthers S G, Klein G J. Acceleration of ventricular response during atrial fibrillation in the Wolff-Parkinson-White syndrome after verapamil. Circulation 1982; 65:348–54.

30. Cranefield P F. The conduction of the cardiac impulse. Mt. Kisco, NY: Futura, 1975.

31. Dangman K H. Cardiac effects of cibenzoline. J Cardiovasc Pharmacol 1984; 6:300–11.

32. Hoffman B F, Cranefield P F. Electrophysiology of the heart. New York: McGraw-Hill, 1960.

33. Dangman K H, Miura D S. Cibenzoline. In: Scriabine A, ed. New cardiovascular drugs 1986. New York: Raven Press, 1986:107–28.

34. Steiner C, Kovalik A T W. A simple technique for production of chronic complete heart block in dogs. J Appl Physiol 1968; 25:631–2.

35. Raehl C L, Patel A K, Leroy M. Drug-induced torsades de pointes. Clin Pharm 1985; 4:675–90.

36. Brachmann J, Scherlag B J, Rosenstraukh L V, Lazzara R. Bradycardia dependent triggered activity: relevance to drug induced multiform ventricular tachycardia. Circulation 1983; 68:846–56.

37. Levine J H, Spear J F, Guarini T, Weisfelt M L, deLangen C D J, Becker L C, Moore E N. Cesium chloride induced long QT syndrome: demonstration of afterdepolarizations and triggered activity in vivo. Circulation 1985; 72:1092–103.

38. Poser R F, Podrid P J, Lombardi F, Lown B. Aggravation of arrhythmias induced with antiarrhythmic drugs during electrophysiologic testing. Am Heart J 1985; 110:9–16.

39. Podrid P J. Aggravation of ventricular arrhythmias. A drug-induced complication. Drugs 1985; 29 (Suppl. 4):33–44.

40. Velebit V, Podrid P, Lown B, et al. Aggravation and provocation of ventricular arrhythmias by antiarrhythmic drugs. Circulation 1982; 65:886–94.

41. Rae A P, Kay H R, Horowitz L N, et al. Proarrhythmic effects of antiarrhythmic drugs in patients with malignant ventricular arrhythmias evaluated by electrophysiologic testing. J Am Coll Cardiol 1988; 12:131–9.

42. Podrid P J, Lampert S, Graboys T B, Blatt C M, Lown B. Aggravation of arrhythmia by antiarrhythmic drugs—incidence and preditors. Am J Cardiol 1987; 59:38E–44E.

43. Garratt C, Camm A J. Arrhythmias caused by antiarrhythmic drugs. Hosp Ther 1989; 14:41–8.

44. Dessertenne F, Fabiato A, Coumel P. Les variations progressives de l'amplitude de l'eletrocardiogramme. Acta Cardiol Angiol Int 1966; 15:241–58.

45. Horowitz L N, Josephson M E. Torsades-de-pointes. In: Surawicz B, Reddy C P, Prystowsky E N, eds. Tachycardias. Boston: Martinus Nijhoff, 1984:283–91.

46. Kay G N, Plumb V J, Arciniegas J G, et al. Torsades-de-pointes: the long-short initiating sequence and other clinical features. Observations in 32 patients. J Am Coll Cardiol 1983; 2:806–17.

47. Lewis B H, Antman E M, Graboys T B. Detailed analysis of 24 hr ambulatory electrocardiographic recordings during ventricular or torsades de pointes. J Am Coll Cardiol 1983; 2:426–36.

48. Krikler D M, Curry P V L. Torsades de pointes, an atypical ventricular tachycardia. Br Heart J 1976; 38:117–20.

49. Bigger J T. Definition of benign versus malignant ventricular arrhythmias. Am J Cardiol 1983; 52:47C–54C.

50. Panidis I P, Morganroth J. Sudden death in hospitalized patients: cardiac rhythm disturbances detected by ambulatory electrocardiographic monitoring. J Am Coll Cardiol 1983; 2:798–805.

51. Kempf J C, Josephson M E. Cardiac arrest recorded on ambulatory electrocardiograms. Am J Cardiol 1984; 53:1577–82.

52. Smirk F H, Ng J. Cardiac ballet. Repetitions of complex electrocardiographic patterns. Br Heart J 1969; 31:426–34.

53. Topol E J, Lerman B B. Hypomagnisemic torsades de pointes. Am J Cardiol 1983; 52:1367–8.

54. Schweitzer P, Mark H. Delayed repolarization syndrome. Am J Med 1983; 75:393–401.

55. Tzivoni D, Keren A, Stern S. Torsades de pointes versus polymorphus ventricular tachycardia. Am J Cardiol 1983; 52:639–40.

56. Dessertenne F. La tachycardie ventriculaire a deux foyers opposes variables Arch Mal Coeur 1966; 59:263–72.

57. Bardy G H, Ungerleider R M, Smith W M, Ideker R E. A mechanism of torsades de pointes in a canine model. Circulation 1983; 67:52–59.

58. D'alnoncourt C N, Zierhut W, Luderitz B. Torsades de pointes tachycardia: re-entry or focal activity? Br Heart J 1982; 48:213–6.

59. Roden D M, Hoffman B F. Action potential prolongation and induction of abnormal automaticity by low quinidine concentrations in canine Purkinje fibers. Relationship to potassium and cycle length. Circ Res 1985; 56: 857–67.

60. Roden D M, Thompson K A, Hoffman B F, Woosley R L. Clinical features and basic mechanisms of quinidine-induced arrhythmias. J Am Coll Cardiol 1986; 8:73A–8A.

61. Nayebpour M, Solymoss B C, Nattel S. Cardiovascular and metabolic effects of a caesium chloride injection in dogs— limitations as a model for the long QT syndrome. Cardiovasc Res 1989; 23:756–66.

62. Hanley S P, Hampton J R. Ventricular arrhythmias associated with lidoflazine: side effects observed in a randomized trial. Eur Heart J 1983; 4:889–93.

63. Smith W M, Gallagher J J. Les torsades de pointes; an atypical ventricular arrhythmia. Ann Intern Med 1980; 93:578–84.

64. Jackman W M, Clark M, Friday K J, et al. Ventricular tachyarrhythmias in the long QT syndrome. Med Clin North Am 1984; 68:1079–109.

65. Nhon N, Hope R R, Kabell G, Scherlag B J, Lazzara R. Torsades de pointes; electrophysiology of atypical ventricular tachycardia (abstract). Am J Cardiol 1980; 45:494.

66. Horowitz L N, Greenspan A M, Spielman S R, Josephson M E. Torsades de pointes: electrophysiologic studies in patients without transient pharmacologic or metabolic abnormalities. Circulation 1981; 63:1120–8.

67. Bhandari A K, Scheinman M. The long QT syndrome. Mod Concepts Cardiovasc Dis 1985; 54:45–50.

17

Cellular Basis for Arrhythmias in Cardiac Hypertrophy and Cardiomyopathy

Ronald S. Aronson

Albert Einstein College of Medicine
Bronx, New York

INTRODUCTION

It is generally agreed that ventricular tachycardia or fibrillation is the proximate cause of death in patients with a wide variety of cardiac diseases. Ventricular arrhythmias are undoubtedly the cause of sudden death in many patients with ischemic heart disease (1) and hypertrophic cardiomyopathy (2). Left ventricular hypertrophy is associated with an increased incidence of both sudden death (3) and ventricular arrhythmias (4), suggesting a link between cardiac hypertrophy and the development of life-threatening arrhythmias. Furthermore, sudden death occurs in many patients with congestive heart failure of various etiologies in whom there is no evidence of hemodynamic or clinical deterioration preceding death (5).

Despite the obvious clinical importance of arrhythmias associated with cardiac hypertrophy and cardiomyopathy, the mechanism or mechanisms underlying the development of these potentially lethal rhythm disorders remains unclear. As we see in the discussion that follows, the most consistent abnormality associated with cardiac hypertrophy is prolongation of the action potential duration. Afterpotentials have also been observed in tissues from some experimental models as well as in tissues removed from diseased human hearts.

In principle there are various mechanisms whereby the prolonged time course of repolarization and the occurrence of afterdepolarizations could provoke abnormal rhythmic activity in the heart. Those possibilities are discussed after a review of the relevant experimental observations, which follows.

EXPERIMENTAL CARDIAC HYPERTROPHY INDUCED BY PRESSURE OVERLOAD

Cardiac hypertrophy induced by pressure overload in a number of models has been universally associated with some degree of prolongation of the action potential. Experimental right ventricular hypertrophy has been produced in cats by banding the pulmonary artery (6–8), and experimental left ventricular hypertrophy has been produced by induction of sustained systemic hypertension in rats (9–14) and by banding the ascending aorta in guinea pigs (15,16). Regardless of the method

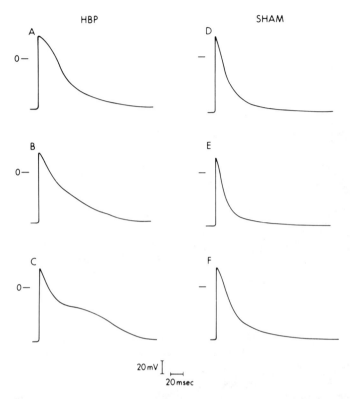

Figure 1 Configurations of action potentials recorded in hypertrophied (HBP) papillary muscles from rats with renal hypertension (caused by constriction of the left renal artery) and in normal papillary muscles from control rats (SHAM; i.e., sham operated). The action potentials in hypertrophied preparations show a marked prolongation of repolarization and considerable variability in the time course of repolarization. The horizontal bars in each panel show the zero potential level.

used to create cardiac hypertrophy, a consistent finding has been a prolonged duration of repolarization (Figure 1). Recent studies in single myocytes isolated from hypertrophied right ventricles of cats (17) and hypertrophied left ventricles of guinea pigs (15,16) have shown that the prolonged duration persists in the isolated hypertrophied cells. These results indicate that the prolonged repolarization is caused by an effect of hypertrophy on individual myocytes rather than by hypertrophy-induced alterations in syncytial structure or electrical interactions. Thus, prolonged repolarization appears to be a primary cellular response to cardiac hypertrophy.

Our own work has also shown that prolongation of the action potential at the cellular level is associated with characteristic changes in the QRS and T waves of the surface electrocardiogram recorded in rats with left

ventricular hypertrophy induced by renal hypertension (Figure 2) (13). We have also shown that hypertrophied ventricular muscle from rats is susceptible to developing afterdepolarizations that can lead to triggered activity (11). Under appropriate conditions papillary muscles isolated from hypertrophied hearts can develop either early or delayed afterdepolarizations, which could lead in turn to self-sustained electrical activity.

We have also found that the effective membrane capacitance is decreased by almost 40% in hypertrophied left ventricular tissue from rats with renal hypertension (14). A recent study in single myocytes isolated from hypertrophied tissue in the same model showed that the membrane capacitance of normal and hypertrophied cells was similar (18). In contrast, we have recently found that the membrane capacitance of single cells isolated from

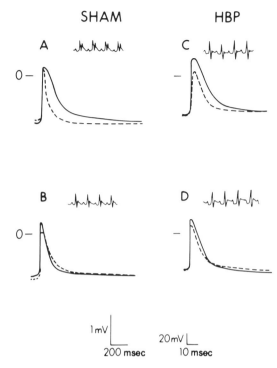

Figure 2 Records of action potentials and lead II of the electrocardiogram. HBP indicates rats with cardiac hypertrophy induced by renal hypertension (caused by constriction of the left renal artery) and SHAM (i.e., sham operated) indicates normal rats. Records were obtained from the same HBP and SHAM animals. The solid tracings show action potentials from an endocardial preparation, and the interrupted tracings show action potentials from an epicardial preparation. (A) The electrocardiographic tracing shows large peaked T waves associated with a wide disparity in the duration of the epicardial and endocardial action potentials. (B) The electrocardiographic tracing shows smaller T waves associated with little difference in duration between epicardial and endocardial action potentials. (C) The electrocardiographic records show practically no T waves despite the wide disparity in duration between epicardial and endocardial action potentials. (D) The electrocardiographic records show small, slow T waves even though there is little difference in the duration of epicardial and endocardial action potentials. Thus although cardiac hypertrophy in the rat is associated with a reproducible decrease in T wave magnitude, there is no simple or consistent correlation between the shape of the T wave and regional differences in the transmembrane action potentials across the wall of the heart. The time and voltage calibrations on the left apply to the electrocardiograms and those on the right to the action potentials.

hypertrophied guinea pig left ventricles is significantly higher than the membrane capacitance of normal left ventricular myocytes (16). The reduced effective membrane capacitance of intact preparations of hypertrophied muscle in the face of either increased or unchanged capacitance of individual hypertrophied myocytes suggests that a portion of the added membrane capacity is not charged in the intact preparation. On the one hand, the reduced effective membrane capacitance of the intact preparation may be useful as a way to enhance conduction along hypertrophied bundles of cardiac tissue, since decreasing the effective membrane capacitance reduces the amount of current required for propagation. On the other hand, the lack of depolarization of areas of membrane in hypertrophied cells may reduce the amount of membrane excited below the optimum required for effective excitation-contraction coupling. It is also possible that various degrees of uncoupling of cells or alterations in extracellular composition and structure influence the spread of current in the intact tissue, whereas the capacity of single cells is not influenced by such factors.

With respect to other passive membrane properties that may have an effect on conduction, we found that R_i was not significantly different in normal and hypertrophied rat myocardium whereas the effective R_m was significantly lower in hypertrophied than in normal myocardium (14). The overall effect of those changes in passive membrane properties on conduction velocity is difficult to predict. The fall in effective R_m in the presence of unchanged R_i would tend to reduce conduction velocity since the length constant would be shorter. On the other hand, the fall in effective C_m would tend to increase conduction velocity, as would the increased cell diameter characteristic of hypertrophy. Thus, at least with compensatory cardiac hypertrophy, it does not seem likely that changes in passive membrane properties are sufficient to cause slowing of conduction to the point that reentry is encouraged to develop.

We have also found, however, that in hypertrophied rat myocardium the distribution of electrical changes in the action potential is not

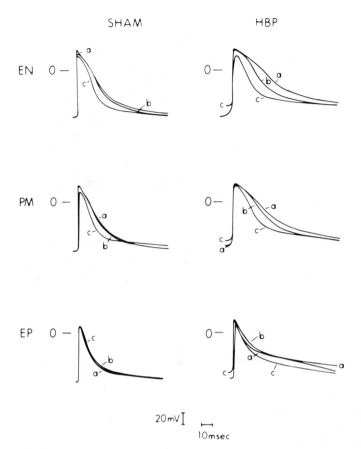

SHAM   HBP

EN   0 —

PM   0 —

EP   0 —

20mV

10msec

Figure 3 Tracings of representative action potentials recorded in endocardial (EN), papillary muscle (PM), and epicardial (EP) preparations from control hearts of normal rats (SHAM; i.e., sham operated) and from hypertrophied hearts (HBP) of rats with renal hypertension (caused by constriction of the left renal artery). The preparations were driven at three cycle lengths: 1000 msec (a), 300 msec (b), and 150 msec (c). The entire time course of repolarization in endocardial and papillary muscle action potentials was clearly longer in HBP than in SHAM preparations at all cycle lengths. In epicardial preparations only the latter half of repolarization was prolonged in HBP fibers.

uniform across the wall of the heart (12). The action potentials recorded from the endocardial surface of hypertrophied myocardium were significantly longer than those recorded from the endocardial surface of control hearts (Figure 3). In contrast, the action potentials recorded from the epicardial surface of hypertrophied hearts were prolonged only during the terminal phase of repolarization compared to normal epicardial action potentials. There is thus a "gradient" in the duration of the action potential from endocardium to epicardium, the action potentials in the endocardium being substantially longer than those in the epicardium in hypertrophied myocardium. The

endocardial-epicardial gradient in action potential duration was substantially more marked in hypertrophied than in normal myocardium. Since some investigators have proposed that disparity in refractoriness could predispose to the development of reentry (19), it is possible that the marked difference in duration between endocardial and epicardial action potentials could encourage the development of reentrant arrhythmias as a consequence of a greater dispersion in the refractoriness of the ventricular tissue.

Another possible mechanism for the generation of abnormal rhythms in hypertrophied muscle is the development of delayed afterde-

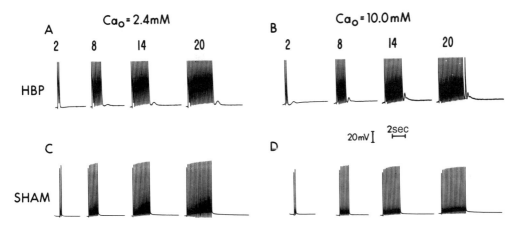

Figure 4 Delayed afterdepolarizations and triggered activity in hypertrophied myocardium. The upper records are from an hypertrophied papillary muscle (HBP) from a rat with renal hypertension (caused by constriction of the left renal artery). The lower records are from a normal papillary muscle taken from a control rat (SHAM; i.e., sham operated). The number above each pair of records indicates the number of driven responses evoked at a cycle length of 200 msec. (A) During exposure to 2.4 mM Ca$_o$ the delayed afterdepolarizations became larger and faster as the number of preceding driven responses increased. (B) Increasing Ca$_o$ to 10 mM enhanced the effects of increasing the number of preceding driven responses, so that after 20 driven responses the delayed afterdepolarization became large enough to evoke a triggered (nondriven) response. (C, D) Under the same conditions the control preparation did not develop either afterdepolarizations or triggered activity.

polarizations in hypertrophied fibers (11). We have found that afterdepolarizations can be induced selectively in hypertrophied myocardium from rats with renal hypertension (Figure 4). Thus, delayed afterdepolarizations and triggered activity could be evoked after a period of rapid drive in hypertrophied papillary muscles exposed to increased Ca$_o$ (7.2–12.0 mM) or to tetraethylammonium chloride (TEA, 10–30 mM). A burst of triggered activity could be evoked in 8 of 15 preparations exposed to high Ca$_o$ and in 10 or 11 exposed to TEA. In contrast, normal papillary muscles exposed to the same conditions did not develop either afterpotentials or triggered activity. Preparations exposed to TEA also showed early afterdepolarizations, especially if they were driven after a long period of quiescence. A number of non-driven upstrokes arose during the early afterdepolarization. In some preparations, after repolarization to more negative levels of potentials following the early afterdepolarization, a burst of triggered activity developed that eventually terminated with

a delayed afterdepolarization, suggesting that the activity originally arose as the result of a delayed afterdepolarization (Figure 5). As in other situations in which delayed afterdepolarizations occur, the magnitude of the delayed afterdepolarizations observed in the hypertrophied preparations increased as either the drive rate or the number of preceding driven beats increased.

Hypertrophied myocardium thus shows a range of rate-dependent afterdepolarizations, some of which could readily provoke abnormal rhythms in the intact heart. For example, an increase in heart rate may provoke triggered activity by enhancing the delayed afterdepolarizations to a degree sufficient to reach threshold and thus produce a train of nondriven impulses. Alternatively, a group of fibers in an area of variable entry block may remain quiescent for a period of time until being invaded by an impulse, at which time the invading impulse could evoke triggered activity arising from an early afterdepolarization (20).

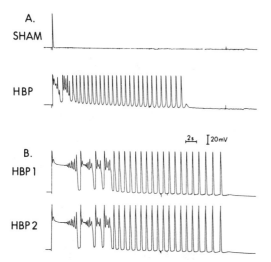

A.
SHAM

HBP

B.
HBP 1

HBP 2

2s. ⌐20mV

Figure 5 Triggered activity arising from early afterdepolarizations in hypertrophied rat papillary muscles exposed to Tyrode's solution containing 20 mM TEA. Hypertrophy was induced by renal hypertension caused by constriction of the left renal artery. (A) After a quiescent period of 2 min, the same external stimulus was applied simultaneously to the normal muscle from a control rat (SHAM; i.e., sham operated) and the hypertrophied muscle (HBP). The control muscle responded with a single driven action potential, whereas an early afterdepolarization interrupted repolarization of the action potential in the hypertrophied muscle. Following a complex series of oscillations, full repolarization was followed by a long burst of triggered (nondriven) activity, presumably sustained by delayed afterdepolarizations since it finally ended with a subthreshold delayed afterdepolarization. (B) Simultaneous records were obtained from two sites, separated by 1.5 mm, in the same hypertrophied muscle. A single driven action potential was evoked after a quiescent period of 2 min. Repolarization of the driven action potential was interrupted by an early afterdepolarization, which after initial quiescence gave rise to progressively larger oscillatory responses. The first burst of activity ceased when the membrane repolarized to a sufficiently negative level, following which a nondriven upstroke occurred, perhaps arising from a delayed afterdepolarization. Repolarization of this action potential was again interrupted by nondriven activity at a positive level of resting potential. A similar sequence was repeated twice more, and after the fourth burst of activity the membrane repolarized to a negative level of potential but nondriven activity followed, again presumably caused by delayed afterdepolarizations. The diastolic potentials during

EXPERIMENTAL HYPERTROPHY INDUCED BY OTHER MEANS

Afterpotentials and aftercontractions have been found in papillary muscles removed from rats in which cardiac hypertrophy was induced by treating unilaterally nephrectomized rats with deoxycorticosterone acetate (DOCA) (21,22). As in hypertrophy induced by pressure overload, preparations from DOCA-treated rats showed longer action potentials, longer contraction times, and longer electrical and mechanical refractory periods than control preparations. However, no bursts of triggered activity were observed.

Prolonged action potentials have also been found in hypertrophied muscle from a strain of spontaneously hypertensive rats (23,24). Hypertrophied papillary muscles from spontaneously hypertensive rats also developed exaggerated delayed afterdepolarizations and aftercontractions (24).

STREPTOZOTOCIN-INDUCED DIABETES IN RATS

As in hypertrophied myocardium, preparations of cardiac muscle taken from hearts of rats made diabetic by injection of streptozotocin show prolonged action potentials (Figure 6) (25,26). The degree of prolongation tends to be less marked than in hypertrophied myocardium but is a consistent finding in diabetic myocardium. Furthermore, myocardium from diabetic animals shows a peculiar susceptibility to develop delayed afterdepolarizations and triggered activity (26) when exposed to ouabain (5×10^{-5}) and to increased levels of Ca_o (Figure 7). As Ca_o was increased, the incidence of delayed afterdepolarizations and triggered activity also increased. At the same time, the action potential of fibers from the

the activity became gradually more negative, and the rate slowed before the activity terminated with a small delayed afterdepolarization. The nearly synchonous changes in membrane potential at two recording sites separated by more than a length constant effectively excludes reentry as a mechanism for the repetitive activity.

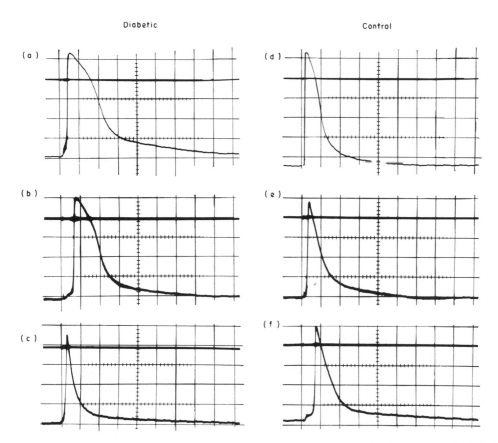

Figure 6 Transmembrane action potentials recorded in papillary muscles from rats made diabetic (a–c) by injection with streptozotocin and in control papillary muscles (d–f). (a,d) Control conditions. (b,e) After exposure to ouabain (10^{-6} M) for 30 min. (c,f) After exposure to ouabain (10^{-5} M) for 30 min. The continuous horizontal trace in each panel shows zero membrane potential. Calibrations: vertical, 20 mV per major division; horizontal, 20 msec per major division. The action potential in the diabetic papillary muscle was much more sensitive to the shortening action of ouabain than was the control action potential.

diabetic hearts shortened, whereas the action potentials in normal fibers were affected little, if at all. Those results suggest that diabetic myocardium had a predilection to develop abnormal rhythmic activity induced by delayed afterdepolarizations under conditions that tend to increase intracellular calcium, such as ischemia or digitalis intoxication.

STREPTOZOTOCIN-INDUCED DIABETES AND HYPERTENSION IN RATS

The combination of experimental diabetes and renal hypertension in rats appears to produce a more severe form of myocardial disease than the imposition of either abnormality alone (27). Thus, in a group of animals that were made diabetic and hypertensive, the mortality rate was 43–55%. Mortality did not correlate with blood pressure, serum glucose concentration, body weight, or serum creatinine, the vast majority of the animals having died suddenly, probably as a consequence of arrhythmias.

Papillary muscles removed from hypertensive diabetic rats showed a remarkable increase of almost 400% in the action potential duration (27). The entire time course of repolarization was dramatically increased in the

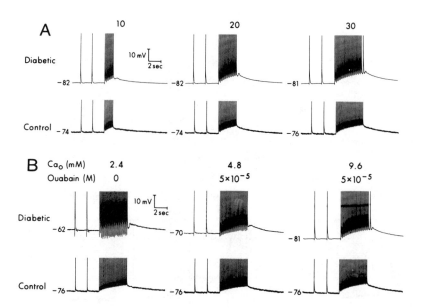

Figure 7 Delayed afterdepolarizations and triggered activity in papillary muscles from rats made diabetic by injection with streptozotocin. (A) The effect of the number of preceding action potentials on diastolic electrical activity in papillary muscles from hearts of control and diabetic rats. The number above each pair of records indicates the number of driven action potentials evoked at a cycle length of 150 msec. The external solution contained 9.6 mM Ca_o and 5×10^{-5}M ouabain. The first two action potentials in each record were the last of 10 responses elicited at a basic cycle length of 2000 msec. The number at the lower left of each record indicates the resting membrane potential (mV). The diabetic muscle developed a small delayed afterdepolarization after 10 driven action potentials. After 20 driven action potentials the delayed afterdepolarization was larger and its time course was more rapid. After 30 driven action potentials a triggered response occurred and was followed by a delayed afterdepolarization. The control preparation, under the same conditions, did not develop either afterdepolarizations or triggered activity. (B) The effects of increasing Ca_o and ouabain on the diastolic electrical activity in papillary muscles from diabetic and control hearts. In each record the period of rapid stimulation consisted of 30 responses evoked at a cycle length of 150 msec. The first two driven action potentials were the last of 10 responses evoked at the basic cycle length of 2000 msec. The number at the lower left of each record indicates the resting membrane potential (mV). The diabetic muscle developed small delayed afterdepolarizations with 2.4 mM Ca_o in the absence of ouabain, and a similar response occurred with 4.8 mM Ca_o in the presence of ouabain. With ouabain still present and Ca_o increased to 9.6 mM, a single triggered action potential developed and was followed by a delayed afterdepolarization. Under the same experimental conditions the control muscle did not develop either delayed afterdepolarizations or triggered activity.

hypertensive diabetic animals (Figure 8). The dramatic increase in action potential duration was substantially reversed after treatment of hypertension and diabetes. The maximum upstroke velocity of the action potential was also reduced significantly in hypertensive diabetic preparations, an abnormality that also reversed after treatment. The amplitude and resting potential of preparations from hypertensive diabetic animals was lower than in control preparations. The reduction in maximal up-

stroke velocity, resting potential, and amplitude may be attributable to diabetes, since all these parameters were also reduced in tissue from purely diabetic animals, whereas none of these parameters were altered significantly in purely hypertensive animals.

No mention is made of afterdepolarizations in preparations from hypertensive diabetic animals (27). However, this study was not designed to evoke either delayed or early afterdepolarizations. It would not be surpris-

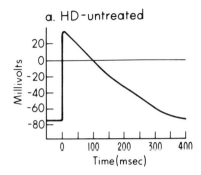

a. HD-untreated

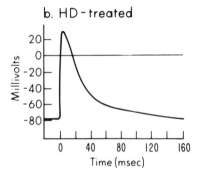

b. HD-treated

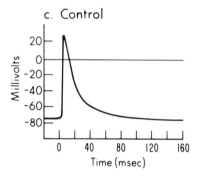

c. Control

Figure 8 Representative transmembrane action potentials recorded in papillary muscles removed from normal rats (control), hypertensive-diabetic rats (HD-untreated), and hypertensive diabetic rats in which treatment was given for hypertension and diabetes (HD-treated). Diabetes was produced by injection of streptozotocin, and hypertension was produced by constriction of the left renal artery. Note the different calibration for the time scale in untreated hypertensive diabetic rats (a) and both treated hypertensive diabetic rats and control rats (b,c). The dramatic increase in duration of the action potential recorded in the muscle from the hypertensive diabetic animals partially reversed after animals were treated for these combined diseases.

ing, however, if tissue with such long action potentials developed triggered activity arising from early afterdepolarizations (20).

HEREDITARY CARDIOMYOPATHY IN SYRIAN HAMSTERS

An inbred strain of Syrian hamsters has been identified in which a genetically transmitted cardiomyopathy develops (28). Some strains develop a progressive form of cardiomyopathy that eventually leads to cardiac decompensation with congestive heart failure, cardiomegaly, and edema. The animals progress through a stage in which compensatory hypertrophy develops, but eventually the heart dilates and fails. Some strains of hamsters with cardiomyopathy do not appear to progress to the stage of heart failure.

This genetic model of heart disease has been known for almost 20 years, and a number of studies have identified biochemical abnormalities and a peculiar susceptibility to develop calcium-dependent cellular necrosis (see Reference 29 for references). In contrast, there is a surprising lack of studies on electrophysiologic abnormalities associated with cardiomyopathy in the Syrian hamster. Various nonspecific electrocardiographic abnormalities have been described (30,31). In one study in which high-frequency, high-fidelity recordings of the electrocardiogram were obtained during progressive development of cardiomyopathy in the hamster model, high-frequency "notches" were recorded during the QRS complex in animals that developed extensive focal myocardial fibrosis (32). The presence of such high-frequency components was believed to result from impaired conduction due to myocardial fibrosis in the cardiomyopathic hearts (32). In this same very brief report, the authors noted that electrocardiographic signs of left ventricular hypertrophy were often absent and, when present, occurred at a much later stage of the disease.

To our knowledge there has been only one study of the cellular electrophysiologic properties of isolated preparations from the cardiomyopathic hamster (33). The major finding in this study was that the action potential duration was increased in papillary muscles removed from the hearts of the cardiomyopathic animals. As is true in hypertrophied muscle from animals with pressure overload, neither the maximum velocity of the upstroke nor the resting membrane potential was reduced in the cardiomyopathic preparations. However, the action potential overshoot was significantly greater in the myopathic tissue. No mention was made of the presence of afterpotentials, even though the preparations from both normal and myopathic hearts were driven at rates ranging from 1 to 8 Hz.

CATECHOLAMINE-INDUCED FOCAL NECROSIS IN RATS AND GUINEA PIGS

A form of cardiac disease in which focal hemorrhage and necrosis develop can be induced by administration of large doses of catecholamines. Such lesions were induced in rats and guinea pigs by the subcutaneous injection of epinephrine (34). Myocardium removed from the animals 24 hr after the injection showed various electrical abnormalities, among which were bursts of electrical activity that, judging by the presence of early and delayed afterdepolarizations, may well have been triggered.

DISEASED CANINE ATRIAL FIBERS

Action potentials recorded from atrial tissue removed from dogs with left atrial enlargement due to mitral insufficiency were not different from those recorded in tissue taken from normal-sized right atria or normal-sized left atria from control dogs (35). Despite the fact that the dogs with left atrial enlargement had intermittent atrial arrhythmias, triggered activity could not be easily induced in tissue removed from enlarged left atria, even after exposure to norepinephrine. Neither the slow-response type of action potentials nor automatic activity was found with any frequency (35). Because enlarged left atria had a number of structural abnormalities, including cellular hypertrophy and proliferation of connective tissue, the arrhythmias observed in the diseased canine hearts were attributed to the effects of the abnormal architecture of the tissue.

DISEASED HUMAN ATRIAL TISSUE

Diseased human atrial fibers removed from the hearts of patients undergoing surgical procedures, mainly for atherosclerotic and congenital heart disease (36), showed two kinds of self-sustained rhythmic activity. In some preparations the abnormal rhythmic activity appeared to depend on ordinary slow diastolic depolarization (phase 4 depolarization). In other preparations triggered activity arising from a delayed afterdepolarization occurred either spontaneously or after treatment with epinephrine. In some fibers self-sustained rhythmic activity that began with a phase 4 depolarization could, as the spontaneous rate of discharge increased and led to the development of delayed afterdepolarizations, give rise to triggered activity.

DISEASED HUMAN VENTRICULAR TISSUE

The action potential recorded in myocardium taken from a patient with hypertrophic cardiomyopathy was found to be prolonged (37), as has been described in hypertrophied myocardium from the experimental models just discussed.

Ventricular preparations removed from seven patients who had ischemic heart disease (left ventricle) and one patient who had "primary electrical disease" (right ventricle) showed a variety of electrical abnormalities, among which were various degrees of loss of resting potential, slowed action potential upstrokes, and abnormal conduction (38). Bursts of triggered activity could be evoked by one or more driven action potentials, the bursts of triggering being followed by a typical subthreshold delayed afterdepolarization.

CELLULAR ELECTRICAL ABNORMALITIES AND THE GENERATION OF ARRHYTHMIAS

We have seen that myocardium from models of cardiac disease and tissue isolated from diseased human hearts can show abnormal cellular electrical activity that could lead to arrhythmias. However, the relationship between those electrical abnormalities and the development of potentially lethal arrhythmias is not yet well understood. One could suppose that arrhythmias arise from an early afterdepolarization or that a delayed afterdepolarization reaches threshold and thereby induces an arrhythmia. Yet, even in pathologic preparations, it is often necessary to alter the ionic environment or the mode of stimulation to provoke afterpotential-dependent triggered activity.

The prolonged duration of repolarization consistently associated with cardiac hypertrophy may represent an adaptive response that could contribute to the development of abnormal rhythmic activity under conditions of physiologic stress (e.g., increased heart rate, hypokalemia, catecholamines, or digitalis intoxication) or when hypertrophy progresses to myocardial failure. In the adaptive phase of pure myocardial hypertrophy, the prolonged depolarization may represent a "compensatory" change that maintains an adequate amount of activator calcium in hypertrophied cells by allowing sufficient influx of calcium via the slow inward current channels and/or by increasing the release of calcium from the sarcoplasmic reticulum (SR) (39). However, this compensatory mechanism carries with it the potential for generating abnormal rhythmic activity in several ways.

The available experimental evidence suggests that afterpotentials develop in cardiac fibers in which the myoplasmic calcium concentration is caused to rise above physiologic levels (see Reference 20 for a complete discussion and references). The precise relationship between a pathologic rise in myoplasmic calcium and the development of afterpotentials is not yet entirely clear. It has been suggested that the increased myoplasmic calcium concentration could provoke delayed afterdepolarizations either by activating a nonspecific cation channel in the sarcolemma or by causing the electrogenic sodium-calcium exchange mechanism in the sarcolemma to generate a net inward current during electrical diastole. However, Cranefield and Aronson (20) have pointed out that a number of other mechanisms that are equally possible have not yet been excluded. In any case, it certainly appears that afterdepolarizations and triggered activity occur under conditions that are also associated with an increase in the myoplasmic calcium level.

The most obvious situation in which hypertrophied fibers are likely to develop triggered activity is thus under conditions that are likely to raise the level of myoplasmic calcium beyond the "optimum" level characteristic of the adaptive phase of hypertrophy. For example, increasing external calcium could further enhance calcium influx through the slow inward current channels and thereby raise the level of calcium above the optimum range for tension development. Many studies have demonstrated that once myoplasmic calcium exceeds a critical level, "spontaneous" and "induced" oscillations of current, voltage, and tension develop in cardiac fibers (see Reference 20). Some forms of spontaneous current oscillation associated with increased myoplasmic calcium may represent an elemental form of the induced oscillations that correspond to delayed afterdepolarizations, whereas other kinds of spontaneous oscillations may themselves cause abnormal rhythmic activity (40). Thus, any conditions that increase myoplasmic calcium concentration, such as increased heart rate, treatment with digitalis or catecholamines, or exposure to low potassium, could provoke delayed afterdepolarizations, which could lead to arrhythmias by the same basic mechanisms.

On the other hand, the long duration of the action potential characteristic of hypertrophied myocardium could lead to arrhythmias arising from early afterdepolarizations. Cranefield and Aronson (20) have pointed out that the kind of electrical response that occurs in conjunction with an early afterdepolarization depends on the balance between inward and outward currents (Figure 9). Thus, if the net outward current is normal, repolarization proceeds along its normal time course. If the inward and outward currents are exactly equal, then there is no net current across the membrane and the membrane potential becomes stable at a low level of resting potential (e.g., -60 mV). However, if after a brief period of zero net current the current becomes net inward, a second upstroke or even a burst of

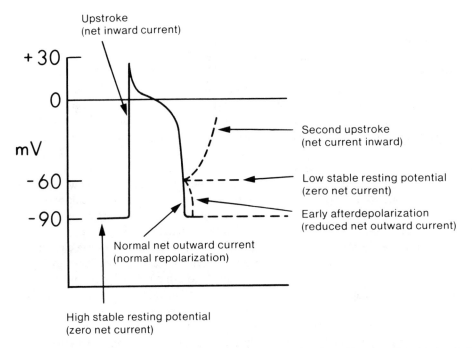

Figure 9 The type of electrical response that occurs at the time that an early afterdepolarization may appear. The type of response depends on the balance between inward and outward currents. If the net outward current is normal, repolarization proceeds along its normal course to the normal level of resting potential (-90 mV). If the inward and outward currents are equal so that there is no net current across the membrane, then the membrane potential becomes stable at a low level of resting potential (-60 mV). If after a brief period of zero net current the current becomes net inward, a second upstroke or even a burst of rhythmic activity occurs, arising from a positive level of maximum diastolic potential (-60 mV). If after a brief period of zero net current the current becomes net outward, retardation of repolarization, that is, an early afterdepolarization, results before the membrane potential returns to its high stable level. Cardiac hypertrophy is associated with an increase in action potential duration, which indicates the presence of an increased amount of net inward current during repolarization. Thus the action potential in hypertrophied fibers may be more susceptible to develop a second upstroke, since only a small amount of additional inward current is necessary to provoke one.

rhythmic activity occurs, usually arising from a level of maximum diastolic potential around -60 mV. Finally, if after a brief period of zero net current the current becomes net outward, repolarization is retarded before the membrane potential returns to its normal stable level of -90 mV. This last case represents an early afterdepolarization without the development of a second upstroke or nondriven response.

The prolonged duration of repolarization in hypertrophied fibers must be caused by an increase in net inward current. Whether this increase is the result of an increase in inward current or a decrease in outward current, or a combination of both, remains to be determined. Moreover, the ionic mechanism underlying the prolonged duration of the action potential need not be the same in all cases; the mechanism may well vary according to the species, model, and degree of hypertrophy. Regardless of the cause of the increase in net inward current, the action potential in hypertrophied fibers should be more susceptible to develop a second upstroke during the prolonged course of repolarization, since only a small additional amount of inward current is required to provoke a second upstroke.

A particularly interesting situation in which an early afterdepolarization may give rise to repetitive activity is when a focus of hypertrophied cells is isolated from the rest of the myocardium by variable entrance block (Figure

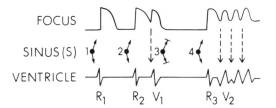

Figure 10 Diagram of the way in which fibers in a focus with variable entry block could lead to the appearance of an early afterdepolarization and initiation of ventricular tachycardia. No account is taken of possible sinus reset, nor is any effort made to show T waves or their possible prolongation by the early afterdepolarization. The timing and duration are strictly schematic. R indicates a QRS complex of sinus origin; V indicates a QRS complex of ectopic origin. The second sinus impulse evokes, in the focus, an action potential that gives rise to a second upstroke, which causes V_1. The next sinus impulse is blocked in the refractory period (compensatory pause). As a result of the pause, the next sinus impulse evokes, in the focus, an action potential in which an early afterdepolarization leads to a burst of activity. Such a situation if it develops in the hypertrophied heart, could allow a small group of cells to produce even longer action potentials and afterdepolarizations, which could lead to triggered activity.

10) (20,41). Under such circumstances the fibers within the focus remain quiescent until, for one reason or another, entry block is dissipated. The invading impulse then excites cells that were quiescent. The resulting action potentials would have a prolonged time course that would tend to favor the development of early afterdepolarizations and triggered activity.

As myocardial hypertrophy decompensates into cardiac failure, other factors may enhance the propensity to develop afterdepolarizations. First, there are conditions that tend to increase myoplasmic calcium to a level high enough to induce oscillatory diastolic electrical activity. Those conditions include (1) augmented transmembrane influx of calcium during extraordinarily prolonged action potentials like those we observed in the cardiomyopathy associated with hypertension and diabetes (27); and (2) the development of a concomitant defect in the subcellular regulation of calcium, like the reduced rate of calcium uptake by the SR in ventricular muscle from diabetic rats (42). Thus, with more advanced myocardial disease, only a small additional increase in myoplasmic calcium may be required to reach the level necessary to provoke oscillatory afterpotentials and, presumably, arrhythmias. Accordingly, myocardium from hearts of animals with more severe myocardial disease may be more sensitive to conditions that tend to increase myoplasmic calcium (e.g., changes in the rate of stimulation, treatment with digitalis or catecholamines, and exposure to low potassium). On the other hand, maneuvers or agents that tend to reduce myoplasmic calcium levels (e.g., calcium antagonists) may prevent such abnormal processes from developing.

The development of afterdepolarizations in hypertrophied fibers, whether due to elevated myoplasmic calcium levels or not, need not necessarily induce abnormal rhythmic activity. The net inward current that generates afterdepolarizations amounts to a form of current noise against which ventricular muscle tends to be stable because of its normally high potassium conductance during diastole (20,43). To depolarize the membrane to threshold, the inward current that generates the afterdepolarization must be large enough to overcome the high resting conductance (43). Therefore, loss of the normally high diastolic membrane conductance may be an important arrhythmogenic factor in decompensated hypertrophied cells.

A recent computer model (44) indicates that in guinea pig ventricular myocardium only a small number of cells need generate delayed afterdepolarizations to provoke triggered activity in the whole heart. For example, as few as three cells generating delayed afterdepolarizations can evoke propagated action potentials under conditions in which these abnormal cells are connected by two gap junctions with increased resistance (10–15MΩ, the normal value being 2–5 MΩ) to the surrounding "normal" tissue. Thus in the hypertrophied or failing heart only a few cells need develop afterpotentials to generate abnormal rhythmic activity in the entire heart, provided other conditions coexist (i.e., reduced number of cell-to-cell couplings and modestly increased resistance of cell-to-cell couplings). In the severely diseased heart it is not difficult to envision those conditions being created by the development of disruptive fibrotic tissue.

In addition to afterpotentials, other electrical abnormalities in diseased myocardium may operate to cause arrhythmias. For example, Han and Moe (19) suggested that nonuniform recovery following excitation favors the development of fractionated impulses arising during the relatively refractory period and thereby increases the chance of reentry. As described earlier, we have found (12) a wide disparity in the action potential durations from endocardium to epicardium in hypertrophied myocardium, a nonuniform distribution that may encourage the development of reentry. Areas of slow conduction, which are a necessary requirement for the development of reentry, may occur in foci of myocardial tissue with reduced upstroke velocity, as has been observed in preparations from diabetic (25) and hypertensive diabetic animals (27). In the adaptive stage of hypertrophy, it does not appear that the changes in passive membrane properties (14) are sufficient to account for significant slowing or interruption of conduction. However, if cell death and fibrosis occur as myocardial disease becomes more severe, then it seems likely that disruption of intercellular connections and the development of fibrous tissue interfere with conduction of the cardiac impulse and could encourage the development of re-entry.

It does not appear that ordinary automaticity dependent on spontaneous phase 4 depolarization occurs very often in hypertrophied or failing myocardium. Although some diseased atrial fibers appear to develop phase 4-dependent automaticity, this kind of activity appears to provoke tachycardias by inducing triggered activity dependent on delayed afterdepolarizations (36). Alterations in the intrinsic automaticity of the diseased heart may be important in provoking arrhythmias, however. For example, excessive tachycardia or bradycardia in the hypertrophied or diseased heart could encourage the development of triggered activity dependent on delayed and early afterdepolarizations, respectively. Automaticity may thus interact with afterpotential-dependent processes to cause arrhythmias in the diseased myocardium.

In summary, cardiac hypertrophy is associated with a variety of electrical abnormalities that could predispose to the development of arrhythmias. Which, if any, of these mechanisms operates in the intact diseased human heart remains to be determined. However, the close correspondence between the abnormal electrical activity in animal models and in the few studies in isolated diseased human tissues is encouraging. With further studies of improved models we can look forward to a better understanding of the cellular mechanisms responsible for arrhythmias in the diseased heart and it is hoped, to the development of more specific and effective therapy directed to those causes.

REFERENCES

1. Greenberg H M, Dwyer E M Jr, eds. Sudden coronary death. New York: New York Academy of Sciences, 1982.
2. Maron B J, Roberts W C, Epstein S E. Sudden death in hypertrophic cardiomyopathy 1982; 65:1388–94.
3. Kannel W B, Sorlie P. Left ventricular hypertrophy in hypertension: prognostic and pathogenetic implications (The Framingham Study). In: Strauer B E, ed. The heart in hypertension. New York: Springer-Verlag, 1981: 223–42.
4. McLenachan J M, Henderson E, Morris K I, Dargie H J. Ventricular arrhyrthmias in patients with hypertensive left ventricular hypertrophy. N Engl J Med 1987; 317:787–92.
5. Packer M. Sudden unexpected death in patients with congestive heart failure: a second frontier. Circulation 1985; 72:681–5.
6. Bassett A, Gelband H. Chronic partial occlusion of the pulmonary artery in cats: charges in ventricular action potential configuration during early hypertrophy. Circ Res 1973; 32:15–26.
7. Gelband H, Bassett A. Depressed transmembrane potentials during experimentally induced ventricular failure in cats. Circ Res 1973; 32:625–34.
8. Tritthart H, Leudeke H, Bayer R, Stierle H, Kaufmann R. Right ventricular hypertrophy in the cat—an electrophysiological and anatomical study. J Mol Cell Cardiol 1975; 7:163–74.

9. Gulch R W, Baumann R, Jacob R. Analysis of myocardial action potential in left ventricular hypertrophy of Goldblatt rats. Basic Res Cardiol 1979; 74:69–82.

10. Aronson R S. Characteristics of action potentials of hypertrophied myocardium from rats with renal hypertension. Circ Res 1980; 47:443–54.

11. Aronson R S. Afterpotentials and triggered activity in hypertrophied myocardium from rats with renal hypertension. Circ Res 1981; 48:720–7.

12. Keung ECH, Aronson R S. Non-uniform electrophysiologic properties and electronic interaction in hypertrophied rat myocardium. Circ Res 1981; 49:150–8.

13. Keung ECH, Aronson R S. Transmembrane action potentials and the electrocardiogram in rats with renal hypertension. Cardiovasc Res 1981; 11:611–4.

14. Keung ECH, Keung C S, Aronson R S. Passive electrical properties of normal and hypertrophied rat myocardium. Am J Physiol 1982; 243:H917–26.

15. Nordin C, Siri F, Aronson R S. Electrical properties of ventricular myocytes isolated from guinea pig hearts (abstract). Clin Res 1987; 35:574A.

16. Nordin C, Siri F, Aronson R S. Electrophysiologic characteristics of single myocytes isolated from hypertrophied guinea pig hearts. J Mol Cell Cardiol 1989; 21:724–39.

17. Kleiman R B, Houser S R. Calcium currents in normal and hypertrophied feline ventricular myocytes. Am J Physiol 1988; 255:H1434–42.

18. Keung E C. Calcium current is increased in isolated adult myocytes from hypertrophied rat myocardium. Circ Res 1989; 64:753–63.

19. Han J, Moe G K. Nonuniform recovery of excitability in ventricular muscle. Circ Res 1964; 14:44–60.

20. Cranefield P F, Aronson R S. Cardiac arrhythmias: the role of triggered activity and other mechanisms. Mount Kisco, NY: Futura, 1988.

21. Heller L J. Augmented aftercontractions in papillary muscles from rats with cardiac hypertrophy. Am J Physiol 1979; 237:H649–54.

22. Heller L J, Stauffer E K. Membrane potentials and contractile events of hypertrophied rat cardiac muscle (41036). Proc Soc Exp Biol Med 1981; 166:141–7.

23. Hayashi H, Shibata S. Electrical property of cardiac cell membrane of spontaneously hypertensive rats. Eur J Pharmacol 1974; 27: 355–9.

24. Heller L J, Stauffer E K. Altered electrical and contractile properties of hypertrophied cardiac muscle (SHR and DOCA-treated WKY) (abstract). Fed Proc 1979; 38:975.

25. Fein R S, Aronson R S, Nordin C, Miller-Green B, Sonnenblick E H. Altered myocardial response to ouabain in diabetic rats: mechanics and electrophysiology. J Mol Cell Cardiol 1983; 15:769–84.

26. Nordin C, Gilat E, Aronson R S. Delayed afterdepolarizations and triggered activity in ventricular muscle from rats with streptozotocin-induced diabetes. Circ Res 1985; 57:28–34.

27. Fein F S, Capasso J M, Aronson R S, Cho S, Nordin C, Miller-Green B, Sonnenblick E H, Factor S M. Combined renovascular hypertension and diabetes in rats: a new preparation of congestive cardiomyopathy. Circulation 1984; 70:318–30.

28. Bajusz E, Baker R, Nixon C W, Homburger F. Spontaneous, hereditary myocardial degeneration and congestive heart failure in a strain of Syrian hamsters. Ann NY Acad Sci 1969; 156:105–29.

29. Markiewicz W, Zhao S W, Parmley W W, Higgins C B, Sievers R, James T L, Wikman-Coffelt J, Jasmin G. Evaluation of the hereditary Syrian hamster cardiomyopathy by ^{31}p nuclear magnetic resonance spectroscopy: improvement after acute verapamil therapy. Circ Res 1986; 59:597–604.

30. Laird C W. Developmental electrocardiography in inbred perinatal hamsters. Adv Cardiol 1974; 13:250–69.

31. Lossnitzer K, Grewe N, Konrad A, Adler J. Electrocardiographic changes in cardiomyopathic Syrian hamsters (strain B10 8262). Basic Res Cardiol 1977; 72:421–35.

32. Angelakos E T, Daniels J, Robinson S, Bajusz E. Electrocardiographic changes during a progressive focal myocardiopathy in hamsters. In: Bajusz E, Rona G, Brink A J, Lockner A, eds. Recent advances in studies on cardiac structure and metabolism, Vol. 2, Cardiomyopathies. Baltimore: University Park Press, 1973:507.

33. Rossner K L, Sachs H G. Electrophysiological study of Syrian hamster hereditary cardiomyopathy. Cardiovasc Res 1978; 12:436–43.

34. Gilmour R F, Zipes D P. Electrophysiological characteristics of rodent myocardium dam-

aged by adrenaline. Cardiovasc Res 1980; 14: 582–9.

35. Boyden P A, Tilley L P, Pham T D, Liu S-K, Fenoglio J J, Wit A L. Effects of left atrial enlargement on atrial transmembrane potentials and structure in dogs with mitral valve fibrosis. Am J Cardiol 1982; 49:1896–908

36. Mary-Rabine L, Hordorf A J, Danilo P, Malm J R, Rosen M R. Mechanisms for impulse initiation in isolated human atrial fibers. Circ Res 1980; 47:267–77.

37. Coltart D J, Meldrum S J. Hypertrophic cardiomyopathy. An electrophysiological study. Br Med J 1970; 4:217–8.

38. Gilmour R F, Heger J J, Prystowsky E N, Zipes D P. Cellular electrophysiologic abnormalities of diseased human ventricular myocardium. Am J Cardiol 1983; 51:137–44.

39. Capasso J M, Aronson R S, Sonneblick E H. Reversible alterations in excitation-contraction coupling during myocardial hyper-

trophy in rat papillary muscles. Circ Res 1982; 51:189–95.

40. Aronson R S, Nordin C. Unpublished observations.

41. Cranefield P F, Aronson R S. Torsade de pointes and other pause-induced ventricular tachycardias: the short-long-short sequence and early afterdepolarizations. PACE 1988; 11:670–8.

42. Penpargkul S, Fein F S, Sonnenblick E H, Scheuer J. Depressed cardiac sarcoplasmic reticular function from diabetic rats. J Mol Cell Cardiol 1981; 13:303–9.

43. Aronson R S, Nordin C. Arrhythmogenic interaction between low potassium and ouabain in isolated guinea-pig ventricular myocytes. J Physiol (Lond) 1988; 400:113–34.

44. Nordin C. A computer model for analysis of syncytial effects of localized transient inward currents in ventricular myocardium (abstract). Biophys J 1988; 53:425a.

18

Animal Models of Naturally Occurring Arrhythmias

Philip R. Fox

The Animal Medical Center, Speyer Hospital, and Caspary Research Institute
New York, New York

INTRODUCTION

In contrast to human electrocardiography, for which the clinical applications were recognized by at least 1913 (1), veterinary electrocardiography has come into its own only during the last two decades. A few descriptions of arrhythmias appeared in the veterinary literature from the 1920s through the 1940s (2–4). However, it was not until after Lannek's 1949 thesis (5) that electrocardiographic assessment of heart disease in animals started in earnest. The first authoritative textbooks for canine electrocardiography appeared in 1970 (6) and 1975 (7). The subject became well defined by other authors (8–10). Feline electrocardiograms were initially performed in anesthetized cats (12–14). They were soon applied to nonanesthetized healthy animals (15–17). Electrocardiography rapidly developed as a clinical diagnostic modality that found large application in congenital heart diseases and cardiomyopathies (8–11,18–25).

Electrocardiographic assessment of cardiac diseases has been widely applied to other mammalian and avian species. Intraspecies variation is often significant. In the horse, alterations in ECG values occur in relation to age, breed, and sex (26–32). Cardiac arrhythmias are common (33–41). Dysrhythmias and P-QRS-T abnormalities have also been reported in other species, including the cow (33, 41–43), ferret (44, 45), hamster (46), and various avians (47–50).

RECORDING AND INTERPRETING THE CANINE AND FELINE ELECTROCARDIOGRAM

Clinical electrocardiographic evaluation of heart disease in the dog and cat utilizes bipolar standard leads, augmented unipolar limb leads, and unipolar precordial chest leads (Table 1). A modified orthogonal lead system is sometimes used to infer cardiac chamber enlargement or to generate a vectorcardiogram (7–10,51). The standard recording position involves placing the dog or cat in right lateral recumbancy with forelimbs held perpendicular to the long axis of the body. Improper positioning, especially forelimb displacement, can distort the mean QRS electrical axis (51). Sternal positioning is used with vicious or dyspneic animals. Copper electrode clips are

Table 1 Electrocardiographic Lead Systems for the Dog and Cat[a]

Lead system	Lead	Positive electrode	Negative electrode
Bipolar standard	I	Left arm	Right arm
	II	Left leg	Right arm
	III	Left leg	Left arm
Augmented unipolar limb leads	aVR	Right arm	Central terminal
	aVL	Left arm	
	aVF	Left leg	
Unipolar precordial chest leads	$rV_2(CV_6RL)$	R5 ICS near sternal edge	
	$V_2(CV_6LL)$	L6 ICS at chostochondral junction (CCJ)	Central terminal
	$V_4(CV_6LU)$	L6 ICS at CCJ	
	V_{10}	Over dorsal spinal process of seventh 7th thoracic vertebra	
Modified orthogonal	X	Lead I	
	Y	Lead aVF	
	Z	V_{10}	

[a]Electrode clip placement: RA, LA, caudal aspect of proximal olecrenon; RL, LL, anterior aspect, over patellar ligament.
Source: From Reference 8.

attached directly to the animal's skin and moistened with conductive gel or paste. Intracardiac and esophageal leads are occasionally used to enhance rhythm diagnosis when information from other electrocardiograph leads is inconclusive. These are especially suitable for demonstrating atrial activity in complex arrhythmias, for pacing to facilitate diagnosis, or for therapy (19).

Conventionally, a paper speed of 50 mm/sec is used to record at least 30 sec of electrical activity. In dogs a recording speed of 25 mm/sec may be advantageous to permit easier identification of deflections with low amplitude and short duration. However, P and PQ durations (but not QRS or QT durations) are underestimated at the slower paper speed (53).

The approach to analysis of the canine and feline electrocardiogram is similar to that performed in the human. Heart rate, rhythm, P-QRS-T complexes, and mean electrical axis are assessed. A summary of normal values is provided for heart rate, mean electrical axis, P-QRS-T complexes, and intervals for the dog (Table 2) and cat (Table 3) (8).

SPONTANEOUS CANINE ARRHYTHMIAS

The incidence of naturally occurring arrhythmias in dogs has been reported in several studies (54–56). In 3000 consecutive clinical cases at one veterinary college in Philadelphia, 15 different arrhythmias were diagnosed in 95 dogs over an 18 month period (Table 4) (54). In another survey of 2000 canine arrhythmias transmitted transtelephonically from 42 states to a commercial service (Cardiopet Inc, Brooklyn, NY), 18 different arrhythmias were documented in 396 dogs (55) (Table 4). The higher arrhythmia incidence in the latter study reflects a sampling bias made to conform clinically suspected arrhythmias or to evaluate the efficacy of antiarrhythmic therapy.

Table 2 Electrocardiographic Parameters for the Normal Dog

Rate
  70–160 beats/min for adult dogs
  Up to 180 beats/min for toy breeds
  Up to 220 beats/min for puppies
Rhythm
  Normal sinus rhythm
  Sinus arrhythmia
  Wandering SA pacemaker
Measurements (lead II, 50 mm/sec, 1 cm = 1 mV)
  P wave
    Width: maximum 0.04 sec
    Height: maximum 0.4 mV
  P-R interval
    Width: 0.06–0.13 sec
  QRS complex
    Width: Maximum 0.05 sec in small breeds
    maximum 0.06 sec in large breeds
    Height of R wave[a] Maximum 3.0 mV in large breeds
    Maximum 2.5 mV in small breeds
  S-T segment
    No depression: no more than 0.2 mV
    No elevation: not more than 0.15 mV
  T wave
    Can be positive, negative, or biphasic
    Not greater than one-fourth amplitude of R wave
  Q-T interval
    Width 0.15–0.25 sec at normal
    heart rate; varies with heart rate (faster rates have
    shorter Q-T intervals and vice versa)
Electrical axis (frontal plane): 40–100°
Precordial chest leads (values of special importance)
  CV_5RL (rV_2): T wave positive
  CV_6LL (V_2): S wave not greater than 0.8 mV (eight boxes),
    R wave not greater than 2.5 mV[a]
  CV_6LU (V_4): S waves not greater than 0.7 mV, R
    wave not greater than 3.0 mV[a]
  V_{10}: negative QRS complex, T wave negative except in chi-
    huahua

[a]Not valid for thin deep-chested dogs under 2 years of age.
Source From Tilley, LP. "Essentials of canine and feline electrocardiography. Philadelphia: Lea & Febizer, 1985, with permission.

Spontaneous arrhythmias accompany innumerable cardiac and extracardiac conditions (8–11,56). These include acid-base and electrolyte derangements, autonomic imbalances, systemic and metabolic diseases, endocrinopathies, ischemia, pulmonary disease, neoplasia, and acquired and congenital heart diseases.

Sinus rhythms, often with wandering sinus pacemakers, are most common. Normal sinus rates vary between 70 and 160 beats/min in the adult dog but vary greatly between breeds. Small and toy breeds may have rates as high as 180; in large and giant breed rates are often between 70 and 120. Puppies may display heart rates up to 220 beats/min.

Sinus arrhythmia is more common than regular sinus rhythm (8). This occurs when the variation between R-R intervals exceeds

Table 3 Electrocardiographic Parameters for the Normal Cat

Rate
 Range 160–240 beats/min
 Mean 197 beats/min
Rhythm
 Normal sinus rhythm
 Sinus tachycardia (physiologic reaction to excitement)
Measurements (lead II, 50 mm/sec, 1 cm = 1 mV)[a]
 P wave
  Width: maximum 0.04 sec
  Height: maximum 0.2 mV
 P-R interval
  Width 0.05–0.09 sec
 QRS complex
  Width: maximum 0.04 sec
  Height of R wave: maximum 0.9 mV
 S-T segment
  No marked depression or elevation
 T wave:
  can be positive, negative, or biphasic; most often positive
  Maximum amplitude 0.3 mV
 Q-T interval:
  width 0.12–0.18 sec (6–9 boxes) at normal heart rate
   (range 0.07–0.20 sec, 3½–10 boxes); varies with heart
   rate (faster rates, shorter Q-T intervals, and vice versa)
Electrical axis (front plane):
 0–160°
Precordial chest leads
 No well-established normal values to date
 CV_6LU (V_4): R wave not greater than 1.0 mV

Source: From Tilley LP. Essentials of canine and feline electrocardiography. Philadelphia: Lea & Febizer, 1985, with permission.

± 10% (57). Small brachycephalic breeds are especially prone to upper and lower respiratory disorders that increase vagal tone and influence sinoatrial nodal discharge. Other conditions enhancing sinus arrhythmia include gastrointestinal disorders (especially with emesis) and central nervous system derangements. Escape beats sometimes intervene during prolonged sinus pauses, although hypotension associated with these pauses is rare.

Sinus bradycardia usually indicates vagotonia from various disorders, including neurologic (increased cerebrospinal fluid pressure, brainstem lesions, and head trauma) gastrointestinal, endocrine (hypothyroidism), or metabolic. Hypoxia or hypothermia may be contributory. Sinus bradycardia may also be associated with organic heart disease (10).

Sinus tachycardia most commonly indicates increased sympathetic tone from fright, pain, excitement, shock, or systemic or metabolic disease. It is variably present as a compensatory response with congestive heart failure due to myocardial or acquired valvular diseases (8,10).

Supraventricular premature complexes (atrial or junctional) and tachycardia have a variety of cardiac and noncardiac associations. Atrial enlargement secondary to acquired chronic atrioventricular valvular disease is the most common cause (54,58–61), and dilated cardiomyopathy is the second most frequent condition (62,63). Congenital cardiac disorders, such as shunts (e.g., patent ductus arteriosus) or mitral valve malformation, occur less frequently (64,65). Atrial tumors

Table 4 Frequency and Incidence of Canine Arrhythmias

Arrhythmia	No. dogs[a]	No. dogs[b]
Supraventricular		
Sinoatrial standstill	1	
Atrial premature complexes	111	14
Paroxysmal atrial tachycardia	13	3
Atrial flutter	1	2
Atrial fibrillation	63	13
Atrioventricular junction		
AV junctional premature complexes		3
AV dissociation		3
Ventricular		
Ventricular premature complexes	101	43
Ventricular tachycardia	11	8
Sinoatrial arrest or block[c]	27	
Persistent atrial standstill	1	
Atrial standstill	1	
AV block		
First degree	30	12
Second degree	35	12
Third degree (complete)	5	2
Preexcitation (Wolff-Parkinson-White)	1	1
Parasystole	1	
Total no. (%) dogs with arrhythmias: 95 (3.2%)	396 (20)	95 (3.2)

= Transtelephonic ECG recordings
[a]Sample size, 2000 dogs (55).
[b]Sample size, 3000 dogs (54).
[c]Affected dogs displayed SA block or SA arrest compatible with sick sinus syndrome; secondary escape beats often recorded.

(especially hemangiosarcoma), pericarditis, bacterial endocarditis, and heartworm disease are occasionally causative. Noncardiac conditions include increased sympathetic tone, hypoxia, toxemia, dysautonomia, and hypokalemia (8, 10, 56). Atrial flutter is rare (7,8,66).

Atrial fibrillation is common and is associated with severe atrial enlargement. The most frequent condition is idiopathic dilated cardiomyopathy of large and giant breed dogs (8, 63). The second most common cause is atrial enlargement accompanying chronic acquired atrioventricular disease in small breeds (10, 54,67,68). Third, it occurs from uncorrected congenital heart disorders (65,69,70). Least commonly, it may accompany systemic or metabolic disease (hypoadrenocorticism or hypothyroidism) (71) or be idiopathic in giant breed dogs with echocardiographically normal cardiac structure and function. In the presence of organic heart disease atrial fibrillation is associated with a 6 month mortality rate of 74–85% (70,72,73).

Ventricular arrhythmias are very prevalent, especially premature ventricular complexes whose causes vary greatly (7–10,55,56,60, 62,63,65,67,71,74–77). They are commonly associated with organic heart disease (e.g., ventricular dilatation from any cause), especially in the company of heart failure and hypoxia. Associated conditions include systemic, metabolic, electrolyte, acid-base, autonomic, neoplastic, inflammatory, and infectious derangements. They may be recorded from structurally normal hearts or arise secondary to blunt trauma. The boxer breed is predisposed to ventricular tachycardia, especially older animals.

Idioventricular tachycardias between 60 and 120 beats/min are common, usually benign, and often transient in the dog (56). These may be greatly influenced by autonomic tone.

Conduction disturbances are frequently identified. Atrial conduction abnormalities often result from hyperkalemia due to renal failure, hypoadrenocorticism, or urethral obstruction (71). They are the most common causes of temporary atrial standstill. Sick sinus syndrome occurs most often in adult, female miniature schnauzer dogs. Rarely, a fascioscapulohumeral type of muscular dystrophy causes persistent atrial standstill, especially in English springer spaniels (80,81).

Atrioventricular block is often recognized. It is usually incomplete and occurs secondary to vagotonia, AV nodal or bundle branch disease, cardiomyopathy, or chronic volume overload. Second-degree AV block is common in brachycephalic breeds that exhibit marked respiratory sinus arrhythmia (8,82). Occasionally, complete AV block occurs as a result of inflammation or infiltration of the AV conduction system or bundle branches; it may also be associated with acquired valvular or myocardial disease, hyperkalemia, hypokalemia, or hypothyroidism or it may be idiopathic (8,10,71).

Ventricular preexcitation is rare but well documented (8). In one series of six dogs it was associated with reciprocating supraventricular tachycardia and was thought to involve bundle of Kent accessory pathways (83). Other cases have been documented by endocardial mapping (84,85).

Several spontaneous cardiovascular diseases are commonly observed in dogs. A discussion of arrhythmias pertaining to these disorders follows.

Acquired Chronic Valvular Disease in Dogs (Mitral Valve Prolapselike Syndrome)

The most common cause of heart failure in dogs results from chronic atrioventricular (AV) valvular disease (CVD) associated with mitral regurgitation (MR). This is caused by myxomatous degeneration of the AV valve leaflets and chordae tendoneae (54,59,60,61,84). Epidemiologic studies report increasing incidence with progressive age. One study reported 10% of dogs 5–8 years old, 20–25% of dogs 9–12 years old, and 30–35% over 13 years to be affected (85–88). The Necropsy incidence of CVD varies from 11 to 42% (86–88). The male-female ratio is 1.5:1 (84,85). Small and toy breed dogs are usually affected, although CVD is occasionally observed in large breeds.

Pathophysiologic changes may occur in one or both AV valves. In one study the mitral valve alone was affected 62%, mitral and tricuspid 32.5%, and tricuspid alone, 1.3%. Aortic and/or pulmonic involvement is rare (59). Similar findings have been reported in other studies (84,85,87). Histopathologic descriptions of lesions are similar to those in human mitral valve prolapse syndrome. In the dog, endocardiosis has been commonly used to describe valvular lesions. More recently, mucoid valvular degeneration and myxomatous transformation of the AV valves have been used to more closely describe changes that parallel human changes (61).

The valvular spongiosa layer sustains the deposition of increased extracellular matrix in which glycosaminoglycans (formerly mucopolysaccharides) play a major role. Resultant nodular thickening of valves and chordae involves progressive structural distortions of the mitral valve complex. In advanced cases AV valves may become billowing or parachutelike (89). Disorders of collagen synthesis, content, or organization may be important in myxomatous transformation of human mitral valve prolapse (90), and this had led to similar suspicions in the dog.

Hemodynamic derangements result from progressive mitral insufficiency. Most affected small breed dog atria display great compliance and a capacity to dilate to accommodate progressive volume overload. Eccentric left ventricular hypertrophy occurs as one of several compensatory responses to normalize wall stress while maintaining ventricular performance. Heart failure supervenes when compensatory mechanisms fail.

Electrocardiographic changes are common, especially in advanced disease. Left heart enlargement is reflected by p-mitrale and left ventricular enlargement (wide QRS complexes or increased R wave amplitude); the mean electrical axis (frontal plane) usually remains normal (6–8). Supraventricular premature complexes are the most common associated rhythm disturbance. Paroxysmal or sustained atrial tachycardia, ventricular premature complexes, and especially sinus tachycardia may accompany cardiac decompensation. Atrial fibrillation usually represents an end-stage rhythm disturbance associated with severe left atrial enlargement. Microelectrode studies of dogs with atrial arrhythmias and left atrial enlargement (endocardiosis) suggest that atrial ultrastructural changes rather than dramatic cellular electrophysiologic alterations may be important in the genesis of atrial arrhythmias (68).

Myocardial Disease

Primary and secondary cardiomyopathies comprise the second most common category of heart failure and arrhythmias in dogs (Table 5). Dilated idiopathic cardiomyopathy (DCM) is most frequently encountered, but hypertrophic idiopathic cardiomyopathy is rare (62,63). Secondary myocardial diseases may be caused by anthracycline toxicity (doxorubicin) (91), acute viral myocarditis (parvovirus) (92), myocardial hypoxia or ischemia (93), Chagas' disease (94), bacterial infections (95), and carnitine-linked defects of myocardial metabolism (96).

Idiopathic DCM affects young (6 months to 14 years; mean 1–4 to 6 years), predominantly male, large and giant breed dogs. The principle functional defect is severe depression of myocardial performance (systolic failure) accompanied by dilatation of all four cardiac chambers. Ventricular dilatation causes geometric distortion of the atrioventricular valve apparatus and subsequent insufficiency. Poor forward stroke volume produces low-output failure and congestion behind the failing ventricles. Atrial and ventricular chamber enlargement predisposes to corresponding tachyarrhythmias (62,63).

Electrocardiographic changes include left atrial and ventricular enlargement patterns,

Table 5 Causes of Canine Myocardial Disease

Primary (idiopathic) cardiomyopathy
Dilated
Hypertrophic
Secondary myocardiopathies
Metabolic
Thyrotoxicosis
Hypothyroidism
Hyperadrenocorticism
Carnitine deficiency
Infiltrative
Neoplasia
Glycogen storage diseases
Fibroplastic: Endocardial fibroelastosis
Physical agents: hyperpyrexia
Hypersensitivity
Trauma
Toxins
Doxorubicin
Catecholamines
Inflammatory
Infectious
Viral
Bacterial
Protozoal
Fungal
Algal
Rickettsial
Noninfectious
Collagen diseases
Miscellaneous
Ischemia
Muscular dystrophies

Source: From References 10 and 11.

conduction abnormalities (especially left bundle branch block), and arrhythmias (Table 6). The most common dysrhythmia is atrial fibrillation (Figure 1A). It typically coincides with initial cardiac decompensation. Less frequently, paroxysmal atrial or sinus tachycardia, ventricular extrasystoles, or ventricular tachycardia is noted (63). A rather consistent variation in disease presentation and progression occurs among several dog breeds in comparison to the "classic" pattern just described (Table 6).

Boxer cardiomyopathy is distinguished by the absence of severe cardiac chamber dilation and the histologic presence of active myocardial changes (focal myocytolysis, myofiber degeneration, and mild mononuclear cellular

Table 6 Breed-Related Features of Canine Idiopathic Dilated Cardiomyopathy[a]

Clinical features	Large or Giant breeds (classic form)	Doberman pinscher	Boxer	English Cocker spaniel
Age	6 months–14 years (4–6 years average)	2.5–14.5 years (6.5 years average)	6 months to 15 years (8 years average)	10 months to 9 years (5–6 years average)
Sex	Predominantly male	Predominantly male	Approximately equal	Approximately equal; male predisposition in one study
Electrocardiography	Atrial fibrillation common; LVE; ventricular ectopia	Sinus, LVE, or LBBB pattern; ventricular arrhythmias common; atrial fibrillation in 20%	Ventricular arrhythmias common (LBBB pattern)	RII, aVF > 3.0 mV (early changes); deep Q waves leads II, aVF; APC common in one study
Radiography	Generalized cardiomegaly; biventricular heart failure	LAE; acute severe pulmonary edema; pleural effusion mild, uncommon	N or cardiomegaly	Generalized cardiomegaly; pulmonary edema
Echocardiography	Ventricular dilation; reduced contractility (FS)	Ventricular dilation, reduced contractility (FS); B shoulder inconsistent; asymptomatic cases— excessive EPSS most sensitive (LV dimensions may be almost N; Ao wall excursion N before onset of CHF)	N to ventricular dilation; contractility N to depressed	LV dilation (usually); one-fourth with N contractility (FS)
Other		Cardiogenic shock common during CHF	Clinical categories I. Asymptomatic with arrhythmias II. Syncope with arrhythmias III. CHF with arrhythmias Arrhythmias often refractory	Chronic AV valvular disease (endocardiosis) common; long asymptomatic period common (usually with ECG evidence of LVE)
Prognosis	6 month survival, 25–40%; some survive more than 24 months	Grave; most die within 6–8 weeks	Category I. 2 years II. 1–2 years III. <6 months, sudden death possible	Guarded

[a]Much overlap occurs between findings, and breed characteristics should not be considered pathognomonic. (Data from References 6, 8, 13, 16, 18, 20, 26, and 58.)
APC, atrial premature complexes; AV, atrioventricular; CHF, congestive heart failure; ECG, electrocardiogram; EPSS, mitral valve E-point (interventricular) septal separation; FS, fractional shortening; LAE, left atrial enlargement; LBBB, left bundle branch block (i.e., QRS > 0.07 secs, upright leads II, aVF); LVE, left ventricular enlargement; N, normal; Ao, aorta.
Source: From Fox PR. Canine myocardial disease. In: Fox PR, ed. Canine and feline cardiology. New York: Churchill-Livingstone, 1988 with permission.

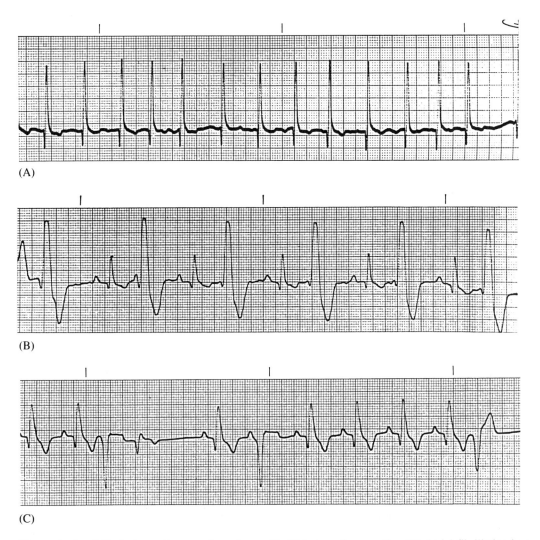

(A)

(B)

(C)

Figure 1 Lead II electrocardiograms from dogs with dilated cardiomyopathy. (A) Atrial fibrillation in a 6-year-old male Great Dane. Left ventricular enlargement is present. Aberrant ventricular conduction is evident in some complexes. (B) Ventricular bigeminy in a 9-year-old female boxer. (C) Left bundle branch block and ventricular premature complexes in a 3-year-old male Doberman pinscher. Paper speed, 50 mm/sec; 1 cm = 1 mV.

infiltration), as well as by chronic alterations (myofiber atrophy, fibrosis, and fatty degeneration). Arrhythmias commonly include ventricular ectopia, which usually arise from the right ventricle, forming a left bundle branch pattern (Figure 1B). Supraventricular arrhythmias are also recorded (Table 7) (62,78).

Doberman pinscher cardiomyopathy is typified by severe left atrial enlargement, fulminating pulmonary edema, cardiogenic shock, and a grave prognosis. Electrocardiographic

changes frequently include sinus tachycardia, left ventricular enlargement or left bundle branch block, and ventricular arrhythmias (Figure 1C) (63,97,98).

English cocker spaniel cardiomyopathy is usually associated with sinus rhythm, tall R wave amplitude (lead II), and supraventricular arrhythmias (99). The disease in this breed is often associated with a long, preclinical asymptomatic period, which is quite different from that in other breeds already described.

Table 7 Clinical Signs and Electrocardiographic Findings in Boxer Cardiomyopathy

Clinical findings	Harpster (N = 63)		Fox (N = 103)	
	N	%	N	%
Age, years (mean)	1–15 (8.2)		0.5–15 (8.0)	
Male	36	57.8	53	51.4
Female	27	42.2	50	48.5
Syncope	22	34.3	36	34.9
Cough	15	23.4	26	25.2
Dyspnea	8	12.4	13	12.6
Weight loss	7	10.9	12	11.6
Electrocardiographic findings				
Sinus rhythms				
Normal sinus rhythm	20	31.7	7	6.8
Sinus arrhythmia	NR[a]		32	31.1
Sinus tachycardia	11	17.5	15	14.6
Atrial arrhythmias				
Supraventricular premature				
complexes	7	11.1	6	5.8
Paroxysmal atrial tachycardia	4	6.3	1	0.9
Atrial fibrillation	7	11.1	2	1.9
Ventricular arrhythmias				
Ventricular premature				
complexes				
Rare/occasional	23	36.5	15	14.6
Frequent	22	34.9	14	13.6
Ventricular tachycardia	27	42.9	12	11.6
Other findings				
QRS interval > 0.07 sec	9	14.3	9	8.7
RII > 3.0 mV	7	11.1	3	2.9

[a] Not reported.
Source: From Fox, PR. Canine myocardial disease. In: Fox PR, ed. Canine and feline cardiology. New York: Churchill-Livingstone, 1988, with permission.

Sick Sinus Syndrome

Sick sinus syndrome is a common disorder of middle-aged or geriatric female miniature schnauzers (79). Affected dogs display alternating brachycardia-tachycardia characterized by paroxysmal atrial tachycardia or fibrillation-flutter, punctuated by long intervals of sinoatrial block without escape complexes. Syncope occurs during these arrhythmias. Pacemaker implantation is the usual therapeutic modality.

SPONTANEOUS FELINE ARRHYTHMIAS

Cardiac arrhythmias in cats are generally associated with myocardial diseases. A survey of 4933 consecutive feline necropsies reported an 8.5% incidence of cardiomyopathy compared with a 1.9% occurrence of congenital heart diseases in the same population (100). The clinical prevalence of myocardial disease has been estimated at 12–15% when including secondary cardiomyopathies (101).

The overall incidence of feline arrhythmias has not been documented in the general population. A comparison of ECG findings in 73 cardiomyopathic cats recorded 12 types of rhythm disorders totaling 77 arrhythmias (24). Ventricular dysrhythmias comprised over half of the abnormalities (Table 8). In a study of 131 cats with spontaneous feline thyrotoxicosis, 10 types of arrhythmias were recorded totaling 116 rhythm disturbances. Sinus tachy-

Table 8 Electrocardiographic Changes in 131 Cats with Hyperthyroidism

ECG finding	No. of cats	% of Cats
Tachycardia	87	66
Increased R wave amplitude (lead II)	38	29
Prolonged QRS duration	23	18
Short Q-T interval	13	10
Atrial premature complexes	9	7
Left anterior fascicular block	8	6
Ventricular premature complexes	3	2
Right bundle branch block	2	2
First-degree atrioventricular block	2	2
Second-degree atrioventricular block with ventricular escape complexes	2	2
Atrial tachycardia	1	1
Ventricular tachycardia and bigeminy	1	1
Ventricular preexcitation	1	1

Source: From Peterson ME, Kilntzer PP, Cavanagh PG, et al. Feline hyperthyroidism: pretreatment clinical and laboratory evaluation of 131 cases. J Am Vet Med Assoc 1983; 183:103, with permission.

cardia was most frequently represented (Table 9) (102).

Normal sinus rhythm predominates in the cat (8). The most common arrhythmia is physiologic sinus tachycardia (>240 beats/min). This is usually associated with pain, fright, excitement, or systemic or metabolic disease. Sinus tachycardia is not a common sequela of congestive heart failure unless thyrotoxicosis is the underlying cause. Unlike the dog, sinus arrhythmia is rare. When present, it usually accompanies upper respiratory infections or other causes of vagotonia. It may demonstrate brief periods of sinus arrest or pause (23). Sinus bradycardia frequently accompanies extracardiac conditions, such as severe systemic or metabolic disorders, shock, hypothermia, and hyperkalemia. Organic heart disease, such as dilated cardiomyopathy and severe congestive heart failure, may also be associated with depressed sinoatrial nodal discharge (8,23,24).

Atrial arrhythmias include atrial premature complexes, atrial and junctional tachycardia, and atrial fibrillation. These are sometimes present with secondary disorders, such as thyrotoxicosis (101,102), sepsis or endocarditis (95), trauma (62,63), neoplasia, and ventricular preexcitation pathways (83). Congenital heart anomalies associated with extensive volume overloads may be causative (104). Most commonly, atrial arrhythmias result from atrial enlargement associated with myocardial diseases (8,10,23).

Cellular electrophysiologic and structural characteristics of affected left atria were studied in cats with atrial arrhythmias due to spontaneous idiopathic feline cardiomyopathies (105). Diseased atria displayed marked structural derangements that included interstitial fibrosis, cellular hypertrophy, basement membrane degeneration, and thickening with marked dilation. These changes were more severe with marked atrial dilation; electrophysiologic abnormalities were related to atrial size.

Ventricular ectopias represent the most common feline arrhythmias (Figure 2) (106). They are associated with a wide variety of conditions similar to those described in the dog (8,24,62,103). Singular, uniform, occasional ventricular premature complexes are of-

Table 9 Comparison of the Electrocardiographic Findings in 73 Cats with Three Forms of Cardiomyopathy

ECG findings	Hypertrophic (31), No. (%)	Intermediate (11), No. (%)	Dilatative (31), No. (%)
P wave–lead II			
>0.04 sec	3 (9.7)	3 (27.3)	6 (19.4)
≥0.2 mV	6 (19.4)	1 (9.1)	2 (6.5)
QRS interval > 0.04 sec	11 (35.5)	6 (54.5)	22 (71.0)
LVH pattern	12 (38.7)	3 (27.3)	12 (38.7)
Conduction disturbances			
Sinoatrial block	—	1 (9.1)	1 (3.2)
Left axis deviation[a]	8 (25.8)	—	—
Left anterior hemiblock[a]	4 (12.9)	1 (9.1)	—
Left bundle branch block	—	—	1 (3.2)
Right bundle branch block	—	—	1 (3.2)
Other intraventricular	2 (6.5)	1 (9.1)	1 (3.2)
Wolff-Parkinson-White pattern	1 (3.2)	—	1 (3.2)
Total (all types)	15 (48.4)	3 (27.3)	5 (16.1)
Arrhythmias[b]			
Supraventricular			
Premature beats	4 (12.9)	3 (27.3)	3 (9.7)
Paroxysmal tachycardia	1 (3.2)	—	1 (3.2)
Atrial fibrillation	1 (3.2)	2 (18.2)	—
Ventricular			
Premature beats	11 (35.5)	5 (45.5)	15 (48.4)
Paroxysmal tachycardia[c]	4 (12.9)	2 (18.2)	4 (12.9)
AV dissociation	1 (3.2)	1 (9.1)	2 (6.5)
Total (all types)	17 (54.8)	7 (63.6)	19 (61.3)

[a]Electrocardiographic differentiation between left axis deviation (normal ≤ 0.04 sec) and left anterior hemiblock (prolonged to > 0.04 sec) was based on the duration of the QRS interval.
[b]More than one arrhythmia was recorded in 12 (16.4%) cats.
[c]The criterion for this category was the occurrence of two or more repetitive ventricular premature beats.
Source: From Harpster NK. The cardiovascular system. In: Holzworth J, ed. Diseases of the cat. Medicine and surgery, Vol. I. Philadelphia: W. B. Saunders, 1987, with permission.

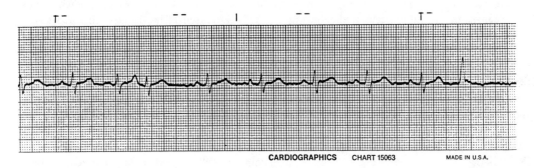

Figure 2 Lead II electrocardiogram from a 7-year-old male domestic short-hair cat with hypertrophic cardiomyopathy. Atrial and ventricular premature complexes are present. Paper speed, 25 mm/sec; 1 cm = 1 mV.

ten recorded in old cats, especially those with left ventricular hypertrophy due to thyrotoxicosis, systemic hypertension, restrictive or hypertrophic cardiomyopathy, heart failure of any etiology, hypoxia, toxemia, anemia, uremia, neoplasia, and myocardial infarction.

Abnormalities of impulse conduction are frequent. Incomplete AV block, temporary atrial standstill associated with hyperkalemia, and left anterior fascicular blocks are commonly encountered. First-degree AV block occurs often with dilated cardiomyopathy in cats with extreme acid-base or electrolyte disturbance, vagotonia from any cause, and shock. Second-degree and complete AV block is uncommon and occurs in cats with AV conduction system degeneration or inflammation, especially in older animals. Hyperkalemia is a frequent consequence of feline urologic syndrome. In this condition urine struvite precipitates, cause urethral obstruction, acute postrenal failure, and hyperkalemia. Atrial standstill with sinoventricular rhythm results and may progress to ventricular fibrillation in untreated individuals (107,108).

Left anterior fascicular block characterized by a frontal plan deviation in the cranial left quadrant and by qR complexes in leads I and aVL is often recorded in cats with severe left ventricular hypertrophy. Associated conditions include aortic stenosis and idiopathic hypertrophic or restrictive cardiomyopathy (8,23, 109).

Right bundle branch block is sometimes observed in normal cats and in animals with congenital endocardial cushion defects, severe right ventricular enlargement, cor pulmonale, excessive left ventricular moderator bands, and hyperthyroidism (8,23–25,104).

Ventricular preexcitation has been recorded in isolated cats with cardiomyopathy, thyrotoxicosis, and congenital cardiac anomalies and in normal individuals (8,23,83). Patterns consistent with Wolff-Parkinson-White syndrome are usually recorded.

Several specific cardiovascular disorders cause spontaneous arrhythmias. Primary and secondary cardiomyopathies represent the majority of naturally occurring feline heart diseases (Table 10) (62,63).

Table 10 Causes of Feline Myocardial Diseases

Primary (idiopathic) cardiomyopathies
  Hypertrophic
Dilated (congestive)
  Restrictive
  Intermediate
Secondary cardiomyopathies
  Metabolic
    Endocrine
      Thyrotoxicosis
      Acromegaly
      Uremia[a]
    Nutritional
      Taurine deficiency
      Selenium or vitamin E deficiency[a]
  Infiltrative
    Neoplasia
    Glycogen storage diseases[a]
    Mucopolysaccharidosis[a]
Leukemia
  Fibroplastic
    Endomyocardial fibrosis
    Endocardial fibroelastosis
  Hypersensitivity[a]
  Physical agents
    Hyperpyrexia
    Hypothermia
  Toxic: doxorubicin
  Inflammatory
    Infectious
      Viral[a]
      Bacterial
      Protozoal
      Fungal
      Algal
    Noninfectious collagen diseases[a]
  Genetic
    Hypertrophic cardiomyopathy[a]
  Dilated cardiomyopathy[a]
  Miscellaneous
    Ischemia
    Muscular dystrophy[a]
    Excessive left ventricular moderator bands[b]

[a]Suspected.
[b]Association and contribution to myocardial diseases unclear.
Source: From References 62 and 63.

Myocardial Diseases

Dilated cardiomyopathy was the most common cause of myocardial failure in the cat. Severely depressed ventricular contractility performance usually results in cardiogenic shock. Sinus rhythm was present in about half of affected cats, and sinus bradycardia occurred in about 20–25% (24,62). In one report supraventricular arrhythmias (atrial premature complexes) were recorded in about 10% and ventricular premature complexes in approximately 50% of affected cats (Table 8) (24). An association has recently been found between myocardial failure and low serum taurine concentrations. Taurine is an essential amino acid for felines. Oral supplementation of taurine in deficient cats produced a reversal of the morphologic changes (i.e., resolution of left ventricular dilatation) and normalization of systolic function during a 4–8 week period (110). Commercial supplementation of cat foods with taurine has, since mid-1988, vastly reduced the incidence of spontaneous feline DCM (63).

Hypertrophic cardiomyopathy (HCM) is now the most common feline myocardial disease. Idiopathic HCM is a disorder of diastolic dysfunction affecting cats between 5 months and 17 years old (mean age 4.8–7 years). Males are more commonly affected, and the Persian breed seems to be overrepresented. The Siamese and Burmese breeds, which are predisposed to DCM, are rarely observed with HCM (23–25, 101, 106, 109). Ventricular extrasystoles are the most common arrhythmias recorded with HCM (Table 8). Left anterior fascicular block occurs in about 13% of affected cats. It is a very specific but insensitive marker of severe left ventricular hypertrophy (8,62).

Restrictive cardiomyopathy is the least common form of primary myocardial disease. Its morphologic hallmarks are advanced left ventricular endocardial or endomyocardial fibrosis and hypertrophy with severe left atrial enlargement. This myocardiopathy has the highest incidence of atrial fibrillation, which is undoubtedly associated with massive left atrial dilatation (62,105).

Thyrotoxicosis is rare in dogs but represents the most common feline endocrinopathy. It results from overproduction of thyroxine (T_4) and triodothyronine (T_3) by benign functional thyroid adenoma (or adenomatous hyperplasia) of one or both thyroid lobes. Thyroid carcinomas are rare in the cat. Hyperthyroid cats range from 6 to 20 years of age (mean 13 years). There is no breed or sex predilection (24,25,62,63,102). Thyrotoxicosis results in a high cardiac output state. Congestive heart failure has been reported in about 20% of affected cats (102). Structural and functional cardiac changes include eccentric left ventricular hypertrophy, supranormal fractional shortening, and left atrial enlargement (111).

Electrocardiographic changes are common with hyperthyroidism (Table 9). Most arrhythmias as well as left ventricular enlargement patterns are reversible after a euthyroid state has been maintained. Therapeutic modalities include antithyroid drugs, surgical removal of affected thyroid lobes, or radioactive iodine therapy.

REFERENCES

1. Lewis T. Clinical electrocardiography. New York: Shaw & Sons, 1913.
2. Roos J. Auricular fibrillation in the domestic animals. Heart 1924; 11:1.
3. Zanzucchi A. Le aritmie cardiache mel cane. Richerche di Electrocardiografia Clinica. Profilassi 1937; 10:136.
4. Fried K J. Fibrillation and tachysystole of auricles and ventricles in dogs. Cas Cesk Vet 1949; 5:98.
5. Lannek N. A clinical and experimental study on the electrocardiogram in dogs. Thesis. Stockholm: Royal Veterinary College, 1949.
6. Ettinger S J, Suter P F. Canine cardiology. Philadelphia: W. B. Saunders, 1970.
7. Bolton GR. Handbook of canine electrocardiography. Philadelphia: W. B. Saunders, 1975.
8. Tilley L P. Essentials of canine and feline electrocardiography, 2nd ed. Philadelphia: W. B. Saunders, 1985.
9. Edwards NJ. Bolton's handbook of canine and feline electrocardiography, 2nd ed. Philadelphia: W. B. Saunders, 1987.
10. Fox P R (ed.). Canine and feline cardiology. New York: Churchill Livingstone, 1988.
11. Ettinger S J. Cardiac arrhythmias. In: Ettinger S J, ed. Textbook of veterinary internal medicine, Vol I, 2nd ed. Philadelphia: W. B. Saunders, 1983:980.

12. Blok J, Boeles J T F. The electrocardiogram of the normal cat. Acta Physiol Pharmacol 1957; 6:95.

13. Hamlin R L, Smetzer D L, Smith C R. The electrocardiogram, phonocardiogram and derived ventricular activation process of domestic cats. Am J Vet Res 1963; 24:792.

14. Calvert C A, Coulter D W. Electrocardiographic values for anesthetized cats in the lateral and sternal recumbancies. Am J Vet Res 1981; 42:1453.

15. Robertson B T, FIgg, F A, Ewell W M. Normal values for the electrocardiogram in the cat. Feline Pract 1976; 2:20.

16. Tilley L P, Gompf R E. Feline electrocardiography. Vet Clin North Am 1977; 7:257.

17. Gompf R E, Tilley L P. Comparison of lateral and sternal recumbant position for electrocardiography of the cat. Am J Vet Res 1979; 40:1483.

18. Tilley L P. Feline cardiac arrhythmias. Vet Clin North Am 1977; 7:273.

19. Tilley L P. Advanced electrocardiographic techniques. Vet Clin North Am 1983; 13:365.

20. Fox P R, Tilley, L P, Liu S K. The cardiovascular system. In: Pratt P W, ed. Feline medicine. Am Vet Pub 1983:249.

21. Gompf R E (Chmn). Cardiac diseases in the dog and cat: a diagnostic handbook. Criteria Committee, American Academy of Veterinary Cardiology. Am Anim Hosp Assoc, 1986.

22. Miller M S, Tilley L P. Electrocardiography. In: Fox P R, ed. Canine and feline cardiology. New York: Churchill Livingstone, 1987:43.

23. Fox P R, Kaplan P. Feline arrhythmias. Contemp Issues Small Anim Pract 1987; 7:251.

24. Harpster N K. The cardiovascular system. In: Holzworth J, ed. Diseases of the cat, Vol. 1. Philadelphia: W. B. Saunders, 1987:820.

25. Bonagura J D. Cardiovascular diseases. In: Sherding R G, ed. The cat: diseases and clinical management, Vol. I. New York: Churchill Livingstone, 1989:649.

26. Detweiler D K, Patterson D F. The cardiovascular system. In: Catcott E J, Smithcors JF, eds. Equine medicine and surgery, 2nd ed. Santa Barbara, Cal: Am Vet Pub, 1972; 277.

27. Steel J D. Studies of the electrocardiogram of the racehorse. Sydney, Australia: Australian Medical Publishing, 1963.

28. Fregin G F. Electrocardiography. Vet Clin North Am: Equine Practice 1985; 1:419.

29. Fregin G F. The equine electrocardiogram with standardized body and limb positions. Cornell Vet 1982; 72:304.

30. Buss D D, Rawlings C A, Bisgard G E. The normal electrocardiogram of the domestic poney. J Electrocardiol 1969; 2:229.

31. Landgrea S, Rugquist L: Electrocardiogram of normal cold blooded draft horses after work. Nord Vet Med 1953; 5:905.

32. Vibe-Peterson G, Nielsen K. Electrocardiography in the horse (a report of 138 cases). Nord Vet Med 1980; 32:105.

33. Brooijmans A W M. Electrocardiography in horses and cattle. Collected Papers from Laboratory of Veterinary Physiology, State University of Utrecht, Netherlands, 1957.

34. Holmes J R, Alps B J. The effect of exercize on rhythm irregularities in the horse. Vet Rec 1966; 78:672.

35. White N A, Rhode E A. Correlation of electrocardiographic findings to clinical disease in the horse. J Am Vet Med Assoc 1974; 164:46.

36. Hillwig R W. Cardiac arrhythmias in the horse. J Am Vet Med Assoc 1977; 170:153.

37. Deem D A, Fregin G F. Atrial fibrillation in horses: a review of 106 clinical cases, with considertion of prevalence, clinical signs and prognosis. J Am Vet Med Assoc 1982; 180:261.

38. Hilwig R W. Cardiac arrhythmias. In: Robinson N E, ed. Current therapy in equine medicine. Philadelphia: W. B. Saunders, 1983:131.

39. Holmes J R. Equine electrocardiography: some practical hints of technique. Equine Vet J 1984; 16:477.

40. McGuirk S M, Muir W W. Diagnosis and treatment of cardiac arrhythmias. Vet Clin North Am: Equine Pract 1985; 1:353.

41. Miller M S, Bonagura J D. Normal cardiac rhythms. J Equine Vet Sci 1985; 5:157.

42. McGuirk S M, Muir W W, Sams R A, et al. Atrial fibrillation in cows: clinical findings and theraputic considerations. J Am Vet Med Assoc 1983; 182:1380.

43. Deroth L. Electrocardiographic parameters in the normal lactating hostein cow. Can Vet J 1980; 21:271.

44. Smith S H, Bishop S P. The electrocardiogram of normal ferrets and ferrets with right ventricular hypertrophy. Lab Anim Sci 1985; 35:268.

45. Andrews P L R, Bower A J, Illman O. Some aspects of the physiology and anatomy of the cardiovascular system of the ferret *Mustela putorius furo*. Lab Anim 1979; 13:215.

46. Hoffman R A, Robinson P F, Magalaes H (eds.). The golden hampster: its biology and use in medical research. Ames, I A: Iowa State Univ Press, 1968.

47. Zenoble R D, Graham D L. Electrocardiography of the parakeet, parrot and owl. Prac Annu Meet Am Assoc Zoo Vet 1979:42.

48. Mitchell B W, Brugh M. Comparison of electrocardiograms of chickens infected with viscerotropic velogenic Newcastle disease virus and virulent avian influenza virus. Am J Vet Res 1982; 43:2274.

49. Miller M S. Electrocardiography. In: Harrison G J, Harrison L R, eds. Clinical avian medicine and surgery. Philadelphia: W. B. Saunders, 1986:286–92.

50. Sturkie P D. Heart: contraction, conduction and electrocardiography. In: Sturkie P D, ed. Avian physiology. New York: Springen-Verlag, 1986:167.

51. Hill J D. The significance of foreleg position in the interpretation of electrocardiograms and vectorcardiograms from research animals. Am Heart J 1968; 75:518.

52. Coulter D B, Calvert C A. Orientation and configuration of vectorcardiographic QRS loops from normal cats. Am J Vet Res 1981; 42:282.

53. Hamlin R L, Stalnaker PS. 25 Versus 50 mm/sec paper speed for canine electrocardiography. J Am Anim Hosp Assoc 1989:25:40.

54. Patterson D F, Detweiler D K, Hubben K, et al. Spontaneous abnormal cardiac arrhythmias and conduction disturbances in the dog (a clinical and pathological study of 3,000 dogs). Am J Vet Res 1961; 22:355.

55. Tilley L P. Transtelephonic analysis of cardiac arrhythmias in the dog. Vet Clin North Am 1983; 13:395.

56. Bonagara J D, Muir W W. Antiarrhythmic therapy. In: Tilley L P, ed. Essentials of canine and feline electrocardiology, 2nd ed. Philadelphia: W. B. Saunders, 1985:281.

57. Hahn A W (Chmn), Hamlin R L, Patterson D F. Standards for canine electrocardiography. Academy of Veterinary Cardiology Committee Report, 1977.

58. Buchanan J W. Spontaneous arrhythmias and conduction disturbances in domestic animals. Ann NY Acad Sci 1965; 127:224.

59. Buchanan J W. Valvular disease (endocardiosis in dogs). Adv Vet Sci Contemp Med 1979; 21:75.

60. Sisson D. Acquired valvular heart disease in dogs and cats. Contemp Issues Small Anim Pract 1987; 7:59.

61. Keene B W. Chronic valvular disease in dogs. In: Fox P R, ed. Canine and feline cardiology. New York: Churchill-Livingstone, 1988:409.

62. Fox P R. Canine myocardial disease. In: Fox P R, ed. Canine and feline cardiology. New York: Churchill-Livingstone, 1988:467.

63. Fox P R. Myocardial disease. In: Ettinger S J, ed. Textbook of veterinary internal medicine, 3rd ed. Philadelphia: W. B. Saunders, 1989:

64. Liu S K, Tilley L P. Malformation of the mitral valve complex. J Am Vet Med Assoc 1975; 167:465.

65. Olivier N B. Congenital heart disease in dogs. In: Fox P R, ed. Canine and feline cardiology. New York: Churchill-Livingstone, 1988:357.

66. Fox P R, Cohen R B. ECG of the Month. J Am Vet Med Assoc 1980; 177:142.

67. Hilwig R W. Cardiac arrhythmias in the dog: detection and treatment. J Am Vet Med Assoc 1976; 169:789.

68. Boyden P A, Tilley L P, Pham T C, et al. Effects of left atrial enlargement on atrial transmembrane potentials and structure in dogs with mitral valve fibrosis. Am J Cardiol 1982; 49:1896.

69. Liu S K, Tilley L P. Dysplasia of the tricuspid valve in the dog and cat. J Am Vet Med Assoc 1976; 169:623.

70. Bohn F K, Patterson D F, Pyle R L. Atrial fibrillation in dogs. Br Vet J 1971; 127:485.

71. Fox P R, Nichols C E R. Cardiac involvement in systemic and metabolic disease. In: Fox P R, ed. Canine and feline cardiology. New York: Churchill-Livingstone, 1988:565.

72. Bonagara J D, Ware W A. Atrial fibrillation in the dog: clinical findings in 81 cases. J Am Anim Hosp Assoc 1986; 22:111.

73. Thomas R E. Atrial fibrillation in the dog: a review of eight cases. J Small Anim Pract 1984; 25:421.

74. D'Agrasa L S. Cardiac arrhythmias of sympathetic origin in the dog. Am J Physiol 1977; 233:H535.

75. Zenoble R D, Hill B L. Hypothermia and associated cardiac arrhythmias in two dogs. J Am Vet Med Assoc 1979; 180:739.

76. Muir W W. Gastric dilation-volvulus in the dog, with emphasis on cardiac dysrhythmias. J Am Vet Med Assoc 1982; 180:739.

77. Macintire D K, Snider T G. Cardiac arrhythmias associated with multiple trauma in dogs. J Am Vet Med Assoc 1984; 184:541.

78. Harpster N K. Boxer cardiomyopathy. In: Kirk R W, ed. Current veterinary therapy: small animal practice, Vol. 8. Philadelphia: W. B. Saunders, 1983;329.

79. Hamlin R L, Smetzer D L, Breznock E M. Sinoatrial syncope in miniature schnauzers. J Am Vet Med Assoc 1972; 161:1022.

80. Tilley L P, Liu S K. Persistent atrial standstill in the dog with muscular dystrophy (Abstract). Proc Am Coll Vet Intern Med 1983; 43.

81. Teraj K, Ogburn P N, Edwards W D, et al. Atrial standstill, myocarditis and obstruction of cardiac conduction system: clinicopathologic correlation in a dog. Am Heart J 1980; 99:185.

82. Branch C E, Robertson B J, William J C. Frequency of second degree atrioventricular heart block in dogs. Am J Vet Res 1975; 36:925.

83. Hill, B L, Tilley L P. Ventricular pre-excitation is seven dogs and nine cats. J Am Vet Med Assoc 1985; 187:1026.

84. Detweiler D K, Patterson D F. The prevalence and types of heart disease in dogs. Ann N Y Acad Sci 1965; 127:481.

85. Detweiler DK, Luginbuhl H, Buchanan J W, et al. The natural history of acquired cardiac disability in the dog. Ann N Y Acad Sci 1968; 147:18.

86. Stunzi H. Zurpathogenese der endocarditis valvularis. Schweiz Arch Tierheilk 1962; 104:135.

87. Das K M, Tachjian R J. Chronic mitral valve disease in the dog. Vet Med 1965; 60:1209.

88. Jones T C, Zook B C. Aging changes in the vascular system of animals. Ann N Y Acad Sci 1965; 127:671.

89. Whitney J C. Observations of the effect of age on the severity of heart valve lesions in the dog. J Small Anim Pract 1974; 15:571.

90. King B D, Clark M A, Baba N, et al. Myxomatous mitral valves: collagen dissolution as the primary defect. Circ 1982; 66:288.

91. Van Vleet J F, Ferrans V, Weirich W. Pathological alterations in congestive cardiomyopathy of dogs. Am J Vet Res 1981; 42:416.

92. Robinson W F, Huxtable C R, Pass D A. Canine parvovirus myocarditis: a morphological description of the natural disease. Vet Pathol 1980; 17:282.

93. Meierhenry E F, Liu S K. Atioventricular bundle degeneration associated with sudden death in the dog. J Am Vet Med Assoc 1978; 712:1418.

94. William G D, Adams L G, Yaeger R G, et al. Naturally occurring trypanosomiasis (Chagas' disease) in dogs. JAMA 1977; 171:171.

95. Calvert C A. Endocarditis and bacteremia. In: Fox P R, ed. Canine and feline cardiology. New York: Churchill-Livingstone, 1988: 419.

96. Keene B W, Panciera D L, Regitz V, et al. Carnitine-linked defects of myocardial metabolism in canine dilated cardiomyopathy (abstract). Proc Fourth Annu Vet Med Forum, Am Coll Vet Int Met Vol. II 1986:54.

97. Harpster N K. Feline myocardial diseases. In: Kirk R W, ed. Current veterinary therapy, Vol. 9. Philadelphia: W. B. Saunders, 1986: 380.

98. Calvert C A, Chapman W L, Toal R L. Congestive cardiomyopathy in doberman pinscher dogs. J Am Vet Med Assoc 1982; 181:598.

99. Thomas R E. Congestive cardiac failure in young cocker spaniels (a form of cardiomypathy?): details of eight cases. J Small Anim Pract 1987; 28:265.

100. Trusk. Pathology of feline heart diseases. Vet Clin North Am 1977; 7:323.

101. Bond B R, Fox P R. Advances in feline cardiomyopathy. Vet Clin North Am 1984; 14:1021.

102. Peterson M E, Kintzer P C, Cavanagh P G, et al. Feline hyperthyroidism: pretreatment clinical and laboratory evaluation of 131 cases. J Am Vet Med Assoc 1983; 183:013.

103. Tilley L P, Bond B R, Patnaik A K, et al. Cardiovascular tumors in the cat. J Am Anim Hosp Assoc 1981; 17:1009.

104. Fox P R. Congenital feline heart disease. In: Fox P R, ed. Canine and feline cardiology. New York: Churchill-Livingstone, 1988:391.

105. Boyden P A, Tilley L P, Albola M S, et al. Mechanisms for atrial arrhythmias associated with cardiomyopathy: a study of feline hearts with primary myocardial disease. Circulation 1984; 69:1036.

106. Harpster N K. Feline cardiomyopathy. Vet Clin North Am 1977; 7:355.

107. Coulter D B, Duncan R J, Sander P D. Effects of asphyxia and potassium on canine

and feline electrocardiograms. Can J Comp Med 1975; 39:442.

108. Schaer M. Hyperkalemia in cats with ure-thral obstruction: electrocardiographic abnor-malities and treatment. Vet Clin North Am 1977; 7:407.

109. Tilley L P, Liu S K, Gilbertson S R, et al. Primary myocardial disease in the cat: a model for human cardiomyopathy. Am J Pathol 1977; 87:493.

110. Pion P D, Kittleson M D, Rogers Q R, et al. Myocardial failure in cats associated with low plasma taurine: a reversible cardiomyo-pathy. Science 1987; 237:697.

111. Bond B R, Fox P R, Peterson M E, et al. Echocardiographic findings in 103 cats with hyperthyroidism. J Am Vet Med Assoc 198; 192:1546.

IV

MECHANISMS AND APPLICATIONS OF CARDIOVASCULAR PHARMACOLOGY: CARDIOTONIC AND ANTIARRHYTHMIC AGENTS

This section consists of seventeen chapters on cardiovascular pharmacology. The first three chapters of this section deal with drugs that function to improve contractility of the heart. The next ten chapters discuss various aspects of local anesthetic (class I) antiarrhythmic drugs. This is followed by chapters on class II, III, and IV antiarrhythmic drugs. The final chapter deals with antifibrillatory agents.

Although digitalis has been available for clinical use for at least two centuries, the narrow therapeutic-toxic ratio of digitoxin and digoxin (the cardiac glycosides obtained from digitalis) leads to limited utility for treatment of patients with congestive heart failure. Many patients treated with cardiac glycosides develop ''digitalis toxicity,'' which can present as a life-threatening arrhythmia. The search for a new effective positive inotropic drugs that are free of many of the side effects of digitalis has therefore been intense for several decades. The drugs that have been considered for development as clinical inotropic agents include various catecholamines, semisynthetic digitalis derivatives, and phosphodiesterase inhibitors, such as amrinone and milrinone. The first three chapters in this section should give the student background information that will be helpful to evaluate further developments in this expanding field of cardiovascular pharmacology.

Much of the information in this section addresses drugs that are useful for the treatment of cardiac arrhythmias and/or reducing the likelihood of sudden cardiac death. Some 20 years ago, Vaughan-Williams proposed a simple classification system for antiarrhythmic drugs. The known antiarrhythmic drugs were grouped according to one or more of the following three effects on transmembrane action potentials recording from myocardial cells:

1. Such drugs as quinidine, procainamide, phenytoin, and lidocaine all had depressant effects on the maximum rate of depolarizaton during phase 0 of the Purkinje fiber and working myocardial cell action potential.
2. Propranolol was found to exert significant antiarrhythmic effects and was known to inhibit the effects of catecholamines on β-adrenergic receptors.
3. Bretylium was known to prolong action potential duration.

These three actions led to the idea that three different classes of antiarrhythmic drugs could exist. That is, "class I" drugs exert local anesthetic effect, "class II" drugs blocked adrenergic stimulation, and "class III" drugs prolonged repolarization and refractoriness. Then, in 1974, verapamil was found to exert antiarrhythmic effects. Its primary mechanism of action was found to involve a decrease in the secondary inward (calcium) current. This led Singh and Vaughan-Williams to recognize verapamil as the prototype of a fourth class of antiarrhythmic drug in the classification system.

More recently, the class I drugs have been subdivided into groups A, B, and C. Group IA includes procainamide, quinidine, and disopyramide. These drugs decreased phase 0 depolarization and show use-dependent block with moderately slow onset. They slow conduction in the heart and prolong QRS duration and QT interval. The group IB drugs include lidocaine, mexilitine, and tocainide. These drugs also decrease phase 0 depolarization and do so in a use-dependent fashion with rapid onset. They do not lengthen action potential duration, QRS duration, or QT interval. Group IC drugs, such as flecainide, encainide, ethmozine, and propafenone, are very potent local anesthetics that have slow use-dependent kinetics. They markedly reduce phase 0 depolarization and prolong QRS duration. These agents may shorten action potential duration in Purkinje fibers and prolong it in ventricular muscle cells. These are discussed in the chapter on antiarrhythmic drug toxicity.

The existing antiarrhythmic drug classification system can be used as a guide to the general mechanisms of action of the different agents. Most drugs exhibit several actions and thus may be placed in one or more of the classes. For example, propranolol is the proto-type of β-adrenergic receptor blocking drugs. In concentrations of 10^{-8} M or higher it inhibits catecholamine effects in ventricular tissues. However, propranolol (in slightly higher concentrations) also exhibits class IA activity by decreasing phase 0 depolarization and conduction velocity in the heart. Thus each agent should be viewed as a unique entity.

Because none of the known antiarrhythmic drugs are always efficacious and because the drugs within a class can in fact exert quite diverse actions, the failure of one agent to produce the desired therapeutic effect in a patient does not preclude the use of other agents within the same class. In addition, one should be aware that many of the agents have varying effects based upon dose, drug levels, and so on. Therefore, the classification scheme is exactly that: it is merely a retrospective guide to the initial choice of agent. It does not present a hierarchy of efficacy. It does not suggest sequence of use. It does not predict side effects. A wise clinician chooses the appropriate agent based upon clinical experience. Knowledge of the mechanism of action of the drug, as well as the cellular mechanism of the arrhythmia, if known, is also useful. For example, arrhythmias associated with an acute myocardial infarction appear to be caused by increased ectopic automaticity, often resulting from β-adrenergic stimulation. Such agents as lidocaine or propranolol may be appropriate. Chronic arrhythmias associated with old myocardial infarctions due to a reentrant mechanism do not respond well to the previous two agents but rather respond to agents that slow or abolish reentrant mechanisms.

Until classification schemes are devised based upon a clearer understanding or knowledge of specific arrhythmias, the clinician is left with only good medical judgment as the guide to the practice of medicine.

α-Adrenergic Receptor-Effector Coupling

Susan F. Steinberg and Michael R. Rosen

College of Physicians and Surgeons, Columbia University
New York, New York

INTRODUCTION

Cardiac electrical and mechanical activity are modulated importantly by catecholamines. Although a vast literature describes the β-agonist effects of adrenergic amines on the heart, understanding of the α-adrenergic component of myocardial catecholamine responses is both more recent and less complete. Nonetheless we have learned that activation of myocardial α_1-adrenergic receptors induces specific physiologic changes in the heart through mechanisms that are distinct from those coupled to the β-adrenergic receptor. Our own research over the past several years has identified certain associations between innervation of the heart and the nature of the α_1-adrenergic pharmacologic response. Our studies probing the molecular mechanisms underlying the α_1-adrenergic response using this model are the subject of this chapter.

Probably the earliest appreciation of the fact that α-adrenergic agonists might modify cardiac rhythm came from studies of repolarization in Purkinje and myocardial fibers (e.g., References 1 and 2). These experiments demonstrated that adrenergic amines could prolong the duration of phases 2 and 3 of the action potential, an effect that was attenuated by α- but not by β-adrenergic blockade. Subsequently it was found that α-adrenergic stimulation decreased the rate of impulse initiation in adult canine Purkinje fibers (3,4). This is not a uniform finding but is characteristic of approximately two-thirds of any randomly selected group of adult canine fibers. In contrast, fibers selected from neonatal dogs in the first 24 hr of life usually show an increase in automaticity in response to α-agonists (4,5). Within the first few weeks of life this response converts to the preponderant decrease in automaticity that is characteristic of adult fibers. The increase in automaticity, like the decrease, is blocked by prazosin but not by propranolol or yohimbine and is interpreted as α_1-adrenergic (6). Hence, with development of the dog heart, the response to α-adrenergic stimulation qualitatively changes from an increase to a diametrically opposed decrease in impulse initiation. This observation raised several questions, including those related to the ubiquity of the α-adrenergic response among mammalian species, as well as the mechanisms responsible for it.

α_1-Adrenergic responsiveness was examined more recently in the rat. Our studies indicate that a similar conversion of the α-adrenergic chronotropic response from positive to negative occurs in the rat heart (7). Moreover, in both the dog and the rat the acquisition of the inhibitory α_1-adrenergic chronotropic response coincides with the maturation of functional sympathetic innervation of the heart (5,7). This prompted the suggestion that sympathetic innervation of the heart itself induced the change in cardiac responsiveness to α_1-adrenergic catecholamines (5). This hypothesis was tested initially in a rat model, chosen because the rat ventricle lacks any evidence of sympathetic innervation in the first week after birth and thus provides a convenient source of extrauterine cardiac tissue that is noninnervated (8,9). Primary myocardial cell cultures were prepared from 2-day-old rat ventricles and maintained alone or in the presence of sympathetic neurons to directly assess the importance of sympathetic innervation in the development of the mature α_1-adrenergic pharmacologic response (7). The results of these studies are summarized in Figure 1. Neonatal rat ventricular myocytes when cultured alone express a positive chronotropic response to the α_1-adrenergic agonist phenylephrine. Myocytes cocultured with and innervated by sympathetic neurons show a predominantly negative chronotropic response to the same concentrations of phenylephrine. Both the increase in automaticity in the pure myocyte cultures and the decrease in automaticity in the nerve-muscle cocultures are inhibited by the α_1-adrenergic antagonist prazosin. Furthermore, both the increase and the decrease in automaticity persist in the presence of atropine, propranolol, and adenosine deaminase, indicating that they do not result from a presynaptic α_1-adrenergic action to release a muscarinic, β-adrenergic, or purinergic agonist (7).

BIOCHEMICAL MEDIATORS

The developmental and neuronal induction of an inhibitory α_1-adrenergic chronotropic response provides an opportunity to attempt the

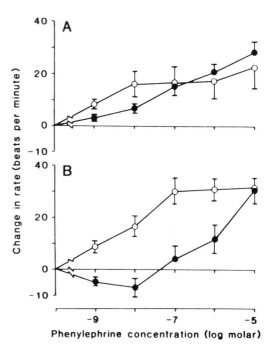

Figure 1 Effects of phenylephrine on the automatic rate of neonatal rat ventricular myocytes in tissue culture alone (A) or in coculture with sympathetic neurons (B). The black circles indicate the response of cultures and cocultures unexposed to pertussis toxin. The myocytes alone show an α_1 increase in automaticity (A); the cocultures show an α_1-mediated decrease at 10^{-9} and 10^{-8} M phenylephrine and an increase at higher agonist concentrations (B). Following incubation with pertussis toxin, 0.5µg/ml for 16–20 h (white circles), there was no change in the response of the ventricular myocytes (A). However, the cocultures showed a uniform increase in automaticity (B). See text for further discussion.(Modified after Reference 14.)

identification of the biochemical mediators of the response. In this regard the α_1-adrenergic receptor belongs to the family of plasma membrane receptors that are coupled to guanine nucleotide binding regulatory proteins (G proteins) (10,11). These receptors are multicomponent membrane-bound complexes consisting of at least three macromolecular entities—the receptor-recognition site, the effector-response mechanism, and the G protein—interposed physically and functionally between the receptor and the effector molecules. Changes in the availability or properties of any of these com-

Table 1 Developmental Changes in α_1-Receptor [(^{125}I)] IBE 2254

	Rat		Dog			
	B_{max} (fmol/mg protein)	K_d (pM)	B_{max} (fmol/mg protein)		K_d	
			Site 1	Site 2	Site 1 (pM)	Site 2 (nM)
Neonate	168 ± 10	124 ± 29	14 ± 10	1710 ± 440	8 ± 6	1.9 ± 0.67
Adult	124 ± 13*	140 ± 34	25 ± 5	510 ± 155*	13 ± 9	1.3 ± 0.43

Values from rat courtesy of Dr. Amy Han.
Values for dog taken from Buchthal et al., Reference 12.
*$P<0.05$ compared with neonate.

ponents as a result of innervation or development could lead to alterations in the α_1-adrenergic response.

We focused initially on the properties of the α_1-adrenergic receptor per se in the context of the changing chronotropic response to phenylephrine. Our studies indicated that the α_1-adrenergic receptor number decreases during development in both the dog (12) and the rat (13) without any changes in the affinity of the receptor for antagonists (Table 1). This developmental decline in α_1-adrenergic receptor number was not temporally correlated with the change in automaticity and did not provide an obvious molecular mechanism for the alteration in autonomic responsiveness.

A second mediator of the modulatory effects of α_1-adrenergic catecholamines that might be affected by innervation is the G protein, which couples the hormone-occupied receptor to an effector response (10,11). We proposed that alterations in the amount or species of G protein as a result of innervation could result in linkage of the α_1-adrenergic receptor to a different effector response. To examine the biochemical and functional properties of myocardial G proteins, we took advantage of the action of certain bacterial exotoxins to catalyze the transfer of ADP-ribose from NAD to G proteins. By providing radiolabeled NAD as the substrate for this ADP-ribosylation reaction, the G proteins can be covalently tagged, identified, and quantified.

Moreover, ADP-ribosylation of certain G proteins by pertussis toxin results in the complete loss of G protein function. This property of pertussis toxin to selectively inactivate certain G proteins and, thereby, mechanisms coupled by those G proteins provides a powerful means to establish a role for specific G proteins in receptor-mediated functions. Using this approach we demonstrated that noninnervated myocyte cultures have a small amount of an approximately 41 kD G protein that is a substrate for pertussis toxin-catalyzed ADP-ribosylation (14). That these cultures respond to acetylcholine with a decrease in automaticity suggests strongly that at least a component of this 41 kD band is the G protein coupled to the muscarinic cholinergic receptor. Clearly, the G protein that may be responsible for the α_1-adrenergic decrease in automaticity is not present in any critical concentration in pure myocyte cultures. In innervated myocyte cultures there is a two- to threefold increase in the amount of pertussis toxin-sensitive G protein in temporal association with the acquisition of a negative chronotropic response. Functional linkage of this pertussis toxin-sensitive G protein to the α_1-adrenergic negative chronotropic response in innervated myocardial cultures is indicated by the observation that pertussis toxin, which ADP-ribosylates and inactivates this G protein, completely reverses the α_1-adrenergic chronotropic response in innervated myocytes from negative to positive (Figure 1). Hence, in a setting where sympathetic innervation was controlled carefully, it was established that a pertussis toxin-sensitive GTP regulatory protein functionally induced by innervation is central in the qualitative change of α responsiveness from excitation to inhibition of automaticity (14).

A similar result was observed in several other experimental models in which in vivo innervation is associated with a change in the pharmacologic response to phenylephrine. Thus both the dog and the rat ventricle acquire a pertussis toxin-sensitive G protein in association with innervation and a change in the α_1-adrenergic response from positive (immature) to negative (mature) chronotropy (14, 15). A relationship between the pertussis toxin-sensitive G protein and an α_1-adrenergic negative chronotropic effect was also observed in adult canine Purkinje fibers (16). Previous studies (3–5) indicated that these fibers can be categorized according to the nature of their α_1-adrenergic chronotropic response (see earlier). Although α_1-adrenergic agonists usually decrease the spontaneous beating rate, one-third of adult canine Purkinje fibers retain an immature α_1-adrenergic positive chronotropic response. We quantified the amount of pertussis toxin-sensitive G protein in individual, isolated adult canine Purkinje fibers whose α_1-adrenergic chronotropic response was characterized as either positive or negative. Our studies indicated that the amount of pertussis toxin-sensitive G protein in Purkinje fibers that respond to α_1-adrenergic agonists with a decrease in automaticity is about twofold greater than that present in fibers responding with an increase in automaticity. Furthermore, pertussis toxin, which functionally inactivates this protein, inhibits the α_1-adrenergic negative chronotropic response, further emphasizing the importance of the pertussis toxin-sensitive G protein in α_1-adrenergic inhibition of chronotropy (16).

The importance of innervation in the maturation of the α_1-adrenergic chronotropic response is underscored by recent studies in which abnormalities of sympathetic innervation were induced using nerve growth factor

(NGF) and NGF antibody (17,18). We demonstrated that the normal development of cardiac sympathetic innervation in the rat could be modified by daily injection of NGF or NGF antiserum during the first 10 days of life. At the end of the 10 day treatment interval, the cardiac α_1-adrenergic response was characterized as stimulating or inhibiting automaticity, and the amount of pertussis toxin-sensitive G protein in ventricular myocardial membranes was measured. Ventricular septa from saline-injected 10-day-old rats express a mixed α_1-adrenergic autonomic response. Of the septa, 58% show an α_1-adrenergic decrease in automaticity, whereas 42% demonstrate an α_1-adrenergic increase in automaticity. In contrast, the effect of NGF antiserum to retard sympathetic innervation is associated with diminished levels of the pertussis toxin-sensitive G protein and a predominantly positive α_1-adrenergic chronotropic response. The effect of NGF to hasten sympathetic innervation is associated with higher levels of the pertussis toxin-sensitive G protein and a largely negative α_1-adrenergic chronotropic response. These studies further emphasize the importance of in vivo sympathetic innervation in the acquisition of a pertussis toxin-sensitive G protein and a negative α_1-adrenergic chronotropic response.

The G protein linkage of the α_1-adrenergic receptor can be deduced from careful studies of the α_1-adrenergic receptor itself. In this regard, properties of the α_1-adrenergic receptor as characterized by antagonist ligands do not necessarily reflect differences in the receptor-agonist interaction. However, it is well established that the presence of G proteins and their linkage to receptors results in changes in the affinity of the receptor for agonists. Specifically, G proteins increase the affinity of the receptor for agonists. Binding of GTP (or a suitable analog) to the G protein leads to a decrease in the affinity of the receptor for agonists reflecting dissociation of a high-affinity agonist-receptor-G protein complex (19,20). Thus, the presence of high-affinity agonist binding, which is reversed by GTP, is compelling evidence for the linkage of a G protein to a receptor. Although our previous studies im-

Table 2 G Protein Linkage of Neonatal and Adult Cardiac α_1-Adrenergic Receptors[a]

	Hill coefficient	
	- Gpp(NH)p	+Gpp(NH)p
Neonate, $n = 5$	0.74 ± 0.01	0.98 ± 0.06[*]
Adult, $n = 6$	0.68 ± 0.03	0.96 ± 0.01

[a]Myocardial membranes were incubated for 30 min at 37°C with 60 pM[^{125}I]IBE 2254 and increasing concentrations of *l*-epinephrine in the absence or presence of 500 μM Gpp(NH)p. Separation of bound from free ligand was achieved by rapid vacuum filtration of the entire assay volume through Gelman A/E glass fiber filters. The Hill coefficient was calculated from the slope of a plot of log [%B/(100 - %B)] versus log [l-epinephrine], where %B is the percentage of radioligand binding displaced by l-epinephrine.
[*]$P<0.05$ compared to value without Gpp(NH)p.
Source: From Reference 13.

plicated a pertussis toxin-sensitive G protein in the adult cardiac α_1-adrenergic chronotropic response, there remained a paucity of information regarding the mechanism of signal transduction at the α_1-adrenergic receptor in the newborn heart. We therefore, used radioligand binding techniques to investigate a potential G protein linkage of the α_1-adrenergic receptor in the newborn (13). Our studies indicated that the competition curve for agonists binding to the α_1-adrenergic receptor in neonatal myocardial membranes is shallow, consistent with a mixed population of α_1-adrenergic receptors with high and low affinities for agonists (Table 2) (13). The agonist competition curve is similar to that obtained in the adult heart and is steepened and shifted rightward by guanine nucleotides in a manner consistent with the redistribution of receptors from a higher to a lower affinity state. These results provide the first evidence that a G protein participates in signal transduction at the α_1-adrenergic receptor in the neonatal heart in a manner analogous to that occurring in the adult heart. To examine the identity of the G protein coupled to the α_1-adrenergic receptor at each developmental stage, binding studies were performed on cardiac membranes prepared from pertussis

toxin-treated rats (13). ADP-ribosylation of certain G proteins by pertussis toxin interferes with their ability to couple to receptors and form the GTP-sensitive high-affinity binding complex for agonists. Therefore, following exposure to pertussis toxin, the binding affinity of agonists to receptors coupled to a pertussis toxin-sensitive G protein is reduced; agonist-receptor interactions at other receptors are unaffected. Our studies revealed that pertussis toxin reduced the agonist binding affinity of the adult α_1-adrenergic receptor but had no effect on agonist binding to the α_1-adrenergic receptor in neonatal membranes (13). Thus, receptor binding experiments indicate that the mechanism of signal transduction at the α_1-adrenergic receptor involves a G protein in both neonatal and adult hearts. However, the G protein linkage of the cardiac α_1-adrenergic receptor changes from a pertussis toxin-sensitive G protein in the neonatal heart to a pertussis toxin-sensitive G protein in the adult heart.

EFFECTOR RESPONSES ACTIVATED BY α-ADRENERGIC RECEPTORS

We next focused on the effector responses activated by α_1-adrenergic receptors in neonatal and adult myocardium. Our aim was to define the biochemical and ionic mechanisms that underlie α_1-adrenergic modulation of automaticity. An important mechanism activated by α_1-adrenergic catecholamines in many tissues is phospholipase C-dependent hydrolysis of membrane phosphoinositides (21). This effector response results in the accumulation of at least two intracellular second messenger molecules. Inositol triphosphate (IP$_3$) mobilizes calcium from intracellular vesicular stores, whereas diacylglycerol activates protein kinase C. In the myocyte culture model we demonstrated that α_1-agonists stimulate the rapid formation of IP$_3$. Of note, α_1-adrenergic-dependent IP$_3$ formation is not inhibited by pertussis toxin, indicating that this effector response is not coupled to a pertussis toxin-sensitive G protein (Table 3) (22). It is

Table 3 Norepinephrine-Dependent $1,4,5$-IP_3 Formation In Cultured Rat Ventricular Cardiomyocytes[a]

	- PT	+ PT
Basal	91 ± 8	79 ± 7
Norepinephrine	267 ± 78	277 ± 38

[a][^{3}H]myoinositol-labeled myocyte cultures were maintained in the presence of vehicle or pertussis toxin (100 ng/ml) for 24 hr before initiating experimental protocols. This treatment regimen was shown previously to completely ADP-ribosylate and inactivate the pertussis toxin-sensitive G protein in the culture. Myocytes were incubated with 10µM norepinephrine for 10 sec, and inositol phosphates in the aqueous phase were separated by high-pressure liquid chromatography on a Whatman Partisil 10 SAX column according to the method of Irvine et al. (22). Results are expressed as radioactivity in the $1,4,5$-IP_3 peak (cpm/5 × 10^5; mean ± SEM) for duplicate determinations from three seperate experiments.
Source: Modified from Reference 22.

therefore unlikely that intermediates generated via α_1-adrenergic-dependent phosphoinositide hydrolysis play a role in the pertussis toxin-sensitive α_1-adrenergic negative chronotropic response. On the other hand, a causal relationship between α_1-adrenergic receptor-dependent phosphoinositide hydrolysis and the α_1-adrenergic positive chronotropic response, which is also insensitive to pertussis toxin, is possible. That phospholipase C, the enzyme involved in hydrolysis of phosphotidylinositol, is in its own right capable of inducing an increase in automaticity was recently demonstrated (23). In experiments in which phospholipase C was superfused over cardiac Purkinje fibers, not only was a clear increase in automaticity induced, but this was potentiated by lithium (23) at a concentration that effectively inhibits the breakdown of IP_3 (24) but does not itself have any measureable effects on electrophysiologic parameters (23). In contrast, phorbol esters had no effect on automaticity. Fluorescence microscopy studies with the calcium-sensitive probe fura-2 indicated that phospholipase C increases intracellular free calcium levels (25). Both ryanodine, which blocks sarcoplasmic reticulum (SR) calcium release, and verapamil, which blocks transsarcolemmal calcium currents, were found to decrease the phospholipase C-induced increase in automaticity, suggesting that an increase in intracellular calcium was central to the increase in automaticity (23, 25). Hence, although conclusive experiments are yet to be performed, there is much circumstantial biochemical and electrophysiologic evidence relating phosphatidylinositol metabolism to an α_1-adrenergic increase in automaticity that is not dependent on a pertussis toxin-sensitive G protein.

Studies probing the precise ionic mechanism underlying the α_1-adrenergic-dependent decrease in automaticity in the adult heart have been more definitive. In experiments on disaggregated adult canine Purkinje myocytes, Shah et al. (26) used a whole-cell voltage clamp to demonstrate that phenylephrine increases an outward current. This increase in outward currents occurs in the presence of Ba^{2+} (precluding the possibility that the current is an inwardly rectifying K current), and it is blocked by prazosin, but not propranolol, indicating it is α_1-adrenergic. Very importantly, the current does not occur in the presence of dihydroouabain, suggesting it is carried by the Na/K pump. Moreover, the α_1-adrenergic-dependent increase in this current does not occur in myocytes pretreated with pertussis toxin (26). These studies indicate that a pertussis toxin-sensitive G protein couples the α-receptor to activation of the Na/K pump. Enhanced Na/K pump activity would decrease automatic rate

Independent evidence favoring a direct rather than indirect linkage of the α_1-adrenergic receptor to the Na/K pump was obtained in studies examining the effect of α_1-adrenergic agonists on intracellular Na^+ activity in intact Purkinje fiber bundles (27). We reasoned that an effect of α_1-agonists to decrease aNa_i would be consistent with direct receptor activation of the Na/K pump. In contrast, an increase in aNa_i following stimulation with α_1-agonists would suggest that the α_1-adrenergic dependent increase in Na/K pump activity was a compensatory mechanism rather than a primary response. Our studies indicated that α_1 stimulation concurrently decreases aNa_i and automaticity (27). Moreover,

aNa$_i$ decreased in two-thirds of adult fiber bundles in a setting in which the drive rate was held constant. This experiment was important because of the possibility that changes in stimulus rate, in their own right, modify aNa$_i$. Finally, the decrease in aNa$_i$ was blocked by prazosin but not propranolol, identifying it as an α-adrenergic process (27).

α-Agonists also decreased a K current that appeared to be iK$_1$ in isolated Purkinje myocytes (26). This action, which would be anticipated to increase automaticity, was also abolished by pertussis toxin. Hence, α-adrenergic-dependent ionic mechanisms that could either increase or decrease automaticity are blocked by pertussis toxin. We can only speculate that the magnitude of an α-adrenergic effect on automaticity reflects a balance between these disparate pathways in a pacemaker tissue. These mechanisms, in turn, are distinct from any potential pertussis toxin-insensitive α-adrenergic effect to modulate automaticity via intermediates generated through phosphoinositide hydrolysis, already referred to.

STUDIES OF DISEASED TISSUES

To this point we have considered developmental changes in α-adrenergic modulation of automaticity in normal cardiac tissues. Another area that warrants consideration is the effect of α-agonists on diseased or abnormally depolarized tissues. For example, in studies using current injection (28) or barium superfusion (29) to depolarize cardiac Purkinje fibers, α-agonists do not alter automaticity, or they increase it. Moreover, Sheridan et al. (30) have shown that in cats whose coronary arteries are ligated and then reperfused, there is an increase in ventricular ectopy that is blocked by α- but not β-adrenergic antagonists. This increase in ectopy is associated with an increase in myocardial α-adrenergic receptors, which are presumed to be coupled to an arrhythmogenic response mechanism (30,31). However, the precise identity of the electrophysiologic process coupled to the α$_1$-adrenergic receptor in ischemic myocardium is uncertain since available evidence supports the presence of several arrhythmogenic mechanisms in this setting, including automaticity, triggered activity and reentry. With respect to automaticity, a change in receptor-effector coupling may be induced by depolarization of ischemic cells (as mentioned, in cells depolarized with current injection or barium α-agonists tend to increase automaticity). Our own studies indicate that when Purkinje fibers are superfused with "ischemic" solutions, α-agonists increase automaticity (32). Moreover, this response persists during reperfusion with nonischemic solutions if the [Ca^{2+}] in the superfusate is elevated (32). Hence it is apparent that the same α-adrenergic receptor-effector system that under conditions of normal innervation and maturation is expected to decrease automaticity and suppress automatic rhythms has exactly the opposite effect under conditions of ischemia. Although the effects of ischemia on receptor number and physiologic responses have been described (e.g., References 30–32), the sequence of intermediary steps activated by the receptor (G protein and effector responses) in this setting remains to be defined.

CONCLUSIONS

Studies to date have demonstrated links between sympathetic nerves, GTP regulatory proteins, and the response of cardiac tissues to α$_1$-adrenergic stimulation. The α response is tissue and membrane potential specific in that it occurs in atrial and ventricular myocardium but not in depolarized tissues like sinus node. Depending on the presence or absence of a pertussis toxin-sensitive regulatory protein, the developmental state of the individual, the status of innervation, and the presence of a normal or pathologic environment, variations on the α response may be seen that are antiarrhythmic or arrhythmogenic. Continuing investigation of the steps in receptor-effector coupling in various tissues under normal physiologic conditions and in disease should afford a greater understanding of the biochemical and ionic determinants of α responsiveness. The information gained through these studies should be of use in synthesizing a holistic picture of the mechanisms that modulate cardiac-autonomic interactions.

ACKNOWLEDGMENTS

The research referred to was supported in part by USPHS-NHLBI Grants HL-28958 and HL-28223.

REFERENCES

1. Ledda F, Marchetti P, Manni A. Influence of phenylephrine on transmembrane potentials and effective refractory period of single Purkinje fibers of sheep heart. Pharmacol Res Commun 1971; 3:195–205.
2. Giotti A, Ledda F, Mannaioni P F. Effects of noradrenaline and isoprenaline, in combination with alpha- and beta-receptor blocking substances, on the action potential of cardiac Purkinje fibers. J Physiol (Lond) 1973; 299: 99–113.
3. Posner P, Farrar E L, Lambert C R. Inhibitory effects of catecholamines in canine cardiac Purkinje fibers. Am J Physiol 1976; 231:1415–20.
4. Rosen M R, Hordof A J, Ilvento J, Danilo P Jr. Effects of adrenergic amines on electrophysiologic properties and automaticity of neonatal and adult canine cardiac Purkinje fibers. Circ Res 1977; 40:390–400.
5. Reder R, Danilo P Jr, Rosen M R. Developmental changes in alpha adrenergic effects on canine Purkinje fiber automaticity. Dev Pharmacol Ther 1984; 7:94–108.
6. Rosen M R, Weiss R M, Danilo P Jr. Effects of alpha adrenergic agonists and blockers on Purkinje fibers transmembrane potential and automaticity in the dog. J Pharmacol Exp Ther 1984; 231:566–71.
7. Drugge E D, Rosen M R, Robinson R B. Neuronal regulation of the development of the alpha adrenergic chronotropic response in the rat heart. Circ Res 1985; 57:415–23.
8. Glowinski J, Axelrod J, Kopin I, Wurtman R B. Physiological disposition of [^{3}H]norepinephrine in the developing rat. J Pharmacol Exp Ther 1964; 146:48–53.
9. Lipp J A M, Rudolph A M. Sympathetic nerve development in the rat and guinea pig heart. Biol Neonate 1972; 21:76–82.
10. Gilman A G. G proteins: transducers of receptor-generated signals. Annu Rev Biochem 1987; 56:615–49.
11. Spiegel A M. Signal transduction by guanine nucleotide binding proteins. Mol Cell Endocrinol 1987; 49:1–16.
12. Buchthal S D, Bilezikian J P, Danilo P Jr. Alpha$_1$-adrenergic receptors in the adult, neonatal, and fetal canine heart. Dev Pharmacol Ther 1987; 10:90–9.
13. Han H M, Steinberg S F, Robinson R B, Bilezikian J P. Developmental changes in coupling alpha$_1$ adrenergic receptors to GTP binding regulatory proteins in the rat heart. FASEB J 1988; 2:A620.
14. Steinberg S F, Drugge E D, Bilezikian J P, Robinson R B. Acquisition by innervated cardiac myocytes of a pertussis toxin-specific regulatory protein linked to the alpha$_1$ receptor. Science 1985; 230:186–8.
15. Rosen M R, Danilo P, Robinson R, Shah A, Steinberg S. Sympathetic neural and alpha-adrenergic modulation of arrhythmias. In: Valdes daPena M, Southall D, Schwartz P, eds. (The sudden infant death syndrome) Ann NY Acad Sci 1988; 533:200–9.
16. Rosen M R, Steinberg S F, Chow Y-K, Bilezikian J P, Danilo P Jr. The role of a pertussis toxin sensitive protein in the modulation of canine Purkinje fiber automaticity. Circ Res 1988; 62:315–23.
17. Malfatto G, Rosen T, Sun L, Steinberg S, Danilo P, Rosen M R. Sympathetic innervation in neonatal rats induces a GTP regulatory protein that modulates alpha adrenergic effects on ventricular automaticity. Pediatr Res 1988; 23(Suppl. I):1401.
18. Malfatto G, Steinberg S F, Rosen T S, Sun L S, Rosen M R. Long Q-T interval and abnormal alpha adrenergic receptor-effector coupling. Circulation 1988; 78:II-557.
19. Limbird L E, Gill D m, Lefkowitz R J. Agonist promoted coupling of the beta-adrenergic receptor with the guanine nucleotide regulatory protein of the anedylate cyclase system. Proc Natl Acad Sci USA 1980; 77:775–9.
20. Rodbell M. The role of hormone receptors and GTP-regulatory proteins in membrane transduction. Nature 1980; 284:17–22.
21. Berridge M J, Irvine R F. Inositol triphosphate, a novel second messenger in cellular signal transduction. Nature 1984; 312:315–21.
22. Irvine R F, Anggard E E, Letcher A J, Downes C P. Metabolism of inositol 1,4,5-trisphosphate and inositol 1,3,4-trisphosphate in rat paratid glands. Biochem J 1985; 227: 505–11.

23. Molina Viamonte V, Rosen M R. Modulation of Purkinje fiber automaticity by phospholipase C. Circulation 1987; 76:IV–14.

24. Berridge M J, Downes C P, Hanley M R. Lithium amplifies agonist-dependent phosphatidylinositol responses in brain and salivary glands. Biochem J 1982; 206:587–95.

25. Molina Viamonte V, Steinberg S F, Chow Y-K, Robinson R B, Rosen M R. Phospholipase C modulates automaticity of canine cardiac Purkinje fibers. J Pharm Exp Ther submitted.

26. Shah A, Cohen I S, Rosen M. Stimulation of cardiac alpha$_1$ receptors increases Na/K pump activity via pertussis toxin sensitive pathway. Biophys J 1988; 54:219–25.

27. Zaza A, Kline R P, Rosen M R. Effects of alpha-adrenergic stimulation on intracellular Na activity. Circulation 1987; 76:IV–62.

28. Hewett K W, Rosen M R. Developmental changes in the rabbit sinus node action potential and its response to adrenergic agonists. J Pharmacol Exp Ther 1985; 235:308–12.

29. Amerini S, Piazzesi G, Giotti A, Mugelli A. Alpha-adrenoceptor stimulation enhances automaticity in barium-treated cardiac Purkinje fibers. Arch Int Pharmacodyn Ther 1984; 270:87–105

30. Sheridan D J, Penkoske P A, Sobel B E, Corr P B. Alpha adrenergic contributors to dysrhythmia during myocardial ischemia and reperfusion in cats. J Clin Invest 1980; 65:161–71.

31. Corr P B, Shayman J A, Kramer J B, Kipnis R J. Increased alpha adrenergic receptors in ischemic cat myocardium: a potential mediator of electrophysiologic derangements. J Clin Invest 1981; 67:1232–6.

32. Hamra M, Rosen M R. α-Adrenergic receptor stimulation during simulated ischemia and reperfusion in canine cardiac Purkinje fibers. Circulation 1988; 78:1495–502.

Positive Inotropic Drugs
Part I. Principles of Action

Eduardo Marban

The Johns Hopkins University School of Medicine
Baltimore, Maryland

Stefan Herzig

University of Kiel
Kiel, Germany

INTRODUCTION

The history of positive inotropic drug therapy is one of promise tempered by disappointment. Although the benefit of short-term support with potent positively inotropic drugs is well established for the treatment of acute, reversible myocardial dysfunction (1), there is no such consensus regarding the value of long-term therapy in chronic congestive heart failure. The cardiotonic steroids known collectively as digitalis illustrate well the ambivalent clinical experience with chronic therapy. Digitalis has been prescribed for congestive heart failure for more than two centuries in Western medicine. It was long used empirically with little regard for its mechanism of action, although in the 1920s the observation was made that digitalis can increase the force of contraction of heart muscle, at least when administered in high dosages. Despite considerable enthusiasm following the first large clinical series (2), the popularity of digitalis has waxed and waned over the years as its inconsistent benefit, and its pronounced toxicity, have become broadly recognized.

Whether digitalis exerts a significant positive inotropic effect at ''therapeutic'' concentrations remains a topic of considerable debate. The question of its efficacy has two facets. First is the narrow issue of the efficacy of digitalis in congestive heart failure, given the restricted dosage range that patients can tolerate. This controversy falls outside the scope of this review but has been discussed thoroughly elsewhere (3). The second doubt focuses on the more fundamental question of whether the chronically failing heart may be ill-served by forcible long-term augmentation of its contractile state by *any* inotropic drug. A patient's sense of well-being is likely to benefit temporarily from an augmentation of cardiac output and improved cardiac reserve, but optimism has been tempered by fear (4) that such therapy may accelerate the underlying myocardial dysfunction, the net effect being no improvement (or even a decrease) in survival. No positive inotropic agent has thus far been demonstrated to increase the survival of patients with failing hearts. Nevertheless, drugs with novel and fundamentally different effects on excitation-contraction coupling may

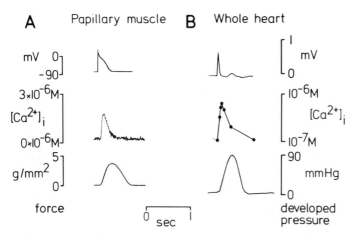

Figure 1 Cardiac electromechanical coupling as illustrated by data from isolated papillary muscle (A) and from the whole heart (B) (unpublished data, kindly provided by H. Kusuoka and Y. Koretsune), both from ferret. In the upper row the electrical events are represented by an action potential recorded by an intracellular microelectrode (A, rearranged from Reference 158) and by the electrocardiogram recorded by leads placed on the cardiac surface (B). The lower row illustrates the mechanical responses, that is, the transient in tension (A, rearranged from Reference 159) or developed pressure (B). The crucial mediator between electrical excitation and mechanical response is the transient increase in free cytoplasmic calcium (middle row). This can be measured by the luminescence from the injected photoprotein aequorin (A, rearranged from Reference 159) or by obtaining ^{19}F-NMR spectra using the NMR-visible calcium indicator 5,5'-difluoro-BAPTA loaded into the intact heart (B; for details, see Reference 160). The Ca^{2+} transient in B was obtained from a different heart than were the electrical and mechanical events.

vary in their long-term efficacy, so that the experience to date does not necessarily augur ill for the future.

The first of our two chapters reviews the principles that underlie the action of inotropic agents, with the emphasis on pathways that are obvious candidates for pharmacologic modulation. Chapter 21 reviews specific agents at various stages of development, including those already in clinical use. We focus throughout on basic mechanisms of drug action; the reader is referred elsewhere (e.g., Reference 5) for discussion of pharmacokinetics and other considerations for the use of these agents in clinical practice.

MYOCARDIAL EXCITATION-CONTRACTION COUPLING

Figure 1 summarizes the major steps of excitation-contraction coupling in a piece of isolated ventricular muscle (Figure 1A) and in the intact heart (Figure 1B). Depolarization (by external stimulation, as in Figure 1, or by

endogenous pacemaker activity in vivo) leads to a regenerative change in the electrical potential across the surface membrane known as the action potential (Figure 1 A, upper row). Such electrical events in heart cells produce small perturbations of the extracellular electrical potential that can be measured on the surface of the heart or on the body surface as the electrocardiogram (Figure 1 B, upper row). These cycles of depolarization and repolarization repeat some 2 billion times in a human life and result from the ensemble behavior of a number of transmembrane proteins that are discussed in detail below.

During depolarization the membrane becomes transiently permeable to calcium, which is otherwise excluded from the cell. Calcium ions enter the cell by diffusion from the extracellular space, where they are 10,000 times as concentrated (~ 1 mM) as in the cytoplasm ($\sim 10^{-7}$ M during diastole) (6). As shown in the middle row of Figure 1, the cytoplasmic concentration of Ca^{2+} ($[Ca^{2+}]_i$) rises quickly during depolarization and decays

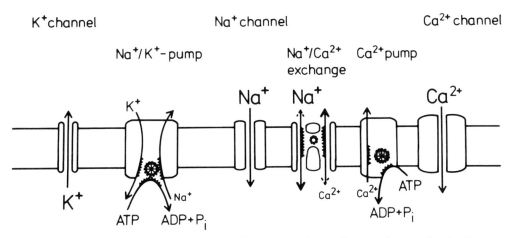

Figure 2 Membrane proteins involved in ion fluxes across the cardiac sarcolemma. For details see text.

more slowly; this fundamental cellular event, measured by aequorin in Figure 1A and by gated nuclear magnetic resonance (NMR) in Figure 1B, is called the Ca^{2+} transient. The Ca^{2+} transient acts as a chemical signal to initiate the cross-bridge cycling that generates force (lower row). Because calcium is the central messenger in myocardial contraction, the remainder of this chapter is divided into sections focusing on individual aspects of cytosolic Ca^{2+} regulation: (1) how the movements of calcium across the myocardial cell membrane are mediated; (2) how intracellular structures regulate $[Ca^{2+}]_i$; and (3) how calcium induces the changes in the contractile proteins that lead to mechanical activity. In each section physiologic regulatory pathways are described. Those steps that may represent targets for modulation by positive inotropic drugs are emphasized.

The Cardiac Action Potential: Channels, Exchangers, and Pumps

The action potential of the myocardial cell membrane (Figure 1A) propagates the wave of electrical excitation throughout the heart (see Reference 7). Membrane depolarization also fulfills an important transducing function as the physiologic trigger of contractile activity of cardiac cells, the first step in the series of events called excitation-contraction coupling. Accordingly, many maneuvers that alter the properties of the surface membrane lead to changes in the electrical as well as the mechanical properties of heart cells. Since the phasic increase in $[Ca^{2+}]_i$ during systole (Figure 1, middle row) is a major determinant of contractile activity, changes in the transmembrane movement of calcium ions are of special importance. The homeostasis of the different cations is strongly interrelated, however, as a result of coupled ion transport processes. Thus we cannot neglect the active and passive movements of other ion species, particularly sodium and potassium, even when their direct effects are minor.

A schematic overview of the most important transmembrane proteins in given in Figure 2. All three major categories of transmembrane proteins providing pathways for ion movement are represented: channels, exchangers, and pumps. Channels are proteins that form selective pores in the sarcolemma when they open; ions move through by electrodiffusion (see Reference 8). Thus channels consume no energy directly. They are unique in their ability to support enormous fluxes (greater than 10 million ions per sec per molecule). Exchangers, as the name implies, utilize the electrochemical potential gradient of one species of molecule, for example an ion, to move another one in the opposite direction. They display much lower transport rates [of the order of 1000 ions per sec (e.g. Reference 9)]. Once again, ATP is not consumed directly, although of course exchanger function depends on the maintenance of ion gradients by other mechanisms. Pumps are the molecules that ultimately maintain electrochemical gradients, and they do so by directly coupling the energy of ATP hydrolysis to the transmembrane transport of ions at a rate of about 100 cycles/sec (e.g., Reference 10). In the biochemical literature pumps are most often called ATPases. The properties and regulation of the major ion channels, exchangers, and pumps are reviewed in detail next.

Calcium Channels

L-Type Channels. Ringer first realized in 1883 (11) that calcium ions must be present in the extracellular medium for the heart to generate force. Sarcolemmal calcium channels constitute the major pathway for calcium entry into the cell. The existence of a calcium-selective current in heart muscle has been recognized for more than 20 years (12). Two distinct types of channels with high selectivity for calcium ions are now known to coexist in myocardial tissue (13,14). The two types of channels can be discriminated on the basis of their gating properties (i.e., the pattern of opening and its voltage dependence) and their pharmacologic sensitivity. We first consider the "traditional" calcium current of heart muscle, which is sensitive to modulation by a variety of drugs. This current flowing though so-called L-type channels ["L" for large and long-lasting (14)] is well characterized with respect to its role in cardiac excitation-contraction coupling. Even though the amount of calcium entering the cell during a single action potential through L channels appears to be too small to account fully for contractile activation (15), calcium influx through these channels is a necessary prerequisite for the initiation of contraction (16–19).

Several organic L-channel inhibitors exist and are called calcium antagonists. The classic members of this drug family come in three chemical groups: the phenylalkylamines (e.g., verapamil), the benzothiazepines (e.g., diltiazem), and many compounds of the dihydropyridine series, including nifedipine and nitrendipine (see, e.g., Reference 20). Exposure to any of the calcium antagonists can abolish contractile force in isolated myocardial preparations because the flux of calcium into the cell via L-type calcium channels is interrupted. There is good evidence that the high-affinity binding sites for these compounds are located on the α_1-subunit of the L-type calcium channel (21).

Interestingly, some compounds belonging to the dihydropyridine series produce effects contrary to those obtained with calcium antagonists. The so-called calcium channel agonists, such as Bay K 8644, exert positive inotropic effects (22) that are mediated by an enhanced probability that L channels open upon depolarization (23). At the single-channel level, the pattern of gating changes such that markedly prolonged openings, which are rare in the absence of drug, occur quite frequently. These effects are stereoselective, in that one enantiomer tends to promote, whereas the other inhibits, calcium current and contractile force (24,25), although even a single enantiomer can exert contrary effects depending on the drug concentration and on the membrane potential (26,27). The net effect of the calcium channel agonists generally turns out to be stimulatory, which renders these drugs candidates for a new class of positive inotropic therapeutic agents (28), particularly if their tendency to promote vasospasm by their action on calcium channels in vascular smooth muscle could be overcome.

β-Adrenergic Regulation of Ca Channels. L-type calcium channels are subject to a rich repertoire of physiologic regulation. Notably, the positive inotropic response to β-adrenergic stimulation is attributable to an enhancement of this current (29–31). Upon occupancy of cardiac β-receptors by an agonist, a series of events takes place, as illustrated in Figure 3. The occupied β-receptor activates a second membrane protein called G protein (for its ability to bind and to split GTP). The activated α-subunit of G protein in turn stimulates the membrane-bound enzyme adenylate cyclase. Biologic membranes contain several types of G proteins (see References 32 and 33). The type that mediates stimulation of adenylate cyclase carries the subscript *s* to discrimi-

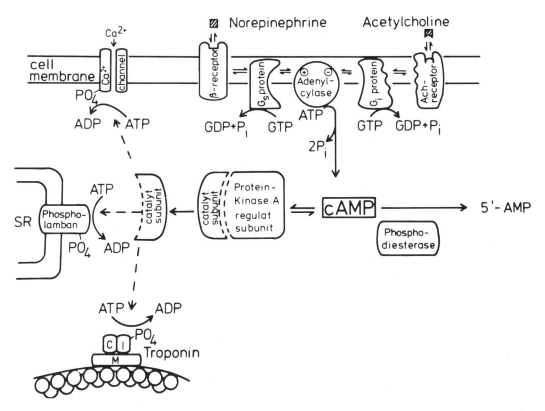

Figure 3 Overview of cardiac cAMP metabolism and targets of cAMP-dependent phosphorylation. β-Adrenergic receptor stimulation enhances, whereas muscarinic receptor stimulation reduces, the activity of adenylate cyclase, both effects being mediated via distinct G proteins. After the regulatory subunit of protein kinase A binds cAMP, the catalytic subunit dissociates and phosphorylates different target proteins. The sarcolemmal L-type calcium channel is thereby affected, as are phospholamban (a protein located in the sarcoplasmic reticular membrane) and troponin (a part of the contractile machinery).

nate it from others of inhibitory (G_i) or unrelated (G_o) function. The enzyme adenylate cyclase catalyzes the formation of cyclic adenosine 3',5'-monophosphate (cAMP) from ATP, tending to increase the cellular content of cAMP (see, e.g., Reference 30). The cAMP concentration is also determined by the rate of its degradation by phosphodiesterase. Cyclic AMP regulates a number of cellular functions by promoting selective protein phosphorylation, initiated by the binding of cAMP to the regulatory subunit of cAMP-dependent protein kinase (protein kinase A). The binding of cAMP liberates the catalytic subunit of the enzyme, which then phosphorylates a variety of cellular proteins (see Reference 34). The cardiac L-type calcium channel appears to be a partic-

ularly important substrate for phosphorylation by protein kinase A, based on evidence primarily from functional studies (31,35,36).

The evidence available to date hints strongly that calcium channels, when phosphorylated by β-adrenergic stimulation, are considerably more active than in the unphosphorylated state, thus producing an increase in the amount of calcium that enters the cell during each action potential(31,35,37). At the single-channel level the increase in current turns out to be attributable to an increase in the probability that any given channel will open upon depolarization, as shown in Figure 4. The left-hand panel shows unitary currents flowing through an L-type calcium channel in the control state. Openings are relatively

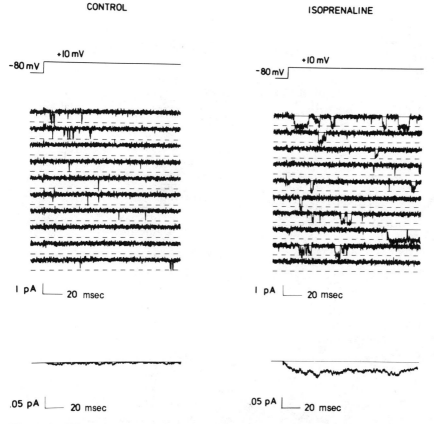

Figure 4 Effect of isoprenaline (2 μm) added together with an inhibitor of phosphodiesterase, isobutyl-methylxanthine (20 μm), on a single cardiac L-type calcium channel. Under control conditions (left), depolarizing voltage steps (upper panels) elicit few, brief channel openings (middle panels; hatched line indicates open channel current level). Not every depolarizing step leads to detectable openings. The ensemble current (lower panel, averaged from 500 sweeps) is relatively small. Upon drug addition (right) the corresponding ensemble current (lower panel) is enhanced severalfold. Examination of the individual sweeps (middle panels) reveals that the fraction of sweeps containing channel activity is higher. In addition, within these active sweeps openings are longer and more frequent. (Unpublished data, obtained by authors in collaboration with D. T. Yue.)

sparse and brief. During exposure to isoproterenol (Figure 4, right) the overall open state probability of the channel is increased. In addition to an increase in the fraction of depolarizing pulses that elicit activity, the mean time the channel remains open is prolonged, and the mean time it dwells in closed states is shortened. The ensemble current flowing through the channel (lower row), averaged from many sweeps, increases greatly upon β-adrenoceptor stimulation.

Thus a complex chain of molecular events ultimately leads to an enhanced calcium delivery to the cytoplasm and to positive inotropy.

It is not surprising that several pharmacologic interventions mimic, or interfere with, this pathway. A number of drugs can bind to and stimulate cardiac β_1-adrenoceptors. Some are useful therapeutic agents in acute myocardial failure (e.g., dopamine and dobutamine); others have been investigated with regard to their possible value in treating chronic myocardial failure (e.g., betaxolol, pirbuterol, and prenalterol).

The downstream elements of the cascade are also directly accessible. The function of G proteins can be probed with the toxins produced naturally by cholera and pertussis bacteria. Both are enzymes that lead to a covalent modification of G protein α-subunits by catalyzing the addition of an ADP-ribose group to a specific site. This causes irreversible activation of the α_s-subunit in the case of cholera toxin (38) and persistent inhibition of the α_i-subunit by pertussis toxin (39). Both interventions are expected to facilitate the elevation of cAMP in the myocardium and, hence, to enhance contractile force. Because of the ubiquitous presence and importance of G proteins and the lack of tissue specificity of these bacterial enzymes, however, they are highly toxic and of interest only as experimental tools.

The enzyme adenylate cyclase can also be activated directly without receptor occupancy or G protein activation. Forskolin is an alkaloid from the Indian plant *Coleus forskohli* that directly activates adenylate cyclase and thereby elevates tissue cAMP levels (see Reference 40), leading to an increase in cardiac contractile force (41). Although forskolin is widely used as an experimental probe, its action on different tissues is so indiscriminate that adverse effects predominate at positively inotropic concentrations. Another strategy for elevating cAMP in the myocardial cell is inhibition of its degradation. The methylxanthines, including theophylline and caffeine, as well as a series of new compounds, including amrinone and milrinone, are capable of elevating myocardial cAMP levels by phosphodiesterase inhibition. Their pharmacologic properties are discussed in Chapter 21.

Recently it has become clear that G proteins can directly influence the activity of ion channels, even in the absence of second messengers such as cAMP. Exposure to a purified preparation of activated G_s α-subunits increases the likelihood that L-type calcium channels in bilayers will open (42). Such cell-free experiments are consistent with the idea that part of the β-adrenergic stimulation of calcium channels is mediated directly by G proteins, but the fact that cAMP and its derivatives mimic the effects of β-agonists on calcium currents in intact cells implies that G proteins are not required. Nevertheless, the recognition of direct ion channel gating by G proteins opens the novel possibility of drugs that may act on this G protein link, rather than on the more conventional second-messenger–mediated cascade.

In sum, a number of compounds presumably affect cardiac contractility by direct or indirect interaction with L-type calcium channels, molecules that play a crucial role in excitation-contraction coupling.

T Type Channels. This second type of calcium channel is relatively sparsely distributed in ventricular cells (14), a morphologic feature that hints they are not vital in excitation-contraction coupling, although a minor role has not yet been excluded. T channels can be discriminated on the basis of their gating properties: they open only briefly and do so at rather negative potentials (< -20 mV) and thus underlie a transient current elicited by small depolarizations from the resting potential level. L-type channels, on the other hand, support a long-lasting current (particularly with barium as the charge carrier), the activation of which requires stronger depolarizations. The physiologic role of T-type channels is most likely pacemaker impulse generation (43), given their relatively high density in SA and AV nodal tissue (44) and the voltage range of their activation and inactivation.

Data on T channel pharmacology are sparse so far (45). β-adrenergic stimulation does not influence T channel currents (46,47). Amiloride and its derivative 3, 4-dichlorobenzamil have a powerful but not specific inhibitory effect on neuronal T channels (48,49). Cardiac T channels are at least partially blocked by flunarizine in concentrations also causing L channel inhibition (50). Block of T channels by divalent cations such as cadmium is rather unselective as well. Nickel ions, however, exhibit some preference for T channels (44) but also block L channels at higher concentrations. Thus, no pharmacologic tool studied to date is well suited to dissect out the effect of selective T channel modulation on cardiac contractile force. Although T channels appear not to function physiologically in excitation-contraction coupling, it would be of theoretical interest whether agents that enhance T channel currents [e.g., neuraminidase (51)] increase the force of contraction.

Sodium Channels

The main function of cardiac sodium channels is to mediate fast conduction of the cardiac impulse (see Reference 7). In so doing, the channels allow a sizable influx of sodium into cells during depolarization. Since myocardial calcium homeostasis depends on the electrochemical sodium gradient across the cell membrane (52), any change in the net transmembrane movements of sodium can alter contractile force. Thus a reduction in the sodium gradient, either by reduction of the extracellular sodium ion concentration or by elevation of intracellular sodium, can cause a positive inotropic effect.

A number of drugs that enhance force do so by increasing the amount of sodium flowing through sodium channels during each depolarization (see Reference 53). Indeed, sodium channels are popular targets for naturally occurring toxins that act to keep the channels open longer than normal. Among these are plant alkaloids like veratridine (Veratrum album) or aconitine (Aconitum napellus), and peptide toxins such as those from sea anemone (54). New synthetic compounds, most notably the inotropic agent DPI 201-106 (55, 56), are also capable of increasing the ion flux through sodium channels. The various compounds apparently bind to different sites of the sodium channel (see Reference 8). Patch clamp studies have shown that they induce unusually long-lasting openings of single sodium channels (57,58). An augmentation of sodium influx through these highly active sodium channels elevates cytosolic sodium concentration (59), thus reducing the driving force for calcium extrusion via sodium-calcium exchange (see Reference 60). Although an action on Na channels is the most obvious mechanism for the positive inotropic effect of these substances, other actions have been suggested for some of the drugs [e.g., myofibrillar sensitization by DPI 201-106 (55,61,62)].

Potassium Channels

A rich variety of potassium channels are present in myocardial tissue (see References 63–65). Their main function is to repolarize the action potential, which is characteristically long-lasting in heart cells. The action potential duration is determined by the balance of inward (predominantly calcium) and outward (predominantly potassium) currents. Since the amount of current is rather small during the plateau phase, the time course of repolarization is a very sensitive function of both components. The action potential is generally prolonged by blockade of potassium currents. An increase in action potential duration can lead to a positive inotropic effect, as has been observed (66) with the potassium channel blocking agent tetraethylammonium. On the other hand, the relationship between action potential duration and contractile force is steep only at rather short action potential durations, flattening out in the physiologic range (67). Thus blockade of potassium channels and consequent broadening of the action potential per se do not consistently provide a useful strategy to increase contractile force. Agents that shorten the action potential significantly tend to limit the influx of calcium and thereby produce marked negative inotropy. For instance, the decline in force observed with toxic digitalis concentrations is at least partially attributable to action potential shortening (68). So far, no drug has been shown to increase myocardial contractility by interacting specifically with potassium channels.

Sodium-Calcium Exchange

The recognition of a sarcolemmal mechanism whereby calcium ions can be transported at the expense of the sodium gradient (52) led to prompt recognition of its implications for the regulation of inotropy (69,70). Evidence for the existence of such a mechanism comes from tracer flux measurements (52,71) (see Reference 72) and, more recently, from current measurements in heart cells (73,74). Several lines of evidence point to an important role for this carrier in the regulation of myocardial calcium homeostasis, such as the steep relationship between intracellular sodium ion activity and contractile force (e.g., References 75 and 76). Energetic calculations assuming a stoichiometry of three sodium ions transported for each calcium ion reveal that the net direction of transport is to extrude calcium, even at submicromolar intracellular concentrations, when the membrane potential is negative to about -40 mV. At more positive potentials the net direction of calcium movement can be inward. Most of the cellular extrusion of calcium is probably mediated by sodium-calcium exchange, although an ATP-dependent calcium pump is also present in cardiac sarcolemma (77). The capacity of this transport mechanism is small compared to that of sodium-calcium exchange. This tentative conclusion, however, depends upon whether data obtained in vitro have been correctly extrapolated to in vivo conditions (78,79).

Despite attempts to purify the sodium-calcium exchange molecule, its structure is not known as of 1989 (80,81) and its pharmacology is disappointingly sparse. Indeed, attempts at purification have been hindered by the lack of selective high-affinity ligands. Amiloride and its derivatives inhibit the exchange (82,83), which may account for the positive inotropy seen in isolated preparations after the addition of high amiloride concentrations (84). Nevertheless, doxorubicin, which inhibits sodium-calcium exchange in vitro (85), has predominantly negative inotropic effects on the myocardium (e.g., Reference 86). In summary, the direct inhibition of sodium-calcium exchange theoretically represents an attractive pharmacologic means to increase contractile force, but evaluation of this possibility must await the development of a specific inhibitor.

Sodium/Potassium Pump

The sodium/potassium pump maintains the concentration gradients of sodium and potassium across the cell membrane. Thus it indirectly maintains the resting membrane potential and preserves membrane excitability. Biochemically the pump corresponds to the membrane-bound enzyme Na^+,K^+-ATPase (see, e.g., References 87–89). Since the pump transports three sodium and two potassium ions per cycle, it generates a net outward current. As a result of the coupling between cellular sodium and calcium homeostasis, sodium/potassium pump activity also indirectly keeps $[Ca^{2+}]_i$ at its very low diastolic levels. Accordingly, a strong inhibition of the sodium/

potassium pump, as in digitalis toxicity, leads to disturbances of excitability and signs of calcium overload (see also Chapter 12).

Under physiologic conditions pump activity is feedback-regulated by the cytosolic sodium ion concentration, which normally lies in the range of half-maximal activation for the intracellular cation binding site. For instance, an increase in beat frequency leads to a slight intracellular accumulation of sodium (90), which in turn enhances pump activity to offset the elevated passive sodium influx (e.g., References 91–93). On a longer time scale, the number of sodium-potassium pump sites in the sarcolemma is subject to physiologic regulation (see References 94 and 95). Under conditions of increased sodium influx or reduced external potassium concentration (96), more pump molecules are incorporated into the cell membrane to cope with the required transport work. It has also been hypothesized than an endogenous factor with digitalis-like properties exists and figures in the pathogenesis of essential hypertension (97). Although many reports indicate the recovery of digitalis-like material from several organs, the molecular structure of such compounds is still unknown (see Reference 98). Furthermore, the question of whether such material exerts quantitatively significant effects on the sodium/potassium pump in vivo is unresolved.

The pharmacology of the sodium/potassium pump is dominated by the fact that digitalis glycosides and related compounds are specific inhibitors of this enzyme (99,100) (see References 101–103). Although many other agents inhibit Na^+,K^+-ATPase (see Reference 104), they have not found application as inotropic agents. The common view of how cardiac glycosides enhance myocardial contractile force is known as the "sodium pump lag" hypothesis: inhibition of sodium/potassium pump leads to an increment of the cytosolic sodium ion concentration and a consequent reduction in calcium extrusion via sodium-calcium exchange (69). Even a small increase in $[Ca^{2+}]_i$ can help replenish the intracellular stores of calcium such that more is available to be released during each beat. At low digitalis concentrations the sodium/potassium pump is only partially inhibited and a new steady state of intracellular sodium is reached, since the elevated cytosolic sodium ion concentration enhances the pump activity of the unoccupied sodium/potassium pump molecules. Conversely, at a higher degree of sodium/potassium pump occupancy and inhibition, sodium outward transport does not suffice to maintain the sodium gradient. Ionic homeostasis deteriorates, and toxicity takes place. Thus an intimate coupling between sodium/potassium pump inhibition and positive inotropy is predicted by this model. This hypothesis explains why a narrow therapeutic range has been observed with all cardiotonic steroids investigated so far.

The development of new drugs in the digitalis family could only lead to safer therapeutic agents if the mechanism of inotropic action of digitalis were not simply one of pump inhibition. Proposals to that effect have indeed been made (105,106), but direct evidence for these alternative ideas is scanty. Not surprisingly, improvements in the safety of digitalis therapy have so far been limited to changes in the pharmacokinetic rather than pharmacodynamic properties of these drugs.

Control of Activator Calcium: The Function of the Sarcoplasmic Reticulum

In skeletal muscle the sarcoplasmic reticulum (SR) has been generally accepted as the predominant source of activator calcium (107, 108). The role of the SR in myocardial excitation-contraction coupling, however, has been subject to substantial uncertainty. Ultrastructural comparison with skeletal muscle reveals that cardiac SR occupies a much smaller fraction of the intracellular volume (e.g., References 105 and 109). Furthermore, the mechanism of signal transduction coupling the cell membrane and the terminal cisternae of the SR is still incompletely understood. As complicating factors, substantial differences have been reported regarding the contribution of SR calcium in atrial as opposed to ventricular tissue, between mammalian and lower vertebrate hearts, and even among ventricles from different mammalian species (110).

In contrast to membrane structures embedded in the sarcolemma, functional proteins located in the SR cannot be studied directly under physiologic conditions. The integrity of the cell must be disrupted, for example by "skinning" or by preparing vesicular membrane fractions from the SR. At the intact cellular level the evidence for the contribution of SR to activator calcium is still indirect: agents that inhibit SR Ca release can markedly reduce contractility, but drugs causing release of calcium from SR can activate contraction. Functional studies (e.g., References 17 and 18) suggest that in the intact cell calcium release from the SR is triggered by the increase of $[Ca^{2+}]_i$ initially produced by the slow inward current. Such observations support the mechanism of calcium-induced calcium release from the SR, first described in skinned preparations (see Reference 111). Finally, other sources of activator calcium, particularly the calcium current, or calcium released from putative potential-dependent plasmalemmal binding sites (105,112), have not been shown to be sufficient quantitatively to account for the Ca transients recorded in mammalian muscle. Thus several lines of evidence point to the SR as the primary site of origin for activator calcium in mammalian heart muscle (e.g., Reference 113). Interestingly, the SR seems to lose its capability to regulate diastolic calcium tightly when the cell is "calcium overloaded." Under these conditions the SR releases calcium spontaneously and asynchronously (114,115). The resultant mechanical inhomogeneity contributes to the negative inotropy observed when the calcium loading of the cell is excessive, as in digitalis toxicity (116).

At the molecular level biochemical techniques and recent single-channel studies have provided more direct evidence to improve our understanding of SR function and pharmacology. At least two proteins are directly involved in calcium transport across the SR membrane: an ATP-dependent pump (see References 117 and 118) and a calcium release channel (119–121). The physiologic function of the calcium pump is to lower the cytosolic calcium ion concentration by allowing the SR to take up Ca during diastole. The calcium pump is subject to physiologic regulation: activation of the cAMP-dependent protein kinase leads to phosphorylation of phospholamban, another protein located in the SR membrane, which then increases the activity of the calcium pump (122,123). This mechanism may participate in the acceleration of relaxation observed upon adrenergic stimulation. Thus all pharmacologic interventions leading to an elevated cAMP level should affect this particular function of the SR. According to a recent study (124), phospholamban itself may function as a calcium pore. This indicates the possibility that cAMP may lead to an increment of both calcium loading and the calcium release capability of the SR. Since phospholamban can also be phosphorylated by other protein kinases, the situation may be even more complex. Pharmacologic agents that exclusively affect the SR calcium pump have not yet been discovered.

The calcium release channel serves as the pathway for the sudden systolic delivery of calcium from the SR to the cytosol, putatively triggered by the increment in cytosolic calcium itself and facilitated by the presence of ATP. This molecule has recently been purified from skeletal and cardiac muscle SR (119–121) by several laboratories using procedures that exploit the high affinity of this channel to the plant alkaloid ryanodine. The ryanodine-binding protein has been characterized electrophysiologically as a channel passing calcium ions and, with a severalfold lower permeability, potassium ions. It can be blocked by the dye ruthenium red. Ryanodine changes the properties of the channel in a complex manner, producing long-lasting openings of low conductance at nanomolar ryanodine concentrations. Thus it causes a continuous leakage of calcium out of the SR, which consequently loses its ability to store and release calcium phasically in the intact cell. Accordingly, a negative inotropic effect is observed in intact myocardial preparations. At higher concentrations ryanodine appears to block the Ca release channel.

Since ryanodine acts effectively to dissociate the SR from excitation-contraction cou-

pling (125,126), it has been widely used as an experimental tool (110,127,128). A homologous mode of action has been proposed for high (millimolar) concentrations of caffeine, which induce a contracture in heart muscle preparations due to a sudden release of calcium, causing calcium depletion of the SR. The anthracycline cytostatic agent doxorubicin has been proposed to affect cardiac contractility by such a mechanism (129–131). In contrast to ryanodine, caffeine and doxorubicin exert a number of additional effects. A specific positive inotropic drug has not yet been found to act by interfering with SR calcium release, although this pathway has emerged as a promising target for rational drug design now that the specific molecular components are becoming increasingly well defined.

In contrast to observations made in other tissues (132,133), it appears unlikely that calcium release in cardiac SR is primarily triggered by the second messenger inositol triphosphate (IP_3), although a modulatory role cannot be excluded. IP_3 is produced by hydrolysis of the membrane phospholipid phosphatidylinositol biphosphate, catalyzed by the enzyme phospholipase C. A variety of agonists can activate phospholipase C in the heart (see Reference 134). In particular, the molecular basis of the positive inotropic effect of α_1-adrenergic stimulation may involve this pathway (see Reference 135). Nevertheless, the inotropic effects of α-adrenergic stimulation are usually quite small and differ among species (136,137).

Calcium and the Contractile Proteins: Regulation of the Ultimate Steps in Excitation-Contraction Coupling

The final event in excitation-contraction coupling is the interaction of the contractile proteins actin and myosin, resulting in muscle shortening and the generation of tension. This interaction takes place at the expense of ATP hydrolysis and is initiated by a rise in the cytosolic calcium ion concentration (see Reference 138). In addition to actin and myosin, striated muscle contains two additional myofilament proteins, troponin and tropomyosin.

The latter is a filamentous structure positioned at the double chain consisting of the globular actin monomers. Tropomyosin prevents the actin-myosin interaction under resting conditions, possibly by steric inhibition of the association between myosin heads and actin filaments. When calcium is elevated it binds to regulatory sites on one of the three subunits of troponin, called TnC. This results in a conformational change of the whole troponin-tropomyosin complex, disinhibiting actin-myosin interaction and thus allowing cross-bridge cycling to occur. This mechanism holds true for myocardial as well as for skeletal muscle contraction.

In smooth muscle, which lacks functionally active troponin, another series of events takes place: the elevation of cytosolic free calcium (see Reference 139) leads to formation of Ca^{2+}-calmodulin complexes, which activate the enzyme myosin light-chain kinase (MLCK). This kinase phosphorylates the light chains of myosin, rendering the myosin capable of binding to actin (see References 140 and 141). Even though this mechanism may exist in myocardium as well, it takes place over too slow a time course to be significant for contractile activation on a beat-to-beat basis.

Even when the comparison is limited to cardiac and skeletal muscle, calcium regulation of the contractile proteins differs, albeit more subtly: the ascending limb of the length-tension curve is considerably steeper in the heart. The classic theory of length-dependent tension development as a function of the degree of overlap between actin and myosin (142) does not account fully for the "Frank-Starling effect" in myocardium. Indeed, in intact and skinned cardiac fibers the apparent calcium affinity of TnC increases with increasing length (143–145). This effect is predicted to result in greater contractile force at any given cytosolic calcium level. It was recently found that this component of the Frank-Starling mechanism is accentuated when activation occurs by calcium binding to cardiac, compared to skeletal muscle, troponin (146). The existence of this mechanism points out that it is entirely possible under physiologic conditions that an increment in contrac-

tile force can be achieved without a primary alteration of cellular calcium metabolism, that is, by enhancing the sensitivity of the contractile apparatus. Because of the major differences among the three muscle types with respect to the modes of activation by calcium, even a selective pharmacologic influence on heart muscle may be feasible (147).

As in previous steps of excitation-contraction coupling, cAMP-dependent protein kinase figures prominently in the regulation of myofilament activation. It phosphorylates the inhibitory subunit of troponin I (TnI), which then reduces the affinity of TnC for calcium (see Reference 148). Thus the sensitivity of the contractile proteins is reduced, presumably as a result of enhanced dissociation of calcium. The consequences include a lower degree of force development at a given free calcium concentration (149) and a faster relaxation upon removal of calcium from the cytosol. Whereas the former effect can be effectively negated by an enhanced supply of calcium, the latter seems to contribute significantly to the accelerated relaxation that is observed upon β-adrenergic stimulation of the heart (150). Again, any pharmacologic agent capable of modifying cAMP levels may be expected to alter the properties of the contractile elements in the described fashion, although compartmentalization of cAMP has been postulated (151,152) to account for different patterns of cellular responses in the face of similar increments in bulk tissue cAMP content evoked by different drugs.

Another significant influence on the contractile proteins is exerted by intracellular protons. A drop in pH reduces, whereas an increment increases, myofilament calcium sensitivity. Although the idea that protons inhibit calcium binding to the regulatory sites of TnC is a simple explanation (153,154), the actual mechanism may be more complex (155). Conversely, an increase in myofilament responsiveness to Ca^{2+} may constitute a means of elevating contractile force without primarily affecting the amount of activator Ca^{2+}. Such a mechanism has been proposed to underlie the positive inotropic effect that can sometimes be observed upon α-adrenergic stimulation. The evidence comes from simultaneous measurements of cytosolic Ca^{2+} transients and contractile force (156). The molecular basis of this apparent enhancement of calcium sensitivity is still not clear.

Various new positive inotropic agents have been demonstrated in vitro to enhance the sensitivity of actomyosin activation by calcium. Such a principle has even been postulated to be the main mode of action of some of these compounds (157), although none of them appears to act solely by this mechanism. Since this type of inotropic drug has been claimed to exemplify a promising new therapeutic concept, the pharmacology of these agents is discussed in greater detail in Chapter 21.

REFERENCES

1. Goldstein R A, Passamani E R, Roberts R. A comparison of digoxin and dobutamine in patients with acute infarction and cardiac failure. N Engl J Med 1980; 303:846–50.
2. Withering W. An account of the foxglove and some of its medical uses: with practical remarks on dropsy and other diseases. Birmingham, 1795.
3. Smith T W, Antman E A, Friedman P L, Blatt C M, Marsh J D. Digitalis glycosides: mechanisms and manifestation of toxicity. Prog Cardiovasc Dis 1984; 26:413–41, 495–523; 27:21–56.
4. Katz A M. A new inotropic drug: its promise and a caution. N Engl J Med 1978; 1409–10.
5. Hoffman B F, Bigger J T. Digitalis and allied cardiac glycosides. In: Goodman Gilman A, Goodman L S, Rall T W, Murad F, eds. The pharmacologic basis of therapeutics, 7th ed. New York: Macmillan, 1985: 716–47.
6. Blinks J R, Wier W G, Hess P, Prendergast F G. Measurement of Ca^{2+} concentrations in living cells. Prog Biophys Mol Biol 1982; 40:1–114.
7. Hoffman B F, Cranefield P F. Electrophysiology of the heart. New York: McGraw-Hill, 1960:20–42.
8. Hillie B. Ionic channels of excitable membranes. Sunderland, M.: Sinauer, 1984
9. Cheon J, Reeves J P. Site density of the sodium-calcium exchange carrier in reconsti-

tuted vesicle from bovine cardiac sarcolemma (abstract). Biophys J 1988; 53:142a.
10. Jorgensen P L. Isolation and characterization of the components of the sodium pump. Rev Biophys 1975; 7:239–74.
11. Ringer S. A further contribution regarding the influence of the different constituents of the blood on the contraction of the heart. J Physiol (Lond) 1883; 4:29–42.
12. Reuter H. The dependence of slow inward current in Purkinje fibres on the extracellular calcium-concentration. J Physiol (Lond) 1967; 192:479–92.
13. Bean B P. Two kinds of calcium channels in canine atrial cells. J Gen Physiol 1985; 86:1–30.
14. Nilius B, Hess P, Lansman J B, Tsien R W. A novel type of cardiac calcium channel in ventricular cells. Nature 1985; 316:443–6.
15. Fabiato A, Baumgarten C M. Methods for detecting calcium release from the sarcoplasmic reticulum of skinned cardiac cells and the relationships between calculated transsarcolemmal calcium movements and calcium release. In: Sperelakis N, ed. Physiology and pathophysiology of the heart. Boston: Martinus Nijhoff, 1984:215–54.
16. London B, Krueger J W. Contraction in voltage clamped, internally perfused single heart cells. J Gen Physiol 1986; 88:475–505.
17. Beuckelmann D J, Wier W G. Mechanism of release of calcium from sarcoplasmic reticulum of guinea-pig cardiac cells. J Physiol (Lond) 1988; 405:233–55.
18. Näbauer N, Callewaert G, Cleeman L, Morad M. Regulation of calcium release is gated by calcium current, not gating charge, in cardiac myocytes. Science 1989; 244:800–3.
19. Valdeolmillos M, O'Neill S C O, Smith G L, Eisner D A. Calcium-induced calcium release activates contraction in intact cardiac cells. Pflügers Arch 1989; 413:676–8.
20. Hosey M M, Lazdunski M. Calcium channels: molecular pharmacology, structure and regulation. J Membr Biol 1988; 104:81–105.
21. Tanabe T, Takeshima H, Mikami A, Flockerzi V, Takahashi H, Kangawa K, Kojima M, Matsuo H, Hirose T, Numa S. Primary structure of the receptor for calcium channel blockers from skeletal muscle. Nature 1987; 328:313–8.
22. Schramm M, Thomas G, Towart R, Franckowiak G. Novel dihydropyridines with posi-

tive inotropic action through activation of Ca^{2+} channels. Nature 1983; 303:535–7.

23. Hess P, Lansman J B, Tsien R W. Different modes of Ca channel gating behaviour favoured by dihydropyridine Ca agonists and antagonists. Nature 1984; 311:538–44.

24. Kokubun S, Prod'hom B, Becker C, Porzig H, Reuter H. Studies on Ca channels in intact cardiac cells: voltage-dependent effects and cooperative interactions of dihydropyridine enantiomers. Mol Pharmacol 1986; 30:571–84.

25. Damarowsky M, Lüllmann H, Ravens U. The dihydropyridine derivative 202-791: interpretation of the effects of the racemate considering inverse agonistic enantiomers. Br J Pharmacol 1988; 95:1125–32.

26. Kass R S. Voltage-dependent modulation of cardiac calcium current by optical isomers of Bay K: implications for channel gating. Circ Res 1987; 61 (suppl.I):1–5.

27. Kamp T J, Sanguinetti M C, Miller R J. Voltage- and use-dependent modulation of cardiac calcium channels by the dihydropyridine (+) -202-791. Circ Res 1989; 64:338–51.

28. Bechem M, Hebisch S, Schramm M. Ca^{2+} agonists: new, sensitive probes for Ca^{2+} channels. Trends Pharmacol Sci 1988; 9:261–4.

29. Reuter H, Scholz H. The regulation of calcium conductance of cardiac muscle by adrenaline. J Physiol (Lond) 1977; 246:49–62.

30. Tsien R W. Cyclic AMP and contractile activity in heart. Adv Cyclic Nucleotide Res 1977; 8:363–420

31. Brum G, Osterrieder W, Trautwein W. β-adrenergic increase in the calcium conductance of cardiac myocytes studies with the patch clamp. Pflugers Arch 1984; 401:111–8.

32. Neer E J, Clapham D E. Role of G protein subunits in transmembrane signalling. Nature 1988; 333:129–34.

33. Robishaw J D, Foster K A. Role of G proteins in the regulation of the cardiovascular system. Annu Rev Physiol 1989; 51:229–44.

34. Tada M, Katz A M. Phosphorylation of the sarcoplasmic reticulum and the sarcolemma. Annu Rev Physiol 1982; 44:401–23.

35. Kameyama M, Hescheler J, Hofmann F, Trautwein W. Modulation of Ca current during the phosphorylation cycle in the guinea pig heart. Pflügers Arch 1986; 407:123–8.

36. Hescheler J, Mieskes G, Rüegg J C, Takai A, Trautwein W. Effects of a protein phosphatase inhibitor, okadaic acid, on membrane currents of isolated guinea-pig myocytes. Pflügers Arch 1988; 412:248–52.

37. Meinertz T, Nawrath H, Scholz H. Dibutyryl cyclic AMP and adrenaline increase contractile force and ^{45}Ca uptake in mammalian cardiac muscle. Naunyn-Schmiedebergs Arch Pharmacol 1973; 277:107–22.

38. Gill D M, Meren R. ADP-ribosylation of membrane proteins catalyzed by cholera toxin: basis of the activation of adenylate cyclase. Proc Natl Acad Sci USA 1978; 75:3050–4.

39. Katada T, Ui M. ADP ribosylation of the specific membrane protein of C6 cells by islet-activating protein associated with modification of adenylate cyclase activity. J Biol Chem 257:7210–6.

40. Seamon K B, Daly J W. Forskolin: a unique diterpene activator of cyclic AMP-generating systems. J Cyclic Nucleotide Res 1981; 8:201–24.

41. Lindner E, Dohadwalla A N, Bhattacharya B K. Positive inotropic and blood pressure lowering activity of a diterpene derivative isolated from Coleus forskohli: forskolin. Arzneim-ittel-Forsch 1978; 28:284–9.

42. Yatani A, Codina J, Imoto Y, Reeves JP, Birnbaumer L, Brown AM. A G protein directly regulates mammalian cardiac calcium channels. Science 1987; 238:1288–92.

43. Doerr T, Denger R, Trautwein W. Calcium currents in a single SA nodal cells of the rabbit heart studies with action potential clamp. Pflugers Arch 1989; 413:599–603.

44. Hagiwara N, Isisawa H, Kameyama M. Contribution of the two types of calcium currents to the pacemaker potentials of rabbit sino-atrial node cells. J Physiol (Lond) 1988; 395:233–53.

45. Hess P. Elementary properties of cardiac calcium channels: a brief review. Can J Physiol Pharmacol 1988; 66:1218–23.

46. Tytgat J, Nilius B, Vereecke J, Carmeliet E. The T-type Ca channel in guinea-pig ventricular myocytes is insensitive to isoproterenol. Pflugers Arch 1988; 411:704–6.

47. Bean B P. Classes of calcium channels in vertebrate cells. Annu Rev Physiol 1989; 51:367–84.

48. Tang C-M, Presser F, Morad M. Amiloride selectively blocks the low threshold (T) calcium channel. Science 1988; 240:213–5.

49. Suarez-Kurtz G, Kaczorowski G J. Effects of dichlorbenzamil on calcium currents in clonal GH$_3$ pituary cells. J. Pharmacol Exp Ther 1988; 247:248–53.

50. Tytgat J, Vereecke J, Carmeliet E. Differential effects of verapamil and flunarizine on cardiac L-type and T-type Ca channels. Naunyn-Schmiedebergs Arch Pharmacol 1988; 337:690–2.

51. Yee H F, Weiss J N, Langer G A. Neuraminidase selectively enhances the transient (T) calcium channel current in cardiac ventriculocytes (abstract). Circulation 1988; 78:II-260.

52. Reuter H, Seitz N. The dependence of calcium efflux from cardiac muscle on temperature and external ion composition. J Physiol (Lond) 1968; 195:451–70.

53. Honerjäger P. Cardioactive substances that prolong the open state of sodium channels. Rev Physiol Biochem Pharmacol 1982; 92:1–74.

54. Isenberg G, Ravens U. The effects of the *Anemonia sulcata* toxin (ATX II) on membrane currents of isolated mammalian myocytes. J Physiol (Lond) 1984; 357:127–49.

55. Scholtysik G, Salzmann R, Berthold R, Herzig J W, Quast U, Markstein R. DPI 201-106, a novel cardiotonic agent. Combination of cAMP-independent positive inotropic, negative chronotropic, action potential prolonging and coronary dilatory properties. Naunyn-Schmiedebergs Arch Pharmacol 1985; 329:316–25.

56. Buggisch D, Isenberg G, Ravens U, Scholtysik G. The role of sodium channels in the effects of the cardiotonic compound DPI 201-106 on contractility and membrane potentials in isolated mammalian heart preparations. Eur J Pharmacol 1985; 118:303–11.

57. Kohlhardt M, Froebe U, Herzig J W. Modification of single cardiac Na$^+$ channels by DPI 201-106. J Membr Biol 1986; 89: 163–72.

58. Nilius B. Calcium block of guinea-pig heart sodium channels with and without modification by the piperazinylindole DPI 201-106. J Physiol (Lond) 1988; 399:537–58.

59. Brill D M, Wasserstrom J A. Intracellular sodium and the positive inotropic effect of veratridine and cardiac glycoside in sheep Purkinje fibers. Circ Res 1986; 58:109–19.

60. Mullins L J. Ion transport in heart. New York: Raven Press, 1981.

61. Hajjar R J, Gwathmey J K, Briggs, G M, Morgan J P. Differential effects of DPI 201-106 on the sensitivity of the myofilaments to Ca^{2+} in intact and skinned trabeculae from control and myopathic human hearts. J Clin Invest 1988; 82:1578–84.

62. Kihara Y, Gwathmey J K, Grossman W, Morgan J P. Mechanisms of positive inotropic effects and delayed relaxation produced by DPI 201-106 in mammalian working myocardium: effects on intracellular calcium handling. Br J Pharmacol 1989; 96:927–39.

63. Pelzer D, Trautwein W. Currents through ionic channels in multicellular cardiac tissue and single heart cells. Experientia 1987; 43:1153–62.

64. Cook N S. The pharmacology of potassium channels and their therapeutic potential. Trends Pharmacol Sci 1988; 9:21–8.

65. Moczydlowksi E, Lucchesi K, Ravindran A. An emerging pharmacology of peptide toxins targeted against potassium channels. J Membr Biol 1988; 105:95–111.

66. Acheson G H, Moe G K. Some effects of tetraethyl ammonium on the mammalian heart. J Pharmacol Exp Ther 1945; 84:189–95.

67. Morad M, Trautwein W. The effect of the duration of the action potential on contraction in the mammalian heart muscle. Pflugers Arch 1968; 299:66–82.

68. Lüllmann H, Ravens U. The time courses of the changes in contractile force and in transmembrane potentials induced by cardiac glycosides in guinea-pig papillary muscle. Br J Pharmacol 1973; 49:377–90.

69. Baker P F, Blaustein M P, Hodgkin A L, Steinhardt RA. The influence of calcium on sodium efflux in squid axons. J Physiol (Lond) 1969; 200:431–58.

70. Langer G A. Effects of digitalis on myocardial ionic exchange. Circulation 1972; 46: 180–7.

71. Reeves J P, Sutko J L. Sodium calcium ion exchange in cardiac membrane vesicles. Proc Natl Acad Sci USA 1979; 76:590–4.

72. Philipson K D. Sodium calcium exchange in plasma membrane vesicles. Annu Rev Physiol 1985; 47:561–71.

73. Kimura J, Miyamae S, Noma A. Identification of sodium-calcium exchange current in single ventricular cells of guinea-pig. J Physiol (Lond) 1987; 384:199–222.

74. Egan T M, Noble D, Noble S J, Powell T, Spindler A J, Twist V W. Sodium-calcium

exchange during the action potential in guinea-pig ventricular cells. J Physiol (Lond) 1989; 411:639–61.

75. Sheu S-S, Fozzard H A. Transmembrane Na$^+$ and Ca^{2+} electrochemical gradients in cardiac muscle and their relationship to force development. J Gen Physiol 1982; 80:325–51.

76. Eisner D A, Lederer W J, Vaughan-Jones RD. The quantitative relationship between twitch tension and intracellular sodium activity in sheep cardiac Purkinje fibers. J Physiol (Lond) 1984; 355:251–66.

77. Caroni P, Carafoli E. An ATP-dependent Ca^{2+} pumping system in dog heart sarcolemma. Nature 1980; 283:756–7.

78. Lüllmann H, Peters T, Ravens U. Pharmacological approaches to influence cardiac inotropism. Pharmacol Ther 1983; 21:229–45.

79. Philipson K D, Ward R. Ca^{2+} transport capacity of sarcolemmal Na$^+$-Ca^{2+} exchange. Extrapolation of vesicle data to in vivo conditions. J Mol Cell Cardiol 1986; 18:943–51.

80. Longoni S, Coady M J, Ikeda T, Philipson K D. Expression of cardiac sarcolemmal Na$^+$-Ca^{2+} exchange activity in Xenopus laevis oocytes. Am J Physiol 1988; 255:C870–3.

81. Hale C C, Kleiboeker S B, Carlton C G, Rovetto M J, Jung C, Kim H D. Evidence for high molecular weight Na-Ca exchange in cardiac sarcolemmal vesicles. J Membr Biol 1988; 106:211–8.

82. Schellenberg G D, Anderson L, Swanson P D. Inhibition of Na$^+$-Ca^{2+} exchange in rat brain by amiloride. Mol Pharmacol 1983; 24:251–8.

83. Siegl P K S, Cragoe E J, Trumble M J, Kaczorowski G J. Inhibition of Na$^+$/Ca^{2+} exchange in membrane vesicle and papillary muscle preparations from guinea pig heart by analogs of amiloride. Proc Natl Acad Sci USA 1984; 81:3238–42.

84. Kennedy R H, Berlin J R, Ng Y-C, Akera T, Brody T M. Amiloride: effects on myocardial force of contraction, sodium pump and Na$^+$/Ca^{2+} exchange. J Mol Cell Cardiol 1986; 18:177–88.

85. Caroni P, Villani F, Carafoli E. The cardiotoxic antibiotic doxorubicin inhibits the Na$^+$/Ca^{2+} exchange of dog heart sarcolemmal vesicles. FEBS Lett 1981; 130:184–6.

86. Höfling B, Bolte H D. Acute negative inotropic effect of adriamycin (doxorubicin).

Naunyn-Schmiedebergs Arch Pharmacol 1981; 317:252–6.

87. Glynn I M, Karlish S D J. The sodium pump. Annu Rev Physiol 1975; 37:13–55.

88. Glitsch H G. Electrogenic sodium pumping in the heart. Annu Rev Physiol 1982; 44:389–400.

89. Eisner D A. The Na-K pump in cardiac muscle. In: Fozzard H A, Haber E, Jennings R B, Katz A M, Morgan H E, eds. The heart and cardiovascular system. New York: Raven Press 1986:489–507.

90. Cohen C J, Fozzard H A, Sheu S-S. Increase in intracellular sodium ion activity during stimulation in mammalian cardiac muscle. Circ Res 1982; 50:651–62.

91. Herzig S, Lüllmann H, Mohr K. On the cooperativity of ouabain binding to intact myocardium. J Mol Cell Cardiol 1985; 17:1095–104.

92. Herzig S, Lüllmann H, Mohr K, Schmitz R. Interpretation of [^{3}H]ouabain binding in guinea pig ventricular myocardium in relation to sodium pump activity. J Physiol (Lond) 1988; 396:105–20.

93. Sejersted O M, Wasserstrom J A, Fozzard H A. Na,K pump stimulation by intracellular Na in isolated, intact sheep cardiac Purkinje fibers. J Gen Physiol 1988; 91:445–66.

94. Fambrough D M, Wolitzki B A, Tamkun M M, Takeyasu K. Regulation of the sodium pump in excitable cells. Kidney Int 1987; (suppl.): 32S-97–112.

95. Pressley T A. Ion concentration-dependent regulation of Na,K-pump abundance. J Membr Biol 1988; 105:187–95.

96. Kim D, Marsh J D, Barry W H, Smith T W. Effects of growth in low potassium medium of ouabain on membrane Na,K-ATPase, cation transport, and contractility in cultured chick heart cells. Circ Res 1984; 55:39–48.

97. Blaustein M P. Sodium ions, calcium ions, blood pressure regulation, and hypertension: a reassessment and a hypothesis. Am J Physiol 1977; 232:C165–73.

98. Cloix J F. Endogenous digitalislike compounds. A tentative update of chemical and biological studies. Hypertension 1987; 10(suppl):I-67–70.

99. Schatzmann H J. Herzglykoside als hemmstoffe für den aktiven kalium und natriumtransport durch die erythrocytenmembran. Helv Physiol Acta 1953; 11:346–54.

100. Skou J C. The influence of some cations on adenosine triphosphatase of peripheral nerves. Biochim Biophys Acta 1957; 23:349–401.

101. Akera T, Brody T M. The role of Na^+, K^+-ATPase in the inotropic action of digitalis. Pharmacol Rev 1978; 187–220.

102. Hansen O. Interaction of cardiac glycosides with $(Na^+ + K^+)$-activated ATPase. A biochemical link to digitalis-induced inotropy. Pharmacol Rev 1984; 36:143–62.

103. Marban E, Smith T W. Digitalis. In: Fozzard H A, Haber E, Jennings R B, Katz A M, Morgan H E, eds. The heart and cardiovascular system. New York: Raven Press 1986:1573–95.

104. Schwartz A, Lindenmayer G E, Allen J C. The sodium-potassium adenosine triphosphatase: pharmacological, physiological and biochemical aspects. Pharmacol Rev 1975; 27:3–134.

105. Lüllmann H, Peters T. Action of cardiac glycosides on the excitation-contraction coupling in heart muscle. Prog Pharmacol 1979; 2:1–58.

106. Noble D. Review: mechanism of action of therapeutic levels of cardiac glycosides. Cardiovasc Res 1980; 14:495–514.

107. Huxley A F, Taylor R E. Local activation of striated muscle fibers. J Physiol (Lond) 1958; 144:426-41.

108. Schneider M F, Chandler W K. Voltage dependent charge movement in skeletal muscle: a possible step in excitation-contraction coupling. Nature 1973; 242:244–6.

109. Fawcett D W, McNutt N S. The ultrastructure of the cat myocardium. I. Ventricular papillary muscle. J Cell Biol 1969; 42:1–45.

110. Bers D. Ca influx and sarcoplasmic reticulum Ca release in cardiac muscle activation during postrest recovery. Am J Physiol 1985; 248:H366–81.

111. Fabiato A. Calcium-induced release of calcium from the cardiac sarcoplasmic reticulum. Am J Physiol 1983; 245:C1–14.

112. Bers D M, Allen L H, Kim Y. Calcium binding to cardiac sarcolemmal vesicles: potential role as a modifier of contraction. Am J Physiol 1986; 251:C861–71.

113. Jorgensen A O, Broderick R, Somlyo A P, Somlyo A V. Two structurally distinct calcium storage sites in rat cardiac sarcoplasmic reticulum: an electron microprobe analysis study. Circ Res 1988; 63:1060–9.

114. Wier W G, Kort A A, Stern M D, Lakatta E G, Marban E. Cellular calcium fluctuations in mammalian heart: direct evidence from noise analysis of aequorin signals in Purkinje fibers. Proc Natl Acad Sci USA 1983; 80:7367–71.

115. Wier W G, Cannell M B, Berlin J R, Marban E, Lederer W J. Cellular and subcellular heterogeneity of $[Ca^{2+}]_i$ in single heart cells revealed by fura-2. Science 1987; 235:325–8.

116. Eisner D A, Valdeolmillos M. A study of intracellular calcium oscillations in sheep cardiac Purkinje fibers measured at the single cell level. J Physiol (Lond) 1986; 372:539–56.

117. Tada M, Yamamoto T, Tonomura Y. Molecular mechanism of active calcium transport by sarcoplasmic reticulum. Physiol Rev 1978; 58:1–79.

118. Inesi G. Mechanism of calcium transport. Annu Rev Physiol 1985; 47:573–601.

119. Inui M, Saito A, Fleischer S. Isolation of the ryanodine receptor from cardiac sarcoplasmic reticulum and identity with the feet structures. J Biol Chem 1987; 262:15637–42.

120. Smith J S, Imagawa T, Ma J, Fill M, Campbell K P, Coronado R. Purified ryanodine receptor from rabbit skeletal muscle is the calcium-release channel of sarcoplasmic reticulum. J Gen Physiol 1988; 92:1–26.

121. Anderson K, Lai F A, Liu Q Y, Rousseau E, Erickson H P, Meissner G. Structural and functional characterization of the purified cardiac ryanodine receptor-Ca^{2+} release channel complex. J Biol chem 1989; 264:1329–35.

122. Tada M, Kirchberger M A, Repke D I, Katz AM. The stimulation of calcium transport in cardiac sarcoplasmic reticulum by adenosine $3':5'$-monophosphate-dependent protein kinase. J Biol Chem 1975; 249:6147–80.

123. Tada M. Kirchberger M A, Katz A M. Phosphorylation of a 22,000-dalton component of the cardiac sarcoplasmic reticulum by adenosine $3':5'$-monophosphate-dependent protein kinase. J Biol Chem 1975; 250:2640–7.

124. Kovacs R J, Nelson M T, Simmerman H K B, Jones L R. Phospholamban forms Ca^{2+}-selective channels in lipid bilayers. J Biol Chem 1988; 263:18364–8.

125. Sutko J L, Willerson J T, Templeton J H, Jones L R, Besch H R. Ryanodine: its alter-

ation of cat papillary muscle contractile state and responsiveness to inotropic interventions and a suggested mechanism of action. J Pharmacol Exp Ther 1979; 209:37–47.

126. Sutko J L, Kenyon J L. Ryanodine modification of cardiac muscle responses to potassium-free solutions. Evidence for inhibition of sarcoplasmic reticulum calcium release. J Gen Physiol 1983; 82:385–404.

127. Stemmer P, Akera T. Concealed positive force-frequency relationships in rat and mouse cardiac muscle revealed by ryanodine. Am J Physiol 1986; 251:H1106–10.

128. Marban E, Kusuoka H, Yue D T, Weisfeldt M L, Wier W G. Maximal Ca^{2+}-activated force elicited by tetanization of ferret papillary muscle and whole heart: mechanism and characteristics of steady state contractile activation in intact myocardium. Circ Res 1986; 59:262–9.

129. Zorzato F, Salviati G, Facchinetti T, Volpe P. Doxorubicin induces calcium release from terminal cisternae of skeletal muscle. A study on isolated sarcoplasmic reticulum and chemically skinned fibers. J Biol Chem 1985; 260:7349–55.

130. Hagane K, Akera T, Berlin J R. Doxorubicin: mechanism of cardiodepressant actions in guinea pigs. J Pharmacol Exp Ther 1988; 246:655–61.

131. Kim D H, Landry A B, Lee Y S, Katz A M. Doxorubicin-induced calcium release from cardiac sarcoplasmic reticulum vesicles. J Mol Cell Cardiol 1989; (in press).

132. Berridge M J, Irvine R F. Inositol triphosphate, a novel second messenger in cellular signal transduction. Nature 1984; 312:315–21.

133. Ehrlich B E, Watras J. Inositol 1,4,5-triphosphate activates a channel from smooth muscle sarcoplasmic reticulum. Nature 1988; 336:583–6.

134. Grupp G. Selective updates on mechanisms of action of positive inotropic agents. Mol Cell Biochem 1987; 76:97–112.

135. Mügge A. a-Adrenozeptoren am myokard: vorkommen und funktionelle bedeutung. Klin Wochenschr 1985; 63:1087–97.

136. Jakob H, Nawrath H, Rupp J. Adrenoceptor-mediated changes of action potential and force of contraction in human isolated ventricular heart muscle. Br J Pharmacol 1988; 94:584–90.

137. Hescheler J, Nawrath H, Tang M, Trautwein W. Adrenoceptor-mediated changes of exci-

138. Rüegg J C. Calcium in muscle activation. A comparative approach. Berlin: Springer, 1986.

139. Somlyo A P. Excitation-contraction coupling and the ultrastructure of smooth muscle. Circ Res 1985; 57:497–507.

140. Kamm K E, Stull J T. The function of myosin and light chain kinase phosphorylation in smooth muscle. Annu Rev Pharmacol Toxicol 1985; 25:593–620.

141. Himpens B. Matthijs G, Somlyo A V, Butler T M, Somlyo A P. Cytoplasmic free calcium, myosin light chain phosphorylation, and force in phasic and tonic smooth muscle. J Gen Physiol 1988; 92:713–29.

142. Gordon A M, Huxley A F, Julian F J. The variation in isometric tension with sarcomere length in vertebrate muscle fibers. J Physiol (Lond) 1966; 184:170–92.

143. Allen D G, Kurihara S. The effects of muscle length on intracellular calcium transients in mammalian myocardium. J Physiol (Lond) 1982; 327:79–94.

144. Hibberd M G, Jewell B R. Calcium- and length-dependent force production in rat ventricular muscle. J Physiol (Lond) 1982; 329:527–40.

145. Allen D G, Kentish J C. Calcium concentration in the myoplasm of skinned ferret muscle following changes in muscle length. J Physiol (Lond) 1988; 407:489–503.

146. Babu A, Sonnenblick E, Gulati J. Molecular basis for the influence of muscle length of myocardial performance. Science 1988; 240:74–6.

147. Herzig J W. Contractile proteins: possible targets for drug action. Trends Pharmacol Sci 1984; 5:296–300.

148. Winegrad S. Regulation of cardiac contractile proteins. Correlations between physiology and biochemistry. Circ Res 1984: 55:565–74.

149. Marban E, Rink T J, Tsien R W, Tsien R Y. Free calcium in heart muscle at rest and during contraction measured with Ca^{2+}-sensitive microelectrodes. Nature 1980; 286:845–50.

150. Morad M, Rolett E L. Relaxing effects of catecholamines on mammalian heart. J Physiol (Lond) 1972; 224:537–58.

151. Weishaar R E, Kobylarz-Singer D C, Quade M M, Kaplan H R. Role of cyclic AMP

in regulating muscle contractility: novel pharmacological approaches to modulating cyclic AMP degradation by phosphodiesterase. Drug Dev Res 1988; 12:119–29.

152.   Rapundolo S T, Solaro R J, Kranias E G. Inotropic responses to isoproterenol and phosphodiesterase inhibitors in intact guinea pig hearts: comparison of cyclic AMP levels and phosphorylation of sarcoplasmic reticulum and myofibrillar proteins. Circ Res 1989; 64:104–11.

153.   Katz A M, Hecht H H. The early ''pump'' failure of the ischemic heart. Am J Med 1969; 47:497–502.

154.   Blanchard E M, Solaro R J. Inhibition of the activation and troponin calcium binding of dog cardiac myofibrils by acidic pH. Circ Res 1984; 55:382–91.

155.   El-Saleh S C, Solaro R J. Troponin I enhances acidic pH-induced depression of Ca^{2+} binding to the regulatory sites in skeletal troponin C. J Biol Chem 1988; 263: 3274–8.

156.   Blinks J R, Endoh M. Modification of myofibrillar responsiveness to Ca^{++} as an inotropic mechanism. Circulation 1986; 73 (suppl.III):85–97.

157.   Van Meel J C, Zimmermann R, Diederen W, Erdmann E, Mrwa U. Increase in calcium sensitivity of cardiac myofibrils contributes to the cardiotonic action of sulmazole. Biochem Pharmacol 1988; 37:213–20.

158.   Wier W G, Yue D T, Marban E. Effects of ryanodine on intracellular Ca^{2+} transients in mammalian cardiac muscle. Fed Proc 1985; 44:2989–93.

159.   Yue D T. Intracellular $[Ca^{2+}]$ related to rate of force development in twitch contraction of heart. Am J Physiol 1987; 252:H760–70.

160.   Marban E, Kitakaze M, Chacko V P, Pike M M. Ca^{2+} transients in perfused hearts revealed by gated ^{19}F NMR spectroscopy. Circ Res 1988; 63:673–78.

21

Positive Inotropic Drugs
Part II. Specific Therapeutic Agents

Stefan Herzig

University of Kiel
Kiel, Germany

INTRODUCTION

The cardiac contraction can be modulated by many physiologic and pharmacologic stimuli. Some important basic mechanisms that may serve as molecular targets for positive inotropic drugs have been outlined in the previous chapter. In this chapter specific therapeutic agents are considered, focusing on drugs that are in clinical use or under current investigation. They are discussed by pharmacologic categories according to their presumed main mode of action.

INHIBITION OF THE NA$^+$,K$^+$-ATPASE: DIGITALIS AND RELATED COMPOUNDS

A large number of naturally occurring and synthetic drugs with a cyclopentanoperhydrophenanthrene nucleus possess positive inotropic properties and are therefore called cardioactive steroids or cardiac glycosides (Figure 1). The steric ring orientation in these compounds is different from the configuration found in the steroid hormones. A lactone ring in position C17 is important for cardiac activity, as well as a OH substitution at C14. The sugar molecules linked by a glycosidic bond to the steroid nucleus influence the physicochemical properties and, thus, the pharmacokinetic behavior of these drugs. They are not essential for cardioactivity. Detailed descriptions of the structure-activity relationships of cardioactive steroids are given elsewhere (1–3). The clinically most important members of this large family are the glycosides from the foxglove, *Digitalis purpurea*, digoxin and digitoxin, commonly referred to as digitalis, which are distinguished only by one OH group present at the C12 position of digoxin (Figure 1). Nevertheless, the pharmacokinetic properties differ considerably between those two classic therapeutic agents, the elimination of digitoxin being much slower but less dependent on renal function. For detailed considerations textbooks of pharmacokinetics and therapeutics should be consulted (e.g., Reference 4).

Another important member of this group of compounds is the *Strophanthus* glycoside ouabain, which is frequently used as an experimental tool. Because of its high affinity, together with a comparatively high degree of hydrophilicity, it is well suited as a radioactive

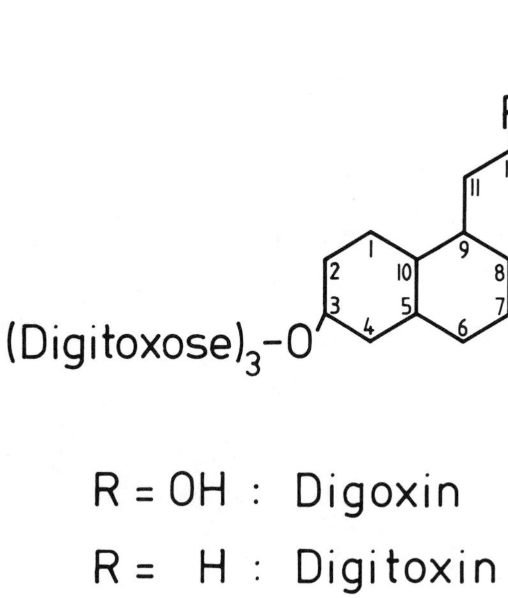

R = OH : Digoxin

R = H : Digitoxin

Figure 1 Chemical structure of digoxin and digitoxin, which are the clinically most important members of the cardiac glycoside drug family.

ligand to probe cardiac glycoside receptors. These are, as outlines in the Chapter 20, identical to the surface membrane enzyme Na^+,K^+-ATPase. The positive inotropic potency of all cardiac steroids explored so far correlates well with their ability to bind to ouabain binding sites and to inhibit Na^+,K^+-ATPase, the individual compounds differing in their effective concentration ranges by several orders of magnitude (e.g., Reference 5). Since the function of the Na^+,K^+-ATPase is of basic importance in most cells, it is not astonishing that in many kinds of isolated tissue preparations functional changes can be elicited by cardiac glycosides. In vivo, however, only a few sites of action are of importance for the nontoxic effects of digitalis, also depending on the presence or absence of heart disease. Besides the positive inotropic effect on the myocardium, vascular and particularly neural effects are worth discussing.

Possibly as a result of a similar mechanism as in heart muscle, digitalis enhances vascular smooth muscle tone, responsible for the increase in vascular resistance observed upon acute administration of cardiac glycosides (6). In fact, in healthy animals and in human sub-

jects a rise in arterial blood pressure precedes the development of the inotropic response upon intravenous administration of rapidly acting glycosides. A constriction of the coronary vessels may also be observed (7,8). In contrast, patients in heart failure usually respond with a decrease in peripheral vascular resistance due to a relaxation of arterial smooth muscle. In addition there is a dilation of venous capacitance vessels. This venous blood pooling was once believed to decrease appreciably the congestive symptoms by reducing the preload of the heart. Many of the vascular effects in patients with congestive heart failure, however, appear to be secondary changes (see Reference 9). Because of the primary improvement in cardiac function, the previously enhanced sympathetic tone of the vascular system is reduced toward normal values. Additional direct glycoside effects on the smooth muscle cell, or on the autonomic nervous control of the blood vessels, are difficult to assess exactly under these pathophysiologic conditions.

Another complex contribution to the profile of the cardiovascular effects of digitalis emerges from the nervous system. At the molecular level Na^+,K^+-ATPase in nervous tissue can be inhibited by cardiac glycosides. However, several isoforms of this enzyme with markedly different glycoside sensitivity have been found (10), which are encoded by three different genes found in the brain (11) (see Reference 12), but also in other tissues (13) (see Reference 14). These more recent findings may be interesting for future drug development, since they may offer a novel opportunity for cardiac glycosides to affect more selectively the Na^+,K^+-ATPases in different tissues, or brain regions, depending on their relative affinities toward the various isozymes, but at the present time this is merely a speculative outlook. At the cellular level cardiac steroids can interfere with the presynaptic release as well as with the postsynaptic sensitivity toward neurotransmitters, such as acetylcholine and norepinephrine (see References 15 and 16). This appears to explain their influence on the autonomic nervous system. At the functional level a vast diversity of experimental observations has been made, involving many different parts of the brain and the peripheral nervous system (see Reference 17). Few of these effects are probably relevant at therapeutic plasma levels of digitalis, but some of them figure essentially in the clinical picture of the drug response. There are the so-called vagotonic effects (see Reference 18), leading to a reduction in heart rate, which turns out to be beneficial in many cases of congestive heart failure. In cases of atrial fibrillation with a high ventricular rate, the slowing of atrioventricular (AV) conduction, which is mainly neurally mediated, is in fact the most important reason for the administration of digitalis. The role of the nervous system in digitalis toxicity may be even more diverse but is not within the scope of this chapter (see, e.g., Reference 17).

In sum, the most important primary effects of digitalis administration to a patient with congestive heart failure are the positive inotropic effect due to the action on myocardial tissue and the cardiac slowing due to an enhanced vagal tone. As functional consequences there are a reduction in end-diastolic volume due to the improved contractile force

at a given diastolic fiber length. The reduction in systolic chamber volume leads to more economical work, since systolic wall tension translates more effectively into pressure development at a lower chamber diameter. The reduction in heart rate is beneficial in many cases and allows improved coronary perfusion to take place as a result of the longer period of time spent in diastole. This in turn may elevate a pathologically lowered diastolic compliance and, therefore, facilitate ventricular filling at a given preload. Secondarily, the abnormally high sympathetic tone in heart failure is reversed, which reduces the increased arteriolar resistance and the sodium and water retention by the kidneys. These changes observed in heart disease contrast markedly with the effects in healthy subjects, in whom neural and vascular effects counteract the increase in cardiac contractile force, which may even lead to a drop in cardiac output.

In conclusion, the acute action of sufficiently high doses of digitalis in congestive heart failure suggests that it should be capable of exerting a *strong* positive inotropic effect, as seen in isolated myocardial tissue. Here the contractile force can be increased to levels comparable to those achieved by catecholamines (Figure 2). Furthermore, the maximal inotropic effect that can be obtained in tissue preparations from diseased human myocardium is even higher compared to that of many other positive inotropic drugs (19–21) (see Reference 22). This observation may stimulate the search for new digitalis compounds with possibly wider margins of safety (see, e.g., Reference 23). Currently it is obviously the toxicity of digitalis that limits the extent of positive inotropy that can be clinically attained. Accordingly, in patients, the dose range between therapeutic and toxic effects is rather narrow and the doses individually required may vary appreciably. Thus it may be quite difficult to induce a marked and sustained positive inotropic effect in the clinical setting (see Reference 24). Accordingly, the question of whether an improvement in cardiac function can be maintained with chronic digitalis treatment of congestive heart failure, at least in cases without atrial fibrillation, is

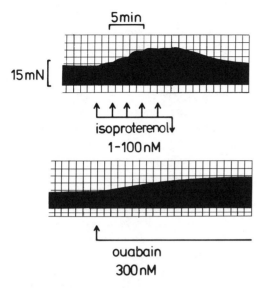

Figure 2 Isometric contractile force of an isolated, electrically driven left atrial muscle from guinea pig heart (Herzig and Mohr, unpublished data; for method see Reference 93). After addition of cumulative concentrations of isoproterenol (1, 3, 10, 30, and 100 nM, at upward arrows in the upper panel), a maximum inotropic effect was attained, and finally the β-adrenoceptor agonist was washed out (downward arrow). When contractile force again declined to baseline, the cardiac glycoside ouabain (300 nM) was applied (lower panel). Note that a positive inotropic effect of rather similar magnitude could be elicited, but it developed more slowly.

still subject to debate. The controlled studies conducted so far have revealed differing results (see References 25 and 26). A certain subgroup of patients, however, certainly benefits from long-term digitalis treatment (27), including cases of moderate cardiac dysfunction (28,29). There is still much to be learned about the factors determining whether chronic digitalis administration is useful in a given patient.

PHOSPHODIESTERASE INHIBITION: OLD AND NEW DRUGS

The methylated xanthine derivatives theophylline (1,3–dimethylxanthine), caffeine (1,3,7-trimethylxanthine), and theobromine (3,7-dimethylxanthine) are widely distributed in nature as plant alkaloids. Their use as constituents of beverages made from *Thea sinensis, Coffea arabica, Theobroma cacao*, or *Cola acuminata* dates from ancient history to the present. Theophylline has an additional role as a therapeutic agent in the treatment of asthmatic disorders. It displays a variety of functional effects, such as relaxing smooth muscle, stimulating diuresis, arousing the nervous system, and affecting the heart. With respect to the cardiovascular system, a vasodilation in most organs, except in the brain, is prominent. In the heart a positive inotropic effect can be observed, and positive chronotropic and arrhythmogenic responses are evoked, which limit the dose of theophylline in the treatment of severe bronchoconstriction. A number of molecular mechanism have been detected in vitro for methylxanthines, and only some of them seem to be involved in the pattern of drug responses observed in vivo since they take place at reasonably low concentrations. Among those, there is an inhibition of the enzyme phosphodiesterase and the antagonistic action on adenosine receptors. Both can explain a positive inotropic action, the former leading to elevated cAMP levels (see Reference 30), the latter because it would prevent a negative inotropic effect possibly elicited by adenosine. Increments in cardiac peak contractile force were also explained by a sensitization of the contractile proteins toward calcium exerted by theophylline (31). Even so, the reported inhibition of calcium reuptake into the SR (e.g., Reference 32) could serve to increase cardiac tension. Both the latter two molecular actions, however, take place at millimolar concentrations of caffeine, or theophylline, in excess of therapeutic plasma levels. In any case, the methylxanthines are not used as primary therapeutic agents in heart failure. The risks and side effects emerging from their stimulating effect on the nervous system and on cardiac rhythm outweigh the benefits of the positive inotropy. Thus inhibition of phosphodiesterase was largely abandoned as a molecular mechanism valuable for positive inotropic agents. The situation changed more recently, however, when several isoforms of this enzyme were discovered and when a new group of drugs with a more specific inhibitory activity was developed. There are now at least three known isozymes, referred to as phosphodiesterase (PDE) I through III, which differ in specificity for cAMP versus cGMP hydrolysis, affinities and capacities for these substrates, susceptibility to stimulation by calmodulin, and their abundance in different tissues (see Reference 33). Of particular interest is PDE III, which has been characterized as a cAMP-specific, calmodulin-independent, high-affinity, and low-capacity enzyme that is inhibited by cGMP. It may be located in part in cellular membranes, not only in the cytosol (34).

The classic PDE inhibitors, the methylxanthines, seem to inhibit all isozymes with about equal potencies, unlike some newer compounds (Figure 3). Among these are the bipyridines amrinone and milrinone and the imidazolone derivatives fenoximone and piroximone, as well as the imidazopyridines sulmazole and isomazole, which are structurally related to the benzimidazole derivative pimobendan. All these compounds are referred to as "non-digitalis, noncatecholaminelike" positive inotropic agents since they enhance contractile force in cardiac preparations, regardless of the presence of adrenergic receptor blocking agents, and since they do not act like cardiac glycosides. A common molecular feature of these and several other new compounds is that they preferentially inhibit the PDE III isoform of cardiac phosphodiesterase (35–37). Their main functional effects in humans are positive inotropy and arterial vasodilation (see References 38 and 39). Even though at least some of them may also have additional molecular modes of action, such as adenosine antagonism (40,41) (see later), they all differ from the classic methylxanthines with respect to their pattern of functional effects. This may indeed be related to the differences outlined with respect to their biochemical effects (e.g., Reference 42).

Many clinical studies have already been conducted on the hemodynamic changes induced by the new PDE inhibitors in patients with congestive heart failure. Both the reduction in afterload and the increment in myocardial contractility seemed to be very effective, at least in the early, uncontrolled short-term settings. The first of the drugs, amrinone, was available for a period of time as an oral medication in the United States, but the occurrence of severe side effects led to its withdrawal. Nowadays amrinone is recommended only for intravenous therapy in very severe cases of heart failure resistant to the usual therapy. Since some of the major side effects of amrinone, thrombocytopenia and hepatic marker enzyme increase, do not appear to be related to the primary mode of action, there has been considerable hope that other compounds of this class may turn out to be better tolerated. In particular, milrinone, fenoximone, piroximone, and pimobendan are currently being tested in phase III clinical trials in some countries. Their efficacy seems not to wear off as fast as observed with β-adrenergic stimulants but is sustained in studies conducted over several weeks. Whether there is lasting benefit for patients receiving continued oral treatment, however, is still controversial. Controlled long-term studies on amrinone have not shown an improvement in outcome (43), and long-term milrinone treatment has been shown to be less effective than digoxin therapy (29). These disappointing results recall the caution that chronic inotropic stimulation of the heart by agents like amrinone may worsen the prognosis and even shorten the survival time in congestive heart failure (44,45) by exhausting the degree to which the diseased heart can supply metabolic energy. With respect to the PDE III inhibitors, the effect on myocardial energy consumption appears to differ among drugs (26) in the clinical setting. Myocardial economy, that is, the ratio between work output and energy expenditure, may be worse compared to digitalis, at least as measured in isolated hearts (46), where the vasodilator properties cannot contribute to the overall effect. The latter effects (e.g., Reference 47) may well be an important reason for the apparently impressive short-term benefit seen with these drugs, resembling those with the so-called direct vasodilators (see Reference 48). These questions remain to be resolved but apparently will require more controlled, prospective studies.

MODULATION OF ION CHANNEL FUNCTION: A THERAPEUTIC PRINCIPLE?

As outlined several times in Chapter 20, drug-induced changes in the function of cardiac ion channels can potentially lead to a positive inotropic effect, which sometimes, however, cannot be recruited therapeutically. For instance, the L-type calcium channel opening effect of agents like Bay K 8644 induces an increase in force of isolated papillary muscles. In the intact animal this effect may be blunted by a pronounced smooth muscle constriction in the coronary vasculature, which lowers perfusion and thus counteracts the direct effect on the myocardial cell. The vasoconstriction is brought about by a stimulation of calcium inward current in vascular smooth muscle cells (49). As a second example, the administration of the sodium channel modulator veratridine leads to a positive inotropy in isolated preparations, whereas in the whole animal a stimulation of cardiac vagal afferent nerve fibers occurs, which triggers a reflex leading to a marked drop in heart rate and blood pressure (see Reference 50). The problem appears in both cases to be the lack of tissue specificity of these agents, that is, the failure to modulate especially the channels of cardiac cells. This may be easily intelligible, because ion channels are largely conserved throughout evolution, revealing striking similarities among different tissues and species (see Reference 51).

There are, on the other hand, some examples of at least a partial tissue selectivity among agents affecting channels. For instance, the sodium channel blocking poison tetrodotoxin is very potent in neurons, but cardiac sodium channels are several orders of magnitude less sensitive (see, e.g., References 52 and 53). In contrast, the drug lidocaine inhibits sodium inward current in heart cells at considerably lower concentrations (54) than those necessary for local anesthesia. The molecular

basis of such a preferential efficacy of a compound on a particular tissue may reside in small differences of the molecular structure of channels, as may be suspected for tetrodotoxin. Also, the way the electrical properties of the whole cell membrane govern the behavior of a particular channel may be important: drugs that have varying affinities to channels in different voltage-dependent states may be more likely to become bound at more depolarized membrane potentials or at a very high frequency of action potentials (55,56). Thus a pathologic situation confined to certain cells may be the basis for them to be rather selective targets for drugs, as proposed for phenytoin in epileptic foci (57–60), in digitalis-poisoned myocardial tissue (e.g., Reference 61), or for some calcium antagonists in ischemic cerebral tissue (e.g., Reference 62). Likewise, the particular shape of the cardiac action potential may predispose certain drugs to act in this organ (see Reference 63).

These issues have been extensively studied so far only for blockers, for instance of sodium and calcium channels. Currently, however, there is only scanty evidence for any positive inotropic channel modulator to be selective for cardiac tissue. The new inotropic drug DPI 201–106 (Figure 3) may turn out to be a first example. It prolongs the action potential by slowing the inactivation of the sodium current (64), favoring a state of the sodium channel characterized by unusually long, repetitive openings (65,66). Although a mechanism of action involving the contractile proteins has also been put forward (67–69), the positive inotropy can be abolished by tetrodotoxin, suggesting that the action on sodium channels is of major importance. Another aspect of its efficacy may be calcium channel blocking activity (70), which could account for its vasodilator action. Since DPI 201–106 combines positive inotropic and coronary dilating effects (67), its properties seem promising with respect to clinical application. Among the other inotropic drugs currently investigated, there are some that prolong the duration of cardiac action potentials. For instance, OPC 8212 (Figure 3) (71) and the bipyridine saterinone (72) have been claimed to exert this effect by blocking potassium channels. At least part of their inotropic activity, however, seems to result from PDE III inhibition (e.g., Reference 73). It is therefore not easy to assess a possible role of potassium channel blockade in their mode of inotropic action. The last example to be mentioned is the racemic compound 202–791, a dihydropyridine, the (+)-enantiomer of which exerts calcium channel agonistic, and the (−)-enantiomer, calcium antagonistic properties. The former effect prevails in myocardial tissue, whereas the latter appears to dominate in the vascular smooth muscle cell (74). Thus, unlike Bay K 8644 or other calcium agonistic dihydropyridines, 202–791 can increase contractile force in the heart without appreciable coronary vasoconstriction. Although this compound in fact represents a drug combination, in that it contains two enantiomers, its effects should stimulate further research on substances acting specifically on cardiac ionic channels, which might be achieved by an action on the rather unique electrical behavior of the cardiac membrane potential (see, e.g., Reference 46). In sum, however, the success in developing a clinically useful inotropic agent that acts by direct ion channel modulation is still scant.

SENSITIZATION OF THE CONTRACTILE PROTEINS TOWARD CALCIUM

All the drugs discussed so far exert their inotropic effect by an increase in the cytosolic calcium ion concentration $[Ca^{2+}]_i$. This mechanism inherently bears the risk of cellular calcium overload, which then may deteriorate cardiac function and metabolism (e.g., Reference 75). An attractive alternative approach could be to increase the force at a given $[Ca^{2+}]_i$ (see Reference 76). Beginning with sulmazole (ARL 115 BS) (77,78), a number of positive inotropic agents (Figure 3), for instance pimobendan (see Reference 79), APP 201–533 (80), and DPI 201–106 (67), are currently believed to exert their effects at least partially by enhancement of the sensitivity of the contractile proteins toward calcium. More precisely, the dissociation of calcium ions from the regulatory site at TnC is assumed to be slowed, which would lead to a higher degree of calcium binding at a given calcium ion concentration. Indirect evidence suggests that these drugs exert their effects by binding themselves to TnC (79). In skinned fibers of cardiac muscle they shift the calcium activation curve for force development to lower calcium concentrations. In intact muscle fibers they increase peak tension at any given level of the intracellular calcium transient (31). Because of the differences between the contractile proteins in different types of muscle (see Reference 81), the proposed mechanism of action may indeed preferentially affect cardiac muscle (82,83). Unfortunately, no drug has so far been shown to act exclusively on the contractile proteins. Sulmazole inhibits PDE III as well as Na^+K^+-ATPase (84); pimobendan and APP 201–533 are also phosphodiesterase inhibitors. The idea that the action on the contractile machinery is important in their overall effect comes from several observations. They elevate cAMP to a smaller extent at a given force increment compared to other drugs inhibiting PDE III (e.g., Reference 85). Additionally, the effect of the enantiomers of sulmazole on the contractile elements displays stereoselectivity, as does its positive inotropic effect. On the other hand, with respect to PDE inhibition, both (+)- and (−)-sulmazole are equipotent (86). Also for the enantiomers of pimobendan, a certain degree of stereoselectivity of their inotropic and calcium-sensitizing effects could be demonstrated (87).

A fundamental problem of calcium sensitization as an inotropic mechanism may reside in the fact that a slowed dissociation of calcium from TnC should not only enhance peak force but also delay the time course of relaxation. It is not entirely clear whether such an effect would not worsen the economy and dynamic efficiency of the cardiac pump function in situ. It is also unknown whether the positive inotropic effects persist during prolonged therapy. Currently, pimobendan is in phase III clinical investigation, whereas studies in humans with sulmazole have been suspended be-

name	code name	structural formula	proposed mechanism(s) of action
Amrinone	Win 40680	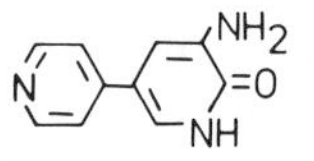	PDE II inhibitor adenosine antagonist
Milrinone	Win 47203	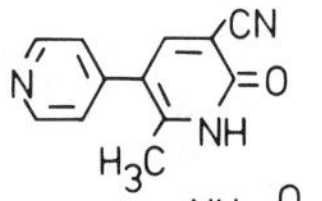	PDE II inhibitor
Piroximone	MDL 19205	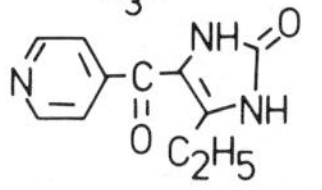	PDE II inhibitor
Fenoximone	MDL 17043	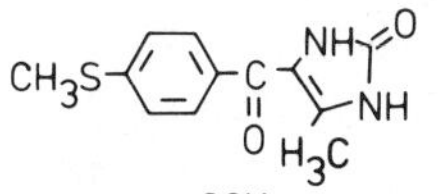	PDE II inhibitor
Sulmazole	ARL 115 BS	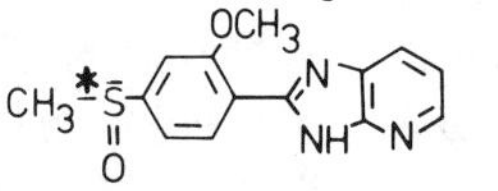	Ca^{2+}-sensitizer PDE II inhibitor
Pimobendan	UD-CG 115	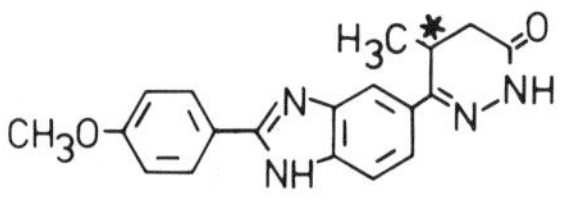	Ca^{2+}-sensitizer PDE II inhibitor
	OPC 8212	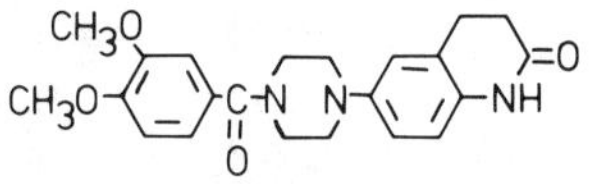	PDE II inhibitor K^{+}-channel blocker
	MCI 154	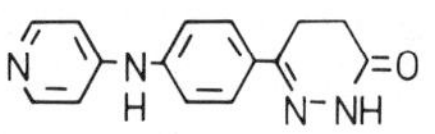	PDE II inhibitor Ca^{2+}-sensitizer
	DPI 201-106	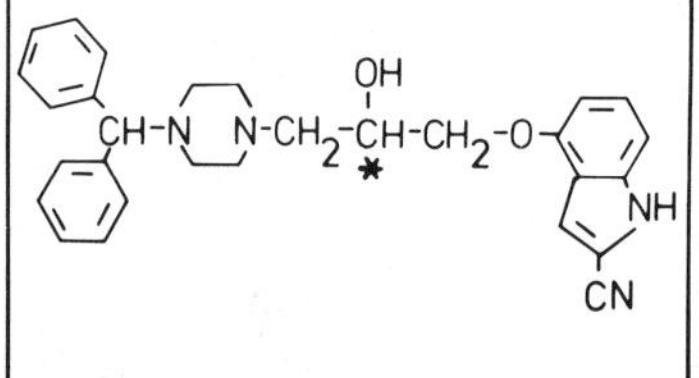	Na^{+} channel opener Ca^{2+}-sensitizer

Figure 3 Structural formulas of various novel positive inotropic agents, which act like neither digitalis nor catecholamine. Often-raised proposals concerning their molecular modes of action are given in the right column. In case of racemic compounds the center of asymmetry is marked by an asterisk.

cause of the toxic side effects of this compound. Another new compound is the pyridazinone derivative MCI 154 (Figure 3), which appears to enhance not only the affinity of the troponin toward calcium, but also the maximal tension generated by actomyosin in vitro (88), by a completely unknown mechanism. Besides this, it also has PDE inhibitory activity.

To date it is not possible to predict the likely clinical benefit of drugs revealing an action on the actomyosin system, since this question would have to be resolved with a drug that lacks additional mechanisms of action. It is theoretically feasible that the hemodynamic changes associated with a retarded relaxation would even be detrimental to the failing heart. On the other hand, it has been argued that these compounds may merely normalize a pathologically reduced myofilament calcium sensitivity (e.g., References 82 and 88), as has been found in hypoxic and ischemic myocardial tissue (see Reference 89). This hypothesis is based on observations of the myofilament sensitivity made in isolated preparations rather than in diseased human heart. Even if this is valid for the failing human heart, however, one might ask whether it is good advice to restore calcium affinity, and thus elevate ATP consumption, under conditions in which the myocardial energy supply can be severely impeded.

ROLE OF POSITIVE INOTROPIC DRUGS IN THE TREATMENT OF CHRONIC HEART FAILURE

It is dangerous to generalize regarding the potential value of positive inotropic agents in the treatment of chronic myocardial failure, in view of the rapidly growing number of new inotropic compounds and of the gain of knowledge about their molecular mechanisms. Furthermore, alternative pharmacologic approaches to treat the failing heart, such as drugs lowering pre- and afterload, and even cardiac transplantation, figure more prominently in the spectrum of the available therapeutic options. Drugs with arterial vasodilator properties seem to be a quite promising measure. Those specifically interfering with the reflex mechanisms that underlie the increased peripheral resistance observed in decompensated heart failure appear to be particularly effective in long-term therapy, that is, the α-adrenergic blockers like prazosin and the angiotensin converting enzyme inhibitors, such as captopril and enalapril (28,90) (see Reference 91). This success contrasts with the recent clinical results with inotropic drug therapy. To date, the only inotropic agents recommended for widespread use are the digitalis compounds (e.g., Reference 92). Ironically, new insights regarding their possible benefits have emerged from studies using digoxin as a reference for comparison against the recently developed drugs (e.g., References 28 and 29). With regard to the new inotropic agents, how-

ever, results from the first well-controlled long-term studies seem to temper the euphoria elicited by the initial trials (29,43). Although this need not lead to pessimism about new inotropics in general, predictions about future progress are virtually impossible. This is because of the multiplicity of effects the new compounds reveal both at the molecular level (Figure 3) and in the whole cardiovascular system, as exemplified by the combined inotropic and vasodilator properties of the phosphodiesterase inhibitors. Finally, one may ask whether there is good reason to expect a prolongation of survival from any inotropic drug: Is restoring the contractile force by whatever mechanism anything but symptomatic therapy, unless it would somehow directly revert the fundamental processes leading to reduced contractility? As long as we are not able to understand, or to specifically interfere with, those pathophysiologic factors, it is difficult to imagine a causal, and thus more satisfying and more definitely successful, form of drug therapy.

ACKNOWLEDGMENTS

The author has been supported by a research fellowship from the Deutsche Forschungsgemeinschaft (He 1578 2–1). The excellent help of Mrs. Andrea Overbeck in preparing the figures for this and the preceding chapter is gratefully acknowledged.

REFERENCES

1. Yoda A, Yoda S. Association and dissociation rate constants of the complexes between various cardiac aglycones and sodium- and potassium-dependent adenosine triphosphatase formed in the presence of magnesium and phosphate. Mol Pharmacol 1977; 13:352–61.
2. Güntert T W, Linde H H A. Chemistry and structure-activity relationships of cardioactive steroids. In: Greeff K, ed. Handbook of experimental pharmacology, Vol. 56/1. Cardiac glycosides. Berlin: Springer, 1981:13–24.
3. Schönfeld W, Weiland J, Lindig C, Masnyk M, Kabat, M M, Kurek, A, Wicha J, Repke K R H. The lead structure in cardiac

glycosides is 5β,14β-androstane-3β,14-diol. Naunyn-Schmiedebergs Arch Pharmacol 1985; 329:414–26.

4. Hoffman B F, Bigger J T. Digitalis and allied cardiac glycosides. In: Goodman Gilman A, Goodman L S, Rall T W, Murad F, eds. The pharmacologic basis of therapeutics, 7th ed. New York: Macmillan, 1985:716–47.

5. Brown L, Erdmann E, Thomas, R. Digitalis structure-activity relationship analyses. Conclusions from indirect binding studies with cardiac (Na$^+$+K$^+$)-ATPase. Biochem Pharmacol 1983; 32:2767–74.

6. Mason D T, Braunwald E. Studies on digitalis. X. Effects of ouabain on forearm vascular resistance and venous tone in normal subjects and in patients in heart failure. J Clin Invest 1964; 43:532–43.

7. Bloor C M, Walker D E, Pensinger R R. Ouabain induced primary coronary constriction. Proc Soc Exp Biol Med 1972; 140:1409–13.

8. Schwartz J S, Bache R J. Effect of ouabain on large coronary artery diameter. J Cardiovasc Pharmacol 1988; 11:608–13.

9. Mason D T. Effects of cardiac glycosides on vascular system. In: Greeff K, ed. Handbook of experimental pharmacology, Vol. 56/1. Cardiac glycosides. Berlin: Springer, 1981: 497–515.

10. Sweadner K J. Two molecular forms of the Na$^+$,K$^+$-ATPase alpha subunit from rat brain. J Biol Chem 1979; 254:6060–7.

11. Shull G E, Greeb J, Lingrel J B. Two molecular forms of (Na$^+$+K$^+$)-stimulated ATPase in brain. Biochemistry 1986; 25:8125–32.

12. Jørgensen P L, Andersen J P. Structural basis for E_1-E_2 conformational transitions in Na,K-pump and Ca-pump proteins. J Membr Biol 1988; 103:95–120.

13. Orlowski J, Lingrel J B. Tissue-specific and developmental regulation of rat Na,K-ATPase catalytic alpha isoform and β-subunit mRNAs. J Biol Chem 1988; 263:10436–42.

14. Sweadner K J. Isozymes of the Na$^+$/K$^+$-ATPase. Biochim Biophys Acta 1989; 988:185–220.

15. Powis D A. Cardiac glycosides and autonomic neurotransmission. J Auton Pharmacol 1983; 3:127–54.

16. Herzig S, Lüllmann H. Effects of cardiac glycosides at the cellular level. In: Vaughan-Williams E M, ed. Handbook of experimental pharmacology, Vol. 89. Antiarrhythmic drugs. Berlin: Springer 1989:545–63.

17. Gillis R A, Quest J A. The role of the nervous system in the cardiovascular effects of digitalis. Pharmacol Rev 1980; 31:19–97.

18. Lendle L. Digitaliskörper und verwandte Substanzen (Digitaloide). In: Häubner W, Schüller L, eds. Handbook of experimental pharmacology (suppl. Vol. 1). Berlin: Springer 1935:11–241.

19. Brown L, Näbauer M, Erdmann E. Additive positive inotropic effects of milrinone, ouabain and calcium in diseased human myocardium. Klin Wochenschr 1986; 64:708–12.

20. Brown L, Lorenz B, Erdmann E. Additive and non-additive positive inotropic effects in human and guinea-pig myocardium. In: Erdmann E, Greeff K, Skou J C, eds. Cardiac glycosides 1785–1985. Biochemistry-pharmacology-clinical relevance. Darmstadt: Steinkopff 1986:195–205.

21. Feldman M D, Copelas L, Gwathmey V M D, Phillips P, Warren S E, Schoen F J, Grossman W, Morgan J P. Deficient production of cyclic AMP: pharmacologic evidence of an important cause of contractile dysfunction in patients with end-stage heart failure. Circulation 1987; 75:331–9.

22. Grupp G. Selective updates on mechanisms of action of positive inotropic agents. Mol Cell Biochem 1987; 76:97–112.

23. Lüllmann H. Cardiac glycosides: drugs out of fashion. Prog Pharmacol 1990; 7:1–9.

24. Smith T W, Antman E A, Friedman P L, Blatt C M, Marsh J D. Digitalis glycosides: mechanisms and manifestation of toxicity. Prog Cardiovasc Dis 1984; 26:413–41, 495–523; 27:21–56.

25. Lipkins D P, Poole-Wilson P A. Treatment of chronic heart failure: a review of recent drug trials. Br Med J 1985; 291:993–6.

26. Weber K T, Gill S K, Janicki J S, Maskin C S, Jain M C. Newer inotropic agents in the treatment of chronic cardiac failure. Current status and future directions. Drugs 1987; 33:503–19.

27. Dobbs S M, Kenyon W, Dobbs R J. Maintenance digoxin after an episode of heart failure: placebo-controlled trial in outpatients. Br Med J 1977; I:749–52.

28. The Captopril-Digoxin Multicenter Research Group. Comparative effects of therapy with captopril and digoxin in patients with mild to moderate heart failure. JAMA 1988; 259:539–44.

29. DiBianco R, Shabetai R, Kostuck W, Moran J, Schlant R C, Wright R, for the Milrinone

Multicenter Trial Group. A comparison of oral milrinone, digoxin, and their combination in the treatment of patients with chronic heart failure. N Engl J Med 1988; 320:677–83.

30. Scholz H. Inotropic drugs and their mechanisms of action. J Am Coll Cardiol 1984; 4:389–97.

31. Blinks J R, Endoh M. Modification of myofibrillar responsiveness to Ca^{++} as an inotropic mechanism. Circulation 1986; 73 (suppl. III):85–97.

32. Hess P, Wier W G. Excitation-contraction coupling in cardiac Purkinje fibers. Effects of caffeine on the intracellular $[Ca^{2+}]$ transient, membrane currents, and contraction. J Gen Physiol 1984; 83:417–33.

33. Weishaar R E, Cain C H, Bristol J A. A new generation of phosphodiesterase inhibitors: multiple molecular forms of phosphodiesterase and the potential for drug selectivity. J Med Chem 1985; 28:537–45.

34. Kaufmann R H, Crowe V G, Utterback B G, Robertson D W. LY 195115: a potent, selective inhibitor of cyclic nucleotide phosphodiesterase located in the sarcoplasmic reticulum. Mol Pharmacol 1986; 30:609–16.

35. Farah A E, Alousi A A, Schwartz R P. Positive inotropic agents. Annu Rev Pharmacol Toxicol 1984; 24:275–328.

36. Weishaar R E, Kobylarz-Singer D C, Quade M M, Kaplan H R. Role of cyclic AMP in regulating muscle contractility: novel pharmacological approaches to modulating cyclic AMP degradation by phosphodiesterase. Drug Dev Res 1988; 12:119–29.

37. Brunkhorst D, V der Leyden H, Meyer W, Nigbur R, Schmidt-Schumacher C, Scholz H. Relation of positive inotropic and chronotropic effects of pimobendan, UD-CG 212 C1, milrinone and other phosphodiesterase inhibitors to phosphodiesterase III inhibition in guinea-pig heart. Naunyn-Schmiedebergs Arch Pharmacol 1989; 339:575–83.

38. Colucci W S, Wright R F, Braunwald E. New positive inotropic agents in the treatment of congestive heart failure. Mechanism of action and recent clinical developments. N Engl J Med 1986; 314:290–9, 349–58.

39. Andersson K E. Some new positive inotropic agents. Acta Med Scand 1986; 707(suppl): 65–73.

40. Dorigo P, Maragno I. Interaction of amrinone with endogenous adenosine in guinea pig atria. Br J Pharmacol 1986; 87:623–9.

41. Parsons W J, Rankumar V, Stile G L. The new cardiotonic agent sulmazole is an A_1 adenosine receptor antagonist and functionally blocks and inhibitory regulator, G_i. Mol Pharmacol 1988; 33:441–8.

42. Harrison S A, Reifsnyder D H, Gallis B, Cadd G G, Beavo J A. Isolation and characterization of bovine cardiac muscle cGMP-inhibited phosphodiesterase: a receptor for new cardiotonic drugs. Mol Pharmacol 1986; 29:506–14.

43. Massie B, Bourassa M, DiBianco R, Hess M, Konstam M, Likoff M, Pacuer M. (The Amrinone Multicenter Trial Group). Long-term oral administration of amrinone for congestive heart failure: lack of efficacy in a multicenter trial. Circulation 1985; 71:963–71.

44. Katz A M. A new inotropic drug: its promise and a caution. N Engl J Med 1978; 299:1409–10.

45. Katz A M. Potential deleterious effects of inotropic agents in the therapy of chronic heart failure. Circulation 1986; 73(suppl. III): 184–8.

46. Bechem M, Hebisch S, Schramm M. Ca^{2+} agonists: new, sensitive probes for Ca^{2+} channels. Trends Pharmacol Sci 1988; 9:261–4.

47. Cody R J, Müller F S, Kubo S H, Rutman H, Leonard D. Identification of the direct vasodilator effects of milrinone with an isolated limb preparation in patients with congestive heart failure. Circulation 1986; 73:124–9.

48. Packer M. Selection of vasodilator drugs for patients with severe chronic heart failure. An approach based on a new classification. Drugs 1982; 24:64–74.

49. Bean B P, Sturek M, Hermsmeyer K. Calcium channels in muscle cells isolated from rat mesenteric arteries: modulation by dihydropyridine drugs. Circ Res 1986; 59:229–35.

50. Krayer O, Acheson G H. The pharmacology of the veratrum alkaloids. Physiol Rev 1946; 26:383–446.

51. Hille B. Ionic channels of excitable membranes. Sunderland, MA: Sinauer, 1984.

52. Narahashi T. Chemicals as tools in the study of excitable membranes. Physiol Rev 1974; 54:813–89.

53. Cohen C J, Bean B P, Colatsky T J, Tsien R W. Tetrodotoxin block of sodium channels in rabbit Purkinje fibers. J Gen Physiol 1981; 78:383–411.

54. Bean B P, Cohen C J, Tsien R W. Lidocaine block of cardiac sodium channels. J Gen Physiol 1983; 81:613–42.

55. Strichartz G R. The inhibition of sodium currents in myelinated nerve by quaternary derivatives of lidocaine. J Gen Physiol 1973; 62:37–57.

56. Courtney K R. Mechanism of frequency-dependent inhibition of sodium currents in frog myelinated nerve by the lidocaine derivative GEA 968. J Pharmacol Exp Ther 1975; 195:225–36.

57. Matsuki N, Quandt F N, Ten Eick, R E, Yeh J Z. Characterization of the block of sodium channels by phenytoin in mouse neuroblastoma cells. J Pharmacol Exp Ther 1984; 228:523–30.

58. Willow M, Gonoi T, Catterall W A. Voltage clamp analysis of the inhibitory actions of diphenylhydantoin and carbamazepine on voltage-sensitive sodium channels in neuroblastoma cells. Mol Pharmacol 1985; 27:549–58.

59. Quandt F N. Modification of slow inactivation of single sodium channels by phenytoin in neuroblastoma cells. Mol Pharmacol 1988; 34:557–65.

60. Tomaselli G, Marban E, Yellen G. Sodium channels from human brain RNA expressed in *Xenopus* oocytes. Basic electrophysiologic characteristics and their modification by diphenylhydantoin. J Clin Invest 1989; 83:1724–32.

61. Lüllmann H, Weber R. Über die wirkung von phenytoin auf digitalis-bedingte arrhythmien. Ärztl Forsch 1969; 22:49–55.

62. Scriabine A, Schuurman T, Traber J. Pharmacological basis for the use of nimodipine in central nervous system disorders. FASEB J 1989; 3:1799–806.

63. Hondeghem L M, Katzung B G. Time- and voltage-dependent interactions of antiarrhythmic drugs with cardiac sodium channels. Biochim Biophys Acta 1977; 472:373–98.

64. Buggisch D, Isenberg G, Ravens, U, Scholtysik G. The role of sodium channels in the effects of the cardiotonic compound DPI 201–106 on contractility and membrane potentials in isolated mammalian heart preparations. Eur J Pharmacol 1985; 118:303–11.

65. Kohlhardt M, Froebe U, Herzig J W. Modification of single cardiac Na$^+$ channels by DPI 201–106. J Membr Biol 1986; 89:163–72.

66. Nilius B. Calcium block of guinea-pig heart sodium channels with and without modification by the piperazinylindole DPI 201–106. J Physiol (Lond) 1988; 399:537–58.

67. Scholtysik G, Salzmann R, Berthold R, Herzig J W, Quast U, Markstein R. DPI 201–106, a novel cardiotonic agent. Combination of cAMP-independent positive inotropic, negative chronotropic, action potential prolonging and coronary dilatory properties. Naunyn-Schmiedebergs Arch Pharmacol 1985; 329:316–25.

68. Hajjar R J, Gwathmey J K, Briggs G M, Morgan J P. Differential effects of DPI 201–106 on the sensitivity of the myofilaments to Ca^{2+} in intact and skinned trabeculae from control and myopathic human hearts. J Clin Invest 1988; 82:1578–84.

69. Kihara Y, Gwathmey J K, Grossman W, Morgan JP. Mechanisms of positive inotropic effects and delayed relaxation produced by DPI 201–106 in mammalian working myocardium: effects on intracellular calcium handling. Br J Pharmacol 1989; 96:927–39.

70. Siegl P K S, Garcia M L, King V F, Scott A L, Morgan G, Kaczorowski G J. Interactions of DPI 201–106, a novel cardiotonic agent, with cardiac calcium channels. Naunyn-Schmiedebergs Arch Pharmacol 1988; 338: 684–91.

71. Iijima T, Taira M. Membrane current changes responsible for the positive inotropic effect of OPC-8212, a new positive inotropic agent, in single ventricular cells of the guinea pig heart. J Pharmacol Exp Ther 1987; 240:657–62.

72. Iven H, Brasch H, Armah B I. Electrophysiological effects of saterinone and milrinone in the isolated guinea pig myocardium. Arzneimittelforsch 1988; 38:1298–302.

73. Rapundalo S T, Lathrop D A, Harrison S A, Beavo J A, Schwartz A. Cyclic AMP-dependent and cyclic AMP-independent actions of a novel cardiotonic agent, OPC-8212. Naunyn-Schmiedebergs Arch Pharmacol 1988; 338:692–8.

74. Hof R P, Rüegg U T, Hof A, Vogel A. Stereoselectivity at the calcium channel: opposite actions of the enantiomers of a 1,4-dihydropyridine. J Cardiovasc Pharmacol 1985; 7:689–93.

75. Kitakaze M, Weisman H F, Marban E. Contractile dysfunction and ATP depletion after transient calcium overload in perfused ferret hearts. Circulation 1988; 77:685–95.

76. Wetzel B, Hauel N. New cardiotonic agents—a promising approach for treatment of heart failure. Trends Pharmacol Sci 1988; 9:166–70.

77. Herzig J W, Feile K, Rüegg J C. Activating effects of AR-L 115 BS on the Ca^{2+} sensitive force, stiffness and unloaded shortening velocity (V_{max}) in isolated contractile structures from mammalian heart muscle. Arzneimittelforsch 1981; 31:188–91.

78. Solaro R J, Rüegg J C. Stimulation of Ca^{2+} binding and ATPase activity of dog cardiac myofibrils by AR-L 115 BS, a novel cardiotonic agent. Circ Res 1982; 51:290–4.

79. Fujino K, Sperelakis N, Solaro R J. Sensitization of dog and guinea pig heart myofilaments to Ca^{2+} activation and the inotropic effect of pimobendan: comparison with milrinone. Circ Res 1988; 63:911–22.

80. Salzmann R, Bormann G, Herzig J W, Markstein R, Scholtysik G. Pharmacological action of APP 201–553, a novel cardiotonic agent. J Cardiovasc Pharmacol 1985; 7:588–96.

81. Rüegg J C. Calcium in muscle activation. A comparative approach. Berlin: Springer, 1986.

82. Herzig J W. Contractile proteins: possible targets for drug action. Trends Pharmacol Sci 1984; 5:296–300.

83. Rüegg J C, Pfitzer G, Eubler D, Zeugner C. Effects on contractility of skinned fibres from mammalian heart and smooth muscle by a new benzimidazole derivative, 4,5-dihydro-6-[2-(4-methoxyphenyl)-1H-benzimidazole-5-yl]-5-methyl-3(2H)-pyridazinone. Arzneimittelforsch 1984; 34:1736–8.

84. Honerjäger P, Klockow M, Schönsteiner G, Jonas R. Imidazopyridines: roles of pyridine nitrogen position and methylsulfinyl oxygen for in vitro positive inotropic mechanism and chronotropic activity. J Cardiovasc Pharmacol 1989; 13:673–81.

85. Endoh M, Yanagisawa T, Morita T, Taira N. Differential effects of sulmazole (AR-L 115 BS) on contractile force and cyclic AMP levels in canine ventricular muscle: comparison with MDL 17,043. J Pharmacol Exp Ther 1985: 234:267–73.

86. Van Meel J C, Zimmermann R, Diederen W, Erdmann E, Mrwa U. Increase in calcium sensitivity of cardiac myofibrils contributes to the cardiotonic action of sulmazole. Biochem Pharmacol 1988; 37:213–20.

87. Fujino K, Sperelakis N, Solaro R J. Differential effects of d- and l-pimobendan on cardiac myofilament calcium sensitivity. J Pharmacol Exp Ther 1988; 247:519–23.

88. Kitada Y, Narimatsu A, Matsumara N, Endo M. Increase in Ca^{++} sensitivity of the contractile system by MCI-154, a novel cardiotonic agent, in chemically skinned fibers from the guinea pig papillary muscles. J Pharmacol Exp Ther 1987; 243:633–8.

89. Allen D G, Orchard C H. Myocardial contractile function during ischemia and hypoxia. Circ Res 1987; 60:153–68.

90. The CONSENSUS Trial Study Group. Effect of enalapril on mortality in severe congestive heart failure. Results of the cooperative north Scandinavian enalapril survival study (CONSENSUS). N Engl J Med 1987; 316:1429–35.

91. Guyatt G H. The treatment of heart failure. A methodological review of the literature. Drugs 1986; 32:538–68.

92. Smith T W. Digitalis: mechanism of action and clinical use. N Engl J Med 1988; 318:358–65.

93. Herzig S, Lüllmann H, Mohr K, Seemann B. Acrihellin, a cardioactive steroid escaping from the organ bath. Naunyn-Schmiedebergs Arch Pharmacol 1987; 335:326–30.

22

Characteristic Local Anesthetic Actions of Antiarrhythmic Drugs

Gary A. Gintant

Masonic Medical Research Laboratory
Utica, New York

INTRODUCTION

It is well known that many antiarrhythmic agents reduce the fast inward sodium current responsible for the action potential upstroke of most myocardial fibers. This local anesthetic effect, by affecting impulse propagation, likely contributes to the antiarrhythmic (and sometimes proarrhythmic) efficacy of many agents. Consequently it is essential to understand the functional characteristics of cardiac sodium channels, the consequences of interactions of local anesthetic-type antiarrhythmic drugs with these channels, how these interactions may be modulated by conditions within the myocardium, and the net effects on impulse conduction. It is the purpose of this review to briefly discuss the aforementioned topics, to provide a framework for understanding the contributions of local anesthetic effects in the actions of antiarrhythmic drugs. Although I limit most discussion to more recent work done on heart tissues, the reader should be aware of the guidance provided by earlier studies done with cardiac as well as nerve tissues.

TECHNIQUES USED TO ASSESS FAST SODIUM CURRENT AND LOCAL ANESTHETIC EFFECTS IN HEART TISSUES

Understanding the local anesthetic effects of drugs in the heart requires an appreciation of the limitations imposed by techniques employed to assess fast sodium current I_{Na}. I_{Na} has been assessed using at least three different techniques, including (1) indirect estimation from the maximum upstroke velocity ($\dot{V}_{max}$) of action potentials, (2) direct measurement of sodium current in multicellular and isolated cell preparations using voltage clamp techniques, and (3) recordings of single-channel currents using patch clamp techniques. All three approaches are unique with regard to the characteristics of the preparations and questions being posed [for a review and listing of selected early literature see Reference (1)].

In general, $\dot{V}_{max}$ studies with syncytial preparations are more likely to be done in (near) physiologic conditions with (it is hoped) minimal alterations in cellular metabolism. Voltage clamp techniques using syncytial

477

preparations require artificially shortened preparations (to reduce series resistance as well as current amplitude), cooling (to slow channel gating), altered extracellular (Na^+) ion concentrations (to minimize current), and pharmacologic blockers (to prevent contamination from other current systems) to obtain the voltage control necessary to directly measure I_{Na}. Patch clamp techniques provide the most detailed analysis of the kinetics of channel gating and drug-channel interactions, but the preparations and necessary experimental conditions (cell isolation with possible membrane alterations, intracellular dialysis-perfusion for whole-cell recordings, membrane "patch" isolation, current "rundown," and shifts in gating voltage dependence) may modify channel behavior as reflected in single-channel and whole-cell current recordings. For example, the sodium channel availability curve (h_∞) is shifted in a hyperpolarized direction following patching or cell break-in (2–5), and gating is affected (6). Ideally, all three approaches should be viewed in unison if we are to understand sodium channel behavior and drug-channel interactions. It should be noted, however, that impulse propagation involves the complex interplay of active and passive membrane properties [see, for example, the matrix approach (7,8)], and that the simplified waveforms used in voltage clamp experiments are not the complex upstrokes of propagating action potentials.

Until recently most studies assessed drug-channel interactions using changes in $\dot{V}_{max}$ to reflect changes in sodium current. The quantitative interpretation of these studies hinge upon the relationship between $\dot{V}_{max}$ and either I_{Na} or available sodium conductance g_{Na}. For a uniform "membrane" (i.e., nonpropagating) action potential, ionic current is proportional to the first derivative of the action potential. Hence peak I_{Na} should be equivalent to $\dot{V}_{max}$ when sodium current predominates. Computer simulations indicate that $\dot{V}_{max}$ should be a linear indicator of g_{Na} if (1) sodium current activation kinetics are rapid compared to inactivation kinetics, and (2) no appreciable interference from non-sodium currents is present (9,10). Experimentally the relation appears

curvilinear [with a 50% decrease in g_{Na} or I_{Na} producing a lesser decrease in $\dot{V}_{max}$ (11,12)], although the nonlinearity appears to decrease with warming from 8 to 27° C (13). This likely results from the different temperature dependencies of activation and inactivation, which at cooler temperatures allow greater channel mobilization with slower upstroke velocities. A decrease in $\dot{V}_{max}$ need not reflect a decrease in the "openness" of sodium channels. Indeed, simulations of sodium current using the Beeler-Reuter model (14) show that decreasing available sodium conductance (g_{Na}) by 50% reduces $\dot{V}_{max}$ appreciably while slightly increasing the product of $m^3 \times h$ (a measure of the "openness" of available channels) because channels open later in the upstroke (Khan and Gintant, unpublished).

Most experimental studies have assessed the $\dot{V}_{max}$ changes in propagating action potentials. The relation between $\dot{V}_{max}$ and g_{Na} (or I_{Na}) under these conditions (assuming constant conduction velocity) is unknown and is complicated by the fact that ionic current and capacitative current (from local circuit currents) both contribute to net membrane current and, further, that the capacitance filled may be frequency dependent. (Indeed, sodium current is just starting to activate when $\dot{V}_{max}$ occurs under conditions of uniform propagation.) In summary, although caution is necessary when interpreting $\dot{V}_{max}$ data, they still provide a convenient (although not necessarily quantitative) index of changes in I_{Na} under physiologic conditions.

CARDIAC SODIUM CHANNELS: BASIC FUNCTIONAL CHARACTERISTICS

Borrowing from the original investigations in nerve by Hodgkin and Huxley, it is useful to consider cardiac sodium channels in terms of three functional states: the resting state, the open (or activated) state, and the inactivated state. Transitions between these three states are thought to reflect conformational changes in the sodium channel structure, which by movement of portions known as "gates" act to open or close the channel pore, thereby allowing the net flow of ions according to their electrochemical gradient. At normally polarized membrane potentials most sodium channels are in the resting state and are available for opening upon depolarization. Upon depolarization the channels briefly open (activate), then quickly inactivate. Inactivation prevents any further flow of ions through the channels. Upon repolarization inactivated channels undergo reactivation, which leaves them in the resting state and available for the next depolarization-repolarization cycle. The three-state model, which forms the basis for most schemes of drug-receptor interactions (see Figure 2), is at present being refined using electrical as well as biochemical techniques. Indeed, multiple openings (reopening) of a channel may occur during a sustained depolarization (3). Further, the different channel states may have multiple substates (15), with different drug-receptor interactions possible. We consider only the three-state model in most discussions.

Early Studies of Sodium Channel Blockade In Vitro

It has been long appreciated that many antiarrhythmic agents affect impulse propagation within the heart and thereby affect cardiac electrical activity. It was not until the pioneering microelectrode studies by Draper and Weidmann, however, that propagation in the heart was firmly linked to inward sodium current (16) and, further, that antiarrhythmic drugs (quinidine and procainamide) slowed propagation by reducing I_{Na} as evidenced by a reduction in the maximum upstroke velocity and overshoot of the action potential (17). These results led Weidmann to comment on the role these agents played in decreasing the "safety factor" for impulse propagation, as well as changes in membrane excitability.

Subsequent work by Johnson and McKinnon (18) and Vaughan Williams (19) demonstrated that the local anesthetic effect of quinidine was modulated by stimulation rate, with a greater reduction in $\dot{V}_{max}$ observed with faster rates. Subsequently the terms "use-dependent" or "frequency-dependent block"

have been used to describe the drug-induced reduction of I_{Na} that is reversibly enhanced by rapid stimulation or activity. Use-dependent block is evident in vitro as a greater reduction of $\dot{V}_{max}$ or I_{Na} of drug-treated tissues when comparing rapid versus slow stimulation rates (Figure 1A). This contrasts with "tonic" or "resting block", terms used to describe the drug-induced reduction of I_{Na} remaining during very slow or infrequent stimulation. Tonic block is most easily represented by constructing "inactivation curves" (h_∞) or "sodium channel availability curves" (plotting resting membrane potential versus I_{Na} or $\dot{V}_{max}$ of upstrokes) at slow stimulation rates. Tonic block is typically manifest as a dose-dependent shift of the inactivation curve in a hyperpolarizing direction (Figure 1B), with in some cases, reduction in the maximum I_{Na}. Both terms (tonic and use-dependent block), borrowed from nerve studies, have been applied to all forms of sodium current measurements ($\dot{V}_{max}$ as well as macroscopic and microscopic recordings).

The reduction in fast inward current depends upon the extent of both tonic and use-dependent block, which vary with drug, drug concentration, experimental conditions, and electrical activity (see later).

Interactions of Local Anesthetic Agents with Cardiac Sodium Channels

Two models have been postulated to account for reduction in I_{Na} by local anesthetic types of antiarrhythmic agents. Both models presume that this effect results from drug binding to sodium channels, which prevents the increase in sodium permeability upon depolarization (i.e., blocks the channel). In particular, use-dependent block is thought to result from the accumulation of drug-associated, blocked (nonconducting) channels when the rate of drug association exceeds drug dissociation during periods of rapid stimulation.

The "modulated receptor hypothesis" postulated by Hille (20) and Hondeghem and Katzung (21) was based extensively upon previous work done in nerve and cardiac tis-

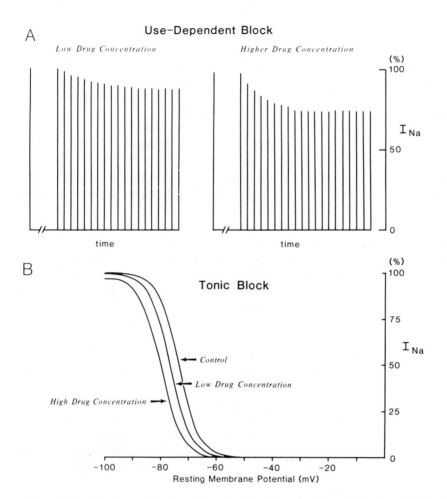

Figure 1 Stylized example of use-dependent block by a local anesthetic type of antiarrhythmic agent. (A, left). Following an abrupt increase in stimulation rate (time axis break), sodium current I_{Na} declines exponentially to a new steady-state value. More rapid stimulation would elicit a further reduction in I_{Na}, but slower stimulation would attenuate the effect. In a drug-free preparation little (if any) alteration in I_{Na} would be evident, unless stimulation was so rapid as to (1) impinge upon the relative refractory period of the tissue, or (2) cause slight depolarization of the resting potential. (Right). Increasing the drug concentration increases the extent of use-dependent block and shortens the time constant describing the approach toward a new steady-state value of I_{Na}. (B) Stylized example of tonic block by a local anesthetic type of antiarrhythmic agent. I_{Na} values were obtained at very slow stimulation rates at which no use-dependent block remains. Curves represent I_{Na} arising from different resting membrane potentials spanning the range of sodium channel inactivation (h_{∞} curve; see text). Sodium current decreases as resting membrane potential is reduced within the range of inactivation (control). Tonic block displaces the relationship in a hyperpolarized direction, which results in a greater depression of I_{Na} of depolarized fibers compared to normally polarized fibers (curve labeled low drug concentration). Displacement of the relationship is also concentration dependent, with greater drug concentrations affecting larger displacement. High drug concentrations may also reduce the maximum amplitude of sodium current (curve labeled high drug concentration).

sues (see also References 22 and 23 for reviews). According to this model there exists a single receptor in one of three different func-

tional (conformational) states (resting, open, or inactivated), with each state having a different affinity for drug [hence a modulated receptor; see Fig. 2 (left)]. For most drugs the affinity of the receptor of either open or inactivated channels in greater than the resting channel receptor. Once drug has bound to the receptor the channel is thought to be in a drug-blocked, nonconducting state, which is not available to conduct ions until drug has left the receptor site. Transitions between conformational states of drug-bound, blocked channels are permitted, although the voltage dependence of these transitions may be altered.

Extending the model to a physical representation, it was suggested that the receptor for local anesthetics was located within the lumen of the sodium channel, beyond the inactivation gating mechanism [see Fig.2(right)]. Drugs may gain access to the receptor via two pathways: a hydrophobic pathway, available for diffusion of drugs to the receptor via the membrane lipids, and a hydrophilic pathway, formed when the channel is open, allowing drug entry into the channel lumen from the cytoplasm (but see References 24 and 25 for different views). Direct drug access from the extracellular space is thought to be blocked by the selectivity filter at the mouth of the channel.

An alternative model, the "guarded receptor" hypothesis, has more recently been proposed by Starmer and colleagues to explain use-dependent block of sodium channels (26). In this model, drug access to the receptor is regulated (or guarded) by channel gates, with resting (closed) channels restricting drug access to the lumen receptor (and possibly trapping drugs inside drug-blocked channels). This model does not require (1) a variable-affinity receptor, or (2) modification of voltage-dependent gating of drug-bound channels, both requirements of the modulated receptor model. One of the strengths of the guarded receptor model is that the number of free variables required to characterize the channel-receptor interactions is reduced.

Both hypothesis will likely be refined as details of sodium channel gating and drug-channel interactions are revealed through the use of patch clamp techniques and single-channel recordings. In general, the macroscopic currents recorded from syncytial and whole-cell preparations reflect the sum of microscopic events at the single-channel level. These single-channel openings are generally described with such characteristics as the probability of channel opening p, the mean channel open time t_o, the time to first latency, and the single-channel conductance I. Alternative mechanisms for drug actions have been postulated based upon data provided at this increased resolution. For example, most studies assume that a lidocaine-bound channel cannot open [reflected in a reduction in p_o (27,28)]; others suggest that such a channel can still open, but with a reduced open time (29). Indeed, the latter study suggests that drugs bind not to the inactivated state of the channel but rather to a preopen channel state. The extent to which differences in species, experimental conditions, and statistical analysis may be responsible for disparate results is unknown. For example, voltage-dependent block of sodium current by lidocaine has been reported in guinea pig ventricular myocytes [whole-cell clamp (30), membrane patches, or fragments (13,29)] but not rabbit Purkinje fibers [two-electrode voltage clamp (31)]. It is comforting to note that nearly all studies report use-dependent block of sodium current by lidocaine.

DRUG CLASSIFICATION SCHEMES

Vaughan-Williams Subclassifications and Ramifications of Different Use-Dependent Block Kinetics

Differences in the local anesthetic effects of various drugs form the basis for a number of drug classification schemes. For example, the four-class classification scheme for antiarrhythmic agents proposed by Singh and Vaughan Williams (32) has been refined by subdividing the class 1 agents (those with prominent local anesthetic effects) into three subcategories (1a, 1b, and 1c), which correspond to the extent of $\dot{V}_{max}$ depression of normal, well-polarized tissues (see Reference 33). These categories generally follow differences in use-dependent block kinetics characterized by the time course of reduction (or recovery)

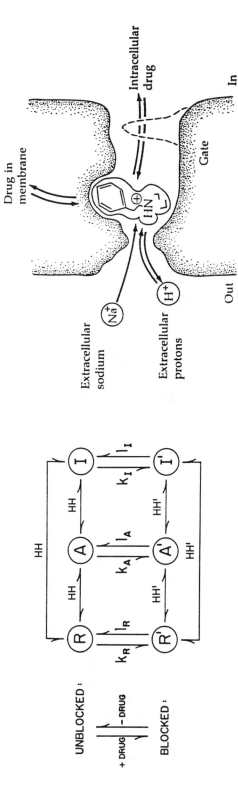

Figure 2 (Left) The modulated receptor hypothesis as a kinetic scheme. Channel blockade is attributed to drug association with a channel receptor that changes as the channel cycles through the resting (R), open (or activated A), and inactivated (I) states according to Hodgkin-Huxley (HH) kinetics. Drugs combine with receptor according to association (k) and dissociation (l) rate constants for the different conformations (i.e., different affinities). Drug-associated channels (denoted by prime symbols) may still undergo conformational changes, although the voltage dependence of these transitions (HH') may be altered. (From Reference 21 with permission of the American Heart Association, Inc.) (Right) Physical model of the modulated receptor hypothesis. A sodium channel with drug located within channel lumen. Drug may gain access to the intrachannel receptor site either via the hydrophilic pathway (formed when the gating structure allows channel opening) or via the hydrophobic pathway (via passage through the lipid membrane). Hydrogen ions may be able to exchange with intrachannel drug via passage through the channel selectivity filter. [From Hille (20), with permission.]

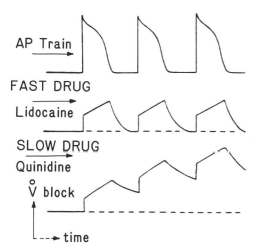

Figure 3 A model comparing use-dependent block with drugs demonstrating fast and slow unblocking kinetics. (Upper panel) The start of a rapid train of action potentials. (Middle panel) Alterations in the extent of channel blockade with lidocaine, a drug with fast unblocking kinetics. Blocked channels accumulate during the upstroke and plateau phases of the action potential but dissipate during diastole, resulting in no incremental block with successive action potentials. However, the excitability of premature beats and closely coupled extrasystoles are affected (not shown). (Lower Panel) For a drug with slow unblocking kinetics (such as quinidine), block accumulates with each successive action potential until a new steady-state value is achieved. (From Reference 46, with permission.)

of $\dot{V}_{max}$ following an abrupt increase (or decrease) in stimulation rate (see, for example, References 34–36). Drugs with fast kinetics of unblock (e.g., lidocaine, mexiletine, and tocainide) cause minimal reduction in $\dot{V}_{max}$ and conduction of normally polarized fibers (type 1b); drugs with intermediate kinetics (e.g., quinidine, procainamide, and disopyramide) causing moderate reductions in $\dot{V}_{max}$ and conduction (type 1a); and drugs with slow kinetics (e.g., flecainide, encainide, and lorcainide) cause marked reductions in $\dot{V}_{max}$ and conduction (type 1c). The correspondence between subdivisions and blocking kinetics is not entirely unexpected (see Figure 3). The rapidity with which use-dependent block develops following alterations in rate may

determine antiarrhythmic efficacy, as in the case of paroxysmal tachyarrhythmias.

Although this classification scheme is useful, its limitations have been recognized (i.e., not necessarily reflecting a drug's actions in depolarized, diseased, or pathologic fibers, different tissue types, or various action potential configurations). For example, for resting potentials near -75 mV, the rate of $\dot{V}_{max}$ recovery with tocainide (fast recovery kinetics) is slowed to that of a quinidine-treated fiber (slow recovery kinetics) at normal diastolic potentials (37).

Classification According to Different Affinities of Channel States

Antiarrhythmic drugs have also been categorized on the basis of their affinity for different states of the channel (i.e., a drug as either an activation, inactivated, or resting channel blocker) within the framework of the modulated receptor hypothesis. For example, a drug [such as amiodarone (38)] is called an inactivation blocker if more drug-induced depression of I_{Na} current occurs from (1) partially depolarized versus hyperpolarized conditioning potentials, (2) after the channels are held in the inactivated state for progressively longer times by depolarizing test pulses or longer action potentials, or (3) the drug causes a hyperpolarizing shift in the sodium channel "availability" or h_∞ curve. Alternatively, a drug [such as quinidine (21,39)] is considered an open channel blocker if depression occurs predominantly during the first few milliseconds of a depolarizing (activating) pulse or action potential upstroke. Some (most?) drugs may be both "inactivation" and "open" channel blockers. For example, two components of sodium channel block by lidocaine have been found, presumably corresponding to drug association to open and inactivated channels (30,31,40).

Complications arise when attempting to classify a drug's actions with this scheme. A drug's characteristics may change under different conditions. For example, an open channel blocker at normally polarized potentials may be considered a mixed open and inactivated channel blocker at partially depolarized potentials and predominantly an inactive channel blocker at more depolarized potentials (at which tonic block predominates). In addition, most class 1 agents are weak bases and thus exist in both charged and uncharged forms at physiologic pH. Alterations in pH may, by changing the proportion of charged to uncharged drug forms, alter the extent of different categories of block. Additional ambiguities are evident. Reduction in I_{Na} by quinidine is strongly voltage dependent, with more block occurring with longer and stronger depolarizations at potentials beyond which inactivation should be complete (102). Using the modulated receptor paradigm this voltage dependence does not appear to be simple binding to inactivated channels. Furthermore, some studies suggest that sodium channels kinetics are quite complex, in that some channels may reopen with sustained depolarization (3). If this is true, then sustained depolarization protocols used to characterize inactivation blockers reflect (re)open and inactivated channel block. To eliminate potential confusion resulting from model-dependent terms, I suggest the more descriptive term ''transient blocker'' be used for those drugs that require short (a few milliseconds) depolarizations to greatly reduce I_{Na} and ''sustained blocker'' for those drugs that cause a greater reduction in I_{Na} with prolonged depolarization in the plateau range of potentials. This categorization describes drug effects with minimal model dependence.

ONE OR MULTIPLE RECEPTOR SITES FOR LOCAL ANESTHETICS AND IMPLICATIONS FOR COMBINATION DRUG THERAPY

Most studies have suggested (or assumed) that drug binding to a single sodium channel receptor or receptor site can account for use-dependent block. Electrophysiologic studies have demonstrated stereospecific effects of quinidine and disopyramide on $\dot{V}_{max}$ measurements (42), consistent with the notion of a receptor site rather than a generalized membrane effect. Evidence also suggests that charged

and uncharged forms of local anesthetics both compete for the same receptor site (43). Other studies using radioligand assay techniques have characterized the binding of type I agents to isolated rat myocytes as saturable, reversible, and occurring at pharmacologically relevant concentrations with a similar ranked order of potency in vitro and in vivo (44), with possibly two stereospecific domains on the receptor (45). Despite this, however, the receptor site must be considered in rather loose terms, as it certainly does not have the specificity evident in other receptors (e.g., nicotinic cholinergeic receptor). Indeed, the drug-receptor interaction may depend more upon molecular weight, lipid solubility, size, or ionization potential imparted by the molecular structure (see References 46 and 47) and the biophysical nature of the membrane environment surrounding the channel (and acting as a ''filter'' for drugs via the hydrophobic pathway) rather than a specific binding site per se.

Different type 1 agents appear to compete for binding to the same receptor site, as demonstrated with lidocaine and either bupivacaine or quinidine (48). Indeed, the addition of lidocaine to a bupivacaine-treated fiber causes a net *increase* in $\dot{V}_{max}$. This effect may be explained in light of the faster recovery kinetics of lidocaine compared to those of bupivacaine. During rapid stimulation, lidocaine displaces bupivacaine from its binding site. During diastole more lidocaine-bound channels recover (due to faster unblocking kinetics) than do bupivacaine-bound channels, resulting in partial relief as seen with subsequent upstrokes. Similar arguments can explain the decreased amount of block observed under certain conditions when glycylxylidide (a deethylated metabolite of lidocaine in the human) is added to lidocaine-treated preparations (49). Of course, this explanation assumes each drug in the pair is equally efficacious in reducing sodium current (binding equivalent to full block of permeability changes), an assumption yet unproven. These results have potential clinical implications in treating drug toxicity.

The different blocking kinetics of drugs may provide a rational basis for combination drug therapy. Indeed, the modulated receptor hypothesis suggests that some drug pairs can enhance block of premature beats to an extent not possible with each individual drug (35). In addition, drug combinations may more specifically target regions of different electrical activity. For example, therapeutic concentrations of tocainide depress $\dot{V}_{max}$ and slow conduction (1) in normally polarized fibers only at rapid heart rates (use-dependent block), and (2) in more depolarized fibers at slower heart rates (tonic block). In contrast, depression of $\dot{V}_{max}$ and conduction by quinidine is mostly use dependent, with little additional tonic block. Thus the addition of tocainide to quinidine-treated fibers (1) causes greater depression of $\dot{V}_{max}$ of depolarized fibers with minimal alteration of $\dot{V}_{max}$ of normally polarized fibers, and (2) produces greater depression of $\dot{V}_{max}$ of early diastolic premature responses without much additional depression at longer coupling intervals (37). Results of this type may provide more selective antiarrhythmic activity through a combination of the different subclasses of type 1 drugs.

Despite these arguments, the possibility of multiple ''receptor'' sites on sodium channels need not be ruled out. For example, altering the shielding of fixed negative charges on the external surface of the membrane [for example, with reduced $[Ca]_o$ produces some effects similar to tonic block (5,17,50)]. Is it not possible that partitioning of local anesthetics in the membrane could lead to alterations in the charge sensed by voltage sensors on the channel, a generalized membrane effect? In canine Purkinje fibers the time course for equilibration of tonic block is much faster than that of use-dependent block measured during superfusion with the quaternary lidocaine analog QX-222 (52). This result is consistent with two different sites of channel interactions with this charged local anesthetic, one for tonic and one for use-dependent block. It should be noted that these results are not common to all local anesthetics, as tonic and use-dependent block with quinidine develop in parallel (Gintant and Goldenson, unpublished observations; see also Reference 53). In a study of propafenone and derivatives a differential time course for washout of tonic and use-dependent block was observed (54). Although other differences between tonic and use-dependent block were noted (most of which could be interpreted using the modulated receptor model), the differential time course for washout was not discussed.

More recently it was shown that use-dependent block predominates when the quaternary lidocaine analog QX-314 is applied to the cytoplasmic membrane surface. Tonic block predominates when the drug is applied to the outer membrane surface, suggesting a second local anesthetic binding site existing outside or near the outside of the sodium channel (55). Considering the complexity now apparent in sodium channel structure (56,57), with at least five known receptor sites for neurotoxins (58), and the influence of the lipid environment surrounding the channel (59), it is likely that different receptor sites (and drugs) will be found and exploited pharmacologically.

FACTORS MODULATING USE-DEPENDENT BLOCK

It is useful to consider those factors that modulate use-dependent block in terms of drug association and dissociation and the accumulation of blocked channels. If, for any given drug, drug concentration, and stimulation rate the dissociation rate is much greater than the association rate, little or no use-dependent block is evident. This likely explains the slight use-dependent block by a drug with fast recovery kinetics, such as lidocaine (40,41,60,61), and the prominent use-dependent block with quinidine [with slow recovery kinetics (62–64); see Figure 3].

Consider further that the drug with the faster dissociation rate has a recovery time constant comparable to the action potential duration. One would expect this drug to markedly prolong the effective refractory period (ERP) and effect excitability of premature stimuli, since channels are recovering during (and soon after) each repolarization. In contrast, the ''slower'' drug is still largely bound to channels throughout diastole, thereby minimally affecting the ERP. Indeed, at physiologic heart rates lidocaine depresses membrane responsiveness primarily during terminal repolarization, whereas quinidine appears to depress responsiveness more uniformly (65). Similar observations have been reported with other drugs (34). Combinations of kinetically different drugs may lead to more specific antiarrhythmic therapy (see *One or Multiple Receptor Sites*).

Drug concentration also modulates use-dependent block, with higher concentrations causing greater block as well as the more rapid exponential decline of sodium current when abruptly changing from a slow to a rapid stimulation rate (for example, References 36, 63, and 66). This effect is due to faster channel blockade, as recovery from block is independent of drug concentration (31, 65–67). Resting membrane potential also modulates use-dependent block. It seems that more use-dependent block is present with modest depolarization (that causing 50% inactivation of sodium channels), but with further depolarization tonic block predominates (35,66,68). Results obtained at modest depolarizations are likely predominated by a decreased rate of recovery from block at depolarized potentials (61,65,69). For open-channel blockers a slight depolarization may increase the number of open sodium channels affected by slower upstrokes (see References 10 and 13), allowing more drug binding per upstroke; stronger depolarization reduces sodium channel availability and prevents open-channel binding. For inactivation channel blockers one might expect a decreased rate of drug association due to the (expected) abbreviation of the action potential duration with modest depolarization (such as with elevated $[K^+]_o$).

pH has also been shown to modulate use-dependent block. Extracellular acidosis causes a further slowing of recovery kinetics of I_{Na} in the presence of lidocaine, but not quaternary analog (31,61). This result has been interpreted by assuming the importance of lipid solubility in the dissociation of the neutral drug form from the receptor. Increasing the ratio of protonated to neutral forms of a drug should affect the recovery kinetics of a lipid-soluble compound (which would normally leave the receptor quite readily) while minimally affecting the dissociation of a largely protonated drug. [Presumably extracellular H^+ ions exchange with the drug (while bound to the receptor) through the channel lumen; see Figure 2B.] Whatever the mechanism, slowing recovery with acidosis may account (in part) for the greater prolongation of the effective refractory period and decreased excitability in regions of myocardial ischemia (but not normal areas) seen with lidocaine (70,71). Acidosis may either enhance or have no effect on $\dot{V}_{max}$ during regular stimulation with either quinidine or lidocaine, depending upon the type of acidosis, preparation, pK_a of the drug, and pH-dependent changes in resting membrane potential (63,72). In these cases, when there is little effect, it is likely that slower recovery from block is offset by decreased channel block per action potential. It should also be noted that buffer and buffering capacity may also affect use-dependent block by affecting recovery kinetics (73,74).

Use-dependent block is also affected by age, although not necessarily for all drugs. Whereas the local anesthetic effects of lidocaine are greater in adult than in neonatal dogs (75), no such difference is found with quinidine (53) or quaternary drugs (76). The effects of various physicochemical properties on use-dependent block were mentioned previously (*One or Multiple Receptor Sites*) and beyond the scope of this review.

MANIFESTATIONS OF BLOCK OF FAST INWARD SODIUM CHANNELS

Most of the studies cited earlier discuss the effects of drugs on I_{Na}, but the clinical importance of their local anesthetic effects involve their modification of impulse propagation. In this regard the following brief discussions comment on the effects of altered I_{Na} on impulse propagation. A discussion of factors affecting discontinuous impulse propagation (i.e., block and reflection) may be found in Chapter 11. The reader is referred to recent reviews that discuss impulse conduction in relation to the genesis and control of arrhythmias (77–83).

Use-Dependent Reduction in Conduction Velocity

It is expected that significantly decreasing I_{Na} would decrease $\dot{V}_{max}$ and conduction velocity. One-dimensional cable theory predicts that $\dot{V}_{max}$ should be proportional to the square of conduction velocity (9,84). Such has been demonstrated in papillary muscle and Purkinje fiber preparations, considered to show one-dimensional propagation (85,86). Indeed, the quadratic relation between $\dot{V}_{max}$ and conduction velocity has been demonstrated with most interventions that reduce I_{Na}, including tetrodotoxin, low $[Na^+]_o$, and different concentrations of lidocaine and quinidine at different rates of stimulation (87,88). Subsequent studies have demonstrated that local anesthetic drugs produce use-dependent changes in conduction time *in vitro* or *in vivo* with kinetics generally comparable to those seen for $\dot{V}_{max}$ changes (88–94). In the human, drug-induced rate-dependent slowing of conduction has been noted (95,96). Of course, conduction in and around areas of ischemia and infarction is much more complex than those studied in the other models (for example, see Reference [97]), and the interplay of cellular geometry, use-dependent block, tonic block, and rate-dependent changes in excitability and conduction pathways must *all* be considered to fully appreciate the actions of local anesthetic types of antiarrhythmic agents.

Use-Dependent Alterations in the Direction of Propagation

Conduction velocity in cardiac muscle is also recognized as direction-dependent (86,98,99), likely resulting from the anatomic organization and the orientation of cell-cell couplings. This complexity leads to directionally dependent effects of antiarrhythmic drugs on conduction. Using an epicardial electrode array on an intact dog heart, Bajaj et al. (100) found that conduction in any direction was frequency independent under drug-free (baseline) conditions. Quinidine increased conduction times at all stimulation frequencies tested, without significant directionality (but see also Reference 93). In the presence of mexiletine, frequency-

dependent increases in conduction times were found at higher stimulation frequencies, and these increases were greater in directions where baseline conduction was most rapid. The directional dependence of these local anesthetic effects support other observations that the drug-induced depression of rapid, longitudinal conduction may be more easily modulated than slower, transverse conduction (93,94,101). This leads to the interesting possibility that the use-dependent blocking kinetics of a drug may act to change not only the speed but the direction of propagation, with implications in establishing or preventing unidirectional block and reentry in anisotropic medium. Clearly, the application of mapping techniques will provide additional possible mechanisms to explain the manifestations of local anesthetic actions.

CONCLUSION

Much is known about the interactions of local anesthetic types of antiarrhythmic agents with cardiac sodium channels and their effects on fast sodium current. Although not discussed here, one must appreciate that these drugs may also affect other current systems (including "slowly inactivating" sodium currents and other, nonsodium currents), as well as produce indirect effects (for example, altering I_{Na}), which may bear directly on their antiarrhythmic (or proarrhythmic) spectrum. The challenge for the research cardiologist is to understand the role of aberrant impulse propagation in the initiation and maintenance of different arrhythmias and to discern the contribution of sodium channel blockade (and resultant effects on conduction) to drug efficacy in the morphologically complex and dynamic setting of an injured or healing heart. This challenge is overshadowed by the benefits reaped from its accomplishment.

ACKNOWLEDGMENTS

Supported in part by Grant HL-37396 from the National Institutes of Health, National Heart, Lung and Blood Institute, and a Grant-in-Aid from the American Heart Association, New York State Affiliate, Syracuse, NY.

REFERENCES

1. Grant A O, Starmer C F, Strauss H C. Antiarrhythmic drug action: blockade of the inward sodium current. Circ Res 1984; 55(4):427–39.
2. Cachelin A B, DePeyer J E, Kokubun S, Reuter H. Sodium channels in cultured cardiac cells. J Physiol (Lond) 1983; 340:389–401.
3. Kunze D L, Lacerda A E, Wilson D L, Brown A M. Cardiac Na currents and the inactivating, reopening, and waiting properties of single cardiac Na channels. J Gen Physiol 1985; 86:691–719.
4. Makielski J C, Sheets M F, Hanck D A, January CT, Fozzard HA. Sodium current in voltage clamped internally perfused canine cardiac Purkinje cells. Biophys J 1987; 52:1–11.
5. Follmer C H, Ten Eick R E, Zeh Y Z. Sodium current kinetics in cat atrial myocytes. J Physiol (Lond) 1987; 384:169–97.
6. Kirsch G E, Brown A M. Kinetic properties of single sodium channels in rat heart and rat brain. J Gen Physiol 1989; 93:85–99.
7. Arnsdorf M F, Wasserstrom J A. Mechanisms of action of antiarrhythmic drugs: a matrical approach. In: Fozzard, HA, et al eds., The heart and cardiovascular system. New York: Raven Press, 1259–316.
8. Arnsdorf M F. Basic understanding of the electrophysiologic actions of antiarrhythmic drugs: sources, sinks, and matrices of information. Med Clin North Am 1984; 68:1247–880.
9. Hunter P J, McNaughton P A, Noble D. Analytical models of propagation in excitable cells. Prog Biophys Mol Biol 1975; 30:99–144.
10. Cohen I, Attwell D, Strichartz G. The dependence of the maximum rate of rise of the action potential upstroke on membrane properties. Proc R Soc Lond [Biol] 1981; 214:85–98.
11. Bean B P, Cohen C J, Tsien R W. Block of cardiac sodium channels by TTX and lidocaine: sodium current and $\dot{V}_{max}$ experiments. In: Conduction in the heart. Normal and abnormal. Paes de Carvalho A, Hoffman BF, M Lieberman, M, eds. Mount Kisco, NY: Futura Press; 1982: 198–209.

12. Cohen C J, Bean B P, Tsien R W. Maximal upstroke velocity ($\dot{V}_{max}$ as an index of available sodium conductance. Comparison of $\dot{V}_{max}$ and voltage clamp measurements of I_{Na} in rabbit Purkinje fibers. Circ Res 1984; 54:636–51.
13. Sheets M F, Hanck D A, Fozzard H A. Nonliner relation between $\dot{V}_{max}$ and I_{Na} in canine cardiac Purkinje cells. Circ Res 1988; 63:386–98.
14. Beeler G W, Reuter H. Reconstruction of the action potential of ventricular myocardial fibres. J Physiol (Lond) 1977; 268:177–210.
15. Grant A O, Starmer C F, Strauss H C. Unitary sodium channels in isolated cardiac myocytes of rabbit. Circ Res 1983; 53:823–9.
16. Draper M H, Weidmann S. Cardiac resting and action potentials recorded with an intracellular electrode. J Physiol (Lond) 1951; 115:74–94.
17. Weidmann S. Effects of calcium ions and local anesthetics on electrical properties of Purkinje Fibres. J Physiol (Lond) 1955; 129:568–82.
18. Johnson E A, McKinnon M C. The differential effect of quinidine and pyrilamine on the myocaridal action potentialat various rates of stimulation. J Pharmacol Exp Ther 1957; 120:460–8.
19. Vaughan Williams E M. The mode of action of quinidine on isolated rabbit atria interpreted from intracellular potential records. Br J Pharmacol 1958; 13:276–87.
20. Hille B. Local anesthetics: hydrophilic and hydrophobic pathways for the drug-receptor reaction. J Gen Physiol 1977; 69:497–515.
21. Hondeghem L M, Katzung B G. Time- and voltage-dependent interactions of antiarrhythmic drugs with cardiac sodium channels. Biochim Biophys Acta 1977; 472:373–98.
22. Hondeghem L M, Katzung B G. Antiarrhythmic agents: the modulated receptor mechanism of action of sodium and calcium channel-blocking drugs. Ann Rev Pharmacol Toxicol 1984; 24:387–423.
23. Hille B. Ionic channels of excitable membranes. Sunderland, MA: Sinauer, 1984.
24. Courtney K R. Why do some drugs preferentially block open sodium channels? J Mol Cell Cardiol 1988: 20:461–4.
25. Rhodes D G, Herbette L G. Discussion of "Why do some drugs preferentially block open sodium channels?": Consideration of

other significant factors in the binding process. J Mol Cell Cardiol 1988; 20:571–2.

26. Starmer C F, Grant A O, Strauss H C. Mechanisms of use-dependent block of sodium channels in excitable membranes by local anesthetics. Biophys J 1984; 46:15–27.

27. Reuter H, Cachelin A B, DePeyer J E, Kokubun S. Whole-cell Na current and single Na channel measurements in cultured cardiac cells. In: Zipes D P, Jalife J, eds. Cardiac electrophysiology and arrhythmias. New York: Grune and Stratton, 1985:13–17.

28. Nilius B, Benndorf K, Markwardt F. Effects of lidocaine on single cardiac sodium channels. J Mol Cell Cardiol 1987; 19:865–74.

29. McDonald T V, Courtney K R, Clusin W T. Use-dependent block of single sodium channels by lidocaine in guinea pig ventricular myocytes. Biophys J 1989; 55:1261–6.

30. Clarkson C W, Follmer C H, Ten Eick R E, Hondeghem L M, Yeh J Z. Evidence for two components of sodium channel block by lidocaine in isolated cardiac myocytes. Circ Res 1988; 63:869–78.

31. Bean B P, Cohen C J, Tsien R W. Lidocaine block of cardiac sodium channels. J Gen Physiol 1983; 81:613–42.

32. Singh B N, Vaughan Williams, E M. A fourth class of anti-dysrhythmic action? Effect of verapamil on ouabain toxicity, on atrial and ventricular intracellular potentials and on other features of cardiac function. Cardiovasc Res 1972; 6:109–19.

33. Vaughn Williams, E M. Subgroups of class 1 antiarrhythmic drugs. Eur Heart J 1984; 5:96–8.

34. Campbell T J. Kinetics of onset of rate-dependent effects of class I antiarrhythmic drugs are important in determining their effects on refractoriness in guinea-pig ventricle, and provide a theoretical basis for their subclassification. Cardiovasc Res 1983; 17:344–52.

35. Hondeghem L M, Katzung B G. Test of a model of antiarrhythmic drug action. Effects of quinidine and lidocaine on myocardial conduction. Circulation 1980; 61:1217–24.

36. Courtney K R. Interval-dependent effects of small antiarrhythmic drugs on excitability of guinea-pig myocardium. J Mol Cell Cardiol 1980; 12:1273–86.

37. Valois M, Sasyniuk B I. Modification of the frequency- and voltage-dependent effects of quinidine when administered in combination with tocainide in canine Purkinje fibers. Circulation 1987; 76(2):427–41.

38. Mason J W, Hondeghem L M, Katzung B G. Block of inactivated sodium channels and of depolarization-induced automaticity in guinea pig papillary muscle by amiodarone. Circ Res 1984; 55:277–85.

39. Colatsky T C. Quinidine block of cardiac sodium channels is rate- and voltage-dependent. Biophys J 1982; 37:343a.

40. Sanchez-Chapula J, Tsuda Y, Josephson I. Voltage- and use-dependent effects of lidocaine on sodium current in rat single ventricular cells. Circ Res 1983; 52:557–65.

41. Weld F M, Bigger J T Jr. Effect of lidocaine on the early inward transient current in sheep cardiac Purkinje fibers. Circ Res 1975; 37:630–9.

42. Mirro J M, Watanabe A M, Bailey J C. Electrophysiological effects of the optical isomers of disopyramide and quinidine in the dog. Dependence on stereochemistry. Circ Res 1981; 48:867–74.

43. Sanchez-Chapula J. Interaction of lidocaine and benzocaine in depressing $\dot{V}_{max}$ of ventricular action potentials. J Mol Cell Cardiol 1985; 17:495–503.

44. Sheldon R S, Cannon N J, Duff H J. Binding of [^{3}H] batrachotoxin A benzoate to specific sites on rat cardiac sodium channels. Mol Pharmacol 1986; 30:617–23.

45. Hill R J, Duff H J, Sheldon R S. Determinants of stereospecific binding of type I antiarrhythmic drugs to cardiac sodium channels. Mol Pharmacol 1989; 34:659–63.

46. Courtney K R. Review: quantitative structure/activity relations based on use-dependent block and repriming kinetics in myocardium. J Mol Cell Cardiol 1987; 19:319–30.

47. Follmer C H, Cullinan C A, Pirozzi C, Colatsky T J. Physico-chemical correlates of resting Na$^+$ block in cardiac myocytes studied in a series of benzene-sulfonamide analogues. J Mol Cell Cardiol 1989; 21(suppl. I):2–112.

48. Clarkson C W, Hondeghem L M. Evidence for a specific receptor site for lidocaine, quinidine, and bupivacaine associated with cardiac sodium channels in guinea pig ventricular myocardium. Circ Res 1985; 56:496–506.

49. Bennett P B, Woosley R L, Hondeghem L M. Competition between lidocaine and

one its metabolites, glycylxylidide, for cardiac sodium channels. Circulation 1988; 78:692–700.

50. Frankenhaeuser B, Hodgkin A L. The action of calcium on the electrical properties of squid axons. J Physiol (Lond) 137:218–24.

51. Pressler M L, Elharrar V, Bailey J C. Effects of extracellular calcium ions, verapamil, and lanthanum on active and passive properties of canine cardiac Purkinje fibers. Circ Res 1982; 51:637–51.

52. Gintant G A, Hoffman B F. The role of local anesthetic effects in the actions of antiarrhythmic drugs. In: Strichartz G R, ed. Handbook of experimental pharmacology, Vol. 81. 1987:213–52.

53. Morikawa Y, Rosen M R. Effects of quinidine on the transmembrane potentials of young and adult canine cardiac Purkinje fibers. J Pharmacol Exp Ther 1986; 236:832–7.

54. Kohlhardt M, Seifert C. Tonic and phasic I_{Na} blockade by antiarrhythmics. Different properties of drug binding to fast sodium channels as judged from $\dot{V}_{max}$ studies with propafenone and derivatives in mammalian ventricular myocardium (with appendix by Hondeghem LM). Pflugers Arch 1983; 396:199–209.

55. Alpert L A, Fozzard H A, Hanck D A, Makielski J C. Is there a second external lidocaine binding site on mammalian cardiac cells. Am J Physiol 1989; 26:H79–84.

56. Noda M, Ikeda T, Kayano T, Suzuki H, Takeshima H, Kurasaki M, Takahashi H, Numa S. Existence of distinct sodium channel messenger RNAs in rat brain. Nature 1986; 320:188–92.

57. Stuhmer W, Conti F, Suzuki H, Wang X, Noda M, Yahagi N, Kubo H, Numa S. Structural parts involved in activation and inactivation of the sodium channel. Nature 1989; 339:597–603.

58. Catterall W A. Structure and function of voltage-sensitive ion channels. Science 1988; 242:50–61.

59. Herbette L G, Vant Erve Y M H, Rhodes D G. Interaction of 1,4-dihydropyridine calcium channel antagonists with biological membranes: lipid bilayer partitioning could occur before drug binding to receptors. J Mol Cell Cardiol 1989;21: 187–201.

60. Davis L D, Temte J V. Electrophysiological actions of lidocaine on canine ventricular muscle and Purkinje fibers. Circ Res 1969; 24:639–55.

61. Grant A O, Strauss L J, Wallace A G, Strauss H C. The influence of pH on the electrophysiological effects of lidocaine in guinea pig ventricular myocardium. Circ Res 1980;47:542–50.

62. Heistracher P. Mechanism of action of antifibrillatory drugs. Naunyn-Schmiedebergs Arch Pharmacol 1971; 269:199–212.

63. Grant A O, Trantham J L, Brown K K, Strauss H C. pH-dependent effects of quinidine on the kinetics of dV/dt_{max} in guinea pig ventricular myocardium. Circ Res 1982; 50:210–217.

64. Weld F M, Coromilas J, Rottman J N, Bigger J T Jr. Mechanisms of quinidine-induced depression of maximum upstroke velocity in ovine cardiac Purkinje fibers. Circ Res 1982; 50:369–76.

65. Chen C-M, Gettes L S, Katzung B G. Effect of lidocaine and quinidine on steady-state characteristics and recovery kinetics of $(dV/dt)_{max}$ in guinea pig ventricular myocardium. Circ Res 1975; 37:20–29.

66. Gintant G A, Hoffman B F, Naylor R E. The influence of molecular form of local anesthetic-type antiarrhythmic agents on reduction of the maximum upstroke velocity of canine cardiac Purkinje fibers. Circ Res 1983; 52:735–46.

67. Sada H, Kojima M, Ban T. Effect of procainamide on transmembrane action potential in guinea pig papillary muscles as affected by external potassium concentration. Naunyn-Schmiedebergs Arch Pharmacol 1980; 309:179–90.

68. Lee K S, Hume J R, Giles W, Brown A M. Sodium current depression by lidocaine and quinidine in isolated ventricular cells. Nature 1981; 291:325–7.

69. Oshita S, Sada H, Kojima J, Ban T. Effects of tocainide and lidocaine on the transmembrane action potential as related to external potassium and calcium concentrations in guinea-pig papillary muscle. Naunyn-Schmiedebergs Arch Pharmacol 316:67–82.

70. Kupersmith J, Hoffman B F. In vivo electrophysiological effects of lidocaine in canine acute myocardial infarction. Circ Res 1975; 36:84–91.

71. Hondeghem L M. Effects of lidocaine, phenytoin, and quinidine on the ischemic canine mycoardum. J Electrocardiol 1976; 9:203–9.

72. Nattel S, Elharrar V, Zipes D P, Bailey J C. pH dependent electrophysiological effects of quinidine and lidocaine on canine cardiac Purkinje fibers. Circ Res 1981; 48:55–61.

73. Courtney K R. Significance of bicarbonate for antiarrhythmic drug action. J Mol Cell Cardiol 1981; 13:1031–4.

74. Stambler B S, Grant A O, Broughton A, Strauss H C. Influence of buffers on dV/dt_{max} recovery kinetics with lidocaine in myocardium. Am J Physiol 1985; 249:H663–71.

75. Morikawa Y, Rosen M R. Developmental changes in the effects of lidocaine on the electrophysiological properties of canine Purkinje fibers. Circ Res 1984; 55:633–41.

76. Spinelli W, Danilo P Jr, Rosen M R. Reduction of $\dot{V}_{max}$ by QX-314 and benzocaine in neonatal and adult canine cardiac Purkinje fibers. J Pharmacol Exp Ther 1988; 245:381–7.

77. Wit A L, Cranefield P F. Reentrant excitation as a cause of arrhythmias. Am J Physiol 1978; 235:H1–17.

78. Spear J F, Moore E N. Mechanisms of cardiac arrhythmias. Ann Rev Physiol 1982; 44:485–97.

79. Janse M J. Reentry rhythms. In: Fozzard H A, Haber E, Jennings R B, Katz A M, Morgan H E, eds. The heart and cardiovascular system. New York: Raven Press, 1986: 1203–38.

80. Antzelevitch, C. Reflection as a mechanism of reentrant cardiac arrhythmias. Prog Cardiol 1988; 1(1):3–16.

81. El-Sherif N. Reentry revisited. PACE 1988; 11:1358–68.

82. Lazzara R, Scherlag B J. Generation of arrhythmias in myocardial ischemia and infarction. Am J Cardiol 1988; 61:20A-26A.

83. Rosen M R. The links between basic and clinical cardiac electrophysiology. Circulation 1988; 77:251–63.

84. Walton M K, Fozzard H A. The conducted action potential: models and comparison to experiments. Biophys J 1983; 44:9–26.

85. Weidmann S. Electrical constants of trabecular muscle from mammalian heart. J Physiol (Lond) 1970; 210:1041–54.

86. Spach M S, Miller W T III, Geselowitz D B, Barr R C, Kootsey J M, Johnson E A. The discontinuous nature of propagation in normal canine cardiac muscle. Evidence for recurrent discontinuities of intracellular resistance that affect the membrane currents. Circ Res 1981; 48:39–54.

87. Buchanan J W Jr, Saito T, Gettes L S. The effects of antiarrhythmic drugs, stimulation frequency, and potassium-induced resting membrane potential changes on conduction velocity and dV/dt_{max} in guinea pig myocardium. Circ Res 1985; 56:696–703.

88. Nattel S. Relationship between use-dependent effects of antiarrhythmic drugs on conduction and $\dot{V}_{max}$ in canine cardiac Purkinje fibers. J Pharmacol Exp Ther 1987; 241:282–8.

89. Wallace A G, Cline R E, Sealey W C, Young W G Jr, Troyer W G Jr. Electrophysiologic effects of quinidine: studies using chronically implanted electrodes in awake dogs with and without cardiac denervation. Circ Res 1966; 19:960–969.

90. Davis J C, Matsubara T, Scheinman M M, Katzung B, Hondeghem L H. Use-dependent effects of lidocaine on conduction in the canine myocardium: application of the modulated receptor hypothesis in vivo. Circulation 1986; 74:205–14.

91. Nattel S. Frequency-dependent effects of amitriptyline on ventricular conduction and cardiac rhythm in dogs. Circulation 1985; 72:898–906.

92. Nattel S. Interval-dependent effects of lidocaine on conduction in canine cardiac Purkinje fibers: experimental observations and theoretical analysis. J Pharmacol Exp Ther 1981; 241:275–81.

93. Spach M S, Dolber P C, Heidlage J F, Kootsey J M, Johnson E A. Propagating depolarization in anisotropic human and canine cardiac muscle: apparent directional differences in membrane capacitance. Circ Res 1987; 60:206–19.

94. Anderson K P, Walker R, Dustman T, Lux R L, Ershler P R, Kates R E, Urie P M. Rate-related electrophysiologic effects of long-term administration of amiodarone on canine ventricular myocardium in vivo. Circulation 1989; 79:948–58.

95. Gang E S, Denton T A, Oseran D S, Mandel W J, Peter T. Rate-dependent effects of procainamide on His-Purkinje conduction in man. Am J Cardiol 1985; 55:1525–9.

96. Morady F, DiCarlo L A, Baerman J M, Krol R B. Rate-dependent effects of intravenous lidocaine, procainamide and amiodarone on intraventricular conduction. J Am Coll Cardiol 1985; 6:179–85.

97. Dillon S M, Allessie M A, Ursell P C, Wit A L. Influence of anisotropic tissue structure on reentrant circuits in the epicardial border zone of subacute canine infarcts. Circ Res 1988; 63:182–206.

98. Sano T, Takayama T, Shimamato T. Directional differences of conduction velocity in cardiac ventricular syncytium studied by microelectrodes. Circ Res 1959; 7:262–

99. Clerc L. Directional differences of impulse spread in trabecular muscle from mammalian heart. J Physiol (Lond) 1976; 255: 335–46.

100. Bajaj A K, Kopelman H A, Wikswo J P, Cassidy F, Woosley R L, Roden D M. Frequency- and orientation-dependent effects of mexiletine and quinidine on conduction in the intact dog heart. Circulation 1987; 75(5):1065–73.

101. Kadish A H, Spear J F, Levine J H, Moore E N. The effects of procainamide on conduction in anisotropic canine ventricular myocardium. Circulation 1986; 74(3):616–25.

102. Furukawa T, Tsujimura Y, Kitamura K, Tanaka H, Habuchi Y. Time- and voltage-dependent block of the delayed K^+ current by quinidine in rabbit sinoatrial and atrioventricular nodes. J Pharmacol Exp Ther 1989; 251:756–63.

23

Quinidine

Dan M. Roden

Vanderbilt University School of Medicine
Nashville, Tennessee

INTRODUCTION

References to the use of extracts of the anti-malarial plant cinchona in antiarrhythmic therapy are said to date back to the middle of the eighteenth century, when De Senac described its efficacy in cases of "rebellious palpitations" (1). Wenckebach (2) related that one of his patients, a Dutch merchant with paroxysmal atrial fibrillation "found that a gram of quinin regularly abolished his irregularity." Frey (3) evaluated the antiarrhythmic efficacy of a variety of cinchona extracts, and quinidine, the d-isomer of quinine, was reported to be the most effective in 1918. Quinidine remains the single most commonly prescribed sodium channel blocking antiarrhythmic in the United States, with quinidine preparations accounting for well over 30% of this market. However, despite the fact that this agent has been in widespread use for over seven decades, several important facets of its pharmacology have only come to light in the past 10 years or so; these include a potential for major drug interactions, a potent α-blocking action, and the mechanisms underlying both its beneficial as well as its detrimental electrophysiologic actions.

BASIC PHARMACOLOGY

> . . . certainly, it is not sufficient to say simply that quinin lengthens the refractory period of the heart.
>
> Wenckebach, 1923

In Vitro Actions

When the technique of recording transmembrane potential from cardiac cells became available in the 1950s, the electrophysiologic actions of quinidine were among the first to be investigated. Weidmann (4,5), Hoffman (6), and Vaughn Williams (7) all reported prototypical "quinidine-like" electrophysiologic changes in the late 1950s. Spontaneous automaticity in Purkinje fibers is slowed by quinidine, without major changes in take off potential or threshold (4–7). Early investigators (4,6,7) described increases in refractoriness in atrial or Purkinje tissue that persisted beyond full repolarization. Vaughn Williams (7) interpreted these findings as suggesting that "quinidine prolongs the effective refractory period by slowing the phase of depolarization, without any change necessarily occurring in half-time for repolarization . . . ".

On the other hand, West and Amory (8) found that quinidine prolonged atrial action potentials in a frequency-independent fashion while decreasing the rate of depolarization only at higher frequencies; they concluded that "the effect of quinidine on the depolarization process was secondary to its effect on the processes of repolarization and recovery." Further studies, outlined here, have clarified the actions of quinidine on atrial, ventricular, and Purkinje tissue: it is now apparent the quinidine both blocks the fast inward sodium current responsible for rapid depolarization in these tissues and delays repolarization to a variable extent, an effect likely due to block of cardiac potassium channel(s).

Actions on the Fast Sodium Current

Johnson and McKinnon (9) found that quinidine block of sodium current, manifest as depression of the maximum upstroke slope of phase 0 ($\dot{V}_{max}$), was more prominent at fast rates than at slow rates. Another major determinant of $\dot{V}_{max}$ depression by antiarrhythmic drugs is takeoff potential: for example, Chen et al. (10) reported that the time constants for recovery from frequency-dependent $\dot{V}_{max}$ depression by drugs were prolonged at depolarized potentials. These rate- and potential-dependent effects of quinidine in cardiac tissue, along with studies of the actions of other drugs in other preparations (11–13), such as squid giant axon, led to the formulation of the "modulated receptor" hypothesis of antiarrhythmic drug action in the late 1970s. Fundamentally, the modulated receptor formulation suggests that drugs bind to specific sites on ion channel proteins and that drug-associated channels do not conduct. Thus as ion channels move through different conformational states as a function of receptor occupancy, voltage, and so on, the affinity of the protein for drug alters; that is, receptor occupancy is modulated by channel state. Characterization of the kinetics of onset of and recovery from frequency-dependent block by quinidine and other sodium channel blockers has provided a convenient framework for classification of drug action (14); in such a

scheme quinidine is generally placed in the Ia subclass, along with procainamide and disopyramide (intermediate recovery kinetics; $\tau \simeq$ 3–10 sec at normal temperature and membrane potential). The modulated receptor hypothesis has been used to correlate the basic electrophysiologic actions of antiarrhythmic agents with their clinical effects. For example, the modulated receptor hypothesis predicts (15) substantially greater block of tachycardias or premature beats, with less depression of normal tissues, when quinidine is combined with lidocaine-like (class Ib; $\tau_{recovery} \simeq 100$–500 msec) properties, and a beneficial clinical effect of such combinations has been reported (16–19). Nattel et al. (20) and Grant et al. (21) have both shown that acidosis enhances the depression of $\dot{V}_{max}$ by quinidine; moreover, Grant et al. demonstrated that acidosis did not alter the time constant for onset of block but almost doubled the time constant for recovery and indicated that protonation could account for the quinidine plus acidosis effect. The modulated receptor hypothesis proposes voltage-dependent rate constants for drug association and disassociation from the channel in its various states, along with a voltage shift of approximately -40 mV for the Hodgkin-Huxley type of state transitions of quinidine-associated (13) states; others have generated data to suggest that the voltage shift may not be necessary to explain the effects of quinidine (22), although this now appears to be a minority view. Most recently, Snyders and Hondeghem (23) have provided evidence validating a major prediction of the modulated receptor hypothesis: after very strong hyperpolarizations, pulsing actually accelerated recovery from drug block. This "use-dependent unblocking" suggested drug dissociation from a channel in the open conformation and has been proposed as strong evidence against the "guarded receptor" hypothesis proposed by Starmer (24).

Action Potential Prolongation

The other major effect of quinidine is increased action potential duration in a variety of cardiac tissues. Mirro et al. (25) demonstrated that prolongation of action potentials in canine cardiac Purkinje tissue by quinidine could be blunted by pretreatment with isoproterenol plus acetylcholine, consistent with a substantial anticholinergic effect of quinidine. The same group also described stereoselective effects of quinidine: quinidine and quinine produced very similar effects on $\dot{V}_{max}$, but quinidine prolonged action potentials in canine cardiac Purkinje tissue and quinine shortened them (26). Viewed in the context of contemporary notions of drug-channel interactions, these data are compatible with a "specific" binding site for drugs on cardiac potassium channel(s).

The mechanism whereby quinidine prolongs action potential has been clarified with the application of voltage clamp techniques. Driot et al. (27) reported that in frog myocardium the delayed rectifier (I_k), an outward (repolarizing) potassium current activated at plateau potentials, was depressed by quinidine. Nawrath (28) found that quinidine depressed sodium, calcium, and potassium currents in guinea pig atrial and ventricular tissues, and the resultant effects on action potential configuration depended on the balance among these effects. Similar findings have been reported in rabbit atrioventricular (AV) node (29). Wong (30) reported that quinidine prolonged action potentials in *Myxicola* giant axons and attributed this effect to a reduction in potassium conductance(s); Colatsky, similarly, attributed increases in action potential duration in rabbit Purkinje tissue by quinidine to block of the delayed rectifier (31). Salata and Wasserstrom (32) found that quinidine depressed sodium current, calcium current, and steady-state outward current in canine ventricular myocytes. On the other hand, Hiraoka et al. (33) suggested that the major effect whereby quinidine prolongs action potentials in guinea pig ventricular myocytes was depression of I_K. We have similarly found that quinidine depresses I_K in disaggregated guinea pig ventricular myocytes and have developed evidence that a modulated receptor type of framework can be used to characterize drug block (34). The delayed rectifier

can be characterized as a series of closed conformational states connected in a catenary fashion to an open state (35,36); quinidine block of outward current was greatest when preparations were held at very negative potentials and was relieved by depolarization (37). Like Salata and Wasserstrom (32) and Hiraoka et al. (33) we have noted a minor effect of quinidine on the inward rectifier I_{K1}, a potassium current thought to contribute primarily to maintenance of the resting potential (38). In single-channel studies quinidine decreased I_{K1} by decreasing the probability of channel opening but mean open time and unitary current were unaltered (38); Sato et al. (39), on the other hand, have reported that the major effect of quinidine was reduction in the unitary current.

In single guinea pig atrial myocytes loaded with GTP, quinidine was a potent inhibitor of adenosine- and acetylcholine-induced potassium current (40). Moreover, in cells in which this potassium current was irreversibly activated by GTP-γS (likely through activation of G proteins), quinidine also suppressed potassium current. Thus in this preparation quinidine appears to inhibit the muscarinic potassium channel itself and/or the G proteins directly involved in its activation.

In addition to these effects on fast inward sodium and on repolarizing currents, quinidine alters other indices of cardiac electrophysiology. Quinidine inhibits isoproterenol-induced normal automaticity (41) as well as depolarization-induced automaticity (42) in guinea pig ventricular myocardium. In sheep Purkinje fibers Carmeliet and Saikawa (43) attributed the reduction in pacemaker current by lidocaine, quinidine, and procainamide to a reduction in the magnitude of the activation curve, with no change in the current's kinetics. Arnsdorf and Sawicki (44) separated the effects of quinidine on cardiac excitability in sheep Purkinje fibers into those related to depression of the sodium current, which were predictable based on the considerations already outlined, and quinidine's effects on passive properties. Interestingly, under normal conditions quinidine actually increased cardiac excitability assessed in this fashion, whereas with hyperkalemia the effect of the drug was less predictable and was based on the balance between these active and passive effects. Quinidine-induced changes in traditional action potential properties were readily reversed by washout, whereas the passive effects were not.

Finally, in canine cardiac Purkinje fibers driven slowly and exposed to lowered concentrations of potassium and/or magnesium, quinidine consistently induces marked abnormalities of terminal repolarization, early afterdepolarizations, and associated triggered activity (45–47). As discussed in further detail later, such triggered activity in association with early afterdepolarizations has been proposed as the major electrophysiologic mechanism underlying polymorphic ventricular tachycardia associated with markedly abnormal repolarization (torsades de pointes), a side effect of quinidine therapy seen in up to 5–10% of patients receiving the drug.

Actions in Syncytial Preparations

The in vivo effects of quinidine on sodium channel-dependent conduction and on repolarization are predictable based on its in vitro actions. Gettes et al. (48) found that quinidine widened the QRS interval (an index of conduction velocity) in isolated rabbit hearts perfused with quinidine; this effect was potentiated by an increase in extracellular potassium, presumably reflecting the dependence of quinidine-induced sodium channel block on membrane potential. Similarly, Hondeghem (49) observed that quinidine increased the threshold stimulation current more in ischemic (depolarized) tissues than in normal tissues. Wallace et al. (50) and Prinzmetal et al. (51) found that the most consistent effect of quinidine in the intact dog heart was slowing of intraventricular conduction; changes in refractoriness and action potential duration were less prominent. Duncan and Nash (52) found that quinidine did not alter threshold or excitability in atrium or ventricle, but it significantly prolonged atrial, AV nodal, and ventricular functional refractory periods and depressed ventricular conduction at therapeu-

tic concentrations in the open chest dog heart. We have documented that, as in experiments in vitro (53), conduction depression by quinidine in the intact dog heart is frequency dependent and that additive effects with mexiletine are seen at very rapid stimulation rates (54). Moreover, conduction depression was more prominent along rather than across cardiac fibers, reflecting the anisotropic nature of conduction in cardiac muscle. Finally, a number of investigators (6,55) have noted that quinidine can impair impulse transmission across ischemic gaps (55) or across the normal or abnormal Purkinje-ventricular muscle junction (6,56). These findings may be of particular relevance in quinidine's actions on reentrant circuits involving electrophysiologically abnormal tissue.

In isolated perfused rabbit hearts quinidine markedly prolonged AV conduction time, particularly in the presence of elevated extracellular potassium (57). Quinidine and high potassium increased action potential amplitude in the nodal and node-His regions of the AV node, and lowering potassium in the presence of quinidine shortened AV conduction by enhancing His-Purkinje-ventricular conduction. Thus the overall effects of quinidine on AV nodal transmission, even in the isolated perfused rabbit heart, vary as a function of the extracellular milieu (potassium); as described further later, quinidine's anticholinergic effect also plays a major role in modulating the net effect the drug produces on AV conduction in the human.

CLINICAL PHARMACOLOGY

Effects on the Normal Human Electrocardiogram

In keeping with its sodium channel blocking and repolarization delaying actions, quinidine alters both QRS and QT durations in the human. Heissenbuttel and Bigger (58) found a good correlation between plasma concentrations of quinidine and the extent of QRS prolongation. In keeping with the concepts of frequency dependence of drug block of cardiac sodium channels already outlined, Morady et al. (59) have reported that the extent of QRS prolongation produced by sodium channel blockers is greater at rapid pacing rates. The changes produced by quinidine on cardiac repolarization have been more difficult to quantify. This reflects the frequent observation that quinidine not only appears to prolong the QT interval to a variable extent, but also to alter the ST segment and to exaggerate the prominence of the U wave (60–64). In their study Heissenbuttel and Bigger (58) found that although QRS correlated well with plasma quinidine, changes in rate-corrected QT did not. Edwards and Hancock (65) similarly found a substantial variability in the relationship between plasma concentrations of quinidine and changes in rate-corrected QT among individuals. They also described the phenomenon of late-peaking QT changes following the administration of quinidine. The finding of such a lag between plasma drug concentrations and pharmacologic effects suggests either a distinct time-dependent myocardial uptake process or time-dependent generation of active metabolites (66); the role of active metabolites during quinidine therapy is discussed later. In dogs, quinidine is avidly taken up by myocardial tissue (67,68). As in the in vitro studies described, quinidine produces substantially more QT prolongation than does quinine (69–71). In some patients even "subtherapeutic" plasma concentrations of quinidine are associated with striking abnormalities of repolarization, including prolongation of the QT interval and very prominent U waves (72–79). Polymorphic ventricular tachycardia (torsades de pointes) is a real risk in such individuals; the underlying explanation for such striking individual sensitivity to low plasma concentrations of quinidine is not known.

Hemodynamic Effects of Quinidine

Intravenous injections of quinidine in dogs or humans results in profound hypotension (80–83). This effect is not a result of depression of cardiac contractility (84,85); rather, a peripheral vascular effect has been implicated in most studies. Secondary sympathetic activation (86) during vasodilation may contribute to the apparent lack of effect of quinidine on measures of left ventricular performance. In normal anesthetized dogs quinidine depressed left ventricular dP/dt to a greater extent than did quinidine + β-blockade (87). On the other hand, in conscious animals with left ventricular volume overload, β-adrenergic blockade appeared to unmask a subtle depression of left ventricular performance produced by intravenous quinidine (88).

Stimulation or block of α or β adrenergic receptors can modify the pharmacologic effects of quinidine (89). The mechanisms underlying these effects have not been completely worked out, although it is clear that quinidine is a competitive α_1- and α_2-receptor antagonist (90–95). In addition, quinidine exerts anticholinergic (vagolytic) actions, possibly by interacting with muscarinic receptors (96). These receptor interactions have clinical consequences. For example, profound hypotension has been reported in patients receiving chronic oral quinidine in whom intravenous verapamil was administered to control arrhythmias (97). As outlined later, quinidine's vagolytic effects may contribute to an increased ventricular response during atrial fibrillation as well as to sinus tachycardia (60,85,86,98). The most straightforward and elegant demonstration that quinidine does not directly depress left ventricular performance in the human was provided by Mason et al. (85), who documented that indices of left ventricular contractility in patients who had received cardiac transplants were unaltered; in their subjects the hemodynamic action of quinidine was most consistent with venodilation. Quinidine has not been evaluated as intensively as some of the newer agents, but congestive heart failure is unusual during chronic oral drug therapy (99), when reflex adrenergic changes are not as prominent as during intravenous drug administration. This may represent one of its major therapeutic advantages even as antiarrhythmic drug treatment enters the 1990s.

Electrophysiologic and Antiarrhythmic Actions of Quinidine in the Human

A number of investigators have demonstrated that single doses of intramuscular or intravenous quinidine produce changes consistent with both sodium channel block and action potential prolongation (100–105). These are manifest as increases in QRS and HV intervals and increases in QT, ventricular effective refractory period, and monophasic action potential, respectively. Changes in repolarization and refractoriness appear to be fairly uniform, suggesting that quinidine usually decreases the heterogeneity of repolarization (104). Intravenous quinidine routinely increases heart rate and shortens AV conduction time (AH interval), effects that are likely attributable to its vagolytic actions and/or sympathetic activation as a consequence of vasodilation; depression of AV conduction has been demonstrated in cardiac transplant recipients (106).

The success with which quinidine therapy controls arrhythmias is, like that of other drugs, a function of the arrhythmia being treated and the criteria with which efficacy are judged; moreover, underlying cardiovascular disease, in particular left ventricular performance, appears to be a major determinant of overall response (19). "Summarizing my own experience and the work done by others, I may say that quinidin has its greatest success in those cases in which there is not much wrong with the heart and in which fibrillation has been present for not too long a time. . . . " (Wenckebach, 1923). The single most common arrhythmia for which antiarrhythmic drugs are prescribed is still atrial fibrillation, and quinidine remains the standard therapy by which other drugs are evaluated. The major factors that appear to determine the outcome of antiarrhythmic therapy for the maintenance of sinus rhythm in patients with recurrent atrial fibrillation are chronicity of the arrhythmia and left atrial size (107,108), although many exceptions to these rough guidelines have been described. Digitalis alone has been reported to cause reversion of acute atrial fibrillation in approximately 50% of patients, no different from reversion rates in patients on placebo (109). Quinidine is somewhat more effective (perhaps 60–70% in trials in which it has been the standard to which newer agents have been compared), and quinidine may be more effective than some newer agents (e.g., flecainide) in patients with atrial fibrillation of greater than 10 days' duration (110–112). It

has been known since the 1920s that ventricular response during atrial fibrillation rises in patients treated with quinidine (60), an effect that, as already outlined, is likely attributable to sympathetic activation and/or the drug's vagolytic actions. The more dramatic clinical problem occurs in patients with atrial flutter in whom quinidine may produce marked incremental increases in ventricular response. The underlying mechanism is quinidine-induced slowing of atrial flutter rate, along with quinidine-induced enhancement of AV conduction. Specifically, an untreated patient may have atrial flutter, at a rate of 300 min^{-1}, with 2:1 AV block and a ventricular response of 150 min^{-1}; treatment with quinidine may slow the atrial flutter rate to 200 min^{-1} but produce 1:1 AV conduction, resulting in a ventricular response of 200 min^{-1}. The treatment for this predictable form of "arrhythmia exacerbation" is to avoid the use of quinidine therapy alone in patients with atrial fibrillation and, most importantly, in patients with atrial flutter unless an AV nodal blocking agent (digitalis, β-blocker, and verapamil) is also used.

Quinidine is also effective in patients with AV nodal reentrant and reciprocating tachycardias; this effect is attributable to depression of ventriculoatrial conduction, a function of the drug's direct rather than its vagolytic actions. (113,114). Interestingly, some of the desired effects of quinidine in patients with accessory AV pathways (Wolff-Parkinson-White syndrome), such as suppression of atrial fibrillation, increases in atrial and bypass tract refractoriness, and conduction slowing in the bypass tract, were partially reversed by epinephrine (114). Whether this reflects a direct antagonism by catecholamines of quinidine's electrophysiologic effects or merely an antagonistic effect of two pharmacologic agents acting at separate sites is unclear; nevertheless this finding suggests that adrenergic stimulation in some patients treated with quinidine may result in the recurrence of arrhythmia.

Quinidine is effective in suppressing chronic, non sustained ventricular arrhythmias. Efficacy rates are approximately 50–70% using 70–80% suppression of ventricular ectopic beat frequency as a criterion for efficacy (115–120). Morganroth and Hunter (121) demonstrated that this effect could be seen with a long-acting once-a-day preparation, a potential advantage for compliance. Whether suppression of ventricular ectopic beats results in decreased mortality following myocardial infarction is currently under intensive study. The class Ic (very long $\tau_{recovery}$ >10 sec) drugs encainide and flecainide resulted in increased postmyocardial infarction mortality despite suppressing non sustained ventricular arrhythmias in the Cardiac Arrhythmia Suppression Trial (CAST) (122). Whether suppression of ventricular ectopic beats by agents with different electrophysiologic characteristics, such as quinidine, might result in a decrease in postmyocardial infarction mortality is not established. In fact, a meta analysis of several series of patients receiving quinidine for atrial fibrillation suggested an increased risk of sudden cardiac death despite apparent arrhythmia control (123). Thus, as in all areas of therapeutics, the physician prescribing antiarrhythmic drugs, including quinidine, must ensure that the benefits of therapy clearly outweigh the risks. The risks of quinidine therapy are discussed later.

Intravenous quinidine in patients with inducible sustained ventricular tachyarrhythmias prevents arrhythmia induction in 40–80% of patients (102,103). Although hypotension is common with intravenous drug, more serious adverse effects, such as heart failure, are unusual. Duff et al. (103) have demonstrated that failure to respond to intravenous quinidine is an excellent predictor of a subsequent failure to respond to oral drug. DiMarco et al. (19) reported that oral quinidine was effective in 38 of 89 patients with inducible sustained ventricular tachycardia and that 32 of 38 of these patients were successfully managed for an average of 2 years with quinidine, alone or in combination with other antiarrhythmic agents.

Clinical Pharmacokinetics

The notion that interindividual variability in response to drugs could be explained in part by variability in drug disposition grew out of

the antimalarial program of World War II (124). Methods to extract and quantify drugs in samples of human blood or urine were then applied to other agents. Therapeutic monitoring of plasma concentrations of quinidine has been recognized as an effective method of reducing some toxicity since the early 1950s (125–127). Initial assay methodologies were not completely specific and included some metabolites (124–128). Thus the "therapeutic range" established by early workers as approximately 3–8 µg/ml has now been revised downward, to approximately 2–5 µg/ml. Despite the inaccuracies of early assay methodologies, good correlations were demonstrated (125,126) between plasma concentrations required for efficacy (generally conversion of atrial fibrillation to sinus rhythm) and plasma concentrations associated with toxicity, such as tinnitus, dizziness, and cinchonism. Establishment of a therapeutic range for a particular drug requires definition of a minimum concentration or range of concentrations likely to be associated with efficacy as well as a concentration or range of concentrations likely to be associated with toxicity. As described later, not all quinidine toxicity is dose related; moreover, at least some workers have described such substantial interindividual variability in minimal effective plasma concentrations that they have advocated omitting routine plasma concentration monitoring and substituting gradual dose escalation if arrhythmias are not controlled and side effects and ominous ECG changes, such as marked QRS or QT prolongations, are absent (117). Most evidence now suggests that arrhythmia control is unlikely to develop at concentrations under 2 µg/ml; an incremental antiarrhythmic response is unlikely at concentrations > 5µg/ml; moreover, at concentrations > 5 µg/ml, dose-related side effects increase in frequency. These concentrations are usually achieved by 800–1600 mg/day of quinidine sulfate or 1–2 g/day of quinidine gluconate in three or four divided doses. Overall, plasma concentration monitoring appears to be a useful adjunct to managing quinidine therapy, although it is no substitute for careful evaluation of the patient and their electrocardiogram during dose titration.

Initial assay methods used fluorometric techniques that were generally quite insensitive (124–128). A number of newer more specific methods, generally based on high-performance liquid chromatography (HPLC), have been described, as well as enzyme immunoassay methods (129–136). The latter may be somewhat less specific than HPLC-based methods (presumably because of cross-reactivity with metabolites), but Drayer et al. (132) proposed that immunoassay-based methods may actually provide better guides to therapeutic drug monitoring than more specific methods because metabolites may, as outlined later, contribute to some of the effects seen during quinidine therapy. As pointed out by Guentert et al. (137), the "therapeutic range" depends largely on the particular assay method used.

In normal volunteers Greenblatt et al. (138) reported that quinidine's elimination half-life was 7.3 ± 0.8 hr and its clearance 3.85 ± 33 ml/kg/min. They also showed that quinidine sulfate was rapidly absorbed with a mean systemic availability of 81%; quinidine gluconate was more slowly absorbed and was only 71% bioavailable. In addition, intramuscular quinidine was rapidly absorbed, painful, and substantially increased serum creatine kinase; therefore they (and most others) have recommended that this route of administration be avoided. Other groups (139–142) have reported similar findings in normal volunteers and in patients, although clearance has generally been found to be higher (4.7–4.9 ml/min/kg), a difference attributed to the lack of sensitivity of the assay used by Guentert et al. (140) Ueda et al. found that quinidine gluconate was 76 ± 11% bioavailable (139). The renal clearance of quinidine is 15–20% of total clearance (0.8–1 ml/kg/min) (141,142). Quinidine disposition appears to be well described by a two-compartment open model following intravenous administration and by two- or three-compartment models following oral administration (140). In patients the elimination half-life has been reported to be 6.3 ± 0.5 and 7.8 ± 0.7 hr (141,143). Kessler et al. reported grossly normal quinidine disposition in patients with congestive heart failure or poor renal function (143), although Conrad et al. (142) found generally higher steady-state plasma concentrations of quinidine in patients with congestive heart failure. A single case report suggests that quinidine and its metabolites are not substantially removed by peritoneal dialysis (144). Urinary alkalization resulted in a 10-fold reduction in the small fraction of quinidine cleared by the kidneys with attendant increases in plasma quinidine and QT intervals, although serum pH was unaltered (145).

Quinidine is 80–90% bound to plasma proteins, both albumin and α_1-acid glycoprotein (146,147). Fremstad et al. (146) showed a positive correlation between the unbound fraction of quinidine and total clearance. Heparin results in substantial increases in the free fraction of quinidine, both in vitro and in vivo (147,148); alteration in the effect of quinidine patients undergoing hemodialysis has been attributed to this mechanism (149). Variability in plasma protein binding can result in substantial changes in the free (pharmacologically active) fraction of quinidine and lead to erroneous management decisions if only total concentrations are considered (150). The free fraction of quinidine is known to fall in patients with recent myocardial infarction or cardiac arrest (151–153). The explanation is thought to relate to substantial increases in plasma α_1-acid glycoprotein, which is an acute-phase reactant. A relationship between free drug concentration and salivary drug concentration has been proposed for other agents, but salivary quinidine concentrations do not correlate well with quinidine effect (154).

The most widely used salts are quinidine sulfate or gluconate, and a number of long-acting quinidine formulations are available (155–160). These contain variable amounts of quinidine base and are generally effective when given once or twice daily (121). In patients in whom long-term arrhythmia control is sought, plasma concentration monitoring should establish the minimal plasma concentration obtained throughout 24 h of dosing; this trough concentration is generally well approximated by the predose value. Evaluations at a single point in time, such as exercise testing or electrophysiology study, should be conducted at the time of expected trough.

Quinidine undergoes oxidation by cytochrome P_{450} to the active metabolites 3-hydroxyquinidine, quinidine N-oxide, 2'-oxoquinidinone, and O-desmethylquinidine; glucuronide conjugates have also been described (161–164). Data in isolated perfused rat livers, as well as in healthy human volunteers, suggest that the rate at which these biotransformations proceed may vary as a function of dose; that is, some elimination pathways may be saturable (161,165,166). Drayer et al. (163) reported that the ratio of plasma 3-hydroxyquinidine to quinidine was >0.5 in 11 of 42 patients receiving chronic oral therapy. Moreover, the plasma protein binding of this metabolite is generally less extensive than that of quinidine; as a result the plasma concentrations of free 3-hydroxyquinidine actually exceeded those of the parent drug in 16% of their series and in 8 of 23 patients studied by Wooding-Scott et al. (167) and 4 of 38 patients reported by Thompson et al. (164) Bowers et al. (168) suggested that the accumulation of 3-hydroxyquinidine may account for the finding that quinidine-related torsades de pointes often occurs at low plasma quinidine concentrations. However, when the plasma concentrations of quinidine, its active metabolites 3-hydroxyquinidine, O-desmethylquinidine, quinidine N-oxide, and 2'-oxoquinidione and that of the commonly found commerical contaminant dihydroquinidine (169) were compared in 19 patients with quinidine-associated torsades de pointes to those observed in 38 patients tolerating quinidine therapy without toxicity, no differences in accumulation of total or free metabolite was observed (164). Moreover, in vitro studies demonstrated that quinidine and dihydroquinidine were roughly equally potent in depressing $\dot{V}_{max}$ and prolonging action potential duration, but the metabolites were somewhat less potent (170).

Drug Interactions

Quinidine-Induced Changes in the Disposition of Other drugs

Quinidine has been widely used for cardiac arrhythmias since the 1920s, and extracts of the foxglove have been used for over two centuries; the two are very commonly combined in the management of atrial fibrillation. As Wenckebach (2) put it, "Among the older generation of clinicians, there was a good number, and I knew some of them, who nearly always gave digitalis in combination with quinin. On being asked why they did it, they could not give me an exact reason for it." However, it was only in the late 1970s that a clinically significant interaction between digitalis and quinidine was first described (171–175). When quinidine therapy is added to therapeutic regimen of patients receiving chronic digoxin, serum digoxin concentrations rise by 0.5 ng/ml or more in about 90% of patients (176,177). The mechanism of this effect appears to be multifactorial, with inhibition of both renal and nonrenal digoxin clearance by quinidine, (175,178). In some studies elimination half-life was not altered despite decreased clearance; this finding indicates a change in digoxin distribution (175). In fact, it has been argued that although digoxin concentrations rise during coadministration of quinidine the cardiac effect of digoxin is not augmented and may, in fact, be blunted, leaving some to suggest that quinidine displaces digoxin from myocardial binding sites (179–183). Most evidence, however, now points to a substantially augmented myocardial digitalis effect, with an attendant increase in the likelihood of arrhythmias related to digitalis toxicity (184–191). Some have suggested that quinidine alters digitalis binding disproportionally in Purkinje tissue and have implicated this finding in arrhythmias seen with the combination (192). The time course of accumulation of digoxin following the initiation of quinidine therapy reflects the elimination half-life of digitalis; that is, the new steady-state is achieved in four to five digoxin elimination half-lives, or roughly 1 week (193–195). The extent of accumulation of digitalis appears to be a function of both the dose of quinidine and the serum digoxin concentration before the initiation of quinidine (193,196). As a rough rule of thumb, the daily administered dose of digoxin should be decreased by approximately 50% when quinidine therapy is initiated. In patients with chronic renal failure a similar increase in serum digoxin has been noted with the initiation of quinidine therapy (one piece of evidence to support the contention that this interaction is not exclusively at the renal level), and a similar recommendation for reduction of digoxin concentrations has been made (186). An initial report suggested that quinidine did not perturb the distribution of digitoxin (197), although when prolonged plasma concentration sampling is carried out an interaction of roughly the same magnitude as the quinidine-digoxin interaction is evident (198). Interestingly, quinine also increases serum digoxin concentrations, although the mechanism underlying this effect has not been as intensively evaluated as that for the quinidine-digoxin interaction (199).

Quinidine has recently been found to be an extremely potent inhibitor of a specific hepatic cytochrome, termed P_{450db1} (200,201). Quinidine is not a substrate for P_{450db1} (162,202); however, for drugs whose disposition depends largely on the presence of functionally active P_{450db1}, quinidine treatment at single doses as low as 50 mg may cause a substantial decrease in clearance and increases in plasma concentration of the second agent. The net result of this interaction depends on whether the effects of the agent metabolized by P_{450db1} are mediated by the parent drug or the metabolites. Substrates whose disposition is largely a function of the presence of a functional P_{450db1} include the antiarrhythmic agents propafenone and encainide, the β-blockers metoprolol and propranolol, and the antihypertensive debrisoquin (203,204). Inhibition of debrisoquin metabolism results in accumulation of parent drug and hypotension (205), and inhibition of metoprolol or propranolol metabolism by low-dose quinidine has resulted in substantially exaggerated heart rate slowing (206–208). A single case report found striking bradycardia when oral quinidine and ophthalmic timolol were combined (209) but no data on any dependence of timolol metabolism on P_{450db1} are available. The effects of propafenone and encainide therapy are mediated to a variable extent by the formation of active metabolites. In the case of propafenone, coadministration of quinidine resulted in a 2½-fold increase in steady-state propafenone concentrations with a corresponding decrease in concentrations of

the active metabolite 5-hydroxypropafenone (210). The extent of QRS prolongation induced by propafenone and the extent of arrhythmia control during propafenone therapy were unaltered, presumably because decreases in 5-hydroxypropafenone were offset by increases in propafenone. For encainide the situation is even more complicated since both encainide metabolism to the extremely potent sodium channel blocker O-desmethylencainide (ODE) and subsequent ODE metabolism to the less potent compund 3-methoxy-ODE (MODE) are mediated by P_{450db1} (204,211). Administration of low-dose quinidine to subjects receiving encainide results in complete inhibition of the ODE → MODE step and partial inhibition of the encainide → ODE step (212,213). The clinical consequences of the interaction therefore depend on the subject's response to the accumulation of encainide and, in some cases, ODE (212,214). The mean concentrations of the procainamide-like agent ajmaline, which is available in Europe, have been reported to rise dramatically (up to 30-fold) during coadministration of quinidine (215), suggesting that ajmaline disposition may be a function of the P_{450db1} phenotype.

The coadministration of quinidine with other agents with electrophysiologic properties, such as β-blockers, calcium channel blockers, or other subclasses of sodium channel blockers, may result in enhanced arrhythmia suppression. There is substantial evidence from theoretical (15), in vitro (15,216,217), and clinical (16–19) points of view that the combination of quinidine with agents with lidocaine-like electrophysiology results in enhanced suppression of early ventricular ectopic beats, marked prolongation of tachycardia cycle lengths and/or suppression of tachycardias, and blunting of potential electrophysiologic toxicity (early afterdepolarizations) produced by quinidine (216,217). Similarly, the combination of quinidine and β-blockers has long been known to provide enhanced efficacy when therapy with the single agents is ineffective in atrial fibrillation (218,219). This effect presumably reflects at least in part the pharmacokinetic ($P450_{db1}$) or the electrophysiologic (quinidine-adrenergic receptor) phenomena already outlined. As well, quinidine and calcium channel blockers may result in enhanced efficacy in atrial fibrillation (220). This effect may also have at least a partial pharmacokinetic basis, outlined later (221,222).

Conditions That May Perturb Disposition of Quinidine

As outlined earlier, renal disease and congestive heart failure do not appear to cause major changes in quinidine disposition (142,143). Food decreases the rate of quinidine absorption, although the extent of absorption is unchanged (223). Moreover, the administration of food results increases plasma binding proteins; as a result the appearance of unbound quinidine in plasma is substantially delayed by the coadministration of food, and side effects are decreased (224). Smoking does not appear to alter the disposition of quinidine (225). Verapamil decreases quinidine clearance (to 3-hydroxyquinidine) and increases quinidine elimination half-life, resulting in increased plasma concentrations of quinidine and increased drug effects during combination therapy (221,222). Conditions resulting in the altered plasma binding of quinidine have been described; e.g., quinidine binding is also decreased in cyanotic congenital heart disease (226).

Induction of hepatic mixed-function oxidase by rifampin, phenytoin, or barbiturates results in marked increase in quinidine clearance and shortened elimination half-life (134,227,228). Anecdotal data (227) attest to a loss of arrhythmia control with the institution of treatment of such hepatic enzyme inducers, providing further evidence that quinidine is more active than its metabolites in arrhythmia suppression. On the other hand, inhibition of hepatic mixed-function oxidase by cimetidine reduced quinidine oral clearance by about 40%, with a concomitant increase in elimination half-life (229). These increased concentrations resulted in increased QT prolongation in normal volunteers, suggesting that an exaggerated quinidine effect could be seen in patients. Cimetidine also decreased quinidine bioavailability, presumably reflecting a reduction in absorption or first-pass hepatic metabolism (230).

SIDE EFFECTS

The major factor limiting chronic quinidine therapy is diarrhea. This occurs in 25–50% of most trials of subacute and chronic oral therapy (112,115,118–121) and is not clearly related to dose or plasma concentration. Occasional patients can be managed by switching formulations or reducing the dose, but these strategies are generally depressingly ineffective. Interestingly, the incidence of diarrhea during therapy with quinidine plus mexiletine was substantially lower than the incidence during quinidine therapy alone (16). The mechanism underlying this effect (e.g., a concomitant constipating effect of mexiletine or a competitive effect on some gastrointestinal ion channel) is completely unknown. In some patients in whom alternative therapy is simply not available antidiarrheal agents, such as imodium, can be used.

Predictable dose- and concentration-related toxicity occurs during quinidine therapy (125–127). This is manifest as "cinchonism," a syndrome characterized by headache, dizziness, and tinnitus. Moreover, high plasma concentrations of quinidine are associated with marked QRS widening (i.e., conduction slowing, reflecting sodium channel block); this electrophysiologic effect has been associated with induction of ventricular tachycardia or coarse ventricular fibrillation (231–234). The infusion of sodium, as sodium lactate or sodium bicarbonate, acutely shortens the QRS in animal models (233) and patients (232). The mechanism underlying this effect is unknown, although changes in pH, osmolarity, or serum potassium do not appear to play a primary role.

The other major side effects observed during quinidine therapy are not dose related (235) and include immunologic reactions as well as induction of torsades de pointes. The former include immune thrombocytopenia (236) as well as the rare occurrence of hepatitis (237). Thrombocytopenia is a result of direct platelet injury by the combination of drug-dependent antibodies, drug (quinidine or quinine), and platelets and resolves rapidly on withdrawal of the offending agent. Bone marrow suppression is not a feature of this syndrome. Quinidine can also cause a lupuslike syndrome, although much less commonly than procainamide (238–240).

Torsades de pointes occurs in approximately 5% of patients receiving quinidine (72,241,242). About half the patients in most series receive the drug for ventricular arrhythmias and about half for management of atrial fibrillation or flutter (72,78,79,241,242). Typically, torsades de pointes develops within 2–3 days of initiation of quinidine therapy, although a minority of cases (approximately 20%) occur in patients receiving chronic quinidine therapy when other exacerbating factors, such as hypokalemia or bradycardia, develop. In patients treated with quinidine for atrial fibrillation torsades de pointes almost inevitably develops after conversion of the arrhythmia to a sinus mechanism, not while the patient is in atrial fibrillation (72). Exacerbating features include hypokalemia and hypomagnesemia (most often associated with diuretic therapy) and bradycardia. A stereotypical series of cycle length changes are almost invariably noted before the onset of a paroxysm: a premature beat or short episode of tachycardia is followed by an appropriate postectopic compensatory pause. The sinus beat that terminates this pause is then followed by markedly abnormal repolarization (marked prolonged QT interval or very prominent U wave), and the initial beat of torsades de pointes develops after the peak of the "late diastolic" wave (64,242). Plasma concentrations of quinidine with the development of torsades de pointes are generally in or in fact below the usual "therapeutic" range of concentrations (72–79), and as mentioned, unusual accumulation of quinidine metabolites or aberrant patterns of quinidine metabolism do not appear to explain this unusually marked sensitivity to the QT-prolonging effects of the drug at low plasma concentrations. Marked QRS widening indicative of excess sodium channel block is not a typical feature of quinidine-associated torsades de pointes, and the arrhythmia appears clinically and etiologically different from that associated with excess sodium channel block due to quinidine or other agents.

The most important factor in the management of quinidine-associated torsades de pointes is recognition of the syndrome based on the marked abnormality of the QT interval, the cycle length changes at onset, and the polymorphic nature of the ventricular tachycardia itself. It should be noted that, particularly over short periods of time and in a single ECG lead, the tachycardia may appear monomorphic. Moreover, drug-associated torsades de pointes may serve as a trigger for sustained monomorphic ventricular tachycardia or ventricular fibrillation in patients susceptible to these rhythms, although the most usual symptom is self-limited syncope. In most patients correction of hypokalemia and withdrawal of quinidine suffices for therapy. There is now ample evidence that intravenous magnesium (1 g over 20 min) is rarely deleterious and may, in fact, prevent further episodes, even in the absence of frank hypomagnesemia (243). Interestingly, the QT interval frequently does not shorten immediately following magnesium therapy, although the arrhythmia is controlled. If the arrhythmia is recurrent, maneuvers to increase the heart rate and shorten the QT interval are then required. These include infusion of isoproterenol in a dose sufficient to raise the ventricular rate to 100–120 beats/min or cardiac pacing. In general, atrial pacing suffices, although ventricular pacing is often preferred because of the stability of temporary lead placement and because of the uncertainty, in some cases, of the adequacy of AV transmission. Lidocaine and other standard antiarrhythmic drugs are generally ineffective; agents that also prolong the QT interval, such as procainamide, should be avoided. Direct current cardioversion is effective for non-self-terminating episodes. It is not known whether patients who develop quinidine-associated torsades de pointes and in whom a clear-cut exacerbating factor, such as marked hypokalemia, has been identified can subsequently receive quinidine safely (244). It seems reasonable to assume that such patients would be at risk again, particularly should an exacerbating factor redevelop; thus reinstitution of therapy with quinidine or any other agent that markedly prolongs the QT interval should be undertaken with caution, if at all. Because of the risk of torsades de pointes, some advocate that therapy with quinidine should only be initiated in inpatients whose cardiac rhythm is monitored.

The electrophysiologic mechanisms underlying the development of torsades de pointes have come under intense scrutiny in the last 5 years. Torsades de pointes has generally been ascribed to marked heterogeneity of repolarization (245–247). More recently it has been shown that quinidine produces very prominent early afterdepolarizations and triggered activity in Purkinje fibers superfused with low extracellular potassium and/or magnesium and driven at slow rates (45–47). The triggered activity seen in this in vitro setting arises during late repolarization, as does torsades de pointes. The parallels between these in vitro findings and the clinical observations have suggested that this form of triggered automaticity accounts for the development of torsades de pointes in patients. It is uncertain whether torsades de pointes arises in the Purkinje network and is then transmitted to ventricular muscle or whether early afterdepolarizations with triggered activity develop in muscle itself (248,249); moreover, the explanation for the polymorphic nature of the tachycardia and the reason that the tachycardia generally self-terminates remain elusive. Interventions that are effective in clinical torsades de pointes, such as raising heart rate, raising extracellular potassium, or adding magnesium, are also effective in reversing triggered activity of this type in vitro. Quinidine metabolites and dihydroquinidine can also produce early afterdepolarizations and triggered activity, but no more frequently than quinidine itself (170). Studies using the monophasic action potential recording technique have demonstrated early afterdepolarizationlike repolarization abnormalities in experimental torsades de pointes [e.g., induced by cesium injection (250,251)] as well as in a patient with the clinical arrhythmia (252).

PLACE OF QUINIDINE IN THERAPY

Despite the explosive increase in the availability of antiarrhythmic entities over the last 10 years, quinidine remains the most widely prescribed antiarrhythmic agent in the United States. Part of its popularity stems from its efficacy in both atrial and ventricular arrhythmias and part stems from familiarity with the drug. Intensive evaluation of the basic and clinical pharmacology of this very old drug has led to considerable advances in contemporary understanding of mechanisms of drug actions: the development of the concepts of state- and voltage-dependent block, the role of early afterdepolarizations in cardiac arrhythmias, and the interactions between quinidine and digitalis glycosides and between quinidine and P_{450db1} substrates are major examples of how continued evaluation of a "familiar" agent may yield striking new insights that are important for both basic understanding of physiologic processes as well as clinical care of patients. Other available drugs carry substantial drawbacks for chronic therapy in many patients: agents with class Ic properties have the CAST shadow; mexiletine and tocainide are not particularly effective as monotherapy and cause frequent side effects; procainamide causes lupus in a high percentage of patients during chronic therapy; disopyramide is associated with substantial risk of urinary retention or heart failure; and amiodarone causes a wide variety of organ toxic side effects during chronic therapy. Thus although quinidine therapy is fraught with difficulties, including a high incidence of dose-related and apparently "idiosyncratic" side effects, its efficacy, in particular its lack of clinically important cardiodepressant properties, has allowed it to retain its preeminence as one of the agents of choice for the chronic management of a wide variety of cardiac arrhythmias.

REFERENCES

1. Willius F A, Keys T E. A remarkably early reference to the use of cinchona in cardiac arrhythmias. Cardiac Clinics XCIV. Mayo Clin Staff Meetings 1942; (May 13):294–7.
2. Wenckebach K F. Cinchona derivates in the treatment of heart disorders. JAMA 1923; 81:472–4.
3. Frey W. Ueber vorhofflimmern beim menschen und seine beseitigung durch chinidin. Berl Klin Wochnschr 1918; 55:417–9.
4. Weidmann S. Effect of the cardiac membrane potential on the rapid availability of

the sodium-carrying system. J Physiol (Lond) 1955; 127:213–24.

5. Weidmann S. Effect of calcium ions and local anaesthetics on electrical properties of Purkinje fibers J Physiol (Lond) 1955; 129:568–82.

6. Hoffman B F. The action of quinidine and procaine amide on single fibers of dog ventricle and specialized conducting system. An Acad Brasil Ciencias 1957; 29:365–8.

7. Vaughn Williams E M. The mode of action of quinidine on isolated rabbit atria interpreted from intracellular potential records. Br J Pharmacol 1958; 13:276–87.

8. West T C, Amory D W. Single fiber recording of the effects of quinidine at atrial and pacemaker sites in the isolated right atrium of the rabbit. J Pharmacol Exp Ther 1960; 130:183–93.

9. Johnson E A, McKinnon M G. The differential effect of quinidine and pyrilamine on the myocardial action potential at various rates of stimulation. J Pharmacol Exp Ther 1956; 117:237–44.

10. Chen C-M, Gettes L S, Katzung B G. Effect of lidocaine and quinidine on steady-state characteristics and recovery kinetics of $(dV/dt)_{max}$ in guinea pig ventricular myocardium. Circ Res 1975; 37:20–9.

11. Armstrong C M. Inactivation of the potassium conductance and related phenomena caused by quaternary ammonium ion injection in squid axons. J Gen Physiol 1969; 54:553–75.

12. Hille B. Local anesthetics: hydrophilic and hydrophobic pathways for the drug-receptor reaction. J Gen Physiol 1977; 69:497–515.

13. Hondeghem L M. Katzung B G. Time- and voltage-interactions of antiarrhythmic drugs with cardiac sodium channels. Biochim Biophys Acta 1977; 472:373–98.

14. Campbell T J. Kinetics of onset of rate-dependent effects of class I antiarrhythmic drugs are important in determining their effects on refractoriness in guinea-pig ventricle, and provided a theoretical basis for their subclassification. Cardiovasc Res 1983; 17:344–52.

15. Hondeghem L, Katzung B. Test of a model of antiarrhythmic drug action: effects of quinidine and lidocaine on myocardial conduction. Circulation 1980; 61:1217–24.

16. Duff H J, Roden D M, Primm R K, Smith R F, Oates J A, Woosley R L. Mexiletine in

the treatment of resistant ventricular tachycardia: enhancement of efficacy and reduction of dose-related side effects by combination with quinidine. Circulation 1983; 67:1124–8.

17. Barbey J T, Thompson K A, Echt D S, Woosley R L, Roden D M. Tocainide plus quinidine for treatment of ventricular arrhythmias. Am J Cardiol 1988; 61:570–3.

18. Greenspan A M, Spielman S R, Webb C R, Sokoloff N M, Rae A P, Horowitz L N. Efficacy of combination therapy with mexiletine and a type Ia agent for inducible ventricular tachyarrhythmias secondary to coronary artery disease. Am J Cardiol 1985; 56:277–84.

19. Dimarco J P, Garan H, Ruskin J N. Quinidine for ventricular arrhythmias: value of electrophysiologic testing. Am J Cardiol 1983; 51:90–5.

20. Nattel S, Elharrar V, Zipes D P, Bailey J C. pH-dependent electrophysiological effects of quinidine and lidocaine on canine cardiac Purkinje fibers. Circ Res 1981; 48:55–61.

21. Grant A O, Trantham J L, Brown K K, Strauss H C. pH-dependent effects of quinidine on the kinetics of dV/dt_{max} in guinea pig ventricular myocardium. Circ Res 1982; 50:210–7.

22. Weld F M, Coromilas J, Rottman J M, Bigger J T Jr. Mechanisms of quinidine-indused depression of maximum upstroke velocity in ovine cardiac Purkinje fibers. Circ Res 1982; 50:369–76.

23. Snyders D J, Hondeghem L M. Use-dependent unblocking of quinidine-blocked sodium channels: slowed activation and inactivation 150. (abstract). Circulation 1987; 76(Suppl. IV): Full manuscript in press; Circ Res 1990.)

24. Starmer C F. Theoretical characterization of ion channel blockade. Biophys J 1987: 52:405–12.

25. Mirro M J, Watanabe A M, Bailey J C. Electrophysiological effects of disopyramide and quinidine on guinea pig atria and canine cardiac Purkinje fibers. Circ Res 1980; 46:660–8.

26. Mirro M J, Watanabe A M, Bailey J C. Electrophysiological effects of the optical isomers of disopyramide and quinidine in the dog: dependence on stereochemistry. Circ Res 1981; 48:867–74.

27. Driot P, Garnier D, Fessard M A. Analyse en courant et voltage imposé des propriétés

antiarythmiques de la quinidine appliqué de la grenouille. CR Acad Sci (Paris) 1972; 274:3421–4.

28. Nawrath H. Action potential, membrane currents and force of contraction in mammalian heart muscle fibers treated with quinidine. J Pharmacol Exp Ther 1981; 216:176–82.

29. Nishimura M, Huan R M, Habuchi Y, Tsuji Y, Nakanishi T, Watanabe Y. Membrane actions of quinidine sulfate in the rabbit atrioventricular node studied by voltage clamp method. J Pharmacol Exp Ther 1988; 244:780–8.

30. Wong B S. Quinidine interactions with myxicola giant axons. Mol Pharmacol 1981; 20:98–106.

31. Colatsky T J. Mechanisms of action of lidocaine and quinidine on action potential duration in rabbit cardiac Purkinje fibers: an effect on steady state sodium currents? Circ Res 1982; 50:17–27.

32. Salata J J, Wasserstrom A. Effects of quinidine on action potentials and ionic currents in isolated canine ventricular myocytes. Circ Res 1988; 62:324–37.

33. Hiraoka M, Sawada K, and Kawano S. Effects of quinidine on plateau currents of guinea-pig ventricular myocytes J Mol Cell Cardiol 1986; 18:10979–1106.

34. Roden D M, Bennett P B, Snyders D J, Balser J R, and Hondeghem L M. Quinidine delays I_K activation in guinea pig myocytes. Circ Res 1988; 62:1055–8.

35. Bennett P B, McKinney L C, Kass R S, Begenisich T. Delayed rectification in the calf cardiac Purkinje fiber: evidence for multiple state kinetics. Biophys J 1985; 48:553–67.

36. Gintant G A, Datyner N B, Cohen I S. Gating of delayed rectification in acutely isolated canine cardiac Purkinje myocytes: evidence for a single voltage-gated conductance. Biophys J 1985; 48:1059–64.

37. Balser J R, Hondeghem L M, Roden D M. Quinidine block of I_K accumulates at negative potentials. American Heart Association 60th Scientific Sessions Circulation 1987; 76:SIV–149.

38. Balser J B, Roden D M, Bennett P B. Quinidine preferentially suppresses a subconductance state of the inward rectifier. American Heart Association, 61st Scientific Session. Circulation 1988; 78:SII–411.

39. Sato R, Hisatome I, Wasserstrom J A, Singer D H. Quinidine blocks the inward-rectifier K+ channel (I_{K1}) from the inside of the membrane in guinea pig ventricular myocytes. Biophys J 1988; 53:642a.

40. Nakajima T, Kirachi Y, Ito H, Takikawa R, Sugimoto T. Anticholinergic effects of quinidine, disopyramide, and procainamide in isolated atrial myocytes: mediation by different molecular mechanisms. Circ Res 1989; 64:297–303.

41. Dangman K H. Effects of procainamide on automatic and triggered impulse imitation in isolated preparations of canine cardiac Purkinje fibers. J Cardiovas Pharmacol 1988; 12:78–87.

42. Grant A O, Katzung B G. The effects of quinidine and verapamil on electrically induced automaticity in the ventricular myocardium of guinea pig. J Pharmacol Exp Ther 1976; 196:407–19.

43. Carmeliet E, Saikawa T. Shortening of the action potential and reduction of pacemaker activity by lidocaine, quinidine, and procainamide in sheep cardiac Purkinje fibers: an effect on Na of K currents? Circ Res 1982; 50:257–72.

44. Arnsdorf M F, Sawicki G J. Effects of quinidine sulfate on the balance among active and passive cellular properties that comprise the electrophysiologic matrix and determine excitability in sheep Purkinje fibers. Circ Res 1987; 61:244–55.

45. Roden D M, Hoffman B F. Action potential prolongation and induction of abnormal automaticity by low quinidine concentrations in canine Purkinje fibers: relationship to potassium and cycle length. Circ Res 1985; 56:857–67.

46. Quantz N A, Nattel S. The ionic mechanism for quinidine-induced early afterdepolarizations. Circulation 1986; 74:SII–420.

47. Davidenko J M, Cohen L, Goodrow R, Antzelevitch C. Quinidine-induced action potential prolongation, early afterdepolarizations, and triggered activity in canine Purkinje fibers. Circulation 1989; 79:674–86.

48. Gettes L S, Surawicz B, Shiue J C. Effect of high K, low K, and quinidine on QRS duration and ventricular action potential. Am J Physiol 1962; 203:1135–40.

49. Hondeghem L M. Effects of lidocaine, phenytoin and quinidine on the ischemic canine myocardium. J Electrocardiol 1976; 9:203–9.

50. Wallace A G, Cline R E, Sealy W C, Young W G, Troyer W G Jr. Electrophysiologic

effects of quinidine: studies using chronically implanted electrodes in awake dogs with and without cardiac denervation. Circ Res 1966; 19:960–9.

51. Prinzmetal M, Ishikawa K, Oishi H, Ozkan E, Wakayama J, Baines J M. Effects of quinidine on electrical behavior in cardiac muscle. J Pharmacol Exp Ther 1967; 157: 659–64.

52. Duncan R J, Nash C B. Dose-response effects of quinidine on electrophysiological properties of the heart. Arch Int Pharmacodyn 1972; 199:358–67.

53. Packer D L, Grant A O, Strauss H C, Starmer C F. Characterization of concentration- and use-dependent effects of quinidine from conduction delay and declining conduction velocity in canine Purkinje fibers. J Clin Invest 1989; 83:2109–19.

54. Bajaj A K, Kopelman H A, Wikswo J R Jr, Woosley R L, Roden D M. Frequency- and orientation-dependent effects of mexiletine and quinidine on conduction in the intact dog heart. Circulation 1987; 75: 1065–73.

55. Shen X, Antzelevitch C. Mechanisms underlying the antiarrhythmic and arrhythmogenic actions of quinidine in a Purkinje fiber-ischemic gap preparation of reflected reentry. Circulation 1986; 73:1342–53.

56. Evans J J, Gilmour R F Jr, Zipes D P. The effects of lidocaine and quinidine on impulse propagation across the canine Purkinje-muscle junction during combined hyperkalemia, hypoxia and acidosis. Circ Res 1984; 455:185–96.

57. Watanabe Y, Dreifus L. Interactions of quinidine and potassium on atrioventricular transmission. Circ Res 1967; 20:434–46.

58. Heissenbuttel R H, Bigger J T Jr. The effect of oral quinidine on intraventricular conduction in man: correlation of plasma quinidine with changes in QRS duration. Am Heart J 1970; 80:453–62.

59. Morady F, DiCarlo L A Jr, Baerman J M, Krol R B. Rate-dependent effects of intravenous lidocaine, procainamide and amiodarone on intraventricular conduction. J Am Coll Cardiol 1985; 6:179–85.

60. Lewis T, Drury A N, Wedd A M, Iliescu C C. Observations upon the action of certain drugs upon fibrillation of the auricles. Heart 1922; 9:207–67.

61. Maher C C, Sullivan C P, Scheribel C P. The effect upon the electrocardiograms of pa-

tients with regular sinus mechanism of quinidin sulphate. Am J Med Sci 1934; 187:23–8.

62. Cheng T O, Sutton G C, Swisher W P, Sutton D C. Effect of quinidine on the ventricular complex of the electrocardiogram with special reference to the duration of the Q-T interval. Am Heart J 1956; 51:417–44.

63. Fieldman A, Beebe R D, Chow M S S. The effect of quinidine sulfate on QRS duration and QT and systolic time intervals in man. J Clin Pharmacol 1977; (Feb–March):134–9.

64. Jackman W M, Friday K J, Anderson J L, Aliot E M, Clark M, Lazzara R. The long QT syndromes: a critical review, new clinical observations and a unifying hypothesis. Prog Cardiovasc Dis 1988; 31:115–72.

65. Edwards I R, Hancock B W. Correlation between plasma quinidine and cardiac effect. Br J Clin Pharmacol 1974; 1:455–9.

66. Holford N H G, Coates P E, Guentert T W, Riegelman S, Sheiner L B. The effect of quinidine and its metabolites on the electrocardiogram and systolic time intervals: concentration—effect relationships Br J Clin Pharmacol 1981; 11:187–95.

67. Scherlis L, Gonzalez L F, Bessman S P. Quinidine: arterial, venous, coronary sinus and myocardial concentrations. J Pharmacol Exp Ther 1960; 60–5

68. Cho Y W. Quantitative correlation of plasma and myocardial quinidine concentrations with biochemical and electrocardiographic changes. Am Heart J 1973; 85:648–54.

69. Klevans L R, Kelly R J, Kovacs J L. Comparison of the antiarrhythmic activity of quinidine and quinine. Arch Int Pharmacodyn 1977; 227:57–68.

70. Phillips R E, Warrell D A, White N J, Looareesuwan S, Karbwang J. Intravenous quinidine for the treatment of severe falciparum malaria. N Engl J Med 1985; 312:1273–8.

71. White N J, Looareesuwan S, Warrell D A. Quinine and quinidine: a comparison of EKG effects during the treatment of malaria. J Cardiovasc Pharmacol 1983; 5:173–5.

72. Roden D M, Woosley R L, Primm R K. Incidence and clinical features of the quinidine-associated long QT syndrome: Implications for patient care. Am Heart J 1986;111:1088–93.

73. Selzer A, Wray H W. Quinidine syncope: paroxysmal ventricular fibrillation occurring

during treatment of chronic atrial arrhythmias. Circulation 1964; 30:17–26.

74. Jenzer H R, Hagemeijer F. Quinidine syncope: torsade de pointes with low quinidine plasma concentrations. Eur J Cardiol 1976; 4:447–51.

75. Koenig W, Schinz A M. Spontaneous ventricular flutter and fibrillation during quinidine medication. Am Heart J 1983; 105:863 5.

76. Seaton A. Quinidine-induced paroxysmal ventricular fibrillation treated with propranolol. Br Med J 1966; 1:1522–3.

77. Koster R W, Wellens H J J. Quinidine-induced ventricular flutter and fibrillation without digitalis therapy. Am J Cardiol 1976; 38:519–23.

78. Bauman J L, Bauernfeind R A, Hoff J V, Strasberg B, Swiryn S, Rosen K M. Torsades de pointes due to quinidine: observations in 31 patients. Am Heart J 1984; 107:425–30.

79. Kay G N, Plumb V J, Arciniegas J G, Henthorn R W, Waldo A L. Torsades de pointes: the long-short initiating sequence and other clinical features: observations in 32 patients. J Am Coll Cardiol 1983, 2: 806–17.

80. Lu G. The mechanism of the vasomotor action of quinidine. J Pharmacol Exp Ther 1951: 441–9.

81. Ferrier M I, Harvey R M, Werkö L, Dresdale D T, Cournand A, Richards D W Jr. Some effects of quinidine sulfate on the heart and circulation in man. Am Heart J 1947; 816–37.

82. Walsh R A, Horwitz L D. Adverse hemodynamic effects of intravenous disopyramide compared with quinidine in conscious dogs. Circulation 1979; 60:1053.

83. Ochs H R, Grube E, Greenblatt D J, Woo E, Bodem G. Intravenous quinidine: pharmacokinetic properties and effects on left ventricular performance in humans. Am Heart J 1980; 99:468–75.

84. Markiewicz W, Winkle R, Binetti G, Kernoff R, Harrison D C. Normal myocardial contractile state in the presence of quinidine. Circulation 1976; 53:101–6.

85. Mason J W, Winkle R A, Ingels N B, Daughters G T, Harrison D C, Stinson E B. Hemodynamic effects of intravenously administered quinidine on the transplanted human heart. Am J Cardiol 1977; 40:99–104.

86. Fenster P E, Dahl C, Marcus F I, Ewy G A. Effect of quinidine on the heart rate and blood pressure response to treadmill exercise. Am Heart J 1982; 104:1244–7.

87. Stern S. Hemodynamic changes following separate and combined administration of beta-blocking drugs and quinidine. Eur J Clin Invest 1971; 1:432–6.

88. Engler R L, Le Winter M M, Karliner J S. Depressant effects of quinidine gluconate on left ventricular function in conscious dogs with and without volume overload. Circulation 1979; 60:828.

89. Berger J E, Mokler C M. The interaction of quinidine with alpha and beta adrenergic receptors in the rat myocardium. J Pharmacol Exp Ther 1969; 165:242–50.

90. Roberts J, Stadter R P, Cairoli V, Modell W. Relationship between adrenergic activity and cardiac actions of quinidine. Circ Res 1962; 11:758–64.

91. Schmid P G, Nelson L D, Mark A L, Heistad DD, Abbound FM. Inhibition of adrenergic vasoconstriction by quinidine. J Pharmacol Exp Ther 1974; 188:124–34.

92. Caldwell R W, Elam J T, Mecca T E, Nash C B. Vascular α-adrenergic blocking properties of quinidine. Eur J Pharmacol 1983; 94:185–92.

93. Motulsky H J, Maisel A S, Snavely M D, Insel P A. Quinidine is a competitive antagonist at α_1- and α_2-adrenergic receptors. Circ Res 1984; 55:376–81.

94. Müller A, Noack E. Additive competitive interaction of verapamil and quinidine at alpha-adrenergic receptors of isolated cardiac guinea pig myocytes and human platelets. Life Sci 1988; 42:667–77.

95. Schipke J, Schulz R, Tölle T, Heusch G, Thämer V. Quinidine attenuates sympathetically induced poststenotic myocardial ischemia. J Cardiovasc Pharmacol 1987; 10:622–6.

96. Waelbroeck M, De Neef P, Robberecht P, Christophe J. Inhibitory effects of quinidine on rat heart muscarinic receptors. Life Sci 1984; 35:1069–76.

97. Maisel A S, Motulsky H J, Insel P A. Hypotension after quinidine plus verapamil. Possible additive competition at alpha-adrenergic receptors. N Engl J Med 1985; 17:167–70.

98. Chassaing C, Duchene-Marullaz P, Paire M. Mechanism of action of quinidine on heart

rate in the dog. J Pharmacol Exp Ther 1982; 222:688–93.

99. Smitherman T C, Gottlich C M, Narahara K A, Osborn R C, Platt M, Rude R E, Lipscomb K. Myocardial contractility in patients with ischemic heart disease during long-term administration of quinidine and procainamide. Chest 1979; 76:552–6.

100. Josephson M E, Seides S F, Batsford W P, Weisfogel G M, Akhtar M, Caracta A R, Lau S H, Damato A N. The electrophysiological effects of intramuscular quinidine on the atrioventricular conducting system in man. Am Heart J 1974; 87:55–64.

101. Hirschfeld D S, Ueda C T, Rowland M, Scheinman M M. Clinical and electrophysiological effects of intravenous quinidine in man. Br Heart J 1977; 39:309–16.

102. Swerdlow C D, Yu J O, Jacobson E, Mann S, Winkle R A, Griffin J C, Ross D L, Mason J W. Safety and efficacy of intravenous quinidine. Am J Med 1983; 75:36–42.

103. Duff H J, Wyse D G, Manyari D, Mitchell L B. Intravenous quinidine: relations among concentration, tachyarrhythmia suppression and electrophysiologic actions with inducible sustained ventricular tachycardia. Am J Cardiol 1985; 55:92–7.

104. Brugada J, Sassine A, Escande D, Masse C, Puech P. Effects of quinidine on ventricular repolarization. Eur Heart J 1987; 8:1340–5.

105. Torres V, Flowers D, Miura D, Somberg J. Intravenous quinidine by intermittent bolus for electrophysiologic studies in patients with ventricular tachycardia. Am Heart J 1984; 1437–42.

106. Mason J W, Winkle R A, Rider A K, Stinson E B, Harrison D C. The electrophysiologic effects of quinidine in the transplanted human heart. J Clin Invest 1977; 59:481–9.

107. Alpert J S, Petersen P, Goldtfredsen J. Atrial fibrillation: natural history, complications, and management. Annu Rev Med 1988; 39:41–52.

108. Brodsky M A, Allen B J, Capparelli E V, Luckett C R, Morton R, Henry W L. Factors determining maintenance of sinus rhythm after chronic atrial fibrillation with left atrial dilation. Am J Cardiol 1989; 63:1065–8.

109. Falk R H, Knowlton A A, Bernard S A, Gotlieb N E, Battinelli N J. Digoxin for converting recent-onset atrial fibrillation to sinus rhythm. Ann Intern Med 1987; 106: 503–6.

110. Hillestad L, Bjerkelund C, Maltau D J, Storstein O. Quinidine in maintenance of sinus rhythm after electroconversion of chronic atrial fibrillation: a controlled clinical study. Br Heart J 1971;33:518–21.

111. Sodermark T, Edhag O, Sjogren A, Jonsson B, Olsson A, Oro L, Danielsson M, Rosenhamer G, Wallin H. Effect of quinidine on maintaining sinus rhythm after conversion of atrial fibrillation or flutter: a multicentre study from Stockholm. Br Heart J 1975; 37: 486–92.

112. Borgeat A, Goy J J, Maendly R, Kaufmann U, Grbic M, Sigwart U. Flecainide versus quinidine for conversion of atrial fibrillation to sinus rhythm. Am J Cardiol 1986; 58: 496–8.

113. Wu D, Hung, J-S, Kuo C-T, Hsu K-S, Shieh W-B. Effects of quinidine on atrioventricular nodal reentrant paroxysmal tachycardia. Circulation 1981; 64:823.

114. Morady F, Kou W H, Kadish A H, Toivonen L K, Kushner J A, Schmaltz S. Effects of epinephrine in patients with an accessory atrioventricular connection treated with quinidine. Am J Cardiol 1988; 62:580–4.

115. Jones D T, Kostuk W J, Gunton R W. Prophylactic quinidine for the prevention of arrhythmias after acute myocardial infarction. Am J Cardiol 1974; 33:655.

116. Gaughan C E, Lown B, Lanigan J, Voukydis P, Besser H W. Acute oral testing for determining antiarrhythmic drug efficacy. Am J Cardiol 1976; 38:677–84.

117. Carliner N H, Fisher M L, Crouthamel W G, Narang P K, Plotnick G D. Relation of ventricular premature beat suppression to serum quinidine concentration determined by a new and specific assay. Am Heart J 1980; 100: 483–9.

118. Panidis I, Morganroth J. Short- and long-term therapeutic efficacy of quinidine sulfate for the treatment of chronic ventricular arrhythmias. J Clin Pharmacol 1982; 22:379–84.

119. Sami M, Harrison D C, Kraemer H, Houston N, Shimasaki C, DeBusk R F. Antiarrhythmic efficacy of encainide and quinidine: validation of a model for drug assessment. Am J Cardiol 1981; 48:147–55.

120. Flecainide-Quinidine Research Group. Flecainide versus quinidine for treatment of chronic ventricular arrhythmias. Circulation 1983; 67:1117–23.

121. Morganroth J, Hunter H. Comparative efficacy and safety of short-acting and sustained release quinidine in the treatment of patients with ventricular arrhythmias. Am Heart J 1985; 110:1176–80.

122. The CAST Investigators. Preliminary report: effect of encainide and flecainide on mortality in a randomized trial of arrhythmia suppression after myocardial infarction. N Engl J Med 1989; 321:406–12.

123. Coplen S E, Antman E M, Berlin J A, Hewitt P, Chalmers T C. Prevention of recurrent atrial fibrillation by quinidine: a metaanalysis of randomized trials. Circulation 1989; 80:SII–633.

124. Brodie B B, Udenfriend S. Estimation of quinine in human plasma, with note on estimation of quinidine. J Pharmacol Exp Ther 1943; 78:154.

125. Sokolow M, Edgar A L. Blood quinidine concentrations as a guide in the treatment of cardiac arrhythmias. Circulation 1950; 1: 576–91.

126. Kalmansohn R W, Sampson J J. Studies of plasma quinidine content. II. Relation to toxic manifestations and therapeutic effect. Circulation 1950; 1:569–75.

127. Sokolow M, Ball R E. Factors influencing conversion of chronic atrial fibrillation with special reference to serum quinidine concentration. Circulation 1956; 14:568–83.

128. Cramer G, Isaksson B. Quantitative determination of quinidine in plasma. Scand J Clin Lab Invest 1963; 15:553–6.

129. Crouthamel W G, Kowarski B, Narang P K. Specific serum quinidine assay by high-performance liquid chromatography. Clin Chem 1977; 23:2030–3.

130. Guentert T W, Coates P E, Upton R A, Combs D L, Riegelman S. Determination of quinidine and its major metabolites by high-performance liquid chromatography. J Chromatogr 1979; 162:59–70.

131. Dextraze, P G, Foreman J, Griffiths W C, Diamond I. Comparison of an enzyme immunoassay and a high performance liquid chromatographic method for quantitation of quinidine in serum. Clin Toxicol 1981; 18: 291–7.

132. Drayer D E, Lorenzo B, Reidenberg M M. Liquid chromatography and fluorescence spectroscopy compared with a homogeneous enzyme immunoassay technique for determining quinidine in serum. Clin Chem 1981; 27:308–10.

133. Patel C P. Liquid chromatological determination of quinidine in serum and urine. Ther Drug Monit 1982; 4:213–7.

134. Pershing L K. An HPLC method for the quantitation of quinidine and its metabolites in plasma: an application to a quinidine-phenytoin drug interaction study. J Anal Toxicol 1982; 6:153–6.

135. Vasiliades J, Finkel J M. Determination of quinidine in serum by spectrofluorometry, liquid chromatography and fluorescence scanning thin-layer chromatography. J Chromatogr 1983; 278:117–32.

136. Bottorff M B, Lalonde R L, Straughn A B. Comparison of high pressure liuid chromatography and fluorescence polarization immunoassay to assess quinidine pharmacokinetics. Biopharm Drug Dispos 1987; 8:213–21.

137. Guentert T W, Upton R A, Holford N H G, Riegelman S. Divergence in pharmacokinetic parameters of quinidine obtained by specific and nonspecific assay methods. J Pharmacokinet Biopharm 1979; 7:303–11.

138. Greenblatt D J, Pfeifer H J, Ochs H R, Franke K, MacLaughlin, D S, Smith T W, Koch-Weser J. Pharmacokinetics of quinidine in humans after intravenous, intramuscular and oral administration. J. Pharmacol Exp Ther 1977; 202:365–78.

139. Ueda C T, Williamson B J, Dzindzio B S. Absolute quinidine bioavailability. Clin Pharmacol Ther 1976; 20:260–5.

140. Guentert T W, Holford N H G, Coates P E, Upton R A, Riegelman S. Quinidine pharmacokinetics in man: choice of a disposition model and absolute bioavailability studies. J Pharmacokinet Biopharm 1979; 7:315–30.

141. Ueda C T, Hirschfeld D S, Scheinman, M M, Rowland M, Williamson B J, Dzindzio B S. Disposition kinetics of quinidine. Clin Pharmacol Ther 1975; 19:30–6.

142. Conrad K A, Molk B L, Chindsey C A. Pharmacokinetic studies of quinidine in patients with arrhythmias. Circulation 1977; 55:1–7.

143. Kessler K M, Lowenthal D T. Warner H, Gibson T, Briggs W, Reidenberg M M. Quinidine elimination in patients with congestive heart failure or poor renal function. N Engl J Med 1974; 290:706–9.

144. Hall K, Meatherall B, Krahn J, Penner B, Rabso J L. Clearance of quinidine during peritoneal dialysis. Am Heart J 1982; 646–7.

145. Gerhardt R E, Knouss R F, Thyrum P T, Luchi R J, Morris J J. Jr. Quinidine excretion
in aciduria and alkaluria. Ann Intern Med
1969; 71:927–33.
146. Femstad D, Nilsen O G, Storstein L, Amlie
J, Jacobsen S. Pharmacokinetics of quinidine
related to plasma protein binding in man.
Eur J Clin Pharmacol 1979; 15:187–92.
147. Guentert T W, Oie S. Factors influencing
the apparent protein binding of quinidine. J
Pharma Sci 1982; 71:325–8.
148. Kessler K M, Leech R C, Spann J F. Blood
collection techniques, heparin and quinidine
protein binding. Clin Pharmacol Ther 1979;
204.
149. Kessler K M, Perez G O. Decreased quinidine plasma protein binding during hemodialysis. Clin Pharmacol Ther 1981; 121.
150. Kessler K M, Wozniak P M, McAuliffe D,
Terracall E, Kozlovskis P, Mahmood I, Zaman L, Trohman R G, Castellanos A, Myerburg R J. The clinical implication of
changing unbound quinidine levels. Am
Heart J 1989; 118:63–9.
151. Kessler K M, Kissane B, Cassidy J, Pefkaros
K C, Kozlovskis P, Hamburg C, Myerburg
R J. Dynamic variability of binding of antiarrhythmic drugs during the evolution of
acute myocardial infarction. Circulation
1984; 70:472–8.
152. Kessler K M, Lisker B, Conde C, Silver J,
Ho-Tung P, Hamburg C. Abnormal quinidine
binding in survivors of prehospital cardiac
arrest. Am Heart J 1984; 107:665–9.
153. Garfinkel D, Mamelok R D, Blaschke T F.
Altered therapeutic range for quinidine after
myocardial infarction and cardiac surgery.
Ann Intern Med 1987; 107:48–50.
154. Narang P K, Carliner N H, Fisher M L,
Crouthamel W G. Quinidine saliva concentrations: absence of correlation with serum
concentrations at steady state. Clin Pharmacol Ther 1983; 34:695–702.
155. Henning R, Nyberg G. Serum quinidine levels after administration of three different
quinidine preparations. Eur J Clin Pharmacol
1973: 6: 239–44.
156. McGilveray I J, Midha K K, Rowe M, Beau-
doin N, Charette C. Bioavailability of 11
quinidine formulations and pharmacokinetic
variation in humans. J Pharma Sci 1981;
70:524–9.
157. Sawyer W T, Pulliam C C, Mattocks A, Foster J, Hadzija B W, Rosenthal H M. Bio-

availability of a commerical sustained
release quinidine tablet compared to oral
quinidine solution. Biopharm Drug Dispos
1982; 3: 301–10.
158. Leizorovicz A, Piolat C, Boissel J P, San-
chini B, Ferry S. Comparison of two long-
acting forms of quinidine. Br J Clin
Pharmacol 1984; 17:729–34.
159. Lehmann C R, Boran K J, Kruyer W B, Van
Reet R E, Scoville G S, Pierson W P, Melikian A P, Crowe J T, Wright G J. Comparison
of sustained-release quinidines given twice
daily to patients with ventricular ectopy. J
Clin Pharmacol 1986; 26:598–604.
160. Wright G J, Melikian A P, Pitts J E, Crowe
J T, Morley E M. Comparative quinidine
plasma profiles at steady state of two
controlled-release products and quinidine
sulfate in solution. Biopharm Drug Dispo
1987; 8:159–72.
161. Palmer K H, Martin B, Baggett B, Wall
M E. The metabolic fate of orally administered quinidine gluconate in humans. Biochem Pharmacol 1969; 18:1845–60.
162. Guengerich F P, Müller-Enoch Blair I A.
Oxidation of quinidine by human liver cytochrome P-450. Mol Pharmacol 1986; 30:
287–95.
163. Drayer D E, Hughes M, Lorenzo B, Reidenberg M M. Prevalence of high (3S)-
3-hydroxyquinidine/quinidine ratios in serum,
and clearance of quinidine in cardiac patients with age. Clin Pharmacol Ther 1980;
27:72–5.
164. Thompson K A, Murray J J, Blair I A,
Woosley R L, Roden D M. Plasma concentrations of quinidine, its major metabolites,
and dihydroquinidine in patients with torsades de pointes. Clin Pharmacol Ther 1988;
43:636–42.
165. Yu V C, Lamirande E D, Horning M G,
Pang K S. Dose-dependent kinetics of quinidine in the perfused rat liver preparation.
Drug Metab Dispos 1982; 10:568–72.
166. Russo J Jr, Russo M E, Smith R A, Pershing
L K. Assessment of quinidine gluconate for
nonlinear kinetics following chronic dosing.
J Clin Parmacol 1982; 22:264–70.
167. Wooding-Scott R A, Visco J, Slaughter R L.
Total and unbound concentrations of quinidine and 3-hydroxyquinidine at steady state.
Am Heart J 1987; 113:302–6.
168. Bowers L D, Nelson K M, Connor R, Lais
C J, Krauss E. Evidence Supporting 3(S)-3-

hydroxyquinidine-associated cardiotoxicity. Ther Drug Monit 1985; 7:308–12.

169. Scott C C, Anderson R C, Chen K K. Comparison of the pharmacologic action of quinidine and dihydroquinidine. J Pharmacol Exp Ther 1945; 84:184–8.

170. Thompson K A, Blair I A, Woosley R L, Roden D M. Comparative electrophysiologic effects of quinidine, its major metabolites and dihydroquinidine in canine cardiac Purkinje fibers. J Pharm Exp Ther 1987; 241:84–90.

171. Leahey E B Jr, Reiffel J A, Drusin R E, Heissenbuttel R H, Lovejoy W P, Bigger J T Jr. Interaction between digoxin, quinidine. JAMA 1978; 240:533–4.

172. Ejvinsson G. Effect of quinidine on plasma concentrations of digoxin. Br Med J 1978; 1:279–80.

173. Doering W, Konig E. Ansteig der digoxin konzentration im serum unter chinidin medikation. Med Clin 1978; 73:1085–8.

174. Doering W. Digoxin-quinidine interaction. N Engl J Med 1979; 301:400–5.

175. Hager W D, Fenster P, Mayersohn M, Perrier D, Graves P, Marcus F I, Goldman S. Digoxin-quinidine interaction N Engl J Med 1979; 300:1238–41.

176. Bigger J T Jr. The quinidine-digoxin interaction. Mod Concepts Cardiovas Dis 1982; 51:73–8.

177. Fichtl B, Doering W. The quinidine-digoxin interaction in perspective. Clin Pharmacokinet 1983; 8:137–54.

178. Angelin B, Arvidsson A, Dahlqvist R, Hedman A, Schenck-Gustafsson K. Quinidine reduces biliary clearance of digoxin in man. Eur J Clin Invest 1987; 17:262–5.

179. Schenck-Gustafsson K, Jogestrand T, Nordlander R, Dahlqvist R. Effect of quinidine on digoxin concentration in skeletal muscle and serum in patients with atrial fibrillation: evidence for reduced binding of digoxin in muscle. N Engl J Med 1981; 305:209–12.

180. Schenck-Gustafsson K, Jogestrand T, Brodin L-A, Nordlander R, Dahlqvist R. Cardiac effects of treatment with quinidine and digoxin, alone and in combination. Am J Cardiol 1983; 51:777–82.

181. Steiness E, Waldorff S, Hansen P B, Kjærgard H, Burch J, Egeblad H. Reduction of digoxin-induced inotropism during quinidine administration. Clin Pharmacol Ther 1980; 27:791.

182. Hirsh P D, Weiner H J, North R L. Further insights into digoxin-quinidine interaction: lack of correlation between serum digoxin concentration and inotropic state of the heart. Am J Cardiol 1980; 46:863.

183. Wilkerson R D, Beck B L. Increase in serum digoxin concentration produced by quinidine does not increase the potential for digoxin-induced ventricular arrhythmias in dogs. J Pharmacol Exp Ther 1987; 240:548–53.

184. Gold R L, Bren G B, Katz R J, Varghese P J, Ross A M. Independent and interactive effects of digoxin and quinidine on the atrial fibrillation threshold in dogs. J Am Coll Cardiol 1985; 6:119–23.

185. Warner N J, Barnard J T, Bigger J T Jr. Tissue digoxin concentrations and digoxin effect during the quinidine-digoxin interaction. J Am Coll Cardiol 1985; 5:680–6.

185. Warner N J, Leahey E B Jr, Hougen T J, Bigger J T Jr, Smith TW. Tissue digoxin concentrations during the quinidine-digoxin interaction. Am J Cardiol 1983; 51:1717–1921.

186. Fenster P E, Hager W D, Perrier D, Powell J R, Graves P E, Michael U F. Digoxin-quinidine interaction in patients with chronic renal failure. Circulation 1982; 66:1277.

187. Goldman S, Hager W D, Olajos M, Perrier D, Mayersohn M. Effect of the ouabain-quinidine interaction on left ventricular and left atrial function in conscious dogs. Circulation 1983; 67:1054.

188. Belz G G, Doering W, Aust P E, Heinz M, Matthews J, Schneider B. Quinidine-digoxin interaction: cardiac efficacy of elevated serum digoxin concentration. Clin Pharmacol Ther 1982; 31:548–54.

189. Leahey E B Jr, Reiffel J A, Heissenbuttel R H, Drusin R E, Lovejoy W P, Bigger J T Jr. Enhanced cardiac effect of digoxin during quinidine treatment. Arch Intern Med 1979; 139:519–21.

190. Williams J F Jr, Mathew B. Effect of quinidine on positive inotropic action of digoxin. Am J Cardiol 1981; 47:1052.

191. Thompson T J, Hanig J P. Quindine enhancement of digoxin toxicity in rats and minipigs. J Cardiovasc Pharmacol 1989; 13:204–9.

192. Somberg J C, Knox S M, Miura D S. Effect of quinidine on differing sensitivities of Purkinje fibers and myocardium to inhibition of monovalent cation transport by digitalis in dogs. Am J Cardiol 1983; 52:1123–6.

193. Leahey E B Jr, Bigger J T Jr, Butler V P Jr, Reiffel J A, O'Connell G C, Schaffidi L E, Rottman J N. Quinidine-digoxin interaction: time course and pharmacokinetics. Am J Cardiol 1981; 48:1141.

194. Kuhlmann J, Dohrmann M, Marcin S. Effects of quinidine on pharmacokinetics and pharmacodynamics of digitoxin achieving steady-state conditions. Clin Pharmacol Ther 1986; 39:288–94.

195. Kuhlmann J. Effects of quinidine, verapamil and nifedipine on the pharmacokinetics and pharmacodynamics of digitoxin during steady state conditions. Arzneimittel-forsch 1987; 37:545–8.

196. Friedman H S, Chen T-S. Use of control steady-state serum digoxin levels for predicting serum digoxin concentration after quinidine administration. Am Heart J 1982; 104:72–6.

197. Ochs H R, Pabst J, Greenblatt D J, Dengler H J. Noninteraction of digitoxin and quinidine. N Engl J Med 1980; 303:672–4.

198. Garty M, Sood P, Rollins D E. Digitoxin elimination reduced during quinidine therapy. Ann Intern Med 1981; 94:35–7.

199. Wandell M, Powell J R, Hager W D, Fenster P E, Graves P E, Conrad K A, Goldman S. Effect of quinine on digoxin kinetics. Clin Pharmacol Ther 1980; 28:425.

200. Otton S V, Inaba T, Kalow W. Competitive inhibition of sparteine oxidation in human liver by β-adrenoceptor antagonists and other cariovascular drugs. Life Sci 1984; 34:73–80.

201. Speirs C J, Murray S, Boobis A R, Seddon C E, Davies D S. Quinidine and the identification of drugs whose elimination is impaired in subjects classified as poor metabolizers of debrisoquine. Br J Clin Pharmacol 1986; 22:739–43.

202. Otton S V, Brinn R U, Gram L F. In vitro evidence against the oxidation of quinidine by the sparteine/debrisoquine monooxygenase of human liver. Drug Metab Dispos 1988; 16:15–7.

203. Eichelbaum M. Defective oxidation of drugs: pharmacokinetic and therapeutic implications. Clin Pharmacokinet 1982; 7:1–22.

204. Roden D M. Encainide and related antiarrhythmic drugs. ISI Atlas Sci 1988; 374–80.

205. Brosen K, Gram L F, Haghfelt T, Bertilsson L. Extensive metabolizers of debrisoquine become poor metabolizers during quinidine treatment. Pharmacol Toxicol 1987; 60: 312–4.

206. Lennard M S, Silas J H, Freestone S, Trevethick J. Br J Clin Pharmacol 1982; 14:301–3.

207. Zhou H H, Anthony L B, Roden D, Wood A J J: Cardiac interaction of propranolol and quinidine combination. Clin Res 1989; 37:342A.

208. Zhou H H, Anthony L B, Roden D, Wood A J J. Stereoselective alteration of propranolol disposition by quinidine. Clin Res 1989; 37:343A.

209. Dinai Y, Sharir M, Naveh N, Halkin H. Bradycardia induced by interaction between quinidine and ophthalmic timolol. Ann Intern Med 1985; 103:890–1.

210. Funck-Brentano C, Kroemer H K, Woosley R L, Roden D M. Genetically-determined interaction between propafenone and low dose quinidine: role of active metabolites in modulating net drug effect. Br J Clin Pharmacol 1989; 27:435–44.

211. Barbey J T, Thompson K A, Echt D S, Woosley R L, Roden D M. Antiarrhythmic activity, electrocardiographic effects and pharmacokinetics of the encainide metabolites O-desmethyl encainide and 3-methoxy-O-desmethyl encainide in man. Circulation 1988; 77:380–91.

212. Funck-Brentano C, Turgeon J, Woosley R L, Roden D M. Effect of low dose quinidine on encainide pharmacokinetics and pharmacodynamics: influence of genetic polymorphism. J Pharmacol Exp Ther 1989; 249: 134–42.

213. Turgeon J, Funck-Brentano C, Pavlou H, Woosley R L, Roden D M. Differential sensitivity of $P450_{db1}$ substrates to inhibition by quinidine in man. IV World conference on clinical pharmacology and therapeutics. Eur J Clin Pharmacol 1989; 36:A41.

214. Turgeon J, Pavlou H, Funck-Brentano C, Roden D M. Genetically-determined interaction of encainide and quinidine in patients with arrhythmias. Accepted for presentation, 62nd Annual Scientific Sessions, American Heart Association. Circulation 1989; 80:SII–326.

215. Hori R, Okumura K, Inui K-I, Yasuhara M, Yamada K, Sakurai T, Kawai C. Quinidine-induced rise in ajmaline plasma concentration. J Pharm Pharmacol 1984: 36:202–4.

216. Roden D M, Iansmith D H S, Woosley R L. Frequency-dependent interactions of mexilet-

ine and quinidine in canine cardiac Purkinje fibers. J Pharmacol Exp Ther 1987; 243:1218–24.

217. Valois M, Sasyniuk B I. Modification of the frequency- and voltage-dependent effects of quinindine when administered in combination with tocainide in canine Purkinje fibers. Circulation 1987; 76:427–41.

218. Dreifus L S, Lim H F, Watanabe Y, McKnight E, Frank M N. Propranolol and quinidine in the management of ventricular tachycardia. JAMA 1968; 204:190–1.

219. Stern S. Treatment and prevention of cardiac arrhythmias with propranolol and quinidine. Br Heart J 1971; 33:522–5.

220. Theisen K, Scheininger M. Electrophysiological effects of quinidine alone and of the combination quinidine-verapamil on AV conduction in humans. Clin Cardiol 1983; 6:405–11.

221. Trohman R G, Estes D M, Castellanos A, Palomo A R, Myerburg R J, Kessler K M. Increased quinidine plasma concentrations during administration of verapamil: a new quinidine-verapamil interaction. Am J Cardiol 1986; 57:706–7.

222. Edwards D J, Lavoie R, Beckman H, Blevins R, Rubenfire M. The effect of coadministration of verapamil on the pharmacokinetics and metabolism of quinidine. Clin Pharmacol Ther 1987; 41:68–73.

223. Ace L N, Jaffe J M, Kunka R L. Effect of food and an antacid on quinidine bioavailability. Biopharm Drug Dispos 1983; 4:183–90.

224. Woo E, Greenblatt D J. Effect of food on enteral absorption of quinidine. Clin Pharmacol Ther 1980; 27:188.

225. Edwards D J, Axelson J E, Visco J P, van Every S, Slaughter R L, Lalka D. Lack of effect of smoking on the metabolism and pharmcokinetics of quinidine in patients. Br J Clin Pharmacol 1987; 23:351–4.

226. Pickoff A S, Kessler K M, Wolff G S, Tamer D, Garcia O L, Gelband H. The effect of age and cyanosis on the protein binding of quinidine in the pediatric patient (abstract). Am J Cardiol 1981; 47:440.

227. Data J L, Wilkinson G R, Nies A S. Interaction of quinidine with anticonvulsant drugs. New Engl J Med 1976; 294:699–702.

228. Twum-Barima Y, Carruthers S G. Quinidine-rifampin interaction. N Engl J Med 1981; 304:1466–9.

229. Hardy B G, Zador I T, Golden L, Lalka D, Schentag J J. Effect of cimetidine on the pharmacokinetics and pharmacodynamics of quinidine. Am J Cardiol 1983; 52:172–5.

230. MacKichan J J, Boudoulas H, Schaal S F. Effect of cimetidine on quinidine bioavailability. Biopharm Drug Dispos 1989; 10:121–5.

231. Wetherbee D G, Holzman D, Brown M G. Ventricular tachycardia following the administration of quinidine. Am Heart J 1951; 89.

232. Wasserman F, Brodsky L, Dick M M, Kathe J H, Rodensky P L. Successful treatment of quinidine and procaine amide intoxication. Report of three cases. N. Engl J Med 1958; 259:797–802.

233. Cox A R, West T C. Sodium lactate reversal of quinidine effect studied in rabbit atria by the microelectrode technique. J Pharmacol Exp Ther 1961; 131:212–22.

234. Luchi R J, Helwig J Jr, Conn H L Jr. Quinidine toxicity and its treatment. Am Heart J 1963; 65:340–8.

235. Lyon A F, DeGraff A C. Antiarrhythmic drugs. Part III. Quinidine toxicity. Am Heart J 1965; 70:139–41.

236. Christie D J, Mullen P C, Aster R H. Fab-mediated binding of drug-dependent antibodies to platelets in quinidine- and quinine-induced thrombocytopenia. J Clin Invest 1985; 75:310–4.

237. Herman J E, Bassan H M. Liver injury due to quinidine. JAMA 1975; 234–310–1.

238. West S G, McMahon M, Portanova J P. Quinidine-induced lupus erythematosus. Ann Intern Med 1984; 100:840–2.

239. Bari-El Y, Shimoni Z, Flatau E. Quinidine-induced lupus erythematosus. Am Heart J 1986; 111:1209–10.

240. Cohen M G, Kevat S, Prowse M V, Ahern MJ. Two distinct quinidine-induced rheumatic syndromes. Ann Intern Med 1988; 108:369–71.

241. Radford M D, Evans D W. Long-term results of DC reversion of atrial fibrillation. Br Heart J 1968; 30:91–6.

242. Ejvinsson G, Orinius E. Prodromal ventricular premature beats preceded by a diastolic wave. Acta Med Scand 1980; 208:445–50.

243. Tzivoni D, Banai S, Schugar C, Benhorin J, Keren A, Gottlieb S, Stern S. Treatment of torsade de pointes with magnesium sulfate. Circulation 1988; 77:392–7.

244. Clark M, Friday K, Anderson J, Jackman W, Aliot E, Lazzara R. Drug induced torsades

de pointes: high concordance rate among type IA antiarrhythmic drugs and amiodarone. J Am Coll Cardiol 1985; 5:450.

245. Surawicz B, Knoebel SB. Long QT: good, bad or indifferent? J Am Coll Cardiol 1984; 4:398–413.

246. Kuo C S, Reddy C P, Munakata K, Surawicz B. Mechanism of ventricular arrhythmias caused by increased dispersion of repolarization. Eur Heart J 1985; 6:63–70.

247. Schwartz P J. Idiopathic long QT syndrome: progress and questions. Am Heart J 1985; 399–411.

248. El-Sherif N, Zeiler R H, Craelius W, Gough W B, Henkin R. QTU prolongation and polymorphic ventricular tachyarrhythmias due to bradycardia-dependent early afterdepolarizations. Circ Res August 1988;

249. Balser J R, Roden D M. Inhibitory effect of ventricular muscle on induction of early af-

terdepolarizations in canine false tendons. American Federation for Clinical Research, 1987. Clin Res 1987; 35:260A.

250. Brachmann J, Scherlag B J, Rosenshtraukh L V, Lazzara R. Bradycardia-dependent triggered activity: relevance to drug-induced multiform ventricular tachycardia. Circulation 1983; 68:846–56.

251. Levine J H, Spear J F, Guarnieri T, Weisfeldt M L, De Langen C D J, Becker L C, Moore E N. Cesium chloride-induced long QT syndrome: demonstration of afterdepolarizations and triggered activity in vivo. Circulation 1985; 72:1092–103.

252. El-Sherif N, Bekheit S S, Henkin R. Quinidine-induced long QTU interval and torsade de pointes: role of bradycardia-dependent early afterdepolarizations. J Am Coll Cardiol 1989; 14:252–7.

24

Procainamide

Elsa-Grace V. Giardina

College of Physicians and Surgeons, Columbia University
New York, New York

HISTORY

The development of procainamide, an analog of procaine hydrochloride, the local anesthetic, was initiated following the observation that procaine hydrochloride administered intravenously exerts an antiarrhythmic action on the heart (1). Stimulatory effects on the central nervous system and rapid inactivation by hydrolysis to *p*-aminobenzoic acid and diethylaminoethanol, however, limited the applicability of procaine as an antiarrhythmic agent. In the late 1940s a series of derivates of diethylaminoethanol were synthesized in the expectation that activity of the alcohol could be enhanced without a comparable increase in toxicity. The most promising compound of the series was the amide analog of procaine. Since 1951, when introduced clinically (2), procainamide has been used for the treatment of supraventricular and ventricular arrhythmias in millions of patients.

BASIC PHARMACOLOGY: ELECTROPHYSIOLOGIC EFFECTS ON ISOLATED CARDIAC TISSUES

The electrophysiologic effects of procainamide have been studied extensively by standard microelectrode techniques on atria, atrioventricular (AV) nodal, normal and ischemic Purkinje fibers, normal and ischemic ventricular muscle, and areas of myocardial infarction in numerous animal species (3–17). Several reports use drug concentrations considerably higher than those expected to be therapeutic in humans, that is, 30–200 mg/L (3–12); others have studied concentrations ranging from 5–10 mg/L (13,16), approximating the therapeutic plasma concentration range. Variability in drug effect dependent on tissue type, tissue state, and drug concentration is underscored by these studies. Procainamide, like other drugs with a local anesthetic action, depresses the responsiveness of cardiac cells (3–17). Procainamide's effects are concentration dependent: in atrial, ventricular, and His-Purkinje fiber it decreases the $(dV/dt)_{max}$ (3,5,8) in a rate-dependent manner, slows conduction velocity (1,3), prolongs the effective refractory period and action potential duration (4–6,8), and shifts the membrane responsiveness curve down and to the right (Table 1) (6). In therapeutic concentrations, it does not affect the resting or maximum diastolic potential of normal cardiac fibers, but at high concentrations it decreases these. The decrease in

Table 1 Electrophysiologic and Electrocardiographic Effects of Procainamide and N-Acetylprocainamide[a]

Effect	Procainamide	N-acetyl procainamide
Electrophysiologic (Purkinje fiber)		
Normal automaticity	↓	NC
Membrane responsiveness	↓	NC
Action potential duration	↑	↑
Effective refractory period	↑	NC/↑
Conduction velocity	↓	NC
Afterdepolarizations	NC	↑
Electrophysiologic intervals		
SCL	±	±
SNRT	±	±
AH	↑	NC
HV	↑↑	±
AERP	↑↑	↑
AFRP	↑↑	↑
NFRP	↑↑	↑
VERP	↑↑	↑
VFRP	↑↑	↑
Electrocardiographic intervals		
PR	↑	NC
QRS	↑	NC
QTc	↑	↑↑

[a]NC = no change; SCL = sinus cycle length; SNRT = sinus node recovery time; AH = interval from the beginning of the atrial depolarization (A) to the beginning of the bundle of HIS electrogram (H); HV = His bundle to ventricular activation time; AERP = atrial effective refractory period; AFRP = atrial functional refractory period; NFRP = atrioventricular nodal functional refractory period; VERP = ventricular effective refractory period; VFRP = ventricular functional refractory period.

responsiveness appears to result from a direct effect on the mechanism controlling the voltage- and time-dependent increase in sodium conductance. The decrease in responsiveness is enhanced by elevating extracellular potassium (14). Recent studies (13) indicate that therapeutic concentrations of procainamide exert selective effects on action potentials in partially depolarized zones of infarct and may explain procainamide's effectiveness against some reentrant arrhythmias. For example (13), in normal subendocardial Purkinje fiber (10 mg/L), procainamide significantly decreases $(dV/dt)_{max}$, but does not affect the action potential duration (APD) at -20 mV. At 10 mg/L in normal muscle cells from left ventricular endocardium it increased only APD 100%. The effect of procainamide on partially

depolarized Purkinje fiber varies. In normal subendocardial Purkinje fiber preparations procainamide slightly decreased action potential amplitude and increased APD at -60 mV, whereas in 24 h infarct zone Purkinje fibers procainamide decreased action potential amplitude and $(dV/dt)_{max}$ and prolonged APD 100%. Recently emphasis has been placed on the observation that many antiarrhythmic agents produce use-dependent decreases in $(dV/dt)_{max}$ (9,10,12). It appears that much of procainamide's effect is "tonic" over the range of physiologic cycle length, and use dependence only increases the degree of block modestly at a cycle length of 300 msec over that which occurs at 1000 msec (12). It has therefore been concluded that use-dependent decreases in $(dV/dt)_{max}$ by procainamide are not important to the reduction in ectopic impulse formation (12).

Studies to evaluate procainamide's effects on automaticity indicate that it suppresses normal and abnormal automaticity in isolated canine Purkinje fiber preparations (4–6,12). It decreases the slope of phase 4 depolarization and slows the rate of automatic firing to account for its effects. Rosen et al. (5,6) observed that relatively low doses of procainamide regularly reduced automaticity even before other changes in action potential were observed and suggested that suppression of automaticity may account for procainamide's mechanism of action at low doses. Dangman (12) suggested that procainamide slows normal automaticity by increasing the threshold potential for inward Na^+ current and phase 0 and that it exerts only modest effects on transmembrane currents that control the voltage-time course of early diastole. Studies in feline infarct zones in vitro suggest procainamide interferes with abnormal impulse conduction by reducing repetitive ventricular responses and reentry (7,18). To what extent procainamide's effects on automaticity account for its mechanism of action against clinical arrhythmias is not clear. There is limited information on how procainmide influences other forms of impulse initiation, that is, early or delayed afterdepolarizations. Procainamide exerts relatively weak effects on triggered activity in infarct zone Purkinje fiber (13); however, in ouabain-toxic canine Purkinje fibers it has been reported to decrease the amplitude of delayed afterdepolarizations and increase the coupling interval between the last driven beat (13a). Another study of normal Purkinje fibers showed that triggered activity at low membrane potentials was suppressed by procainamide (13b). These results may reflect differences between normal tissue and ischemia or ouabain-induced delayed afterdepolarizations.

Procainamide's effects on the components of excitability and refractoriness have been studied in the intact animal and in isolated tissue. In 1953 Woske et al. (15) showed that procainamide decreases excitability in the mammalian heart. Subsequent studies also described procainamide-induced prolongation in refractoriness, threshold, and action potential configuration in Purkinje fibers (6,16) and in isolated heart muscle. Utilizing microelectrode techniques in sheep Purkinje fiber, Arnsdorf and Bigger (16) showed that procainamide decreases excitability primarily by reducing sodium conductance, and procainamide's effect to increase or decrease excitability depended on the relative contribution of the drug-induced alterations in passive and active membrane properties. Procainamide delays repolarization and increases the duration of refractoriness in canine atrial and ventricular muscle fibers and Purkinje fibers but shortens the action potential of sheep Purkinje fibers. The increase in action potential duration is more marked at low rates and is attenuated by catecholamines (14). Investigators have used models of experimental ischemia and reperfusion in isolated feline ventricular myocardium to quantitate different drug effects on the time course of repolarization of ventricular muscle (18,19). Procainamide decreases differences in refractoriness between tissue types by prolonging action potential duration and refractoriness most markedly in acutely ischemic cells with the shortest action potential duration and refractoriness and least in chronically injured cells with the longest action potential duration and refractoriness; intermediate drug changes occur in normal cells (18). The effective refractory period of all cell types increase more than would be expected from changes in duration of the action potential. It was originally suggested by Weidmann (3) that a principal mode of action of procainamide is prolongation of the effective refractory period of Purkinje fibers out of proportion to any increase in action potential duration, and this property has been stressed as accounting for procainamide's mechanism of action. The greater increase in effective refractory period than drug-induced lengthening of the action potential duration has been attributed to a decrease in membrane responsiveness. Because of reduced responsiveness, repolarization must proceed to a more negative value before excitation can occur, resulting in a prolongation of refractoriness independent of any change in action potential duration (7). However, this is only true in those fibers whose action potential duration is not altered by procainamide at physiologic K^+ concentrations. In blood-perfused Purkinje fibers Rosen and associates (5,6) found that the increase in effective refractory period tended to lag behind the increase in action potential duration at therapeutic concentrations of drug and that membrane responsiveness was not altered.

BASIC PHARMACOLOGY: ANTIARRHYTHMIC EFFECTS IN EXPERIMENTAL ANIMALS

Procainamide does not significantly modify arterial blood pressure as studied in the models of the anesthetized (5,20) or conscious dogs (21,22). Woske et al. showed (15) that in anesthetized dogs procainamide caused an initial fall in blood pressure that was related more closely to the speed with which drug was administered than the total amount of drug administered. A vasodilatory effect, presumably resulting from inhibition of ganglionic transmission, has also been described (23).

There are conflicting data in electrophysiologic studies regarding procainamide's effects on heart rate. Bagwell et al. (24) and Amlie et al. (25) found a decrease in heart rate after injection of procainamide in pentobarbital-anesthetized dogs. Using isolated rat atria Refsum et al. (26) showed a decrease in the spontaneous atrial rate. Jaillon and Winkle (20) speculated that the effect on sinus node fuction may result from a dual action; that is, at low drug concentrations there is a predominant vagolytic action, and at higher concentrations an overriding direct depressant effect occurs. In anesthetized dogs procainamide in a concentration-dependent manner significantly prolongs atrionodal conduction time and His-Purkinje conduction and the effective and functional refractory period of the atria, AV nodal, and ventricular muscle tissue (20). In a dog model of digitalis intoxication procainamide terminates arrhythmias induced by high

concentrations of digitalis (27–29); however, a high incidence of atrioventricular conduction delay is seen when procainamide is used in digitalis-induced arrhythmias. In a dog model of infarction procainamide decreases excitability and prolongs the refractoriness of abnormal myocardium, preventing inducible ventricular arrhythmias and increasing the cycle length of inducible ventricular arrhythmias (30). Yoon et al. (31) showed that procainamide increased the ventricular fibrillation threshold in both normal and ischemic ventricle; this increase was maintained at a high value even while plasma concentrations decreased. The change in ventricular fibrillation threshold in the ischemic ventricle was not as pronounced as that in normal ventricle, however, and the drug failed to reverse completely the decreased fibrillation threshold to the normal value during ischemia. In contrast, lidocaine reverts the decreased ventricular fibrillation threshold well above the normal value during coronary occlusion (32). Lown and Wolf (33) and Weissel et al. (34), however, reported that procainamide offers a greater degree of protection than lidocaine, quinidine, or propranolol against ventricular fibrillation in dogs during coronary occlusion, and Gamble and Cohn (35) showed that procainamide was more effective than lidocaine in abolishing repetitive premature beats in cats following coronary artery ligation.

CLINICAL PHARMACOLOGY

Effects on Normal Human Electrocardiogram

There is much interindividual variability in the changes induced in the intervals of the surface electrocardiogram after procainamide. As expected from its effects on the electrical activity of single cardiac cells, procainamide causes dose-dependent changes observed from a standard 12-lead electrocardiogram. Within the therapeutic plasma concentration range some prolongation of the PR, QRS, and QTc intervals can be expected; on the other hand, procainamide has no significant effect on the R-R interval (36). Procainamide is classified as a class IA drug, and like others in its class, quinidine and disopyramide, it characteristically causes some prolongation of the QRS and QT intervals on the surface electrocardiogram. Such drugs as quinidine and procainamide, which have intermediate time constants for recovery from sodium channel blockade, tend to widen the QRS slightly at usual doses but may markedly increase the QRS at faster rates or at high plasma concentrations, and rate-dependent QRS widening of the electrocardiogram has been demonstrated (37). Progressive prolongation of the QRS as plasma procainamide concentration increases is frequently used to assess the myocardial effect, and widening of the QRS interval >25% has been recommended as an end point to procainamide dosing. As the plasma drug concentration increases, the coupling interval of ventricular premature depolarizations (VPD) is prolonged, indicating progressive prolongation of His-Purkinje conduction (38). Both procainamide and its metabolite, N-acetylprocainamide, prolong the effective refractory period, and hence QT interval prolongation is commonly seen. Along these lines, procainamide prolongs total electrical systole of ventricular premature depolarizations such that the QRS and QTc of the VPD are also prolonged, compatible with prolongation of the action potential duration and effective refractory period of ventricular muscle (39). The effect of procainamide on PR and QRS duration is less marked than with class IC antiarrhythmic agents, such as encainide (40), flecainide (41), and indecainide (42). High plasma procainamide concentrations have been associated with atrioventricular block, asystole, intraventricular conduction defects, and ventricular arrhythmias, including increased VPD frequency, ventricular tachycardia, and ventricular fibrillation.

Acute Effects in Humans: Programmed Extrastimulation Studies

The effects of low-dose procainamide on sinus rate in normal patients studied in the clinical electrophysiology laboratory (43,44) are variable, although a slight increase in heart rate (7%) has been reported. Intravenous procainamide produces a significant decrease in sinus cycle length, uncorrected sinus recovery time, and sinoatrial conduction time (45). Since the report by Short in 1954 (46) describing sinus node dysfunction aggravated by procainamide only a few studies have evaluated the effect of procainamide in patients with sinus node disease. In patients with sinus node dysfunction the corrected sinus recovery time lengthens, which could aggravate preexisting sinus node dysfunction, particularly in patients with the bradycardia-tachycardia syndrome (47,48). Occasional patients without sinus node disease have been noted to have significant sinus node depression after procainamide (47). The recommendation has been made that patients with suspected sinus node dysfunction undergo electrophysiologic study before receiving procainamide (43).

Procainamide is associated with increased atrial refractoriness in humans (43,44). The effects on conduction time through normal and impaired atrioventricular conduction have been described after low and high doses (43,44). In the human, at therapeutic concentrations, it causes slight prolongation of AV conduction and causes variable effects of the effective and functional refractory period of the AV node; a vagolytic effect has been invoked to account for such variability. On the other hand, it significantly increases His-Purkinje conduction time and His-Purkinje functional and relative refractory periods. Even at very low doses procainamide prolongs His-Purkinje conduction, although its effects on the AV node are minimal. In patients with intraventricular conduction defects procainamide causes prolongation of H-V of about 18% (47); however, of interest is the relatively safe and high degree of AV block and asystole or malignant arrhythmias have not been commonly observed, even in these patients.

Electrophysiologic Studies of Ventricular Arrhythmias

The value of procainamide in managing patients with sustained ventricular arrhythmias has been reported in a number of clinical electrophysiologic studies (49–56). Efficacy in terminating ventricular tachycardia (VT) or preventing induction of ventricular tachycardia by programmed electrical stimulation ranges from 15 to 50% (49,52,53). In the clinical electrophysiology laboratory incremental procainamide increases tachycardia cycle length, increases the effective refractory period of the ventricles, and potentiates rate-dependent prolongation (49,56) of QRS duration. Procainamide increases the cycle length of VT; this is not predictive of the inability to induce ventricular tachyarrhythmias, however, and some patients are more easily induced or more difficult to have inducible ventricular tachycardia terminated after procainamide (49,53). It has been suggested that procainamide's effectiveness can be enhanced when used in combination with other agents with different electrophysiologic effects, such as class IB drugs, phenytoin (57), and lidocaine or mexiletine (58), although combination therapy with procainamide has not been extensively studied. Some suggest it is possible to use intravenous procainamide to predict the response to other conventional antiarrhythmic agents during electrophysiologic studies (54); others have found that intravenous procainamide does not predict the response to oral procainamide or other oral drugs, such as quinidine, and therefore electrophysiologic studies should be conducted during the appropriate treatment (59). Greater concordance between intravenous and oral drug administration may be achieved when the plasma drug concentrations are similar (60).

Proarrhythmic events (13–16%) have been recorded in the electrophysiology laboratory associated with the use of procainamide in patients with sustained ventricular arrhythmias, including new onset of monomorphic and polymorphic ventricular tachycardia (61,62). In some patients with chronic recurrent VT, procainamide can facilitate initiation of VT, sometimes even at faster rates, which is not predictable from the baseline rate of VT (63,64). In a prospective study using programmed ventricular stimulation, procainamide in the plasma drug concentration range 3.6–14.3 μ/ml was associated with proarrhythmic responses in 8% of patients without known previous ventricular tachycardia (64).

Studies During Chronic Antiarrhythmic Therapy

Atrial Arrhythmias

Procainamide when given in adequate doses is effective in suppressing premature atrial depolarizations, paroxysmal atrial tachycardia, and atrial fibrillation and flutter (2). Early studies indicated it was more effective against ventricular than supraventricular arrhythmias; however, it approximates the effectiveness of quinidine against supraventriculr arrhythmias (65–67). Procainamide is effective in converting atrial fibrillation to sinus rhythm in patients with normal left atrial size (68), in reducing the frequency of premature atrial depolarizations, and in treating ectopic atrial tachycardia and atrial echo beats (65–67,69). Procainamide's effect on atrial flutter has been described in the electrophysiology laboratory, where it increases flutter cycle length, increases atrial refractoriness, and prolongs atrial conduction (70). It has been used successfully with atrial pacing to convert atrial flutter to normal sinus rhythm (71), and early studies suggested it was useful in combination with quinidine to convert atrial fibrillation to sinus rhythm (72). The mechanism of action of procainamide against supraventricular arrhythmias has been inferred from its electrophysiologic properties. Procainamide increases the effective refractory period of atrial fibers (by decreasing the ability of incompletely repolarized fibers to generate an active response and by delaying completion of repolarization), which may in part account for its antifibrillatory effects (1–4). Since the atrial rate in fibrillation and flutter decreases, procainamide probably slows the maximum repetition rate for a cell until it is not possible for a circulating wavefront of excitation to find a mass of excitable cells (4).

Wolff-Parkinson-White Syndrome

Procainamide has been used to treat arrhythmias associated with the Wolff-Parkinson-White syndrome. Wellens and associates (73) evaluated the influence of procainamide in identifying patients with a short refractory period and an accessory pathway in an antegrade direction. Intravenous procainamide (10 mg/kg body weight) produced complete antegrade block in the accessory pathway in more than 50% (20 of 39) of patients with Wolff-Parkinson-White syndrome. They concluded that intravenous procainamide is a reliable and rapid method of identifying patients with Wolff-Parkinson-White syndrome at risk for circulatory insufficiency or sudden death with atrial fibrillation (74) Proarrhythmic effects, such as incessant orthodromic atrioventricular tachycardia induced by prolonged refractoriness in the accessory pathway, should be guarded against, however (75).

Ventricular Arrhythmias

Procainamide has been in clinical use for almost 40 years against ventricular arrhythmias (1,76,77). Patients with chronic stable VPD (78–81), postmyocardial infarction patients (82,83), and those with lethal and potentially lethal ventricular arrhythmias have been treated (49–60). It has been reported to reduce or abolish ventricular arrhythmias in the acute setting in up to 90% of patients with VPD and 80% of patients with nonsustained ventricular tachycardia (1,36,76). In a double-blind study by Koch-Weser et al. (82) the prophylactic effect of procainamide was evaluated in 70 patients with uncomplicated myocardial infarction. Procainamide gave significant protection against all types of ventricular arrhythmias without major adverse effects. On the other hand, other studies do not support these beneficial effects. Kosowsky et al. (83) found no statistically significant difference in VPD frequency between control and treated groups (39 patients), although advanced grades of arrhythmia were diminished (62). Koch-Weser and Klein (81) found that in 65% of 218 patients with chronic ventricular arrhythmias procainamide had an antiarrhythmic effect. Other studies have shown similar results in patients with chronic ventricular arrhythmias (84,85). Many studies assessing procainamide's efficacy were conducted before strict criteria for judging antiarrhythmic efficacy were established (86–88). Investigators have commented on the length of drug-free monitoring and percentage of VPD suppression required to judge antiarrhythmic efficacy. Since

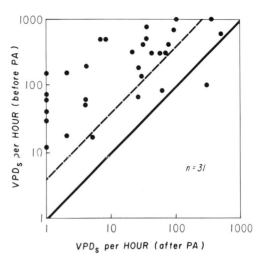

Figure 1 The antiarrhythmic effect of sustained-release procainamide in patients with frequent ventricular premature depolarizations (VPD) who received from 3.0 to 7.5 g/day. The solid line is a line of identity; that is, if there is no arrhythmia suppression the data points fall on or close to this line. The broken line demarcates ≥ 80% efficacy; thus data points representing more than 80% improvement fall above the line and those less than 80% fall between the broken and solid lines. In 25 (81%) patients there was more than 80% VPD suppression.

much data regarding procainamide's antiarrhythmic effect antedated these recent reports, procainamide has not been subjected to as rigorous testing as many new antiarrhythmic drugs in clinical trials (40–42, 88–90). However, the efficacy of a sustained-release procainamide formulation against chronic stable and potentially lethal VPD found 76% of patients had at least a 75% reduction in VPD frequency and complex features (80) when treated with 3.0–7.5 g/ day (Figure 1). Procainamide's overall efficacy for patients with potentially lethal VPD is probably less, that is, 65%, than seen with class IC drugs, such as encainide, flecainide, or indecainide (40–42).

The therapeutic antiarrhythmic plasma concentration range of procainamide against acute VPD ranges from 4 to 12 mg/L (Table 2) (36,81). This range may vary among patients and in different clinical situations, and to achieve and maintain an effective concentra-

Table 2 Clinical Pharmacology of Procainamide and *N*-Acetylprocainamide

	Procainamide	*N*-acetyprocainamide
Bioavailability, %	75– 95	85– 95
Peak concentration, hr	0.5–1.5	0.5–1.5
Volume of distribution, L/kg	1.5–2.5	1.2–1.7
Plasma protein binding, %	10– 20	10– 15
Effective concentration, mg/L	4– 12	9– 20
Half-time elimination, hr	3– 5	4– 15
Total body clearance, ml/min	400–700	200–300
Excretion unchanged drug, %	40– 70	60– 80

tion requires individualization of dosage. The typical or average dose may lead to ineffective arrhythmia control in some patients and untoward adverse effects in others or may result in a wide range of plasma drug concentrations. The average plasma concentration required for suppression of chronic stable VPD is higher than for acute arrhythmias following myocardial infarction, that is, range 2–17 mg/L (80), and the average plasma concentration that prevents initiation of sustained ventricular tachyarrhythmias is even higher, that is, 14.0 mg/L; range of 5–32 mg/L (50). However, Myerburg et al. (91) suggested that even when drug levels are not very high and VPD suppression is less than 70% (mean 36%) there is still a beneficial effect from procainamide that may be important in preventing sudden death. Accordingly, even relatively low plasma concentrations of procainamide are associated with a reduction in the frequency of complex ventricular arrhythmias, including ventricular tachycardia, before VPD frequency is significantly reduced (80). It may be that the suppression of complex features with procainamide is sufficient to protect against a malignant outcome in some patients.

The mechanism of action of procainamide against ventricular premature depolarizations is dependent on the genesis of the arrhythmia. Arrhythmias due to altered automaticity may be interrupted by suppression of phase 4 depolarization in conjunction with a shift in the level of threshold potential toward zero (4–6). Arrhythmias that have their genesis in depressed conduction and unidirectional block, that is, reentrant arrhythmias, may be suppressed by other mechanisms. If premature de-

polarizations result from reentry it is possible that procainamide depresses conduction in a reentrant circuit such that unidirectional block is converted to bidirectional block (14). In support of this view, as the plasma procainamide concentration rises the coupling interval of reentrant VPD progressively lengthens until VPD are completely abolished. This clinical observation suggests that reentrant arrhythmias are suppressed by converting unidirection to bidirectional block (38). Termination may also result from prolongation of the effective refractory period in tissues proximal to the site of reentry.

Pharmacokinetics

Experimental Animal Studies

The pharmacokinetics of procainamide are variable among species. Both the human and the monkey metabolize procainamide to *N*-acetylprocainamide; however, the monkey is more efficient in this regard, with only a trace of unchanged procainamide found in the urine. Although as much as 50–60% of a dose may be found in the urine of humans or dogs as procainamide, the dog eliminates five other compounds; although *N*-acetylprocainamide is the major metabolite of the monkey and the human, it does not appear in the urine of dogs (92,93). The monkey further metabolizes *N*-acetylprocainamide to *p*-acetoamidobenzoic acid and to a minor metabolite. Humans also metabolize procainamide to *N*-acetylprocainamide and then to another metabolite with an alteration in an aromatic amino group, but it is otherwise unchanged. Thus, although the human and the monkey both form the same metabolic intermediate, deethylation, the favored subsequent process in the monkey, does not occur in the human (92,93).

Clinical Studies

The bioavailability of orally administered procainamide ranges from 75 to 95% (Table 2) (78,79). Peak plasma concentration is reached relatively rapidly, that is, within 0.5–1.5 hr. An advantage of sustained-release formulations of procainamide is that the "peak" concentration is attenuated because of prolonged absorption from the gastrointestinal tract (78,79,94). A small amount of procainamide is protein bound, that is, 10–20%; however, binding to the acute-phase reactant α1-acid glycoprotein, which increases following myocardial infarction (95), does not appear to alter the effect of procainamide as it may for other strong basic drugs, such as lidocaine. Procainamide is a weak base, and it follows urine pH-dependent excretion in dogs but not in humans (96,97). The apparent volume of distribution is very large, ranging from 1.5 to 2.5 L/kg body weight (97). However, the volume of distribution can be significantly reduced in such conditions as congestive heart failure or cardiogenic shock resulting in high concentrations from a relatively small dose. At steady state the myocardium-plasma procainamide concentration ratio is 3:1. Procainamide is metabolized by the liver, and at least three metabolites have been recognized and two identified (78). Approximately 7–24% of the major cardioactive metabolite *N*-acetylprocainamide is recovered in the urine after a single dose. The metabolite, desethyl-*N*-acetylprocainamide, is less well characterized (78). The $t_{1/2}$ elimination of the parent compound ranges from 3 to 5 hr, this can be significantly prolonged in patients with diminished renal function or low-output states, however. In particular, patients on continuous dialysis or those with end-stage renal disease have a markedly prolonged elimination half-life and reduced clearance (95–97,99,100). These patients require significantly less procainamide or less frequent dosing intervals than patients with normal renal function (100). The active metabolite, *N*-acetylprocainamide, which is renally excreted,

accumulates to an even greater extent in renal failure (101,103). Even conventional doses in elderly patients with severe renal dysfunction may cause extremely high *N*-acetylprocainamide concentrations related to marked and delayed accumulation and elimination (103). Cardiotoxicity associated with *N*-acetylprocainamide concentration of >40 μg/ml may manifest as progressive widening of the QRS and QTc intervals, induction of polymorphic ventricular tachycardia, severe depression of left ventricular function, and death. Use of lower procainamide doses and careful monitoring of serum concentration of procainamide and *N*-acetylprocainamide are essential in these patients.

Available data on procainamide pharmacokinetics in pregnancy are limited. Transplacental procainamide passage has been documented, and the fetal-maternal plasma concentration ration is 0.28–1.32. The milk-plasma ratio is 4.30 (*N*-acetylprocainamide, 3.8), indicating that nursing mothers preferably should not use procainamide. Because of limited data and the potentially serious adverse effects of procainamide, it should not be recommended for use in pregnancy (98,104).

Methods of Administration. Procainamide is a very versatile agent since it may be given orally, intravenously, or intramuscularly (Table 3). Oral administration is most widely used for the treatment of chronic stable VPD. In general, 500–1500 mg every 4–6 hr has been shown to be a satisfactory schedule for many patients taking conventional procainamide (81,82). This dosing interval was established based on the half-life of elimination of procainamide, that is 3–5 hr. However, many cardiac patients have significantly longer half-lives of elimination than normal subjects as a result of decreased renal function and/or low cardiac output states. Moreover, since *N*-acetylprocainamide has antiarrhythmic effects (105–109) and may contribute to a sustained antiarrhythmic effect, longer dosing intervals are allowed than predicted from the half-life of the parent compound. To improve patient compliance and avoid peak and nadir plasma concentrations, sustained-release formulations (79,80,94) based on delayed gastrointestinal

Table 3 Oral and Intravenous Dosing for Procainamide

Method of administration	Conventional Drug	Sustained release
1. Oral		
Total daily dose, mg	2000–6000	3000–7500
Dosing interval, hr	3–5	6–8
Time to peak, hr	0.5–1.5	1–2
Time to steady state, days	1	1
2. Intravenous, intermittent		
Dose, mg	100	—
Dosing interval, min	5	—
Maximum dose, mg	1000	—
3. Intravenous, constant-rate infusion		
Rate mg/min	1.5–5.5	—
μg/kg/min	20–80	—
Time to 90% plateau, hr	12	—

absorption have been developed. Doses ranging from 3 to 7.5 g daily (three or four times a day) result in ≥75% VPC suppression in >75% of patients. With the sustained-release formulation the effective procainamide plasma concentration ranges from 7 to 10 mg/L and N-acetylprocainamide from 9 to 12 mg/L (107,108). Although not widely used, the intramuscular administration of procainamide is possible (17). Approximately 90–100% of an intramuscular dose is absorbed; however, intramuscular absorption offers little advantage over oral therapy since absorption time, time to peak, and plasma concentrations are approximately the same.

In acute situations in which drug therapy must be administered rapidly, *intermittent intravenous* procainamide can be given as 100 mg over 5 min through an indwelling intravenous catheter to a maximum of 1000 mg (36). With this method blood pressure is measured every 5 min following a dose, and continuous electrocardiographic monitoring of ECG intervals accompanies the intravenous injection. This method results in a graded decrease in frequency of VPD and a predictable increase in plasma procainamide concentration (36). The formula $Y = 0.84 + 0.73X$ describes the relationship between plasma procainamide concentration (Y) and dose of procainamide administered in mg/kg (X) and allows one to predict the plasma procainamide concentration after this method of drug administration if weight and total dose of procainamide are

known. This method has been useful in treating patients with chronic stable VPD, as well as those with life-threatening ventricular arrhythmias. With intermittent intravenous injection of procainamide significant hypotension is unusual, in contrast to the hypotension observed following the intravenous injection of quinidine. Very high plasma concentrations of procainamide reached rapidly, however, can diminish myocardial performance and induce hypotension, particularly in patients with pre-existing reduced left ventricular performance and low ejection fraction. An alternative method of procainamide administration for rapid control of arrhythmias is to administer drug via a *rapid* constant-rate infusion, that is, to administer the same dose but at a constant-rate infusion, 10–20 mg/min.

After controlling the acute arrhythmia, begin a constant rate intravenous infusion to maintain effective plasma concentrations. The infusion rate can be estimated as the product of the desired plasma concentration (4–12 mg/L) and estimated total clearance of procainamide (400–700 ml/min). For example, if procainamide clearance is estimated as 500 ml/min and the desired plasma concentration is 8 mg/ml, 4.0 mg/min is infused.

Drug Interactions. Only a few pharmacokinetic drug-drug interactions between procainamide and other drugs have been described. In contrast to quinidine, procainamide does not interact with digoxin (110); however, treatment with amiodarone results in increased procainamide concentrations (111). Drug interactions with cimetidine (112) and ranitidine (113) are noteworthy. Procainamide, cimetidine, and ranitidine are secreted by an active transport mechanism in the proximal tubule, and cimetidine and ranitidine may decrease the systemic clearance of procainamide in part by inhibiting its active secretion by the kidneys. Hence inhibition of renal clearance and prolongation of the half-life of elimination of procainamide and its metabolite are possible, resulting in higher than predicted procainamide concentrations. These findings indicate that a reduction of the procainamide dose may be necessary for patients who require cimetidine and ranitidine. There is conflicting evidence regarding the effects of procainamide in combination with β-blockers. One report indicates β-blockers have no significant effect on the kinetics of procainamide or N-acetylprocainamide (114); another reports that the half-life of elimination is increased and clearance decreased when procainamide and propranolol are administered (115). Under these circumstances care should be individualized and the patient observed carefully when both are used for treatment. Ethanol causes a significant reduction in the half-life and increases the total clearance of procainamide without effecting either the volume of distribution or the renal clearance, which could account for the unpredictably low plasma drug concentration in patients whose alcohol intake is increased (116). Ethanol also increases the percentage of N-acetylprocainamide measured in blood and urine.

Pharmacodynamic interactions of procainamide may be important when treating arrhythmias in patients with conduction system disease in combination with other drugs that effect sinus, AV nodal, or His-Purkinje conduction, such as quinidine, disopyramide, encainide (40), flecainide (41), indecainide (42), tricyclic antidepressants (117), or calcium channel antagonists. Since effects on conduction could be potentiated it may be reasonable to reduce the dose of each drug used in combination or to use procainamide in combination with lidocaine or phenytoin (28,29), which have less profound effects on AV and

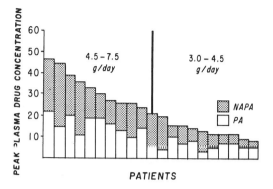

Figure 2 Variability in the plasma concentration of procainamide (PA) and N-acetylprocainamide (NAPA) after treatment with 4.5–7.5 g/day (left) and 3.0–4.5 g/day (right) of sustained-release procainamide. As expected, higher doses were associated with higher total concentrations of procainamide and N-acetylprocainamide; moreover, there is much interindividual variability in the concentration. The six patients with the highest concentrations received from 6.0 to 7.5 g/day. (Reprinted with permission, Reference 139.)

His-Purkinje conduction, particularly in patients with preexisting conduction disease.

Metabolism

Although procainamide was introduced in 1950, in 1976 the major metabolite of procainamide (78), N-acetylprocainamide, and two other peaks, $R_f = 0.0$ and $R_f = 0.3$, were quantified in human plasma and urine. There is wide interindividual variability in the amount of procainamide and N-acetylprocainamide recovered after a dose of procainamide, which is dependent on genetic predisposition but also on factors that affect drug metabolism and excretion and differences in volume of distribution and clearance (Figure 2).

The discovery of N-acetylprocainamide was underscored by the finding it had electrophysiologic properties in humans and other animals (118,119); however, the electrophysiologic effects of N-acetylprocainamide contrast with those procainamide (119). In isolated Purkinje fibers N-acetylprocainamide prolongs action potential duration but does not alter phase 0 upstroke or phase 4 depolarization. In dogs N-acetylprocainamide has no consistent effect on intraventricular or His-Purkinje conduction times but does prolong ventricular refractoriness and QT intervals. Findings in animals parallel changes on the electrocardiogram that show that N-acetylprocainamide prolongs the QTc interval but does not alter PR or QRS duration. Marked QT prolongation and torsade de pointes have been associated with the accumulation of N-acetylprocainamide (120). In the clinical electrophysiology laboratory N-acetylprocainamide prolongs the QTc interval but does not significantly change heart rate, mean arterial blood pressure, ECG intervals, or AH and HV intervals (118).

The kinetics of N-acetylprocainamide have been studied in a small number of normal and cardiac patients (Table 2) (105,106,108,121). The majority is excreted unchanged (60–80%) in the urine; the half-life varies between 4 and 15 hr and total body clearance is 200–300 ml/min, about 2.5 times less than that of the parent compound. Net deacetylation of N-acetylprocainamide to procainamide is minimal (122). Renal clearance of N-acetylprocainamide is decreased in patients with cardiac disease (122), and in functionally anephric patients it may be more than 40 hr; however, N-acetylprocainamide is cleared by hemodialysis (122). The effective N-acetylprocainamide concentration is 9–20 mg/L (105). Initial reports were optimistic about the antiarrhythmic effects of N-acetylprocainamide (107), and its pharmacokinetics, with a mean half-life of elimination of 7.5 hr, suggested it may be useful in enhancing patient compliance. N-acetylprocainamide demonstrates antiarrhythmic effects in patients with sustained ventricular tachycardia, but it has been only moderately successful even when the mean serum concentration level is >15 mg/L (118). Long-term use has been disappointing because of recurrent arrhythmias and, also, a relatively high incidence of minor adverse effects, which are primarily gastrointestinal (105).

One area of particular interest has been the use of N-acetylprocainamide for patients who developed a syndrome similar to systemic lupus erythematosus (SLE). A number of independent investigators (105–109) observed that N-acetylprocainamide could be used to treat patients with ventricular arrhythmias in whom the potential for developing the SLE-like syndrome was high. Remission of procainamide-induced lupus when treatment is changed to N-acetylprocainamide and failure of N-acetylprocainamide to induce the SLE-like syndrome suggest that the aromatic amino group on the procainamide molecule incites drug-induced lupus.

TOXICOLOGY

Toxic Effects in Experimental Animals and Tissues

The cardiopulmonary effects of procainamide have been studied in the anesthetized intact dog (123). Rapid and large intravenous injections of procainamide cause systemic hypotension, a decrease in pulmonary vascular resistance, a fall in pulmonary artery pressure, local vasodilation, and a fall in cardiac output (124). Low-dose intravenous procainamide has a positive ionotropic effect, but high doses are associated with marked myocardial depression in the intact animal (123). Procainamide slows both AV conduction and intraventricular conduction in digitalized and undigitalized dogs (125). In a model of complete heart block procainamide depresses both ventricular and sinus automaticity and changes ventricular tachycardia induced by digitalis to a slower, multifocal ventricular rhythm with widened complexes (125).

Clinical Toxicology

A number of extracardiac effects have been reported, including gastrointestinal symptoms (anorexia, nausea, and vomiting); central nervous symptoms (headache, dizziness, psychosis, hallucinations, and depression); fever, rash, myalgias, digital vasculitis, and Raynaud's phenomenon (83). Recent reports indicate that agranulocytosis is more common after procainamide than previously thought, particularly following administration of the sustained-release formulation (126,127). The possibility of agranulocytosis in a febrile patient receiving procainamide should be considered and the drug withdrawn and, when necessary, treatment with appropriate antibiotics started (126,127). Toxic concentrations can diminish myocardial performance, and large intravenous doses have been associated with significant hypotension (128). However, radionuclide studies of patients treated with customary doses indicate that the chronic use of procainamide only slightly decreases left ventricular function, but this should be evaluated periodically (129).

A worrisome adverse effect associated with procainamide is the systemic lupuslike syndrome (130,131). This syndrome was originally thought to occur relatively late after administration of procainamide and to be associated with large doses. Kosowsky and associates (83), however, reported that more than 50% of patients taking procainamide develop this complication. Antinuclear antibodies (ANA) are present in many patients receiving procainamide (132). In a prospective study, 27% (9 of 33) of patients using a sustained-release formulation had the ANA convert from negative to positive, and one of these developed the full-blown lupuslike syndrome (80). Many possible serologic changes associated with procainamide administration include antihistone antibodies (133), in vivo complement activation (134), and positive direct antiglobulin (Coombs) test due to the production of red cell autoantibody indistinguishable from that seen in warm, autoimmune hemolytic anemia. High levels of IgG antiguanosine antibodies have been reported primarily in patients with arthritis, pleuritis, and pericarditis after procainamide, suggesting a strong association between IgG antiguanosine antibodies and major manifestation of procainamide-induced SLE (132).

Efforts by a number of investigators have been made to determine if the potential for developing the SLE-like syndrome is predictable (135–138). First, investigators focused on the rate of acetylation to assess whether slow or fast acetylators are more likely to develop adverse effects. This approach was based on the observation that hydralazine (acetylated by the enzyme with a bimodal distribution) is more likely to cause SLE in slow than fast acetyla-

tors. The relationship between the fraction of N-acetylprocainamide in urine and plasma samples versus acetylation phenotype determined with isoniazid (INH), dapsone, or sulfamethazine has been reported. However, the acetylation phenotype determined from the fraction of N-acetylprocainamide recovered in timed urine or plasma samples can be misleading. A subject who is a phenotypic slow acetylator but has a prolonged rate of renal excretion due to congestive heart failure or renal disease can excrete a very large fraction as N-acetylprocainamide. It has been reported (137) that slow acetylators, in addition to the SLE-like syndrome, develop positive antinuclear antibody more rapidly and at a lower procainamide dose than fast acetylators. However, acetylation phenotype does not reliably predict the incidence of adverse effects; that is, fast acetylators develop adverse effects with the same frequency as slow acetylators (139). Thus slow acetylators are at risk for developing the SLE-like syndrome, but the fast acetylation phenotype does not offer protection from other adverse effects.

Proarrhythmia

The difficulty in assessing proarrhythmia is associated with the baseline variability of many arrhythmias. It has been widely held that events considered proarrhythmic, such as an increase in the frequency of VPD, faster rates of VT, and longer runs of VT, should probably not be considered proarrhythmic if they occur within 72 hr of acute myocardial infarction or following changes in the physiologic state of the patient, such as worsening heart failure, hypokalemia or hypomagnesemia, or hypoxia. Proarrhythmia or worsening of ventricular arrhythmias has been observed in 3–12% of patients taking procainamide and is similar to the incidence of proarrhythmic events following treatment with quinidine or disopyramide (140). Proarrhythmia and nonfatal cardiac arrest do not appear as common with procainamide as with the class IC drugs, encainide and flecainide, in postinfarction patients. Further studies with a postinfarction population are required to confirm this.

SUMMARY

Procainamide is a versatile class IA antiarrhythmic agent for supraventricular and ventricular arrhythmias, and it has been used in millions of patients over the course of 40 years. In contrast to newer agents, classified as IC drugs, it appears to be a less potent antiarrhythmic agent, and its adverse effects on cardiac conduction and left ventricular function are significantly less. For the most part the cardiodepressant effects of procainamide are related to the size of the dose and the method of administration; when given orally procainamide is well tolerated hemodynamically. The major adverse effects of procainamide are related to the systemic lupus-like syndrome, and more recently, the incidence of agranulocytosis, particularly with the sustained-release formulation, has been noted. It remains a first-line drug for acute arrhythmias because of its spectrum of efficacy against supraventricular and ventricular arrhythmias and versatility of administration.

REFERENCES

1. Burstein C L. The utility of intravenous procaine in the anesthetic management of cardiac disturbances. Anesthesiology 1949; 10:133–5.
2. Kayden J H, Steele J M, Mark L, Brodie B B. The use of procainamide in cardiac arrhythmias. Circulation 1951; 4:13–22.
3. Weidmann S. Effects of calcium ions and local anaesthetics on electrical properties of Purkinje fibres. J Physiol (Lond) 1955; 129.368–82.
4. Hoffman B F. The action of quinidine and procaine amide on single fiber of dog ventricle and specialized conducting system. An Acad Bras Cienc 1958; 29:365–8.
5. Rosen M R, Gelband H, Hoffman B F. Canine electrocardiographic and cardiac electrophysiologic changes induced by procainamide. Circulation 1972; 46:528–36.
6. Rosen M R, Merker C, Gelband H, Hoffman B F. Effects of procainamide on the electrophysiologic properties of the canine ventricular conducting system J Pharmacol Exp Ther 1973; 185:438–46.
7. Sasyniuk B I, Ogilvie R I. Antiarrhythmic drugs: electrophysiological and pharmacoki-

netic considerations. Annu Rev Pharmacol 1975; 15:131–55.
8. Toyama J, Furuta T. The electrophysiological action of lidocaine on ischemic ventricular muscle as compared with procainamide. Jpn Circ J 1983; 47:82–91.
9. Nattel S. Relationship between use-dependent effects of antiarrhythmic drugs on conduction and V max in canine cardiac Purkinje fiber. J Pharmacol Exp Ther 1987; 241:282–8.
10. Varro A, Elharrar V, Surawicz B. Frequency dependent effects of several class I antiarrhythmic drugs on V_{max} of action potential upstroke in canine cardiac Purkinje fibers. J Cardiovasc Pharmacol 1985; 7:482–92.
11. Colatsky T J, Bird L B, Jurkiewicz N K, Wendt T L. Cellular electrophysiology of the new antiarrhythmic agent recainam (Wy-42,362) in canine cardiac Purkinje fibers. J Cardiovasc Pharmacol 1987; 9:435–44.
12. Dangman K. Effects of procainamide on automatic and triggered impulse initiation in isolated preparations of canine cardiac Purkinje fibers. J Cardiovasc Pharmacol 1988; 12:78–87.
13. Dangman K H, Miura D S. Effect of therapeutic concentrations of procainamide on transmembrane action potentials of normal and infarct zone Purkinje fibers and ventricular muscle cells. J Cardiovasc Pharmacol 1989; 13:846–52.
13a. Hewett K, Gessman L, Rosen M R. Effects of procaine amide, quinidine and ethmozin on delayed afterdepolarizations. Eur J Pharmacol 1983; 96:21–8.
13b. Arnsdorf M F. The effect of antiarrhythmic drugs on triggered sustained rhythmic activity in cardiac Purkinje fibers. J Pharmacol Exp Ther 1977; 201:689–700.
14. Hoffman B F, Rosen MR, Wit AL. Electrophysiology and pharmacology of cardiac arrhythmias. VII. Cardiac effects of quinidine and procaine amide. Am Heart J 1975; 90:117–22.
15. Woske H, Belford J, Fastier F N, Brooks C M C. The effect of procaine amide on excitability, refractoriness and conduction in the mammalian heart. J Pharmacol Exp Ther 1953; 107:134–40.
16. Arnsdorf M, Bigger J T. The effects of procainamide on components of excitability in long mammalian cardiac Purkinje fiber. Circ Res 1976; 38:115–22.

17. Hoffman B F, Bigger J T. Antiarrhythmic drugs. In: Di Palma J., ed. Drill's pharmacology in medicine New York: McGraw-Hill, 1971: Chapter 40.

18. Myerburg R J, Basset A L, Epstein K, Gaide M, Kozlovskis P, Wong S, Castellanos A, Gelband H. Electrophysiological effects of procainamide in acute and healed experimental ischemic injury of cat myocardium. Circ Res 1982; 50:386–93.

19. Kimura S, Bassett A, Saoudi N, Cameron J, Kozlovskis P, Myerburg R. Cellular electrophysiologic changes and "arrhythmias" during experimental ischemia and reperfusion in isolated cat ventricular myocardium. J Am Coll Cardiol 1986: 7(4):833–42.

20. Jaillon P, Winkle R A. Electrophysiologic comparative study of procainamide and N-acetylprocainamide in anesthetized dogs: concentration-response relationships. Circulation 1979; 60:1386–93.

21. O'Rourke R A, Bishop V S, Stone H L, Rapaport E. Lack of effect of procainamide on ventricular function of conscious dogs. Am J Cardiol 1969; 23:238.

22. Mandel W J, Laks M M, Arieff A I, Obayaski K, Hayakawa H, McCullen A. Cardiorenal effects of lidocaine and procainamide in the conscious dog. Am J Physiol 1975; 228:1440–5.

23. Schmid P G, Nelson L D, Heistad D D, Mark A L, Abboud R. Vascular effects of procainamide in the dog. Circ Res 1974; 35:948–60.

24. Bagwell E E, Walle T, Drayer D E, Reidenberg M M, Pruett J K. Correlation of the electrophysiological and antiarrhythmic properties of the n-acetyl metabolite of procainamide with plasma and tissue concentrations in the dog. J Pharmacol Exp Ther 1976; 197:38–48.

25. Amlie J P, Nesje O A, Frislid K, Lunde P K M, Landmark K H. Serum levels and electrophysiologic effects of n-acetyl procainamide as compared with procainamide in the dog heart in situ. Acta Pharmacol Toxicol (Copenh) 1978; 42:280–6.

26. Refsum H, Frislid K, Lunde P K M, Landmark K H. Effects of n-acetylprocainamide as compared with procainamide in isolated rat atria Eur J Pharmacol 1975; 33:47–52.

27. Mosey L, Tyler M D. The effect of diphenylhydantoin sodium, procaine hydrochloride, procainamide hydrochloride and quinidine hydrochloride upon ouabain-induced ventricular tachycardia in unanesthetized dogs. Circulation 1954; 10:65–70.

28. Helfant R H, Scherlag B J, and Damato A N. The electrophysiological properties of diphenylhydantoin sodium as compared to procaine amide in the normal and digitalis intoxicated heart. Circulation 1967; 36:108–18.

29. Scherlag B J, Helfant R H, Damato A N. The contrasting effects of diphenylhydantoin and procaine amide on AV conduction in the digitalis-intoxicated and the normal heart. Am Heart J 1968; 75:200–5.

30. Michaelson E L, Spear J F, Moore E N. Effects of procainamide on strength interval in normal and chronically infarcted canine myocardium. Am J Cardiol 1981; 47:1223–32.

31. Yoon M S, Han J, Goel B G, Cramer P. Effect of procainamide on fibrillation threshold of normal and ischemic ventricles. Am J Cardiol 1974; 33:238–342.

32. Spear J F, Moore E N, Gerstenblith G. Effects of lidocaine on the ventricular fibrillation threshold in the dog during acute ischemia and premature ventricular contractions. Circulation 1972; 46:64–73.

33. Lown B, Wolf M. Approaches to sudden death from coronary heart disease. Circulation 1971; 44:130–42.

34. Weissel A B, Moschos C B, Passannante A J, Khan M I, Regan T J. Relative effectiveness of three antiarrhythmic agents in the treatment of ventricular arrhythmias in experimental acute myocardial ischemia. Am Heart J 1971; 81:503–10.

35. Gamble O W, Cohn K. Effect of propranolol, procainamide, and lidocaine on ventricular automaticity and reentry in experimental myocardial infarction. Circulation 1972; 46:498–506.

36. Giardina E G V, Heissenbuttel R H, Bigger J T. Intermittent intravenous procainamide to treat ventricular arrhythmias: correlation of plasma concentration with effect on arrhythmia, electrocardiogram, and blood pressure. Ann Intern Med 1973; 78:183–93.

37. Morady F, DiCarlo L A, Baerman J M, Krol R B,. Rate dependent effects of intravenous lidocaine, procainamide, and amiodarone on intraventricular conduction. J Am Coll Cardiol, 1985; 6:179–85.

38. Giardina E G V, Bigger J T. Procainamide against reentrant ventricular arrhythmias. Circulation 1973; 48:959–68.

39. Giardina E G V, Bigger J T Jr. Effect of procainamide and lidocaine on total electrical systole of ventricular premature depolarizations. Am J Med 1975; 59:405–9.

40. Roden D M, Reele S B, Higgins S B, Mayol R F, Gammans R E, Oates J A, Woosley R L. Total suppression of ventricular arrhythmias by encainide. N Engl J Med 1980; 302:877–82.

41. Anderson J L, Stewart J R, Perry B A, Hamersveld D D V, Johnson T A, Conrad G J, Chang S F, Kvam D C, Pitt B. Oral flecainide for the treatment of ventricular arrhythmias. N Engl J Med 1981; 305:473–7.

42. Giardina E G V, Zaim S, Saroff A L, Kirschenbaum M. Comparison of indecainide with quinidine in patients with chronic stable ventricular arrhythmias secondary to coronary artery disease or cardiomyopathy. Am J Cardiol 1987; 60:584–9.

43. Josephson M E, Caracta A R, Ricciutti M A, Lau S H, Damato A N. Electrophysiologic properties of procainamide in man. Am J Cardiol 1974; 33:596–603.

44. Ogunkelu J B, Damato A N, Akhatar M, Reddy C P, Caracta A R, Lau S H. Electrophysiologic effects of procainamide in subtherapeutic to therapeutic doses on human atrioventricular conduction system. Am J Cardiol 1976; 37:724–31.

45. Wyse D G, McAnulty J H, Rahimtoola S H. Influence of plasma drug level and the presence of conduction disease on the electrophysiologic effects of procainamide. Am J Cardiol 1979; 43:619–26.

46. Short D S. The syndrome of alternating bradycardia and tachycardia. Br Heart J 1954; 16:208–14.

47. Scheinman M M, Weiss A N, Strafton E, Benowitz N, Rowland M. Electrophysiologic effects of procainamide in patients with intraventricular conduction delay. Circulation 1974; 49:522–9.

48. Goldberg D, Reiffel J A, Davis J C, Gang E, Livelli F, Bigger J T. Electrophysiologic effects of procainamide on sinus node function in patients with and without sinus node disease. Am Heart J 1982; 103:75–9.

49. Morady F, Di Carlo L A, de Buitleir M, Krol R B, Baerman J M, Kou W H. Effects of incremental doses of procainamide onventricular refractoriness, intraventricularconduction, and induction of ventricular tachycardia. Circulation 1986; 74:1355–64.

50. Horowitz L N, Josephson M E, Kastor J A. Intracardiac electrophysiologic studies as a method for the optimization of drug therapy in chronic ventricular arrhythmia. Prog Cardiovas Dis 1980; 23:81–98.

51. Greenspan A M, Horowitz, L N, Spielman S R, Josephsohn M E. Large does procainamide therapy for ventricular tachycardia. Am J Cardiol 1980; 46:453–62.

52. Wynn J, Torres V, Flowers D, Mizruchi M, Keefe D, Miura D, Somberg J. Antiarrhythmic drug efficacy at electrophysiologic testing; predictive effectiveness of procainamide and flecainide. Am Heart J 1986; 111:632–8.

53. Roy D, Waxman H L, Buxton L H, Marchlinski F E, Cain M E, Gardner M J, Josephson M. Termination of ventricular tachycardia: role of tachycardia cycle length. Am J Cardiol 1982; 50:1346–50.

54. Waxman L H, Buxton A E, Sadowski L M, Josephson M E. The response to procainamide during electrophysiologic study for sustained ventricular tachyarrhythmias predicts the response to other medications. Am J Cardiol 1983; 51:1175–81.

55. Rae A P, Sokoloff N M, Webb C R, Spielman S R, Greenspan A M, Horowtiz L N. Limitations of failure of procainamide during electrophysiologic testing to predict response to other medical therapy. J Am Coll Cardiol 1985; 6:410–6.

56. Kastor J, Josephson M E, Guss S B, Horowitz L. Human ventricular refractoriness. II. Effects of procainamide. Circulation 1977; 56:462–7.

57. Bigger J T Jr, Giardina E G V. Rational use of drugs alone and in combination. In: Melmon K, ed. Cardiovascular drug therapy. Philadelphia: F. A. Davis, 1974: 103–17.

58. Greenspan A M, Spielman S R, Webb C R, Sokoloff N M, Rae A P, Horowitz L N. Efficacy of combination therapy with mexiletine and a type IA agent for inducible ventricular tachyarrhythmias secondary to coronary artery disease. Am J Cardiol 1985; 56:277–84.

59. Oseran D S, Gang E S, Rosenthal M E, Mandel W J, Peter T. Electropharmacologic testing in sustained ventricular tachycardia associated with coronary heart disease: value of the response to intravenous procainamide in predicting the response to oral procainamide and oral quinidine treatment. Am J Cardiol 1985; 56:883–6.

60. Marchlinski F E, Buxton A E, Vassallo J A, Waxman H L, Cassidy D M, Doherty J,

Josephson M E. Comparative electrophysiologic effects of intravenous and oral procainamide in patients with sustained ventricular arrhythmias. J Am Coll Cardiol 1984; 4:1247–54.

61. Torres V, Flowers D, Somberg J C. The arrhythmogenicity of antiarrhythmic agents. Am Heart J 1985; 109:1090–7.

62. Poser R F, Podrid P J, Lombardi F, Lown B. Aggravation of arrhythmia induced with antiarrhythmic drugs during electrophysiologic testing. Am Heart J 1985; 110:9–16.

63. Kang P S, Gomes J A, El-Sherif N. Procainamide in the induction and perpetuation of ventricular tachycardia in man. PACE 1982; 5(3):311–22.

64. Au P K, Bhandari A K, Bream R, Schreck D, Siddiqi R, Rahimtoola S. Proarrhythmic effects of antiarrhythmic drugs during programmed ventricular stimulation in patients without ventricular tachycardia. J Am Coll Cardiol 1987; 10:389–97.

65. Schack J A, Hoffman I, Vesell H. The response of arrhythmias and tachycardias of supraventricular origin to oral procainamide. Br Heart J 1952; 14:465.

66. Schaffer A I, Blumenfeld S M, Pittman E R, Dix J H. Procainamide: its effect on auricular arrhythmias. Am Heart J 1951; 42:115.

67. Miller H, Nathanson M H, Griffith G C. The action of procainamide in cardiac arrhythmias. JAMA 1951; 146:1004–10.

68. Halpern S W, Ellrodt G, Singh B N, Mandel W J: Efficacy of intravenous procainmide infusion in converting atrial fibrillation to sinus rhythm; relation to left atrial size. Br Heart J 1980; 44:589–95.

69. McCord M C, Taguchi J R. A study of the effect of procainamide hydrochloride in supraventricular arrhythmias. Circulation 1951; 4:387.

70. Josephson M E, Caracta M E, Ricciutti M A, Lau S, Damato A N. Electrophysiologic properties of procainamide in man. Am J Cardiol 1974; 33:596–603.

71. Olshansky B, Okumura K, Hess P, Henthorn R, Waldo A L. Use of procainamide with rapid atrial pacing for successful conversion of atrial flutter to sinus rhythm. J Am Coll Cardiol 1988; 11(2):359–64.

72. Goldman M J. Combined quinidine and procaine amide treatment for chronic atrial fibrillation. Am Heart J 1957; 54:742–5.

73. Wellens H J, Braat P, Gorgels A P, Bar F W. Use of procainamide in patients with Wolff-Parkinson-White syndrome to disclose a short refractory period of the accessory pathway. Am J Cardiol 1982; 50:1087–9.

74. Brugada P, Dassen W R, Braat P, Gorgels A P, Wellens H J. Value of the ajmaline-procainamide test to predict the effect of long-term oral amiodarone on the antegrade effective refractory period of the accessory pathway in the Wolff-Parkinson-White syndrome. Am J Cardiol 1983; 52:70–72.

75. Eldar M, Ruder M A, Davis J C, Abbot J A, Seger J, Griffin J C, Scheinman M. Procainamide induced incessant supraventricular tachycardia in the Wolff-Parkinson-White syndrome. PACE 1986; 9:652–9.

76. Kayden H J, Brodie B B, Steele J M. Procainamide: a review. Circulation 1957; 15:118–26.

77. McCord M C, Taguchi J T. A study of the effect of procaine amide hydrochloride in supraventricular arrhythmias. Circulation 1951; 4:387–93.

78. Giardina E G V, Dreyfuss J, Bigger J T, Shaw J T, Schreiber E C. Metabolism of procainamide in normal and cardiac subjects. Clin Pharmacol Ther 1976; 19:339–51.

79. Graffner C, Johnsson G, Sjogren J. Pharmacokinetics of procainamide intravenously and orally as conventional and slow-release tablets. Clin Pharmacol Ther 1975; 17:414–23.

80. Giardina E G V, Fenster P E, Bigger J T, Mayersohn D, Marcus F I. Efficacy, plasma concentrations and adverse effects of a new sustained release procainamide preparation. Am J Cardiol 1980; 46:855–61.

81. Koch-Weser J, Klein S M. Procainamide dosage schedules, plasma concentrations and clinical effects. JAMA 1971; 215:1454–60.

82. Koch-Weser J, Klein S W, Foo-Canto LL, Kastor J A, DeSanctis R W. Antiarrhythmic prophylaxis with procainamide in acute myocardial infarction. N Engl J Med 1969; 218:1253–60.

83. Kosowsky B D, Taylor J, Lown B, Ritchie. Long-term use of procaine amide following acute myocardial infarction. Circulation 1973; 42:1204–10.

84. Karlsson, E. Procainamide and phenytoin. Comparative study of their antiarrhythmic effects at apparent therapeutic plasma levels. Br Heart J 1975; 3:731–40.

85. Jelinek M V, Lohrbauer L, Lown B. Antiarrhythmic drug therapy for sporadic ventricular arrhythmias. Circulation 1974; 49:659–66.

86. Winkle R A. Antiarrhythmic drug effect mimicked by spontaneous variability of ventricular ectopy. Circulation 1978; 57:1116–21.

87. Morganroth J, Michelson E L, Horowitz L N, Josephson ME, Pearlman AS, Dunkman WB. Limitations of routine long-term electrocardiographic monitoring to assess ventricular ectopic frequency. Circulation 1978; 58:408–14.

88. Sami M, Harrison D C, Kramer H, Houston N, Shimasaki C, Debusk RF. Antiarrhythmic efficacy of encainide and quinidine: validation of a model for drug assessment. Am J Cardiol 1981; 48:147–56.

89. Zipes D, Troup P J. New antiarrhythmic agents. Am J Cardiol 1978; 41:1005–24.

90. Podrid P J, Lyakishev A, Lown B, Mazur. Ethmozine, a new antiarrhythmic drug for suppressing ventricular premature complexes. Circulation 1980; 61:450–7.

91. Myerburg R J, Kessler K M, Kiem I, Pefkaras K C, Conde C A, Cooper D, Castellanos A. Relationship between plasma levels of procainamide, suppression of premature ventricular complexes and prevention of recurrent ventricular tachycardia. Circulation 1981; 64:280–9.

92. Dreyfuss J, Bigger J T, Cohen A I, Schreiber E C. Metabolism of procainamide in rhesus monkey and man. Clin Pharmacol Ther 1972; 13(3):366–71.

93. Dreyfuss J, Ross J J, Schreiber E C. Absorption, excretion, and biotransformation of procainamide $_{14}C$ in the dog and rhesus monkey. Arzneimittelforsch 1971; 21:948–51.

94. Karlsson, E. Plasma levels of procaine amide after administration of conventional and sustained-release tablets. Eur J Clin Pharmacol 1973; 6:245–50.

95. Giardina E G V, Raby K, Freilich D, Vita J, Brem R, Louie M. Time course of alpha-1-acid glycoprotein and its relation to myocardial enzymes. Am J Cardio 1985; 56:262–5.

96. Galeazzi R L, Sheiner L B, Lockwood T, Benet L. The renal elimination of procainamide. Clin Pharmacol Ther 1976; 19:55–62.

97. Weily H S, Genton E. Pharmacokinetics of procainamide. Arch Intern Med 1972; 130:366–9.

98. Dumeric DA, Silverman N H, Tobias S, Golbus M S. Transplacental cardioversion of fetal supraventricular tachycardia with procainamide. N Engl J Med 1982; 307:1128–31.

99. Ruo T, Thenot J P, Stec G, Atkinson A J. Plasma concentrations of desethyl N-acetylprocainamide in patients treated with procainamide and N-acetylprocainamide. Ther Drug Monit 1981; 3(3):231–7.

100. Raehl C L, Moorthy A V, Beirne G J. Procainamide pharmacokinetics in patients on continuous ambulatory peritoneal dialysis. Nephron 1986; 1944(3):191–4.

101. Drayer D E, Lowenthal D T, Woosley R L, Nies A S, Schwartz A, Reidenberg M M. Cumulation of N-acetylprocainamide, an active metabolite of procainamide in patients with impaired renal function. Clin Pharmacol Ther 1977; 22:63–9.

102. Strong J M, Dutcher J S, Lee W K, Atkinson A J. Pharmacokinetics in man of the N-acetylated metabolite of procainamide. J Pharmacokinet Biopharm 1975; 3:223–35.

103. Vlasses P H, Ferguson R K, Rocci M L, Raja R M, Porter R S, Greenspan A M. Lethal accumulation of procainamide metabolite in severe renal insufficiency. Am J Nephrol 1986; 6(2):112–6.

104. Lima J J, Kuritzky P M, Schentag J J, Jusko W J. Fetal uptake and neonatal disposition of procainamide and its deacetylated metabolite: a case report. Pediatrics 1978; 61:491–3.

105. Roden D M, Reele S B, Higgins R F, Wilkinson G R, Smith R F, Oates J A, Woosley R L. 1980. Antiarrhythmic efficacy, pharmacokinetics and safety of N-acetylprocainamide in human subjects: comparison with procainamide. Am J Cardiol 1980; 46:463–8.

106. Dutcher J S, Strong J S, Lucas S V, Lee W K, Atkinson A J. Procainamide and N-acetylprocainamide kinetics investigated simultaneously with stable isotope methodology. Clin Pharmacol Ther 1977; 22:447–57.

107. Atkinson A J, Lee W K, Qui M L, Kusher W, Nevin M J, Strong J M. Dose-ranging trial of N-acetylprocainamide in patients with premature ventricular contractions. Clin Pharmacol Ther 1977; 21:575–87.

108. Winkle R A, Jaillon P, Kates R E, Peters F. Clinical pharmacology and antiarrhythmic efficacy of N-acetylprocainamide Am J Cardiol 1981; 47:123–30.

109. Kluger J, Leech S, Reidenberg M M, Lloyd V, Drayer D E. Long-term antiarrhythmic therapy with acetylprocainamide. Am J Cardiol 1981; 48:1124–32.

110. Leahey E B, Reiffel J A, Giardina E G V, Bigger J T. The effect of quinidine and other oral antiarrhythmic drugs on serum digoxin: a prospective study. Ann Intern Med 1980; 92:605–8.

111. Windle J, Prystowsky E N, Miles W M, Heger J J. Pharmacokinetics and electrophysiologic interactions of amiodarone and procainamide. Clin Pharmacol Ther 1987; 41.603–10.

112. Christian C D, Meredith C G, Speeg K V. Cimetidine inhibits renal procainamide clearance. Clin Pharmacol Ther 1984; 36(2):221–7.

113. Somogyi A, Bochner F. Dose and concentration dependent effect of ranitidine on procainamide disposition and renal clearance in man. Br J Clin Pharmacol 1984; 18(2):175–81.

114. Ochs H R, Carstens G, Roberts G M, Greenblatt DJ. Metoprolol or propranolol does not alter the kinetics of procainamide. J Cardiovasc Pharmacol 1983; 5:392–5.

115. Weidler D J, Garg D C, Jallard N S, McFarland M A. The effect of long-term propranolol administration on the pharmacokinetics of procainamide in humans Clin Pharmacol Ther 1981; 29:289.

116. Olsen H, Mørland J. Ethanol-induced increase in procainamide acetylation in man. Br J Clin Pharmacol 1982; 13:203–8.

117. Giardina E G V. Tricyclic antidepressants in the 80s: electrocardiographic and antiarrhythmic effects of imipramine in patients treated for ventricular arrhythmias. Cardiovasc Rev Rep 1987; 8(9):21–5.

118. Wynn J, Miura D S, Torres V, Flowers D, Keefe D, Williams S, Somberg J C. Electrophysiologic evaluation of the antiarrhythmic effects of N-acetylprocainamide for ventricular tachycardia secondary to coronary artery disease. Am J Cardiol 1985; 56(13):877–81.

119. Dangman K H, Hoffman B F. In vivo and in vitro antiarrhythmic and arrhythmogenic effects of N-acetylprocainamide. J Pharmacol Exp Ther 1981; 217:851–62.

120. Chow M J, Piergies A A, Bowsher D J, Murphy J J, Kushner W, Ruo T I, Asada A, Talano J V, Atkinson A J. Torsade de pointes induced by N-acetylprocainamide. J Am Coll Cardiol 1984; 4:621–4.

121. Ludden T M, Crawford M H, Kennedy G. N-acetylprocainamide kinetics during intravenous infusions and subsequent oral doses in patients with coronary artery disease and ventricular arrhythmias. Pharmacotherapy 1985; 5:11–5.

122. Connolly S J, Kates R A. Clinical pharmacokinetics of N-acetylprocainamide. Clin Pharmacokinet 1982; 7(3):206–20.

123. Austen W G, Moran J M. Cardiac and peripheral vascular effects of lidocaine and procainamide. Am J Cardiol 1965; 16:701–7.

124. Folle L, Aviado D. The cardiopulmonary effects of quinidine and procainamide. J Pharmacol Exp Ther 1966; 154:92–101.

125. Helfant R H, Scherlag B, Damato A N. Use of diphenylhydantoin sodium to dissociate the effects of procainamide on automaticity and conduction in the normal and arrhythmic heart. Am J Cardiol 1967; 20:820–5.

126. Reidy T J, Upshaw J D. Procainamide-induced agranulocytosis. South Med J 1984; 77(12):1582–4.

127. Ellrodt A G, Murata G H, Riedinger M S, Stewart M E, Mochizuki C, Gray R. Severe neutropenia associated with sustained-release procainamide. Ann Intern Med 1984; 100(2):197–201.

128. Bellet S, Hamdan G, Somlyo A, Lara R. A reversal of the cardiotoxic effects of procaine amide by molar sodium lactate. Am J Med Sci 1959; 237:177–89.

129. Wisenberg G, Zawadowski A G, Gebhardt V A, Pratof S, Goddard M D, Nichol P M, Rechnitzer P A, Gryte-Becker B. Effects on ventricular function of disopyramide, procainamide, and quinidine as determined by radionuclide angiography. Am J Cardiol 1984; 53:1292–7.

130. Ladd A T. Procainamide induced lupus erythematosus. N Engl J Med 1962; 67:1357–8.

131. London B L, Pincus I. Reversible lupus-like illness induced by procainamide. Am Heart J 1966; 71:806–8.

132. Weisbart R H, Yee W S, Colburn K K, Whang S H, Heng M D, Boucek R J. Antiguanosine antibodies: a new marker for procainamide-induced systemic lupus erythematosus. Ann Intern Med 1986; 104(3):310–3.

133. Rubin R L, Nusinow S R, Johnson A D, Rubenson D S, Curd J G, Tan E M. Serologic changes during induction of lupus-like disease by procainamide. Am J Med 1986; 80(5):999–1002.

134. Kleinman S, Nelson R, Smith L, Goldfinger D. Positive direct antiglobulin tests and immune hemolytic anemia in patients receiving procainamide. N Engl J Med 1984; 311(13):809–12.

135. Giardina E G V, Stein R M, Bigger J T. The relationship between the metabolism of procainamide and sulfamethazine. Circulation 1977; 55:388–94.

136. Reidenberg M M, Drayer D E, Levy M M, Warner H. Polymorphic acetylation of procainamide in man. Clin Pharmacol Ther 1975; 17:722–30.

137. Woosley R L, Drayer D E, Reidenberg M M, Nies A S, Carr K, Oates J A. Effect of acetylator phenotype on the rate at which procainamide induces antinuclear antibodies and the lupus syndrome. N Engl J Med 1978; 298:1157–9.

138. Alarcon-Segovia D. Drug-induced lupus syndromes. Mayo Clin Proc 1969; 44:664–81.

139. Giardina E G V. Procainamide: clinical pharmacology and efficacy against ventricular arrhythmias. Ann NY Acad Sci 1984; 432: 177–89.

140. Velebit V, Podrid P, Lown B, Cohen B, Graboys T. Aggravation and provocation of ventricular arrhythmias by antiarrhythmic drugs. Circulation 1982; 65:886–94.

25

Disopyramide

Betty I. Sasyniuk

McGill University Faculty of Medicine
Montreal, Quebec, Canada

Teresa Kus

Hôpital du Sacre-Coeur de Montréal
Montreal, Quebec, Canada

INTRODUCTION

Disopyramide was developed in the course of a screening program designed to develop a new antiarrhythmic agent as an alternative to quinidine or procainamide, which were the main agents available in 1962. Mokler and Van Arman (1) first studied the pharmacology of this new agent, and Sekiya and Vaughan Williams (2) were the first to test its electrophysiologic actions in isolated cardiac tissue. Even at this early stage it was known that the effects of disopyramide on the heart depend critically upon the autonomic tone present at the time the drug is administered. Its main electrophysiologic effects in slowing the upstroke velocity of the action potential, lengthening the terminal phase of repolarization, and depressing automaticity were also established early. Disopyramide has been classified as a class 1A antiarrhythmic drug together with quinidine and procainamide (3,4). It is important to recognize, however, that although all three drugs have many electrophysiologic characteristics in common disopyramide differs in many important respects.

BASIC PHARMACOLOGY: ELECTROPHYSIOLOGIC EFFECTS ON ISOLATED CARDIAC TISSUES

SA Node

Disopyramide has dual actions on sinus nodal cells: a direct depressant action, causing a slowing of heart rate, and an indirect acceleratory action mediated by disopyramide's anticholinergic action (5–9). The response to these dual actions depends on the underlying cholinergic tone of the tissue and on the concentration of drug. Katoh et al. (7) found that disopyramide has a direct depressant effect on normal rabbit sinus nodal cells at the upper therapeutic and toxic levels that is enhanced during cholinergic blockade, while disopyramide's acceleratory action appears at much lower concentrations and only during cholinergic stimulation. Similar dual actions were observed by Mirro et al. (10) in guinea pig right atrial preparations.

Large doses of disopyramide injected directly into the cannulated sinus node artery of the isolated dog atrium produced a relatively mild negative chronotropic effect when compared to other antiarrhythmic drugs (8). The major mechanisms of sinus slowing in all species are a marked prolongation of sinus nodal action potential duration and a reduction in the slope of diastolic depolarization (5,7).

The depressant effect on the sinus node has been shown to be mediated largely by a reduction in the magnitude of the potassium outward current and a reduction in the magnitude and slowing of the kinetics of the slow inward current (5). The hyperpolarization-activated inward current (pacemaker current) was also reduced (5). Alteration in atrial cyclic AMP has been proposed to partly mediate the depression of automaticity (9).

The direct depressant effects of disopyramide on sinus automaticity are much less pronounced than its effects on sinoatrial conduction and refractoriness (11).

Atrial Muscle

Disopyramide has dual actions on pacemaker activity in right atrial preparations (10). Moklar and Van Arman (1) showed that disopyramide abolishes the effects of vagal stimulation to slow the atrial rate in anesthetized dogs and blocks the negative chronotropic effects of acetylcholine in isolated perfused rabbit hearts. Studies in isolated guinea pig atria suggest that the anticholinergic properties of disopyramide can be accounted for by a direct interaction with muscarinic receptors similar to but less potent than that of atropine (10). Mirro et al. (10) showed that disopyramide antagonized the negative chronotropic effects of muscarinic receptor activation. This anticholinergic effect, which increased automaticity, predominated over the direct rate slowing effect. Nakajima et al. (12) examined the effects of disopyramide on acetycholine (ACh)-induced K^+ channel current in isolated atrial myocytes and concluded that the most likely mechanism for its anticholinergic effect was a specific blockade of agonist binding to the muscarinic acetylcholine receptor. Both Nakajima et al. (12) and Mirro et al. (10) showed that the anticholinergic effects occur at concentrations well within the range achieved in plasma of patients treated with this drug and

lower than those required to produce a direct membrane effect.

Disopyramide has been shown to significantly depress impulse conduction and to increase action potential duration and effective refractory period in rabbit atria (13,14). Prolongation of action potential duration in atrial tissue is much more pronounced than in either Purkinje or ventricular muscle fibers. In atrial muscle the plateau of the action potential is unaltered; only the terminal phase of repolarization is prolonged. Lowering the extracellular potassium concentration does not alter the effects of disopyramide on upstroke velocity in atrial fibers but enhances its effects on duration (14). The anticholinergic effect in atrial tissue prevents the marked shortening of action potential duration and effective refractory period produced by acetylcholine. Thus both the direct and indirect effects are to increase the action potential duration and effective refractory period.

AV node

The direct effect of disopryamide is to slow the rate of spontaneously beating rabbit atrioventricular (AV) nodal pacemakers (13). This effect is due largely to a prolongation of action potential duration and partly to a reduction in the slope of diastolic depolarization. Disopyramide also slows conduction and prolongs the functional refractory period in the AV node (15). Its indirect effect antagonizes its direct effects on the node.

Ventricular Conduction Tissue and Working Myocardium

Effects on $\dot{V}_{max}$

The primary antiarrhythmic effect of disopyramide in ventricular tissue is block of sodium channels. Disopyramide, like other class 1 antiarrhythmic drugs, depresses the maximum rate of depolarization $\dot{V}_{max}$ in Purkinje fibers and ventricular muscle in a frequency-and voltage-dependent manner (16–18). Both refractory period and conduction time are prolonged at therapeutic concentrations and normal heart rates.

The modulated receptor hypothesis was proposed by Hondeghem and Katzung (19,20) to explain the antiarrhythmic actions of class 1 drugs based on their interactions with sodium channels. According to this hypothesis the actions of these drugs are modulated by different binding affinities to various states of the sodium channel. The channels cycle through three states: a rested state during diastole when the channels are available for activation but have not yet opened; an activated state during the upstroke of the action potential when the channels are open allowing sodium ions to pass; and an inactivated state during the plateau of the action potential when the channels are closed and unavailable for activation until the resting state is assumed. Drugs bind to the channels intermittently as they cycle through the three states. Sodium channel blocking drugs have different affinities for the various states of the channel. An alternative model, called the guarded receptor hypothesis, assumes that the drug-receptor affinity is constant but access to the receptor depends on the state of the channel gates (21). The channel gates restrict access to the binding sites.

In rabbit Purkinje fibers therapeutic concentrations of disopyramide did not cause resting (tonic) block at membrane potentials ranging from -100 to -65 mV (22). Thus as with most antiarrhythmic drugs (20) disopyramide has a low affinity for the rested state of the channel.

Several lines of evidence suggest that disopyramide predominantly blocks activated Na channels. In voltage-clamped rabbit Purkinje fibers the time course of development of use-dependent block was not significantly influenced by the duration of the depolarizing pulse (22). In single guinea pig ventricular myocytes multiple short clamp pulses caused a greater $\dot{V}_{max}$ reduction than a single prolonged clamp pulse in the presence of disopyramide (23,24). No block was observed in the absence of stimulation even when the membrane was depolarized by conditioning prepulses. These data suggest that most of the use-dependent block by disopyramide is associated with activation.

Studies in cell-attached membrane patches in rabbit ventricular myocytes provide further support for block of activated channels (25).

Intracellular forms of antiarrhythmic drugs can gain access to the activated channel via an aqueous pathway during depolarization (during the brief period of the upstroke of the action potential). During maintained depolarization (during the plateau of the action potential) drugs can access the receptor site through the hydrophobic or lipid membrane phase (26). Two different hypotheses have been advanced to explain this phase of drug access. According to the modulated receptor hypothesis (20) this represents block of the inactivated state of the sodium channel. According to the guarded receptor hypothesis (21) this represents blocking access to channels whose m gates are open. Courtney (27) suggested that drug access through the lipid membrane phase is limited by size. Kodama et al. (23,24) found that all the activation blockers tended to be larger molecules than inactivation blockers. Both quinidine and disopyramide are among the largest of the class I drugs. Only class IC drugs are larger. Existing evidence suggests that class IC drugs are also activation blockers (23,24). The pathway accessible during maintained depolarization may not be able to accomodate drugs of a large dimension, such as disopyramide.

Diastolic recovery from disopyramide block occurs slowly. The recovery time constant of $\dot{V}_{max}$ in multicellular tissue preparations has been variously reported to range from 12 sec to as long as 197 sec (16,17,22,28–32). Disopyramide has a peculiar voltage dependence of recovery from block that may account for the discrepancies in the time constants reported in the literature. Block by antiarrhythmic drugs is generally assumed to be relieved by hyperpolarization, as has been demonstrated for lidocaine (33) and quinidine (34). However, the opposite is true for disopyramide. Gruber and Carmeliet (22) showed that recovery from use-dependent block is slowed at membrane potentials more negative than -75 mV. The time constant of recovery ranged from approximately 75 sec at -95 mV to approximately 10 sec at -75 mV. Kojima et al. (28) showed that the time constant of $\dot{V}_{max}$ recovery decreased from an average of 197 sec to an average of 28 sec when the extracellular potassium concentration was increased from 2.7 to 8.1 mM potassium in guinea pig ventricular tissue. Recovery of $\dot{V}_{max}$ has also been shown to be a function of pH (22). Recovery is accelerated when the pH of the external solution is increased. For disopyramide, unblocking may occur predominantly via the hydrophilic pathway, as has been suggested for quaternary drugs (35). Gruber and Carmeliet (22) showed that not only blocking of sodium channels by disopyramide but also unblocking is facilitated by opening of the sodium channels. Recovery from use-dependent block is slower at hyperpolarized potentials but can be accelerated by repeating the depolarizing pulse, suggesting that unblocking of sodium channels is also activation dependent. Activation trapping and activation unblocking have now been shown to occur with a number of different drugs, most of which have extremely long time constants of diastolic recovery (34,36–38).

The opening of sodium channels plays a role in the modulation of the time courses of both block development and recovery for a number of different disopyramide analogs (37,38).

Based on its recovery kinetics disopyramide must be considered as belonging to the kinetically slow group of drugs. At clinical heart rates unblocking from the closed state must be a relatively unimportant route of unblocking with disopyramide since the slow recovery process yields too little unblocking during one diastolic interval. Thus activation unblocking must be significant under clinical conditions. Activation blocking and unblocking would endow disopyramide with at least one potentially useful feature. The drug produces greater block of sodium channels during tachycardias than at normal heart rates. However, the potential exists for enhanced toxicity. Small changes in membrane potential can markedly alter activation unblock. A therapeutic concentration of drug at a given heart rate and membrane potential can easily become toxic at an increased heart rate or serum potassium since availability for activation unblocking decreases with depolarization. This may partly account for instances of marked widening of the QRS complex and precipitation of ventricular tachycardia during therapy.

Effects on Action Potential Duration

Disopyramide exerts complex effects on action potential duration in Purkinje fibers depending on the proximity of the fibers to ventricular muscle (initial action potential duration value) and external potassium concentration (39,40). The drug prolongs total duration in fibers that have short durations to begin with and are closely apposed to ventricular muscle and tends to shorten durations in gate Purkinje fibers, which are most remote from ventricular muscle. Thus action potential durations become more uniform throughout the ventricles. This action is less apparent at low extracellular potassium concentrations (40). The drug has a tendency to equalize action potential durations between normal and infarcted areas in infarcted ventricular preparations (41,42). Like other class I antiarrhythmic drugs, disopyramide shifts the curve describing the restitution of action potential duration in canine Purkinje fibers (43). However, unlike the class IB drugs, it lengthens the premature action potential duration without changing the effective refractory period or the kinetics of restitution. This effect was postulated to reduce the differences in duration of action potentials during propagation of early premature impulses.

The variable effects of disopyramide on action potential duration are probably due to its effects on a variety of ionic currents that determine action potential duration. Disopyramide has been shown to depress both the calcium current and the delayed outward potassium current at therapeutic concentrations (32). At very high concentrations disopyramide decreases the transient outward current and reduces the tetrodotoxin (TTX)-sensitive slow component of the sodium current (44). Since the contribution of these currents to the generation of the action potential varies from one tissue to another this may account for the unpredictable effects of disopyramide in both shortening and prolonging duration. Disopyram-

DISOPYRAMIDE 5 μM

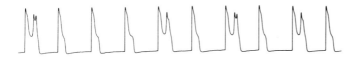

pacing   DISOPYRAMIDE 5 μM + MND 10 μM

2 sec

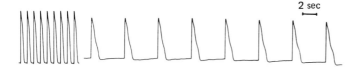

Figure 1 Typical example of triggered activity due to high membrane potential early afterdepolarizations induced by 5 μM disopyramide in canine Purkinje fibers in the presence of hypokalemia (2.7 mM) and extreme bradycardia. (Top) Early afterdepolarizations and triggered activity after 1 min of steady-state stimulation at a basic cycle length of 5 sec. Pacing at a cycle length of 1 sec abolished triggered activity (bottom left). When disopyramide was combined with its metabolite, MND, triggered activity did not occur even after 5 min of stimulation at a cycle length of 5 sec.

ide also causes prolongation of slow-response action potentials in neonatal rat ventricular cells (45).

Disopyramide exerts its anticholinergic effects in the ventricular conducting system as well. This action is manifest only on action potential duration. Acetylcholine normally antagonizes the actions of isoproterenol to shorten action potential in canine Purkinje fibers. Mirro et al. (46) showed that this effect of acetylcholine was antagonized by disopyramide at therapeutic concentrations. Quinidine had similar effects but only at very high concentrations.

The manifestation of the class III action of disopyramide in both Purkinje fibers and ventricular muscle is favored by low concentrations of drug, low extracellular potassium concentrations, and low stimulation rates (the reverse of its class I actions) (16,29,40,47).

Torsade de pointes arrhythmias have been attributed to drug-induced early afterdepolarizations and triggered activity in association with prolongation of action potential duration in cardiac Purkinje fibers by class IA and III drugs (48,49). Disopyramide has been shown to induce early afterdepolarizations and triggered activity in Purkinje fibers in association

with hypokalemia and slow heart rates (49,47). Early afterdepolarizations, like torsade de pointes, arose during terminal repolarization and were readily reversed by increasing the stimulation rate (Fig. 1). Exposure to mexiletine or to mono-N-dealkylated disopyramide (MND), the major metabolite of disopyramide, either prevented or decreased the incidence of triggered activity (49,50). Opposite effects on action potential duration of MND to that of the parent compound may account for the lessor incidence of torsade de pointes with this drug than with quinidine (48). The major metabolites of quinidine are all capable of inducing triggered activity in canine Purkinje fibers (51).

Stereospecificity

Disopyramide is commercially available as a racemic mixture of two optical isomers, R(-) and S(+). Mirro et al. (52) and Kidwell et al. (53) compared the electrophysiologic effects of these enantiomers in canine cardiac Purkinje fibers and observed directionally opposite effects on action potential duration but similar effects on depolarization. The R(-)-isomer shortened action potential duration and refractoriness, but the S(+)-isomer prolonged duration. Kidwell et al. (54) obtained indirect evidence to suggest that the increase in action potential duration by the $S(+)$-enantiomer was mediated by a stereospecific inhibition of an outward repolarizing current. In the study of Mirro et al. (52), racemic disopyramide prolonged action potential duration to the same extent as its $S(+)$ optical isomer. They suggested that the $S(+)$-isomer associates with higher affinity with a membrane site that results in repolarization delay.

Mirro et al. (46) also reported stereospecific interactions of disopyramide with muscarinic cholinergic receptors in atrium and ventricular muscle fibers. The $S(+)$-isomer was approximately three times more potent than the $R(-)$-isomer in antagonizing the electrophysiologic effects of cholinergic stimulation in isolated guinea pig right atria. A similar potency was observed in receptor binding studies. In anesthetized closed-chest dogs l-disopyramide was more potent than d-disopyramide in prolonging sinus cycle length and AV nodal refractoriness (55). This is consistent with the increased anticholinergic effect of the d-enantiomer, which antagonizes its direct effects. Thus the stereochemistry of disopyramide appears to influence both the direct effect of disopyramide on repolarizing current and its indirect anticholinergic effects.

The depression of upstroke velocity and conduction in Purkinje fibers are not stereodependent (52,53). Depression of left ventricular function is also not stereodependent (54) Racemic disopyramide and its enantiomes produced similar negative inotropic effects in the canine blood superfusion model (54).

Effects on Pacemaker Activity

Disopyramide depresses automaticity in normal spontaneously beating Purkinje fibers (39). The drug produces a concentration-dependent decrease in the slope of diastolic depolarization and a lengthening of action potential duration in automatic fibers. The drug also depresses automaticity in depolarized Purkinje fibers surviving on the endocardial surface of transmural infarcts 24 hr after coronary artery occlusion (41).

Electrophysiologic Effects of MND, the Major Metabolite of Disopyramide

Electrophysiologic studies of MND have demonstrated that it is an active compound in cardiac muscle. It has been shown to reverse experimentally induced atrial fibrillation in dogs (56) and to diminish the maximal pacing frequency of canine atrial tissue (57,58). In canine Purkinje fibers MND produced a rate-dependent depression of $\dot{V}_{max}$ and conduction at clinically relevant concentrations and stimulation rates (50,59). The recovery time constant was much faster than that of disopyramide (50,59). Like disopyramide, MND did not produce any voltage shift in the $\dot{V}_{max}$-membrane potential relationship. Unlike the parent compound, MND shortens action potential duration in Purkinje fibers. In ventricular muscle action potential duration as well as effective refractory period is prolonged.

MND probably plays a significant role in both the antiarrhythmic and toxic effects of disopyramide. Both compounds have an additive effect on $\dot{V}_{max}$ and effective refractory period. These actions should be beneficial in the abolition and prevention of reentrant ventricular arrhythmias. However, MND may contribute to toxicity if sodium channel block is excessive. At clinically relevant heart rates unblocking from sodium channels is minimal for both disopyramide and MND. An increase in the concentration of metabolite can readily lead to a marked slowing of conduction. Opposite effects of the metabolite on action potential duration may considerably reduce the incidence of disopyramide-induced torsade de pointes arrhythmias.

BASIC PHARMACOLOGY: ANTIARRHYTHMIC EFFECTS IN EXPERIMENTAL ANIMALS

Disopyramide has significant effects against a variety of experimental arrhythmias of both atrial and ventricular origin.

Atrial Arrhythmias

Mokler and Van Arman (1) showed that disopyramide is two to three times more potent than quinidine in abolishing atrial arrhythmias induced by aconitine and electrical stimulation. Bertrix et al. (60) compared the efficacy of disopyramide with that of verapamil and propranolol on atrial fibrillation induced in the dog heart by combined electrical stimulation and intraaortic injection of acetylcholine. Only disopyramide prevented atrial fibrillation and reversed the effects of acetylcholine on the monophasic action potential.

Ventricular Arrhythmias

Mokler and Van Arman (1) showed that disopyramide was more potent than quinidine in abolishing ventricular arrhythmias induced by ouabain.

The drug has been studied in the acute, subacute, and chronic phases of ischemia. Kus and Sasyniuk (61) showed that disopyramide is effective in abolishing ventricular arrhythmias in a conscious canine myocardial infarction model in which infarction was the result of an occluding thrombus.

Disopyramide decreases the inhomogeneity of refractoriness between normal and infarcted myocardium in the dog during early ischemia (62). Studies on ventricular tissue from both normal and infarcted regions of canine hearts obtained 24–48 hr after coronary artery occlusion showed that disopyramide has different membrane effects on Purkinje fibers from normal and infarcted myocardium, the net effect being a more homogenous repolarization within the infarcted area and a decrease in the disparity of refractoriness between normal and infarcted tissue (42). Whenever disopyramide prolonged refractory periods more in normal regions than in infarcted regions, thereby reducing the difference in refractory periods between normal and infarcted areas, it prevented initiation of reentrant responses in infarcted preparations. Whenever conduction was slowed through the infarcted region much more than refractory period was prolonged in the normal region, disopyramide was ineffective and allowed reentry to occur, albeit at longer coupling intervals (42). Thus the effectiveness or lack thereof of disopyramide is highly dependent upon a balance between its

effect on conduction versus its effect on refractoriness. This may explain the facilitation by low concentrations of drug of reentrant ventricular arrhythmias resulting from programmed electrical stimulation in the presence of chronic myocardial ischemia (63,64).

The drug was not very effective in preventing reentrant arrhythmias resulting from programmed electrical stimulation in the presence of chronic myocardial ischemia at therapeutic concentrations in conscious dogs (63–65). In this model of chronic infarction disopyramide selectively increased refractoriness and depressed conduction in the ischemic area. Disopyramide prevented the induction of VT in only 20–40% of animals and increased the tachycardia cycle length in others.

Disopyramide significantly lowered the incidence of reperfusion arrhythmias as well as the incidence of arrhythmias occurring in the occlusion period preceding reperfusion. In these experiments the drug was administered before occlusion and serum levels above the normal therapeutic range were necessary for efficacy (66).

CLINICAL PHARMACOLOGY

Effects on Normal Human Electrocardiogram

The effects of disopyramide on the normal human electrocardiogram are variable and minor. Usual oral doses have been reported to have little effect on the normal resting sinus rate (67–69). Variable increases in the PR interval and QRS or QT duration have been observed (1,67,70). However, the increase in QRS duration rarely exceeds 20% at concentrations in the therapeutic range and the increase in QTc interval is of lesser magnitude than that produced by quinidine (71).

Acute Effects in Humans: Programmed Extrastimulation Studies

Effects of disopyramide on the electrophysiologic properties of supraventricular tissue are the result of a direct depressant action and its indirect anticholinergic effects. Thus when given intravenously (1–2 mg/kg) to patients with various types of heart disease, the sinus node recovery time was shortened, the atrial effective and functional refractory periods were prolonged, and there was little effect on or a shortening of the refractory period of the AV node (68,72–76). When administered after atropine pretreatment (0.025 mg/kg intravenously), however, disopyramide prolonged sinus node recovery time and spontaneous sinus cycle length, lengthened the effective refractory period of the atrium, and prolonged the AH interval and the functional refractory period of the AV node (15).

In patients with sinus node dysfunction (75,77) disopyramide can prolong the sinus node recovery time dramatically (by 81–544%). This effect was seen, however, only in the subgroup of patients who manifested spontaneous sinus pauses and sinoatrial block (75).

In the presence of first-degree AV block, disopyramide has been reported to further depress retrograde but not anterograde conduction (78). Similarly, only retrograde conduction was decreased by drug in cases of dual AV nodal pathways. Anterograde slow and fast pathway conduction was unchanged (79).

In patients with paroxysmal atrial fibrillation in whom a programmed electrophysiologic stimulation technique was used to assess drug efficacy in preventing induction of arrhythmia, disopyramide (2 mg/kg intravenously) prolonged atrial effective and functional refractory periods. Furthermore, prolongation of refractory period was greater in the group (18 of 40 patients) in whom disopyramide completely prevented the electrical induction of atrial fibrillation (80).

Disopyramide has also been shown to be useful in the electrical termination of atrial flutter (81,82). In patients in atrial flutter, intravenous administration (3 mg/kg over 1 hr) prolonged the atrial effective refractory period. The drug prolonged the cycle length of the flutter by a greater amount, however, thus increasing the duration of the excitable gap by 55% (82). This suggests that the drug exerts its effect on atrial flutter cycle length predominantly by depressing conduction velocity

rather than by prolonging refractoriness. Furthermore, the widening of the excitable gap facilitates penetration of the reentry circuit and termination of the arrhythmia by overdrive pacing.

In patients with accessory atrioventricular pathways, disopyramide slows both anterograde and retrograde conduction through the pathway (83–86). It increases the cycle length of orthodromic reciprocating tachycardia primarily by its depressant effect on retrograde conduction (85,86). The drug also prolongs accessory pathway refractoriness and thus increases the minimum R-R interval of preexcited complexes during atrial fibrillation (84,85,87).

Induction of atrioventricular nodal reentry tachycardia by programmed stimulation is also prevented by disopyramide (79,86).

In the ventricle, disopyramide minimally but significantly prolongs His-Purkinje conduction time as reflected in the HV interval (68,88). Others have reported no change in the mean HV interval (15,67,73,83), but this result may reflect the small patient population or different drug doses used. An early study (88) reported no significant adverse effects of disopyramide in patients with bundle branch block. However, more recent work (89) in patients with bifascicular block with a history of syncope has demonstrated that in this setting intravenous disopyramide (2 mg/kg) can markedly prolong the AV interval (43%) and result in intra- or infra-Hisian second- or third-degree AV block, possibly requiring temporary pacing. Furthermore, the positive predictive value of such a result for later spontaneous development of high-grade AV block was 80%.

Finally, disopyramide variably prolongs (up to 20%) right ventricular effective and functional refractory periods (15,67,68,71,74, 75,83,88,90,91). Using the technique of monophasic action potential (MAP) recording during programmed stimulation, Endresen et al. (92) have reported that disopyramide increases the duration of MAP signals and also the right ventricular effective refractory period. This effect is greater on early premature action potentials than on steady-state action potentials. Conduction time through the ventricles of both normal and premature beats is also significantly prolonged.

Programmed extrastimulation studies assessing the acute efficacy of either intravenous or oral disopyramide administration in preventing ventricular tachycardia induction have found in general a similar efficacy compared to other class IA agents. Thus Benditt et al. (93) and Breithardt et al. (94) found disopyramide to be effective in 5 of 12 patients and Lerman et al. (95) demonstrated efficacy in 17 of 50 patients. However, there is not a good correlation between the efficacy of other class IA drugs and that of disopyramide. For example, although significant concordance of response and nonresponse was observed between procainamide and quinidine, neither of these agent's effects predicted the response to disopyramide against the induction of ventricular tachycardia or fibrillation (96). Similarly, in a recent study by Wyse et al. (71), the efficacy of quinidine or procainamide was not necessarily predictive of disopyramide efficacy against ventricular tachycardia induction. The cycle length of ventricular tachycardia, still inducible despite disopyramide therapy, is lengthened in comparison to control, however. This prolongation is linearly related to serum drug level (71,91).

Studies During Chronic Antiarrhythmic Therapy

Supraventricular Arrhythmias

The long-term efficacy of disopyramide administered chronically to patients with paroxysmal supraventricular tachycardia or paroxysmal atrial fibrillation was demonstrated by Bauman et al. (97) in patients responding initially to drugs as assessed by Holter monitoring or electrophysiologic study. Prevention of arrhythmia recurrence was maintained (23±16 months) in two-thirds of the population. Even higher long-term success against recurrence of paroxysmal atrial fibrillation (12 of 13 patients) was seen by Ito et al. (80) in those patients in whom drug prevented programmed stimulation induction of arrhythmia.

No significant difference in efficacy has been observed between quinidine and disopyramide against atrial ectopy (98). Similarly, no difference in efficacy over 6 months was seen between disopyramide and quinidine in maintaining sinus rhythm after cardioversion of atrial fibrillation (99); however, neither drug was much more effective than placebo. Low-dose disopyramide (300 mg) and procainamide (750 mg) were equally effective in preventing recurrences of paroxysmal supraventricular tachycardia in a double-blind crossover trial (100). Finally, disopyramide was less effective than amiodarone in maintaining asymptomatic status but not sinus rhythm in patients followed for up to 2 years for paroxysmal atrial flutter or fibrillation (101).

Ventricular Premature Contractions

As reviewed by Heel et al. (102), disopyramide in 17 uncontrolled studies was effective in reducing ventricular premature beat frequency in 65% of the studied population. In a crossover single-blind study with placebo, disopyramide was more effective in diminishing the number of premature ventricular beats (103). In comparison with other agents, oral disopyramide (600 mg daily) in short-term trials of 3–10 days has demonstrated efficacy equal to that of quinidine, procainamide, mexiletine, perhexilene, atenolol, tocainide, propafenone, and prajmaline but it was less effective than flecainide, dehydroquinidine, and ethmozine [as cited in reviews by Brogden and Todd (104) and Wilson and Wallace (105)]. Similar efficacy to propafenone in a randomized double-blind crossover trial with placebo of greater duration (2 weeks per treatment) was recently confirmed by Rabkin et al. (106). Furthermore, combination therapy with disopyramide and mexiletine has been shown (107) to be more effective (in 62% of patients) in smaller and better tolerated doses than individual drug administration (24% of patients receiving disopyramide alone and 14% receiving mexiletine alone).

Controlled-release formulations are comparable in efficacy to conventional capsules when crossed over with placebo (108). Maintained efficacy, tolerance, and patient compliance have been reported (109) against complex premature ventricular contractions.

Ventricular Tachycardia

Disopyramide administered chronically is effective in preventing the recurrence of spontaneous ventricular tachycardia. Thus in uncontrolled studies in which patients presented with frequent episodes of recurrent ventricular tachycardia and in which invasive electrophysiologic testing was not used to verify noninducibility on drug, disopyramide was nevertheless reported to diminish the recurrence rate or to eliminate further episodes (110–112). Follow-up of patients receiving disopyramide only following invasive electrophysiologic demonstration of noninducibility on drug therapy have confirmed its long-term efficacy. Thus, 4 of 5 patients in one study (93) and 9 of 11 patients in another (96) had no recurrence of ventricular tachycardia over 18 and 19 months, respectively. Long-term therapy with a combination of disopyramide and mexiletine shown effective in acute oral invasive testing in 7 of 12 patients prevented recurrence in 5 of these 7 over a follow-up of 42 ± 23 weeks (94).

Ventricular Arrhythmias Following Myocardial Infarction

The utility of disopyramide administration in patients presenting with myocardial infarction was recently reviewed by Brogden and Todd (104). Although disopyramide diminished the frequency of ventricular premature beats in comparison to placebo, it failed to decrease the incidence of ventricular tachycardia and fibrillation or of mortality in patients with acute myocardial infarction treated in coronary care units. A single study reported in 1977 (113) of patients admitted to an open ward with myocardial infarction demonstrated a significant decrease in in-hospital mortality in those patients receiving disopyramide compared to placebo. These results have not yet been confirmed by other investigators. Finally, the use of disopyramide as a prophylactic agent against sudden death following myocardial infarction after hospital discharge has not been addressed in long-term studies.

Pharmacokinetics

Experimental Animal Studies

Absorption and Bioavailability. The pharmacokinetics and steady-state myocardial uptake of disopyramide were determined in dogs after oral and intravenous administration of the phosphate salt (114,115). Both disopyramide and MND are rapidly absorbed and have a high absolute bioavailability (>70%) similar to that in humans.

Distribution and Protein Binding. Disopyramide is widely distributed in the body. In the dog heart the steady-state ventricular concentrations were twice those in plasma but in atrium they were similar to those in plasma (114). However, Patterson et al. (64) found disopyramide concentrations in canine myocardial tissue to be approximately four times the plasma concentration. In the rat the drug is rapidly taken up in the placenta and fetus and excreted in appreciable amounts in milk (116). Disopyramide concentrations in the placenta are six times that in maternal plasma but concentrations in the fetal heart are half the maternal plasma level 30 min after an intravenous dose. Drug levels in milk are three times higher than in plasma.

The apparent volume of distribution in the dog is about three times that in the human reflecting higher tissue uptake probably related to the high proportion of unbound drug present in the plasma (114).

Disopyramide is a basic antiarrhythmic drug that is almost exclusively bound to α_1-acid glycoprotein (117). Consequently it has been used as a model probe to study the behavior of α_1-acid glycoprotein and/or the plasma protein binding of basic drugs in certain disease states (118,119).

The pharmacologic effects of disopyramide are dependent upon free (unbound) drug concentrations (120). Disopyramide is unusual in that it exhibits saturable (nonlinear) protein binding in the therapeutic range of plasma concentrations (121). Thus the unbound fraction increases with total concentration. In the pig, free and total concentrations could be described by a two-compartment model with a

$T_{1/2}$ of approximately 2 hr. The free concentrations better estimated the kinetic parameters.

Serum protein binding of disopyramide is stereoselective. Stereoselective binding is species dependent (117). In gorilla, pig, and sheep the binding of $S(+)$-disopyramide is higher than that for $R(-)$-disopyramide. The opposite is true in cow serum. No stereoselective binding occurs in serum from the horse or goat. This has been attributed to a binding site located on albumin, in contrast to other species, including the human.

Metabolism and Elimination. Disopyramide is metabolized by N-dealkylation and arylhydroxylation to mono-N-dealkylated disopyramide and a pyrrolidone derivative. The former is the major pathway in dog; the latter occurs predominantly in the rat (114,122). In the dog both disopyramide and MND show similar pharmacokinetic characteristics. The metabolic process follows nonlinear kinetics.

Besides species differences in the metabolic pathway, stereoselective metabolism has also been established in laboratory animals (123–126). In the dog, the $S(+)$-disopyramide enantiomer metabolized more completely on first pass (123,124). The clearance of the $S(+)$-enantiomer is significantly greater than that of $R(-)$-enantiomer. The steady-state volumes of distribution of the two compounds were similar, resulting in a longer half-life for the $R(-)$-enantiomer. Different rates of clearance for the two enantiomers have also been demonstrated in the rabbit (125,126). In the pig, clearance of drug was three times greater than in the human. Otherwise the kinetics were similar to those in humans (121).

Clinical Studies

The clinical pharmacokinetics of disopyramide have been reviewed most recently by Brogden and Todd (104), Siddoway and Woosley (127), Karim et al. (128), and Campbell (128a).

Absorption and Bioavailability. Following oral administration of either the free base (Norpace, Searle) or phosphate salt (Rhythmodan, Roussel), absorption of disopyramide occurs rapidly and is essentially complete, and in general it appears that the two preparations are similar [see Brogden and Todd (104)]. The fraction of an oral dose compared with intravenous administration that reaches the systemic circulation is approximately 85%, reflecting a "first-pass" effect of 15% through the liver (129).

In healthy subjects peak plasma concentrations are achieved 1–2 hr following an oral dose using conventional capsules. Using a controlled-release preparation bioavailability is not significantly different, but peak levels occur 3–5 hrs following ingestion and there seems to be less intersubject variability in absorption (104,127). Administered to patients with cardiac arrhythmias, a low ratio of maximal concentration to trough concentration has been observed with the controlled-release preparation, suggesting the improved stability of plasma levels with this formulation (130). Peak plasma concentrations are lower in patients within the first 24 hr of acute myocardial infarction. This has been in part attributed to lower gastrointestinal absorption, possibly due to concurrent therapy with narcotic analgesics and antiemetics (104,131).

Distribution and Protein Binding. Disopyramide is widely distributed throughout the body. Following intravenous administration distribution is rapid, with a half-life of 3–15 mins (128). According to animal studies disopyramide is concentrated in fat, liver, spleen, and myocardial tissue, is taken up by the placenta and fetus, and is secreted in saliva and milk. The human fetal-maternal ratio of disopyramide has been estimated as about 0.80 (132). Disopyramide levels in human milk are also approximately equivalent to those in maternal plasma. However, *N*-monodesalkyldisopyramide, the major metabolite of disopyramide, tends to accumulate to levels sixfold greater than in maternal plasma (104,133,134).

The steady-state volume of distribution for total drug varies among normal subjects (0.5–1.2 l/kg), is dose and age dependent, and is diminished in congestive heart failure and, possibly, in end-stage renal failure (104,134). This variability in part reflects the interaction of disopyramide and serum proteins. Disopyramide binds almost exclusively to α_1-acid glycoprotein (AAG) and in minor amounts to albumin (135). Plasma protein binding is also stereoselective in humans (136,137). The binding of $S(+)$-disopyramide is higher than that of $R(-)$-disopyramide at similar unbound concentrations. Since binding is saturable (non-linear) in the therapeutic range of concentrations, the fraction of free (unbound) disopyramide increases with rising total concentration (138). Thus the amount of drug exerting a pharmacologic effect on body tissues can increase in excess of modest augmentation in dose. Furthermore, the concentration of AAG, being an acute-phase reactant, increases with acute myocardial infarction (139) and chronic renal failure requiring dialysis (140). Thus although total plasma concentration increases, the free fraction of drug is diminished (141). In contrast AAG concentration is less in cirrhosis (142,143) and during an exacerbation of nephrotic syndrome (144). The free fraction of drug is therefore increased. The mono-N-dealkylated metabolite, furthermore, binds competitively to AAG (69,145), thus displacing the more antiarrhythmically active parent compound. These interactions demonstrate the necessity of monitoring free rather than total drug concentration and the caution required in augmenting the dose to avoid a disproportionate increase in electrophysiologic or toxic effect.

Metabolism and Elimination. In the human, disopyramide is metabolized primarily by N-dealkylation to mono-N-dealkyldisopyramide. Significant accumulation occurs at doses greater than 3 mg/kg, and in some patients the plasma concentration of metabolite can exceed that of the parent drug (69,145). Metabolism is increased in patients receiving such hepatic microsomal enzyme inducers as rifampicin, phenytoin (146), and phenobarbitone (147). In these cases plasma levels of parent drug are markedly decreased. In contrast, in hepatic cirrhosis or following alcohol ingestion, metabolite formation is decreased (146). The major route of elimination is through the kidneys, and in the healthy human approximately 50% of drug is excreted unchanged, 20% as the mono-N-dealkylated metabolite, and 10% as other minor metabolites (69). The elimination half-life has been reported as 4–10 hr in normal subjects (148,149). This is prolonged in

elderly subjects (150). In patients with renal failure the renal clearance of disopyramide is correlated with creatinine clearance (151,152). Furthermore, nonrenal metabolic clearance may also be decreased (up to twofold) in inverse relation to the increase in AAG in this disease state (153). Finally, hemodialysis removes very little (less than 2.4%) of a dose of disopyramide (154). As a result of all these factors, the elimination half-life can be significantly prolonged (up to fourfold) in patients with creatinine clearance less than 40 ml/min (155) and necessitates a reduction in drug dose. Individual dose adjustment based on measurement of free disopyramide plasma concentration is necessary, however, because of the complexity and variability of disopyramide pharmacokinetics in renal failure. The clearance of disopyramide is not significantly affected by congestive heart failure uncomplicated by severe renal failure (156). After acute myocardial infarction, however, the clearance of disopyramide is initially high and diminishes with time following the acute event, possibly reflecting the increase in AAG and consequent decrease in free fraction of drug (157).

Elimination of disopyramide can be enhanced by resin (158) or by charcoal (159) hemoperfusion when necessary in cases of drug overdose. Gastrointestinal dialysis by means of multiple-dose administration of oral activated charcoal has also been demonstrated in healthy volunteers to markedly diminish plasma levels of both parent drug and metabolite and decrease their elimination half-life (160).

The importance of stereoselectivity in the disposition of disopyramide has recently been emphasized in humans (161–163). Both the unbound renal clearance and the nonrenal (hepatic metabolic clearance was greater for the $S(+)$-enantiomer following oral administration of the drug to healthy subjects (162).

These clinical studies further demonstrated the role of stereoselectivity in antiarrhythmic activity. The enantiomers had different antiarrhythmic activity in patients with reproducible inducible atrial flutter (161). Only the $S(+)$-enantiomer prevented the inducibility of atrial flutter, suggesting that the antiarrhythmic activity against atrial flutter associated with racemic disopyramide resides with the S(+)-enantiomer. In patients with ventricular arrhythmias, however, there was no difference between the racemic compound and R(-)-disopyramide in reducing the frequency of ventricular extrasystoles (163). This may imply that the sodium channel blocking properties of the drug, which are nonstereoselective, may be important for its antiarrhythmic action against ventricular arrhythmias but its anticholinergic and phase 3 actions, which are stereoselective, may be important in atrial arrhythmias.

TOXICOLOGY

Toxic Effects in Experimental Animals and Tissues

Arrhythmogenic Effects

The electrophysiologic mechanism of the arrhythmogenic properties of disopyramide are not yet well defined. As discussed earlier, disopyramide-induced early afterdepolarizations and triggered activity in Purkinje fibers may be the mechanism of torsades de pointes arrhythmias. Marked slowing of conduction as a result of combined effects of both the parent compound and its metabolite in blocking sodium channels may account for facilitation of a reentrant arrhythmia.

Hemodynamic Effects

Negative inotropic effects have been identified in animal experiments (1,164–166). In anesthetized dogs the most prominant hemodynamic effect of intravenous disopyramide is a fall in cardiac output accompanied by a transient increase in total peripheral resistance (1,164). Abdollah et al. (164) found no temporal correlation between the hemodynamic effects and either total serum concentration or free fraction of drug. This may relate to a delay in the distribution of drug into myocardial tissue. Depression of left ventricular function and peripheral vasoconstriction accompanied by increases in heart rate also occur in conscious dogs (166). In dogs overdosed with

disopyramide death was due to myocardial failure rather than arrhythmogenesis (167). Treatment with isoproterenol was found to restore the failing circulation.

In addition to its important cardiac effects, disopyramide causes significant side effects on organs other than the heart as a result of its anticholinergic actions. These actions are the cause of the majority of side effects observed with disopyramide and frequently necessitate discontinuation of therapy with this drug. Konishi et al. (168) found that bethanechol can counteract the anticholinergic effects of disopyramide on the dog urinary bladder without reducing its direct effect on the canine ventricle. However, bethanechol may counteract the beneficial effects of disopyramide on atrial tissue and should therefore be used with caution in the treatment of atrial arrhythmias.

Hypoglycemic Effects

The occurrence of hypoglycemia is being increasingly recognized as one of the most serious complications of disopyramide treatment (169–174). Studies in rats and in the in situ canine pancreas suggest that the hypoglycemic effect is brought about through the facilitation of insulin release (171–173). The mechanism of this action has not yet been elucidated but may be mediated via inhibition of potassium channels in insulin-secreting cells.

Clinical Toxicology. Disopyramide is relatively well tolerated on chronic administration. In an 8 week trial (175) comparing its efficacy against ventricular premature contractions with that of quinidine, the dropout rate due to adverse effects in the disopyramide group (10%) was much less than that in the quinidine group (36%). Side effects were more frequently reported (in 70% of patients) in long-term follow-up (23±16 months) of patients receiving disopyramide for symptomatic tachyarrhythmias (98). However, they were usually mild and necessitated drug discontinuation in less than a third of these patients. The most common side effects (105) result from the anticholinergic properties of disopyramide and include dry mouth (40% of patients), urinary hesitancy (16%), blurred vision (3–9%), nausea and vomiting (3–9%), and urinary retention (2%). These effects can be minimized by concomitant administration of pyridostigmine (176) without affecting either antiarrhythmic activity or electrophysiologic effect. Although the N-dealkylated metabolite has greater anticholinergic activity, only a loose correlation has been observed between side-effect score and unbound disopyramide concentration and none with that of metabolite (177).

Disopyramide also exerts a negative inotropic effect [see reviews by Di Bianco et al. (178) and Block and Winkle (179)] resulting in humans in a modest (10–30%) depression of cardiac contractility and cardiac index and prolongation of the pre-ejection period index. These effects are quantitatively greater than those produced by quinidine or procainamide. They are accompanied by an increase in systemic vascular resistance, an effect that tends to maintain blood pressure but further compromises cardiac performance. The negative inotropic effect of disopyramide is more pronounced when loading doses (e.g., intravenous) are used, when there is a preexistent history of heart failure, or when the maintenance dose is not appropriately decreased (e.g., renal failure). Thus disopyramide has been reported to worsen symptoms of heart failure (in up to 55% of patients), especially if inadequately treated, and even occasionally to precipitate symptoms in patients with cardiac disease without previously suspected failure. Whether the more pronounced effect of disopyramide on already diminished cardiac contractility is solely a result of a greater negative inotropic effect in damaged tissue and/or a result of the greater plasma levels achieved with decreased volume of distribution and clearance of drug in heart failure (180) is not clear.

It is recommended that cardiac performance be optimized (e.g., digitalization and vasodilator therapy) before disopyramide is administered, that oral or intravenous loading doses be avoided, and that the plasma concentration of drug be monitored to avoid an inappropriately high dosage regimen in patients with altered disopyramide pharmacokinetics.

Like all other antiarrhythmic drugs, disopyramide can aggravate the frequency or severity of arrhythmias. Podrid et al. (181), in a review of the effects of antiarrhythmic drugs monitored using noninvasive means, found that disopyramide produced a proarrhythmic effect in 6% of cases (6 of 102 patients). That is, there was a 4-fold increase in the frequency of ventricular premature beats, a 10-fold increase in repetitive forms, or the appearance of a new sustained ventricular tachycardia. Using invasive programmed stimulation testing for ventricular tachycardia, disopyramide was proarrhythmic in 1 of 21 cases. Although the numbers of patients are small (especially in the invasive study), disopyramide tended to be less proarrhythmic than the class IC agents and caused a similar or lesser aggravation of arrhythmia than the class IA or IB drugs.

In common with other antiarrhythmics, which prolong the QT interval, disopyramide has also been reported to produce typical "torsade de pointes." Casedevant and Sabaut (182) were the first to report a case of torsades de pointes associated with disopyramide therapy. Since then, several cases of abnormal prolongation of the QT interval complicated by torsade de pointes have been reported in the literature (183–194). These cases, like "quinidine syncope," have occurred at the usual therapeutic doses and in some instances have been associated with hypokalemia or bradycardia, but in all there was significant to marked prolongation of the QT interval. In addition, ventricular tachycardia or fibrillation with excessive QT interval prolongation has also occurred on disopyramide therapy (195–197). Elimination of these arrhythmias required discontinuation of disopyramide therapy, correction of hypokalemia, and, if necessary, temporary pacing or isoproterenol administration (188). As a preventive measure it is recommended that QT prolongation by disopyramide of 25% or greater be avoided.

Gastrointestinal side effects, such as nausea, vomiting, or diarrhea, have occasionally been reported. Rarely, cases of intrahepatic cholestasis have been attributed to disopyramide, but other causes were not necessarily ruled out in these reports (104).

Finally, disopyramide can reduce blood glucose levels slightly in normal subjects, but an increasing number of cases of symptomatic hypoglycemia and even death have been reported, usually in aged patients or those with impaired renal or hepatic function (169–171,174).

SUMMARY

Few aspects of the pharmacology of disopyramide are simple. Its frequency-dependent interactions with both the sodium and potassium channels are modified by powerful anticholinergic actions. It blocks the sodium channel in its activated state. Thus it is more likely to be effective in arrhythmias occurring at rapid heart rates. Its efficacy against supraventricular and ventricular arrhythmias is approximately equivalent to that of other class IA drugs. However, in individual cases the effects of quinidine or procainamide do not necessarily predict disopyramide efficacy. Its role in the treatment of ventricular arrhythmias in comparison with the newer agents is not well defined. The pharmacokinetics of disopyramide are complex. Its disposition is complicated by variable binding to plasma proteins, the concentration of which fluctuates widely in disease states. Elimination kinetics are concentration dependent. The electrophysiologic, hemodynamic, and anticholinergic effects, as well as the antiarrhythmic efficacy, correlate best with free disopyramide concentrations. Like quinidine, disopyramide occasionally causes ventricular tachycardia with prolongation of the QT interval. The likely mechanism of this proarrhythmic effect is the induction of early afterdepolarizations under conditions of hypokalemia and bradycardia. Thus disopyramide should be used with caution in patients with contributing abnormalities, such as mild hypokalemia, bradycardia-tachycardia syndrome, underlying heart disease, or congestive heart failure. Patients who have this complication with another class IA agent or with a class III agent should not be given disopyramide. The side-effect profile of disopyramide makes it more easily tolerated than quinidine or procainamide. However, its negative inotropic effects limit its use to patients with a well-preserved cardiac inotropic state. The safe, effective clinical use of disopyramide depends on recognition of its complex electrophysiology, hemodynamics, and disposition kinetics.

REFERENCES

1. Mokler C M, Van Arman C G. Pharmacology of a new antiarrhythmic agent, γ-disopropylamino-α-phenyl-α-(2-pyridyl)-butyramide (SC-7031). J Pharmacol Exp Ther 1962; 136:114–24.
2. Sekiya A, Vaughan Williams E M. A comparison of the antifibrillatory actions and effects on intracellular cardiac potentials of pronethalol, disopyramide and quinidine. Br J Pharmacol 1963; 21:473–81.
3. Vaughan Williams E M. A classification of antiarrhythmic actions reassessed after a decade of new drugs. J Clin Pharmacol 1984; 24:129–47.
4. Campbell T J. Kinetics of onset of rate dependent effects of class 1 antiarrhythmic drugs are important in determining their effects on refractoriness in guinea-pig ventricle, and provide a theoretical basis for their subclassification. Cardiovasc Res 1983; 17:344–52.
5. Kotake H, Hasegawa J, Hata T, Mashiba H. Electrophysiological effect of disopyramide on rabbit sinus node cells. J Electrocardiol 1985; 18:377–83.
6. Campbell T. Differing electrophysiological effects of class IA, IB, and IC antiarrhythmic drugs on guinea-pig sinoatrial node. Br J Pharmacol 1987; 91:395–401.
7. Katoh T, Karagueuzian H S, Jordan J, Mandel W J. The cellular electrophysiologic mechanism of the dual actions of disopyramide on rabbit sinus node function. Circulation 1982; 66:1216–24.
8. Chiba S, Kobayashi M, Furukawa Y. Effects of disopyramide on SA nodal pacemaker activity and contractility in the isolated blood-perfused atrium of the dog. Eur J Pharmacol 1979; 57:13–9.
9. Mirro M J. Effects of quinidine, procainamide and disopyramide on automaticity and cyclic AMP content of guinea-pig atria. J Mol Cell Cardiol 1981; 13:641–53.
10. Mirro M J, Watanabe A M, Bailey J C. Electrophysiological effects of disopyramide and quinidine on guinea pig atria and canine cardiac Purkinje fibers. Circ Res 1980; 46:660–8.

11. Kirchhof C J H J, Bonke F I M, Allessie M A. Effects of verapamil, diltiazem and disopyramide on sinus function: a comparison with bepridil. Eur J Pharmacol 1989; 160:369–76.

12. Nakajima T, Kurachi Y, Ito H, Takikawa R, Sugimoto T. Anticholinergic effects of quinidine, disopyramide, and procainamide in isolated atrial myocytes: mediation by different molecular mechanisms. Circ Res 1989; 64:297–303.

13. Vaughan Williams E M. Disopyramide. Ann NY Acad Sci 1984; 432:189–200.

14. Winslow E, Campbell J K, Marshall R J. Comparative electrophysiological effects of disopyramide and bepridil on rabbit atrial, papillary, and Purkinje tissue: modification by reduced extracellular potassium. J Cardiovasc Pharmacol 1986; 8:1208–16.

15. Birkhead J S, Vaughan Williams E M. Dual effect of disopyramide on atrial and atrioventricular conduction and refractory periods. Br Heart J 1977; 39:657–60.

16. Flemming M A, Sasyniuk B I. Frequency- and voltage-dependent effects of disopyramide in canine Purkinje fibers. Can J Physiol Pharmacol 1989; 67:710–21.

17. Campbell T J. Kinetics of onset of rate-dependent effects of class 1 antiarrhythmic drugs are important in determining their effects on refractoriness in guinea-pig ventricle, and provide a theoretical basis for their subclassification. Cardiovasc Res 1983; 17:344–52.

18. Campbell T J. Resting and rate-dependent depression of maximum rate of depolarization (V_{max}) in guinea pig ventricular action potentials by mexiletine, disopyramide, and encainide. J Cardiovasc Pharmacol 1983; 5:291–6.

19. Hondeghem L M, Katzung B G. Time- and voltage-dependent interactions of antiarrhythmic drugs with cardiac sodium channels. Biochim Biophys Acta 1977; 472:373–98.

20. Hondeghem L M, Katzung B G. The modulated receptor mechanism of action of sodium and calcium channel blocking drugs. Annu Rev Pharmacol Toxicol 1984; 24:387–423.

21. Starmer C F, Grant A O, Strauss H C. Mechanism of use-dependent block of sodium channels in excitable membranes by local anesthetics. Biophys J 1984; 46:15–27.

22. Gruber R, Carmeliet E. The activation gate of the sodium channel controls blockade and deblockade by disopyramide in rabbit Purkinje fibres. Br J Pharmacol 1989; 97:41–50.

23. Kodama I, Honjo H, Kamiya K, Toyama J. Two types of sodium channel block by class I antiarrhythmic drugs studied by using V_{max} of action potential in single ventricular myocytes. J Mol Cell Cardiol 1990; 22:1–12.

24. Kodama I, Toyama J, Takanaka C, Yamada K. Block of activated and inactivated sodium channels by class I antiarrhythmic drugs studied by using maximum upstroke velocity (V_{max}) of action potential in guinea pig cardiac muscles. J Mol Cell Cardiol 1987; 19:367–77.

25. Grant A O. Evolving concepts of cardiac sodium channel function. J Cardiovasc Electrophsiol 1990; 1:53–67.

26. Hille B. Local anesthetics: hydrophilic and hydrophobic pathways for the drug-receptor interaction. J Gen Physiol 1977; 69:497–515.

27. Courtney K R. Why do some drugs preferentially block open sodium channels? J Mol Cell Cardiol 1988; 20:461–4.

28. Kojima M, Ban T, Sada H. Effects of disopyramide on the maximum rate of rise of action potential (V_{max}) in guinea-pig papillary muscles. Jpn J Pharmacol 1982; 32:91–102.

29. Kojima M. Effects of disopyramide on transmembrane action potentials in guinea-pig papillary muscles. Eur J Pharmacol 1981; 69:11–24.

30. Varro A, Elharrar V, Surawicz B. Frequency-dependent effects of several class I antiarrhythmic drugs on V_{max} of action potential upstroke in canine cardiac Purkinje fibers. J Cardiovasc Pharmacol 1985; 7:482–92.

31. Elharrar V. Recovery from use-dependent block of V_{max} and restitution of action potential duration in canine cardiac Purkinje fibers. J Pharmacol Exp Ther 1988; 246:235–42.

32. Hiraoka M, Kuga K, Kawano S, Sunami A, Fan Z. New observations on the mechanisms of antiarrhythmic actions of disopyramide on cardiac membranes. Am J Cardiol 1989; 64:15J–19J.

33. Bean B P, Cohen C M, Tsien R W. Lidocaine block of cardiac sodium channels. J Gen Physiol 1983; 81:613–42.

34. Weld F M, Coromilas J, Rottman J N, Bigger J T Jr. Mechanisms of quinidine induced depression of maximum upstroke velocity in

ovine cardiac Purkinje fibers. Circ Res 1982; 50:369–76.

35. Yeh, J Z, Tanguy J. Na channel activation gate modulates slow recovery from use-dependent block by local anesthetics in squid giant axons. Biophys J 1985; 47:685–94.

36. Anno T, Hondeghem L M. Interactions of flecainide with guinea pig cardiac sodium channels. Importance of activation unblocking to the voltage dependence of recovery. Circ Res 1990; 66:789–803.

37. Yeh J Z, Ten Eick R E. Molecular and structural basis of resting and use-dependent block of sodium current defined using diso-pyramide analogues. Biophys J 1987; 51:123–35.

38. Carmeliet E. Activation block and trapping of penticainide, a disopyramide analogue, in the Na$^+$ channel of rabbit cardiac Purkinje fibers. Circ Res 1988; 63:50–60.

39. Kus T, Sasyniuk B I. Electrophysiological actions of disopyramide phosphate on canine ventricular muscle and Purkinje fibers. Circ Res 1975; 37:844–54.

40. Kus T, Sasyniuk B I. The electrophysiological effects of disopyramide phosphate on canine ventricular muscle and Purkinje fibers in normal and low potassium. Can J Physiol Pharmacol 1978; 56: 139–49.

41. Sasyniuk B I, Kus T. Cellular electrophysiologic changes induced by disopyramide phosphate in normal and infarcted hearts. J Int Med Res 1976; 4(Suppl. 1):20–5.

42. Sasyniuk B I, McQuillan J. Mechanisms by which antiarrhythmic drugs influence induction of reentrant responses in the subendocardial Purkinje network of 1-day old infarcted canine ventricle. In: Zipes D P, Jalife J, eds. Cardiac electrophysiology and arrhythmias. New York: Grune & Stratton, 1985:389–96.

43. Nakaya Y, Varro A, Elharrar V, Surawicz B. Effect of altered repolarization course induced by antiarrhythmic drugs and constant current pulses on duration of premature action potentials in canine cardiac Purkinje fibers. J Cardiovasc Pharmacol 1989; 14:908–18.

44. Coraboeuf E, Deroubaix E, Escande D, Coulombe A. Comparative effects of three class I antiarrhythmic drugs of plateau and pacemaker currents of sheep cardiac Purkinje fibres. Cardiovasc Res 1988; 22:375–84.

45. Schanne O F, Bkaily B, Dumais B, Boutin L. Disopyramide phosphate effects on slow and depressed fast responses. Can J Physiol Pharmacol 1986; 64:487–91.

46. Mirro M J, Manalan A S, Bailey J C, Watanabe A M. Anticholinergic effects of disopyramide and quinidine on guinea pig myocardium. Circ Res 1980; 47:855–65.

47. Danilo P, Hordof A J, Rosen M R. Effects of disopyramide on electrophysiologic properties of canine cardiac Purkinje fibers. J Pharm Exp Ther 1977; 201:701–10.

48. Roden D. Clinical features of arrhythmia aggravation by antiarrhythmic drugs and their implications for basic mechanisms. Drug Dev Res 1990; 19:153–72.

49. Sasyniuk B I, Valois M, Toy W. Recent advances in understanding the mechanisms of drug-induced torsades de pointes arrhythmias. Am J Cardiol 1989; 64:29J–32J.

50. Toy W, Sasyniuk B I. Electrophysiological interactions between disopyramide and its major metabolite, mono-N-dealkyldisopyramide, in canine ventricular tissue (abstract). Eur J Pharmacol 1990; 83:1238.

51. Thompson K A, Blair I A, Woosley R L, Roden D M. Comparative in vitro electrophysiology of quinidine, its major metabolites and dihydroquinidine. J Pharmacol Exp Ther 1987; 241:84–90.

52. Mirro M J, Watanabe A M, Bailey J C. Electrophysiological effects of the optical isomers of disopyramide and quinidine in the dog. Circ Res 1981; 48:867–74.

53. Kidwell G A, Schaal S F, Muir W W III. Stereospecific effects of disopyramide enantiomers following pretreatment of canine cardiac Purkinje fibers with verapamil and nisoldipine. J Cardiovasc Pharmacol 1987; 9:276–84.

54. Kidwell G A, Lima J J, Schaal S F, Muir W W III. Hemodynamic and electrophysiologic effects of disopyramide enantiomers in a canine blood superfusion model. J Cardiovasc Pharmacol 1989; 13:644–55.

55. Giacomini J C, Giacomini K M, Nelson W L, Harrison D C, Blaschke T F. Electrophysiology of the enantiomers of disopyramide in dogs. J Cardiovasc Pharmacol 1985; 7:884–90.

56. Baines M W, Davies J E, Kellet D N, Munt P L. Some pharmacological effects of disopyramide and a metabolite. J Int Med Res 1976; 4(Suppl. 1):5–7.

57. Grant A M, Marshall R J, Ankier S I. Some effects of disopyramide and its N-dealkylated metabolite on isolated nerve and cardiac muscle. Eur J Pharmacol 1978; 49:389–94.

58. Dubray C, Boucher M, Paire M, Pinatel H, Duchene-Marullaz P. Comparative effects of disopyramide and its mono-N-dealkylated metabolite in conscious dogs with chronic atrioventricular block: plasma concentration-response relationships. J Cardiovasc Pharmacol 1986; 8:1229–34.

59. Toy W, Sasyniuk B I. Frequency and voltage dependent effects of mono-N-dealkyldisopyramide, the major metabolite of disopyramide, in canine ventricular tissue. J Pharmacol Exp Ther 1990; 254.

60. Bertrix L, Timour Chah Q, Lang J, Lakhal M, Bouzouita K, Faucon G. Efficacy of diopyramide in comparison with verapamil and propranolol in the prevention of acetylcholine induced atrial fibrillation in the dog. Arch Int Pharmacodyn 1985; 274:97–110.

61. Kus T, Sasyniuk B I. Effects of disopyramide phosphate on ventricular arrhythmias in experimental myocardial infarction. J Pharmacol Exp Ther 1975; 196:665–75.

62. Levites R, Anderson G J. Electrophysiologic effects of disopyramide phosphate during experimental myocardial ischemia. Am Heart J 1979; 98:339–44.

63. Patterson E, Gibson J K, Lucchesi B R. Electrophysiologic effects of disopyramide phosphate on reentrant ventricular arrhythmia in conscious dogs after myocardial infarction. Am J Cardiol 1980; 46:792–9.

64. Patterson E, Stetson P, Lucchesi B R. Disopyramide plasma and myocardial tissue concentrations as they relate to antiarrhythmic activity. J Cardiovasc Pharmacol 1979; 1:541–50.

65. Cobbe S M, Hoffmann E, Ritzenhoff A, Brachmann J, Kubler W, Senges J. Actions of disopyramide on potential reentrant pathways and ventricular tachyarrhythmias in conscious dogs during the late post-myocardial infarction phase. Am J Cardiol 1984; 53:1712–8.

66. Chagnac A, Pelleg A, Belhassen B, Lubliner J, Vidne B, Laniado S. Effects of disopyramide on reperfusion arrhythmias in dogs. J Cardiovasc Pharmacol 1982; 4:994–8.

67. Josephson M E, Caracta A R, Lau S H, Gallagher J J, Damato A N. Electrophysiological evaluation of disopyramide in man. Am Heart J 1973; 86:771–80.

68. Marrott P K, Ruttley M S T, Winterbottam J T, Muir J R. A study of the acute electrophysiological and cardiovascular action of disopyramide in man. Eur J Cardiol 1976; 4:303–12.

69. Hinderling P H, Garrett E R. Pharmacodynamics of the antiarrhythmic disopyramide in healthy humans: correlation of the kinetics of the drug and its effects. J Pharmacokinet Biopharm 1976; 4:231–42.

70. Mathur P. Cardiovascular effects of a newer antiarrhythmic agent, disopyramide phosphate. Am Heart J 1972; 84:764–70.

71. Wyse D G, Mitchell L B, Duff H J. Procainamide, disopyramide and quinidine: discordant antiarrhythmic effects during crossover comparison in patients with inducible ventricular tachycardia. J Am Coll Cardiol 1987; 9:882–9.

72. Caracta A. The electrophysiology of Norpace. Part III. Angiology 1975; 26(Suppl.1): 120–3.

73. Befeler B, Castellanos A, Wells D E, Vagueiro M C, Yeh BK. Electrophysiologic effects of the antiarrhythmic agent disopyramide phosphate. Am J Cardiol 1975; 35:282–7.

74. Ross D, Vohra J, Cole P, Hunt D, Sloueman G. Electrophysiology of disopyramide in man. Aust NZ J Med 1978; 8:377–83.

75. La Barre A, Strauss H C, Scheinman M M, Evans G T, Bashore T. Electrophysiologic effects of disopyramide phosphate on sinus node function in patients with sinus node dysfunction. Circulation 1979; 59:226–35.

76. Pimenta J, Pereira C B. Electrophysiologic effects of disopyramide in Chagas disease with bundle branch block. Int J Cardiol 1984; 5:364–6.

77. Seipel L, Breithardt G. Sinus recovery time after disopyramide phosphate (letter). Am J Cardiol 1976; 37: 1118.

78. Wilkinson P R, Desai J, Hollister J, Gonzalez R, Abbott J A, Scheinman M M. Electrophysiologic effects of disopyramide in patients with atrioventricular nodal dysfunction. Circulation 1982; 66:1211–6.

79. Sethi K K, Jaishankar S, Khalilullah M, Gupta M P. Selective blockade of retrograde fast pathway by intravenous disopyramide in paroxysmal supraventricular tachycardia mediated by dual atrioventricular nodal pathways. Br Heart J 1983; 49:532–43.

80. Ito M, Onodera S, Hashimoto J, et al. Effect of disopyramide on initiation of atrial fibril-

lation and relation to effective refractory period. Am J Cardiol 1989; 63:561–6.

81. Camm J, Ward D, Spurrell R. Response of atrial flutter to overdrive atrial pacing and intravenous disopyramide phosphate, singly and in combination. Br Heart J 1980; 44:240–7.

82. Della Bella P, Marenzi G, Tondo C, et al. Effects of disopyramide on cycle length, effective refractory period and excitable gap of atrial flutter, and relation to arrhythmia termination by overdrive pacing. Am J Cardiol 1989; 63:812–6.

83. Spurrell R A J, Thorburn C W, Camm J, Sowton E, Deuchar D C. Effects of disopyramide on electrophysiological properties of specialized conduction system in man and on accessory atrioventricular pathway in Wolff-Parkinson-White syndrome. Br Heart J 1975; 37:861–7.

84. Bennett D H. Disopyramide in patients with the Wolff-Parkinson-White syndrome and atrial fibrillation. Chest 1978; 74:624–8.

85. Kerr C R, Prystowsky E N, Smith W M, Cook L, Gallagher J J. Electrophysiologic effects of disopyramide phosphate in patients with Wolff-Parkinson-White syndrome. Circulation 1982;65:869–78.

86. Swiryn S, Bauernfeind R A, Wyndham C R C Dhindra R C, Palileo E, Strasberg B, Rosen K M. Effects of oral disopyramide phosphate on induction of paroxysmal supraventricular tachycardia. Circulation 1981; 64:169–75.

87. Fujimura O, Klein G J, Sharma A D, Yee R, Szabo T. Acute effect of disopyramide on atrial fibrillation in the Wolff-Parkinson-White syndrome. J Am Coll Cardiol 1989; 13:1133–7.

88. Desai J M, Scheinman M, Peters R W, O'Young J. Electrophysiological effects of disopyramide in patients with bundle branch block. Circulation 1979; 59:215–25.

89. Bergfeldt L, Rossenqvist M, Vallin H, Edhag O. Disopyramide induced second and third degree atrioventricular block in patients with bifascicular block. An acute stress test to predict atrioventricular block progression. Br Heart J 1985; 53: 328–34.

90. Spurrell R A J. The effects of disopyramide on the human heart: an electrophysiological study. J Int Med Res 1976; 4(Suppl. 1):31–6.

91. Duff H J, Mitchell L B, Nath C F, Manyari D E, Baynton R, Wyse D G. Concentration-

response relationships of disopyramide in patients with ventricular tachycardia. Clin Pharmacol Ther 1989; 45:542–7.

92. Endresen K, Amlie J P, Forfang K. Effects of disopyramide on repolarization and intraventricular conduction in man. Eur J Clin Pharmacol 1988; 35:467–74.

93. Benditt D G, Pritchett E L C, Wallace A G, Gallagher J J. Recurrent ventricular tachycardia in man: evaluation of disopyramide therapy in intracardiac electrical stimulation. Eur J Cardiol 1979; 9:255–76.

94. Breithardt G, Seipel L, Abendroth R R. Comparison of the antiarrhythmic efficacy of disopyramide and mexiletine against stimulus-induced ventricular tachycardia. J Cardiovasc Pharmacol 1981; 3:1026–37.

95. Lerman B B, Waxman H L, Buxton A E, Josephson M E. Disopyramide: evaluation of electrophysiologic effects and clinical efficacy in patients with sustained ventricular tachycardia or ventricular fibrillation. Am J Cardiol 1983; 51:759–64.

96. Swiryn S, Bauernfeind R A, Strasberg B, Palileo E, Iverson N, Levy P S, Rosen K M. Prediction of response to class I antiarrhythmic drugs during electrophysiologic study of ventricular tachycardia. Am Heart J 1982; 104:43–50.

97. Bauman J L, Gallastegui J, Strasberg B, et al. Long-term therapy with disopyramide phosphate: side effects and effectiveness. Am Heart J 1986; 111:654–60.

98. Arif M, Laidlaw J C, Oshrain C, Willis P W, Nissen C H. A randomized, double-blind, parallel group comparison of disopyramide phosphate and quinidine in patients with cardiac arrhythmias. Angiology 1983; 34:393–400.

99. Lloyd E A, Gersh B J, Forman R. The efficacy of quinidine and disopyramide in the maintenance of sinus rhythm after electroconversion from atrial fibrillation. S Afr Med J 1984; 65: 367–9.

100. Millar M W, Raftery E B. A double-blind trial of disopyramide, procainamide and digoxin in paroxysmal supraventricular tachycardia. Clin Cardiol 1979; 2:179–84.

101. Martin A, Benbow L J, Leach C, Bailey R J. Comparison of amiodarone and disopyramide in the control of paroxysmal atrial fibrillation and atrial flutter (interim report). Br J Clin Pract 1986; 40(Suppl. 4):52–60.

102. Heel R C, Brogden R N, Speight T M, Avery G S. Disopyramide: a review of its

pharmacological properties and therapeutic
use in treating cardiac arrhythmias. Drugs
1978; 15:331–68.

103. Smith W S, Vismara L, Kalmansohn R B, et
al. Clinical studies of Norpace. Angiology
1975; 26(Suppl. 1):124–53.

104. Brogden R N, Todd P A. Disopyramide. A
reappraisal of its pharmacodynamic and
pharmacokinetic properties, and therapeutic
use in cardiac arrhythmias. Drugs 1987;
34:151–87.

105. Wilson R R, Wallace A G. Disopyramide:
six years experience. Angiology 1983; 34:
367–74.

106. Rabkin S W, Boroomand-Rashti K, McKinnon J, Rotem C E. Comparison of propafenone and disopyramide in the treatment
of ventricular premature complexes: a randomized double blind crossover placebo controlled trial. Can J Cardiol 1987; 3:105–10.

107. Kim S G, Mercando A D, Tam S, Fisher
J D. Combination of disopyramide and
mexiletine for better tolerance and additive
effects for treatment of ventricular arrhythmias. J Am Coll Cardiol 1989; 13:659–64.

108. Ekelund L G, Nilsson E, Walldius G. Efficacy of and adverse effects of disopyramide.
Comparison of capsules, controlled release
tablets and placebo in patients with chronic
ventricular arrhythmias. Eur J Clin Pharmacol 1986; 29:673–7.

109. Paulk E A. Long-term use of controlled-
release disopyramide in patients with severe
ventricular arrhythmias. Angiology 1987;
38:198–204.

110. Puech P. Treatment of cardiac arrhythmias
with disopyramide. Minerva Med 1970;
61:3763–8.

111. Vismara L A, Vera Z, Miller R R, Mason
D T. Efficacy of disopyramide phosphate in
the treatment of refractory ventricular tachycardia. Am J Cardiol 1977; 39:1027–34.

112. Denes P, Wu D, Wyndham C, et al. Chronic
long-term electrophysiologic study of paroxysmal ventricular tachycardia. Chest 1980;
77:478–87.

113. Zainal N, Griffiths J W, Carmichael D J S,
et al. Oral disopyramide for the prevention
of arrhythmias in patients with acute myocardial infarction admitted to open wards.
Lancet 1977; 2:887–9.

114. Karim A, Cook C, Novotney R L, Zagarella
J, Campion J. Pharmacokinetics and steady
state myocardial uptake of disopyramide in
the dog. Drug Metab Dispos 1978; 6:338–45.

115. Cook C S, Gwilt P R, Kowalski K, Gupta S,
Oppermann J, Karim A. Pharmacokinetics of
disopyramide in the dog. Drug Metab Dispos
1990; 18:42–9.

116. Karim A, Kook C, Campion J. Placental and
milk transfer of disopyramide and metabolites. Drug Metab Dispos 1978; 6:346–8.

117. Lima J J. Species dependent binding of disopyramide enantiomers. Drug Metab Dispos
1988; 16:563–7.

118. Pedersen L E, Hermansen K, Olsen H O,
Rasmussen N. The influence of surgery on
the elimination kinetics of disopyramide in
pigs. Acta Pharmacol Toxicol (Copenh)
1986; 59:86–8.

119. Pedersen L E, Bonde J, Graudal N A,
Backer N V, Hansen J E S, Kampmann J P.
Quantitative and qualitative binding characteristics of disopyramide in serum from patients with decreased renal and hepatic
function. Br J Clin Pharmacol 1987; 23:41–
6.

120. Huang J, Oie S. Effect of altered disopyramide binding on its pharmacologic response
in rabbits. J Pharmacol Exp Ther 1982;
223:468–71.

121. Pedersen L E, et al. The pharmacokinetics
and protein binding of disopyramide in pigs.
Acta Pharmacol Toxicol (Copenh) 1986;
58:282–8.

122. Karim A, Ranney R E, Kraychy S. Species
differences in the biotransformation of a new
antiarrhythmic drug. J Pharmacol Sci 1972;
61:888–93.

123. Cook C S, Karim A, Sollman P. Stereoselectivity in the metabolism of disopyramide
enantiomers in rat and dog. Drug Metab Dispos 1981; 10:116–21.

124. Giacomini K M, Giacomini J C, Swezey
S E, Harrison D C, Nelson W L, Burke
T R, Jr, Blaschke T F. The stereoselective
disposition of disopyramide in the dog. J
Cardiovasc Pharmacol 1980; 2:825–32.

125. Huang J, Oie S. Comparison of electrocardiographic response and disposition of R-
and S-disopyramide in the rabbit. Res Commun Chem Pathol Pharmacol 1983; 41:227–
41.

126. Huang J D. Stereoselective gastrointestinal
clearance of disopyramide in rabbits treated
with activated charcoal. J Pharm Sci 1988;
77:959–62.

127. Siddoway L A, Woosley R L. Clinical pharmacokinetic of disopyramide. Clin Pharmacokinet 1986; 11:214–23.

128. Karim A, Nissen C, Azarnoff D L. Clinical pharmacokinetics of disopyramide. J Pharmacokinet Biopharm 1982; 10:465–94.

128a. Campbell R W F. Disopyramide: pharmacology. In: Katz A M, ed. Disorders of cardiac rhythm—focus on disopyramide. Auckland: Adis Press Ltd, 1986: 101–20.

129. Henderling P H, Garrett E R. Pharmacokinetics of the antiarrhythmic disopyramide in healthy humans. J Pharmacokinet Biopharm 1976; 4:199–230.

130. Capparelli E V, DiPersio D M, Zhao H, Kluger J, Chow M S. Clinical pharmacokinetics of controlled-release disopyramide in patients with cardiac arrhythmias. J Clin Pharmacol 1988; 28:306–11.

131. Pentikainen P J, Huikuri H, Jounela A J, Wilen G. Disopyramide pharmacokinetics in patients with acute myocardial infarction. Eur J Clin Pharmacol 1985; 28:45–51.

132. Echizen H, Saotome T, Minoura S, Ishizaki T. Plasma protein binding of disopyramide in pregnant and postpartum women, and in neonates and their mothers. Eur J Pharmacol 1990; 183:634.

133. Ellsworth A J, Horn J R, Raisys V A, Miyagawa L A, Bell J L. Disopyramide and N-monodesalkyl disopyramide in serum and breast milk. Drug Intell Clin Pharm 1989; 23:56–7.

134. Roberto P, Vitaliano B, Donatella P, Raffaella M, Sergio B, Gabriella C. Disopyramide pharmacokinetics in the elderly after single oral administration. Pharmacol Res Commun 1988; 20: 1025–34.

135. Bredesen J E, Kierulf P. Relationship between alpha-1-acid glycoprotein and plasma binding of disopyramide and mono-N-dealhyldisopyramide. Br J Clin Pharmacol 1984; 18:779–84.

136. Lima J J, Jungbluth G L, Devine T, Robertson L W. Stereoselective binding of disopyramide to human plasma protein. Life Sci 1984; 35:835–9.

137. Lima J J, Boudoulas H, Shields B J. Stereoselective pharmacokinetics of disopyramide enantiomers in man. Drug Metab Dispos 1985; 13:572–7.

138. Chen B H, Taylor H, Pappas A A. Total and free disopyramide by fluorescence polarization immunoassay and relationship between free fraction and alpha-1 glycoprotein. Clin Chim Acta 1987; 163:75–80.

139. Piafsky K M, Sellers E M, Strauss H, Woolneer B. Plasma binding of lidocaine, disopyramide and propranolol in acute myocardial infarction. In: Turner P, Padgham C, eds. World conference on clinical pharmacology and therapeutics. London: MacMillan 1980:Abstract 0346.

140. Haughey D B, Kraft C J, Matzke G R, Keane W F, Halstenson C F. Protein binding of disopyramide and elevated alpha-1-acid glycoprotein concentrations in serum obtained from dialysis patients and renal transplant recipients. Am J Nephrol 1985; 5:35–9.

141. Bredesen J E, Kierulf P. Relationship between a_1-acid glycoprotein and distribution of disopyramide and mono-N-dealkyldisopyramide in whole blood. Br J Clin Pharmacol 1986; 22: 281–6.

142. Echizen H, Saima S, Umeda N, Ishizaki T. Protein binding of disopyramide in liver cirrhosis and in nephrotic syndrome. Clin Pharmacol Ther 1986; 40:274–80.

143. Bonde J, Graudal N A, Pedersen L E, et al. Kinetics of disopyramide in decreased hepatic function. Eur J Clin Pharmacol 1986; 31:73–7.

144. Echizen H, Saima S, Ishizaki T. Disopyramide protein binding in plasma from patients with nephrotic syndrome during the exacerbation and remission phases. Br J Clin Pharmacol 1987; 24:199–206.

145. Bredesen J E, Pike E, Lunde P K M. Plasma binding of disopyramide and mono-N-dealkyldisopyramide. Br J Clin Pharmacol 1982; 14:673–6.

146. Aitio M L, Maasury L, Tala E, Haataja M, Aiio A. The effect of enzyme induction on the metabolism of disopyramide in man. Br J Pharmacol 1981; 11: 279–85.

147. Kapil R P, Axelson J E, Mansfield IL, et al. Disopyramide pharmacokinetics and metabolism: effect of inducers. Br J Clin Pharmacol 1987; 24:781–91.

148. Karim A. The pharmacokinetics of Norpace. Angiology 1975; 26(Suppl. 1):85–98.

149. Bryson S M, Whiting B, Lawrence J R. Disopyramide serum and pharmacologic effect kinetics applied to the assessment of bioavailability. Br J Clin Pharmacol 1978; 6:409–19.

150. Bonde J, Pedersen L E, Bodtker S, et al. The influence of age and smoking on the elimination of disopyramide. Br J Clin Pharmacol 1985; 20:453–8.

151. Johnson A, Henry J A, Warrington S J, Hamer N A J. Pharmacokinetics of oral diso-

pyramide phosphate in patients with renal impairment. Br J Clin Pharmacol 1980; 10:245–8.

152. Burk M, Peters U. Disopyramide kinetics in renal impairment: determinants of interindividual variability. Clin Pharmacol Ther 1983; 34:331–40.

153. Braun J, Storgel F, Gluth W P, Oie S. Does alpha 1-acid glycoprotein reduce the unbound metabolic clearance of disopyramide in patients with renal impairment? Eur J Clin Pharmacol 1988; 35:313–7.

154. Sevka M J, Matthews S J, Nightingale C H, et al. Disopyramide hemodialysis and kinetics in patients requiring long-term hemodialysis. Clin Pharmacol Ther 1981; 29:322–6.

155. Shen D D, Cunningham J L, Shudo I, Azarnoff D L. Disposition kinetics of disopyramide in patients with renal insufficiency. Biopharm Drug Dispos 1980; 1:133–40.

156. Lima J J, Haughey D B, Leier C V. Disopyramide pharmacokinetics and bioavailability following the simultaneous administration of disopyramide and ^{14}C-disopyramide. J Pharmacokin Biopharm 1984; 12:289–313.

157. Elliott H L, Thomson A H, Bryson S M. Disopyramide in acute myocardial infarction: problems with changing pharmacokinetics. Eur J Clin Pharmacol 1986; 30:345–7.

158. Gosselin B, Mathieu D, Chopin C, et al. Acute intoxication with disopyramide: clinical and experimental study by hemoperfusion or Amberlite XAD 4 resin. Clin Toxicol 1980; 17:438–49.

159. Holt D W, Helliwell M, O'Keeffe B, et al. Successful management of serious disopyramide poisoning. Postgrad Med J 1980; 56:256–60.

160. Arimori K, Kawano H, Nakano M. Gastrointestinal dialysis of disopyramide in healthy subjects. Int J Clin Pharmacol Ther Toxicol 1989; 27:280–4.

161. Lima J J, Wenzke S C, Boudoulas H, Schaal S F. Antiarrhythmic activity and unbound concentrations of disopyramide enantiomers in patients. Ther Drug Monit 1990; 12:23–8.

162. Le Corre P, Gibassier D, Sado P, Le Verge R. Stereoselective metabolism and pharmacokinetics of disopyramide enantiomers in humans. Drug Metab Dispos 1988;16:858–64.

163. Le Corre P, Gibassier D, Descaves C, Sado P, Daubert J C, Le Verge R. Clinical pharmacokinetics of levorotatory and racemic disopyramide, at steady state, following oral administration in patients with ventricular arrhythmias. J Clin Pharmacol 1989; 29:1089–96.

164. Abdollah H, Brien J F, Armstrong P W. Pharmacokinetic-hemodynamic studies of disopyramide. J Cardiovasc Pharmacol 1984; 6:28–34.

165. Beltrame J, Aylward P E, McRitchie R J, Chalmers J P. Comparative haemodynamic effects of lidocaine, mexiletine, and disopyramide. J Cardiovasc Pharmacol 1984; 6:483–90.

166. Walsh R A, Horwitz L D. Adverse hemodynamic effects of intravenous disopyramide compared with quinidine in conscious dogs. Circulation 1979; 60:1053–8.

167. O'Keeffe B, Hayler A M, Holt D W, Medd R K. Cardiac consequences and treatment of disopyramide intoxication: experimental evaluation in dogs. Cardiovasc Res 1979; 13:630.

168. Konishi T, Kadoya M, Ikeguchi S, Sakai K, Tamamura T, Kawai C. Combined effect of disopyramide and bethanechol: use of bethanechol to prevent anticholinergic side effects of disopyramide without reduction of antiarrhythmic efficacy. J Cardiovasc Pharmacol 1989; 14:341–350.

169. Semel J D, Wortham E, Karl D M. Fasting hypoglycemia associated with disopyramide. Am Heart J 1983; 106:1160–1.

170. Croxson M S, Shaw D W, Henley P G, Gabriel H D. Disopyramide induced hypoglycemia and increased serum insulin. NZ Med J 1987; 100:407–8.

171. Nakabayashi H, Ito T, Igawa T, Imamura T, Seta T, Kawato T, Usukura N, Takeda R. Disopyramide induces insulin secretion and plasma glucose diminution: studies using the in situ canine pancreas. Metabolism 1989; 38:179–83.

172. Kimura F et al. Effects of disopyramide on insulin secretion in the perfusion of isolated rat pancreas in situ. Nippon Ika Daigaku Zasshi 1987; 54:339–45.

173. Means J R, et al. The effects of disopyramide phosphate on serum glucose and glucose counterregulation in the dog. Fundam Appl Toxicol 1985; 5:539–45.

174. Series C. Hypoglycemia induced or facilitated by disopyramide. Rev Med Int 1988; 9:528–9.

175. Oshrain C, Arif M, Laidlaw J C, Cook W R, Willis P. A double-blind comparison

of disopyramide phosphate and quinidine sulphate as antiarrhythmic agents. Report from Scientific Exhibit, 40th Scientific Sessions, American Heart Association, Miami, Florida, Nov. 15–18, 1976.

176. Teichman S L, Ferrick A, Kim S G, Matos J A, Waspe L E, Fisher J D. Disopyramide-pyridostigmine interaction: selective reversal of anticholinergic symptoms with preservation of antiarrhythmic effect. J Am Coll Cardiol 1987; 10:633–41.

177. Ilett K F, Tjokrosetio R R, Benzie J L. Correlation of disopyramide and N-desalkyl disopyramide plasma levels with anticholinergic side effects. Aust J Hosp Pharm 1982; 13:142–5.

178. Di Bianco R, Gottdiener J S, Singh S N, Fletcher R D. A review of the effects of disopyramide phosphate on left ventricular function and the peripheral circulation. Angiology 1987; 38:174–83.

179. Block P J, Winkle R A. Hemodynamic effects of antiarrhythmic drugs. Am J Cardiol 1983; 52:14C–23C.

180. Landmark K, Bredesen J E, Thaulow E, Simonsen S, Amlie JP. Pharmacokinetics of disopyramide in patients with imminent to moderate cardiac failure. Eur J Clin Pharmacol 1981; 19:187–92.

181. Podrid P J, Lampert S, Braboys T B, Blatt C M, Lown B. Aggravation of arrhythmia by antiarrhythmic drugs—incidence and predictors. Am J Cardiol 1987; 59:38E–44E.

182. Casedevant B, Sabaut D. Syncopes par torsades de pointe en rapport avec la prise de disopyramide. Nouv Presse Med 1975; 4:2339.

183. Commeerford P J, Beck W. Ventricular tachycardia with torsade de pointes morphology induced by oral disopyramide. S Afr Med J 1980; 58:447–8.

184. Rothman M T. Prolonged QT interval, atrioventricular block, and torsade de pointes after antiarrhythmic therapy. Br Med J 1980; 280:922–3.

185. Tzivoni D, Keren A, Stern S, Gottlieb S. Disopyramide-induced torsade de pointes. Arch Intern Med 1981; 141:946–7.

186. Croft C H, Kennelly B M. Ventricular tachyarrhythmias induced by disopyramide and other similar antiarrhythmic drugs. S Afr Med J 1981; 59:871–3.

187. Wald R W, Waxman M B, Colman J M. Torsade de pointes ventricular tachycardia. A complication of disopyramide shared with quinidine. J Electrocardiol 1981; 14:301–7.

188. Keren A, Tzivoni D, Golhman J M, Corcos P, Benhorin J, Stern S. Ventricular pacing in atypical ventricular tachycardia. J Electrocardiol 1981; 14:201–6.

189. Ko P T, Gulamhusein S, Kostuk W, Klein G J. Torsades de pointes, a common arrhythmia, induced by medication. Can Med J 1982; 127:368–72.

190. Schweitzer P, Mark H. Torsade de pointes caused by disopyramide and hypokalemia. Mt Sinai J Med 1982; 49:110–4.

191. Santinelli V, Chiariello M, Condorelli M. Torsade de pointes (letter). Circulation 1982; 66:250–1.

192. Riccioni N, Castiglioni M, Bartolomei C. Disopyramide-induced QT prolongation and ventricular tachyarrhythmias. Am Heart J 1983; 105:870–1.

193. Kay G N, Plumb V J, Arciniegas J G, Henthorn R W, Waldo A L. Torsade de pointes: the long-short initiating sequence and other clinical features. Observations in 32 patients. J Am Coll Cardiol 1983; 2:806–17.

194. Nguyen P T, Scheinman M M, Seger J. Polymorphous ventricular tachycardia: clinical characterization, therapy and the QT interval. Circulation 1986; 74: 340–9.

195. Meltzer R S, Robert E W, McMorrow M, Martin R P. Atypical ventricular tachycardia as a manifestation of disopyramide toxicity. Am J Cardiol 1978; 42:1049–53.

196. Nicholson W J, Martin C E, Gracey J G, Knoch H R. Disopyramide-induced ventricular fibrillation. Am J Cardiol 1979; 43:1053–5.

197. Lo K S, Gantz K B, Stetson P L, Lucchesi B R, Pitt B. Disopyramide-induced ventricular tachycardia. Arch Intern Med 1980; 140:413–4.

26

Lidocaine

Jonathan C. Makielski and Morton F. Arnsdorf

The University of Chicago
Chicago, Illinois

INTRODUCTION

Lidocaine hydrochloride was developed in 1946 as a local anesthetic agent and was used as an antiarrhythmic agent for the first time in 1950 (1). It has subsequently become the most commonly used antiarrhythmic drug for the treatment of emergent ventricular arrhythmias. The drug has found favor because of its ease of use, rapidity of effect, and relatively few bioelectric and other complications.

BASIC PHARMACOLOGY: ELECTROPHYSIOLOGIC EFFECTS ON ISOLATED CARDIAC TISSUES

The Hypothesis of Altered Excitability

We suggested in 1977 that excitability must be rendered abnormal for dangerous ventricular arrhythmias to arise. We called this the hypothesis of altered excitability (2). Cardiac excitability connotes the ease with which cells undergo individual and sequential regenerative depolarization and repolarization, communicate with each other, and propagate in a normal and abnormal manner (3–5). Normal excitability results in a coordinated spread of electrical excitation and contraction and an efficient cardiac output. Arrhythmias appear when excitability is rendered abnormal.

In the sections that follow, we develop the three premises that underly the hypothesis of altered excitability. The first premise is that cardiac excitability depends on the interaction among the determinants of the resting potential and both the active and passive cellular properties, which in turn can be considered elements in an electrophysiologic matrix. The second is that the normal matrix must be altered by arrhythmogenic influences that affect one or more components of excitability to produce abnormal excitability, which in turn may influence impulse propagation, alter automaticity, and affect repolarization singly or in combination, thereby resulting in arrhythmias. The third is that the normal matrix or the matrix deformed by arrhythmogenic influences may interact with antiarrhythmic drugs, resulting in yet another matrix configuration. The predominant drug action or actions may differ in time depending on the matrix encountered, perhaps resulting in yet another matrix configuration that theoretically may be antiarrhythmic, antifibrillatory, or proarrhythmic.

Effect of Lidocaine on Active Cellular Properties

Active cellular properties relate to the opening and closing of channels that carry the currents responsible for the ionic currents that in turn are responsible for rapid depolarization and repolarization of the action potential. The channels are selectively permeable to different ionic species and are controlled by gates that open and close as a function of voltage, time, or, sometimes, binding by a hormone, drug, or other ligand.

The TTX-Sensitive Sodium Channel

Lidocaine is both an antiarrhythmic agent and a local anesthetic. The mechanism of action and its relative selectivity for heart can largely be explained by its action on active cellular properties, in particular the block of the sodium channel. The interested reader is directed to a review of the role of local anesthetic properties in the mechanism of antiarrhythmic drugs by Gintant and Hoffman (6).

Lidocaine blocks sodium current I_{Na} in cardiac tissue as well as in nerve and skeletal muscle. The action of lidocaine on the sodium channel has been most thoroughly investigated in nerve and skeletal muscle because these preparations were most amenable to study. Initial studies in heart depended upon indirect measures of I_{Na}, such as maximal upstroke velocity of the action potential $\dot{V}_{max}$ and conduction. Weidmann (7) showed a reduction in $\dot{V}_{max}$ by the local anesthetic cocaine in Purkinje fibers. Lidocaine has little effect on $\dot{V}_{max}$ or conduction in normal atrial, Purkinje, or ventricular tissues (8–11). Lidocaine may increase $\dot{V}_{max}$ in partially depolarized tissues, presumably by hyperpolarizing the cell and removing some inactivation of the sodium channel. Lidocaine can decrease $\dot{V}_{max}$ and slow conduction in depolarized, acidotic, and ischemic tissues (12–22). More recently, the block of I_{Na} by lidocaine has been measured directly in cardiac voltage clamp preparations (23–25).

The development and recovery of lidocaine block of I_{Na} has a complex dependence upon pH and membrane potential. Lidocaine is a

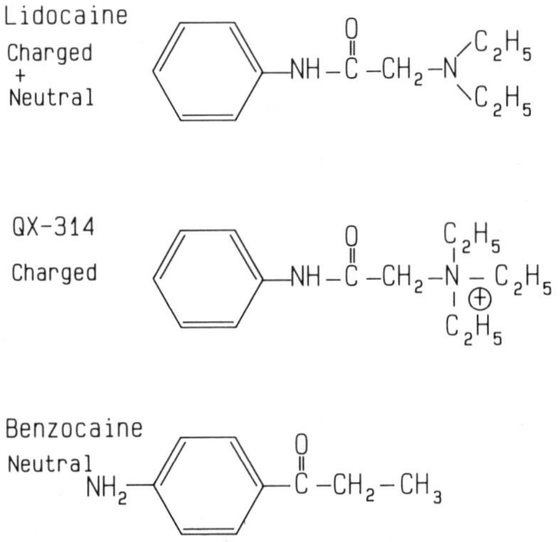

Figure 1 Local anesthetic structures. Lidocaine, a tertiary amine, has a pK_a of 7.9 and therefore exists in both the charged and neutral species. QX-314, a quaternary amine, is permanently charged. Benzocaine is always neutral.

tertiary amine (Fig. 1) with a pK_a of about 7.9 so that at physiologic pH more than half of the drug exists as the charged species. Neutral lidocaine partitions rapidly into the membrane, but charged lidocaine does not (26). Lidocaine is thought to block the sodium channel by binding to site inside the pore (27), thus rendering the channel nonconductive. The idea that lidocaine when bound completely blocks each channel is supported by recent patch clamp studies that show single-channel current levels are not affected by lidocaine (28). The charged drug can only get to the binding site through the aqueous route from the inside of the cell (Fig. 2). This route may not be available when the channel is in the closed state; that is, the channel must first be opened for the drug to block. Neutral drug, on the other hand, can reach the binding site and, perhaps more importantly, leave the binding site, through the membrane. This view of the sodium channel was derived mainly from voltage clamp studies in nerve (26,29,30) and skeletal muscle (31). The permanently charged lidocaine analog QX-314 blocked sodium channels only from the inside and blocked only the open state of the channel. This model has been presumed to hold for heart as well,

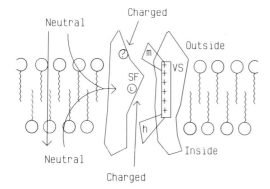

Figure 2 The way in which charged and neutral local anesthetics may interact with the sodium channel. The channel consists of an aqueous pore formed by a channel protein through the membrane. The channel has a selectivity filter (SF) and a voltage sensor (VS) that moves the gates (m and h) in response to changes in the transmembrane potential. The local anesthetic site (L) can be reached by charged drug from the inside only. Neutral drug can cross the membrane and also access the receptor from the lipid phase. Also shown is a putative binding site on the outside (?) that may be unique to cardiac sodium channels. This site is suggested by studies showing block on the outside of Purkinje cells (32).

but QX-314 has been shown to block I_{Na} from the outside of Purkinje cells (Fig. 3) (32) and $\dot{V}_{max}$ from the outside of Purkinje fibers (33,34). Perhaps cardiac sodium channels have an additional outside site (Fig. 2) that may be exploited to design drugs selectively targeted for the cardiac sodium channel.

Lidocaine causes both rest block and use-dependent block (35). Lidocaine binding to the channel can best be thought of in terms of the modulated receptor model (Fig. 4) (36) (in Ref. 26, see Introduction by Gintant). During the cardiac cycle sodium channels at rest (R) open briefly (A), on the order of about 1 msec, and then inactivate (I). The channel stays in the inactivated conformation (I) until repolarization of the membrane, at which time they revert to the resting state (R). Lidocaine binds most avidly to the states present during a depolarization (A and I) and then unbinds from the resting state (R). The binding to the open and inactivated states during each depolarization produces block that wears off during diastole. If recovery is incomplete subsequent pulses exhibit a decrease in current, until after

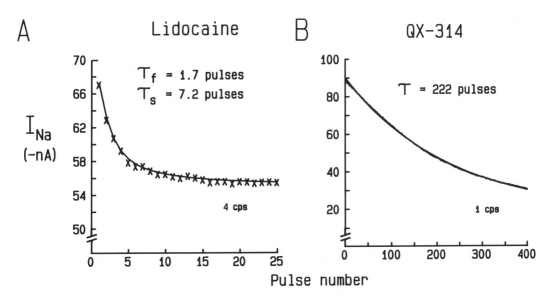

Figure 3 Use-dependent block of I_{Na} by lidocaine. Peak I_{Na} plotted for each depolarizing pulses in a train in internally perfused voltage-clamped Purkinje cells. (A) The fall in peak current for 50×10^{-6}M lidocaine is biexponential. (B) The fall in 10×10^{-6}M QX-314 applied inside is a single exponential. (16°C, external Na 45 mM, internal Na 0 mM, holding potential -150 mV, depolarizations to -10 mV lasting 100 msec in at 4 Hz lidocaine and 10 msec at 1 Hz in QX-314.)

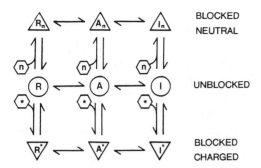

Figure 4 The state transitions in the modulated receptor model of drug action, with block by neutral drug and charged drug. At negative potentials the channel exists in the resting state (R). In response to a depolarization it enters an activated state (A), which conducts current and then enters the inactivated state (I). When the membrane is repolarized the channel recovers (IR). Drug-bound channel states are indicated by an asterisk (*) for charged drugs and neutral drugs by n. Not all transitions shown neccessarily occur with high probability (e.g., binding of changed drug to the resting state RR*), and for clarity of illustration some transitions (e.g., IR) are not shown.

a number of pulses the amount of drug binding during the pulse is equal to the recovery and a "steady state" is achieved (Fig. 3). Lidocaine has a relatively fast onset and recovery from block (37), with steady state achieved after only a few pulses. The level of block also increases with longer depolarizations and with depolarizations that are subthreshold for opening channels but sufficient to inactivate channels (24). Although lidocaine avidly blocks the open channel (38,39), lidocaine is known as primarily an inactivated state blocker because this property accounts for the majority of its important effects. Another factor that contributes to the accumulation of block is the hyperpolarizing shift in the recovery gating kinetics of the drug-bound channels (the transitions between the starred states in Fig. 4), which is predicted by the modulated receptor model. This shift causes channels to accumulate in the drug-bound inactivated state, with greater accumulation at depolarized potentials. Although the necessity for the assumption of altered drug-bound channels has been questioned in the guarded receptor hypothesis (40),

experiments show that depolarization favors increased block (24,41).

Lidocaine exists as both a charged and uncharged species. Which species accounts for the block? The permanently charged lidocaine derivative QX-314 shows use-dependent block (Fig. 3); the neutral derivative benzocaine shows only rest block. QX-314 block also develops very slowly and does not increase when the depolarization is lengthened. This suggests that the charged form binds primarily to the open state and comes off very slowly. That benzocaine shows only rest block suggests that if it binds preferentially to the open and inactivated states it comes off so quickly no block is evident on the following pulse. The development of lidocaine block is at least biexponential (Fig. 3). The fast exponential may be caused by neutral drug coming off and the slower exponential by charged drug unbinding. The slow time constant for lidocaine is faster than for QX-314 because lidocaine can deprotonate (42,43) and escape as the neutral species. This makes the recovery rates pH dependent, with recovery slower at more acid pH (44).

These complex actions at the sodium channel can explain many of the mechanisms that are important for lidocaine's action as an antiarrhythmic agent. How does lidocaine act preferentially on heart over nerve and skeletal muscle? The cardiac sodium channel may have an intrinsically higher affinity for lidocaine, but much if not all of the preference can be explained by the greater block that develops to the inactivated state during the longer cardiac action potentials. This also may explain the much greater effectiveness against arrhythmias developing in the ventricle and Purkinje system, where action potentials are longer than in the atria.

How does lidocaine act against arrhythmias but not against normal excitability? The more acid pH and the depolarized membrane potential found in ischemia or damaged tissue both favor greater block. This is considered in more detail in a later section.

By blocking Na^+ influx lidocaine can reduce intracellular sodium activity in vitro (3,45). Reduced intracellular sodium activity can lead to reduced intracellular calcium activity through the sodium-calcium exchange mechanism. This reduced calcium activity causes reduced contractility, thus providing a mechanism for the negative inotropy seen with lidocaine. The same mechanism, however, can be beneficial in ameliorating calcium overload conditions, which have been implicated in causing afterdepolarizations and arrhythmias caused by triggered automaticity (45).

Another interesting effect of the modulated receptor model explains how the faster drug lidocaine competes with the slower acting local anesthetic bupivacaine (46), causing a reduction in the block by bupivacaine. Lidocaine binds to the channel, displacing bupivacaine during a depolarization, but because it recovers quickly it allows more channels to open on the subsequent pulse that if they were bound by bupivacaine.

Effect on Other Membrane Currents

Changes in potassium and calcium conductances have been suggested by the effects of lidocaine on the action potential duration and upon resting membrane resistance. Both block (47) and lack of effect (48) by lidocaine have been reported in voltage clamp studies. Effects on these currents have been shown for quinidine (49,50). Lidocaine increased ^{42}K flux in Purkinje and ventricular tissues but not in atrial tissues (51). In voltage-clamped Purkinje fibers, however, no effect was found on potassium conductances, but rather block of the "pacemaker current" (i_f), carried by sodium ions, was found (52). The effects of lidocaine on currents other than the tetrodotoxin (TTX)-sensitive rapid Na^+ require further study because of their possible importance in automaticity, repolarization, and refractoriness.

Most explanations of mechanism assume that lidocaine results from direct actions on the myocardial cell membrane. Because lidocaine is also active against channels in nerves, the possibility that at least some of its action may result from change in autonomic activity must be considered (53).

Repolarization and Refractoriness

Lidocaine shortens the action potential duration and effective refractory period in normal Purkinje fibers and ventricular muscle (8,10). The levels of lidocaine achieved during bolus administration, however, may prolong the refractory period (54). Wittig et al. (55) reported that the effect is greatest in the distal Purkinje fibers, where the action potential is the longest. Lidocaine does not affect the action potential duration a effective refractory period of atrial tissues (9).

A number of investigators attributed the action potential shortening after lidocaine to a drug-induced decrease in a TTX-sensitive inward current during the plateau (45,52,56). Bennet (57) in patch clamp studies suggested that lidocaine preferentially blocks late Na channel openings. Other membrane currents may also play a role in this action, as may the accumulation of extracellular potassium. The duration of refractoriness is prolonged more than is the action potential, presumably because lidocaine delays reactivation of the fast sodium channel (19,23,24,58). This tends to eliminate very early ventricular activation.

"Membrane responsiveness" is a useful screening approach to assessing the effect of a drug on inactivation and reactivation of the sodium system. $\dot{V}_{max}$, used as an index of sodium current, is plotted as a function of V_m at the time of activation by a premature depolarization introduced during phase 3 of a train of basic cycles. An S-shaped relationship results that can provide an estimation of the inactivation variable. In Figure 5 the membrane responsiveness is shown after three concentrations of lidocaine at $[K+]_o$ of 3.0 mM (10). In Figure 5A the higher concentrations of lidocaine (5×10^{-5} and 1×10^{-4} M) decreased $\dot{V}_{max}$ and shifted the curve rightward and downward. The lower concentration (1×10^{-5} M), however, increased $\dot{V}_{max}$ and the curve was steeper. Although it was not commented upon in this article, the increased $\dot{V}_{max}$ may have resulted from hyperpolarization of the resting cell after lidocaine with removal of some inhibition of the sodium channel. Figure 5B shows the reversibility of lidocaine's effect.

Repolarization may fail to occur normally in a variety of settings, resulting in prolongation of the action potential or in the failure of

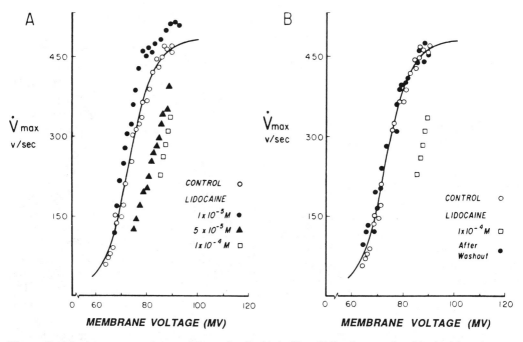

Figure 5 Membrane responsiveness in a canine Purkinje fiber. Following a train of basic driven beats at a constant cycle length, a premature test beat is introduced into electrical diastole. The test beat is made increasingly premature until it encroaches into the refractory period of the last basic driven beat. $\dot{V}_{max}$ of the premature action potential is plotted as a function of the membrane voltage at which activation occurs. (A) The effect of three concentrations of lidocaine on membrane responsiveness. The control shows the typical S-shaped curve. Lidocaine at 1×10^{-5} M shifts the curve to the left, makes it steeper, and increases $\dot{V}_{max}$. Lidocaine at 5×10^{-5} M shifts the curve downward and to the right and decreases $\dot{V}_{max}$. Lidocaine at 1×10^{-4} shifts the curve farther to the right and further depresses $\dot{V}_{max}$. Note the change in the minimal membrane activation voltage at which a response could be elicited. (B) Reversibility of lidocaine-induced depression of membrane responsiveness 1 hr after washout. [Reproduced from Bigger and Mandel (101), with permission.]

normal repolarization with the establishment of a quiescent stable steady state at the plateau voltage or in triggered activity at a low V_m, and lidocaine has been shown capable of normalizing such action potentials (59–62). Examples are shown in Figures 6 and 7.

Effect of Lidocaine on Passive Cellular Properties

In the mid nineteenth century Kelvin developed equations to describe the decrement in signal carried by the transatlantic telegraph cable. The cell has a low-resistance myoplasm that is surrounded by a membrane that has both capacitative elements and a high resistance, analogous to a telegraph cable with a low-resistance core and a high-resistance insu-

lation. As recently reviewed (4,5), the cable equations have been modified for the heart and describe experimental observations quite well. Cells are connected and communicate with each other through gap junctions that normally have a low resistance to ionic flow. With injury, gap junctional resistance may increase and cells may uncouple, actions mediated by changes in pH and intracellular calcium activity. The membrane insulation is imperfect, so current leaks throughout. This current loss results in less current being available as a function of distance for the longitudinal flow of ions through the myoplasm and the gap junctions.

Electrical analogs are shown in Figures 8B and 8C. The terms in the modified cable equations can be assessed experimentally, permit-

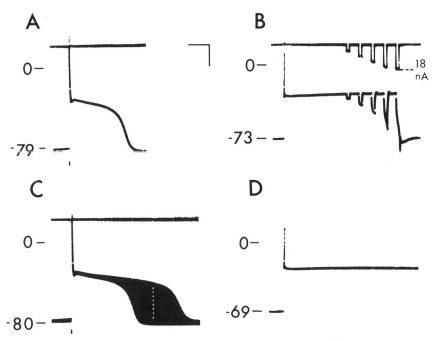

Figure 6 Failed repolarization after exposure of a sheep Purkinje fiber to lysophosphatidylcholine (LPC), a putative metabolite of ischemia, and normalization of the action potential by lidocaine. (A) Control with a V_r of -79 mV and an action potential duration of 290 msec. (B) After exposure to LPC, one steady state was observed at a V_r of -73 mV and a second steady state was observed at the plateau potential. Intracellular hyperpolarizing currents of increasing strength were applied with 18 nA, finally causing attainment of the repolarization "threshold" and a return to V_r. If current is not applied V_m remains at the plateau indefinitely. (C) After exposure to lidocaine the action potential duration progressively shortened to a normal value of 300 msec and V_r became somewhat more negative at -80 mV. (D) Washout of lidocaine during continued LPC superfusion caused a return to two stable steady states and a less negative V_r. [From Sawicki and Arnsdorf (62), with permission.]

ting determination of specific longitudinal resistance (R_i, Ω/cm) that is determined by myoplasmic and gap junctional resistance, specific membrane resistance (R_m, Ω/cm^2), membrane capacitance (C_m, μF/cm^2), the time constant (τ_m, msec) that describes the charging of the capacitor and the effects of R_m, and the length distance constant (λ, mm) that describes the interactions between cells in terms of the distance over which one cell may electrotonically influence another. Figure 8B shows the drop-off in V_m as a function of distance, and λ is defined as the distance at which V_m falls to $V_o e^{-1}$, which is about 37% of its value at the point of stimulation V_o.

Lidocaine has little effect on R_i and C_m but decreases R_m, λ, and τ_m in normal cardiac Purkinje fibers (63,64). The effect on R_m as assessed in multicellular preparations differs

from that in the isolated myocyte (48) for reasons that are unclear. Lidocaine also has little effect on resting potential V_r in the atria, His-Purkinje system, and ventricular muscle.

Effect of Lidocaine on Electrophysiologic Properties Dependent on Both Active and Passive Cellular Properties: Liminal Length and Impulse Propagation

Liminal length is the amount of tissue that must be raised above threshold so that the inward depolarizing current from one region is greater than the repolarizing influences of the adjacent tissues to permit regenerative depolarization of neighboring tissues (65). The liminal length is directly proportional to the charge developed by the active cellular proper-

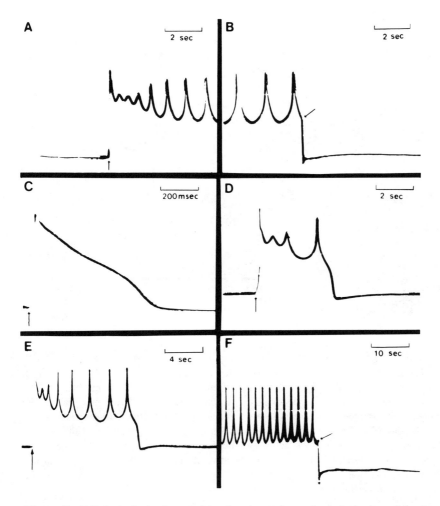

Figure 7 Failed repolarization resulting in triggered sustained rhythmic activity in a sheep cardiac Purkinje fiber with normalization of the action potential by lidocaine. (A, B) An intracellularly applied current resulted in a relatively normal phase 0 that was followed by a failure of normal repolarization and the appearance of oscillatory activity at a low V_m. The triggered sustained rhythmic activity persisted indefinitely until terminated by a intracellularly applied hyperpolarizing current (arrow in B) that permitted attainment of the repolarization "threshold" and a return to V_r. (C) Lidocaine caused almost immediately attainment of the repolarization threshold and normalization of the action potential. (D–F) After washout of lidocaine triggered sustained rhythmic activity reappeared rapidly. By the time the photograph in F was taken, an intracellularly applied hyperpolarizing current was required to return the action potential to V_r. [From Arnsdorf and Friedlander (61), with permission.]

ties and inversely proportional to the membrane capacitance and the length constant.

Referring again to Figure 8B, if the liminal length requirements of element A-B are fulfilled, this influences its neighboring element, C-D. If the electrotonic influence from membrane element A-B is sufficient to bring membrane element C-D up to threshold (or, more properly, to fulfill its liminal length requirements), regenerative depolarization and an ac-

tion potential result in element C-D. If the electrotonic influence is insufficient the current continues to decay exponentially. Quite clearly, the ability of a cell to attain threshold depends both on the current strength due to active cellular properties and on the sink of the tissue's cable properties. Lidocaine decreases R_m and λ. As a result the electrotonic current produces smaller changes in V_m for a given current than normal, resulting in less ef-

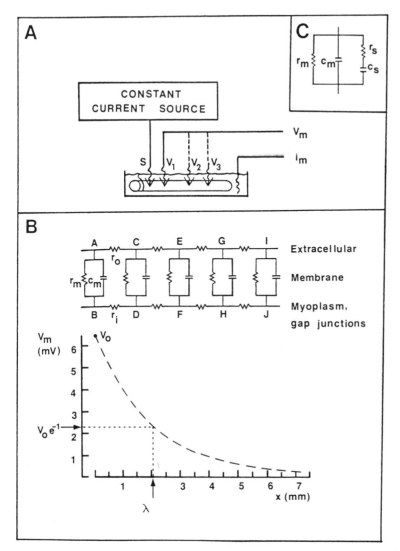

Figure 8 (A) Experimental arrangement for cable analysis in which constant current is injected intracellularly through a microelectrode (S) positioned near the ligated end of a cardiac Purkinje fiber so that all the current passes longitudinally in one direction to the right. The response in V_m is recorded by microelectrodes positioned at several points along the cablelike Purkinje fiber (V_1, V_2, and V_3). Measurements of current I are obtained from the bath ground. (B,top) The electrical analogs of the resistance of the extracellular space r_o, the resistance and capacitance of the cell membrane r_m and c_m, respectively, and the longitudinal or internal resistance r_i that results from the major effect of the gap junction and the lesser effect of the myoplasm. (Bottom) V_m plotted as a function of the distance x between the stimulating and recording microelectrodes. (C) A more complex electrical analog that includes series resistance and capacitance r_s and c_s, respectively. [From Arnsdorf (169), with permission.]

fect on neighboring elements. This may result in neighboring tissue elements failing to have their liminal length requirements fulfilled with failure of excitation.

Assuming that element C-D fulfills the liminal length requirements of unit E-F, the action potential propagates one until further, and so on. Impulse propagation thus depends on both active and passive cellular properties. The safety factor for impulse propagation depends on the excess of current source over the drain due to passive properties, the sink, so that the liminal length requirements of one cell after another are met. A decrease in the intensity of the active properties generally reduces conduction velocity.

Lidocaine in concentrations equivalent to antiarrhythmic plasma levels has little effect on conduction in normal tissues (8,10,66). Lidocaine may improve conduction in tissues injured by stretch or ischemia (10,63), presumably as a result of V_r more toward normal in depolarized tissue, thereby removing inactivation of the sodium system. As discussed earlier, lidocaine may normalize repolarization, which in turn normalizes conduction (2,60,62). These mechanisms may interrupt reentry by abolishing the area of unidirectional block in the reentrant circuit.

Lidocaine slows conduction in depolarization, hyperkalemic, acidotic, and ischemic tissues (12–18,22,67), and this slowing is use dependent (68,69). This is presumably related to the increased binding affinity for the inactivated state of the sodium channels that occurs at lower V_m, which has been discussed. Moreover, a lower pH increases the ionization of lidocaine (16,70). We found that lidocaine decreases conduction velocity in tissues exposed to lysophosphatidylcholine (LPC), a putative metabolite of ischemia, by affecting both active and passive properties, that is, both by decreasing sodium conductance and by decreasing R_m and λ (62,64). Slowing of conduction could interrupt reentrant arrhythmias by converting an area of unidirectional block into one of bidirectional block.

Cardiac Excitability, Arrhythmogenic Influences, and the Action of Lidocaine

The first premise, then, seems well supported. Cardiac excitability depends on the interaction among the determinants of the resting potential and both the active and passive cellular properties. This can be depicted as an electrophysiologic matrix (Fig. 9). The second premise is that the normal matrix must be altered by arrhythmogenic influences that affect one or more components of excitability to produce abnormal excitability. Experimentally, LPC, a putative metabolite of ischemia, may increase or decrease excitability by affecting the balance among active and passive proper-

ties and creating a proarrhythmic matrix configuration (upper and lower pathways in Fig. 9) (62,71).

The third premise was that the normal matrix or the matrix deformed by arrhythmogenic influences may interact with antiarrhythmic drugs resulting in yet another matrix configuration. Experimentally, lidocaine has been found to have different predominant actions depending on whether the electrophysiologic matrix was normally configured (middle pathway) or deformed by LPC to increase of decrease excitability (lower and upper pathways, respectively) (62). This demonstration that the predominant drug action or actions may differ in time depending on the matrix encountered highlights the limitations of rigid drug classifications, such as that by Vaughan Williams (72).

Automaticity

Lidocaine has no significant effect on sinus node automaticity. In awake dogs lidocaine affected neither sinus nodal function nor atrioventricular conduction (73). As is discussed, the same holds true in humans.

Lidocaine can increase the maximum diastolic potential in an automatic fast-response tissue, which would cause a decrease in the rate of firing (60,63,64,74). Lidocaine also suppresses the rate of isoproterenol-enhanced automaticity (75). Lidocaine can decrease the slope of phase 4 depolarization. This probably occurs through a depression of inward depolarizing current as assessed by ^{42}K flux (51) and electrophysiologic measurements (63). The apparent voltage threshold for depolarization does not seem to be much changed by lidocaine.

Cellular calcium loading, whether caused by digitalis, catecholamines, or other methods, leads to the development of delayed afterdepolarizations. Lidocaine suppresses such afterdepolarizations, presumably by depressing the inward sodium current (45,76–79) or perhaps by hyperpolarizing the cell and decreasing excitability. Lidocaine has been reported to elevate the ventricular fibrillation threshold in the Langendorff-perfused rabbit

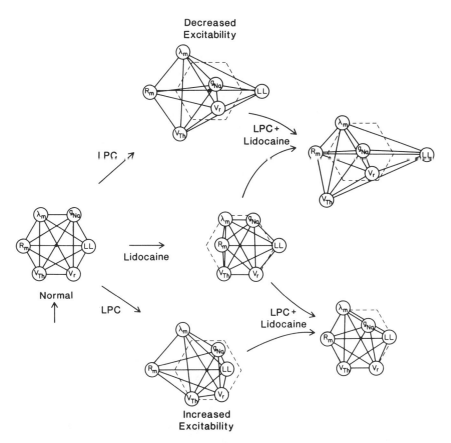

Figure 9 Drugs may have multiple actions depending on the matrix encountered. A simplified normal electrophysiologic matrix composed of active and passive cellular properties relevant to cardiac excitability. The determinants include the resting potential V_r, threshold voltage V_{th}, sodium conductance g_{Na}, membrane resistance R_m, the length constant λ, and as a measure of overall excitability the liminal length (LL). Each in turn has its own determinants, but these contain broad descriptions of the resting potential and its several determinants; active generator properties and the relevant gates; passive cellular properties that determine transmembrane and longitudinal current flow; and the net excitability. The bonds between the determinants suggest interactions and mutual dependencies. The normal state is depicted by the hexagon. A shift toward the center of the hexagon indicates a decrease in the quantity; a shift away from the center of the hexagon an increase in the quantity. After exposure to lysophosphatidylcholine (LPC) excitability may be increase (lower pathway) due largely to an increase in R_m and λ despite a decrease in g_{Na} or decrease (upper pathway) due primarily to depression of g_{Na}. Lidocaine slightly decreases R_m in normal tissues (middle pathway). In the lower pathway lidocaine decreases excitability and returns liminal length to nearly its normal value by decreasing R_m and λ despite some decrease in g_{Na}. Note that the effects on passive properties are primarily responsible for the near normalization of the matrix. In the upper pathway lidocaine decreases excitability by further depressing g_{Na} and making V_{th} less negative rather than by affecting passive properties. [Reproduced with permission from Arnsdorf and Wasserstrom (3).]

heart and to protect against ouabain-induced arrhythmias (80).

Early afterdepolarizations (EAD) are a form of triggered automaticity associated with a prolonged action potential plateau that arise before complete repolarization. EAD have been implicated in the genesis of long QT interval-related polymorphic ventricular tachycardia (torsades de pointes). Lidocaine eliminates EAD induced by Cs (81) or Bay K 8644 (82). It has been postulated that lidocaine eliminates EAD indirectly by blocking the inward sodium current during the plateau, which shortens the action potential and diminishes recovery of the inward calcium current that causes the EAD (83).

Effect of Specific Tissues

Much of this material has been covered in the general discussion and the citations in the preceding sections.

Sinoatrial Node

Lidocaine has little direct effect on the electrophysiologic properties of the normal sinoatrial node, nor does it indirectly affect the sinus node through the autonomic nervous system.

Atrial Muscle

Lidocaine has little effect on the active properties of the atria. As mentioned, the short action potential duration characteristic of atrial tissue is disadvantageous to a drug, such as lidocaine, that preferentially binds during the inactivated state of the sodium channel. Kabela (51) found that lidocaine little affected $^{42}K^+$ flux in the atria.

AV Node

Lidocaine has little effect on the slow inward current responsible for phase 0 depolarization in the AV node or on the autonomics that mediate AV nodal conduction.

Ventricular Conduction Tissue and the Working Myocardium

Much of the individual work has been cited. In summary, lidocaine causes a use- and voltage-dependent decrease in $\dot{V}_{max}$ primarily by binding with the sodium channel in the inactivated state. Lidocaine shortens the action potential duration, and the mechanism is thought to be by decreasing a TTX-sensitive inward current during the plateau. Lidocaine may normalize the action potentials of tissues in which some influence has prolonged the action potential duration or caused a failure of normal phase 3 repolarization. In the multicellular tissue of the Purkinje system lidocaine decreases R_m and shortens the length constant. In single ventricular myocytes lidocaine may increase R_m. As discussed, lidocaine under

some circumstances may improve conduction in these fast-response tissues. Lidocaine slows conduction in depolarized, acidotic, and ischemic tissues. Kabela found that lidocaine increased ^{42}K flux in Purkinje and ventricular tissues. The importance of this observation is uncertain, although it may be related to lidocaine's effect to move V_r closer to the normal resting and equilibrium potentials in depolarized tissues, thereby lessening inactivation of the sodium system, and may play a role in decreasing the slope of phase 4 depolarization (63). Lidocaine has little effect on the canine electrocardiogram (84). Issues regarding ischemia are discussed in the next major section.

Developmental Changes

Infants have been noted to be resistant to the actions of some antiarrhythmics (85). These effects may be explained by a developmental change in the sensitivity of sodium channels to block by the drugs. This effect has been demonstrated by showing that the decrease in $\dot{V}_{max}$ caused by lidocaine is greater in Purkinje fibers from adult dogs than those from young dogs (86,87).

BASIC PHARMACOLOGY: ANTIARRHYTHMIC EFFECTS IN EXPERIMENTAL ANIMALS

Atrial Arrhythmias

Lidocaine has little effect on the normal sinus node or on the electrophysiologic properties of the normal atrium. In a canine model of atrial flutter, lidocaine was not effective in converting the arrhythmia (88). Lidocaine may be useful in treating supraventricular arrhythmias due to digitalis toxicity.

Ventricular Arrhythmias

There is a large experimental literature. The drug is useful against arrhythmias following experimental myocardial infarction, reperfusion, and digitalis toxicity. Lidocaine has little effect on conduction in normal tissues in vitro or in vivo (8,10,66,73,89).

To briefly review some of the literature on ischemia, some studies have found lidocaine to be antiarrhythmic in this setting. Avitall et al. (90) assessed the effect of lidocaine on cardiac excitability in dogs during occlusion and reperfusion of coronary arteries using strength-duration curves and conduction times. The peak occurrence of ligation arrhythmias occurred, with a leftward shift of the strength-duration curve and with prolongation of conduction time. Lidocaine shifted the strength-duration curve upward, rendering the preparation less excitable. Other studies suggest that lidocaine does not reduce the incidence of ventricular arrhythmias during coronary artery ligation (91–93). Hope et al. (93) found that ischemic zone activation delay always preceded ventricular tachycardia, and the effect was heightened by rapid pacing. Lidocaine hastened the ischemic zone activation delay but in this study showed no significant effect on the ventricular tachycardia. Epstein et al. (94) also found early arrhythmias associated with ischemia to be relatively resistant to lidocaine. Yet other studies suggest that lidocaine may be proarrhythmic during acute ischemia in dogs (95), cats (96), and pigs (97). Lidocaine, however, may depress automaticity in the first 24 hr after occlusion (96,98). An increase in the ventricular fibrillation threshold has been reported during acute ischemia in the dog and rat (99–101).

The situation in late infarction is somewhat different. El-Sherif et al. (14) reported on studies done 3–7 days following ligation of the anterior descending coronary artery in dogs. They found that lidocaine consistently prolonged the refractoriness of potential reentrant pathways as assessed by a composite electrode, preferentially depressed conduction in the ischemic zone, and by these mechanisms abolished reentrant ventricular arrhythmias. Lidocaine increased the H-V time and could result in advanced block, including block in the His bundle and right bundle branch, 4–6 days after anterior septal artery ligation in a dog (66). Lidocaine may prolong the effective refractory period in depolarization ventricular muscle (14,15,102).

Reperfusion arrhythmias may represent yet another issue. Again, some studies show that lidocaine reduces ventricular fibrillation in a reperfusion model (101). Several canine studies have found lidocaine to have little effect against reperfusion ventricular arrhythmias (91,92,103). Bergey et al. (104) found that lidocaine pretreatment effectively prevented ventricular fibrillation in rats but increased the incidence of reperfusion-induced ventricular fibrillation in dogs and pigs. Avitall et al. (90) found that, during reperfusion, there were initially a downward shift in the strength-interval curve and conduction times were shorter than in the control. Lidocaine increased excitability by reducing excitation thresholds and exaggerated the effect of reperfusion on conduction. One study has suggested that lidocaine may reduce the size of experimental myocardial infarction in a model that employed 40 min of coronary occlusion followed by 5 hr of reperfusion (105).

Ilvento et al. (106) produced an accelerated idioventricular rhythm by injecting formalin into the His bundle. The accelerated idioventricular rhythm lasts for about 3 days, following which a slow idioventricular rhythm assumes control of the ventricles. Lidocaine suppressed the slow, but not the rapid idioventricular rhythm. Of interest, ethmozin suppressed the fast but not the slow idioventricular rhythm. The results suggest that lidocaine can suppress normal idioventricular pacemaker activity but not the abnormal type that is sensitive to ethmozin.

CLINICAL PHARMACOLOGY

Effects on Normal Human Electrocardiogram

Lidocaine little affects the normal sinus node directly or through autonomic mediation, so sinus rhythm is generally not disturbed. Because lidocaine has little effect on conduction in the atrium, AV node, His-Purkinje system, or ventricles in the normal heart, the drug has no significant effect on the P wave, the PR interval, or the QRS complex. Even though lidocaine shortens the action potential duration, changes in the QT duration are difficult to detect.

Acute Effects in Humans: Programmed Extrastimulation Studies

Lidocaine has no consistent effect on the sinus rate or the sinoatrial (SA) nodal recovery time in patients with the sick sinus syndrome (107). There is an occasional report of sinus arrest following lidocaine, presumably due to associated sinus nodal disease (e.g., Refs. 108 and 109).

Studies using His bundle recordings indicate that lidocaine has little effect on intratrial conduction and atrial refractoriness, on AV nodal conduction and refractoriness, on conduction in the His bundle branch-terminal Purkinje specialized conduction system, or on conduction or refractoriness in the ventricle (Refs. 110–112 among others). Rarely, infranodal block has been reported after lidocaine (113,114).

Lidocaine may somewhat increase antegrade refractoriness in accessory AV pathways (115). Akhtar et al. (116), however, reported that lidocaine either had no effect or actually enhance the ventricular response through accessary AV pathways during atrial fibrillation.

Tenczer et al. (117) studied the effects of overdrive atrial pacing and lidocaine on AV junctional rhythms in the human. Overdrive atrial pacing suppressed the AV junctional rhythm in some patients but increased it in others. Lidocaine decreased the rate and recovery time of the junctional rhythm in the group that showed overdrive suppression but had little effect on the rate or recovery time of the rhythm in the group that showed overdrive acceleration of the rhythm. The authors considered their study the clinical extension of the investigation by Ilvento et al. (106) in dogs already discussed and suggested that the AV junctional rhythm was due to normal automaticity in the group with overdrive suppression and to abnormal automaticity in the group with overdrive acceleration of the junctional rhythm. Another study showed that lidocaine had varying effects on AV junctional rhythms (Kuo and Reddy, Ref. 118).

Studies During Antiarrhythmic Therapy

The literature concerning the use of lidocaine clinically is vast, and we focus on a few articles. The primary use of lidocaine is for the control of prevention of ventricular arrhythmias in the setting of an acute myocardial infarction or during hospitalization and acutely in patients with recurrent life-threatening arrhythmias.

Lidocaine is effective in suppressing ventricular premature beats (VPB) and ventricular arrhythmias after acute myocardial infarction (Refs. 119–123 among others). Recalling the basic science literature suggesting that early arrhythmias may be resistant to lidocaine, it was not surprising that there is a substantial body of clinical literature that has questioned the efficacy of lidocaine in the first hours after a myocardial infarction (Refs. 124–130 among others). Clinical experience, however, suggests that the dosage and plasma levels of lidocaine determine efficacy in controlling ventricular arrhythmias associated with acute myocardial infarction (131,132). The recommendation has been made that prophylactic therapy may be useful (119,133).

Because of the high risk of arrhythmic death in the prehospital phase of myocardial infarction, therapy with lidocaine has been advocated in the field. Goldreyer and Wyman (134) reported a 89% response rate to lidocaine for ventricular premature beats within an hour of an acute myocardial infarction. Valentine et al. (135) did a double-blind investigation of 269 patients with acute myocardial infarction and found 8 of 113 patients died in the control group and 3 of 156 patients treated with 300 mg lidocaine IM died ($p < 0.03$). Others have reported IM lidocaine to be effective in the prehospital phase of myocardial infarction (136,137), but Bleifield et al. (138) found the drug not to be protective.

The prophylactic use of lidocaine during the in-hospital phase of acute myocardial infarction has been debated for years. Most studies have not shown much benefit. Lie et al. (139), however, found prophylactic therapy with lidocaine to be useful. A double-blind study was performed in 212 consecutive patients within 6 hr of acute myocardial infarction. Lidocaine was given in a 100 mg IV bolus followed by a 3 mg/min infusion, and 11 control patients and none of those receiving lidocaine experienced ventricular fibrillation. Of interest was that there were 10 deaths in the control group and 8 in the drug group, suggesting that the ultimate outcome was not affected by drug intervention since only 1 patient could not be resuscitated using direct current (DC) countershock. The drug may have reduced the morbidity associated with the resuscitative procedure, however. The protocol Lie et al. used, however, may have left a period of time between the bolus and the establishment of a stable drug level during which suboptimal plasma levels were present. High-dose lidocaine therapy, however, is associated with a high incidence of undesirable side effects, particularly those involving the central nervous system, such as convulsions. In general, antiarrhythmic prophylaxis with an appropriate administration of lidocaine for 2–3 days after acute myocardial infarction may be a reasonable approach to preventing primary ventricular fibrillation (133), and this has been suggested by the Bethesda Task Force on critical care. Lidocaine is relatively safe, and inotropic depression is rarely a problem.

Lidocaine has also been used in survivors of out-of-hospital ventricular fibrillation after myocardial infarction and was found effective in patients under 70 years of age within 6 hr of the onset of symptoms (140).

Lidocaine has been reported to be effective against a variety of digitalis-induced arrhythmias, including atrial tachycardia with block and bidirectional tachycardia (141).

Pharmacokinetics

Experimental Animal Studies
Animal studies have suggested important interactions between lidocaine and other commonly used drugs. Lidocaine is metabolized and cleared very efficiently in the liver. A decrease in hepatic blood flow, such as caused by propranolol, metoprolol, norepinephrine, or hemorrhage, decreases the clearance of

lidocaine and increases the plasma level (142–146). Conversely, increasing hepatic blood flow with isoproterenol or glucagon increases lidocaine clearance (142,144). Induction of microsomal enzymes by phenobarbital also increases hepatic clearance of lidocaine (147). Cimetidine also blocks some hepatic enzymes and may decrease hepatic blood flow, resulting in increased plasma lidocaine levels (148). Ranitidine, however, another H_2-antagonist that also decreases hepatic blood flow, does not effect the clearance of lidocaine (149).

Clinical Studies
The plasma half-life or half-time is the time required for the plasma concentration of lidocaine to decrease by one-half ($T_{1/2}$). In a two-compartment system, the disappearance of drug is biexponential, with a rapid distribution phase and a longer elimination phase, and the respective half-times are termed $T_{1/2}$ α and $T_{1/2}$ β. $T_{1/2}$ β is directly proportional to the volume of distribution and inversely proportional to the clearance.

The initial intravenous bolus of lidocaine is administered directly into the central compartment from which it transferred to the peripheral compartment. The $T_{1/2}$ α of lidocaine is 8–10 min, and $T_{1/2}$ β normally is about 100 min (150,151). This means that the plasma concentration of an initial bolus will fall below the clinically effective antidysrhythmic range of 1.5–5 µg/ml in 10–50 min depending on a variety of factors, such as the initial dose and the volume of the central compartment. An intravenous infusion begun at the time of the initial bolus produces only about 30% of the desired steady-state concentration in 1 hr and about 90% in 5 hr (i.e., three cycles of $T_{1/2}$ β or 300 min). Inadequate blood levels may be present for several hours in a regimen that employs a single bolus followed by a constant infusion.

Many regimens have been suggested for giving lidocaine. We have been pleased with the schedule of Benowitz et al. (150), which employs small loading doses and a constant-rate infusion. Given the $T_{1/2}$ α of 9 min, a total loading dose of 3.9 mg/kg is given as four injections at 8 min intervals, the first dose being 1.5 mg/kg and the subsequent doses being

0.8 mg/kg. The rate of administration of a bo-lus should be no more than 50 mg/min to minimize the chances for acute toxicity. Alter-natively, and initial bolus of 1.0 mg/kg fol-lowed by boli at 8–10 min of 0.8 mg/kg to a total of 200 or 300 mg can be used. After the last dose the plasma half-life approaches $T_{1/2}$ β, and a constant-rate intravenous infusion can maintain the plasma concentration. Various rates of infusion have been recommended in the literature, ranging from 20 to 50 μg/kg per min (about 1–5 mg/min). The rationale is that the plasma clearance is about 10 ml/kg per min in patients with normal hepatic blood flow, so the infusion rate required to maintain a plasma concentration of 3 μg/ml is 30 μg/kg per min. In the absence of heart failure and hepatic dysfunction, we generally recommend a dose of 30 μg/ml (about 3 mg/min) or more for the constant infusion. The $T_{1/2}$ β of 100 min also means that 5–8 hr is required for a change in the rate of infusion to produce a new steady-state plasma concentration. If an acute increase in the plasma concentration is required, boli of 25 mg or less should be ad-ministered every 15 min, the response titrated, and the infusion rate changed. Several varia-tions on this approach have been proposed by others. Wyman et al. (152) recommended a multiple-bolus technique that consists of a 75 mg bolus initially followed by 50 mg bolus in-jections every 5 min to total 225 mg depend-ing on the response. Intravenous lidocaine is also given, 2 mg/min initially and increased by 1 mg/min after each additional bolus to a maximum of 4 mg/ml. The investigators re-ported little toxicity with this regimen.

Alternatively, double-infusion techniques can be employed. Woosley and Shand (153) employed a rapid infusion of 120 μg/kg per min for 25 mins followed by a maintenance level of 32.7 μg/kg per min. The method of Benowitz has simplicity to recommend it.

A third half-life of about 4 hr has been de-scribed in patients after an acute myocardial that resulted in the toxic accumulation of lidocaine in patients at 48 hr or later after the beginning of lidocaine infusion (154,155).

The recommended regimens produce plasma levels of lidocaine that often are close to toxicity. Congestive heart failure may re-duce the central compartment volume as well as the total volume of distribution and de-crease hepatic blood flow, thereby reducing the clearance of lidocaine (156,157). Conges-tive heart failure may reduce the volume of the central compartment and the total volume of distribution and, by decreasing hepatic blood flow, reduce the clearance of lidocaine (156,157). Patients without congestive heart failure have a mean apparent volume of distri-bution of 1.32 L/kg and a mean clearance of 780 ml/min. Patients with moderate conges-tive heart failure have a smaller mean appar-ent volume of distribution of 0.88 L/kg and a lower mean clearance of 443 ml/min. Of inter-est, the $T_{1/2}$ β may be unchanged or prolong only by 30 min or so in patients with conges-tive heart failure. Congestive heart failure may also reduce enzymatic activity. In gen-eral, a 50–60% decrease in the infusion rate is required in the presence of a moderately re-duced cardiac output. This is equivalent to an initial bolus of 0.75 mg/kg and to an infusion rate of 20 μg/kg per min. Often, multiple boli are not required.

Hepatic dysfunction does not much affect the central compartment volume but may re-duce the drug clearance by some 40–60%. There is, however, great individual variability. Renal dysfunction little affects lidocaine levels since less than 10% appears unchanged in the urine. Drugs that affect hepatic blood flow or enzymatic activity were discussed in the pre-ceding section.

The use of intramuscular lidocaine in the prehospital phase of myocardial infarction has been mentioned. In the absence of shock an injection of 250 mg lidocaine reaches a plasma concentration of 1 μg/ml or more within 5–10 min and 2.0–2.5 μg/ml within 15–30 min (158).

Metabolism

Hepatic metabolism involves microsomal en-zymes (159–162). Lidocaine is deethylated and hydrolyzed in the liver. Lidocaine has two active metabolites, glycinexyldide and mono-ethylglyinexylidide, but the electrophysiologic effects are less than for the parent drug (162).

The metabolites, however, may accumulate during administration (163). Competitive displacement of lidocaine from sodium channels by glycinexylidide has been demonstrated in vitro (164), but the clinical significance of this interaction is unknown. Lidocaine is about half bound. It has an affinity to α_1-acid glycoprotein, which is an acute-phase reactant and increases after acute myocardial infarction (165).

Normally the clearance of lidocaine approximates hepatic blood flow, and less than 10% appears in the urine. The effect of congestive heart failure and certain drugs on clearance and metabolism was discussed in the preceding section.

Only 35% of lidocaine is absorbed if taken orally, and doses of 250–500 mg result in subtherapeutic plasma levels (166). Once absorbed, lidocaine passes via the portal vein into the liver, where 50% or more is cleared. Metabolites build up and toxicity is usual.

Toxicology

Toxic Effects in Experimental Animals and Tissues

Lidocaine and its two major metabolites, glycinexyldide and monethylglycinexyldide, may induce convulsions, muscular fasciculations, respiratory arrest, and other manifestations of neurotoxicity in animals. In experimental animals large doses of lidocaine may produce ventricular arrhythmias, including ventricular fibrillation and cardiac arrest.

Clinical Toxicology

The most common adverse reactions are neurotoxicity, including dizziness, drowsiness, slurred speech, blurred vision, seizures, muscular fasciculations, and respiratory arrest. Rarely, sinus nodal arrest and conduction disturbances may result. On occasion lidocaine may facilitate atrioventricular conduction, particularly through an accessory AV pathway, and increase the ventricular response to atrial fibrillation or atrial flutter. Hypersensitivity to lidocaine is rare, perhaps because it is an amide type rather than an ester type of local anesthetic. The negative inotropic effect is usually of little significance, although transient myocardial depression may follow intravenous lidocaine in some patients with congestive heart failure (131,167,168).

SUMMARY: THE ROLE OF LIDOCAINE IN THERAPEUTICS

Lidocaine is the most useful antiarrhythmic drug in the treatment of emergent ventricular arrhythmias. It is very effective against ventricular arrhythmias regardless of etiology and has been particularly useful in the setting of acute myocardial infarction and recurrent ventricular arrhythmias. Lidocaine is also effective against both supraventricular and ventricular arrhythmias due to digitalis toxicity, although other therapies, such as the use of digoxin antibodies, should be considered. Its efficacy against reperfusion arrhythmias is uncertain.

The drug is easily administered intravenously and intramuscularly. Clinically effective antiarrhythmic plasma levels can be achieved rapidly and quite easily. Toxicity can usually be avoided by judicious administration of the drug, and the hemodynamic and bioelectric complications of the drug are usually insignificant.

ACKNOWLEDGMENTS

Supported in part by a Physician Scientist Award K11-HL01572 (Makielski) and USPHS Merit Grant R37 HL 21788 (Arnsdorf) from the National Heart, Lung and Blood Insitute. We thank Mrs. Clarice Connor for her help in the preparation of this manuscript.

REFERENCES

1. Southworth J L, McKusick V A, Pierce E C, Rawson F L Jr. Ventricular fibrillation precipitated by cardiac catheterization. JAMA 1950; 143:717–20,
2. Arnsdorf M F. Membrane factors in arrhythmogenesis: concepts and definitions. Prog Cardiovasc Dis 1977; 19:413–29.
3. Arnsdorf M F, Wasserstrom J A. Mechanisms of action of antiarrhythmic drugs: a matrical approach. In: Fozzard H A, Haber

E, Jennings R B, Katz A M, Morgan H E, eds. The heart and cardiovascular system. New York: Raven Press 1986:1259–316.

4. Arnsdorf M F, Wasserstrom J A. A matrical approach to the basic and clinical pharmacology of antiarrhythmic drugs. Rev Clin Basic Pharmacol 1987; 6:131–88.

5. Arnsdorf M R. A matrical perspective of cardiac excitability: cable properties and impulse propagation. In: Sperelakis N, ed. Physiology and pathophysiology of the heart, 2nd ed. Boston: Mastinus Nijhoff 1989:133–74.

6. Gintant G A, Hoffman B F. The role of local anesthetic effects in the actions of antiarrhythmic drugs. In: Strichartz G R, ed. Handbook of experimental pharmacology. Berlin: Springer-Verlag 1987:213–51.

7. Weidmann S L. Effects of calcium ions and local anesthetics on electrical properties of Purkinje fibers. J Physiol (Lond) 1955; 129:568–82.

8. Davis L D, Temte J V. Electrophysiologic actions of lidocaine on cardiac ventricular muscle and Purkinje fibers. Circ Res 1969; 34:639–55.

9. Mandel W J, Bigger J T. Electrophysiologic effects of lidocaine on isolated canine and rabbit atrial tissue. J Pharmacol Exp Ther 1971; 178:81–102.

10. Bigger J T Jr, Mandel W T. Effect of lidocaine on transmembrane potentials of ventricular muscle and Purkinje fibers. J Clin Invest 1970; 49:63–77.

11. Bigger J T Jr, Mandel W T.- The effect of lidocaine on conduction in canine Purkinje fibers and at the ventricular muscle-Purkinje fiber junction. J Pharmacol Exp Ther 1970; 172:239–54.

12. Brennan F J, Cranefield P F, Wit A L. Effects of lidocaine on slow response and depressed fast response action potentials of canine cardiac Purkinje fibers. J Pharmacol Exp Ther 1982; 204:312–24.

13. Cardinal R, Janse M J, van Eeden I. et al. The effects of lidocaine on intracellular and extracellular potentials, activation and ventricular arrhythmias during acute regional ischemia in the isolated porcine heart. Circ Res 1981; 49:792–806.

14. El-Sherif N, Scherlag, Lazzara R, Hope R R. Re-entrant ventricular arrhythmias in the late myocardial infarction period. 4. Mechanism of action of lidocaine. Circulation 1977; 56:395–402.

15. Kupersmith J, Antman E M, Hoffman B F. In vivo electrophysiologic effects of lidocaine in canine acute myocardial infarction. Circ Res 1975; 36:84–91.

16. Nattel S, Elharrar V, Zipes D P, Baily J C. pH-dependent electrophysiologic effects of quinidine and lidocaine on canine cardiac Purkinje fibers. Circ Res 1981; 48:55–61.

17. Sasyniuk B I, Kus T: Comparison of the effects of lidocaine on electrophysiologic properties of normal Purkinje fibers and those surviving acute myocardial infarction. Fed Proc 1974; 33:476.

18. Singh B N, Vaughan Williams E M. Effect of altering potassium concentration on the action of lidocaine and diphenylhydantoin on rabbit atrial and ventricular muscles. Circ Res 1971; 29:286–95.

19. Chen C M, Gettes L C, Katzung B G. Effects of lidocaine and quinidine on steady-state characteristics and recovery kinetics (dV/dt_{max}) in guinea pig ventricular myocardium. Circ Res 1975; 37:20–9.

20. Hondeghem L M. Effects of lidocaine, phenytoin, and quinidine on ischemic canine myocardium. J Electrocardiol 1976; 9:203–9.

21. Hondeghem L M, Katzung B G. Test of a model of antiarrhythmic drug action: effects of quinidine and lidocaine on myocardial conduction. Circulation 1980; 61:1217–24.

22. Lazzara R, Hope R R, El-Sherif N, et al. Effects of lidocaine on hypoxia and ischemic cardiac cells. Am J Cardiol 1978; 41:872–9.

23. Lee K S, Hume J, Giles W, Brown A M. Sodium current depression by lidocaine and quinidine in isolated ventricular cells. Nature 1981; 291:325–7.

24. Bean B P, Cohen C J, Tsien R W. Lidocaine block of cardiac sodium channels. J Gen Physiol 1983; 81:613–42.

25. Sanchez-Chapula J, Tsuda Y, Josephson I R. Voltage and use-dependant effects of lidocaine on sodium current in rat single ventricular cells. Circ Res 1983; 52:557–65.

26. Hille B. Local anesthetics: Hydrophilic and hydrophobic pathways for the drug-receptor reaction. J Gen Physiol 1977; 69:497–515.

27. Hille B. Ionic channels of excitable membranes. Sunderland, MA: Sinauer Associates 1984.

28. Nilius B, Benndorf K, Markwardt F. Effects of lidocaine on single cardiac sodium channels. J Mol Cell Cardiol 1987; 19:965–74.

29. Strichartz G R. The inhibition of sodium currents in myelinated nerve by quaternary derivatives of lidocaine. J Gen Physiol 1973; 62:37–57.

30. Frazier D T, Narahashi T, Yamanda M. The site of action and active form of local anesthetics. II. Experiments with quaternary compounds. J Pharmacol Exp Ther 1970; 171:45–51.

31. Schwarz W, Palade P T, Hille B. Local anesthetics: effect of pH on use-dependent block of sodium channels in frog muscle. Biophy J 1977; 20:343–68.

32. Makielski J C, Alpert L A, Hanck D A, Fozzard H A. An externally accessible receptor for lidocaine block of sodium current in canine cardiac Purkinje cells. Biophys J 1988; 53:540a.

33. Gintant G, Hoffman B F, Naylor R E. The influence of molecular form on the interactions of local anesthetic-type antiarrhythmic agents with canine cardiac Na+ channels. Circ Res 1983; 52:735–46.

34. Gintant G A, Hoffman B F. Use-dependent block of cardiac sodium channels by quaternary derivatives of lidocaine. Pflugers Arch 1984; 400:121–9.

35. Courtney K R. Mechanisms of frequency-dependent inhibition of sodium currents in the frog myelinated nerve by the lidocaine derivative GEA 968. J Pharmacol Exp Ther 1975; 195:225–36.

36. Hondeghem L M, Katzung B G. Time and voltage-dependent interactions of antiarrhythmic drugs with cardiac sodium channels. Biochim Biophys Acta 1977; 474:373–98.

37. Courtney K R. Review: quantitative structure/activity relations on use-dependent block and repriming kinetics in myocardium. J Mol Cell Cardiol 1987; 19:319–30.

38. Matsubara T, Clarkson C, Hondeghem L. Lidocaine blocks open and inactivated cardiac sodium channels. Naunyn Schmiedebergs Arch Pharmacol 1987; 336:224–31.

39. Alpert L A, Makielski J C, Hanck D A, Fozzard H A. Lidocaine block of sodium currents in single canine cardiac Purkinje cells (abstract). Circulation 1987; 76(Part II):IV-149.

40. Starmer C F, Grant A O, Strauss H. Mechanisms of use-dependent block of sodium channels in excitable membranes by local anesthetics. Biophys J 1984; 46:15–27.

41. Payet M D. Effect of lidocaine on fast and slow inactivation of sodium current in rat ventricular cells. J Pharmacol Exp Ther 1982; 223:235–40.

42. Moorman J R, Yee R, Bjornsson T, Starmer C F, Grant A O, Strauss H C. pK_a does not predict pH potentiation of sodium channel blockade by lidocaine and W6211 in guinea pig ventricular myocardium. J Pharmacol Exp Ther 1986; 238:159–66.

43. Starmer C F, Courtney K R. Modeling ion channel blockade at guarded binding sites: application to tertiary drugs. Am J Physiol 1986; 251:H840–56.

44. Courtney K. pH and voltage dependence of I_{Na} recovery kinetics in atrial cells exposed to lidocaine. Am J Physiol 1988; 255(Heart Circ Physiol 24):H1554–7.

45. Sheu S S, Lederer W J. Lidocaine's negative inotropic and antiarrhythmic actions. Dependance on shortening of action potential duration and reduction of intracellular sodium activity. Cir Res 1985; 57:578–90.

46. Clarkson C W, Hondeghem L M. Evidence for a specific receptor site for lidocaine, quinidine, and bupivicaine associated with cardiac sodium channels in guinea pig ventricular myocardium. Circ Res 1985; 56:496–506.

47. Josephson I. Lidocaine blocks Na, Ca, and Na currents of chick ventricular myocytes. J Mol Cell Cardiol 1988; 20:593–604.

48. Wasserstrom J A, Salata J J. Basis for tetrodotoxin and lidocaine effects on action potentials in dog ventricular myocytes. Am J Physiol 1988; 254(Heart Circ Physiol 23):H1157–66.

49. Hiraoka M, Sawada K, Kawano S. Effects of quinidine on plateau currents of guinea-pig ventricular myocytes. J Mol Cell Cardiol 1986; 18:1097–106,

50. Salata J J, Wasserstrom J A. Effects of quinidine on action potentials and ionic currents in isolated canine ventricular myocytes. Circ Res 988; 62:324–37.

51. Kabela E. The effect of lidocaine on potassium efflux from various tissues of dig heart. J Pharmacol Exp Ther 1973; 184:611–8.

52. Carmeliet E. Saikawa T. Shortening of the action potential and reduction of pacemaker activity by lidocaine, quinidine and procainamide in cardiac Purkinje fibers: An effect on Na or K currents? Circ Res 1982; 50:257–72.

53. Miller B D, Thames M D, Mark A L. Inhibition of cardiac sympathetic nerve activity during intravenous administration of lidocaine. J Clin Invest 1983; 71:1247–53.

54. Martins J B, Kelly K J. Prolongation of refractoriness and activation time in normal canine ventricular myocardium following bolus administration of lidocaine. Am Heart J 1985; 109:533–9.

55. Wittig J, Harrison L A, Wallace A G. Electrophysiological effects of lidocaine on distal Purkinje fibers of canine heart. Am Heart J 1973; 86:69–78.

56. Colatsky T. Mechanisms of action of lidocaine and quinidine on action potential duration in rabbit cardiac Purkinje fibers: an effect on steady-state sodium currents? Circ Res 1982; 50:17–27.

57. Bennet P B. Mechanisms of antiarrhythmic drug action: block of sodium channels in voltage clamped cardiac cell membranes. J Appl Cardiol 1987; 2:463–88.

58. Weld F M, Bigger J T Jr. Effect of lidocaine on the early inward transient current in sheep cardiac Purkinje fibers. Circ Res 1975; 37:630–9.

59. Arnsdorf M F. The effect of antiarrhythmic drugs on triggered sustained rhythmic activity in cardiac Purkinje fibers. J Pharmacol Exp Ther 1977; 201:689–700.

60. Arnsdorf M F, Mehlman D J. Observations on the effects of selected antiarrhythmic drugs on mammalian cardiac Purkinje fibers with two levels of steady-state potential. J Pharmacol Exp Ther 1978; 207:983–91.

61. Arnsdorf M F, Friedlander I. The electrophysiologic effects of tolamolol (UK-6558-01) on the passive membrane properties of mammalian cardiac Purkinje fibers. 1976; J Pharmacol Expt Ther 199:601–10.

62. Sawicki G J, Arnsdorf M F. Electrophysiologic actions and interactions between lysophosphatidylcholine and lidocaine in the nonsteady state: the match between multiphasic arrhythmogenic mechanisms and multiple drug effects in cardiac Purkinje fibers. J Pharmacol Exp Ther 1985: 235:829–38.

63. Arnsdorf M F, Bigger J T Jr. The effect of lidocaine hydrochloride on membrane conductance in mammalian cardiac Purkinje fibers. J Clin Invest 1972; 51:2252–63.

64. Arnsdorf M F, Bigger J T Jr. The effect of procaine amide on components of excitability in long mammalian Purkinje fibers Circ Res 1976; 38:115–21.

65. Fozzard HA, Schoenberg M. Strength-duration curves in cardiac Purkinje fibers: effects of liminal length and charge distribution. J Physiol (Lond) 1972; 226:593–618.

66. Gerstenblith G, Scherlag B J, Hope R R, Lazzara R. Effect of lidocaine on conduction in the ischemic His-Purkinje system of dogs. Am J Cardiol 1978; 42:587–91.

67. Obayaski H, Hayakawa H, Mandel W J. Interrelationships between external potassium concentration and lidocaine: effects on the canine Purkinje fibers. Am Heart J 1975; 89:221–6.

68. Morady F, DiCarlo L A, Baerman J M, Krol R B. Rate-dependent effects of intravenous lidocaine, procainamide, and amiodarone on intraventricular conduction. J Am Coll Cardiol 1985; 6:179–85.

69. Davis J, Matsubara T, Scheinman M M, Katzung B, Hondeghem L M. Use-dependent effects of lidocaine on conduction in canine myocardium: application of the modulated receptor hypothesis in vivo. Circulation 1986; 74:205–14.

70. Grant A O, Strauss L J, Wallace A G, Strauss HC. The influence of pH on the electrophysiologic effects of lidocaine in guinea pig ventricular myocardium. Circ Res 1980; 47:542–50.

71. Arnsdorf M F, Sawicki G J. The effects of lysophosphatidylcholine, a toxic metabolite of ischemia, on the components of cardiac excitability in sheep Purkinje fibers. 1981; Circ Res 49:16–30.

72. Vaughan-Williams E M. A classification of antiarrhythmic actions reassessed after a decade of new drugs. J Clin Pharmacol 1984; 24:129–35.

73. Sugimoto T, Schaal S F, Dunn N M, Wallace A G. Electrophysiologic effects of lidocaine in awake dogs. J Pharmacol Exp Ther 1969; 166:146–50.

74. Gadsby D C, Cranefield P F. Two levels of resting potential in cardiac Purkinje fibers. J Gen Physiol 1977; 70:725–46.

75. Dangman K H. Effects of procainamide on automatic and triggered impulse in isolated preparations of canine cardiac Purkinje fibers. J Cardiovasc Pharmacol 1988; 12:78–87.

76. Eisner D A, Lederer W J. A cellular basis for lidocaine's antiarrhythmic action. J Physiol (Lond) 1979; 295:25P–26P.

77. Rosen M R, Danilo P. Effects of tetrodotoxin, lidocaine, verapamil and AHR-2666 on ouabain-induced delayed afterdepolarization in canine Purkinje fibers. Circ Res 1980; 46:117–24.

78. Mitchell M R, Plant S. Effects of lidocaine on action potentials, currents, and contractions in the absence and presence or ouabain in guinea-pig ventricular cells. J Exp Physiol 1988; 73:379 90.

79. Henning B, Zehender M, Meinertz T, Just H. Effects of tetrodotoxin, lidocaine, and quinidine on the transient inward current of sheep Purkinje fibers. Basic Res Cardiol 1988; 83:176–89.

80. Almotrefi A A, Baker J B. The antifibrillatory potency of aprindine, mexiletine, tocainide and lignocaine compared on Langendorff-perfused hearts of rabbits and guinea-pigs. J Pharm Pharmacol 1980; 32(11):746–50.

81. Roden D M, Hoffman B F. Action potential prolongation and induction of abnormal automaticity by low quinidine concentrations in canine Purkinje fibers. Relationship to potassium and cycle length. Circ Res 1985; 56:857–67.

82. January C T, Riddle J M, Salata J J. A model for early after depolarizations: induction with the Ca^{++} channel agonist Bay K 8644. Circ Res 1988; 62:563–71.

83. January C T, Riddle J M. Early afterdepolarizations: mechanism of induction and block. A role for L-type Ca^{++} current. Circ Res 1989; 64:977–90.

84. Rosen M R, Merker C, Pippenger C E. The effects of lidocaine on canine ECG and electrophysiologic properties of Purkinje fibers. Am Heart J 1976; 91:191–202.

85. Gelband H, Steeg C N, Bigger J R. Use of massive dose of procainamide in treatment of ventricular tachycardia in infancy. Pediatrics 1971; 48:110–5.

86. Morikawa Y, Rosen M. Developmental changes in the effects of lidocaine on the electrophysiological properties of canine Purkinje fibers. Circ Res 1984; 55:663–41.

87. Spinelli W, Danilo P Jr, Rosen M R. Reduction of V_{max} by QX-314 and benzocaine in neonatal and adult canine cardiac Purkinje fibers. J Pharmacol Exp Ther 1988; 245:381–7.

88. Feld G K, Venkatesh N, Singh B N. Pharmacologic conversion and suppression of experimental canine atrial flutter: differing effects of d-sotalol, quinidine, lidocaine and significance of changes in refractoriness and conduction. Circulation 1986; 74:197–204.

89. Lieberman N A, Harris R S, Katz R J, et al. The effects of lidocaine on the electrical and mechanical activity of the heart. Am J Cardiol 1968; 22:375–80.

90. Avitall B, Naimi S, Levine H J, et al. Time course of changes in ventricular excitability and conduction during myocardial ischemia and reperfusion in the dog: effect of lidocaine. J Electrocardiol 1979; 12:271–7.

91. Naito M, Michelson E L, Kmetzo J J, et al. Failure of antiarrhythmic drugs to affect epicardial delay during acute experimental coronary artery occlusion and reperfusion: correlation with lack of antiarrhythmic efficacy. J Pharmacol Exp Tther 1981; 218(2):475–80.

92. Naito M, Michelson E L, Kmetzo J J, et al. Failure of antiarrhythmic drugs to prevent experimental reperfusion ventricular fibrillation. Circulation 1981; 63:70–9.

93. Hope R R, Williams D O, El-Sherif N, et al. The efficacy of antiarrhythmic agents during acute myocardial ischemia and the role of heart rate. Circulation 1974; 50:507–14.

94. Epstein S E, Beiser G D, Rosing D R et al. Experimental acute myocardial infarction: characterization and treatment of malignant premature contraction. Circulation 1973; 47:446–54.

95. Stephenson S E, Cole R K, Parris T F, et al. Ventricular fibrillation during and after coronary artery occlusion. Am J Cardiol 1960; 5:77–85.

96. Gamble O W, Cohn K. Effect of propranolol, procainamide and lidocaine on ventricular automaticity and reentry in experimental myocardial infarction. Circulation 1972; 46:498–506.

97. Carson D L, Cardinal R, Savard P, et al. Relationship between an arrhythmogenic action of lidocaine and its effects on excitation patterns in acutely ischemic porcine myocardium. J Cardiovasc Pharmacol 1986; 8(1):126–36.

98. Davis J, Glassman R, Wit A L. Method of evaluating the effects of antiarrhythmic drugs on ventricular tachycardias with different electrophysiologic characteristics and different mechanisms in the infarcted canine heart. Am J Cardiol 1982; 49:1176–84.

99. Gerstenblilth G, Spear J F, Moore E N. Quantitative study of the effect of lidocaine on the threshold for ventricular fibrillation in the dog. Am J Cardiol 1972; 30:242–7.

100. Spear J F, Moore E N, Gerstenblith G. Effect of lidocaine on the ventricular fibrillation threshold in the dog during acute ischemia and premature ventricular contractions. Circulation 1972; 46:65–73.

101. Uematsu T, Vozeh S, Ha H R, et al. Coronary ligation-reperfusion arrhythmia models in anesthetized rats and isolated perfused rat hearts concentration-effect relationships of lidocaine. J Pharmacol Methods 1986; 16(1):53–61.

102. Gettes L S, Reuter H. Slow recovery from inactivation of inward currents in mammalian myocardial fibers. J Physiol (Lond) 1974; 240:703.

103. Bonaduce D, Ferrara N, Abete P, et al. Effect of mexiletine on reperfusion-induced ventricular arrhythmias: comparison with lidocaine. Arch Int Pharmacodyn Ther 1986; 284:19–29.

104. Bergey J L, Nocella K, McCallum J D. Acute coronary artery occlusion-reperfusion-induced arrhythmias in rats, dogs and pigs: antiarrhythmic evaluation of quinidine, procainamide and lidocaine. Eur J Pharmacol 1982; 81(2):205–16.

105. Nasser F N, Walls J T, Edwards W D. Lidocaine-induced reduction in size of experimental myocardial infarction. Am J Cardiol 1980; 46:967–75.

106. Ilvento J P, Provet J, Danilo P, Rosen M R. Fast and slow indioventricular rhythms in the canine heart: a study of their mechanism using antiarrhythmic drugs and electrophysiologic testing. Am J Cardiol 1982; 49:1909–16.

107. Roos J C, Dunning A J. Effects of lidocaine on impulse formation and conduction defects in man. Am Heart J 1975; 89:686–99.

108. Chang T O, Wadhwa K. Sinus standstill following intravenous lidocaine administration JAMA 1968; 223:790–2.

109. Lippestad C T, Forfang K. Production of sinus arrest by lignocaine. Br Med J 1971; 1:537.

110. Josephson M E, Caracta A R, Lau S H, Gallagher J J, Damato A N. Effects of lidocaine on refractory periods in man. Am Heart J 1972; 84:778–86.

111. Kunkel F, Rowland M, Scheinman M M. The electrophysiologic effects of lidocaine in patients with intraventricular conduction defects. Circulation 1974; 49:894–9.

112. Rosen K M, Lau S H, Weiss M B, Damato A N. The effect of lidocaine on atrioventricular and intraventricular conduction in man. Am J Cardiol 1970; 25:1–5.

113. Lichstein E, Chadda K D, Gupta P K. Atrioventricular block with lidocaine therapy. Am J Cardiol 1973; 31:277–81.

114. Gupta P K, Lichstein E, Dhadda K D. Lidocaine-induced heart block in patients with bundle branch block. Am J Cardiol 1974; 33:487–92.

115. Rosen K M, Barwolf D, Ehsani A, Rahimtoola S H. Effects of lidocaine and propranolol on the normal and anomalous pathways in patients with pre-excitation. Am J Cardiol 1972; 30:801–9.

116. Akhtar M, Gilbert C J, Shenasa M. Effect of lidocaine on atrioventricular response via the accessory pathway in patients with Wolff-Parkinson-White syndrome. Circulation 1981: 63:435–41.

117. Tenczer J, Littmann L, Rohla M, Fenyvesi T. The effects of overdrive pacing and lidocaine on atrioventricular junctional rhythm in man: the role of abnormal automaticity. Circulation 1985; 72;480–6.

118. Kuo C, Reddy C P. Effect of lidocaine on escape rate in patients with complete atrioventricular block. B. Proximal His bundle block. Am J Cardiol 1981; 47:1315–20.

119. Bigger J T Jr, Dresdale R J, Heissenbutel RH, et al. Ventricular arrhythmias in ischemic heart diseases: mechanism, prevalence, significance and management. Prog Cardiovasc Dis 1977; 4:255–300.

120. Jewitt D E, Kisbon Y, Thomas M. Lidocaine in the management of arrhythmias after acute myocardial infarction. Lancet 1968; I:266–70.

121. Lown B, Vassaux C. Lidocaine in acute myocardial infarction. Am Heart J 1968; 69:586–7.

122. Malach M, Kostis J B, Fischetti J L. Lidocaine for ventricular arrhythmias in acute myocardial infarction. Am J Med Sci 1969; 257:52–60.

123. Pitt A, Lipp H, Anderson S T. Lignocaine given prophylactically to patients with acute myocardial infarction. Lancet 1971; 1:612–6.

124. Adgey A A J, Allen J D, Geddes J S, et al. Acute phase of myocardial infarction. Lancet 1971; 2:501–4.

125. Bennett M A, Wilner J M, Pentecost BL. Controlled trial of lignocaine in prophylaxis of ventricular arrhythmias complicating myocardial infarction. Lancet 1970; 2:909–11.
126. Chopra M P, Portal R W, Aber C P. Lignocaine therapy after acute myocardial infarction. Br Med J 1969; 1:213–6.
127. Chopra M P, Thadani U, Portal R W, et al. Lignocaine therapy for ventricular ectopic activity after acute myocardial infarction: a double-blind trail. Br Med J 1971; 3:668–70.
128. Darby S, Bennet M A, Cruickshank J C et al. Trial of combined intramuscular and intravenous lignocaine in prophylaxis of ventricular tachyarrhythmias. Lancet 1972; 1:817–9.
129. Morgenson L. Ventricular tachycarrhythmias and lignocaine prophylaxis in acute myocardial infarction: a clinical and therapeutic study. Acta Med Scand [Suppl] 1970; 513:1–80.
130. Pantridge J F. Emergency treatment of cardiac arrhythmias in myocardial infarction. In: Scott D B, Julian D G, eds. Lidocaine in the treatment of ventricular arrhyuthmias. Edinburgh: E S Livingstone 1971:77–81.
131. Gianelly R, Van der Groeben J D, Spivack A P, Harrison D C. Effect of lidocaine on ventricular arrhythmias in patients with coronary heart disease. N Engl J Med 1967; 277:1215–9.
132. Harrison D C, Alderman E L. Relationship of blood levels to clinical effectiveness of lidocaine. In: Scott D B, Julian D G, eds. Lidocaine in the treatment of ventricular arrhythmias. Edinburgh: E S Livingstone, 1971, p. 178.
133. Harrison D C. Should lidocaine be administered routinely to all patients after acute myocardial infarction? Circulation 1978; 58:581–4.
134. Goldreyer B N, Wyman M G. The effect of the first hour hospitalization in myocardial infarction. Circulation 1974; 50 (Suppl.):III-121.
135. Valentine P A, Frew J L, Mashford M L, Sloman J F. Lidocaine in the prevention of sudden death in the pre-hospital phase of acute infarction. N Engl J Med 1974; 291:1327–31.
136. Lie K I, Liem K L, Louridtz W J, et al. Efficacy of lidocaine preventing primary ventricular fibrillation within one hour after a 300 mg intramuscular injection: a double-blind randomized study of 300 hospitalized patients with acute myocardial infarction. Am J Cardiol 1978; 42:486–8.
137. Koster R W, Dunning A F. Intramuscular lidocaine for prevention of lethal arrhythmias in the prehospitalization phase of acute myocardial infarction. N Engl J Med 1985; 313:1105–10.
138. Bleifield W. Merx W. Heinrich K W, et al. Controlled trial of prophylactic treatment with lidocaine in acute myocardial infarction. Eur J Clin Pharmacol 1973; 6:119–26.
139. Lie I K I, Wellens H J, Van Capelle F J, Durrer D. Lidocaine in the prevention of primary ventricular fibrillation. A double-blind randomized study of 212 consecutive patients. N Engl J Med 1974; 291:1324–6.
140. Haynes J R E, Chinn T L, Copass M K, Cobb LA. Comparison of bretylium tosylate and lidocaine in management of out of hospital ventricular fibrillation: a randomized clinical trail. Am J Cardiol 1981; 48:353–6.
141. Castellanos A, Ferreiro J, Pefkaros K, et al. Effects of lignocaine on bidirectional tachycardia and on digitalis-induced atrial tachycardia with block. Br Heart J 1982; 48:27–32.
142. Benowitz N, Forsyth R P, Melmon K L, Rowland ML. Lidocaine disposition in monkey and man. II. Effect of hemorrhage and sympathomimetic drug administration. Clin Pharmacol Ther 1974; 16:99–109.
143. Branch R A, Shand D G, Nies AS. Increase in hepatic blood flow and d-propranolol clearance by glucagon in the monkey. J Pharmacol Exp Ther 1973; 187:581–7.
144. Branch R A, Shand D G, Wilkinson G R, et al. The reduction of lidocaine clearance by d-propranolol: an example of hemodynamic drug interaction. J Pharmacol Exp Ther 1973; 184:515–87.
145. Conrad K A, Byers J M, Finley P R, et al. Lidocaine elimination. Effects of metroprolol and propranolol. Clin Pharmacol Ther 1983; 33:133–38.
146. Ochs H R, Carstens G, Greenblatt D J. Reductions in lidocaine clearance during continuous infusion and by coadminstration of propranolol. N Engl J Med 1980: 303:373–7.
147. DiFazio C A, Brown R E. Lidocaine metabolism in normal and phenobarbital pretreated dogs. Anesthesiology 1972; 36:328–43.
148. Knapp A B, Maguire W, Keren F, et al. The cimetidine-lidocaine interaction. Ann Intern Med 1983; 98:174–7.

149. Jackson J E, Bentley J B, Glass S J, et al. Effects of histamine-2 receptor blockade on lidocaine kinetics. Clin Pharmacol Ther 1985; 37:544–8.

150. Benowitz N L. Clinical applications of the pharmacokinetics of lidocaine. Cardiovasc Clin 1974; 6:77–101.

151. Collinsworth K A, Kalman S M, Harrison D C. The clinical pharmacology of lidocaine as an antiarrhythmic drug. Circulation 1974; 50:1217–30.

152. Wyman M G, Lalka D, Hammersmith, et al. Multiple bolus technique for lidocaine administration during the first hours of an acute myocardial infarction. Am J Cardiol 1978; 41:313–7.

153. Woosley R, Shand D G. Pharmacokinetics of antiarrhythmic drugs. Am J Cardiol 1978; 41:986–95.

154. LeLoner J, Grenon D, Latour G, Caille G, Dumont G, Brosseau A, Solilgnac A. Pharmacokinetics of lidocaine after prolonged intravenous infusions in uncomplicated myocardial infarction. Ann Intern Med 1977; 87:700–2.

155. Prescott L F, Adjepon-Yamoah K K, Talbot R G. Improved lignocaine metabolism in patients with myocardial infarction and cardiac failure. Br Med J 1976; 1:939–41.

156. Stenson R E, Constantino R T, Harrison D C. Interrelationships of hepatic blood flow, cardiac output and blood levels of lidocaine in man. Circulation 1971; 43:205–11.

157. Thomson P D, Melmon K L, Richardson J A, Cohn K, Streinbrunn W, Cudihee R, Rowland M. Lidocaine pharmacokinetics in advanced heart failure, liver disease, and renal failure in humans. Ann Intern Med 1973; 78:499–508.

158. Fehmers M C O, Van Datselaar J J, Dunning A J. Intramusculair en oraal toegediende lidocaine voor de behandeling van kameraritmieen bij het hartinfarct. Ned Tijdschr Geneeskd 1972; 116:1224, as cited in Rosen M R, Hoffman B F, Wit A L. Electrophysiology and pharmacology of cardiac arrhythmias. V. Cardiac antiarrhythmic effects of lidocaine. Am Heart J 1975; 89:526–36.

159. Sung C Y, Truant A P. The physiological disposition of lidocaine and its comparison in some respects with procaine. J Pharmacol Exp Ther 1954; 112:432–43.

160. Hollunger C. On the metabolism of lidocaine. I. The properties of the enzyme system responsible for the oxidative metabolism of lidocaine. Acta Pharmacol Toxicol (Copenh) 1960; 17:356–64.

161. Hollunger C. On the metabolism of lidocaine. II. Biotransformation of lidocaine, hydrolysis of the amide linkage. Acta Pharmacol Toxicol (Copenh) 1960: 17:365–73.

162. Narang P K, Crouthamel W G, Carliner N H. Lidocaine and its active metabolites. Clin Pharmacol Ther 1978; 24:654–62.

163. Drayer D E, Lorenzo B, Werns S, et al. Plasma levels, protein binding and elimination data of lidocaine and active metabolites in cardiac patients of various ages. Clin Pharmacol Ther 1983; 34:14–22.

164. Bennet P, Woosley R L, Hondeghem L M. Competition between lidocaine and one of its metabolites, glycylxylidide, for cardiac sodium channels. Circulation 1988; 78:692–700.

165. Routledge P A, Shand D G, Barchowsky A, et al. Relationship between alpha$_1$-acid glycoprotein and lidocaine disposition in myocardial infarction. Clin Pharmacol Ther 1981; 30:154–7.

166. Boyes R N, Scott D B, Jebson PJ, Godman M J, Julian DG. Pharmacokinetics of lidocaine in man. Clin Pharmacol Ther 1971; 12:105–6.

167. Grossman J I, Cooper J A, Frieden J. Cardiovascular effects of infusion of lidocaine in patients with heart disease. Am J Cardiol 1969; 24:191–7.

168. Schumacher R R, Lieberson A D, Childress R H, Williams J F Jr. Hemodynamic effects of lidocaine in patients with heart disease. Circulation 968; 37:965–72.

169. Arnsdorf M F. Basic understanding of the electrophysiologic actions of antiarrhythmic drugs: sources, sinks and matrices of information. Med Clin North Am 1984; 68:1247–80.

27

Mexiletine and Tocainide

Lawrence H. Frame

University of Pennsylvania School of Medicine
Philadelphia, Pennsylvania

INTRODUCTION

Mexiletine and tocainide are structural analogs of lidocaine. Their electrophysiologic and antiarrhythmic profiles are similar to those of lidocaine, but they each lack significant first-pass metabolism in the liver, making them more suitable for oral administration. Both drugs are approved in the United States for the suppression of symptomatic ventricular arrhythmias, including frequent premature ventricular contractions, uniform or multifocal couplets, and ventricular tachycardia. However, tocainide should be reserved for patients in whom the benefits outweigh the risks, which include the rare but potentially fatal occurrence of hematologic disorders. Their molecular structures are shown in Figure 1. The molecular size of both drugs is small compared with that of lidocaine and most other antiarrhythmic drugs; the molecular weight of mexiletine HCl is 216 and that of tocainide HCl is 229. Despite similarity in electrophysiology antiarrhythmicity and common side effects, mexiletine and tocainide have important differences in pharmacokinetics and the incidence of rare but serious hematologic side effects. A number of reviews provide additional information or perspectives on tocainide (1–3) and mexiletine (4–6).

BASIC PHARMACOLOGY: ELECTROPHYSIOLOGIC EFFECTS ON ISOLATED CARDIAC TISSUES

Therapeutic concentrations are considered to be 4–10 mg/L for tocainide and 0.75–2.0 mg/L for mexiletine. Some experimental studies have investigated the effects of much higher concentration because the electrophysiologic effects of tocainide and mexiletine on normal myocardial tissue are relatively slight at therapeutic concentrations.

Sinoatrial Node

Sinus cycle length is not changed by therapeutic concentrations of mexiletine (7,8) or tocainide (9). At much higher concentrations a slight increase in sinus cycle length may be seen that is much less marked than with class IA antiarrhythmic drugs (10). The mechanism is a decrease in phase 4 depolarization in sinoatrial node cells, although at even higher

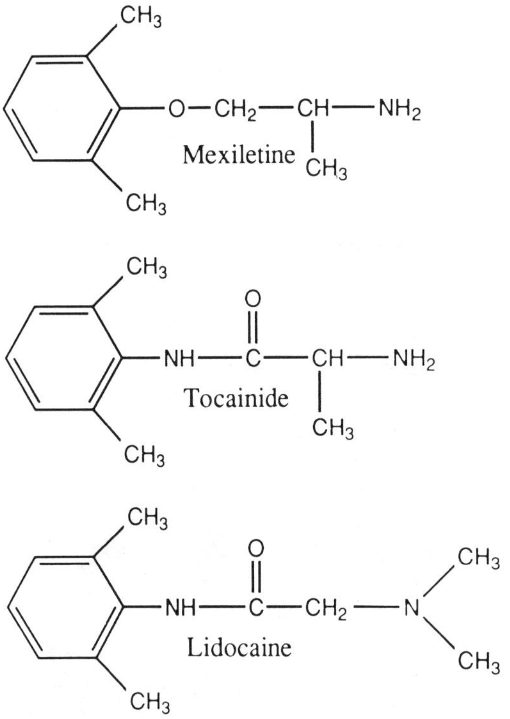

Figure 1 Molecular structures of mexiletine, tocainide, and lidocaine.

concentrations an increase in the duration of the action potential also contributes. Neither tocainide nor mexiletine affects the maximum rate of depolarization during phase 0 or the amplitude of the sinus node action potential (10). Mexiletine has been shown to increase sinoatrial conduction time (8).

Atrial Muscle

Mexiletine at a concentration of 1 mg/L significantly reduced the maximum rate of depolarization $\dot{V}_{max}$ of rabbit atrial muscle, and at a concentration of 3 mg/L it also significantly decreased the amplitude of the action potential, conduction velocity, and contractile amplitude while increasing electrical stimulation threshold. There was no significant change in resting potential or action potential duration (7).

In potassium-depolarized fibers exhibiting slow-response action potentials mexiletine does not decrease the maximum rate of depolarization, suggesting that it does not block the cal-

cium current (11,12). Tocainide's effects on atrial muscle have not been studied.

Atrioventricular Node

Tocainide can slightly increase the atrial-to-His bundle conduction time (AH interval) by 10–40% at high plasma concentration of 20 mg/L (9).

Ventricular Muscle and His-Purkinje Conduction System

In ventricular muscle and Purkinje fibers $\dot{V}_{max}$, action potential amplitude, conduction velocity, membrane responsiveness, and action potential duration are all reduced by mexiletine (7,8,13,14) and tocainide (9,5,16). The magnitude of these effects vary greatly with resting membrane potential and depolarization frequency as well as drug concentration. As with lidocaine, these drugs have little effect on $\dot{V}_{max}$ or conduction velocity at therapeutic concentrations during pacing at slow rates in cells with normal resting potentials. Under these conditions the most prominent effect is a shortening of the action potential duration. However, in depolarized fibers or at faster heart rates significant decreases in $\dot{V}_{max}$ and conduction velocity are seen. The steady-state relationship between $\dot{V}_{max}$ and resting membrane potential is shifted toward more negative voltages (16,17). These characteristics are the basis for classification of tocainide and mexiletine as class IB antiarrhythmic drugs along with lidocaine and phenytoin.

Greater depression of $\dot{V}_{max}$ at faster rates of stimulation is a reflection of the use-dependent block of sodium channels by these drugs. Use-dependence describes the phenomena that depolarization causes an increment in sodium channel blockade and repolarization causes a time-dependent recovery from sodium channel blockade. The modulated receptor hypothesis is the most widely accepted explanation for use-dependence, and it postulates that the affinity of the sodium channel for the drug is greater when it is in the active or inactivated states than in the resting state.

Antiarrhythmic drugs vary widely in the kinetics for the development and recovery from use-dependent block. Tocainide and mexiletine are similar to lidocaine in that they have relatively fast use-dependent kinetics. A good way to compare the relative kinetics of different drugs is with the exponential time constant for recovery from use-dependent block because it is unaffected by drug concentration. The time constant for recovery of $\dot{V}_{max}$ in Purkinje fibers in most studies is between 120 and 350 msec for mexiletine (18–21), but values as long as 750 msec have been reported (22,23). In some studies this time constant was nearly identical for mexiletine and lidocaine (19), whereas in others it was significantly longer. For tocainide most studies report recovery time constants of 300–670 msec (15,24,25), but longer values up to 1.3 sec have been reported (26). Additional slower components of recovery lasting several seconds have also been reported (15,20). When the time constants of mexiletine and tocainide were measured by the same laboratory, the time constants of recovery for tocainide were always longer (15,23). Recovery time constants are prolonged when fibers are depolarized by potassium (15,23).

The time-dependent recovery from use-dependent block also produces a similar time-dependent depression of conduction velocity of early premature beats (21,27). Thus important functional correlates of relatively fast kinetics of use-dependent characteristics of class IB drugs are more interval-dependent conduction slowing of premature beats, faster adaptation of use-dependent effects after a change in rate, and greater selectivity for sodium channel blockade when resting potential is depolarized, such as during ischemia.

Both tocainide and mexiletine shorten action potential duration. The shortening is more prominent in Purkinje fibers (16,28) than in ventricular muscle and more prominent at long cycle lengths than at short cycle lengths (13–16,28–31). The ratio of effective refractory period to action potential duration is increased by both tocainide and mexiletine, especially at fast rates (8,28,29,32). In Purkinje fibers, where action potential duration is markedly shortened, the effective refractory period is decreased as well, but to a smaller extent. In ventricular muscle, where the shortening of action potential duration is less, effective refractory period is usually little changed or may be slightly prolonged.

Studies of electrical restitution of action potential duration have shown that mexiletine blunts the shortening of premature action potentials (19,33). Mexiletine does not further shorten action potentials previously shortened by tetrodotoxin, which suggests that the decrease in action potential duration is due to blockade of the small amount of maintained tetrodotoxin-sensitive sodium current during the plateau of the action potential (31). Thus all the electrophysiologic effects of these two drugs can be explained by sodium channel blockade. There is also no evidence of anticholinergic or β-receptor blocking activity of these drugs.

Mexiletine has been shown to decrease the automaticity of normal well-polarized Purkinje fibers, and Weld et al. (14) reported that the mechanism was a change in threshold potential with no change in the rate of phase 4 depolarization. In depolarized Purkinje fibers showing automatic activity mexiletine decreases the slope of phase 4 depolarization (13). Mexiletine decreases the rate of the idioventricular escape rhythm in dogs with atrioventricular (AV) block (34).

Tocainide has been shown to have a greater depressant effect on $\dot{V}_{max}$ in subendocardial Purkinje fibers surviving in a region of myocardial infarction than in normal fibers (24,28).

The effects on the resting electrocardiogram in experimental animals given tocainide or mexiletine are small. PR interval, QRS duration, and QT interval are not significantly changed (35,36).

BASIC PHARMACOLOGY: ANTIARRHYTHMIC EFFECTS IN EXPERIMENTAL ANIMALS

Atrial Arrhythmias

There is little published information about the effect of mexiletine or tocainide in experimental atrial arrhythmias. We studied the effect of mexiletine in two canine models of rapid atrial tachycardias simulating atrial flutter (Frame and Hoffman, unpublished observations). Mexiletine caused a dose-dependent increase in the cycle length of the tachycardia in both models, but the incidence of termination of the flutter was different. In a model of atrial flutter due to right atrial enlargement secondary to pulmonic stenosis and tricuspid insufficiency, the drug caused termination of tachycardia in every experiment at plasma levels between 2.2 and 9.4 mg/L. In this model reentry has been shown to occur around a functional barrier (37). In the other model of atrial flutter, in which reentry occurs around the tricuspid ring after a surgical incision in the right atrium (38), the drug terminated reentry in only one of six experiments at mexiletine concentrations just above 2 mg/L. The reduced antiarrhythmic efficacy in this model may be due either to lower plasma concentrations or to the fact that this model is due to reentry around the fixed barrier and has a longer cycle length.

Ventricular Arrhythmias

Ventricular ectopic beats produced by toxic infusions of ouabain have been shown to be completely suppressed by mexiletine at 0.6–1.3 mg/L (39) and by tocainide at plasma concentrations of 18.3 mg/L (9). In vitro studies have shown that mexiletine can decrease ouabain-induced triggered activity due to delayed afterdepolarizations (14,40,41) and early afterdepolarizations (14). Mexiletine infusion, 2 mg/kg, can prevent rapid repetitive responses or ventricular fibrillation induced by programmed stimulation during acute ischemia (34).

Both drugs produce a significant partial suppression of ventricular ectopic beats at therapeutic concentrations in the Harris dog model, 24 hr after coronary ligation, and complete suppression of ectopy at higher doses. For tocainide, a 50% decrease in ectopic beats was observed at plasma concentrations of 5 (36) or 18.7 mg/L (9). Complete suppression of ectopic beats was observed at 12 or 43 mg/L in these two studies, respectively. High therapeutic concentrations of mexiletine produced about a 60% reduction in ventricular ectopic activity, with complete suppression of ectopic activity observed at concentrations between 2.2 and 5 mg/L (39).

Tocainide was shown to prevent the induction of ventricular tachycardia 7–30 days after coronary artery ligation in about one-half of the dogs studied (35). Mexiletine was shown to be highly effective in preventing reperfusion-induced ventricular arrhythmias (42).

Ventricular fibrillation threshold is significantly increased in a dose-dependent fashion by therapeutic and higher concentrations of both tocainide (9,43) and mexiletine (39). Furthermore, mexiletine has been shown to prevent the decrease in ventricular fibrillation threshold induced by acute ischemia (34,39).

CLINICAL PHARMACOLOGY

Effects on the Normal Human Electrocardiogram

At therapeutic concentrations tocainide and mexiletine produce little consistent effect on sinus node automaticity and conduction and refractoriness in various parts of the heart. However, clinically significant changes may be seen is some patients, especially at higher concentrations, at faster heart rates, and in the presence of preexisting conduction disease.

Mexiletine produces no consistent effect on sinus rate and sinus node recovery time in normal patients (44) or in patients with cardiac disease (45,46). However, sinoatrial recovery time may increase in patients with sick sinus syndrome (46). There was no consistent effect on atrial effective refractory period (44–46).

No consistent effects on conduction time or effective refractory period of the atrioventricular node are observed at normal heart rates. However, during atrial pacing at faster rates the AH intervals tend to be prolonged and Wenckebach block occurs at a lower heart rate in many patients (46). No significant change or small increase in HV conduction time are observed (44,46). However, when severe AV conduction disease or complete AV block is present, mexiletine should be used with caution because of the possibility of marked suppression of the rate of the junctional escape pacemaker (46). Marked increases in the relative refractory period and the effective refractory period of the His-Purkinje system exceeding 100 msec can be observed.

Mexiletine does not change ventricular effective refractory period (44,45). The refractory period of atrioventricular accessory bypass tract can be either increased (46) or decreased (45) by mexiletine. The conduction time for early ventricular premature beats can be markedly increased by mexiletine (47). It does not significantly alter the PR, QRS, or corrected QT intervals on the electrocardiogram (48–51). Mexiletine may increase the energy required for ventricular defibrillation (52).

In one study, tocainide produced decreases of approximately 20 msec in effective refractory periods of the atrium, AV node, and right ventricle at mean plasma concentrations of 7.4 mg/L. Sinus rate, sinus node recovery time, and Wenckebach cycle length were unchanged. The AH interval was increased slightly at the time of the peak concentration of 11 mg/L. The corrected QT interval was unchanged or slightly decreased during drug infusion (53). In two other studies in which lower plasma concentrations were reached, no significant change in refractory periods or conduction times were observed (54,55). In addition, no significant change in PR, QRS, or QT intervals on the electrocardiogram were observed.

Antiarrhythmic Efficacy Following Acute Administration in Humans

Reported response rates for suppression of ventricular arrhythmias by tocainide and mexiletine range from 6 to 95%. Much of this variability can be explained by differences in the arrhythmia, the clinical setting being studied, the method for evaluating efficacy, and whether patients are preselected as refractory to other antiarrhythmic drugs. The clearest demonstration of antiarrhythmic efficacy comes from placebo-controlled trials and con-trolled comparisons between two or more antiarrhythmic agents on the suppression of premature ventricular contractions (PVC). Such studies clearly show that these drugs can decrease the frequency of PVC and various forms of high-grade ectopy. Although frequent PVC and high-grade ectopy are associated with a higher risk of sudden death in patients with heart disease, there is no evidence that reducing this ectopy confers a lower risk for sudden death. Patients who have experienced syncope or cardiac arrest are at the highest risk of recurrent life-threatening arrhythmias. In these patients efficacy can be measured in terms of the suppression of frequent nonsustained ventricular tachycardia during ambulatory monitoring or by the prevention of inducibility of ventricular tachycardia using programmed stimulation. However, such patients are not enrolled in placebo-controlled long-term follow-up trials that would prove antiarrhythmic efficacy against life-threatening arrhythmias in a particular patient population in a statistically rigorous way. Thus, whereas the most important use of antiarrhythmic drugs is to decrease the risk of life-threatening arrhythmias, the best statistical evidence of patient benefit relates to the suppression of symptoms related to arrhythmias that are not life threatening in themselves.

Arrhythmias Following Acute Myocardial Infarction

In several placebo-controlled trials oral mexiletine begun shortly after the onset of acute myocardial infarction significantly reduced the frequency of PVC, high-grade ectopy, and ventricular tachycardia (56–60). None of these studies demonstrated a significant reduction in ventricular fibrillation or arrhythmic death in the early postinfarction period; however, because of the relatively small incidence of such effect, larger studies are needed to demonstrate such an effect. Horowitz et al. (61) found intravenous mexiletine to be more effective than intravenous lidocaine at suppressing multifocal PVC and nonsustained ventricular tachycardia during the second 24 hr after myocardial infarction, although their effects were similar during the first 24 hr.

A multicenter placebo-controlled trial with 791 patients showed that tocainide administration for 48 hr, begun within 6 hr after the onset of myocardial infarction, did not significantly alter the incidence of primary ventricular fibrillation. There was a significantly higher incidence in the placebo group of ventricular arrhythmias serious enough to warrant withdrawal from the study, which implies that tocainide decreased their frequency (62). Another study showed that lidocaine and intravenous tocainide produced similar reductions in PVC and complex ectopy in patients with these arrhythmias during the first 24 hr following myocardial infarction (63). Most of these studies excluded patients that had cardiogenic shock or AV block. In this patient population both tocainide and mexiletine appeared to be hemodynamically well tolerated during the acute phase of myocardial infarction. Keefe et al. (64) also found intravenous tocainide to be somewhat more effective than lidocaine in suppressing nonsustained ventricular tachycardia and accelerated idioventricular rhythms acutely following myocardial infarction.

Other studies confirm that tocainide and mexiletine continue to decrease high-grade ectopy during the days and months following the acute phase of myocardial infarction, although no effect on the risk of ventricular fibrillation or arrhythmic death has been shown. A randomized placebo-controlled trial of patients with high-grade ectopy during the acute phase of myocardial infarction showed that 77% of patients receiving placebo demonstrated high-grade ectopy or nonsustained ventricular tachycardia during 24 hr electrocardiographic recordings on days 4 and 10 of the study versus 35% of patients receiving procainamide and 32% of patients receiving mexiletine. Ventricular fibrillation did not occur in any group (65). In a similar trial tocainide decreased the frequency of PVC and the incidence of serious ventricular arrhythmias observed on 24 hr ambulatory monitoring at 2, 8, 16, and 24 weeks after myocardial infarction (66).

The effect of these drugs on ventricular fibrillation or sudden death following myocar-

dial infarction was addressed in several studies involving 50–344 patients (58,67). No significant reduction was found. A much larger study involving 630 patients comparing mexiletine treatment to placebo during the first year after infarction further indicates it is unlikely that this agent has any significant effect on ventricular fibrillation following myocardial infarction. In this study the death rate among patients receiving mexiletine was 7.6 versus 4.8% in the placebo-treated group (68). The difference was not statistically significant. This result occurred despite a significant reduction in high-grade ectopy in the mexiletine group during the first 4 months following the infarction. Other, less well controlled studies also confirm that mexiletine can decrease ectopy following infarction (69).

Suppression of Chronic PVC and High-Grade Ectopy

Both tocainide and mexiletine have been shown to be effective in decreasing the frequency complexity of chronic ventricular ectopy in patients with heart disease as assessed by ambulatory electrocardiographic recording (70–81). Their efficacy is comparable to that of other antiarrhythmic drugs such as quinidine, procainamide, disopyramide, and other antiarrhythmic drugs (70,72–75,77,82). Frequent PVC and complex ectopy including frequent nonsustained ventricular tachycardia that is not life threatening by itself are treated either because the symptoms are bothersome to the patient or because such arrhythmias are associated with an increased risk of sudden death in patients with heart disease. However, there is no evidence that reducing the amount of spontaneous complex ectopy by mexiletine, tocainide, or any other antiarrhythmic drug is able to modify the increased risk of sudden death.

The range of efficacy of oral mexiletine for suppression of frequent high-grade ectopy ranges from 27 to 95%. However, most reports estimate the efficacy between 40 and 70%. The wide range can in part be explained by differences in the patient selection, the criteria for demonstrating efficacy, and whether a single dose was administered or doses were titrated to achieve an effective or maximally tolerated dose. In the article by Flaker et al. (76) that reported the lowest efficacy of 27% in suppressing chronic ventricular ectopy, 17 of 22 patients had been refractory to previous antiarrhythmic therapy, and the criteria for efficacy were the most stringent among these studies. These required both a decrease in the number of PVC by 85% and a decrease in the Lown score for grading the severity of efficacy. Of their patients 45% would have been considered effectively treated if the decrease in PVC by 85% was the sole criterion. Another study with a low efficacy of 35% used only a single oral administration of mexiletine, 200 mg, which is unlikely to achieve therapeutic concentrations over several hours because of the large volume of distribution of this drug (70).

An efficacy of 36% was reported among patients refractory to or intolerant of other antiarrhythmic drugs (83). On the other hand, the highest efficacy (95%) was reported in a population that was selected for being responsive to lidocaine. Most of the studies with intermediate efficacy do not report patient responses to other antiarrhythmic drugs, and several of them also use a dose ranging protocol to find the optimal effective and tolerated dose for each patient (71,72,74). In one study reporting an efficacy of only 38%, the study design included a week of therapy to evaluate the long-term tolerance of the drug. Mexiletine was effective after acute testing in 54% of patients, but two of seven patients with an effective response developed intolerable side effects (71).

Controlled studies showed mexiletine to have comparable efficacy to class IA antiarrhythmic drugs. Nearly identical efficacy of mexiletine and quinidine were reported in three studies (71,74,82). Nademanee et al. (72) found mexiletine slightly more effective than procainamide, 43 versus 19%, whereas Jewitt et al. (73) found little difference (52% for mexiletine and 60% for procainamide). A study comparing mexiletine, disopyramide, flecainide, propafenone, and penticainide concluded that there was no statistically significant difference in their efficacy (70). Trimarco

et al. (75) found similar efficacy between mexiletine and disopyramide.

The efficacy for tocainide against chronic high-grade ectopy has been reported between 60 and 80% in most studies (78–81,84). However, one study reported an efficacy of 37% (77). The lower efficacy in the study by Morganroth may have been because most patients had already received antiarrhythmic drug therapy and presumably had been refractory before entering the study. In most of the studies citing higher efficacy, previous drug refractoriness was not reported or not commented on, and in one case patients were selected for the study based on lidocaine responsiveness (79). In a comparative study tocainide, 600 mg every 12 hr, was slightly less effective than quinidine sulfate, 300 mg every 6 hr (38 versus 50%, respectively) (77).

Prevention of Recurrence of Documented Life-Threatening Ventricular Arrhythmias

It is widely believed that tocainide and mexiletine are rarely effective as single agents against sustained ventricular tachycardia and ventricular fibrillation that cause syncope or cardiac arrest. However, there is very little evidence on which to base such a conclusion for patients who are not preselected as refractory to many other antiarrhythmic drugs. Almost all the studies reported in conjunction with the development of these drugs as new antiarrhythmic agents included only patients who had been unresponsive to, or intolerant of, several standard antiarrhythmic agents. Thus a more appropriate conclusion is that patients with life-threatening arrhythmias who have demonstrated unresponsiveness or intolerance to class IA antiarrhythmic drugs by long-term ECG monitoring or programmed stimulation are unlikely to respond to tocainide or mexiletine used as a single agent.

For patients with symptomatic life-threatening ventricular arrhythmias refractory to other antiarrhythmic drugs, the reported efficacy of tocainide as assessed by Holter monitor suppression of nonsustained ventricular tachycardia ranges between 33 and 79% (85–91). In three of the studies reporting the highest efficacy between 61 and 79%, all or most of the patients had been shown to respond to lidocaine, which represents a selection bias for patients more likely to respond to the drug (85–87). Most of the patients in these studies had suffered from syncope or cardiac arrest and had documented ventricular tachycardia or ventricular fibrillation. The studies with the lowest efficacy of 47 and 46% used the strictest criteria for efficacy involving suppression of arrhythmias during exercise testing as well as Holter monitoring (90,91). The use of Holter monitoring to evaluate therapy selects for a group of patients who have a high incidence of nonsustained ventricular tachycardia to provide an end point to evaluate therapy.

For similarly highly symptomatic patients with life-threatening arrhythmias treated with mexiletine, the efficacy judged by the decrease in nonsustained ventricular tachycardia on Holter monitoring ranged from 16 to 41% (50,72,91,92). Although this range of efficacy appears lower than that for tocainide, none of these studies involved a selection of patients based on the response to lidocaine. Patients in all these studies were refractory to previous antiarrhythmic therapy. In one crossover study the efficacies of mexiletine and tocainide assessed by noninvasive criteria were comparable (37 and 47%, respectively) (91).

For patients with life-threatening ventricular tachycardia or fibrillation, the efficacies of mexiletine and tocainide used as single agents are low when evaluated by the ability to prevent the induction of arrhythmias by programmed stimulation. For mexiletine the frequency of suppression of all inducible arrhythmias ranges from 0 to 37% (76,91,93–98). This measure of efficacy was less than 13% in all but two studies, which were from the same center. These studies, showing efficacy of 19 and 37% for overlapping groups of patients, represent the largest single study involving 148 patients (93,94). However, the population also included a higher proportion of patients whose presenting arrhythmia was ventricular fibrillation or nonsustained ventricular tachycardia rather than sustained ventricular tachycardia. Furthermore, a large proportion of the population were patients whose induced arrhythmia was nonsustained

ventricular tachycardia or ventricular fibrillation. They found that such patients had a higher response rate, around 50% (94). Response rates of 10% or less are typical of studies involving patients with a history of recurrent and inducible sustained ventricular tachycardia refractory to other drugs. The efficacy of mexiletine in preventing the induction by programmed stimulation of sustained ventricular tachycardia ranges from 6 to 13% (49,76,96).

For patients with life-threatening sustained ventricular arrhythmias, refractory or intolerant to other antiarrhythmic drugs, tocainide effectively prevented reinduction of the arrhythmia by programmed electrical stimulation in 6–35% of cases (89,91,98,99). In the two studies reporting the highest efficacy of 32 and 35% (89,91) nonsustained rather than sustained ventricular tachycardia was the presenting arrhythmia or induced arrhythmia at the baseline study in some patients. However, in one of these studies comparable efficacy was observed regardless of the presenting or induced arrhythmia (91).

Comparable efficacy has been found against life-threatening ventricular arrhythmias assessed by program stimulation in studies comparing mexiletine with disopyramide (95, 97) and mexiletine with tocainide (91,98). However, there is not a complete concordance between patients who respond to mexiletine and to tocainide (91,98).

There appears to be a very useful, although not perfect, correlation between the response to intravenous lidocaine and the efficacy of either tocainide or mexiletine (87,91,98). The overall predictive accuracy appears to be between 60 and 80%. Thus, whereas the efficacy of mexiletine and tocainide is low in typical patients refractory to IA drugs, it is much better in patients who responded to lidocaine. This not only helps to explain variability in efficacy reported among studies, but also provides a useful tool for identifying patients more likely to respond to mexiletine or tocainide. However, because the correlation is not perfect lidocaine responders may not respond to either tocainide or mexiletine. A somewhat contradictory result is a study that reports that intravenous mexiletine was highly effective (89%) in terminating ventricular tachycardia that did not respond to lidocaine primarily in the postmyocardial infarction period (100). It is possible that the result could represent an additive effect because mexiletine was given rapidly and soon after the lidocaine infusion.

Efficacy of Arrhythmias from Causes Other Than Coronary Disease

In most reports of drug efficacy the predominant cause of heart disease is coronary artery disease, particularly myocardial infarction. However, mexiletine and tocainide have also been reported to be effective in other settings. An efficacy rate of 89% was reported for a variety of ventricular arrhythmias in patients with congenital heart disease (101) and children following repair of tetrology of Fallot (102). Both mexiletine and tocainide useful for the treatment of torsade de pointes (103,104). Tocainide was shown to be highly effective in suppressing high-grade ventricular ectopy and ventricular tachycardia in adult patients following cardiac surgery (105).

Combination Therapy with Mexiletine or Tocainide and a Class IA Agent

Because tocainide and mexiletine are infrequently effective when used by themselves in patients with life-threatening arrhythmias that are refractory to other agents, their greatest utility may be in combination with a class IA antiarrhythmic drug. Several studies have reported efficacy of mexiletine and a class IA agent between 20 and 80% for patients with serious ventricular arrhythmias who were refractory to several antiarrhythmic agents, including mexiletine and the class IA agent given alone (49,95,106–109). Similarly, tocainide and quinidine were effective in 80% of patients as a combination compared with 15 and 30% for tocainide and quinidine alone in a study of patients with high-grade ventricular ectopy and nonsustained ventricular tachycardia assessed by Holter monitoring (110). An important advantaged of combined therapy is that side effects did not seem to be additive so that lower doses can be used with a reduction of side effects as well as an enhancement of efficacy.

Antiarrhythmic Efficacy During Chronic Therapy

Both tocainide and mexiletine continue to be effective antiarrhythmic agents during long-term oral administration when their efficacy was demonstrated in the short term by ambulatory monitoring or programmed stimulation. For high-risk patients in whom inducible sustained ventricular arrhythmias were prevented by either tocainide or mexiletine the incidence of late arrhythmia occurrence ranges from zero to 20% in long-term therapy (86,89,93,94,99). Long-term results when efficacy was assessed by ambulatory electrocardiographic recording are comparable (83,84,90,92,111,112). These results are comparable to those with other antiarrhythmic agents and are presumed to be much better than the natural history of these high-risk patients if they are not treated by drugs. There is also a 10–20% incidence of side effects that require discontinuation of long-term therapy.

Pharmacokinetics

The lack of significant first-pass metabolism through the liver, lack of active metabolites, relatively long half-lives of elimination, high bioavailability, minimal hemodynamic depression, and infrequent occurrence of allergic or delayed side effects make the pharmacokinetics of tocainide and mexiletine favorable for chronic administration as oral antiarrhythmic agents.

Administration, Absorption, and Distribution of Tocainide

After oral administration tocainide is rapidly absorbed, with a bioavailability near 100% and minimal first-pass metabolism in the liver (113). It reaches a peak plasma concentration 0.5–2 hr after oral ingestion (113,114). When tocainide is taken with a meal the peak plasma concentration may be decreased by 40% without affecting the total bioavailability (113). Tocainide is approximately 10–15% bound to plasma proteins (115,116). After intravenous administration the half-life of the rapid distribution phase averaged 7 min in normal subjects and about twice as long in patients after myocardial infarction (114). The apparent volume of distribution has been reported as 1.46 or 2.9 L/kg in normal subjects and 3.2 L/g in patients after myocardial infarction. No significant pharmacokinetic drug interactions have been reported, although the electrophysiologic effects of tocainide and β-adrenergic receptor blockers, such as metoprolol, can be additive, which in patients with sinus node disease can lead to asystole (117).

Metabolism and Elimination of Tocainide

Individuals with normal renal function excrete about 40% of an administered dose unchanged in the urine (113,114). The rest is metabolized in the liver to a glucuronide (118). If the urine is alkalinized the renal excretion is significantly reduced (113). The half-life for elimination was reported as 11–14 hr in healthy subjects (80,113,114) and 15–16 hr in patients with cardiac disease, with an individual variation between 11 and 23 hr (80,81,114). Because of renal excretion the elimination half-life is significantly prolonged in patients with renal disease (119). It can be effectively cleared by hemodialysis but is not cleared by peritoneal dialysis (119,120). Congestive heart failure does not significantly alter the elimination kinetics (121).

Administration, Absorption, and Distribution of Mexiletine

Oral mexiletine has a bioavailability of about 90%, with less than 10% metabolized during the first pass through the liver (122). Since it is nearly all ionized at the normal gastric pH, it is not absorbed until it reaches the small intestine. Therefore, antacids, anticholinergic drugs, and narcotic analgesics, which, for instance, may be given to patients following myocardial infarction, can delay gastric emptying by several hours (122–124). These drugs can delay the peak plasma concentration from 2–4 to 4–6 hr after ingestion. The volume of distribution of mexiletine is 9–10 L/kg, which is unusually high among antiarrhythmic drugs. This prolongs the time to reach steady-state concentration following initiation or change of the drug dose. Plasma binding of mexiletine in serum is about 70% (125).

Metabolism and Elimination of Mexiletine

Approximately 90% of mexiletine is eliminated by transformation to inactive metabolites in the liver. The half-life for elimination ranges from 8 to 12 hr in healthy subjects but increases to a mean of 16.7 hr in patients with acute myocardial infarction (122). The half-life can be markedly prolonged in patients with liver disease, such as those with cirrhosis (126), but is not greatly affected by renal insufficiency (127). However, the fraction that is excreted in the urine may increase if the urine is acidified (128).

Such drugs as phenobarbital, phenytoin, primadone, and rifampin that enhance hepatic enzyme activity can significantly increase the nonrenal clearance of the drug and reduce the elimination half-life by 40% (129,130). On the other hand cimetidine, isoniazid, chloramphenicol, and dicumarol are likely to decrease the hepatic metabolism of mexiletine and prolong its plasma half-life (131). Serum digoxin concentration is not affected by mexiletine (132). Caffeine elimination is reduced 30% by mexiletine (133).

TOXICOLOGY

Noncardiac Side Effects

Mild neurologic and gastrointestinal side effects occur in over 50% of patients starting therapy with tocainide or mexiletine. Common symptoms are dizziness, tremor, nausea, and vomiting. Confusion, paraesthesias, and anorexia are somewhat less common. These symptoms may be transient and are also usually dose related so they may respond to a decrease in the dose or administration of more frequent smaller doses. Taking the dose with food may also decrease the peak plasma concentrations and side effects without decreasing the total drug absorbed. Symptoms have been severe enough to result in discontinuation of the drug in 10–20% of patients treated with tocainide (86,87,111,134,135) and 15–50% of patients receiving mexiletine (48,50,72,92).

The most important of several uncommon but serious side effects produced by tocainide are various blood dyscrasias. These include agranulocytosis, leukopenia, aplastic anemia, and thrombocytopenia. Their incidence is estimated as 0.18% (136–138). Fatalities have occurred. These reactions usually occur in the first 12 weeks of therapy and, if detected early, are usually reversible when therapy is discontinued. It is therefore recommended that blood counts be performed weekly during the first 3 months of therapy and periodically thereafter. Pulmonary fibrosis, interstitial pneuomonitis and fibrosing alveolitis have also been reported with an incidence estimated at 0.11% (139,140). These reactions usually occur between 3 and 18 weeks of therapy. A number of forms of severe dermatologic reactions, including the Stevens-Johnson syndrome, erythema multiforme, and stomatitis, have also been reported, usually during the first 3 weeks of therapy (141). Tocainide has also been implicated in rare cases of paranoid psychosis (142).

The occurrence of fatal blood dyscrasias has led to a modification of the indications for using tocainide, that its use be limited to cases in which in the physician's judgment the benefits outweigh the risk.

Mexiletine induces marked leukopenia or agranulocytosis much less frequently (approximately 0.06%), although thrombocytopenia has been reported (143,144). Elevations of liver enzymes have occurred in 1–2% of patients on mexiletine, and rare cases of severe liver injury have occurred.

Cardiac Side Effects

Tocainide and mexiletine have very slight negative ionotropic effects similar to those of lidocaine and much less than those of other class I antiarrhythmic drugs. Studies of tocainide demonstrate little decrease in cardiac output, although some studies demonstrate a slight increase in peripheral and systemic vascular resistance (111,117,145–147). The incidence of exacerbation of congestive heart failure in an open-label compassionate-use protocol for tocainide was 1.4% (135). Similarly, mexiletine has little depressant effect on cardiac hemodynamics (148–152).

Aggravation of arrhythmias, including the occurrence of ventricular fibrillation and ventricular tachycardia occur with an incidence of 5–10% for patients treated either with tocainide (90,135,153) or mexiletine (92–94,154). The incidence of proarrhythmic effects is comparable to that of other drugs (154). As with other class I drugs the incidence of aggravation of arrhythmias is higher for patients who present with sustained ventricular tachycardia than those with nonsustained ventricular tachycardia or ventricular premature beats (155). Although mexiletine and tocainide have little effect on sinus rate and conduction in normal hearts, they should be used with caution in patients with conduction system disease, including sinus node dysfunction and second- and third-degree AV block.

SUMMARY: THE ROLES OF TOCAINIDE AND MEXILETINE IN THERAPEUTICS

Tocainide and mexiletine have favorable pharmacokinetic and hemodynamic properties for long-term oral antiarrhythmic use and are highly effective in suppressing symptomatic frequent premature ventricular contractions, high-grade ectopy, and nonsustained ventricular tachycardia. However, a correlation with suppression of these arrhythmias and the prevention of sustained ventricular tachycardia, ventricular fibrillation, or sudden death has not been demonstrated. It is not known whether these drugs are effective as first-line therapy against life-threatening ventricular tachycardia or fibrillation. Used as single agents they are rarely effective in patients with life-threatening arrhythmias who have been shown to be intolerant or nonresponsive to several other class I antiarrhythmic drugs. They do, however, seem to be effective when used in combination with another class IA antiarrhythmic drug, even when the patients have failed to respond to each drug individually. Minor gastrointestinal and neurologic symptoms are very common with both tocainide and mexiletine, and although they are usually dose related and may respond to a decrease in the dose, the treatment of life-threatening arrhythmias frequently requires concentrations near the upper end of the therapeutic range, which are associated with a high incidence of intolerable side effects. A 0.18% incidence of potentially life-threatening blood dyscrasias has significantly decreased the use of tocainide when other effective antiarrhythmic agents are available.

REFERENCES

1. Roden D, Woosley R. Drug therapy. Tocainide. N Engl J Med 1986; 315:41–45.
2. Morganroth J, Nestico P, Horowitz L. A review of the uses and limitations of tocainide—a class IB antiarrhythmic agent. Am Heart J 1985; 110:856–63.
3. Kutalek S, Morganroth J, Horowitz L. Tocainide: a new oral antiarrhythmic agent. Ann Intern Med 1985; 103:387–91.
4. Campbell R. Mexiletine. N Engl J Med 1987; 316:29–34.
5. Chew C, Collett J, Singh B. Mexiletine: a review of its pharmacological properties and therapeutic efficacy in arrhythmias. Drugs 1979; 17:161–81.
6. Woosley R, Wang T, Stone W, Siddoway L, Thompson K, Duff H, Cerskus I, Roden D. Pharmacology, electrophysiology, and pharmacokinetics of mexiletine. Am Heart J 1984; 107:1058–65.
7. Singh B, Vaughan Williams E. Investigations of the mode of action of a new antidysrhythmic drug, KÖ 1173. Br J Pharmacol 1972; 44:1–9.
8. Yamaguchi I, Singh B, Mandel W. Electrophysiological actions of mexiletine on isolated rabbit atria and canine ventricular muscle and Purkinje fibres. Cardiovasc Res 1979; 13:288–96.
9. Moore E, Spear J, Horowitz L, Feldman H, Moller R. Electrophysiologic properties of a new antiarrhythmic drug—tocainide. Am J Cardiol 1978; 41:703–9.
10. Campbell T. Differing electrophysiological effects of class IA, IB, and IC antiarrhythmic drugs on guinea-pig sinoatrial node. Br J Pharmacol 1987; 91:395–401.
11. Brown J, Marshall R, Winslow E. Effects of selective channel blocking agents on contractions and action potentials in K^+-depolarized guinea-pig atria. Br J Pharmacol 1985; 86:7–17.
12. Carmeliet E. Mechanisms of arrhythmias and of antiarrhythmic activity, with special reference to mexiletine. Acta Cardiol (Brux) 1980; 25(Suppl.):5–25.
13. Arita M, Goto M, Nagamoto Y, Saikawa T. Electrophysiological actions of mexiletine (Ko1173) on canine Purkinje fibres and ventricular muscle. Br J Pharmacol 1979; 67:143–52.
14. Weld F, Bigger J Jr, Swistel D, Bordiuk J, Lau U. Electrophysiological effects of mexiletine (Ko1173) on ovine cardiac Purkinje fibers. J Pharmacol Exp Ther 1979; 210:222–8.
15. Oshita S, Sada H, Kojima M, Ban T. Effects of tocainide and lidocaine on the transmembrane action potentials as related to external potassium and calcium concentrations in guinea-pig papillary muscles. Naunyn Schmiedebergs Arch Pharmacol 1980; 314: 67–82.
16. Kinnaird A, Man R. The interaction of cycle length with the electrophysiological effect of lidocaine, tocainide and verapamil on canine Purkinje fibers. Eur J Pharmacol 1984; 99:63–71.
17. Hohnloser S, Weirich J, Antoni H. Effects of mexiletine on steady-state characteristics and recovery kinetics of $\dot{V}_{max}$ and conduction velocity in guinea pig myocardium. J Cardiovasc Pharmacol 1982; 4:232–9.
18. Varro A, Elharrar V, Surawicz B. Frequency-dependent effects of several class I antiarrhythmic drugs on $\dot{V}_{max}$ of action potential upstroke in canine cardiac Purkinje fibers. J Cardiovasc Pharmacol 1985; 7:482–92.
19. Elharrar V. Recovery from use-dependent block of $\dot{V}_{max}$ and restitution of action potential duration in canine cardiac Purkinje fibers. J Pharmacol Exp Ther 1988; 246:235–42.
20. Toyama J, Kodama I, Kusunoki T, Ishihara T, Hattori Y, Yamada K. Use-dependent blocking action of newly developed lidocaine-analogs on maximum rate of rise of action potentials in guinea pig papillary muscle. Jpn Heart J 1987; 28:273–85.
21. Nattel S. Relationship between use-dependent effects of antiarrhythmic drugs on conduction and $\dot{V}_{max}$ in canine cardiac Purkinje fibers. J Pharmacol Exp Ther 1987; 241:282–8.
22. Courtney K. Comparative actions of mexiletine on sodium channels in nerve, skeletal and cardiac muscle. Eur J Pharmacol 1981; 74:9–18.

23. Frame L, Gintant G, Hoffman B. Mexiletine and tocainide differ from lidocaine in their use-dependent kinetics. Circulation 1982; 66(II):II-292.
24. Kinnaird A, Man R. Electrophysiological effects of tocainide on canine subendocardial Purkinje fibers surviving infarction. Eur J Pharmacol 1986; 124:135–41.
25. Kodama I, Toyama J, Takanaka C, Yamada K. Block of activated and inactivated sodium channels by class-I antiarrhythmic drugs studied by using the maximum upstroke velocity ($\dot{V}_{max}$) of action potential in guinea-pig cardiac muscles. J Mol Cell Cardiol 1987; 19:367–77.
26. Gintant G, Hoffman B, Naylor R. The influence of molecular form of local anesthetic-type antiarrhythmic agents on reduction of the maximum upstroke velocity of canine cardiac Purkinje fibers. Circ Res 1983; 52:735–46.
27. Bajaj A, Kopelman H, Wikswo J Jr, Cassidy F, Woosley R, Roden D. Frequency- and orientation-dependent effects of mexiletine and quinidine on conduction in the intact dog heart. Circulation 1987; 75:1065–73.
28. Dersham G, Han J, Cameron J, OConnell D. Effects of tocainide on Purkinje fibers from normal and infarcted ventricular tissues. J Electrocardiol 1986; 19:355–9.
29. Campbell T. Kinetics of onset of rate-dependent effects of class I antiarrhythmic drugs are important in determining their effects on refractoriness in guinea-pig ventricle, and provide a theoretical basis for their subclassification. Cardiovasc Res 1983; 17:344–52.
30. Varro A, Nakaya Y, Elharrar V, Surawicz B. Effect of antiarrhythmic drugs on the cycle length-dependent action potential duration in dog Purkinje and ventricular muscle fibers. J Cardiovasc Pharmacol 1986; 8:178–85.
31. Matsuo S, Kishida H, Munakata K, Atarashi H. The effects of mexiletine on action potential duration and its restitution in guinea pig ventricular muscles. Jpn Heart J 1985; 26:271–87.
32. Burke G, Loukides J, Berman N. Comparative electropharmacology of mexiletine, lidocaine and quinidine in a canine Purkinje fiber model. J Pharmacol Exp Ther 1986; 237:232–6.
33. Varro A, Elharrar V, Surawicz B. Effect of antiarrhythmic drugs on the premature action potential duration in canine cardiac Purkinje fibers. J Pharmacol Exp Ther 1985; 233:304–11.
34. Yoon M, Han J. Electrophysiologic effects of mexiletine on normal and ischemic ventricles. J Electrocardiol 1982; 15:109–13.
35. Uprichard A, Allen J, Harron D. Effects of tocainide enantiomers on experimental arrhythmias produced by programmed electrical stimulation. J Cardiovasc Pharmacol 1988; 11:235–41.
36. Aberg G, Ronfeld R, Aberg L, Fitzgerald T, McCollom K, Moller R. Antiarrhythmic effects of tocainide and lidocaine in dogs. Acta Pharmacol Toxicol (Copenh) 1983; 53:146–52.
37. Boyden P. Activation sequence during atrial flutter in dogs with surgically induced right atrial enlargement. I. Observations during sustained rhythms. Circ Res 1988; 62:596–608.
38. Frame L, Page R, Hoffman B. Atrial reentry around an anatomic barrier with a partially refractory excitable gap. A canine model of atrial flutter. Circ Res 1986; 58:495–511.
39. Allen J, Kelly J, James RGG, Shanks RG, Zaidi S. Comparison of the effects of lignocaine and mexiletine on experimental ventricular arrhythmias. Postgrad Med J 1977; 53(Suppl. 1):35–45.
40. Endou K, Yamamoto H, Sato T. Comparison of the effects of calcium channel blockers and antiarrhythmic drugs on digitalis-induced oscillatory afterpotentials on canine Purkinje fiber. Jpn Heart J 1987; 28:719–35.
41. Amerini S, Carbonin P, Cerbai E, Giotti A, Mugelli A, Pahor M. Electrophysiological mechanisms for the antiarrhythmic action of mexiletine on digitalis-, reperfusion- and reoxygenation-induced arrhythmias. Br J Pharmacol 1985; 86:805–15.
42. Bonaduce D, Ferrara N, Abete P, Longobardi G, Leosco D, Canonico V, Morgano G, Rengo F. Effect of mexiletine on reperfusion-induced ventricular arrhythmias: comparison with lidocaine. Arch Int Pharmacodyn Ther 1986; 284:19–29.
43. Schnittger I, Griffin J, Hall R, Meffin P, Winkle R. Effects of tocainide on ventricular fibrillation threshold. Comparison with lidocaine. Am J Cardiol 1978; 42:76–81.
44. Harper R, Olsson S, Varnauskas E. The effect of mexiletine on the electrophysical properties of the intact human heart. Scand J Clin Lab Invest 1977; 37:503–7.

45. McComish M, Kitson D, Robinson C, Jewitt D. Clinical electrophysiological effects of mexiletine. Postgrad Med J 1977; 53(Suppl. 1):85–91.

46. Roos J, Paalman A, Dunning A. Electro-physiological effects of mexiletine in man. Br Heart J 1976; 38:1262–71.

47. Harper R, Olsson S. Effect of mexiletine on conduction of premature ventricular beats in man: a study using monophasic action potential recordings from the right ventricle. Cardiovasc Res 1979; 13:311–9.

48. Campbell N, Shanks R, Kelly J, Adgey A. Long term oral antiarrhythmic therapy with mexiletine. Postgrad Med J 1977; 53(Suppl. 1):143–5.

49. Waspe L, Waxman H, Buxton A, Josephson M. Mexiletine for control of drug-resistant ventricular tachycardia: clinical and electro-physiologic results in 44 patients. Am J Cardiol 1983; 51:1175–81.

50. Heger J, Nattel S, Rinkenberger R, Zipes D. Mexiletine therapy in 15 patients with drug-resistant ventricular tachycardia. Am J Cardiol 1980; 45:627–32.

51. Mehta J, Conti C. Mexiletine, a new antiarrhythmic agent, for treatment of premature ventricular complexes. Am J Cardiol 1982; 49:455–60.

52. Marinchak R, Friehling T, Kline R, Stohler J, Kowey P. Effect of antiarrhythmic drugs on defibrillation threshold: case report of an adverse effect of mexiletine and review of the literature. PACE 1988; 11:7–12.

53. Anderson J, Mason J, Winkle R, Meffin P, Fowles R, Peters L, Harrison D. Clinical electrophysiologic effects of tocainide. Circulation 1978; 57:685–91.

54. Horowitz L, Josephson M, Farshidi A. Human electropharmacology of tocainide, a lidocaine congener. Am J Cardiol 1978; 42:276–80.

55. Waleffe A, Bruninx P, Mary R, Kulbertus H. Effects of tocainide studied with pro-grammed electrical stimulation of the heart in patients with reentrant tachyarrhythmias. Am J Cardiol 1979; 43:292–9.

56. Campbell R, Achuff S, Pottage A, Murray A, Prescott L, Julian D. Mexiletine in the prophylaxis of ventricular arrhythmias during acute myocardial infarction. J Cardiovasc Pharmacol 1979; 1:43–52.

57. Achuff S, Pottage A, Prescott L, Campbell R, Murray A, Julian D. Mexiletine in the

prevention of ventricular arrhythmias in acute myocardial infarction. Postgrad Med J 1977; 1:163–5.

58. Bell J, Thomas J, Isaacson J, Snell N, Holt D. A trial of prophylactic mexiletine in home coronary care. Br Heart J 1982; 48:285–90.

59. Smyllie H, Doar J, Head C, Leggett R. A trial of intravenous and oral mexiletine in acute myocardial infarction. Eur J Clin Pharmacol 1984; 26:537–42.

60. Merx W, Henning B, Franken G, Effert S. Mexiletine in acute myocardial infarction. In: Sandoe E, Julian D, Bell JW, eds. Management of ventricular tachycardia: role of mexiletine. Amsterdam: Excerpta Medica 1978:472–8.

61. Horowitz J, Anavekar S, Morris P, Goble A, Doyle A, Louis W. Comparative trial of mexiletine and lignocaine in the treatment of early ventricular tachyarrhythmias after acute myocardial infarction. J Cardiovasc Pharmacol 1981; 3:409–19.

62. Campbell R, Hutton I, Elton R, Goodfellow R, Taylor E. Prophylaxis of primary ventricular fibrillation with tocainide in acute myocardial infarction. Br Heart J 1983; 49:557–63.

63. Rehnqvist N, Erhardt L, Ericsson C, Olsson G, Svensson G, Sjogren A. Comparative study of tocainide and lidocaine in patients admitted for suspected acute myocardial infarction. Acta Med Scand 1983; 214:21–7.

64. Keefe D, Williams S, Torres V, Flowers D, Somberg J. Prophylactic tocainide or lidocaine in acute myocardial infarction. Am J Cardiol 1986; 57:527–31.

65. Campbell R, Dolder M, Prescott L, Talbot R, Murray A, Julian D. Comparison of pro-cainamide and mexiletine in prevention of ventricular arrhythmias after acute myocardial infarction. Lancet 1975; 1:1257–9.

66. Bastian B, Macfarlane P, McLauchlan J, Ballantyne D, Clark P, Hillis W, Rae A, Hutton I. A prospective randomized trial of tocainide in patients following myocardial infarction. Am Heart J 1980; 100:1017–22.

67. Ryden L, Arnman K, Conradson T, Hofvendahl S, Mortensen O, Smedgard P. Prophylaxis of ventricular tachyarrhythmias with intravenous and oral tocainide in patients with and recovering from acute myocardial infarction. Am Heart J 1980; 100:1006–12.

68. Impact Research Group. International mexiletine and placebo antiarrhythmic coronary

trial. I. Report on arrhythmia and other findings. J Am Coll Cardiol 1984; 4:1148–63.

69. Talbot R, Julian D, Prescott L. Long-term treatment of ventricular arrhythmias with oral mexiletine. Am Heart J 1976; 91:58–65.

70. Priori S, Bonazzi O, Facchini M, Varisco T, Schwartz P. Antiarrhythmic efficacy of penticainide and comparison with disopyramide, flecainide, propafenone and mexiletine by acute oral drug testing. Am J Cardiol 1987, 60:1068–72.

71. Fenster P, Hanson C. Mexiletine and quinidine in ventricular ectopy. Clin Pharmacol Ther 1983; 34:136–42.

72. Nademanee K, Feld G, Hendrickson J, Intarachot V, Yale C, Heng M, Singh B. Mexiletine: double-blind comparison with procainamide in PVC suppression and open-label sequential comparison with amiodarone in life-threatening ventricular arrhythmias. Am Heart J 1985; 110:923–31.

73. Jewitt D, Jackson G, McComish M. Comparative anti-arrhythmic efficacy of mexiletine, procainamide and tolamolol in patients with symptomatic ventricular arrhythmias. Postgrad Med J 1977; 53(Suppl. 1):158–62.

74. Singh J, Rasul A, Shah A, Adams E, Flessas A, Kocot S. Efficacy of mexiletine in chronic ventricular arrhythmias compared with quinidine: a single-blind, randomized trial. Am J Cardiol 1984; 53:84–7.

75. Trimarco B, Volpe M, Ricciardelli B, Sacca L, De Luca N, Rengo F, Condorelli M. Disopyramide and mexiletine: which is the agent of choice in the long term-oral treatment of lidocaine-responsive arrhythmias? Efficacy comparison in a randomized trial. Arch Int Pharmacodyn Ther 1980; 248:251–9.

80. Flaker G, Madigan N, Alpert M, Moser S. Mexiletine for recurring ventricular arrhythmias: assessment of long-term electrocardiographic recordings and sequential electrophysiologic studies. Am Heart J 1984; 108:490–5.

77. Morganroth J, Oshrain C, Steele P. Comparative efficacy and safety of oral tocainide and quinidine for benign and potentially lethal ventricular arrhythmias. Am J Cardiol 1985; 56:581–5.

78. LeWinter M, Engler R, Karliner J. Tocainide therapy for treatment of ventricular arrhythmias: assessment with ambulatory electrocardiographic monitoring and treadmill exercise. Am J Cardiol 1980; 45:1045–52.

79. McDevitt D, Nies A, Wilkinson G, Smith R, Woosley R, Oates J. Antiarrhythmic effects of a lidocaine congener, tocainide, 2-amino-2′, 6′-propionoxylidide, in man. Clin Pharmacol Ther 1976; 19:396–402.

80. Winkle R, Meffin P, Fitzgerald J, Harrison D. Clinical efficacy and pharmacokinetics of a new orally effective antiarrhythmic, tocainide. Circulation 1976; 54:885–9.

81. Woosley R., McDevitt D, Nies A, Smith R., Wilkinson G, Oates J. Suppression of ventricular ectopic depolarizations by tocainide. Circulation 1977; 56:980–4.

82. Morganroth J. Comparative efficacy and safety of oral mexiletine and quinidine in benign or potentially lethal ventricular arrhythmias. Am J Cardiol 1987; 60:1276–81.

83. Rutledge J, Harris F, Amsterdam EA, Skalsky E. Clinical evaluation of oral mexiletine therapy in the treatment of ventricular arrhythmias. J Am Coll Cardiol 1985; 6:780–4.

84. Haffajee C, Alpert J, Dalen J. Tocainide for refractory ventricular arrhythmias of myocardial infarction. Am Heart J 1980; 100:1013–6.

85. Roden D, Reele SB, Higgins S, Carr R, Smith R, Oates J, Woosley R. Tocainide therapy for refractory ventricular arrhythmias. Am Heart J 1980; 100:15–22.

86. Maloney J, Nissen R, McColgan J. Open clinical studies at a referral center: chronic maintenance tocainide therapy in patients with recurrent sustained ventricular tachycardia refractory to conventional antiarrhythmic agents. Am Heart J 1980; 100:1023–30.

87. Winkle R, Mason J, Harrison D. Tocainide for drug-resistant ventricular arrhythmias: efficacy, side effects, and lidocaine responsiveness for predicting tocainide success. Am Heart J 1980; 100:1031–6.

88. Ryan W, Engler R, LeWinter M, Karliner J. Efficacy of a new oral agent (tocainide) in the acute treatment of refractory ventricular arrhythmias. Am J Cardiol 1979; 43:285–91.

89. Hohnloser S, Lange H, Raeder E, Podrid P, Lown B. Short- and long-term therapy with tocainide for malignant ventricular tachyarrhythmias. Circulation 1986; 73:143–9.

90. Podrid P, Lown B. Tocainide for refractory symptomatic ventricular arrhythmias. Am J Cardiol 1982; 49:1279–86.

91. Hession M, Blum R, Podrid P, Lampert S, Stein J, Lown B. Mexiletine and tocainide: does response to one predict response to the other? J Am Coll Cardiol 1986; 7:338–43.

92. Podrid P, Lown B. Mexiletine for ventricular arrhythmias. Am J Cardiol 1981; 47:895–902.

93. DiMarco J, Garan H, Ruskin J. Mexiletine for refractory-ventricular arrhythmias: results using serial electrophysiologic testing. Am J Cardiol 1981; 47:131–8.

94. Schoenfeld M, Whitford E, McGovern B, Garan H, Ruskin J. Oral mexiletine in the treatment of refractory ventricular arrhythmias: the role of electrophysiologic techniques. Am Heart J 1984; 107:1071–8.

95. Breithardt G, Seipel L, Abendroth R. Comparison of the antiarrhythmic efficacy of disopyramide and mexiletine against stimulus-induced ventricular tachycardia. J Cardiovasc Pharmacol 1981; 3:1026–37.

96. Palileo E, Welch W, Hoff J, Strasberg B, Bauernfeind R, Swiryn S, Coelho A, Rosen K. Lack of effectiveness of oral mexiletine in patients with drug-refractory paroxysmal sustained ventricular tachycardia. A study utilizing programmed stimulation. Am J Cardiol 1982; 50:1075–81.

97. Manz M, Steinbeck G, Nitsch J, Luderitz B. Treatment of recurrent sustained ventricular tachycardia with mexiletine and disopyramide. Control by programmed ventricular stimulation. Br Heart J 1983; 49:222–8.

98. Reiter M, Easley A, Mann D. Efficacy of class Ib (lidocaine-like) antiarrhythmic agents for prevention of sustained ventricular tachycardia secondary to coronary artery disease. Am J Cardiol 1987; 59:1319–24.

99. Adhar G, Swerdlow C, Lance B, Clay D, Bardy G, Greene H. Tocainide for drug-resistant sustained ventricular tachyarrhythmias. J Am Coll Cardiol 1988; 11:124–31.

100. Santinelli V, Chiariello M, Stanislao M, Condorelli M. Intravenous mexiletine in management of lidocaine-resistant ventricular tachycardia. Am Heart J 1983; 105:680–5.

101. Moak J, Smith R, Garson A Jr. Mexiletine: an effective antiarrhythmic drug for treatment of ventricular arrhythmias in congenital heart disease. J Am Coll Cardiol 1987; 10:824–9.

102. Garson A Jr, Randall D, Gillette P, Smith R, Moak J, McVey P, McNamara D. Prevention of sudden death after repair of tetralogy of Fallot: treatment of ventricular arrhythmias. J Am Coll Cardiol 1985; 6:221–7.

103. Shah A, Schwartz H. Mexiletine for treatment of torsade de pointes. Am Heart J 1984; 107:589–91.

104. Bansal A, Kugler J, Pinsky W, Norberg W, Frank W. Torsade de pointes: successful acute control by lidocaine and chronic control by tocainide in two patients—one each with acquired long QT and the congenial long QT syndrome. Am Heart J 1986; 112:618–21.

105. Morganroth J, Panidis I, Harley S, Johnson J, Smith E, McVaugh H. Efficacy and safety of intravenous tocainide compared with intravenous lidocaine for acute ventricular arrhythmias immediately after cardiac surgery. Am J Cardiol 1984; 54:1253–8.

106. Duff H, Roden D, Primm R, Oates J, Woosley R. Mexiletine in the treatment of resistant ventricular arrhythmias: enhancement of efficacy and reduction of dose-related side effects by combination with quinidine. Circulation 1983; 67:1124–8.

107. DiMarco J, Garan H, Ruskin J. Quinidine for ventricular arrhythmias: value of electrophysiologic testing. Am J Cardiol 1983; 51:90–5.

108. Rae A, Greenspan A, Spielman S, Sokoloff N, Webb C, Kay H, Horowitz L. Antiarrhythmic drug efficacy for ventricular tachyarrhythmias associated with coronary artery disease as assessed by electrophysiologic studies. Am J Cardiol 1985; 55:1494–8.

109. Greenspan A, Spielman S, Webb C, Sokoloff N, Rae A, Horowitz L. Efficacy of combination therapy with mexiletine and a type IA agent for inducible ventricular tachyarrhythmias secondary to coronary artery disease. Am J Cardiol 1985; 56:277–84.

110. Kim S, Mercando A, Fisher J. Combination of tocainide and quinidine for better tolerance and additive effects in patients with coronary artery disease. J Am Coll Cardiol 1987; 9:1369–74.

111. Winkle R, Meffin P, Harrison D. Long-term tocainide therapy for ventricular arrhythmias. Circulation 1978; 57:1008–16.

112. Stein J, Podrid P, Lampert S, Hirsowitz G, Lown B. Long-term mexiletine for ventricular arrhythmia. Am Heart J 1984; 107:1091–8.

113. Lalka D, Meyer M, Duce B, Elvin A. Kinetics of the oral antiarrhythmic lidocaine congener, tocainide. Clin Pharmacol Ther 1976; 19:757–66.

114. Graffner C, Conradson T, Hofvendahl S, Ryden L. Tocainide kinetics after intravenous and oral administration in healthy subjects

and in patients with acute myocardial infarction. Clin Pharmacol Ther 1980; 27:64–71.

115. Sedman A, Bloedow D, Gal J. Serum binding of tocainide and its enantiomers in human subjects. Res Commun Chem Pathol Pharmacol 1982; 38:165–8.

116. Elvin A, Axelson J, Lalka D. Tocainide protein binding in normal volunteers and trauma patients. Br J Clin Pharmacol 1982; 13: 872–3.

117. Ikram H. Hemodynamic and electrophysiologic interactions between antiarrhythmic drugs and beta blockers, with special reference to tocainide. Am Heart J 1980; 100: 1076–80.

118. Elvin A, Keenaghan J, Byrnes E, Tenthorey P, McMaster P, Takman B, Lalka D, Manion C, Baer D, Wolshin E, Meyer M, Ronfeld R. Tocainide conjugation in humans; novel biotransformation pathway for a primary amine. J Pharm Sci 1980; 69:47–9.

119. Wiegers U, Hanrath P, Kuck K, Pottage A, Graffner C, Augustin J, Runge M. Pharmacokinetics of tocainide in patients with renal dysfunction and during haemodialysis. Eur J Clin Pharmacol 1982; 24:503–7.

120. Raehl C, Beirne G, Moorthy A, Patel A. Tocainide pharmacokinetics during continuous ambulatory peritoneal dialysis. Am J Cardiol 1987; 60:747–50.

121. Mohiuddin S, Esterbrooks D, Hilleman D, Aronow W, Patterson A, Sketch M, Mooss A, Hee T, Reich J. Tocainide kinetics in congestive heart failure. Clin Pharmacol Ther 1983; 34:596–603.

122. Prescott L, Pottage A, Clements J. Absorption, distribution and elimination of mexiletine. Postgrad Med J 1977; 53(Suppl. 1): 50–5.

123. Herzog P, Holtermuller K, Kasper W, Meinertz T, Trenk D, Jahnchen E. Absorption of mexiletine after treatment with gastric antacids. Br J Clin Pharmacol 1982; 14:746–7.

124. Wing L, Meffin P, Grygiel J, Smith K, Birkett D. The effect of metoclopramide and atropine on the absorption of orally administered mexiletine. Br J Clin Pharmacol 1980; 9:505–9.

125. Singh B, Cho Y, Kuemmerle H. Clinical pharmacology of antiarrhythmic drugs: a review and overview, part II. Int J Clin Pharmacol Ther Toxicol 1981; 19:185–99.

126. Pentikainen P, Hietakorpi S, Halinen M, Lampinen L. Cirrhosis of the liver markedly impairs the elimination of mexiletine. Eur J Clin Pharmacol 1986; 30:83–8.

127. Baudinet G, Henrard L, Quinaux N, El AD, de Landsheere C, Carlier J, Dresse A. Pharmacokinetics of mexiletine in renal insufficiency. Acta Cardiol (Brux) 1980; 25 (Suppl.):55–65.

128. Kiddie M, Kaye C, Turner P, Shaw T. The influence of urinary pH on the elimination of mexiletine. Br J Clin Pharmacol 1974; 1:229–32.

129. Pentikainen P, Koivula I, Hiltunen H. Effect of rifampicin treatment on the kinetics of mexiletine. Eur J Clin Pharmacol 1982; 23:261–6.

130. Begg E, Chinwah P, Webb C, Day R, Wade D. Enhanced metabolism of mexiletine after phenytoin administration. Br J Clin Pharmacol 1982; 14:219–23.

131. Bigger J Jr. The interaction of mexiletine with other cardiovascular drugs. Am Heart J 1984; 107:1079–85.

132. Leahey E Jr, Reiffel J, Giardina E, Bigger J Jr. The effect of quinidine and other oral antiarrhythmic drugs on serum digoxin. A prospective study. Ann Intern Med 1980; 92:605–8.

133. Joeres R, Richter E. Mexiletine and caffeine elimination (letter). N Engl J Med 1987; 317:1170.

134. Young M, Hadidian Z, Horn H, Johnson J, Vassallo H. Treatment of ventricular arrhythmias with oral tocainide. Am Heart J 1980; 100:1041–5.

135. Horn H, Hadidian Z, Johnson J, Vassallo H, Williams J, Young M. Safety evaluation of tocainide in the American Emergency Use Program. Am Heart J 1980; 100:1037–40.

136. Volosin K, Greenberg R, Greenspon A. Tocainide associated agranulocytosis. Am Heart J 1985; 109:1392–3.

137. Gertz M, Garton J, Jennings W. Aplastic anemia due to tocainide (letter). N Engl J Med 1986; 314:583–4.

138. True C. Aplastic anemia due to tocainide. N Engl J Med 1986; 314:584.

139. Perlow G, Jain B, Pauker S, Zarren H, Wistran D, Epstein R. Tocainide-associated interstitial pneumonitis. Ann Intern Med 1981; 94:489–90.

140. Braude A, Downar E, Chamberlain D, Rebuck A. Tocainide-associated interstitial pneumonitis. Thorax 1982; 37:309–10.

141. Arrowsmith J, Creamer J, Bosco L. Severe dermatologic reactions reported after treat-

ment with tocainide. Ann Intern Med 1987; 107:693–6.

142. Currie P, Ramsdale D. Paranoid pyschosis induced by tocainide. Br Med J 1984; 288:606–7.

143. Fasola G, Dosualdo F, de Pangher V, Barducci E. Thrombocytopenia and mexiletine (letter). Ann Intern Med 1984; 100:162.

144. Girmann G, Pees H, Scheurlen P. Pseudo-thrombocytopenia and mexiletine (letter). Ann Intern Med 1984; 100:767

145. MacMahon B, Bakshi M, Branagan P, Kelly J, Walsh M. Pharmacokinetics and haemodynamic effects of tocainide in patients with acute myocardial infarction complicated by left ventricular failure. Br J Clin Pharmacol 1985; 19:429–34.

146. Winkle R, Anderson J, Peters F, Meffin P, Fowles R, Harrison D. The hemodynamic effects of intravenous tocainide in patients with heart disease. Circulation 1978; 57:787–92.

147. Swedberg K, Pehrson J, Ryden L. Electrocardiographic and hemodynamic effects of tocainide (W-36095) in man. Eur J Clin Pharmacol 1978; 14:15–9.

148. Pozenel H. Haemodynamic studies on mexiletine, a new antiarrhythmic agent. Postgrad Med J 1977; 1:78–80.

149. Kuhn P, Kroiss A, Klicpera M, Zilcher H, Kaindl F. Antiarrhythmic and haemodynamic effects of mexiletine. Postgrad Med J 1977; 53(Suppl. 1):81–4.

150. Banim S, Da Silva A, Stone D, Balcon R. Observations of the haemodynamics of mexiletine. Postgrad Med J 1977; 53(Suppl. 1):74–7.

151. Stein J, Podrid P, Lown B. Effects of oral mexiletine on left and right ventricular function. Am J Cardiol 1984; 54:575–8.

152. Campbell N, Zaidi S, Adgey A, Patterson G, Pantridge J. Observations on haemodynamic effects of mexiletine. Br Heart J 1979; 41:182–6.

153. Engler R, LeWinter M. Tocainide-induced ventricular fibrillation. Am Heart J 1981; 101:494–6.

154. Velebit V, Podrid P, Lown B, Cohen B, Graboys T. Aggravation and provocation of ventricular arrhythmias by antiarrhythmic drugs. Circulation 1982; 65:886–94.

155. Slater W, Lampert S, Podrid P, Lown B. Clinical predictors of arrhythmia worsening by antiarrhythmic drugs. Am J Cardiol 1988; 61:349–53.

28

Propafenone

Hrayr S. Karagueuzian

Cedars-Sinai Medical Center and UCLA School of Medicine
Los Angeles, California

INTRODUCTION

Propafenone (Fig. 1) was synthesized in 1970, and its hydrochloride salt has been commercially available in Germany since 1977 as Rytmonorm (Knoll AG) for the management of cardiac arrhythmias of various etiologies. Its electrophysiologic actions are not confined to any specific cardiac fiber type, as it has potent electrophysiologic effects on atrial, atrioventricular (AV) nodal, and ventricular tissues. Propafenone can be classified as a "broad-spectrum" antiarrhythmic drug because clinically it is effective against atrial, junctional, and ventricular arrhythmias and against tachyarrhythmias involving anomalous atrioventricular accessory pathways, as in the Wolff-Parkinson-White syndrome. Propafenone is considered a class IC antiarrhythmic agent. It is currently undergoing approval procedures in the United States for clinical use.

CELLULAR ELECTROPHYSIOLOGIC EFFECTS OF PROPAFENONE

Sinoatrial Node

Katoh and associates (1), using a standard microelectrode technique, have shown that propafenone at concentrations up to 7 μg/ml has no significant effect on isolated rabbit sinoatrial node (Fig. 2). Only at higher concentrations (>7 μg/ml) could propafenone cause a significant depression of sinus nodal automaticity (1). This observation is consistent with the results obtained by Satoh and Hashimoto (2), who showed that only high concentrations (i.e., >5 μg/ml) of propafenone could cause significant slowing of sinus nodal automaticity. In these studies, using voltage clamp techniques on isolated rabbit sinoatrial tissue preparations, propafenone caused a concentration-dependent decrease (1–10 μg/ml) in the outward potassium current I_K and in the slow inward current I_s. The decrease in the amplitude of these two currents was caused by a reduction in the maximum conductance of these currents rather than by a change in the voltage-dependent characteristics of these currents (2). The decrease in the outward potassium current could conceivably explain the action potential prolongation of sinus nodal cells (1–3). A prolongation of sinus nodal action potential duration may cause slowing of sinus rate (independently of pacemaker current) because the slowly repolarizing process delays the onset of automatic impulse

(2'-[3-(propylamino)-2-(hydroxy)-propoxy]-3-phenylpropiophenone

MW=377.9

Figure 1 Structural formula of propafenone.

initiation. The depressant effect of propafenone on sinus nodal automaticity was,
however, exaggerated during total pharmacologic autonomic blockage with atropine and
propranolol (Fig. 3 and Table 1) (1). During
cholinergic blockade with atropine alone, propafenone at concentrations of 1.25 μg/ml and
above caused significant depression of sinus
node automaticity. This finding suggests that
propafenone exerts an atropinelike accelerator

effect on sinus node that offsets its direct depressant membrane effects. This property of
propafenone is similar to the effects of disopyramide on rabbit sinus node (4). In contrast,
the effects of incremental concentrations of
propafenone during β-adrenoceptor blockade
with propranolol were essentially similar to
the effects seen in the absence of autonomic
blockade (1). The modest β-adrenoreceptor
blocking property of propafenone (5,6) does
not seem to quantitatively or qualitatively
change the overall depressant effect of propafenone on sinus node automaticity (1).

Atrial Fibers

Propafenone caused a concentration-dependent
decrease in the action potential amplitude of
rabbit atrial fibers with a concomitant decrease in the maximum slope of phase 0

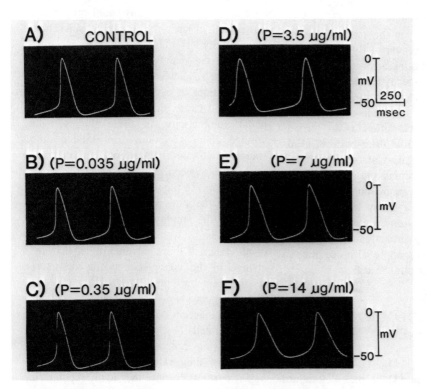

Figure 2 Effects of increasing concentrations of propafenone superfusion with Tyrode's solution (indicated above panels B–F) on rabbit sinus nodal automaticity. It is evident that only high concentrations of
propafenone (i.e., 14 μg/ml) can cause a slight depolarization of sinus nodal cells with a concomitant slight
prolongation of both action potential duration and spontaneous cycle length. (From Ref. 1.)

Table 1 Effects of Propafenone on Action Potential Characteristics of Rabbit Sinus Node[a]

| | Group | Control | Propafenone | | | | | |
			1×10^{-7} M, 0.035 µg/ml	1×10^{-6} M, 0.35 µg/ml	5×10^{-6} M, 1.75 µg/ml	1×10^{-5} M, 3.5 µg/ml	2×10^{-5} M, 7 µg/ml	4×10^{-5} M, 14 µg/ml
SCL, msec	I	484.1 ± 90.1	484.4 ± 94.3	490 ± 98.2	465.6 ± 87.6	472 ± 88.1	497.1 ± 80	662 ± 110[b]
	II	487.3 ± 70.4	513.3 ± 86.4	550 ± 104.1	556.6 ± 102.1[b]	562.1 ± 100[b]	617.6 ± 110[b]	679 ± 125.4[c]
MDP, mV	I	-63.3 ± 3.9	-63.4 ± 3.1	-63.3 ± 3.1	-61.9 ± 4.8	-60.3 ± 6	-57.1 ± 4.5	-54.0 ± 3.1
	II	-63.0 ± 3.6	-62.4 ± 2.6	-62.8 ± 7.2	-61.6 ± 7.2	-61.4 ± 8.6	-58.4 ± 8.6	-56.8 ± 8.2
TP, mV	I	-50.6 ± 6.4	-50.9 ± 6.1	-50.1 ± 5.5	-50.0 ± 5.5	-49.0 ± 5.1	-46.4 ± 3.2	-39.3 ± 9.2
	II	-50.6 ± 5.8	-50.6 ± 7.1	-50.0 ± 6.8	-49.2 ± 8.4	-49.2 ± 6.2	-46.0 ± 8.1	-42.3 ± 8.9
Phase 4 slope, mV/sec	I	56.2 ± 14.4	55.2 ± 13.7	53.0 ± 2.1	49.8 ± 14.8[b]	47.8 ± 13.7[b]	44.0 ± 11.5[b]	26.5 ± 14.5[c]
	II	54.8 ± 12.6	54.4 ± 12.6	54.0 ± 12.5	50.0 ± 18[b]	40.6 ± 17[b]	32.0 ± 16.5[b]	27.5 ± 12.5[b]
ADP$_{50}$, msec	I	120.7 ± 23	120.7 ± 22	121.4 ± 23	122.1 ± 23.4	133.6 ± 23.5[b]	140.7 ± 28[b]	150.0 ± 19.2[b]
	II	120.0 ± 27.1	125.0 ± 29.3	128.0 ± 28.4	131.0 ± 30.1	145.0 ± 34.1[b]	156.0 ± 36.5[c]	168.8 ± 38.5[b]
APD$_{100}$, msec	I	230.0 ± 52	229.3 ± 51	231.4 ± 40.8	240.7 ± 40.8	266.4 ± 43.2[b]	290.0 ± 40.8[c]	312.5 ± 50.1[b]
	II	237.0 ± 48	244.0 ± 50	252.0 ± 48.3	259.0 ± 50.1	284.0 ± 61.2[b]	307.0 ± 61.4[c]	362.5 ± 62.3[b]

[a]Group I during normal Tyrode's superfusion and group II during autonomic blockade 10^{-6} M (atropine + 5×10^{-6} M propranolol). All values are mean ± SD in seven preparations in each group. SCL, sinus cycle length; MDP, maximum diastolic potential; TP, takeoff potential; APD$_{50}$, action potential duration at 50% repolarization; APD$_{100}$, action potential duration at 100% repolarization.

[b]$p < 0.05$.

[c]$p < 0.01$ compared to control (paired tc test).

Source: From Reference 1.

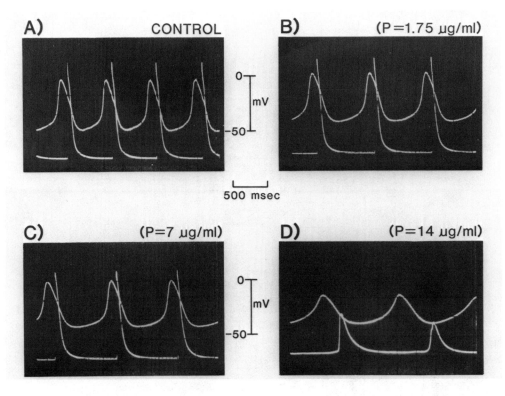

Figure 3 Effects of increasing concentrations of propafenone on simultaneously recorded rabbit sinus nodal cells and adjoining crista terminalis fibers during autonomic blockade with atropine (10^{-6} M) and propranolol (5×10^{-6} M). It is evident that a progressive concentration-dependent increase in the cycle length of sinus nodal automaticity occurs. Note that at 14 µg/ml the action potential amplitude of both crista terminalis fiber and sinus nodal cells is considerably decreased, with only slight depolarization of the resting membrane potential. (From Ref. 1.)

depolarization ($\dot{V}_{max}$) (Table 2) (1,3). These changes occurred in the absence of any significant change in the resting membrane potential, indicating blockade of fast inward sodium current (1,3). At a high propafenone concentration (14 µg/ml), however, a slight but significant decrease in the resting membrane potential with a dramatic decrease in the action potential amplitude occurred (Fig. 3 and Table 2). The action potential duration slightly but significantly increased in a concentration-dependent manner (1.75–14 µg/ml) for both 50 and 90% repolarization (Fig. 4 and Table 2). A slight but significant decrease in conduction velocity in rabbit atrial tissue was also reported by Dukes and Vaughan Williams (3).

Ventricular Muscle Cells

As in atrial fibers propafenone caused a significant concentration-dependent blockade of $\dot{V}_{max}$ and action potential amplitude without significant effect on resting membrane potential (Table 3) (1,2). The depressant effect of propafenone on the $\dot{V}_{max}$ appears to be frequency dependent (use dependent) (7). A greater degree of steady-state depression occurred at faster rates of pacing. However, a slight but significant decrease in the $\dot{V}_{max}$ also occurs at very slow rates of pacing or after a period of rest (tonic blockade) (7). The blockade of fast inward sodium channel by propafenone depend in a critical manner on the resting membrane potential (7,8). A stepwise reduction in the resting membrane potential from -90 to -70 mV by elevation of extracellular potassium ion concentration causes the $\dot{V}_{max}$ blockade to increase significantly (8). Voltage sensitivity of the tonic and the frequency-dependent sodium channel blockades are, however, different. Tonic inhibition

Table 2 Effects of Propafenone on the Transmembrane Potential Characteristics of Rabbit Crista Terminalis[a]

	Group	Control	1×10^{-7} M, 0.035 µg/ml	1×10^{-6} M, 0.35 µg/ml	5×10^{-6} M, 1.75 µg/ml	1×10^{-5} M, 3.5 µg/ml	2×10^{-5} M, 7 µg/ml	4×10^{-5} M, 14 µg/ml
					Propafenone			
RMP, mV	I	81.1 ± 3.5	-81.3 ± 3.4	-81.6 ± 1.8	-80.1 ± 3.6	-80.8 ± 1.8	-78.5 ± 4.3	-69.7 ± 5.4[c]
	II	-82.7 ± 1.7	-82.3 ± 2.4	-80.8 ± 1.1	-79.7 ± 1.6	-78.8 ± 1.9	-78.2 ± 1.1	-70.5 ± 6.2[c]
APA, mV	I	93.6 ± 6.4	93.0 ± 7.2	93.0 ± 7.2	91.5 ± 5.6	88.3 ± 5.4[c]	81.3 ± 10.1[c]	66.1 ± 9.2[c]
	II	94.3 ± 7.6	94.0 ± 7.9	90.7 ± 6.2	88.0 ± 5.4[b]	77.7 ± 11.2[c]	72.0 ± 12.4[c]	60.5 ± 14.1[c]
$\dot{V}_{max}$, V/sec	I	159.4 ± 29	155.6 ± 31	146.3 ± 34	123.9 ± 29.5[c]	80.6 ± 20.2[d]	50.4 ± 25[d]	20.0 ± 12[d]
	II	148.3 ± 32	132.5 ± 38	122.5 ± 40	99.2 ± 36.2[c]	63.0 ± 38.6[c]	37.5 ± 32.4[d]	16.5 ± 14.5[d]
APD$_{50}$, msec	I	50.4 ± 17.9	51.8 ± 6.4	54.0 ± 7.2	56.9 ± 9.1[b]	60.4 ± 9.2[c]	68.1 ± 12.1[d]	78.6 ± 14.5[d]
	II	49.2 ± 6.4	49.2 ± 6.1	50.0 ± 7.1	51.7 ± 7.1	58.3 ± 8.6[c]	70.8 ± 13.4[d]	91.3 ± 20.1[d]
APD$_{90}$, msec	I	94.3 ± 12.5	95.0 ± 17.5	96.0 ± 14.3	98.1 ± 13.5[b]	112.9 ± 14.5[d]	133.6 ± 24.5[d]	162.9 ± 34.8[d]
	II	97.5 ± 14.6	97.5 ± 17.2	100.0 ± 12.3	103.3 ± 15.1[b]	117.5 ± 18.5[d]	145.0 ± 30.1[d]	178.8 ± 46.6[d]

[a]Group I during normal Tyrode's superfusion and group II during autonomic blockade 10^{-6} M (atropine $+ 5 \times 10^{-6}$ M propranolol);
All values are mean ± SD, in seven preparations in each group. RMP, resting membrane potential; APA, amplitude of action potential; $\dot{V}_{max}$, maximum rate of rise of phase 0 depolarization; APD$_{50}$, action potential duration at 50% repolarization; APD$_{90}$, action potential duration at 90% repolarization.
[b]$p < 0.05$.
[c]$p < 0.01$.
[d]$p < 0.005$.
Source: From Reference 1.

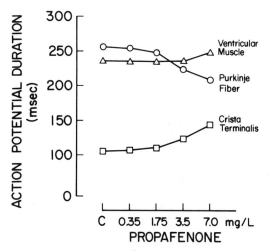

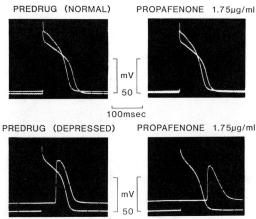

Figure 4 A graphic display of action potential duration (APD) changes to 90% repolarization (*Y* axis) caused by various concentrations of propafenone superfusion (*X* axis) on canine Purkinje and ventricular muscle preparation and on rabbit crista terminalis fiber. A concentration-dependent shortening of APD in Purkinje fiber occurs, as does a progressive lengthening of both ventricular muscle and crista terminalis APD. (From Ref. 1.)

Figure 5 Effects of propafenone (1.7 μg/ml) on simultaneously recorded normal canine Purkinje-ventricular muscle junction conduction time (upper panels) and on normal Purkinje and partially depolarized ventricular muscle junction (lower panels). In the normal preparation the Purkinje fiber resting membrane potential was -84 mV and that of ventricular muscle cell was -78 mV. No conduction delay was caused by 30 min of propafenone superfusion. In contrast, in a depressed preparation the Purkinje fiber resting membrane potential was -79 mV and that of ventricular muscle -63 mV. Conduction time during control condition was 42 msec. After 20 min of propafenone superfusion the conduction time was doubled to 84 msec. Note also a sizable depression of the depressed ventricular muscle action potential amplitude from -63 to -50 mV. (Previously unpublished record.)

increases from 10 to >60% in response to 20 mV depolarization, whereas frequency-dependent blockade increase from 20 to 40% during similar degrees of depolarization (8). Zeiler and associates (9) evaluated the effects of propafenone on canine ischemic surviving subendocardial fibers 1 day after permanent coronary artery occlusion. Ventricular muscle fibers with reduced resting membrane potential (-69 mV) had a significantly greater reduction in their action potential amplitude (43%) and $\dot{V}_{max}$ (70%) during propafenone (2 μg/ml) superfusion than ventricular muscle cells with a resting potential of -79 mV (5 and 29%, respectively) (9). The significance of the greater sensitivity of partially depolarized ventricular muscle cells to the depressant effect of propafenone with respect to conduction velocity is illustrated in Figure 5. In this experiment, conducted in our laboratory, propafenone at concentration of 1.75 μg/ml had no detectable effect on the conduction time at the normal Purkinje fiber-ventricular muscle junction. However, in another preparation in which the ventricular muscle was partially depolarized

the conduction time was appreciably increased. Superfusion with 1.75 μg/ml of propafenone caused a further dramatic increase in conduction time. Such a differential effect of propafenone on partially depolarized ventricular muscle fibers could have important antiarrhythmic implications, namely terminating reentrant tachyarrhythmias and perhaps at times even aggravating an existing reentrant arrhythmia by transforming the nonsustained form to a sustained form of tachycardia. Propafenone causes a concentration-dependent prolongation of action potential duration for both 50 and 90% repolarization (Table 3 and Fig. 6), with a concomitant increase in the duration of the effective refractory period (1,3).

Table 3 Effects of Propafenone on Canine Purkinje Fiber and Ventricular Muscle Transmembrane Potential[a] Properties

		Control	Propafenone			
			1×10^{-6}M, 0.35 µg/ml	5×10^{-6}M, 1.75 µg/ml	1×10^{-5}M, 3.5 µg/ml	2×10^{-5}M, 7 µg/ml
RMP,	PF	-91.0 ± 3.6	-90.8 ± 3.4	-90.4 ± 3.2	-89.9 ± 3.1	-86.3 ± 4.2
mV	VM	-86.8 ± 3.5	-86.4 ± 2.9	-86.6 ± 4.2	-86.6 ± 2.7	-86.0 ± 3.2
APA,	PF	117.0 ± 9.1	116.2 ± 9.8	113.9 ± 10.3	109.8 ± 9.2[d]	96.7 ± 10.1[d]
mV	VM	104.8 ± 9.8	104.2 ± 9.1	104.6 ± 8.9	102.6 ± 8.4	97.8 ± 7.3[b]
$\dot{V}_{max}$,	PF	518.3 ± 130.5	512.5 ± 125.6	475.0 ± 142.5	356.7 ± 145.7[b]	296.0 ± 189.5[c]
V/sec	VM	206.0 ± 68.5	206.0 ± 67.7	206.0 ± 70.4	175.0 ± 52.6[b]	95.0 ± 18.5[d]
APD_{50},	PF	183.0 ± 33.2	181.5 ± 31.4	169.5 ± 26.4[d]	126.5 ± 22.5[d]	100.0 ± 17.5[d]
msec	VM	159.0 ± 31.5	159.0 ± 31.2	158.0 ± 35.6	159.0 ± 37.4	164.0 ± 38.5[b]
APD_{90},	PF	256.0 ± 34.6	254.0 ± 30.5	248.0 ± 32.1[c]	224.5 ± 24.7[d]	209.3 ± 27.3[d]
msec	VM	235.0 ± 30.5	235.0 ± 29.6	235.0 ± 31.5	236.0 ± 28.7	249.0 ± 34.7[c]
DET (mA), msec		1.0 ± 0.08	1.1 ± 0.1	1.05 ± 0.1	1.6 ± 0.2[b]	4.0 ± 1.5[c]

[a]Mean ± SD; $N = 10$. Basic drive cycle = 800 msec. RMP, resting membrane potential; APA, action potential amplitude; $\dot{V}_{max}$, maximum rate of phase 0 depolarization; APD_{50} and APD_{90}, action potential duration at 50 and 90% repolarization, respectively; DET, diastolic excitability threshold, in milliamperes; PF, Purkinje fiber; VM, ventricular muscle.
[b]$p < 0.05$.
[c]$p < 0.01$.
[d]$p < 0.005$.
Source: From Reference 1.

Purkinje Fibers

Propafenone causes a concentration-dependent decrease in the action potential amplitude and $\dot{V}_{max}$ without altering resting membrane potential (1,3,5). As in the ventricular muscle fibers the depressant effect of propafenone on the $\dot{V}_{max}$ and action potential amplitude appeared exaggerated in partially depolarized Purkinje fibers; however, unlike in ventricular muscle cells, these differences failed to reach statistical significance (9). Propafenone causes significant concentration-dependent shortening of both sheep (5) and canine (1,10) free-running Purkinje fibers at 50 and 90% repolarization (Table 3 and Fig.6). This shortening effect eliminates Purkinje fiber-ventricular muscle cell disparity with respect to action potential duration (Fig. 6) and thus removes conduction block of premature impulses propagating in the Purkinje to ventricular muscle direction (Fig. 7). On isolated rabbit Purkinje fibers, however, propafenone had a variable effect on the process of repolarization (3). Slight but significant prolongation occurred for up to 1.3 µg/ml and then a shortening oc-

curred at propafenone concentration of about 2.6 µg/ml (3). This sequence could be caused by differences in the species used (rabbit versus canine and sheep). In larger mammals (sheep and canine) the shortening effects of propafenone appear more uniform and consistent (1,5). The electrophysiologic mechanism(s) of propafenone's differential effects on the repolarization of Purkinje fibers and ventricular muscle cells is unknown. Similar disparate effects on the repolarization process were also observed with propafenone by others (5,9) and also with another newly approved antiarrhythmic drug, flecainide (11). It has been suggested that the plateau phase of the Purkinje fiber action potential is in part regulated by a tetrodotoxin-sensitive steady-state sodium inward current that apparently contributes more to the Purkinje fiber plateau than to that of ventricular muscle fibers, because tetrodotoxin was found to abolish the differences of action potential duration between these two fiber types (12). It is therefore conceivable that propafenone exerts an inhibitory effect on the tetrodotoxin-sensitive

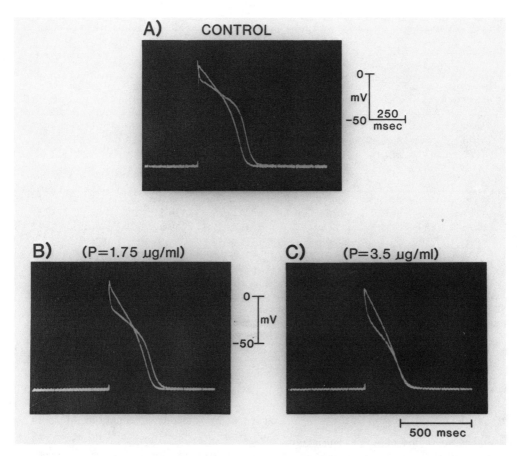

Figure 6 Effects of superfusion of two different concentrations of propafenone, 1.75 and 3.5 µg/ml (B and C, respectively), on simultaneously recorded action potentials from a canine Purkinje fiber-ventricular muscle preparation. During the control condition (A) Purkinje fiber action potential duration (APD) outlasts that of the ventricular muscle APD. Shortening of Purkinje fiber APD occurred in a concentration-dependent manner without much effect on ventricular muscle APD, thus removing APD disparity between these two fiber types (C). (From Ref. 1.)

steady-state inward sodium current, accounting for the observed shortening of the action potential duration of Purkinje fibers and not that of ventricular muscle fibers.

Purkinje Fiber Automaticity

Propafenone has a potent inhibitory effect on enhanced normal spontaneous automaticity in Purkinje fibers (1). In Purkinje fibers with a resting membrane potential of -72 to -84 mV and superfused with 2.7 mM potassium to promote automaticity, propafenone at a concentration of 1.75 µg/ml significantly decreased the rate of automatic impulse initiation (Fig. 8) (1). The slowing of the au-

tomatic discharge rate was caused by a decrease in the slope of spontaneous phase 4 depolarization (Fig. 8). Propafenone superfusion also depressed abnormal automaticity induced by barium chloride (0.25 mM) and hypokalemia (2.7 mM) in a concentration-dependent manner (3–10 µg/ml) (10). Similarly, in partially depolarized Purkinje fibers propafenone at a concentration of 2 µg/ml terminated triggered automatic activity arising from delayed afterdepolarization (9). Termination of triggered automatic activity was caused by a decrease in the rate of rise of the delayed afterdepolarization, which eventually failed to reach threshold potential (9). Such an inhibitory effect on the mechanism of triggered au-

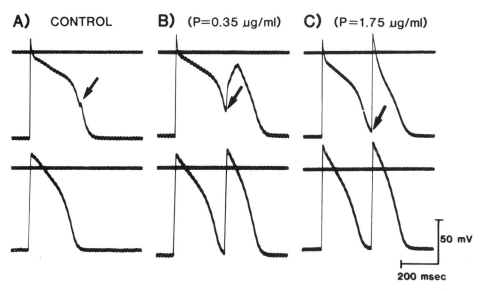

Figure 7 Effects of propafenone on early premature stimuli (arrows) on simultaneously recorded action potentials of canine Purkinje fiber (top recordings) and ventricular muscle (lower recordings). During the control condition (A) a single premature stimulus applied near the Purkinje fiber with a coupling interval of 260 msec blocks and does not conduct to the distal ventricular muscle. Superfusion with 0.35 μg/ml of propafenone (B) causes a slight shortening of Purkinje fiber action potential duration (APD), allowing the same premature stimulus (i.e., coupling interval of 260 msec) to cause a "slow-response" action potential, which conducts to the distal ventricular muscle. Further shortening of Purkinje fiber APD with 1.75 μg/ml of propafenone superfusion (C) allows the induction of full-blown action potential in the Purkinje fiber with the same premature stimulus coupling interval (i.e., 260 msec), which also conducts to the distal ventricular muscle. The preparation is driven at 800 msec cycle length and stimulated with 2 msec duration pulses at twice diastolic current strength for both basic and premature stimuli. (From Ref. 1.)

tomaticity could be caused by the mild calcium channel blocking and β-adrenoceptor blocking properties of propafenone on cardiac fibers (3,5,6,10). This is so because triggered automaticity is readily induced by elevation of intracellular calcium ion concentration (13,14).

ELECTROPHYSIOLOGIC AND HEMODYNAMIC EFFECTS OF PROPAFENONE IN INTACT EXPERIMENTAL ANIMAL MODELS

Electrophysiologic Effects

Table 4 summarizes the salient electrophysiologic properties of propafenone in anesthetized closed-chest dogs and compares its effects to that of a "standard" antiarrhythmic drug, lido-

caine. Propafenone significantly increased ($p < 0.05$) the right ventricular endocardial diastolic excitability threshold for both bipolar and cathodal stimulation (Table 4) (15). Propafenone slowed impulse conduction through the AV node with a concomitant increase in the AV nodal functional refractory period (FRP; Table 4). Propafenone also caused a significant ($p < 0.05$) increase in intraatrial conduction time (Table 4). Lidocaine, in contrast, had no significant effect on any of these parameters (Table 4). Both drugs had no effect on the right ventricular endocardial effective refractory period (ERP), His-Purkinje (HV) conduction time, or the sinus node recovery time (SNRT; Table 4). Propafenone shifted upward the tail portion of the strength-interval curve for both cathodal and bipolar stimulation (Fig. 9). Lidocaine, in contrast, had no effect on the strength-interval curve (15).

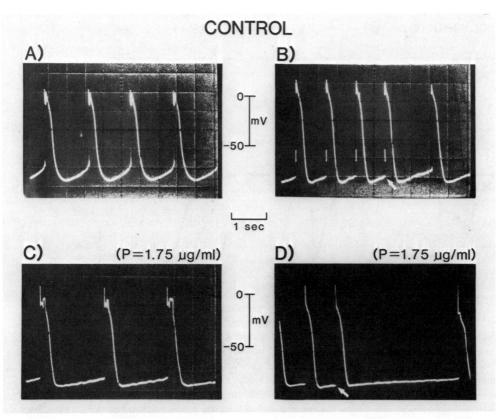

Figure 8 Effects of propafenone superfusion (1.7 µg/ml) on canine Purkinje fiber automaticity induced by superfusion with modified Tyrode's solution containing 2.7 mM potassium. During the control conditions (A and B) spontaneous automatic activity is present with a cycle length of 1160 msec (A), which manifests slight overdrive suppression (return cycle 1290 msec) after overdrive stimulation at 800 msec for 15 sec (arrow in B). Propafenone superfusion increased both the cycle length of spontaneous automatic activity (1743 msec, C) and the return cycle after overdrive (arrow) to 3370 msec (D). (From Ref. 1.)

Hemodynamic Effects

Table 5 summarizes the comparative effects of propafenone and lidocaine on the major hemodynamic parameters in closed-chest anesthetized dogs (15). Although both drugs caused a significant reduction in aortic blood pressure, the effects of propafenone were significantly more pronounced than those of lidocaine. Propafenone, unlike lidocaine, significantly reduced pulmonary systolic pressure and cardiac output during constant atrial pacing. Cardiac output 5–10 min after intravenous administration of propafenone (4 mg/kg) significantly decreased during regular atrial pacing (Table 5) (15).

EFFECTS OF PROPAFENONE AGAINST VENTRICULAR ARRHYTHMIAS IN EXPERIMENTAL ANIMAL MODELS

The efficacy of intravenous propafenone was evaluated against acute ischemic ventricular tachycardias in conscious dogs with either permanent coronary artery occlusion (10,16) or with transient coronary artery occlusion followed by reperfusion (16). The studies were conducted 24 hr after coronary artery occlusion. Propafenone (4 mg/kg over 2 min) suppressed ventricular tachycardias in both models, with greater suppression occurring with tachycardia rates slower than 160 beats/

Table 4 Electrophysiologic Effects of Propafenone and Lidocaine on Anesthetized, Closed-Chest Dogs[a]

Electrophysiologic parameters	Propafenone (4 mg/kg IV, $n = 8$)			Lidocaine (5 mg/kg IV, $n = 8$)	
	Control	5 min	60 min	Control	5 min
H-V, msec	32.6 ± 2.5	32.5 ± 2.6	31.3 ± 2.8	30.7 ± 3.1	32.1 ± 2.7
ERP, msec	128 ± 10.31	131 ± 11.42	128.7 ± 6.07	120.5 ± 7.9	116.4 ± 9.4
DET, mA	1.38 ± 0.62	2.23 ± 0.95[b]	1.48 ± 0.64	1.37 ± 0.53	1.36 ± 0.55
AVNFRP, msec	187.3 ± 16.5	232.8 ± 15.3[b]	187.8 ± 14.7	186.5 ± 11.7	187 ± 12.7
IACT, msec	40.3 ± 8.7	62.7 ± 10.3[b]	36.3 ± 9.3	41.5 ± 9.2	43.2 ± 10.5
SNRT, msec	658.3 ± 210	633.3 ± 96.9	645 ± 184.8	640.5 ± 175.3	660 ± 185.3

[a]Abbreviations: *n*, number of dogs; ERP, effective refractory period of the right ventricle; DET, diastolic excitability threshold (bipolar) of the right ventricle; AVNFRP, atrioventricular nodal functional refractory period; IACT, intra-atrial conduction time; SNRT, sinus node recovery time; H-V, His-Purkinje conduction time during regular atrial drive at 400 msec cycle length (note that this interval was unchanged during premature atrial stimulation either before or after either propafenone or lidocaine administration). Data are presented as mean ± SD.
[b]$p = 0.05$ (Newman-Keul's test).
Source: From Reference 15.

min (16). The lesser efficacy of propafenone seen by Malfatto et al. (10) could be caused by the fact that the dose of propafenone (4 mg/kg IV) was administered over a 45 min instead of 5 min as in the study of Karagueuzian et al. (16). Furthermore, in the Malfatto study (10) it was found that the metabolite of pro- pafenone (5-hydroxypropafenone) had more potent antiarrhythmic efficacy than the parent compound. Unlike its potent effect on acute ischemic ventricular tachycardias, propafenone was much less effective against electrically inducible sustained and nonsustained ventricular tachycardias during the chronic phase of

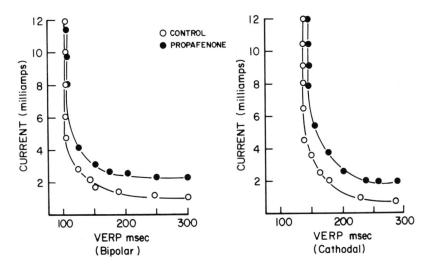

Figure 9 Effects of propafenone, 4 mg/kg IV, on the strength-interval curves constructed from measurements made in a dog with temporary left anterior descending coronary artery occlusion during the 24 hr postinfarction period. Measurements were made during the period of tachycardia, that is, during the control period, and during propafenone-induced normal sinus rhythm. Measurements were made from the right ventricular apex while pacing the ventricle at a cycle length of 300 msec. VERP, ventricular effective refractory period. (From Ref. 16.)

Table 5 Hemodynamic Effects of Propafenone and Lidocaine on Anesthetized, Closed-Chest Dogs[a]

Hemodynamic parameters	Propafenone (4 mg/kg IV, $n = 8$)			Lidocaine (5 mg/kg IV, $n = 8$)		
	Control	5 min	60 min	Control	5 min	60 min
AoSBP, mmHg	156.6 ± 12.82	143.0 ± 9.1[b]	154.3 ± 7.6	156.3 ± 6.2	150.3 ± 4.5[c]	158.4 ± 7.3
AoDBP, mmHg	98.7 ± 13.5	96.0 ± 12.2	101.5 ± 11.9	105.5 ± 4.9	105.6 ± 5.4	104.4 ± 5.7
PSBP, mmHg	32.3 ± 6.9	26.8 ± 5.4[b]	29.3 ± 5.2	28.6 ± 4.9	28.3 ± 6.3	27.9 ± 6.8
PDBP, mmHg	5.0 ± 2.4	3.0 ± 4.37	3.0 ± 4.37	4.3 ± 2.2	5.1 ± 2.7	4.3 ± 2.1
PCP, mmHg	6.5 ± 1.8	8.2 ± 1.5	6.9 ± 2.0	4.0 ± 1.6	5.0 ± 1.8	4.7 ± 1.6
CO, L/min	4.5 ± 1.1	3.86 ± 0.75[b]	4.30 ± 1.15	4.23 ± 1.52	4.05 ± 1.05	4 ± 1.45
HR, (beats/min)	117.0 ± 22.4	137.3 ± 15.2[b]	117.3 ± 21.2	108.8. ± 7.9	118.3 ± 11.8[d]	110.5 ± 8.7

[a]Abbreviations: n, number of dogs, AoSBP and AoDBP, aortic systolic and diastolic blood pressures, respectively; PSBP and PDBP, pulmonary systolic and diastolic blood pressures; PCP, pulmonary capillary pressure; CO, cardiac output measured during atrial drive at 400 msec cycle length; HR, heart rate. Date are presented as mean ± SD.
[b]$p = 0.05$ (Newman-Keul's test).
[c]$p \leq 0.5$ (Wilcoxon paired sample test).
Source: From Reference 15.

myocardial infarction. In a canine model of chronic isolated right ventricular infarction caused by permanent occlusion of the right coronary artery, propafenone could neither prevent tachycardia iducibility nor terminate it once induced (Fig. 10) (17). These studies were conducted in the conscious state 3–10 days after right coronary artery occlusion (17). Propafenone, however, significantly reduced the rate of the inducible sustained tachycardia from a mean of 269 to 230 beats/min (Fig. 10) (17). Propafenone was very effective against accelerated idioventricular rhythm (AIVR) in intact anesthetized closed-chest dogs (Fig. 11) (1). AIVR was promoted in the dogs after complete AV block was induced with electrode catheter ablation of the His bundle (1).

ELECTROPHYSIOLOGIC AND HEMODYNAMIC EFFECTS OF PROPAFENONE IN THE HUMAN

Electrophysiologic Effect

Propafenone administered intravenously (2 mg/kg) (18–20) or given orally (900 mg/day) (21–23) had no effect on sinus cycle length. Similarly corrected sinus node recovery time remained unchanged after either intravenous (18) or oral (22) administration of pro-

pafenone. In an earlier study involving 20 patients Seipel and Breithardt (24) reported a significant increase in sinus cycle length (decreased heart rate) and an increase in sinus nodal recovery time after 2 mg/kg intravenous administration of propafenone. Such a variant effect of propafenone in these series of patients could be caused by an abnormal underlying autonomic nervous system activity. Alboni and associates (25) showed that 2 mg/kg of intravenous propafenone had no effect on either sinus rate or sinus nodal recovery time, consistent with all previously reported studies (18–23). After total pharmacologic autonomic blockade with propranolol and atropine, however, similar intravenous doses of propafenone in the same patients caused a significant decrease in the heart rate and an increase in the sinus nodal recovery time (25). These authors suggested that propafenone has a direct depressant effect on sinus nodal automaticity; however, this effect is counteracted by its autonomically mediated vagolytic effect and because its mild β-adrenoceptor blocking effects are clinically insignificant (25). These observations are consistent with experimental findings on isolated rabbit sinoatrial preparations using the microelectrode technique (1). Sinoatrial conduction time after intravenous propafenone (2 mg/kg) remained unchanged in patients without pharmacologic autonomic

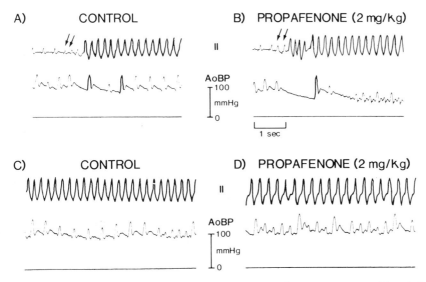

Figure 10 Inability of 2 mg/kg of intravenous propafenone to prevent either inducibility of sustained monomorphic ventricular tachycardia or termination once induced in a conscious dog 5 days after permanent right coronary artery occlusion. (A) Control predrug state of tachycardia inducibility. (B) Tachycardia remains inducible 5 min after the initial propafenone administration. (C) Sustained monomorphic tachycardia is induced again 90 min after the initial propafenone testing, and during this established running tachycardia 2 mg/kg of propafenone (D) does not terminate the tachycardia but causes a slowing in its rate. II, ECG lead; AoBP, aortic blood pressure with 100 mmHg calibration. (From Ref. 17.)

blockade (18,25); after autonomic blockade, however, propafenone significantly slowed it (25). In an earlier series reported by Seipel and Breithardt (24) intravenous propafenone (2 mg/kg) increased sinoatrial conduction time. Propafenone caused a significant prolongation of atrioventricular nodal refractory period after both intravenous (18–20,24) and oral (21,22,26) administration. QRS duration and His-Purkinje conduction time (HV interval) were also significantly increased after both intravenous (18–20) and oral (21,22,26) propafenone administration. Propafenone had no significant effect on the corrected QT interval either after intravenous injection (2 mg/kg) (18,20) or after oral administration (26). However, the study by Connaly et al. (23) showed a modest prolongation of QT interval after oral propafenone in 16 patients from a mean of 402 to 459 msec (25). Such a discrepancy could be caused either by the different patient population or by different methods of computations or both. The slight prolongation of the corrected QT interval in the study of Shen et al. (18) did not reach statistical significance.

Propafenone uniformly prolonged both atrial and ventricular effective refractory periods after intravenous (20,24) and after oral (21,22) administration. Furthermore, propafenone also increased the effective refractory period of anomalous AV pathways after both intravenous (19) and oral administration (22).

Hemodynamic Effects

Acute intravenous propafenone (2 mg/kg) had no significant effect on mean arterial blood pressure (18,20). It slightly increased right atrial, pulmonary artery, and pulmonary capillary wedge pressure however, resulting in a mild depression of the cardiac index (2.6–2.3 L/min per m^2; $p < 0.001$) (18). Propafenone also caused a significant increase in both pulmonary vascular resistance and systemic vascular resistance (18). In a series of five patients, similar doses of propafenone given intravenously had no significant effect on any of these hemodynamic parameters (20). Similar conflicting results were obtained with respect to propafenone's effect on left

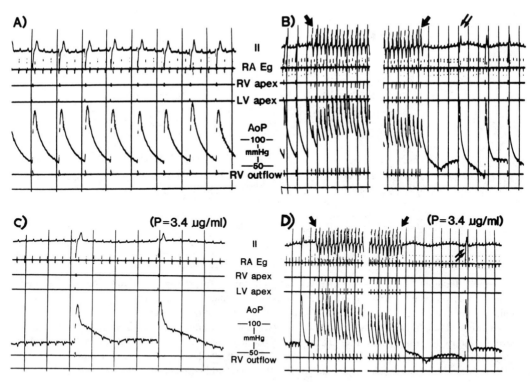

Figure 11 Effects of intravenous propafenone (4 mg/kg) on idioventricular rhythm and on ventricular recovery after overdrive in an anesthetized closed-chest dog with complete AV block. (A–D) The upper recording is a lead II electrocardiogram; RAEg, RV apex, LV apex, and RV outflow are bipolar recordings obtained from high right atrium, right ventricular apex, left ventricular apex, and right ventricular outflow tract, respectively. AoP, aortic pressure with calibration. P in C and D denotes plasma propafenone concentration during the electrophysiologic measurements (i.e., 5 min after injection). (A) An idioventricular rhythm at a cycle length of 1048 msec is shown during the control conditions, with a recovery time (pane B, double arrows) of 4.5 sec after 30 sec overdrive at 150 beats/min (single arrow). (C) After propafenone injection the cycle length of the idioventricular rhythm was 3700 msec, and the recovery time (double arrows) after 30 sec of overdrive at 150 beats/min (single arrow) was 7955 msec. (From Ref. 1.)

ventricular ejection fraction. Podrid and Lown (27) reported that oral propafenone significantly decreases left ventricular ejection fraction in patients with baseline ejection fraction of less than 50%. In patients with ejection fraction greater than 50% propafenone had no significant deleterious hemodynamic effects (27). This differential effect of propafenone was independent of plasma propafenone concentration (27). At variance with these observations is the report of Brodsky et al. (28), who found no significant effect of oral propafenone in patients with ejection fraction of about 30%, and the report of Baker et al. (29), who found a slight but significant decrease in this parameter in patients with baseline ejec-

tion fraction of 52%. These discrepancies could be caused by differences in patient populations and/or by differences in the methodology used, that is, echocardiography in Reference 27 versus radionuclide ventriculography in References 28 and 29. Nevertheless these studies suggest cautious use of propafenone in patients with impaired left ventricular function.

CLINICAL PHARMACOKINETICS OF PROPAFENONE

The disposition kinetics of propafenone were evaluated after both oral administration and intravenous injection in normal subjects and in patients with cardiac arrhythmias. Sensitive high-pressure chromatographic method for propafenone assay in biologic fluids by Harapat and Kates (30) helped greatly to advance our understanding of the pharmacokinetics and pharamacodynamics of this new antiarrhythmic drug.

Absorption

Axelson et al. (31) evaluated oral absorption of 300 mg propafenone in 24 healthy males aged 19–38 years (mean 24.4 years). Food intake significantly increased the oral absorption of propafenone. The area under the concentration-time curve of propafenone after food was significantly larger than after fasting. The peak plasma propafenone level after food intake was also significantly higher than after fasting (0.47 versus 0.31 µg/ml), and it was reached sooner after food intake than after fasting (mean of 1.8 versus 2.8 hr) (31). These authors suggested that patients taking propafenone must maintain a constant relationship with respect to food intake to ensure consistent bioavailability (31). Connolly et al. (32) found a nonlinear relationship between oral propafenone dose and mean steady-state plasma concentration in 13 patients with frequent premature depolarizations. A 3-fold increase in dose of propafenone from 300 to 900 mg caused a 10-fold increase in plasma propafenone levels. Such a nonlinear relationship (dose-dependent kinetics) between dose and plasma concentration could be due to presystemic saturation of a cytochrome P_{450} isoenzyme system (33,34). A saturation of potential first-pass elimination and/or clearance mechanism can cause a drastic increase in drug plasma concentration secondary to a small increase in the dose of oral drug intake. Such situations could have significant clinical implications necessitating reconsideration of propafenone's dosage schedule. Lee et al. (35) found that patients with reduced hepatic function have higher propafenone bioavailability than healthy subjects with normal hepatic function. Reduced presystemic clearance of propafenone caused by hepatocyte malfunction

results in a higher degree of propafenone bioavailability. These authors recommended at least a 50% reduction in propafenone dosage when it is administered to patients with significantly reduced liver function (35).

Distribution

After an intravenous dose of propafenone, plasma concentration-time data were fitted to a two-compartment model (36). The steady-state volume of distribution in patients was 3.12 ± 2.1 L/kg (36), which was significantly higher than in normal healthy subjects (1.2 L/kg) (37). Propafenone is 75–95% bound to human plasma protein (24,37). In the human propafenone appears to concentrate 2–6 times more in the lungs and in the liver than in the heart (38). According to one experimental study conducted on rabbits, myocardial propafenone concentrations were 114 times higher than the concentration in the coronary sinus effluent (39). Mason et al. (40) showed in 24 healthy male subjects that steady-state plasma concentration after oral propafenone could be estimated from saliva propafenone concentration, the latter being about 25% that in the plasma (40).

Metabolism and Elimination

Propafenone is extensively metabolized by the liver by a mechanism involving the cytochrome P_{450} enzyme system (33,41). The two major metabolites of propafenone are 5-hydroxypropafenone (5-OHP) and N-depropylpropafenone (NDPP) (33,41). Both these metabolites have potent electrophysiologic and antiarrhythmic actions (10,42), 5-OHP being more potent than NDPP (10). Less than 1% of propafenone is excreted unchanged in the urine and feces (43). Early clinical experience with propafenone showed that poor metabolizers of the polymorphically metabolized antihypertensive debrisoquine manifested an unusually long propafenone half-life (33). Later systematic study on 28 patients in fact showed that 22 of the patients were extensive metabolizers and 6 were poor metabolizers of debrisoquine (33). The extensive metabolizers had a relatively shorter propafenone half-life (5.5 versus 17.2 hr), lower average plasma concentration (1.1 versus 2.5 µg/ml), and higher oral clearance (1115 versus 264 ml/min) than poor metabolizers (33). These differences were all statistically significant. Furthermore, the active metabolite 5-OHP was detected in 9 of 10 patients in extensive metabolizers and in neither of the two poor metabolizers in whom it was assayed (33). In this study it was concluded that propafenone is metabolized via the same cytochrome P_{450} responsible for debrisoquine's 4-hydroxylation and that its pharmacokinetics are different in patients of different debrisoquine metabolic phenotype (33). Clearance of propafenone decreases with chronic oral therapy (36,44). After 5 (36) to 30 (43) days of oral therapy propafenone half-life was increased from an average of 3.5 hr to about 6.5 hr (36,43). The area under the plasma concentration curve was significantly larger after a single oral dose than after chronic (1 month) therapy (7.6 versus 3.4 µg/ml per hr) (42). Depression of hepatic metabolic function as a result of chronic propafenone therapy was suggested as a possible mechanism (42). Food intake does not affect the bioavailability of propafenone in poor metabolizers (31).

Pharmacodynamics

In seven patients Keller et al. (45) found that after a single oral dose of propafenone the degree of AV nodal conduction slowing, the most consistent electrophysiologic effect of propafenone, was positively correlated with plasma propafenone concentration with a rank correlation of 0.68 (45). At a given plasma concentration of propafenone the PR, QRS, and corrected QT intervals were all increased, with no significant difference in the magnitude of these changes between poor and extensive metabolizers of propafenone (33). In one experimental study on rabbits a linear relationship between myocardial propafenone concentration and QRS prolongation was found, with a large interexperimental variability in the slopes of the myocardial concentration-effect relationship (39).

CLINICAL THERAPEUTIC USE OFPROPAFENONE

Supraventricular Arrhythmias

Atrial Tachyarrhythmias

The efficacy of acute intravenous (2 mg/kg) propafenone against atrial flutter and atrial fibrillation was evaluated in 14 patients recovering from open heart surgery by Connolly et al. (46). Of these 14 patients, 6 (43%) had their arrhythmias converted to normal sinus rhythm and the ventricular response to atrial fibrillation or flutter decreased significantly, with a mean plasma propafenone concentration of 3.5 µg/ml (46). The efficacy of oral propafenone (900 mg/day) against both vagally and adrenergically dependent atrial flutter and atrial fibrillation was evaluated by Coumel et al. (47). Propafenone was found to be less effective against vagally dependent atrial flutter and fibrillation (i.e., tachyarrhythmia induced by slowing of heart rate) than against adrenergically dependent tachyarrhythmias (i.e., induced after acceleration of sinus rate) (47). In the latter case propafenone was found to be more effective than either propranolol or amiodarone (47). In another study chronic (3–6 months) oral propafenone (600–900 mg/day) was also found to be effective in 15 of 20 patients with recurrent atrial flutter and atrial fibrillation (48).

AV Nodal Reentrant Tachyarrhythmias

Intravenous propafenone (1.5 mg/kg) was found to be highly effective against inducible AV nodal reentrant paroxysmal supraventricular tachycardias (49). In seven of nine patients tachycardia could no longer be induced or sustained after propafenone. In these series all patients utilized an AV nodal slow pathway for anterograde conduction and an AV nodal fast pathway for retrograde conduction for the reentry circuit (49). In this study propafenone was found to prevent induction of the tachycardia by depressing retrograde AV nodal fast conduction pathway (49). In a similar study Hammill et al. (50) evaluated the efficacy of intravenous propafenone (2 mg/kg) in six patients against supraventricular tachycardia caused by a reentrant mechanism in the AV node. Propafenone terminated the tachycardias in all six patients and prevented the reinduction in all six (50).

Wolff-Parkinson-White Syndrome (Tachycardia Involving Accessory Pathways)

Ludmer et al. (51) evaluated the efficacy of intravenous (2 mg/kg over 10 min) propafenone in 10 patients with Wolff-Parkinson-White syndrome and in 2 patients with concealed accessory pathway. Sustained AV reentrant tachycardia was inducible in 11 patients at baseline, and propafenone administration promptly terminated the tachycardia in 10 of these 11 patients (51). In this study propafenone's efficacy was most likely caused by a significant increase in the accessory pathway refractory period in both the anterograde and retrograde directions (51). The effect of long-term administration of oral propafenone with a mean daily dosage of 694 mg/day (range 450–1200 mg/day) was evaluated in 8 of these 12 patients (51). Of 8 patients, 6 did not report any episodes of symptomatic recurrences of tachycardia during the follow-up period (12 ± 2 months). In the remaining 2 patients propafenone was not effective (51). In a series of 43 patients with Wolff-Parkinson-White syndrome the long-term efficacy of oral propafenone (2–3 years) was evaluated by Breithardt et al. (22). With an average mean daily dosage of about 800 mg propafenone was effective in 17 of 43 patients with no recurrences of symptomatic tachycardias; in 18 patients tachycardias were nonsustained and self-terminating, and in the remaining patients propafenone had to be discontinued for either lack of efficacy or intolerable side effects. One patient with dilated cardiomyopathy died suddenly (22).

Ventricular Arrhythmias

Ventricular Premature Depolarizations

Propafenone was found to be quite effective in suppressing premature ventricular depolarizations (PVD) in 60–90% of patients (32,52–62). Connolly et al. (32) evaluated the efficacy of oral propafenone (up to 900 mg/day) for 3–7 days in 13 patients with stable

PVDs. Stability of ventricular ectopy was confirmed in this study by the lack of significant difference in the number of PVD (22,503; range 5268–47,791 per 24 hr), pairs (1128; range 2–7681 per 24 hr), or runs of three or more (22; range 0–102) in any of the six drug-free 24 hr ambulatory ECG analyzed (32). Propafenone suppressed ventricular ectopy (greater than 90%) in 10 of these 13 patients. During a randomized, placebo-controlled double-blind study, followed over a 2 week period, propafenone in this same study (32) was effective in 7 of 10 patients studied in suppressing ventricular ectopy. The effective oral doses were 300–900 mg/day) (32). The relation of propafenone's efficacy in relation to the patient's underlying disease entity was not reported in this study (32). The long-term efficacy of oral propafenone against chronic PVD appears to decline with time (57,58). This could be caused by changing electrophysiologic mechanism(s) of the ventricular ectopic activity and/or caused by propafenone hysterisis, as myocardial cells become tolerant to propafenone's effect. Intravenous propafenone (2 mg/kg) was very effective against torsades de pointes (ventricular tachycardia) in 8 10 patients during acute myocardial infarction (63). In these series propafenone was effective in patients with or without QT prolongation (63). In 30 patients the addition of propafenone to either quinidine or procainamide monotherapy resulted in a significantly greater reduction of PVD (62). However, higher propafenone doses were necessary during monotherapy compared to propafenone therapy combined with procainamide or quinidine (730 versus 480 mg/day) (62).

Effects of Propafenone Against Inducible Ventricular Tachycardias by Programmed Electrical Stimulation

Oral propafenone administered in an escalating dosages of 450–900 mg/day had fairly satisfactory therapeutic outcome (21,28,53,56). In a series of 9 patients Podrid and Lown (56) reported efficacy in 7 patients, similarly, in a series of 6 patients with congestive heart failure, propafenone prevented tachycardia inducibility in 5 of these 6 patients (28). Somewhat lesser efficacy with oral propafenone was reported by Chilson et al. (21) and by Heger et al. (53) in a total of 33 patients. In one series propafenone prevented tachycardia inducibility in 3 of 15 patients with significant slowing of tachycardia rate in the remaining 12 patients (21): 10 such patients were discharged on oral propafenone therapy as the response to propafenone was considered satisfactory on the basis of lack of symptoms. With a mean follow-up period of 11 months 8 of these 10 patients remained symptom free (21). The effects of intravenous propafenone, however, were less satisfactory (18,64). Shen et al. (18) found that 1 mg/min of continuous intravenous propafenone was ineffective in preventing induction of tachycardia in 14 patients tested. However, when a 2 mg/min infusion was applied a better therapeutic outcome was obtained. In 11 patients with inducible sustained ventricular tachycardia in the baseline predrug state, intravenous propafenone prevented tachycardia inducibility in 3, made it nonsustained in 3, and had no effect in the remaining 6 patients (18). In 3 patients with nonsustained ventricular tachycardia intravenous propafenone prevented it in 1, made it sustained (aggravation) in another, and had no effect in the third patient (18). Much less efficacy with intravenous propafenone was obtained by Doherty et al. in a series of 14 patients (64). Propafenone had no effect on tachycardia inducibility in 13 of 14 patients studied, and it had an effect on the rate of the induced tachycardia (64). Shen et al. (18) evaluated the efficacy of oral propafenone on 4 patients who did not respond to intravenous propafenone. Of these patients 2 responded favorably to oral propafenone for a mean follow-up period of 15.8 months despite the failure of acute intravenous therapy (18). Should a similar therapeutic outcome be obtained in a larger patient population, then testing the efficacy of acute intravenous propafenone against inducible sustained ventricular tachycardias should be coupled with long-term oral therapy.

Efficacy of Propafenone Against Exercise-Induced Ventricular Arrhythmias

Propafenone appears quite effective in preventing exercise-induced ventricular arrhythmias in patients with various myocardial disease entities (28,56,65). Brodsky et al. (28) observed the occurrence of exercise-induced ventricular tachycardia in 5 of 10 patients with congestive heart failure during the predrug state. Oral propafenone (900 mg/kg) prevented the emergence of tachycardia in all 5 patients (28). Similarly, Podrid and Lown (56), in a series of 21 patients, found that oral propafenone (900 mg/kg) significantly reduced the peak heart rate during exercise from 142 beats/min during control to 119 beats/min. There was also in all patients a significant decrease in PVD, couplets, and ventricular tachycardia (56). Patient tolerance to exercise was unaltered after propafenone (5.9 versus 6.2 min) (56). This was at variance with the study of Cokkinos et al. (65), who found a significant increase in tolerance to exercise after propafenone. In this study, too, there was a significant decrease in exercise-induced ventricular arrhythmias as well as a significant decrease in the mean peak heart rate (65).

Side Effects of Propafenone

In nine published reports (21–23,28,32,49,53, 58,60), involving 266 patients on long-term oral propafenone (900 mg/kg) therapy with propafenone was discontinued in 15% of the total patient population (adjusted percentage). The percentage discontinuation in these studies ranged between 4% (22) and 40% (21). Side effects are classified as cardiovascular, neurologic, and gastrointestinal.

Cardiovascular Side Effects

The major cardiovascular side effects are arrhythmia worsening and exacerbation of symptoms of congestive heart failure. In five published reports (23,32,47,56,64) the reported incidence of arrhythmia aggravation ranged between 11% (47) and 36% (23), with an adjusted rate of 16% involving a total of 139 patients. Exacerbation of the symptoms of heart failure occurs less frequently, ranging between 0% (55,60) and 10% (28,52,55,57), accounting for an adjusted percentage of 4% in a total of 75 patients. This suggests that arrhythmia aggravation constitutes the major reason for discontinuation of propafenone therapy and that all other side effects of propafenone rarely necessitate discontinuation of therapy. Other cardiovascular side effects that can be minimized and/or eliminated altogether with dosage reduction without loss of antiarrhythmic efficacy include hypotension (4–12% of patients) (54,61), sinus bradycardia (8–10% of patients) (52,56), sinoatrial block (less than 10% of the patients), bundle branch block (less than 8% of the patients) (47,52,56), and various degrees of AV block (47,52,57).

Noncardiovascular Side Effects
These can be classified under neurologic and gastrointestinal.
Neurologic   Dizziness is the most common. It occurs in 3–41% of the patients (22,28,36,47, 55,57), with an adjusted occurrence of 13% in a total of 172 patients. Headache and visual disturbances were reported to occur in 7–12% of patients (22,40).
Gastrointestinal   The most common side effect complained of by patients taking propafenone is a bitter metallic taste in the mouth. In almost every study this side effect is reported to occur. In 10 published articles the reported incidence was 10–60%. The adjusted percentage incidence was 24% involving a total of 223 patients (18,32,44,47,53,54, 55,57,60,61). Nausea and vomiting were also reported to occur in 4–12% of the patients (40,49,54,55). In few isolated instances anaphylactic reaction (53), facial acne, and urticarial rash (53), constipation (22), dry mouth (22,32), abdominal and pleuritic chest pain (18,53), fatigue and tremor (21,40,49, 53), dyspnea (28) necessitating cautious use in asthmatic patients (66) An evaluation of antinuclear antibody titer is recommended (18).

DRUG INTERACTIONS

At present only a limited amount of information exists concerning drug interactions with propafenone. Because propafenone is extensively metabolized by liver, it is conceivable that other drugs could change the pharmacokinetic profile of propafenone by altering hepatic enzyme activity. In addition, the high

percentage of (>95%) propafenone bound to plasma proteins can potentially be displaced by coadministration of other medications, or propafenone could in itself displace drugs already bound to plasma protein. Thus careful monitoring of patients is required when a drug is contemplated to be added to a propafenone dosage regimen and/or when propafenone is removed from a multiple-drug dosage regimen.

Warfarin-Propafenone Interaction

Kates et al. (67) observed in eight healthy male volunteers with a mean age of 27.6 years that concurrent oral administration of propafenone (225 mg three times daily) and warfarin (5 mg) for 7 days resulted in an average increase of 38% in plasma warfarin levels. The mechanism for such an increase was suggested by these authors to be due to altered hepatic metabolism induced by propafenone as protein binding of warfarin was unaffected by propafenone (67).

β-Adrenoceptor Blockers, Calcium Channel Blockers, and Propafenone

Coadministration of β-blockers and/or calcium channel blockers with propafenone must be done, if at all, under careful monitoring because of potential AV conduction blockade, especially in patients with abnormalities in the AV conduction system. All three drug types have a potent and consistent depressant effect on the AV node.

Digoxin-Propafenone Interaction

Addition of oral propafenone dosing during steady-state maintenance digoxin therapy was found to increase plasma digoxin concentrations. Coadministration of propafenone to 36 healthy subjects caused a 37% increase (<0.01) in serum levels of digoxin (68). Similar findings were also observed in 5 patients on maintenance digoxin therapy with frequent ventricular premature depolarizations (52). In this study 900 mg propafenone given in three divided dose increased digoxin plasma levels by 83% (from 0.69 to 1.30 ng/ml) 3 days after propafenone treatment (52). If the binding and displacement properties of digoxin by propafenone in patients with ventricular arrhythmias are similar to those found in healthy subjects, it appears that digoxin displacement from its binding sites by propafenone is dose dependent. The toxic arrhythmic manifestations of elevated digoxin plasma levels remain undefined.

Isosorbide Dinitrate-Propafenone Interaction

In the study of Salerno et al. (52) it was observed that a patient complained of dizziness after taking isosorbide dinitrate and propafenone together. Because both drugs have the potential to cause dizziness when taken separately, it is probably that in susceptible patients this interaction may be of clinical significance. More studies are needed to substantiate this interaction.

Amiodarone-Propafenone Interaction

Drug-induced torsades de pointes has been reported for a combination of amiodarone and propafenone (69). The QT interval was prolonged before the onset of the tachycardia (69).

Cimetidine-Propafenone Interaction

In 12 healthy subjects the combination of cimetidine (H_2-receptor antagonist) with propafenone caused a modest but a significant increase in the QRS duration (70). These authors suggested that this is unlikely to have a significant clinical significance, however.

SUMMARY

Propafenone can be considered clinically a well-tolerated antiarrhythmic agent. It has a broad-spectrum antiarrhythmic activity. It can thus be a useful alternative drug when other agents fail to bring cardiac arrhythmias under control. Arrhythmia aggravation appears to be the major and perhaps the only cause for discontinuation, as other side effects are either minor or can be brought under control with

adjustment of dosage regimen. Propafenone's rate of successful control of arrhythmias is variable and as such may be an effective alternative in susceptible patients.

ACKNOWLEDGMENTS

Supported in part by ECHO Cedars-Sinai Research Foundation. The author was a recipient of Research Career Development Award HL-02193-05 from the National Heart, Lung and Blood Institute, Bethesda, Maryland.

REFERENCES

1. Katoh T, Karagueuzian H S, Sugi K, Ohta M, Mandel W J, Peter T. Effects of propafenone on sinus nodal and ventricular automaticity: in vitro and vivo correlation. Am Heart J 1987; 113:941–52.
2. Satoh H, Hashimoto K. Effects of propafenone on the membrane currents of rabbit sino-atrial node cells. Eur J Pharmacol 1984; 99:185–91.
3. Dukes I D, Vaughan Williams E M. The multiple modes of action of propafenone. Eur Heart J 1984; 5:115–25.
4. Katoh T, Karagueuzian H S, Jordan J, Mandel W J. The cellular electrophysiological mechanisms of the dual actions of disopyramide on rabbit sinus node function. Circulation 1982; 44:1216–24.
5. Ledda F, Mantelli L, Manzini S, Amerini S, Mugelli A. Electro-physiological and antiarrhythmic properties of propafenone in isolated cardiac preparations. J Cardiovasc Pharmacol 1981; 3:1162–73.
6. McLeod A A, Stiles G L, Shand D G. Demonstration of beta adrenoceptor blockade by propafenone hydrochloride: clinical pharmacologic, radioligand binding and adenylate cyclase activation studies. J Pharmacol Exp Ther 1983; 228:461–6.
7. Kohlhardt M, Seifert C. Tonic and phasic I_{Na} blockade by antiarrhythmics. Different properties of drug binding to fast sodium channels as judged from $\dot{V}_{max}$ studies with propafenone and derivatives in mammalian ventricular myocardium. Pflugers Arch 1983; 396:199–209.
8. Kohlhardt M. Block of sodium currents by antiarrhythmic agents: analysis of the electrophysiologic effects of propafenone in heart muscle. Am J Cardiol 1984; 54:13D–19D.

9. Zeiler R H, Gough W B, El-Sherif N. Electrophysiologic effects of propafenone on canine ischemic cardiac cells. Am J Cardiol 1984; 54:424–9.

10. Malfatto G, Zaza A, Forster M, Sodowick B, Danilo P Jr, Rosen M R. Electrophysiologic, inotropic and antiarrhythmic effects of propafenone, 5-hydroxypropaphenone and N-depropylpropafenone. J Pharmacol Exp Ther 1988; 246:419 26.

11. Ikeda N, Singh B N, Davis L D, Hauswith O. Effects of flacainide on the electrophysiologic properties of isolated canine and rabbit myocardial fibers. J Am Coll Cardiol 1985; 5:303–12.

12. Coraboeuf E, Deroubaix E. Shortening effect of tetrodotoxin on action potentials of the conducting system in the dogheart. J Physiol (Paris) 1978; 280.

13. Karagueuzian H S, Katzung B G. Voltage clamp studies of transient inward current and mechanical oscillation induced by ouabain in ferret papillary muscle. J Physio (Lond) 1982; 327:255–71.

14. Lederer W J, Tsien R W. Transient inward current underlying the arrhythmogenic effects of cardiotonic steroids in Purkinje fibers. J Physiol (Lond) 1976; 263:73–100.

15. Karagueuzian H S, Katoh T, McCullen A, Mandel W J, Peter T. Electrophysiologic and hemodynamic effects of propafenone, a new anti-arrhythmic agent on the anesthetized, closed-chest dog: comparative study with lidocaine. Am Heart J 1984; 107:418–24.

16. Karagueuzian H S, Fujimoto T, Katoh T, Peter T, McCullen A, Mandel W J. Suppression of ventricular arrhythmias by propafenone, a new anti-arrhythmic agent, during acute myocardial infarction in the conscious dog. Circulation 1982; 66:1190–8.

17. Karagueuzian HS, Sugi K, Ohta M, Meenmann M, Ino T, Peter P, Mandel W J. The efficacy of cibenzoline and propafenone against inducible sustained and nonsustained ventricular tachycardias in conscious dogs with isolated chronic right ventricular infarction: a comparative study with procainamide. Am Heart J 1986; 112:1173–83.

18. Shen E N, Sung R J, Morady F, Schwartz A B, Scheinman M M, DiCarlo L, Shapiro W. Electrophysiologic and hemodynamic effects of intravenous propafenone in patients with recurrent ventricular tachycardia. J Am Coll Cardiol 1984; 5:1291–7.

19. Waleffe A, Mary-Rabine L, DeRijbel R, Soyeur D, Legrand V, Kulbertus H E. Electrophysiological effects of propafenone studied with programmed electrical stimulation of the heart in patients with recurrent paroxysmal supraventricular tachycardia. Eur Heart J 1981; 2:345–52.

20. Feld GK, Nademanee K, Singh B N, Kirsten E. Hemodynamic and electrophysiologic effects of combined infusion of lidocaine and propafenone in humans. J Clin Pharmacol 1987; 27:52–9.

21. Chilson DA, Heger J J, Lipes D P, Browne K F, Prystowsky E N. Electrophysiologic effects and clinical efficacy of oral propafenone therapy in patients with ventricular tachycardia. J Am Col Cardioll 1985; 5:1407–13.

22. Breithardt G, Borggrefe M, Wiebringhaus E, Seipel L. Effect of propafenone in the Wolff-Parkinson-White syndrome: electrophysiologic findings and long-term follow-up. Am J Cardiol 1984; 54:29D–39D.

23. Connolly S J, Kates R E, Lebsack C S, Echt D S, Mason J W, Winkle R A. Clinical efficacy and electrophysiology of oral propafenone for ventricular tachycardia. Am J Cardiol 1983; 52:1208–13.

24. Seipel L, Breithardt B. Propafenone—a new antiarrhythmic drug. Eur Heart J 1980; 1:309–13.

25. Alboni P, Pirani R, Paparella N, Candini G C, Tomasi A M, Masoni A. A method for evaluating different modes of action of an antiarrhythmic drug in man. The effects of propafenone on sinus nodal functions. Int J Cardiol 1985; 7:255–65.

26. Cheriex E C, Krijne R, Brugada P, Heymeriks J, Wellens H J J. Lack of clinically significant beta-blocking effect of propafenone. Eur Heart J 1987; 8:53–6.

27. Podrid P J, Lown B. Propafenone: a new agent for ventricular arrhythmias. J Am Coll Cardiol 1984; 4:117–25.

28. Brodsky M A, Allen B J, Abate D, Henry W L. Propafenone therapy for ventricular tachycardia in the setting of congestive heart failure. Am Heart J 1985; 110:794–9.

29. Baker B J, Dinh H A, Kroskey D, de Soyza N D B, Murphy M L, Franciosa J A. Effect of propafenone on left ventricular ejection fraction. Am J Cardiol 1984; 54:20D–22D.

30. Harapat H J, Kates R E. High performance liquid chromatography analysis of propafenone in human plasma samples. J Chromatog 1982; 230:448–53.

31. Axelson J E, Chan G L Y, Kirsten E B, Mason W D, Lanman R C, Kerr C R. Food increases the bioavailability of propafenone. Br J Clin Pharmacol 1987; 23:735–41.

32. Connolly S J, Kates R E, Lebsack C S, Harrison D C, Winkle R A. Clinical pharmacology of propafenone. Circulation 1983; 68:589–96.

33. Siddoway L A, Thompson K A, McAllister C B, Wang T, Wilkinson G R, Roden D M, Woosley R L. Polymorphism of propafenone metabolism and disposition in man: clinical and pharmacokinetic consequences. Circulation 1987; 75:785–91.

34. Harron D W G, Brogden R N. Propafenone: a review of its pharmacodynamic and pharmacokinetic properties, and therapeutic use in the treatment of arrhythmias. Drugs 1987; 34:617–47.

35. Lee J T, Yee Y G, Dorian P, Kates R E. Influence of hepatic dyfunction on the pharmacokinetics of propafenone. J Clin Pharmacol 1987; 27:384–9.

36. Connolly S, Lebsack C, Winkle R A, Harrison D C, Kates RE. Propafenone disposition kinetics in cardiac arrhythmia. II. Pharmacokinetics, pharmacodynamics, drug interaction. Clin Pharmacol Ther 1984; 36:163–8.II.

37. Hollman M, Brode E, Hotz D, Kaumier S, Kehrhahn O H. Investigation on the pharmacokinetics of propafenone in man. Arzneimittelforsch 1983; 33:763–70.

38. Latini R, Marchi S, Riva E, Cavalli A, Cazzaniga M G, Maggioni A P, Volpi A. Distribution of propafenone and its active metabolite, 5-hydroxypropafenone, in human tissues. Am Heart J 1987; 113:843–4.

39. Gillis A M, Kates R E. Myocardial uptake kinetics and pharmacodynamics of propafenone in the isolated perfused rabbit heart. J Pharmacol Exp Ther 1986; 237:708–12.

40. Mason W D, Lanman R C, Kirsten E B. Plasma and saliva propafenone concentration at steady state. J Pharm Sci 1987; 76:437–40.

41. Kates R E, Yee Y G, Winkle R A. Metabolite cumulation during chronic propafenone dosing in arrhythmia. Clin Pharmacol Ther 1985; 37:610–4.

42. Philipsborn G V, Gries J, Hofman H P, Kreiskott H, Kretzschmar R, Muller C D, Raschack M, Teschendorf H J. Pharmacological studies on propafenone and its metabolite 5-hydroxypropafenone. Arzneimittelforsch 1984; 34:1489–97.

43. Hege H G, Hollman M, Kavmeier S, Lietz H. The metabolic fate of ^{3}H-labelled propafenone in man. Eur J Drug Metab Pharmacokinet 1984; 9:41–55.

44. Giani P, Landolina M, Giudici V, Bianchini C, Ferrario G, Marchi S, Riva E, Latini R. Pharmacokinetics and pharmacodynamics of propafenone during acute and chronic administration. Eur J Clin Pharmacol 1988; 34: 187–94.

45. Keller K, Meyer-Estorf G, Beck O A, Hochrein H. Correlation between serum concentration and pharmacological effect on atrioventricular conduction time of the antiarrhythmic drug propafenone. Eur J Clin Pharmacol 1978; 13:17–20.

46. Connolly S J, Mulji A S, Hoffert D L, Davis C, Shragge W. Randomized placebo-controlled trial of propafenone for treatment of atrial tachyarrhythmias after cardiac surgery. J Am Coll Cardiol 1987; 10:1145–8.

47. Coumel P, Leclercq J F, Assayag P. European experience with the antiarrhythmic efficacy of propafenone for supraventricular and ventricular arrhythmias. Am J Cardiol 1984; 54:60D–66D.

48. Bounhoure J P, Sabot G, Cassagneau B, Calazel J, Dechandol AM. Etude de la propafenone oral dans les arythmies auriculaires rebelles. Ann Cardiol Angiol (Paris) 1985; 34:485–8.

49. Garcia-Civera R, Sanjuan R, Morell S, Ferrero J A, Miralles L, LLavador J, Lopez-Merino V. Effects of propafenone on induction and maintenance of atrioventricular nodal reentrant tachycardia. Pace 1984; 7:649–55.

50. Hamill S C, McLaran C J, Wood D L, Osborn M J, Gersh B J, Holmes D R Jr. Double-blind study of intravenous propafenone for paroxysmal supraventricular reentrant tachycardia. J Am Coll Cardiol 1987; 9:1364–8.

51. Ludmer P L, McGowan N E, Antman E M, Friedman P L. Efficacy of propafenone in Wolff-Parkinson-White syndrome: electrophysiologic findings and long-term follow-up. J Am Coll Cardiol 1987; 9:1357–63.

52. Salerno D M, Granrud G, Sharkey P, Asinger R, Hodges M. A controlled trial of propafenone for treatment of frequent and repetitive ventricular premature complexes. Am J Cardiol 1984; 53:77–83.

53. Heger J J, Hubbard J, Zipes D P, Miles W M, Prystowsky E N. Propafenone treatment of recurrent ventricular tachycardia: comparison of

continuous electrocardiographic recording and electrophysiologic study in predicting drug efficacy. Am J Cardiol 1984; 54:40D–44D.

54. Naccarella F, Bracchetti D, Palmieri M, Marchesini B, Ambrosioni E. Propafenone for refractory ventricular arrhythmias: correlation with drug plasma levels during long-term treatment. Am J Cardiol 1984; 54:1008–14.

55. de Soyza N, Terry L, Murphy L M, Thompson M L, Thompson C H, Doherty J E, Sakhaii M, Dinh H. Effect of propafenone in patients with stable ventricular arrhythmias. Am Heart J 1984; 108:285–9.

56. Podrid P J, Lown B. Propafenone: a new agent for ventricular arrhythmia. J Am Coll Cardiol 1984; 4:117–25.

57. Hodges M, Salerno D, Granrud G. Double-blind placebo-controlled evaluation of propafenone in suppressing ventricular ectopic activity. Am J Cardiol 1984; 54:45D–50D.

58. Hammill S C, Sorenson P B, Wood D L, Sugrue D D, Osborn M J, Gersh B J, Holmes D R. Propafenone for the treatment of refractory complex ventricular ectopic activity. Mayo Clin Proc 1986; 61:98–103.

59. Gaita F, Richiardi E, Bocchiardo M, Asteggiano R, Pinnavaia A, Di Leo M, Rosettani E, Brusca A. Short- and long-term effects of propafenone in ventricular arrhythmias. Int J Cardiol 1986; 13:163–70.

60. Dinh H A, Murphy M L, Baker B J, deSoyza N, Franciosa J A. Efficacy of propafenone compared with quinidine in chronic ventricular arrhythmias. Am J Cardiol 1985: 55: 1520–4.

61. Naccarella F, Bracchetti D, Palmieri M, Cantelli I, Bertaccini P, Ambrosioni E. Comparison of propafenone and disopyramide for treatment of chronic ventricular arrhythmias: placebo-controlled, double-blind, randomized crossover study. Am Heart J 1985; 109:833–40.

62. Klein R C, Huang S K, Marcus F I, Horwitz L, Fenster P E, Rushfort N, Kirsten E B. Enhanced antiarrhythmic efficacy of propafenone when used in combination with procainamide or quinidine. Am Heart J 1987; 114:551–8.

63. Zilcher H, Glogar D, Kaindl. Torsades de pointes: occurrence in myocardial ischaemia as a separate entity. Multiform ventricular tachycardia or not? Eur Heart J 1980; 1:63–9.

64. Doherty J U, Waxman H L, Kienzle M G, Cassidy D M, Marchlinski F E, Buxton A E, Josephson M E. Limited role of intravenous propafenone hydrochloride in the treatment of sustained ventricular tachycardia: electrophysiologic effects and results of programmed ventricular stimulation. J Am Coll Cardiol 1984; 4:378–81.

65. Cokkinos D V, Perrakis C, Argyrakis S, Hatzisavvas J, Papantonakos A. The efficacy of propafenone on exercise-induced ventricular arrhythmias. Eur Heart J 1987; 8(Suppl.):95–8.

66. Hill M R, Gotz V P, Harman E, McLeod I, Hendeles L. Evaluation of the asthmogenicity of propafenone, a new antiarrhythmic drug. Chest 1986; 90:698–702.

67. Kates R E, Yee Y G, Kirsten B. Interaction between warfarin and propafenone in healthy volunteer subjects. Clin Pharmacol Ther 1987; 42:305–11.

68. Steinbach K, Frohner K, Meisl F, Unger G. Interaction between propafenone and other drugs. In: Schlepper M, Olsson B, eds. Cardiac arrhythmias: diagnosis, prognosis, and therapy. Berlin: Springer-Verlag 1983:41–147.

69. Marcus F I. Drug interactions with amiodarone. Am Heart J 1983; 106:924–30.

70. Pritchett E L C, Smith W M, Kirsten E B. Pharmacokinetic and pharmacodynamic interaction of propafenone and cimetidine. J Clin Pharmacol 1988; 28:619–24.

29

Cibenzoline

Dennis S. Miura

Albert Einstein College of Medicine
Bronx, New York

Kenneth H. Dangman

College of Physicians and Surgeons, Columbia University
New York, New York

INTRODUCTION

Cibenzoline succinate [4,5-dihydro-2-(2,2-diphenyl-cyclo-propyl)imidazole butanedioate (1:1) salt] is a new and novel antiarrhythmic agent not chemically related to other known antiarrhythmic agents. Cibenzoline is the first imidazoline derivative reported to have antiarrhythmic activity. Other designations reported for cibenzoline in the literature include Cipralan, Ritmalan, Pracizoline, UP 339.01, and RO 22-796/001. The molecular mass of cibenzoline succinate is 380 daltons. Cibenzoline has been shown to have clinical efficacy in the suppression of ventricular arrhythmias, and it has been noted to have few adverse reactions when given orally. The reported antiarrhythmic mechanism of action is based on laboratory studies in isolated preparations. It appears to prolong the effective refractory period, decrease the rate of rise of the action potential, prolong repolarization, and block the slow inward calcium channel (1–7). These findings have led Vaughan Williams to propose that the drug fits into three of his four categories of antiarrhythmic agents (4,5).

CARDIAC ELECTROPHYSIOLOGY

Cellular Mechanisms

The cardiac electrophysiologic effects of dibenzoline have been described from studies on isolated tissues and whole-animal preparations. The effects of cibenzoline were demonstrated by Millar and Vaughan Williams (4,5) on isolated rabbit sinoatrial node. Cibenzoline slows the isolated tissue sinus node rate in concentrations of 1.3–4.5 μM. This effect did not appear to depend on decreasing the slope of phase 4 depolarization or on a β-receptor blockade. Rather, it appeared to be caused by a dose-dependent increase in the duration of the repolarization phase of the transmembrane action potential. The remainder of the bradycardic effect of cibenzoline appears to be due to the small reduction in the maximum rate and peak amplitude of phase 0 depolarization. Ohta et al. (6) showed that cibenzoline (1.3–39 μM) prolonged action potential duration in the rabbit sinus node pacemaker cells. They similarly found that the drug had no effect on sinus node automaticity. In the Langendorff isolated perfused rabbit heart, 5–40

Table 1 Electrophysiologic Effects of
Cibenzoline[a]

Sinus cycle length	−
AH conduction time	+
HV conduction time	+
Ventricular fibrillation threshold	+
Action potential	

Ventricular muscle	Purkinje fiber
Phase 0 −	Phase 0 —
Phase 1 0	Phase 1 0
Phase 2 +	Phase 2 ±
Phase 3 +	Phase 3 ±
Phase 4 −	Phase 4 —

[a]Decreases (-), increases (+), no effect (0).

μg cibenzoline did not significantly slow heart rate (7); it was also reported that cibenzoline had negligible effects on the sinus rate in anesthetized dogs (8).

Several studies of the electrophysiologic effects of cibenzoline in animal hearts also suggest that the drug may slow atrioventricular conduction. Millar and Vaughan Williams (4,5) reported that 3.1–5.3 μM cibenzoline slowed AH conduction times in the isolated rabbit septum preparation. Verdouw et al. (9), using a pig model, found at 2–5 min after intravenous administration of 0.5–2 mg/kg of cibenzoline the PQ interval increased by 20–35% with only a slight increase in the ST interval. Keren et al. (10,11) found similar effects in the digitalized dog. Cibenzoline at 2.6 ± 0.8 mg/kg increased PR interval by 17 ± 9%. Sassine et al. (8) reported that cibenzoline, either IV (4 mg/kg) or PO (7 or 14 mg/kg/day for 8–16 days), had little or no effect on AH conduction time in the in situ canine heart (see Table 1).

The effects of cibenzoline on the transmembrane action potentials recorded from isolated ventricular tissues from several species have been reported. Cibenzoline 1–40 μM) decreased the maximum rate of depolarization during phase 0 of action potentials recorded from Purkinje fibers and ventricular muscle cells from rabbit (4,5) and dog (1,3,6). The effects of cibenzoline on phase 0 depolarization on rabbit Purkinje fibers appeared to be more prominent than in ventricular muscle fibers (4). Cibenzoline at 1.3 μM decreased the

maximum rate of depolarization of rabbit His bundle fibers by 29%, Purkinje fibers by 31%, and ventricular right papillary muscle by 10%. Dangman (1) observed similar results in canine tissues. Cibenzoline at 3.8 μM caused a decrease in the maximum rate of depolarization of canine Purkinje fibers by 17% and that of ventricular muscle by 12%.

Studies of the effects of cibenzoline on pacemaker activity in cardiac Purkinje fibers have been reported (1,3,6). The effects of cibenzoline on Purkinje fiber pacemaker activity were complex. They appeared to depend on the resting transmembrane potential of the tissues and on the presence or absence of catecholamines. Dangman (1) showed that cibenzoline does not appear to affect automaticity of normal Purkinje fibers caused by superfusion of low-potassium Tyrode's solution. In contrast, cibenzoline has been shown to decrease automaticity of normal Purkinje fibers chronically exposed to 5×10^{-7} M isoproterenol. Cibenzoline did not reduce the increase in spontaneous rate that occurs during acute exposure to isoproterenol. The mean rate increased 14 beats/min in normal fibers after 10–15 min exposure to isoproterenol. After equilibration with cibenzoline the rate increased after a second exposure to isoproterenol to 17 beats/min. The threshold dose of isoproterenol that caused an increase in automaticity was not significantly changed by pretreatment with cibenzoline. This would not have occurred if cibenzoline were a specific β-receptor blocking agent.

The effects of cibenzoline on abnormal automaticity in infarct zone Purkinje fibers obtained 24 hr after a Harris dog preparation (12) have been reported (1). Cibenzoline decreased this automaticity in these fibers in a dose-dependent manner (1). Studies by Millar and Vaughan Williams (4,5) in rabbit pacemaker fibers exhibiting automaticity similar to that of the infarct zone tissues showed that cibenzoline slowed automatic rate by prolongation of the action potential duration and suppression of the upstroke velocity of phase 0. Phase 4 depolarization was not suppressed. These results suggested that the mechanisms for suppression of automaticity by cibenzoline in the sinus node versus partially depolarized Purkinje fibers may be different (1–3).

Antiarrhythmic Effects in Animal Studies

The antiarrhythmic effects of cibenzoline have been studied on multiform ventricular ectopic activity that occurs in Harris dog heart preparations 24 and 48 hr after ligation of the left anterior descending coronary artery (1,12,13). At 24 hr after ligation, 5 mg/kg IV of cibenzoline was shown to significantly increase the percentage of normal sinus beats after drug treatment from 5% during the control period to 81%. These antiarrhythmic effects lasted 20–60 min (1). The sinus cycle length decreased during drug treatment, which was presumably a result of reflex changes (sympathetic stimulation or parasympathetic withdrawal) produced by drug effects on systemic vascular resistance or cardiac contractility.

In dogs with infarctions after 48 hr, 20 mg/kg PO of cibenzoline reduced the number of ventricular premature depolarizations from 80% of the total beats to 20% of the total number of heart beats (1). This decrease in ventricular extrasystoles was sustained for about 3 hr. The overall heart rate declined from approximately 145 beats/min during the control period to about 130 beats/min 2–4 hr after drug administration (1). It was thought that the arrhythmias that occurred 1–2 days after coronary ligation in the infarcted dog heart were caused by enhanced pacemaker activity in partially depolarized subendocardial Purkinje fibers in the infarcted area (12–15). Plasma catecholamine levels are elevated during this period and may contribute to the increase in observed ventricular ectopic activity (12–15). Cibenzoline is thought to abolish these arrhythmias by slowing abnormal automaticity in the partially depolarized Purkinje fibers or by slowing catecholamine-enhanced automaticity in Purkinje fibers.

Cibenzoline has been studied on the ventricular fibrillation threshold in the isolated Langendorff rabbit heart preparation and the in situ infarcted dog heart (1,2,7). It was shown that cibenzoline at 5, 10, 20, and 40 μg

Table 2 Pharmacokinetics of Cibenzoline

Usual dose	PO 130–320 mg/day in divided doses IV 1.0–1.5 mg/kg
Half-life ($t_{1/2}$)	7–8 hr
Absorption	Complete
Elimination	Renal excretion, hepatic metabolism
Metabolites	Inactive

in the Langendorff heart increased ventricular fibrillation threshold by 22, 72, 105, and 150%, respectively. In the infarcted canine heart it was reported that cibenzoline, 5 mg/kg IV followed by 1 mg/kg/hr, decreased induction of ventricular fibrillation by programmed electrical stimulation (2,7,16).

CLINICAL PHARMACOKINETICS

Cibenzoline has been studied in clinical trials to determine its efficacy in suppressing ventricular arrhythmias. Its usual dose orally is 130–325 mg/day in divided doses. The intravenous loading dose is 1.0–1.5 mg/kg. The drug is rapidly and completely absorbed when given orally (Table 2).

The elimination half-life appears to be 7–8 hr; however, this appears to be dependent on the age and general physical status of the patient. Reported elimination times of cibenzoline vary from those reported by Canal et al. (17), approximately 4 hr in normal healthy volunteers, to those reported by Khoo et al. (18), who also reported in normal volunteers kinetic data of 7.3–8.7 hr, which appeared to be independent of dose. Cibenzoline blood levels and kinetic data were reported by Miura et al. (19) for eight patients with ventricular arrhythmias. The half-life was 7.4 hr with a single-phase elimination coefficient of 0.094. The discrepancies between the studies by Canal et al. (17) and Miura et al. (19) may be due to the differences in the patient populations. The healthy volunteers had a mean age of 25.6 years compared to 61.6 years for cardiac patients. Brazell et al. (20,21) supported these observations with reported oral cibenzoline elimination kinetics from 5.9 to 13 hr, which depended upon the age of the patients

Table 3 Electrocardiographic Effects of
Cibenzoline[a]

PR interval	+
QRS duration	++
QTc duration	+
RR interval	±

[a]Decreases (−); increases (+).

and their renal function. The mean was 7 hr, which appeared to increase with patient age.

The metabolic fate of cibenzoline is not entirely known. Loh et al. (22) incubated cibenzoline with rat liver microsomes, which produced a metabolite that was identified as 2-(2,2-diphenylcyclopropyl)-1H-imidazole. This metabolite has been given to Harris preparation dogs with no apparent effect on ventricular ectopy suppression at the same dose as cibenzoline. The metabolite given at four times the cibenzoline effective dose in these animals showed a significant widening of the QRS complex (16). No other metabolites are known at this time.

CLINICAL STUDIES

Effects on the Electrocardiogram

Clinical studies on the electrocardiographic effects of cibenzoline indicate that the drug generally slows conduction velocity within the heart. These effects are predicted from cellular and animal electrophysiologic studies. The effects of cibenzoline on the surface electrocardiogram are therefore predictable (Table 3). Miura et al. (19,23) noted that PR interval increased by an average of 9–10% after acute administration of cibenzoline (1.1–1.2 mg/kg IV). During chronic oral therapy with cibenzoline (260–700 mg/day PO), it was reported that the PR interval increased by about 15% (4,7,9,10,24–26). Invasive studies have shown that electrocardiographically cibenzoline generally slows AV conduction times (19,23,27, 28). Kostis et al. (29,30) reported that the extent of increased PR interval was directly proportional to the plasma concentration of cibenzoline. In addition, the HV interval duration has been reported to increase after acute (15) or chronic oral therapy (26–28) with

cibenzoline. One exception to the general finding of increases in PR interval following clinical cibenzoline treatment was reported by Thizy et al. (31). They noted that during infusion at a rate of 1 mg/kg/min cibenzoline "exerted variable and statistically insignificant effects on the AV conduction time" and the effective refractory period of the AV node.

The QRS duration was repeatedly observed to increase after cibenzoline administration. These increases were observed after either acute intravenous (9,23,32) or chronic oral therapy (27,28,33,34). In most of these studies the increases in QRS duration have been from 14 to 17% over control. Chronic oral cibenzoline therapy has been reported to exert little or no effect on QT interval (25–29,33,34). Other studies, however, have indicated that QT interval increased following acute (18,23,32,36) or chronic (27,30,34) loading therapy with the drug.

In investigational clinical trials it has been reported that chronic oral cibenzoline therapy (325 mg/day) either shortened spontaneous sinus cycle length (28) or did not affect it significantly (35). During studies using acute intravenous administration of the drug, it was found that 1.2 mg/kg IV of cibenzoline did not alter heart rate significantly (19,23) but that cibenzoline infusions at a rate of 1 mg/kg/min "significantly shortened spontaneous [sinus] cycle length" (31). These changes may have been caused by the effects of the drug on cardiac contractility to produce reflex increases in sympathetic tone (9,36). Clinically it was reported that chronic cibenzoline therapy (130–325 mg/day) appeared to have no effect on atrial refractory periods (26,28,35).

Hemodynamic Effects

Clinical reports of the negative hemodynamic effects of cibenzoline follow the reports of the negative inotropic and chronotropic effects of cibenzoline in laboratory studies. A summary is provided in Table 4. Millar and Vaughan Williams (4,5) reported that cibenzoline exerted negative inotropic effects on rabbit myocardium. These observations were also noted by Verdouw et al. (9), who reported that

Table 4 Hemodynamic Effects of Cibenzoline[a]

Heart rate	−
Blood pressure	−
Cardiac index	−
Pulmonary wedge pressure	+
Systemic vascular resistance	+

[a]Decreases (−); increases (+).

cibenzoline at 0.5–2.0 mg/kg given intravenously to the anesthetized pig decreased stroke volume 20–35% in a dose-dependent manner. Verdouw concluded that this may be due to a decrease in cardiac contractility and an increase in systemic vascular resistance. Keren et al. (11) showed that at a total dose of 3.75 mg/kg cibenzoline was an effective antiarrhythmic agent against programmed electrical stimulation induction of ventricular tachycardia in the digitalized dog. At higher doses of cibenzoline of 7.0 mg/kg there was a decrease in contractile force of approximately 15% but mean blood pressure, heart rate, total vascular resistance, and systolic ejection fraction changed by less than 8%.

Clinical hemodynamic effects of cibenzoline were reported in 14 patients with coronary artery disease during routine cardiac catheterization by van den Brand (36). There were significant decreases in left ventricular contraction after infusion of the drug, with a maximal effect 2–5 min after infusion. An increase in heart rate, decrease in left ventricular systolic pressure, decrease in cardiac index, and increase in systemic vascular resistance were noted. The left ventricular end-diastolic pressure was not significantly altered.

Humen et al. (37) reported that patients given cibenzoline, 1.0 or 1.2 mg/kg, had a significant decrease in left ventricular ejection fraction that was sustained for 2 hr. This was associated with a decrease in cardiac output and stroke volume and an increase in pumonary capillary wedge pressure, left ventricular end-diastolic volume, end-systolic volume, heart rate, and systemic vascular resistance.

The effects of cibenzoline at 1.5 mg/kg given intravenously to 20 patient with coronary artery disease undergoing cardiac cathe-

terization were reported by Strom et al. (38). There was a decrease in left ventricular dP/dt, ejection fraction, and cardiac output. Cibenzoline in patients with coronary artery disease acutely increased systemic vascular resistance and had a significant negative inotropic effect. The authors therefore suggest, in view of these effects, that cibenzoline should be used with caution in patients with left ventricular dys function.

Acute Antiarrhythmic Drug Testing

Invasive electrophysiologic methods have been used to evaluate the clinical efficacy of cibenzoline and to determine its effects on the cardiac conduction system. These programmed electrical stimulation techniques have been used by a number of investigators as a rapid method to assess the efficacy of antiarrhythmic drug therapy in patients with serious ventricular tachyarrhythmias. Acute loading of intravenous cibenzoline in 33 patients with symptomatic ventricular tachycardia was reported by Miura et al. (19,23). Programmed electrical stimulation methods were used to provoke sustained ventricular tachycardia in 17 patients (54%) off all antiarrhythmic agents and nonsustained ventricular tachycardia in 14 (45%). The mean rate of ventricular tachycardia induced in this study was 261 ± 14 beats/min. In 16 patients cibenzoline (given 1.0–1.5 mg/kg IV) provided protection against induction of ventricular tachycardia. In the other 17 patients tachycardia could be induced despite higher doses of cibenzoline. Cibenzoline did not change mean heart rate; the mean PR interval increased from 169 ± 9 to 191 ± 12 msec (NS); QRS duration significantly widened from 88 ± 5 to 112 ± 5 msec; and no significant change was noted in duration of QT interval, although the mean QTc was prolonged by 7%. Effective ventricular refractory period was markedly prolonged by cibenzoline administration. The mean blood pressure decreased from 105 ± 7 to 96 ± 8 mmHg. The rate of the tachycardia induced was significantly reduced to 200 ± 16 beats/min. Miura et al. (19), following programmed electrical stimulation studies and serial drug testing,

Table 5 Cibenzoline Adverse Effects

Gastrointestinal	Vomiting, diarrhea, constipation
CNS	Visual disturbances, headaches, tremors
Anticholinergic	Dry mouth, urinary retention
Liver enzymes	Asymptomatic elevation
Cardiac	Decreased cardiac output;
	decreased ejection fraction;
	increased pulmonary capillary wedge pressure;
	increased systemic vascular resistance

discharged the patients on an antiarrhythmic agent that provided protection at acute drug testing. Cibenzoline was given to 13 patients with a mean follow-up of 8.8 months. Chronic oral cibenzoline therapy did not change electrocardiographic parameters. There was a reduction in mean premature ventricular contraction frequency on Holter monitor recordings from 666 to 190 beats/hr. Ventricular tachycardia events per Holter recording decreased from 6 to 0.6.

Browne et al. (28) reported the effects of cibenzoline in 26 patients who had symptomatic ventricular tachycardia. These patients were given oral cibenzoline from 65 mg every 8 hr (2 patients) to 81.25 mg (22 patients) or 97.5 mg (2 patients). Cibenzoline abolished the ventricular tachycardia in 8 of 16 patients; 7 of 22 patients had greater than 83% suppression of their ventricular complexes. Electrocardiographic changes noted included an increase in the PR interval by 14% and increase in QRS duration by 17%, and there was no change in the QT interval. Invasive electrophysiologic studies were performed in 10 patients during a control period and during a maximum cibenzoline dosage given orally. Cibenzoline did not significantly affect AH and HV conduction times; however, it did prolong the ventricular effective refractory period from 223 ± 16 to 241 ± 22 msec. Ventricular tachycardia was induced in 9 of 10 patients, and cibenzoline prevented induction of ventricular tachycardia in 2 patients. The other 7 patients had their tachycardia cycle length increased from 210 to 260 msec. Of these patients 6 were discharged on oral drug; 1 patient died of a myocardial infarction during follow-up; 2 patients discontinued the drug because of recurrence of their symptomatic ven-

tricular tachycardia; and 3 patients continued oral cibenzoline for 10 ± 4 months with arrhythmia control.

Saksena et al. (27) reported 16 patients with refractory ventricular tachycardia. They loaded cibenzoline orally (130, 160, and 190 mg every 12 hr for 3.5–20 days (mean 10.7 days). Cibenzoline prolonged the PR interval, QRS duration, and QTc interval. Programmed electrical stimulation induced sustained ventricular tachycardia in 15 patients during the control study. After cibenzoline, 11 patients were not inducible or an increase in the induced tachycardia cycle length was found.

Chronic Oral Therapy

Long-term follow-up of patients with a history of ventricular tachyarrhythmias who are treated with antiarrhythmic agents guided by electrophysiologic studies appear to have a good prognosis. See Table 6 for a summary of the clinical results reported on chronic oral therapy with cibenzoline. The oral dose of cibenzoline ranged from 130 to 700 mg/day with an efficacy against ventricular premature contractions ranging from 18 to 90%. Holter monitor recordings identified those patients who have either failed their drug therapy or possibly had an increase in ventricular ectopy due to a further deterioration in their underlying disease. Reported electrocardiographic changes did not appear to be a limitation to chronic oral antiarrhythmic therapy. The side effects reported by the investigators limited oral therapy with cibenzoline.

ADVERSE REACTIONS

Most reports have concluded that cibenzoline in clinically effective antiarrhythmic doses has

Table 6 Efficacy of Cibenzoline During Chronic Oral Therapy

Author	Patients	Dose (mg/day)	Effects	Side effect
Baligadoo and Chiche (24)	55	260	a	—
Browne et al (28)	26	81.25 mg every 6 hr	7/26 83% VPC	b
Brazzell et al. (20)	25	325 max	90% VPC	None
Cocco et al. (25)	28	700 max	5/28 eff.	c
Heger et al. (39)	19	65–97.5 mg every 6 hr	5/16 80% VPC	—
Herpin et al. (40)	9	260 twice a day	6/9 90% VPC	None
Klein et al. (33)	20	130 to 125 four times a day	14/19 80% VPC	d
Kostis et al. (30)	20	130–160 twice a day	12/20 79% VPC	e
Kushner et al. (26)	5	—	3/5 85% VPC	f
Magiros et al. (35)	5	130–325	—	g
Miura et al. (19)	33	130–325	16/33 no VT	h
Mohiuddin et al. (41)	20	130 twice a day	16/20 75% VPC	i
Saksena et al. (27)	16	130–190 mg twice a day	11/15 no VT	—
Sander and Giles (34)	13	130–320	8/13 75% VPC	None
Tepper et al. (42)	11	32.5–81.25 every 6 hr	75% VPC	None
Thebaut et al. (43)	8	1 mg/kg IV	5/8 blocked WPW	Pathway
Wasty et al. (44)	13	130–160 twice a day	6/13 75% VPC	—

a Significant VPC reduction.
b Breakthrough VPCs.
c Two patients gastrointestinal, two headaches, two visual, one anticholinergic.
d One patient diarrhea, two elevated transaminases, two tremors.
e Four patients gastrointestinal, one hypotension.
f Two patients gastrointestinal with vomiting and widened QRS.
g Two patients gastrointestinal vomiting.
h One patient blurred vision, two increase in CHF.
i Six patients with dry mouth.

minor side effects that may limit its use (Table 5). The majority of patients who were treated with oral cibenzoline appeared to tolerate the drug as noted in Table 6. Only one report by Cocco et al. (25) found cibenzoline to have low efficacy (18% of patients) and to produce a high incidence of side effects (21% of patients).

Other reported side effects of cibenzoline include a variety of gastrointestinal symptoms (vomiting, diarrhea, and constipation), central nervous system effects (visual disturbances, headache, and tremors), anticholinergic side effects (xerostomia and urinary retention), and asymptomatic elevation of liver transaminase enzymes.

for ventricular arrhythmias. The doses that appear effective are 1.0–1.5 mg/kg IV or from 32.5 to 97.5 mg PO every 6 hr. The oral doses, however, have been divided to twice to three times a day with good effects because of the extended half-life of the agent. Electrocardiographic effects of the agent are well documented, with dose-dependent increases in PR and QRS durations. Those patients with depressed cardiac function and renal insufficiency must be carefully monitored because of the negative inotropic effects and extended clearance of the drug. The majority of patients, however, appear to tolerate oral cibenzoline well with minimal long-term side effects.

SUMMARY

Oral cibenzoline therapy appears to be well tolerated by the majority of patients treated

ACKNOWLEDGMENTS

Supported in part by NIH Grant HL 24354 and a grant from Hoffman-LaRoche, Inc.

REFERENCES

1. Dangman K H. Cardiac effects of cibenzoline. J Cardiovasc Pharmacol 1984;6:300–11.
2. Dangman, K H, Miura D S. Cibenzoline. In: Scriabine A, ed. New drugs annual, Vol. 3. New York: Raven Press, 1985.
3. Ikeda N, Singh B N. Electrophysiologic profile of a new antiarrhythmic drug, cibenzoline, in isolated cardiac tissues. Fed Proc 1983; 42:635.
4. Millar J S, Vaughan Williams E M. Effects on rabbit nodal, atrial, ventricular and Purkinje cell potentials of a new antiarrhythmic drug, cibenzoline, which protects against action potential shortening in hypoxia. Br J Pharmacol 1982; 75:469–78.
5. Millar J S, Vaughan Williams E M. Pharmacological mapping of regional effects in the rabbit heart of some new antiarrhythmic drugs. Br J Pharmacol 1983; 79:701–9.
6. Ohta M, Sugi K, McCullen A, Mandel W J, Peter T, Karaguezian H S. Electrophysiologic effects of cibenzoline, a new antiarrhythmic drug, on isolated cardiac tissue. Circulation 1983; 68(Suppl. III):220.
7. Doorley B M, Hutcheon D E, Dapson S C. The antifibrillatory effects of cibenzoline on Langendorff-perfused rabbit hearts. Fed Proc 1984; 43:961.
8. Sassine A, Masse C, Dufour A, Hirsch J L, Cazes M, Puech P. Cardiac electrophysiological effects of cibenzoline by acute and chronic administration in the anesthetized dog. Arch Int Pharmacodyn 1984; 269:201–18.
9. Verdouw P D, Hartog J M, Scheffer M G, van Bremen R H, Dufour A. The effects of cibenzoline, an imidazoline derivative with antiarrhythmic properties, on systemic hemodynamics and regional myocardial performance. Drug Dev Res 1982; 2:519–32.
10. Keren G, Aogaichi K, Somberg J C, Miura D S. Effects of cibenzoline on ventricular tachycardia induced by programmed electrical stimulation in the dog. Clin Res 1982; 30:633A.
11. Keren G, Tepper D, Butler B, et al. The efficacy of cibenzoline in preventing PES induction of ventricular tachycardia in the dog. J Clin Pharmacol 1984; 24:466–72.
12. Desoutter P, DuFour A, Aymard M F, Haiat R. Etude pharmacocinetique d'un nouvel antiarythmique la cibenzoine a la phase aique d'un infarctus myocardique. Correlations theraputiques. Therapie 1983; 36:237–45.
13. Wit A L, Bigger J T. Possible electrophysiological mechanisms for lethal arrhythmias accompanying myocardial ischemia and infarction. Circulation 1975; 51–52(Suppl.III): 96–115.
14. Richardson J A. Circulating levels of catecholamines in acute myocardial infarction and angina pectoris. Prog Cardiovasc Dis 1963; 6:56–62.
15. Cameron J S, Dersham G H, Han J. Effects of epinephrine on the electrophysiologic properties of Purkinje fibers surviving myocardial infarction. Am Heart J 1982; 104:551–60.
16. Leinweber F J, Loh A C, Szuna A J, et al. Biotransformation of cibenzoline to 2-(2,2-diphenylcyclopropyl)-1H-imidazole. Xenobiotica 1983; 13:287–94.
17. Canal M, Flouvat B, Tremblay D, Dufour A. Pharmacokinetics in man of a new antiarrhythmic drug, cibenzoline. Eur J Clin Pharmacol 1983; 24:509–19.
18. Khoo K C, Szuna A J, Colburn W A, et al. Single dose pharmacokinetics and dose proportionality of oral cibenzoline. J Clin Pharmacol 1984; 24:283–8.
19. Miura D S, Keren G, Torres V, et al. Antiarrhythmic effects of cibenzoline. Am Heart J 1985; 109:827–33.
20. Brazzell R K, Aogaichi K, Heger J J, et al. Cibenzoline plasma concentration and antiarrhythmic effect. Clin Pharmacol Ther 1984; 35:307–16.
21. Brazzell R K, Rees M M C, Khoo K C, et al. Age and cibenzoline disposition. Clin Pharmacol Ther 1984; 36:613–9.
22. Loh A C, Szuna A J, Carbone J J, et al. Identification and pharmacologic activity of a cibenzoline metabolite. Fed Proc Fed Am Soc Exp Biol 1983; 12:912.
23. Miura DS, Torres V, Butler B, et al. Effects of cibenzoline in patients with ventricular tachycardia. J Clin Pharmacol 1984; 24:413.
24. Baligadoo S, Chiche P. Beneficial effects of U.S. 339.01, a new anti-arrhythmic agent, against ventricular premature beats. Circulation 1978; 58(Suppl. II):179.
25. Cocco G, Strozzi C, Pansini R, et al. Antiarrhythmic use of cibenzoline, a new class 1 antiarrhythmic agent with class 3 and 4 properties, in patients with recurrent ventricular tachycardia. Eur Heart J 1984; 5:108–14.
26. Kushner M, Magiros E, Peters R, et al. The electrophysiologic effects of oral cibenzoline. J Electrocardiol 1984; 17:15–24.

27. Saksena S, Rothbart S, Shah Y, Liptak K. Chronic effects of oral cibenzoline in refractory ventricular tachycardia. Clin Pharmacol Ther 1984; 35:271.

28. Browne K F, Prystowsky E N, Zipes D P, Chilson D A, Heger J J. Clinical efficacy and electrophysiological effects of cibenzoline therapy in patients with ventricular arrhythmias. J Am Coll Cardiol 1984; 3:857–64.

29. Kostis J D, Krieger S, Cosgrove N, et al. Cibenzoline in ventricular ectopic activity. Circulation 1983; 68(Suppl.III):274.

30. Kostis J B, Krieger S, Moreyra A, Cosgrove N. Cibenzoline for treatment of ventricular arrhythmias: a double blind placebo controlled study. J Am Coll Cardiol 1984; 4:372–7.

31. Thizy J F, Jandot V, Andre-Fouet X, et al. Etude electrophysiologique de l' UP 339–01 chez l'homme. Lyon Med 1981; 245:119–22.

32. Miura D S, Keren G, Siegel L, et al. Effect of cibenzoline in suppressing ventricular tachycardia induced by programmed stimulation. J Am Coll Cardiol 1983; 1:699.

33. Klein R C, House M, Rushforth N. Efficacy and safety of oral cibenzoline in treatment of ventricular ectopy. Clin Res 1984; 32:9A.

34. Sander G E, Giles T T. The clinical efficacy of oral cibenzoline in the suppression of ventricular ectopy. Clin Res 1983; 31:829A.

35. Magiros E, Kushner M, Peters R, et al. Electrophysiology of oral cibenzoline. Clin Res 1982; 30:674A.

36. Van den Brand M, Serruys P, de Roon Y, et al. Haemodynamic effects of intravenous cibenzoline in patients with coronary heart disease. Eur J Clin Pharmacol 1984; 26:297–302.

37. Humen D P, Lesoway R, Kostuk W J. Cibenzoline: a new antiarrhythmic: hemodynamic effects. Clin Pharmacol Ther 1984; 35:248.

38. Strom J A, Miura D S, Jordan A, Loor S. Effects of cibenzoline on left ventricular performance in patients with coronary artery disease. J Am Coll Cardiol 1985; 5:451.

39. Heger J J, Prystowsky E N, Browne K F, et al. Cibenzoline treatment of patients with chronic ventricular arrhythmias. Clin Res 1982; 30:709A.

40. Herpin D, Gaudeau B, Boutaud P, Amiel A, Tourdias B, Demange J. Clinical trial of a new anti-arrhythmic drug: cibenzoline (cipralan). Curr Ther Res Clin Exp 1981; 30:741.

41. Mohiuddin S M, Hilleman D E, Butler M L, Stengel L A. Efficacy, side effects and plasma concentrations of cibenzoline in patients with ventricular arrhythmias. Drug Intell Clin Pharm 1984; 18:499.

42. Tepper D, Butler B, Keren G, et al. Effects of oral cibenzoline therapy on ventricular ectopic activity. Clin Res 1983; 31:634A.

43. Thebaut J F, Achard F, de Langenhagen B. Etude electrophysiologique chez l'homme d'un nouvel antiarythmique, la cibenzoline, das le syndrome de Wolffe-Parkinson-White. Information Cardiol 1980; 4:393–402.

44. Wasty N, Saksena S, Cappello G, Barr M J. Comparative efficacy and safety of oral cibenzoline and quinidine in ventricular arrhythmias: a randomized cross-over study. Circulation 1984; 70(Suppl.II):442.

30

Amiodarone

Bertram G. Katzung and Michael A. Lee

University of California
San Francisco, California

Jonathan J. Langberg

University of Michigan Medical Center
Ann Arbor, Michigan

INTRODUCTION

Amiodarone, an unusual iodine-containing benzofuran derivative, was introduced into clinical trials in Europe in the 1960s as a potential antianginal agent. Because it was reported to have some antiarrhythmic actions (1), its electrophysiologic effects were studied by Singh and Vaughan Williams (2) in guinea pigs and in isolated rabbit myocardium. These authors found that acute administration of amiodarone protected guinea pigs against ouabain-induced arrhythmias and that pretreatment of rabbits for 6 weeks caused a considerable prolongation of action potential duration in both atrial and ventricular muscle. Subsequent studies by other authors have documented a significant effect on I_{Na}, action potential upstroke, and conduction velocity, as well as on adrenoceptors and calcium channels. Therefore, if the drug is to be classified in the Vaughan Williams system, it must be considered a multiclass agent.

In clinical studies amiodarone has been found to be extremely useful in the treatment of arrhythmias, completely eclipsing its use in angina. Its very significant toxicity prevents its use in patients who can be managed with any other drug, but it has become an essential drug of last resort for some refractory arrhythmias. A review of the amiodarone literature appeared in 1987 (3) and further reviews of the drug's basic and clinical pharmacology in 1988 (4) and 1989 (5).

BASIC PHARMACOLOGY

Amiodarone is a large molecule and, because of its iodine content, an unusually heavy one (molecular weight 646). The drug's pK_a is 8.7 at 37° C. It is extremely lipophilic, demonstrating partition coefficients from 16,500 (6) to 760,000 (7), depending on the circumstances of the determination. It partitions so completely into the lipids of the membrane that it probably exerts little action from the aqueous solution bathing the membrane. Chatelain et al. (8) showed that the drug significantly changes membrane fluidity at 10–20 μM. These effects are probably not relevant to changes in passive membrane electrophysiologic changes in vivo since aqueous concentrations probably never reach such high levels.

However, the very high lipid solubility and hydrophobicity result in two problems for experimental studies. First, in vitro studies of amiodarone are hampered by the drug's extremely low aqueous solubility. Most authors dissolved the drug in a mixture of albumin or serum and physiologic saline or in polysorbate and saline. Second, it is extremely difficult to relate the aqueous concentrations of drug used in studies in vitro to the "effective concentration," that is, the concentration of the drug at its receptors, especially since this concentration changes over time as the drug partitions into the membrane. Chatelain et al. (8) also found that amiodarone inhibits ATPase activity with a K_i of about 20 μM. However, it is not clear that ATPase inhibition is important at the concentrations of drug used in most electrophysiologic studies and in clinical applications.

Electrophysiologic Effects in Isolated Tissue

SA Node

Singh and Vaughan Williams (2) found that amiodarone given intravenously promptly reduced the rabbit sinoatrial (SA) rate from 265 to 223 per min at 50 mg/kg, less at lower doses. A similar depressant effect was found by Goupil and Lenfant (9) and by Gloor et al. (10). Using microelectrode techniques Goupil and Lenfant showed that the action potential duration was prolonged and the slope of diastolic depolarization was reduced in rabbit SA node. In a recent study Yabek et al. (11) found that both amiodarone and its monodesethyl metabolite reduced the rate of diastolic depolarization and slowed the spontaneous rate in SA nodal tissue treated with the drugs in vitro.

Atrial Muscle

Relatively few studies have been carried out using this tissue. In their original paper Singh and Vaughan Williams (2) reported that amiodarone had similar effects in rabbit atrial tissue and ventricular strips. Although measured resting potentials were surprisingly low in their control atrial preparations, they found no change in this variable when animals were treated with the drug for 1, 3, or 6 weeks before isolation of the tissue for study. However, they did find significant decreases from control in the mean rate of rise of the action potentials after 3 weeks or more of treatment and significant prolongation of the action potential. In a more recent study of tissue isolated after chronic treatment for 3 or 6 weeks (12) the drug was shown to progressively increase action potential duration in atrial tissue with increasing duration of treatment, with no change in the well-polarized resting potentials.

Purkinje Tissue

I_{Na}, $\dot{V}_{max}$, and Conduction.   Follmer et al. (13) studied the effects of amiodarone on I_{Na} in both Purkinje and ventricular myocytes. They found that 1.4 μM drug shifted the inactivation curve 16 mV in the hyperpolarizing direction and increased the slope factor (the reciprocal of the steepness, that is, voltage dependence, of the inactivation curve) from 6.6 to 9.3 mV. The drug also produced a "tonic" block (defined as block not removed by prepulses to -140 mV) of about 30% of the control I_{Na}. However, there was no change in the shape of the current-voltage curve and only a modest increase in the time constants of decay of the sodium current. Use-dependent block of sodium current was markedly dependent on clamp duration, with steady-state block achieved by the second pulse when 200 msec pulses were used but requiring four pulses of 20 msec duration and more than 10 pulses of 2 msec duration. The onset of block was biphasic, with 5.4 and 66 msec time constants at 7.3 μM amiodarone. Recovery from block was also biphasic, with 71 and 1430 msec time constants.

Varro et al. (14) found that in vitro exposure to 5 μM amiodarone reduced the $\dot{V}_{max}$ of canine Purkinje fibers, with a rapid onset of use-dependent block and a single exponential recovery with a time constant of 289 msec.

Nattel et al. (15) depolarized isolated canine false tendons with high-potassium solutions and found evidence for significant use-dependent block of isoproterenol-dependent action potentials, suggesting significant slow channel blockade.

Action Potential Duration. In contrast to amiodarone's effect on atrial and ventricular action potential duration, Yabek et al. (11) found that in vitro application of the parent drug or its desethyl metabolite significantly *reduced* the action potential duration of Purkinje fibers from adult dogs. The effect on neonatal Purkinje fibers, although in the same direction, was much smaller and did not reach significance. Varro et al. (14) also reported that acute in vitro administration of amiodarone shortened the action potential duration in dog Purkinje fibers but chronic pretreatment did not change this variable. Aomine (16) reported that in vitro addition of the drug did not increase action potential duration in canine Purkinje fibers from animals that had not been pretreated; concentrations of 4.4×10^{-5} to 4.4×10^{-4} M shortened the duration slightly over the 30 min duration of the experiment. The effect was not frequency dependent.

Ventricular Myocardium

I_{Na}, $\dot{V}_{max}$, *and Conduction.* When added in a soluble or protein-bound form, amiodarone significantly reduces $\dot{V}_{max}$ (11,17–20) and I_{Na} (13). This reduction is frequency (use) dependent. In experiments in which voltage clamp was used to vary the duration of depolarization the block was also dependent on the duration of depolarization, indicating that the drug probably has a high affinity for channels in the inactivated state (18). The time constant for recovery from block was 1630 (18) or 1480 msec (19) at the resting potential, in good agreement with the value of 1430 msec reported by Follmer et al. (13) for whole-cell voltage-clamped Purkinje myocytes. Follmer et al. (13) and Varro et al. (14) also found similar effects in their ventricular preparations. In a patch clamp study of single sodium channels in neonatal rat myocytes, Kohlhardt and Fichtner (21) found that amiodarone reduced the number of channel openings evoked by depolarizing steps (increased proportion of blank sweeps) in a use- and time-dependent manner but did not change the open time, open time distribution, or unitary current size. This observation is also consistent with a high affinity of the drug for the inactivated state of the channel.

Levine et al. (22) treated beagle dogs for 2 weeks with a loading dose of 400 mg/day of amiodarone orally and then 200 mg/day for 3–6 weeks. They then isolated ventricular epicardial slabs and used microelectrodes to study the configuration and conduction velocity of action potentials in vitro. They found that the action potential amplitude was significantly reduced in tissue from the treated animals (from 105 to 92 mV). Although the decrease in $\dot{V}_{max}$ (from 152 to 132 V/sec) was not statistically significant, the decrease in conduction velocity (from 0.56 to 0.41 m/sec) was significant and was correlated with a decrease in the space constant (from 1.05 to 0.69 mm). They concluded that the slowing of conduction velocity, an action assumed to be of major importance in the clinical efficacy of amiodarone, resulted more from changes in passive membrane properties (the decreased space constant) than from changes in sodium current. This provocative finding deserves further study under more controlled conditions.

Action Potential Duration. Singh and Vaughan Williams (2) were the first to report the marked prolongation of action potential duration in both atrial and ventricular muscle, when the drug has been given chronically before tissue isolation, that caused the drug to be classified as a class III agent. This effect has been confirmed in almost every study in ventricular muscle in which action potential duration has been measured. Pallandi and Campbell (19) found that amiodarone increased action potential duration of guinea pig ventricular muscle more than did desethylamiodarone. It is unclear how much of amiodarone's antiarrhythmic action is due to this effect and how much to blockade of sodium channels or other actions relating to conduction velocity (class I). However, since the drug's affinity for sodium channels is greater in the inactivated state, prolongation of the action potential plateau increases the amount of sodium channel block (18). A possible mechanism for the prolongation was described by Neliat (23), who found that the drug decreases the delayed outward current (I_K, the current primarily responsible for repolarization) in these tissues.

In contrast, Aomine (20) found that acute treatment of guinea pig ventricular fibers with concentrations as high as 4.4×10^{-5} M had no effect on action potential duration. Using tissue perfused with an "ischemic solution" high K^+ and CO_2; low glucose and pH) or metabolic inhibitors, Aomine found that amiodarone produced a small transient increase in action potential duration, followed by a decrease.

Ectopic Pacemaker Activity. Mason et al. (17) showed that amiodarone effectively blocks depolarization-induced automaticity. Aconitine-induced automaticity is also suppressed (24). Naumann d'Alnoncourt et al. (25) found that amiodarone prevented high-rate automaticity in Purkinje fibers isolated from guinea pigs previously treated with the drug. Ohta et al. (26) found that triggered automaticity was reduced in rabbit ventricular tissue following chronic treatment of the animals with amiodarone but not following in vitro application of the drug. The amplitude of delayed afterdepolarizations was reduced in both chronic and acute preparations but more so following chronic pretreatment.

Other Electrophysiologic Effects. Aomine (20) reported that after 3–5 hr treatment amiodarone depressed the resting membrane potential from about -82 to -76 mV. Other authors have not observed this effect (11,18,19,22).

Electrophysiologic Effects In Vivo

Nattel (27) found that both single doses and chronic treatment with amiodarone or desethylamiodarone prolonged QRS and QT intervals in anesthetized rats. Amiodarone was more effective in prolonging AV conduction, but its metabolite had more prominent effects on atrial and ventricular conduction. Talajic et al. (28) studied the effects of acutely administered amiodarone and desethylamiodarone in anesthetized dogs. They found that both drugs caused frequency-dependent slowing of atrioventricular and ventricular conduction velocity and increased both atrial and ventricular refractory periods. Amiodarone was more effective than its metabolite in prolonging Wenckebach cycle length, and desethylamiodarone was more effective in increasing QRS

duration and atrial and ventricular refractory periods. They suggested that the delayed portion of amiodarone's clinical efficacy is due to the cumulation of the metabolite during chronic therapy. These two studies suggest that, compared to the desethyl metabolite, amiodarone has a higher affinity for calcium channels and the metabolite has a higher affinity for sodium channels. In another study from the same laboratory (15) the action of acute administration of amiodarone on atrioventricular (AV) node function was studied in open-chest dogs. An interval-dependent slowing was observed. Anderson et al. (29) reported that 3 weeks of amiodarone treatment of dogs resulted in depression of both transverse and longitudinal conduction velocity, sinus rate, and ventricular escape automaticity. It increased the repolarization time and refractory period. The drug had no effect on stimulus threshold current. Epstein et al. (30) found that acute treatment of dogs with doses that produced therapeutic concentrations (1–2.5 µg/ml) caused little use-dependent slowing of HV conduction (measured from the onset of the His deflection to the onset of the surface QRS wave) in dogs, whereas chronic therapy caused significant slowing at the same plasma levels of drug.

Role of the Thyroid

Singh and Vaughan Williams (2) found that concurrent chronic administration of thyroxin and amiodarone could prevent the action of the latter drug on action potential duration in rabbit myocardium. In contrast, Lambert et al. (31) found that amiodarone pretreatment increased the refractory period of ventricular preparations isolated from euthyroid, hypothyroid, and T_3- and T_4-pretreated rats to the same extent and concluded that this effect of amiodarone was independent of thyroid state. Furthermore, administration of triiodothyronine to patients does not abolish amiodarone's therapeutic effects. There is considerable evidence (32,33) that amiodarone facilitates the conversion of thyroxin to reverse T_3. This may explain the reports of both hypo- and hyperthyroidism in patients treated with amiodarone. However, it is not clear how this effect contributes (or whether it contributes) to the therapeutic effects of the drug.

Autonomic Effects of Amiodarone

Early reports on the effects of amiodarone noted its ability to reduce blood pressure and heart rate and attributed these to adrenoceptor blocking effects. However, the drug is only a weak antagonist at α- and β-receptors (34) compared to phentolamine and propranolol. Furthermore, amiodarone can still reduce the heart rate after administration of propranolol (35). However, there is evidence to suggest that amiodarone does noncompetitively interfere with β function by reducing the number of functional β-receptors (36,37) in rabbit and rat myocardium. It is not clear whether this effect is related to the effects of amiodarone on thyroid hormone metabolism.

Other Tissues

Singh and Vaugh Williams (2) found that subcutaneous injections of amiodarone had no local anesthetic effects in guinea pigs. However, Revenko et al. (38) found that the drug produced a use-dependent block of I_{Na} in isolated frog node of Ranvier preparations that was very similar to the block subsequently reported for cardiac preparations. This discrepancy has not yet been explained.

Summary of Cellular and Membrane Actions of Amiodarone

The channel blocking effects of amiodarone are not yet completely understood. There is ample evidence that the drug blocks sodium channels (13,17), with the highest affinity of the drug for its receptor occurring during the inactivated state of the channel. Effects on AV conduction and "slow action potentials" in depolarized tissue indicate an action on calcium channels (15). The drug's effect on action potential duration and evidence from one laboratory (23) suggest that the potassium channels responsible for the delayed outward current are blocked. Because of its very high concentration in the membrane, the drug may modify the lipid bilayer and the passive electrical properties of the membrane. However, attempts to correlate the membrane concentration of amiodarone with its intensity of action

have not been successful to date (39). Finally, amiodarone has poorly understood effects on adrenoceptors and thyroid hormone metabolism.

Antiarrhythmic Effects of Amiodarone in Experimental Animals

Atrial Arrhythmias

Winslow (24) showed that amiodarone stopped the atrial fibrillation caused by the direct application of aconitine to the atria of anesthetized cats.

Ventricular Arrhythmias

The first demonstrations of antiarrhythmic activity in experimental animals were those of Charlier et al. (1). Singh and Vaughan Williams (2) found significant block of ouabain-induced arrhythmias (which were presumably mostly ventricular) at doses as low as 12.5 mg/kg when the amiodarone was given intravenously 5 min before the ouabain infusion. Arredondo et al. (40) reported that a single intravenous dose of 10 mg/kg of amiodarone doubled the fibrillation threshold but had no significant effect on the defibrillation threshold. In contrast, Fain et al. (41) found that acute intravenous amiodarone (10 mg/kg loading followed by 0.03 mg/kg per min maintenance) reduced the defibrillation energy requirement in dogs. However, chronic oral therapy had no effect on the defibrillation energy requirement. Rosenbaum et al. (42) showed that chronic pretreatment could markedly reduce the incidence of ventricular fibrillation in dogs subjected to coronary ligation. Patterson et al. (43) found a reduction of mortality in dogs with a model of sudden coronary death after both acute and chronic amiodarone pretreatment. Similar results were obtained by Nattel et al. (44). In addition to reduction in arrhythmia incidence, pretreatment has been reported to reduce infarct size in experimental animals (45,46).

CLINICAL PHARMACOLOGY

Electrophysiologic Effects

The clinical electrophysiologic effects of amiodarone are complex, due to the interactions already described between its slow and fast sodium channel blocking properties (9,18), use dependency (17,18), α- and β-blocking effects, and effects on thyroid metabolism (5).

Effects on the ECG

Acute Effects in Humans

The intravenous administration of amiodarone in humans is associated with little change in heart rate or mild, transient tachycardia (47). The decrease in rate mediated by the antiadrenergic effects and direct suppression of phase 4 depolarization (9) is offset by sympathetic activation resulting from vasodilation as well as the effects of the ethanol and polysorbate in the diluent (48). The AH interval is increased by 10–20% (12,47), with no significant change in the HV or QRS durations or QTc intervals. Atrial and ventricular effective refractory periods do not change, but the atrioventricular nodal and extranodal accessory pathway refractory periods are increased by approximately 15% (47).

Chronic Effects

The electrophysiologic effects of amiodarone during chronic oral administration are distinctly different from those seen during intravenous administration. Heart rate is deceased by 15–30% (12,47,49–51). Symptomatic sinus bradycardia or sinus arrest may occur, necessitating permanent pacing to allow the continued use of amiodarone (50,52,53). The AH interval may be increased by 20%. Atrial, AV nodal, ventricular, and accessory pathway refractoriness are increased from 10 to 45%. Depressed conduction in the His-Purkinje system is also present, especially in the presence of preexisting bundle branch block (50,54–56).

On the electrocardiogram bradycardia is often present, and the PR interval is usually increased by about 20% above the baseline (50,51,57). The QRS duration is increased by 10–20% at resting rates (47,58) but demonstrates use dependency, with widening up to 40% above pretreatment values at a paced rate of 170 beats/min. The QT interval is invariably prolonged, and T wave abnormalities and prominent U waves are common. (54).

Antiarrhythmic Effects of Amiodarone

Chronic (Oral) Therapy

Ventricular Tachyarrhythmias. Amiodarone is indicated for the treatment of sustained ventricular tachycardia or ventricular fibrillation refractory to other pharmacologic agents.

In a comparison of 5125 patients with coronary artery disease without arrhythmias and 54 patients with coronary artery disease and ventricular tachycardia or ventricular fibrillation treated with amiodarone, Key et al.(59) found that there was a significant increase in mortality at 1 and 2 years in the arrhythmia group before adjustment for comorbidity factors but no change after adjustment. They concluded that amiodarone was able to reduce the mortality of the arrhythmia group down to the risk of the underlying myocardial dysfunction only.

Herre et al. (60) studied 462 patients following an episode of sustained ventricular tachycardia or a caradiac arrest who were treated with amiodarone after the failure of class I antiarrhythmic drugs. Of these, 35 patients (7.6%) either failed to respond to amiodarone or died during the initial oral or intravenous loading phase and the remainder were sent home on amiodarone and followed for up to 98 months. The cumulative incidence of sudden death was 10% at 1 year, 15% at 3 years, and 21% at 5 years. Risk factors for recurrent cardiac arrest included increased age, decreased ejection fraction, and history of previous cardiac arrest. Other studies have shown a 40–100% (mean 70%) incidence of arrhythmia-free survival, with follow-ups ranging from 6 to 36 months (61–65).

The Amiodarone Toxicity Study Group, comprised of eight centers with combined data on 1307 patients followed for a mean of 396 days, reported a 29 and 49% incidence of arrhythmia recurrence at 1 and 3 years, respectively (66).

The rate of recurrent cardiac arrest while on amiodarone therapy was reported as 6–15% by 10–16 months (62,63,67,68). However, DiCarlo et al. (69) reported a recurrence rate of 24%. These differences may be due to differences in the patient populations and in the doses of amiodarone used. Morady et al. (63) reported that adverse effects of amiodarone were common, but 75% of the patients could be continued on the drug with dose adjustments based on clinical response and development of adverse effects.

The Role of Electrophysiologic Testing and Holter Monitoring. The role of electrophysiologic testing to assess the efficacy of amiodarone remains controversial. In a study of 100 consecutive patients Horowitz et al. (70) found no recurrences of ventricular tachycardia or ventricular fibrillation in the group of 20 patients in whom amiodarone suppressed the inducibility of arrhythmias during electrophysiologic study. In contrast, 38 of 80 patients (48%) with continued inducibility on follow-up testing had recurrence of ventricular tachyarrhythmias at 3–21 months follow-up. If the induced ventricular tachycardia was relatively slow and well tolerated hemodynamically, spontaneous recurrences (26 of 56 patients) were nonfatal. If the induced ventricular tachycardia was fast and poorly tolerated, there was a high incidence of sudden death.

In a study of 121 patients treated with amiodarone for malignant ventricular arrhythmias, Kadish et al. (71) reported similar results. Only 3 of 57 patients with well-tolerated ventricular tachycardia induced at electrophysiologic testing had recurrent sudden death, compared with 19 of 47 who had poorly tolerated arrhythmias during electrophysiologic testing. Multivariate analysis showed that the best predictor of recurrent sudden death was the presence of poorly tolerated arrhythmias on follow-up electrophysiologic testing. Other predictors included a younger age, lower ejection fraction, sudden death as the initial presentation, and lack of left ventricular aneurysm.

McGovern et al. (72) also found that electrophysiologic studies performed after 1–2 weeks of amiodarone loading had prognostic significance. At 10 months of follow-up 10 of 23 patients with continued inducibility had recurrent sudden death or sustained ventricular tachycardia, but only 1 of 19 with noninducibility on follow-up testing had recurrence.

The presence of persistent premature ventricular complexes or nonsustained ventricular tachycardia during amiodarone treatment may also be a marker for subsequent sudden death or symptomatic ventricular tachycardia. Marchlinski et al. (73) found that of 21 patients with continued frequent premature ventricular complexes or complex ventricular ectopy on Holter monitoring 11 days after initiation of amiodarone treatment, 11 (52%) had recurrence of cardiac arrest or symptomatic ventricular tachycardia at 13 months follow-up, compared with 6 of 34 patients in whom ectopy was suppressed. The findings of Di-Carlo et al. (69) were similar.

Veltri et al. (74) investigated the value of Holter recordings in 42 patients. The predictive accuracy of arrhythmia suppression was 76, 76, and 79% for 24, 48, and 72 hr recordings. Several authors have recommended that Holter monitoring be used to screen for the persistence of nonsustained ventricular tachycardia after a loading period of 2 weeks or more. Those patients who have significant suppression (or insufficient ectopy on baseline studies) would then have follow-up electrophysiologic testing. Those patients who have a poor response to amiodarone on either Holter monitoring or electrophysiologic testing would then be candidates for nonpharmacologic treatment, such as the automatic defibrillator (75,76).

Supraventricular Tachyarrhythmias. Rosenbaum et al. (42) reported successful conversion of atrial fibrillation or atrial flutter to normal sinus rhythm in 29 of 30 patients (97%). Haffajee et al. (62) reported the elimination of supraventricular tachycardia in 57 of 77 patients. This is similar to the 78% complete success and 6% partial success reported by Graboys et al. (77) from a series of 121 patients with supraventricular tachycardia, including 95 patients with atrial fibrillation alone or atrial fibrillation plus atrial flutter. The success rate of amiodarone in the treatment of tachycardia mediated by an accessory pathway in the Wolff-Parkinson-White syndrome is also high (42,78). At electrophysiologic testing a significant increase in the accessory pathway antegrade effective refractory period was noted, with variable effects on the retrograde effective refractory period (55,56).

Effects of Intravenous Amiodarone

Ventricular Tachyarrhythmias. Kadish and Morady reviewed the intravenous use of amiodarone (79). Helmy et al. (80) described 46 patients with recurrent, drug-refractory, sustained ventricular tachycardia or ventricular fibrillation treated with intravenous amiodarone. In this group 15 patients (33%) responded to intravenous amiodarone within 2 hr, 11 additional patients (23%) responded by 72 hr, and 1 patient after 72 hr. Another 6 patients (13%) responded after changing to oral amiodarone. Of the 27 patients who responded to intravenous amiodarone 6 had recurrences between 6 and 8 days after the beginning of amiodarone therapy. Of these six, 2 died, 1 was controlled by the addition of a second drug, and 3 were eventually controlled and discharged on oral amiodarone alone. Of the 46 patients, 6 had significant adverse effects: 2 patients had hypotension requiring dopamine, 2 had significant bradycardia requiring temporary pacing (1 permanently), and 2 had polymorphous ventricular tachycardia associated with QT prolongation. The dose used was 5 mg/kg as a bolus followed by 1000 mg per 24 hr.

Morady et al. (81) studied 15 patients with ventricular tachycardia refractory to two or more drugs and found that intravenous amiodarone was able to abolish the ventricular tachycardia in 12 patients. No proarrhythmic effects were noted.

Supraventricular Tachyarrhythmias. Supraventricular tachycardias can be successfully treated with intravenous amiodarone. In a study of 100 cases Benaim et al. (82) reported that 30% of patients with atrial fibrillation and 65% of patients with atrial or junctional tachycardia were successfully converted to normal sinus rhythm after the administration of intravenous amiodarone at 5 mg/kg, and a slowing of the ventricular response was noted in 47% of patients. Overall they reported that 80% of patients with supraventricular tachycardia had a beneficial effect.

PHARMACOKINETICS OF AMIODARONE

Experimental Animal Studies

An early study of the drug in several species indicated that it had low bioavailability, slow oral absorption, and slow renal clearance (83). These findings have been confirmed in many studies. Latini et al. (84) measured the pharmacokinetics of amiodarone in dogs. They measured a volume of distribution of approximately 17 L/kg. Connolly et al. (85) found that acute intravenous administration of amiodarone to dogs produced effects that correlated better with tissue concentrations of the drug than with plasma concentrations. Camus and Mehendale (86) found that amiodarone is concentrated rapidly in the isolated perfused rat and rabbit lung, reaching tissue-medium concentration ratios as high as 122. The tissue-medium ratio for the desethylamiodarone metabolite reached 506.

Clinical Studies

Absorption

Amiodarone is absorbed slowly. The time to peak concentration after oral administration is reported as 2–10 hr (mean 4 hr) (87–89). Bioavailability varies from 22 to 86% (90), with an average of 42%.

Distribution

Although approximately 96% of circulating amiodarone is bound to plasma proteins (86), distribution to the tissues is extensive; at steady-state the myocardial concentration is 10–50 times the plasma level and adipose, liver, and lung concentrations are 100–1000 times higher than in plasma (86,88,90). The volume of distribution has been variously calculated as between 0.9 and 148 L/kg (86), from 7 to 21 L/kg (89), and as 5000 L (90). The extraordinary range of these estimates may be the result of distribution to two compartments, a suggestion borne out by the existence of two elimination half-lives.

Elimination

Half-life measurements have varied from 8 to 107 days. Holt et al. (91) reported a 25 day half-life following a single intavenous dose and a mean of 52 days in a group of eight patients after chronic therapy. In fact elimination is probably biphasic, with the first half-life about 2 weeks and the second much longer (3). Clearance is 0.14–0.6 L/min (86). Dialysis does not remove amiodarone (92).

Metabolism

Low bioavailability probably reflects metabolism in the intestinal wall by dealkylation (93). Both monodesethyl and didesethyl metabolites have been recognized in dogs; the monodesethyl product is the dominant metabolite in humans. Its half-life is longer than that of amiodarone. In dogs the monodesethyl metabolite is more potent than the parent compound in prolonging the QRS duration and the atrial and ventricular refractory periods (28). Yabek et al. (94) found that monodesethylamiodarone was less potent than the parent compound in reducing upstroke velocity and prolonging the ventricular refractory period.

Plasma Levels Versus Effect

Falik et al. (95) found that the mean serum concentrations of amiodarone and desethylamiodarone were 2.1 and 1.5 μg/mL, respectively, in patients without adverse effects and 2.6 and 2.0 μg/mL, respectively, in patients with adverse effects.

Amiodarone Dosing Regimens

The dosing regimens most often used for the chronic treatment of ventricular tachyarrhythmias include a loading phase at 800–1200 mg/day in two to three divided doses for 10–14 days, followed by 600–800 mg/day for 4–8 weeks. The maintenance dose is 200–600 mg/day (60,62,96). Maintenance doses of 400–800 mg/day are associated with serum levels of 1.5 ± 0.6 μg/ml (97), but the correlation between serum levels and the daily or cumulative amiodarone dose is variable (98). Serum levels > 1.5 μg/ml are associated with a therapeutic effect on ventricular tachycardia (99), and some investigators reported that levels > 2.5 μg/ml predispose toward a higher incidence of adverse effects (62). However, tissue levels of amiodarone can be as much as 30–300 times greater than serum levels (88) and the correlation between serum levels and either efficacy or toxicity is not very strong. Therefore, measurements of serum levels of amiodarone are of limited clinical utility.

TOXICOLOGY

Biochemical Mechanisms

Chronic treatment with amiodarone results in the formation of intracellular multilamellar inclusion bodies, structures that signal the accumulation of abnormal amounts or types of lipids. This effect is demonstrable in the cells of the lung, cornea, skin, liver, and peripheral nerve in animals and humans (100). These inclusion bodies appear to be the result of lipid accumulation, mostly phospholipids (101). In lungs of rats treated with doses of 100–150 mg/kg for 2 weeks, cholesterol is increased by approximately 20% and phospholipid (mainly phosphatidylcholine) increases by about 70%. In another study in which rats were treated for only 5 days with 150 mg/kg per day, an extraordinary increase of 500% in the phospholipid content of pulmonary macrophages was observed (102). This change probably results from amiodarone accumulation in the lysosomes of pulmonary macrophages and inhibition of phospholipase A_1 in these subcellular structures (103). In fact, both amiodarone and desethylamiodarone are extremely potent inhibitors of this enzyme (104).

Similarly, phospholipase A_2 and phospholipase C of human neutrophils are inhibited by low concentrations of amiodarone (99). Unfortunately, the significance of lamellar bodies in peripheral cells (e.g., circulating neutrophils) is not clear since they may be found in cells of patients without toxicity as well as those with it (105).

Clinical Toxicology

Although amiodarone is the most effective antiarrhythmic agent available at present, it is also by far the most toxic. Adverse effects occur in 45–100% of patients treated with amiodarone (63,64,75,106). Up to 22% of patients are taken off the drug by 1 year (50,105), and 50–80% can no longer tolerate the drug after

5 years (60,107). A general overview of amiodarone toxicity has been presented by Vrobel et al. (108).

Cardiac Effects

The proarrhythmic effects of amiodarone have been reviewed by Mattioni et al. (109). Torsade de pointes has been described in association with amiodarone alone or in combination with other antiarrhythmic agents, including quinidine, procainamide, disopyramide, propafenone, and mexiletine (110–113). It is almost always associated with a long QT interval and may be related to an amiodarone-induced rise in the serum levels of the other antiarrhythmic agents. Symptomatic sinus bradycardia, sinus arrest, or, in patients with underlying conduction system disease, advanced AV block may occur, requiring lowered amiodarone doses or permanent pacemaker implantation.

Pulmonary Toxicity

Pulmonary toxicity is the most serious complication of amiodarone(3,114). It occurs in 0.7–14% of patients after 1 year (51,66,80,115), and the incidence may be as high as 28% after 3 years (66). Mortality rates of 10% have been reported if the drug is not promptly discontinued (116). Toxicity may be related to the cumulative dose (117) and often presents with nonspecific symptoms, including nonproductive cough, pleuritic pain, dyspnea, fever, and weight loss (116,118). Occasionally patients present with acute respiratory failure (119). Physical examination may reveal bilateral rales and pleural friction rubs. Laboratory studies frequently show leukocytosis and an elevated erythrocyte sedimentation rate. The elevation of the latter may be especially useful to help exclude either congestive heart failure or pulmonary emboli, both common diseases with similar presentations in this patient group (112). The chest x-ray almost invariably shows diffuse interstitial infiltrates or a patchy alveolar pattern, or both (115,118,119). Pulmonary function tests demonstrate a decrease in the diffusing capacity for carbon monoxide (D_{LCO}) and total lung capacity (TLC). Kudenchuk (117) has proposed that a diagnosis of

amiodarone pulmonary toxicity be made if two of the following three criteria are met:

1. New (or worsening of) pulmonary symptoms
2. New (or worsening of) chest x-ray findings
3. A decrease in D_{LCO} or TLC by >15%

Additional studies frequently include gallium scans. In the absence of other known causes new areas of gallium uptake compared with the baseline study are consistent with amiodarone pulmonary toxicity (120). Bronchoalveolar lavage or transbronchial biopsy may be useful. The presence of cytoplasmic cell inclusions, giving the cells a foamy appearance, is typical although not pathognomonic: up to 50% of amiodarone patients without pulmonary toxicity may have this finding (112). Two-thirds of patients with amiodarone pulmonary toxicity have increased numbers of CD8+ lymphocytes (T suppressor/cytotoxic) or polymorphonuclear cells present in the lavage fluid.

The treatment of amiodarone pulmonary toxicity includes immediate discontinuation of amiodarone. The role of corticosteroids is uncertain. The pathologic findings suggest a metabolic rather than immunologic mechanism (114,118), but at least some investigators recommend empirical treatment with 40–60 mg prednisone per day if the symptoms are severe, with tapering of dosage over 2–6 months.

Thyroid Effects

Although clinical hyper- or hypothyroidism is rare, laboratory abnormalities of thyroid metabolism are common. In a review of patients on amiodarone treated for an average of 16 months Nademanee et al. (121) reported that 8% were clinically hypothyroid, 3% clinically hyperthyroid, and 89% clinically euthyroid. However, there were significant laboratory abnormalities in the clinically euthyroid group. The changes included a T_4 elevation of 42%, a reverse T_3 elevation of 172%, and a T_3 decrease of 16%. There was no significant effect on the thyroid stimulating hormone (TSH). These changes reached steady state by 3 months and appeared to be unrelated to dose or duration of therapy (111,117). Hyper- or hypothyroidism may be severe and persist for months after discontinuation of amiodarone (122). Thyroid replacement may be given for hypothyroidism without affecting the antiarrhythmic efficacy of amiodarone (123). Hyperthyroidism may present insidiously or as recurrent ventricular tachycardia or angina. Propylthiouracil or methimazole may be used to treat hyperthyroidism, with propylthiouracil the preferred agent because of its ability to block the peripheral conversion of T_4 to T_3. β-Blockers may be useful to control the symptoms and tachycardia (124). Surgical thyroidectomy may be necessary in extreme cases. Administration of ^{131}I is ineffective because of the markedly increased iodine stores present in the body during amiodarone therapy.

Gastrointestinal and Hepatic Effects

Nausea and anorexia occur in 8% of patients, and 15% of patients have an increase in serum aspartate aminotransferase and alanine aminotransferase levels to 1.5–4 times normal, without concomitant rises in serum alkaline phosphatase or bilirubin levels (115). These changes appear to be dose dependent and tend to resolve over time, despite the continued administration of amiodarone. Clinically evident hepatitis, although rare, may also occur. Constipation is common, may be severe, and is often successfully managed with stool softeners.

Ophthalmic Effects

Corneal microdeposits are extremely common. They can be seen as early as 10 days after initiation of therapy and may be found in 100% of patients on slit-lamp examination at 1 month (115). These changes are dose and duration dependent (125). Corneal deposits are usually asymptomatic, and the amiodarone dose does not need to be adjusted. Up to 6% of patients may experience blurred vision or halos. These changes are reversible after discontinuation of the drug (126).

Neurologic Effects

One-third of patients treated with amiodarone experience adverse neurologic effects, including tremor, ataxia, and weakness (65). These changes appear to be dose dependent. A low incidence of peripheral neuropathy has also been described. It does not appear to be dose dependent. This has been associated histologically with segmental demyelination, and Schwann cell lysosomal inclusion bodies (multilamellar bodies) containing lipids. These changes may partially resolve after discontinuation of amiodarone. Decreases in nerve conduction velocity have also been described for amiodarone.

Dermatologic Effects

Photosensitivity is very common with amiodarone, occurring in 50% of patients, and can be severe enough to cause burning, erythema, and swelling in sun-exposed patients (115). A slate gray discoloration is also present in approximately 2% of patients in a dose- and duration-dependent fashion. Biopsies of these areas reveal increased lipofuscin deposition and significant elastin degeneration with decreased melanin deposits (127). Facial pigmentation (visage mauve) is also present in 25% of patients. A history of photosensitivity, as well as increased doses and duration of amiodarone treatment, is associated with this.

Drug Interactions

Amiodarone administration results in increased serum levels of digoxin in a dose-dependent manner. This may be due to decreased elimination of digoxin, and it has been recommended that the dose of digoxin be halved when amiodarone is added (110,128). It can also elevate the levels of most of the class IA antiarrhythmic agents. Saal et al. (129) found that the maintenance requirements for quinidine and procainamide were reduced by 37 and 20%, respectively, when amiodarone was added. A potentiation of the effects of warfarin has also been described (110,130), and the dosage of warfarin should be reduced. Finally, it should be noted that amiodarone may also potentiate the negative chronotropic effects of β-blockers or calcium channel blockers, resulting in severe sinus bradycardia or sinus arrest.

SUMMARY

Oral amiodarone is an extremely effective antiarrhythmic drug. Because of the significant toxicities associated with its use it is generally reserved for the treatment of refractory, life-threatening ventricular tachyarrhythmias. Although there have been no studies comparing noninvasive monitoring and electrophysiologic studies in patients on amiodarone, both these techniques may be useful predictors of the risk of recurrent fatal or nonfatal tachyarrhythmias in patients taking amiodarone. Amiodarone can also be highly effective for the treatment of supraventricular tachyarrhythmias. Intravenous amiodarone, although possessing different electrophysiologic properties, is highly effective for both ventricular and supraventricular tachyarrhythmias.

REFERENCES

1. Charlier R, Delaunois G, Bauthier J, Deltour G. Recherches dans la serie des benzofuranes. XL. Propriete antiarrythmiques de l'amiodarone. Cardiologia 1969; 54:83–90.
2. Singh B N, Vaughan Williams E M. The effect of amiodarone, a new antianginal drug, on cardiac muscle. Br J Pharmacol 1970; 39:657–67.
3. Mason J W. Amiodarone. N Engl J Med 1987; 318:455–66.
4. Nattel S, Talajic M. Recent advances in understanding the pharmacology of amiodarone. Drugs 1988; 36:121–31.
5. Singh B N, Venkatèsh N, Nademanee K, Josephson M A, Kannan R. The historical development, cellular electrophysiology and pharmacology of amiodarone. Prog Cardiovasc Dis 1989; 31:249–80.
6. Chatelain P, Laruel R. Amiodarone partitioning with phospholipid bilayers and erythrocyte membranes. J Pharm Sci 1985; 74:783–4.
7. Trumbore M, Chester D W, Moring J, Rhodes D, Herbette L G. Structure and location of amiodarone in a membrane bilayer as determined by molecular mechanics and quantitative x-ray diffraction, Biophys J 1988; 54:535–43.
8. Chatelain P, Laruel R, Gillard M. Effect of amiodarone on membrane fluidity and Na^+/K^+ ATPase activity in rat brain synaptic membranes. Biochem Biophys Res Commun 1985; 129:148–54.
9. Goupil N, Lenfant J. The effects of amiodarone on the sinus node activity of the rabbit heart. Eur J Pharmacol 1976; 39:23–31.
10. Gloor H O, Urthaler F, James T N. Acute effects of amiodarone upon the canine sinus node and atrioventricular junctional region. J Clin Invest 1983; 71:1457–66.
11. Yabek S M, Kato R, Singh B N. Acute effects of amiodarone on the electrophysiologic properties of isolated neonatal and adult cardiac fibers. J Am Coll Cardiol 1985; 5:1109–15.
12. Ikeda N, Nademanee K, Kannan R, et al. Electrophysiologic effects of amiodarone: experimental and clinical observations relative to serum and tissue concentrations. Am Heart J 1984; 108:890–9.
13. Follmer C H, Aomine M, Yeh J Z, Singer D H. Amiodarone-induced block of sodium current in isolated cardiac cells. J Pharmacol Exp Ther 1987; 243:187–94.
14. Varro A, Nakaya Y, Elharrar V, Surawicz B. Use-dependent effects of amiodarone on V_{max} in cardiac Purkinje and ventricular muscle fibers. Eur J Pharmacol 1985; 112:419–22.
15. Nattel S, Talajic M, Quantz M, DeRoode M. Frequency-dependent effects of amiodarone on atrioventricular nodal function and slow-channel action potentials: evidence for calcium-channel-blocking activity. Circulation 1987; 76:442–9.
16. Aomine M. Acute effects of amiodarone on action potentials of isolated canine Purkinje fibers: comparison with tetrodotoxin effects. Gen Pharmacol 1988; 19:601–7.
17. Mason J, Hondeghem L M, Katzung B G. Amiodarone blocks inactivated cardiac sodium channels. Pflugers Arch 1983; 396:79–81.
18. Mason J W, Hondeghem L M, Katzung B G. Block of inactivated sodium channels and of depolarization-induced automaticity in guinea pig papillary muscle by amiodarone. Circ Res 1984; 55:277–85.
19. Pallandi R T, Campbell T J. Resting, and rate-dependent depression of V_{max} of guinea-pig ventricular action potentials by amiodarone and desethylamiodarone. Br J Pharmacol 1987; 92:97–103.
20. Aomine M. Does acute exposure to amiodarone prolong cardiac action potential duration? Gen Pharmacol 1988; 19:615–9.

21. Kohlhardt M, Fichtner H. Block of single cardiac Na + channel by antiarrhythmic drugs: the effect of amiodarone, propafenone and diprafenone. J Membr Biol 1988; 102:105–19.

22. Levine J H, Moore I N, Kadish A H, et al. Mechanisms of depressed conduction from long-term amiodarone therapy in canine myocardium. Circulation 1988; 78:684–91.

23. Neliat G. Effects of butoprozine on ionic currents in frog atrial and ferret ventricular fibers. Comparison with amiodarone and verapamil. Arch Int Pharmacodyn Ther 1982; 255:237–55.

24. Winslow E. Hemodynamic and arrhythmogenic effects of aconitine applied to the left atria of anesthetized cats: effects of amiodarone and atropine. J Cardiovasc Pharmacol 1981; 3:87–100.

25. Naumann d'Alnoncourt C, Zierhut W, Nitsch J, Luderitz B. Effects of amiodarone on Purkinje fibers. In: Breithardt G, Loogen F, eds. New aspects in the medical treatment of tachyarrhythmias. Role of amiodarone. Munich: Urban & Schwartzenberg 1983:88–90.

26. Ohta M, Karagueuzian H, Mandel W J, et al. Acute and chronic effects of amiodarone on delayed afterdepolarization and triggered automaticity in rabbit ventricular myocardium. Am Heart J 1987; 113:289–96.

27. Nattel S. Pharmacodynamic studies of amiodarone and its active N-desethyl metabolite. J Cardiovasc Pharmacol 1986; 8:771–7.

28. Talajic M, DeRoode M R, Nattel S. Comparative electrophysiologic effects of intravenous amiodarone and desethylamiodarone in dogs: evidence for clinically relevant activity of the metabolite. Circulation 1987; 75:265–71.

29. Anderson K P, Walker R, Dustman T, Lux R L, Ershler P R, Kates R E, Urie P M. Rate-related electrophysiologic effects of long-term administration of amiodarone on canine ventricular myocardium in vivo. Circulation 1989; 79:948–58.

30. Epstein L M, Chin M C, Garcia J A, et al. A comparison of the use-dependent effects of acute and chronic amiodarone administration in vivo (abstract). Circulation 1989; 80:II-136.

31. Lambert C, Cardinal R, Vermeulen M. Lack of relation between the ventricular refractory period prolongation by amiodarone and the thyroid state in rats. J Pharmacol Exp Ther 1987; 242:320–5.

32. Singh B N, Phil D, Nadimanee K. Amiodarone and thyroid function: clinical implications during antiarrhythmic therapy. Am Heart J 1983; 106:857–68.

33. Zipes D P, Prystowsky E N, Heger J J. Amiodarone: electrophysiologic actions, pharmacokinetics, and clinical effects. J Am Coll Cardiol 1984; 3:1059–71.

34. Polster P, Broekhuysen J. The adrenergic antagonism of amiodarone. Biochem Pharmacol 1976; 25:131–8.

35. Charlier R. Cardiac actions in the dog of a new antagonist of adrenergic excitation which does not produce competitive blockade of adrenoceptors. Br J Pharmacol 1970; 39:668–74.

36. Venkatesh N, Padbury J F, Singh B N. Effects of amiodarone and desethylamiodarone on rabbit myocardial beta-adrenoceptors and serum thyroid hormones—absence of relationship to serum and myocardial drug concentrations. J Cardiovasc Pharmacol 1986; 8:989–97.

37. Nokin P, Clinet M, Schoenfeld P. Cardiac beta-adrenoceptor modulation by amiodarone. Biochem Pharmacol 1983; 32:2473–7.

38. Revenko S V, Khodorov B I, Avrutskii M Y. Blocking of inactivated sodium channels by the antiarrhythmic cordarone. M Y Byull Eksper Biol Med 1980; 89:702–4.

39. Venkatesh N, Somani P, Bersohn M, et al. Electropharmacology of amiodarone: absence of relationship to serum, myocardial, and cardiac sarcolemmal membrane drug concentrations. Am Heart J 1986; 112:916–22.

40. Arredondo M T, Guillen S G, Quinteiro R A. Effect of amiodarone on ventricular fibrillation and defibrillation thresholds in the canine heart under normal and ischemic conditions. Eur J Pharmacol 1986; 125:23–8.

41. Fain E S, Lee J T, Winkle R A. Effects of acute intravenous and chronic oral amiodarone on defibrillation energy requirements. Am Heart J 1987; 114:8–17.

42. Rosenbaum M B, Chiale P A, Halpern M S, et al. Clinical efficacy of amiodarone as an antiarrhythmic agent. Am J Cardiol 1976; 38:934–42.

43. Patterson E, Eller B T, Abrams G D, et al. Ventricular fibrillation in conscious canine preparation of sudden coronary death. Prevention by short- and long-term amiodarone administration. Circulation 1983; 68:857–64.

44. Nattel S, Davies M, Quantz M. The antiarrhythmic efficacy of amiodarone and desethylamiodarone, alone and in combination, in dogs with acute myocardial infarction. Circulation 1988; 77:200–8.

45. Chew C Y C, Collet J T, Campbell C, et al. Beneficial effects of amiodarone pretreatment on early ischemic ventricular arrhythmias relative to infarct size and regional myocardial blood flow in the conscious dog. J Cardiovasc Pharmacol 1982; 4:1028–36.

46. DeBoer L W V, Nosta J J, Kloner R A, et al. Studies of amiodarone during experimental myocardial infarction: beneficial effcts on hemodynamics and infarct size. Circulation 1982; 65:508–12.

47. Wellens H J J, Brugada P, Abdollah H, Dassen W R. A comparison of the electrophysiologic effects of intravenous and oral amiodarone in the same patient. Circulation 1984; 69:120–4.

48. Sicart M, Besse P, Choussat A, Bricaud H. Action hemodynamique de l'amiodarone intraveineuse chez l'homme. Arch Mal Coeur 1977; 70:219–27.

49. Petta J M, Zaccheo V J. Comparative profile of L3428 and other antianginal agents on cardiac hemodynamics. J Pharmacol Exp Ther 1971; 176:328–38.

50. Waxman H L, Groh W C, Marchlinski F E, et al. Amiodarone for control of sustained ventricular tachyarrhythmia: clinical and electrophysiologic effects in 51 patients. Am J Cardiol 1982; 50:1066–74.

51. Heger J J, Prystowsky E N, Jackman W M, et al. Amiodarone: clinical efficacy and electrophysiology during long-term therapy for recurrent ventricular tachycardia or ventricular fibrillation. N Engl J Med 1981; 305:539–45.

52. McGovern B, Garan H, Ruskin J N. Sinus arrest during treatment with amiodarone. Br Med J 1982; 284:160–1.

53. Lee T H, Friedman P L, Goldman L, Stone P H, Antman E M. Sinus arrest and hypotension with combined amiodarone-diltiazem therapy. Am Heart J 1985; 109:163–4.

54. Rosenbaum M B, Chiale P A, Ryba D, Elizari M. Control of tachyarrhythmias associated with Wolff-Parkinson-White syndrome by amiodarone hydrochloride. Am J Cardiol 1974; 34:215–23.

55. Wellens H J J, Lie K I, Bar F W, et al. Effect of amiodarone in the Wolff-Parkinson-White syndrome. Am J Cardiol 1976; 38:189–94.

56. Rowland E, Krikler D M. Electrophysiological assessment of amiodarone in the treatment of resistant supraventricular arrhythmias. Br Heart J 1980; 44:82–90.

57. Touboul P, Huerta F, Porte J, Delahaye P. Bases electrophysiologiques de l'action antiarrhythmique de l'amiodarone chez l'homme. Arch Mal Coeur 1976; 69:845.

58. Morady F, DiCarlo L A, Krol R B, Baerman JM, de Buitleir M. Acute and chronic effects of amiodarone on ventricular refractoriness, intraventricular conduction and ventricular tachycardia induction. J Am Coll Cardiol 1986; 7:148–57.

59. Key G N, Pryor D B, Lee K L, et al. Comparison of survival of amiodarone treated patients with coronary artery disease and malignant ventricular arrhythmias with that of a control group with coronary artery disease. J Am Coll Cardiol 1987; 9:877–81.

60. Herre J M, Sauve M J, Malone P, et al. Long-term results of amiodarone therapy in patients with recurrent sustained ventricular tachycardia or ventricular fibrillation. J Am Coll Cardiol 1989; 13:442–9.

61. Rosenbaum M B, Chiale P A, Haedo A, Lazzari J O, Elizari M V. Ten years of experience with amiodarone. Am Heart J 1983; 106:957–64.

62. Haffajee C I, Love J C, Alpert J S, Asdourian G K, Sloan K C. Efficacy and safety of long-term amiodarone in treatment of cardiac arrhythmias: dosage experience. Am Heart J 1983; 106:935–43.

63. Morady F, Sauve M J, Malone P, et al. Long-term efficacy and toxicity of high-dose amiodarone therapy for ventricular tachycardia or ventricular fibrillation. Am J Cardiol 1983; 52:975–9.

64. Kaski J C, Girotti L A, Messuti H, Rutitzky B, Rosenbaum M B. Long-term management of sustained, recurrent, symptomatic ventricular tachycardia with amiodarone. Circulation 1981; 64:273–9.

65. Heger J J, Prystowsky E N, Miles W M, Zipes D P. Clinical use and pharmacology of amiodarone. Med Clin North Am 1984; 68:1339–66.

66. Mason J W and the Amiodarone Toxicity Study Group. Toxicity of amiodarone (abstract). Circulation 1985; 72 (Suppl. III):III–272A.

67. Peter T, Hamer A, Weiss D, Mandel W J. Prognosis after sudden cardiac death without associated myocardial infarction: one year follow-up of empiric amiodarone therapy. Am Heart J 1984; 107:209–14.

68. Nademanee K, Singh B N, Cannom D S, Weiss J, Feld G, Stevenson W G. Control of sudden recurrent arrhythmic deaths: role of amiodarone. Am Heart J 1983; 106:895–901

69. DiCarlo L A, Morady F, Sauve M J, et al. Cardiac arrest and sudden death in patients treated with amiodarone for sustained ventricular tachycardia or ventricular fibrillation: risk stratification based on clinical variables. Am J Cardiol 1985; 55:372–4.

70. Horowitz L N, Greenspan A M, Spielman S R, et al. Usefulness of electrophysiologic testing in evaluation of amiodarone therapy for sustained ventricular tachyarrhythmias associated with coronary heart disease. Am J Cardiol 1985; 55:367–71.

71. Kadish A H, Buxton A E, Waxman H L, Flores B, Josephson M E, Marchlinski F E. Usefulness of electrophysiologic study to determine the clinical tolerance of arrhythmia recurrences during amiodarone therapy. J Am Coll Cardiol 1987; 10:90–6.

72. McGovern B, Garan H, Malacoff R F, et al. Long-term clinical outcome of ventricular tachycardia or fibrillation treated with amiodarone. Am J Cardiol 1984; 53:1558–63.

73. Marchlinski F E, Buxton A E, Flores B T, Doherty J U, Waxman H L, Josephson M E. Value of Holter monitoring in identifying risk for sustained ventricular arrhythmia recurrence on amiodarone. Am J Cardiol 1985; 55:709–12.

74. Veltri E P, Reid P R, Platia E V, Griffith L S C. Amiodarone in the treatment of life-threatening ventricular tachycardia—the role of Holter monitoring in predicting long-term clinical efficacy. J Am Coll Cardiol 1985; 6:806–13.

75. Greene H C. The efficacy of amiodarone in the treatment of ventricular tachycardia or ventricular fibrillation. Prog Cardiovasc Dis 1989; 31:319–54.

76. Winkle R A. Amiodarone and the American way (editorial). J Am Coll Cardiol 1985; 6:822–4.

77. Graboys T B, Podrid P J, Lown B. Efficacy of amiodarone for refractory supraventricular tachyarrhythmias. Am Heart J 1983; 106:870–6.

78. Kopelman H A, Horowitz L N. Efficacy and toxicity of amiodarone for the treatment of supraventricular tachyarrhythmias. Prog Cardiovasc Dis 1989; 31:355–66.

79. Kadish A, Morady F. The use of intravenous amiodarone in the acute therapy of life-threatening arrhythmias. Prog Cardiovasc Dis 1989; 31:281–94.

80. Helmy I, Herre J M, Gee G, et al. Use of intravenous amiodarone for emergency treatment of life-threatening ventricular arrhythmias. J Am Coll Cardiol 1988; 12:1015–22.

81. Morady F, Scheinman M M, Shen E, Shapiro W, Sung R J, DiCarlo L. Intravenous amiodarone in the acute treatment of recurrent symptomatic ventricular tachycardia. Am J Cardiol 1983; 51:156–9.

82. Benaim R, Denizeau J P, Melon J. Les effets antiarythmiques de l'amiodarone injectable: a propos de 100 cas. Arch Mal Coeur 1976; 69:513–22.

83. Bruekhuysen J, Laruel R, Sion R. Recherches dans la serie des benzofurannes. XXXVII. Etude comparee du transit et du metabolisme de l'amiodarone chez diverses especes animales et chez l'homme. Arch Int Pharmacodyn 1969; 177:340–59.

84. Latini R, Connolly S J, Kates R E. Myocardial disposition of amiodarone in the dog. J Pharmacol Exp Ther 1983; 224:603–8.

85. Connolly S J, Latini R, Kates R E. Pharmacodynamics of intravenous amiodarone in the dog. J Cardiovasc Pharmacol 1984; 6:531–5.

86. Camus P, Mehendale H M. Pulmonary sequestration of amiodarone and desethylamiodarone. J Pharmacacol Exp Ther 1986; 237:867–73.

87. Latini R, Tognoni G, Kates R E. Clinical pharmacokinetics of amiodarone. Clin Pharmacokinet 1984; 9:136–56.

88. Andreason F, Agerbaek H, Bjerregaard P, Gotzsche H. Pharmacokinetics of amiodarone after intravenous and oral administration. Eur J Clin Pharmacol 1981; 19:293–9.

89. Haffajee C I, Love J C, Canada A T, Lesko L J, Asdourian G, Alpert J S. Clinical pharmacokinetics and efficacy of amiodarone for refractory tachyarrhythmias. Circulation 1983; 67:1347–55.

90. Riva E, Gerna M, Latini R, Giani P, Volpi A, Maggioni A. Pharmacokinetics of amiodarone in man. J Cardiovasc Pharmacol 1982; 4:264–9.

91. Holt D W, Tucker G T, Jackson P R, Storey G C A. Amiodarone pharmacokinetics. Am Heart J 1983; 106:840–7.

92. Bonati M, Volpe A, Tognoni G. Amiodarone in patients on long-term dialysis (letter). N Engl J Med 1983; 308:906.

93. Berdeaux A, Roche A, Labaille T, et al. Tissue extraction of amiodarone and N-desethylamiodarone in man after a single oral dose. Br J Clin Pharmacol 1984; 18:759–63.

94. Yabek S M, Kato R, Singh B N. Effects of amiodarone and its metabolite, desethylamiodarone, on the electrophysiologic properties of isolated cardiac muscle. J Cardiovasc Pharmacol 1986; 8:197–207.

95. Falik R, Flores B T, Shaw L, Gibson G A, Josephson M E, Marchlinski F E. Relationship of steady-state serum concentrations of amiodarone and desethylamiodarone to therapeutic efficacy and adverse effects. Am J Med 1987; 82:1102–8.

96. Greene H L, Graham R L, Werner J A, et al. Toxic and therapeutic effects of amiodarone in the treatment of cardiac arrhythmia. J Am Coll Cardiol 1983; 2:1114–28.

97. Saksena S, Rothbart S T, Sheh Y, et al. Clinical efficacy and electropharmacology of continuous intravenous amiodarone infusion and chronic oral amiodarone in refractory ventricular tachycardia. Am J Cardiol 1984; 54:347–52.

98. Raeder E A, Podrid P J, Lown B. Side effects and complications of amiodarone therapy. Am Heart J 1985; 109:975–83.

99. Mostow N D, Rakita L, Vrobel T R, et al. Amiodarone: correlation of serum concentration with suppression of complex ventricular ectopic activity. Am J Cardiol 1984; 54:569–74.

100. Shaikh N A, Downar E, Butany J. Amiodarone—an inhibitor of phospholipase activity: a comparative study of the inhibitory effects of amiodarone, chloroquine and chlorpromazine. Mol Cell Biochem 1987; 76:163–72.

101. Chatelain P, Brotelle R. Phospholipid composition of rat lung after amiodarone treatment. Res Commun Chem Pathol Pharmacol 1985; 50:407–18.

102. Reasor M, Ogle C L, Walker E R, Kacew S. Amiodarone-induced phospholipidosis in rat alveolar macrophages. Am Rev Respir Dis 1988; 137:510–8.

103. Hostetler K Y, Reasor M J, Walker E R, Yazaki P J, Frazee B W. Role of phopholipase A inhibition in amiodarone pulmonary toxicity in rats. Biochim Biophys Acta 1986; 875:400–5.

104. Hostetler K Y, Giordano J R, Jellison E J. In vitro inhibition of lysosomal phospholipase A₁ of rat lung by amiodarone and desethylamiodarone. Biochim Biophys Acta 1988; 959:316–21.

105. Somani P, Bandyopadhyay S, Gross S A, Morady F, DiCarlo L A. Amiodarone and multilamellar inclusion bodies. Br J Clin Pharmacol 1987; 24:237–8.

106. Camm A J, Ward D E, Al-Hamde A, et al. The use of oral amiodarone in the control of tachyarrhythmias associated with the Wolff-Parkinson-White syndrome. In: Amiodarone in cardiac arrhythmias, London: Royal Society of Medicine 1979:25–8.

107. Smith W M, Lubbe W D, Whitlock K, et al. Long-term tolerance of amiodarone treatment for cardiac arrhythmia. Am J Cardiol 1986; 57:1288–93.

108. Vrobel T R, Miller P E, Mostow N D, Rakita L. A general overview of amiodarone toxicity: its prevention, detection, and management. Prog Cardiovasc Dis 1989; 31:393–426.

109. Mattioni T A, Zheutlin T A, Dunnington C, Kehoe R F. The proarrhythmic effects of amiodarone. Prog Cardiovasc Dis 1989; 31:439–46.

110. Marcus F I. Drug interactions with amiodarone. Am Heart J 1983; 106:924–30.

111. Keren A, Tzivoni D, Gavish D, et al. Etiology, warning signs and therapy of torsade de pointes: a study of 10 patients. Circulation 1981; 64:1167–74.

112. McComb J M, Logan K R, Khon M M, Geddes J S, Adgey A A J. Amiodarone-induced ventricular fibrillation. Eur J Cardiol 1980; 11:381–5.

113. Tartini R, Kappenberger L, Steinbrunn W, Meyer U A. Dangerous interaction between amiodarone and quinidine. Lancet 1982; 1:1327–9.

114. Dunn M, Glassroth J. Pulmonary complications of amiodarone toxicity. Prog Cardiovasc Dis 1989; 31:447–53.

115. Harris L, McKenna W J, Rowland E, Holt D W, Storey G C A, Krikler D M. Side effects of long-term amiodarone therapy. Circulation 1983; 67:45–51.

116. Martin W J, Rosenow E L. Amiodarone pulmonary toxicity: recognition and pathogenesis. Chest 1988; 93:1067–75.

117. Kudenchuk P J, Pierson D J, Greene H L, Graham E L, Sears G K, Trobaugh G B. Prospective evaluation of amiodarone pulmonary toxicity. Chest 1984; 86:541–8.

118. Marchlinski F E, Gansler T S, Waxman J L, Josephson M E. Amiodarone pulmonary toxicity. Ann Intern Med 1982; 97:839–45.

119. Dean P J, Groshart K D, Porterfield J C, Iansmith D H, Golden E B. Amiodarone-associated pulmonary toxicity. A clinical and pathological study of 11 cases. Am J Clin Pathol 1987; 87:7–13.

120. Dake M D, Hattner R, Warnock M L, Golden J A. Gallium-67 lung uptake associated with amiodarone pulmonary toxicity. Am Heart J 1985; 109:1114–6.

121. Nademanee K, Singh B, Callahan B, Hendrickson J A, Hershman J M. Amiodarone, thyroid hormone indexes and altered thyroid function: long-term serial effects in patients with cardiac arrhythmias. Am J Cardiol 1986; 58:981–6.

122. Jonckheer M H, Block P, Kaivers R, Wyffels G. Hyperthyroidism as a possible complication of the treatment of ischemic heart disease with amiodarone. Acta Cardiol (Brux) 1973; 28:192–200.

123. Poliker R, Goy J, Schlapfer J, et al. Effect of oral triiodothyronine during amiodarone treatment for ventricular premature complexes. Am J Cardiol 1986; 58:987–91.

124. Nademanee K, Piwonka R W, Singh B N, Hershman J M. Amiodarone and thyroid function. Prog Cardiovasc Dis 1989; 31:427–37.

125. Kaplan L J, Cappaert W E. Amiodarone keratopathy. Correlation to dosage and duration. Arch Ophthalmol 1982; 100:601–2.

126. Zipes D P, Troup P J. New antiarrhythmic agents: amiodarone, aprindine, disopyramide, ethmozine, mexiletine, tocainide, verapamil. Am J Cardiol 1978; 41:1005–24.

127. Geerts M L. Amiodarone pigmentation: an electron microscopic study. Arch Belg Dermatol Syphiligr 1971; 27:339–51.

128. Moysey J O, Jaggarao N S V, Grundy E N, Chamberlain D N. Amiodarone increases plasma digoxin concentrations. Br Med J 1981; 282:272.

129. Saal A K, Werner J A, Greene H L, Sears G K, Graham E L. Effects of amiodarone on serum quinidine and procainamide levels. Am J Cardiol 1984; 53:1264–7.

130. Hamer A, Peter T, Mandel W J, Scheinman M M, Weiss D. The potentiation of warfarin anticoagulation by amiodarone. Circulation 1982; 65:1025–9.

31

Moricizine

Dennis S. Miura

Albert Einstein College of Medicine
Bronx, New York

Kenneth H. Dangman

College of Physicians and Surgeons, Columbia University
New York, New York

INTRODUCTION

Recently a new phenothiazine derivative with unique antiarrhythmic properties has been approved for clinical use in the United States. This agent, moricizine (ethmozine), was initially synthesized in the Soviet Union in 1964, with clinical development in that country from 1966 to 1971 (1,2). Moricizine has been noted by a variety of names in the literature, including EN-313, ethmozine, ethmosine, aetmozine, etmosin, ethmozin, ethmosin, and carbazin. Ethmozine was used as the generic name before its approval for clinical use as an antiarrhythmic agent in the United States; now it is the brand name with moricizine as the generic name (3). The chemical structure is noted in Figure 1. The drug appears to have antiarrhythmic efficacy in a wide variety of ventricular as well as supraventricular arrhythmias (4–20).

CARDIAC ELECTROPHYSIOLOGY

Cellular Mechanisms

The effects of moricizine on cardiac tissues have been extensively described in the literature (21–25). It appears to be a class I antiarrhythmic agent with dose-dependent effects on the maximal upstroke velocity (dV/dt_{max}) of phase 0 of the action potential. At high doses there is a slowing of conduction of the cardiac impulse throughout the conduction system and myocardial tissues. These effects appear to be manifest in the ischemic zone of myocardium during acute occlusion of a coronary artery (25). The blockade of the inward sodium channel during phase 0 by moricizine increases with increasing frequency of stimulation rate (24). The excitability of Purkinje fibers is depressed; that is, the threshold potential to initiate the "all-or-none" response is shifted to less negative potentials (26). Moricizine causes a more rapid repolarization of the action potential, leading to a shortening of phase 2 and 3. This results in a decrease in the action potential duration and effective refractory period (21–23). These effects at low doses of drug resemble lidocaine's effects, whereas higher doses of moricizine cause a conduction delay that mimics the effects of both the class Ia and Ic agents.

In spontaneously firing Purkinje fibers moricizine has a marked suppressant effect on

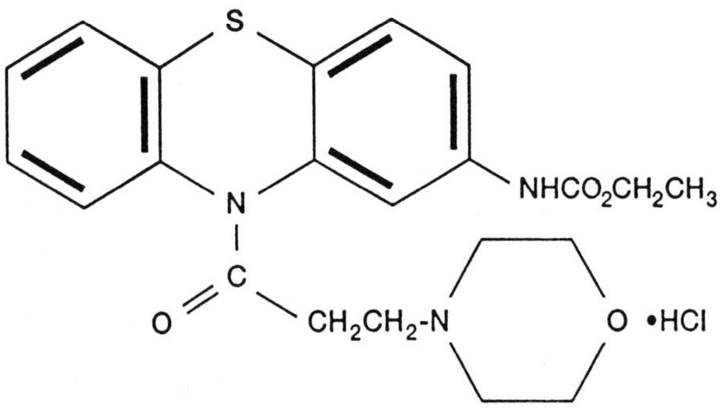

Figure 1 Chemical structure of moricizine.

normal automaticity (22). However, moricizine does not decrease the slope of phase 4 depolarization in normal Purkinje fibers (21–23,27). Thus the decrease in pacemaker activity in normal Purkinje fibers must be caused by a shift of the threshold potential to less negative values (22).

In addition, Dangman and Hoffman (22) studied the effects of moricizine on abnormal automaticity in Purkinje fibers with maximum diastolic potentials between -60 and -45 mV. Two models of abnormal automaticity were studied: the 24 hr infarct zone Purkinje fiber and the barium-depolarized Purkinje fiber. Moricizine slowed and abolished abnormal automaticity in both models (22). The drug exerted this effect by decreasing the slope of diastolic depolarization in the abnormally automatic fibers. In some fibers it also appeared to increase the threshold potential for phase 0. The decrease in phase 4 depolarization could be caused by inhibition of the sodium window current (22). The effects on threshold potential could be caused by inhibition of the inward calcium current by moricizine. In addition, moricizine reduces the amplitude of delayed afterdepolarizations and triggered ac-

tivity caused by ischemia or digitalis toxicity (22).

The cellular electrophysiologic properties of moricizine appear to support the clinical observation of its wide efficacy range. Suppression of arrhythmias, regardless of etiology, has been demonstrated in the laboratory. Suppression of reentrant arrhythmias may be due to dose-dependent effects on phase 0 depolarization and conduction velocity. Suppression of arrhythmias due to early afterdepolarizations may be due to effects on the action potential plateau. Suppression of ischemic arrhythmias caused by abnormal automaticity and delayed afterdepolarizations in partially depolarized cells may also be suppressed by moricizine. The mechanism for this action is probably a decrease in the slope of phase 4 depolarization and a shift of the threshold potential to less negative levels.

Clinical Electrophysiology

The effects of oral moricizine on clinical electrophysiologic parameters are predictable from the cellular studies noted previously (28–30). The effects of moricizine in patients with coronary artery disease and ventricular arrhythmias were to significantly shorten sinus cycle length and prolong PR (20%), QRS (19%), QTc, AH (17%), and HV (26%) intervals (30). The JT interval decreased but the QTc interval increased, which reflected the increase in QRS duration. These changes suggest moricizine classification as a Ib agent at low doses and a Ic agent at higher doses associated with QRS widening (Table 2).

Table 1 Cellular Electrophysiologic Properties of Moricizine

Phase 0	Concentration-dependent decrease
Phase 2	Speeds repolarization; suppresses early afterdepolarizations
Phase 3	Speeds repolarization
Phase 4	No effect on slope; suppresses abnormal automaticity

Table 2 Clinical Electrophysiologic Effects of Moricizine[a]

Parameter	Effect
Sinus cycle length	−
PR interval	+
AH interval	+
HV interval	+
QRS interval	+
QT_c	+
JT interval	−

[a]decrease (−); increase (+)

Table 3 Clinical Pharmacokinetics of Moricizine

Dose	200–400 mg PO three times a day
Bioavailability	38%
Metabolism	Hepatic
Protein binding	95%
Elimination $t_{1/2}$	2–6 hr (84 hr for metabolites)

Studies published in the Soviet Union of the effects of moricizine given intravenously were reviewed by Bigger (30). Various types of cardiac arrhythmias in 235 patients aged 13–77 years were noted in nine studies. In most studies the drug showed intraatrial and AV nodal slowing of conduction. Conduction in aberrant pathways was prolonged. The effects of moricizine on AV reciprocating tachycardias in 16 patients with bypass tracts were reported by Chazov et al. (14) Intravenous moricizine, 1.5–2 mg/kg, terminated inducible sustained supraventricular tachycardia in 9 of 14 patients. The drug prevented induction of the supraventricular tachycardia in 8 patients. The SVT rate was slowed by 10% by moricizine, and it increased PA, AH, and PR intervals. No significant effects were noted on HV, QRS, or QT intervals at doses that terminated the arrhythmia.

The effects of moricizine in patients with sinus node dysfunction were variable. Rozenshtraukh (31) reported that 4 of 10 patients with sinus node dysfunction who were given moricizine (1.5–2.0 mg/kg) had marked increases in sinus cycle time and sinus node recovery times. In addition, 3 of these 4 patients developed second-degree SA block.

Similarly, Rakovec et al. (32) showed marked increases in sinus node recovery times after intravenous moricizine. The other 6 patients in their study had increases in sinoatrial conduction times and sinus cycle length.

CLINICAL PHARMACOKINETICS

Moricizine is approved for clinical use in the treatment of documented ventricular arrhyth-

mias, such as sustained ventricular tachycardia, that in the judgment of the physician are life threatening. Moricizine is an orally active antiarrhythmic agent available in tablets of 200, 250, and 300 mg with usual adult doses of 600–900 mg daily in divided doses on an 8 hr schedule (Table 3) (33–35).

Moricizine is rapidly absorbed after oral administration, with peak blood levels reached in 0.8–2.0 hr. Because of the rapid and extensive metabolism of the drug in the liver, the bioavailability is about 38%. The metabolites of moricizine have not been well studied for their antiarrhythmic activity. The volume of distribution of the agent is about 300 L, suggesting extensive tissue binding. The plasma half-life ($t_{1/2}$) is 1.5–3.5 hr, with a range from 1 to 6 hr in normal volunteers.

Drug Interactions

Drug interactions between moricizine and digoxin have been examined. No significant changes in digoxin concentrations were noted at moricizine doses suppressing ventricular arrhythmias (36,37). A trend toward a slightly higher serum digoxin level was noted during the initial 2 weeks of therapy with moricizine. Although no significant direct drug-drug interactions were seen, the electrophysiologic effects appeared to be additive. There are reports of an increase in PR interval and slowing of conduction through the AV node.

Cimetidine has been reported to decrease moricizine metabolism by 48% and increase mean half-life 35% (38). No changes were reported on the surface ECG, however.

Moricizine, by increasing hepatic metabolism, has been reported to increase the rate of theophylline metabolism (34). Pretreatment of healthy volunteers with moricizine for 2 weeks

Table 4 Moricizine Effect on Hemodynamics and LV Function

Variable	Baseline	Maximum change, mean
Heart rate, beats/min	73	4.8
BP, mmHg		
Systolic	127	3.7
Diastolic	79	1.6
SV, ml	68	-0.5
LVEF, %	47	-0.7
CI, L/min/m^2	3	0.6
SVR, dynes-sec-cm^5	1626	-51
Mean PAP, mmHg	23	1.4
PCWP, mmHg	14	1.0
PVR, dynes-sec-cm^5	234	-23

Source: From Reference 41.

increased clearance of a single oral dose of theophylline by 46–68% and decreased the elimination half-life by 20–34%. These effects have led to the suggestion that concomitantly administered agents that are metabolized in the liver be monitored.

Hemodynamic Effects

Since many patients with serious ventricular tachyarrhythmias have left ventricular dysfunction, the effects of antiarrhythmic agents on left ventricular function is of concern. Moricizine in many studies has been found not to significantly effect left ventricular function (Tables 4 and 5) (39–41). No change in left ventricular ejection fraction (LVEF) was noted in patients evaluated by two-dimensional echocardiography during moricizine therapy (39–41).

LVEF was assessed in patients treated with moricizine, who did not have a significant changes as determined by radionuclide studies

(39). When compared to baseline or placebo, moricizine did not significantly change measured left ventricular hemodynamic parameters (Tables 4 and 5) in 194 patients (39–41). A recent review by Podrid and Bean (40) of 1072 patients treated with moricizine in various clinical trials suggested that congestive heart failure occurred with greater frequency de novo rather than being drug induced (15 versus 0.8%).

ANTIARRHYTHMIC EFFECTS OF MORICIZINE

Ventricular Arrhythmias

The antiarrhythmic efficacy of moricizine in suppression of ventricular arrhythmias was evaluated in clinical trials sponsored by Du-Pont Pharmaceuticals. Morganroth (42) reviewed the data from various clinical trials in 1072 patients treated with moricizine through February 1987. Dose range studies determined that the minimally effective dosage of moricizine was 600 mg/day in divided doses. This was similar to the results reported from the Cardiac Arrhythmia Pilot Study (CAPS) (43). CAPS was a placebo-controlled trial in which patients with ventricular arrhythmias following myocardial infarction were studied with and without antiarrhythmic intervention. One group of patients in this trial received from 600 to 750 mg/day of moricizine, with the optimal dosage range from 600 to 900 mg/day, with

Table 5 Moricizine Effect on LVEF (*N* = 156)

Baseline LVEF (%)	Number of patients	Baseline mean (%)	Moricizine mean (%)
<30	25	22	23
>30–39	26	36	37
>40	105	55	54

Source: From Reference 41.

Table 6 Efficacy of Moricizine During Oral Therapy of Nonmalignant Ventricular Arrhythmias

Author	Patients	Dose	Duration of therapy	Efficacy (%)	Criteria of efficacy (%)
Baker et al. (46)	19	600–1050 mg	4 weeks	5/19 (79)	>80 PVC
Gear et al. (47)	20	600–900 mg	6 months	11/17 (65)	>75 PVC
				7/13 (54)	100 VT
Kennedy et al. (48)	21	300–750 mg	1 week	12/21 (57)	
Kennedy et al. (19)	13	10 mg/kg	2 weeks	10/13 (77)	>90 PVC
				9/10 (90)	>90 VT
Kurbanov and Mazur (49)	44	600–800 mg	5–6 days	29/44 (66)	>100 PVC
				7/8 (88)	>100 VT
Podrid et al. (13)	37	225/600 mg	4–9 days	2/10 (20)	>50 PVC
				14/26 (54)	>50 VT
Pratt et al. (17)	39	300–1500 mg	1 week/6 months	28/39 (72)	>70 PVC
				15/19 (70)	100 VT
Pratt et al. (50)	50	10.0–14.6 mg/kg	3 months	11/22 (50)	>90 PVC
				15/22 (68)	100 VT
Salerno et al. (51)	10	12.4–15.7 mg/kg	10 days	7/8 (88)	>80 PVC
				4/6 (67)	100 VT
Singh et al. (52)	20	6.0–15.0	4 weeks	10/20 (50)	>65 PVC
Yepsen et al. (53)	32	9–15 mg/kg	4 months	22/32 (69)	>75 PVC
				14/19 (74)	100 VT

PVC = premature ventricular contraction; VT = ventricular tachycardia.
Source: From Reference 45.

little increase in efficacy of ventricular arrhythmia suppression above doses of 900 mg/day.

The onset of antiarrhythmic action of moricizine for a 75% suppression of ventricular arrhythmias appears to occur about 16–20 hr after initiation of dosing in a three times per day schedule (42). This effect suggests that there is a minimal concentration versus dose requirement or that metabolites may play a role in its antiarrhythmic efficacy.

A summary of the therapeutic efficacy of moricizine in patients with nonmalignant ventricular arrhythmias is shown in Table 6. Moricizine at 6.0–15.0 mg/kg/day in divided doses showed suppression of greater than 80% of premature ventricular contractions in 50–88% of patients. Nonsustained ventricular tachycardia was abolished in 68–100% of the patients reported. This antiarrhythmic effect of moricizine was maintained in several long-term studies (50,52–54). The efficacy of moricizine in suppression of ventricular arrhythmias in patients following myocardial infarction is being evaluated in the Cardiac

Table 7 Efficacy of Moricizine During Oral Therapy of Malignant Ventricular Arrhythmias

Author	Patients	Dose	Duration of therapy	Efficacy (%)	Criteria of efficacy (%)
Hession et al.(54)	82	600–1200 mg	5 days	31/75 (44)	>90 VT suppression
Calvo et al.(55)	7	11.5 mg/kg	5 days	3/7	—[a]
Doherty et al.(56)	6	10.0 mg/kg	5.6	1/6	—[a]
Hession et al.(54)	12	600–1200	5 days	1/12	—[a]
Mann et al.(57)	10	11.1 mg/kg	3 days	3/10	—[a]
Wyndham et al.(58)	33	10–15 mg/kg	3 days	6/33	—[a]

[a]Noninducible on drug at programmed electrical stimulation study.
Source: From Reference 45.

Table 8 Efficacy of Moricizine During Oral Therapy of Supraventricular Arrhythmias

Author	Patients	Dose	Duration of Therapy	Arrhythmia	Efficacy (% response)
Evans et al.(59)	4	9.75–15 mg/kg	1–12 months	Ectopic atrial tachycardia	75
Zhivoderoy et al.(60)	3	400–600 mg/day	5–9 days	PAC	100
	2			PSVT	50
	4			AF	50
Korkushko et al.(61)	23	300–450	14 days	PAC	52
Mazur et al.(62)	5	7.3–13.6 mg/kg.	3–5 days	PAC	20
	5			PSVT	40
	2			AF	100
	1			AT	100
Morganroth et al.(12)	8	2.4–11.2 mg/kg	7 days	PAC	75
Chazov et al.(14)	9	1.5–2.0 mg/mg IV	—	AVNRT	67
Chazov et al.(15)	14	1.5–2.0 mg/kg IV	—	PSVT in WPW	64
Shugushey et al.(63)	23	150 mg IV	—	PSVT	75
Shugushey et al.(64)	12	2.0 mg/kg IV	—	AVNRT	67

PAC = premature atrial contraction; PSVT = paroxysmal supraventricular tachycardia; AF = atrial fibrillation; AT = atrial tachycardia; AVNRT = AV nodal reentry tachycardia; WPW = Wolff-Parkinson-White syndrome.
Source: From Reference 45.

Arrhythmia Suppression Trial (CAST) (44). Preliminary results suggest that the agent is not as proarrhythmic as flecainide and encainide, class Ic agents, which were terminated in the CAST study in April 1989. These Ic agents, although extremely successful in suppressing ventricular arrhythmias, appeared to increase the incidence of sudden death and total mortality compared to placebo. The results of the moricizine versus placebo limb to assess the efficacy of antiarrhythmic therapy in decreasing long-term mortality will be available within the next 2 years.

Moricizine has been studied in patients with life-threatening ventricular arrhythmis. Several studies, shown in Table 7 evaluated the efficacy of oral moricizine in preventing the inducibility of sustained ventricular tachycardia in the electrophysiology laboratory. Moricizine appears to prevent the induction of these life-threatening arrhythmias in 8–43% of patients (55–59). Using Holter monitoring techniques, Hession et al. (54) reported that moricizine at 600–1200 mg/day has an effi-

cacy of 44%, with >50% suppression of premature ventricular contractions and >90% suppression of ventricular tachycardia.

Supraventricular Arrhythmias

Uncontrolled clinical reports have suggested that moricizine may have efficacy in a variety of supraventricular arrhythmias. A report of the effects on the sinus node function was made by Rakovec et al. (32). They reported increases in sinus node recovery times and sinoatrial conduction times due to intravenous moricizine. Rozenshtraukh (31) noted the moricizine given intravenously suppressed sinus node function, especially in patients with underlying sinus node dysfunction.

Table 8 is a summary of various reports of the efficacy of moricizine in a variety of supraventricular arrhythmias. Short-term studies with moricizine showed greater than 50% suppression of specific atrial arrhythmias in 20–100% of patients. Invasive studies in patients with recurrent reentry atrial dysrhythmias suggest that moricizine is effective in terminating and preventing reinduction of these arrhythmias (14,15,63,64).

ADVERSE EFFECTS

Moricizine appears to be well tolerated in the clinical doses effective against ventricular arrhythmias. The noncardiac side effects summarized in Table 9 are generally mild and resolve on dose reduction or discontinuation. Table 9 summarizes all reported side effects in the data base of 1256 patients (65). Caution should be used in the interpretation of these data since a very small percentage of patients actually had the drug discontinued because of the adverse side effects reported. The best indication of the incidence of adverse reactions was reported in the CAPS in which the adverse reactions of moricizine were compared to those of placebo (Table 10). The incidence of adverse reactions in the placebo group was surprisingly high in all categories reported.

Table 9 Moricizine Side Effects

Adverse effect	Reported, $n = 1256$ (%)
Dizziness	15.1
Nausea	9.6
Headache	8.0
Fatigue	5.9
Palpitations	5.8
Dyspnea	5.7
Sustained VT	4.3
Hypesthesia	3.5
Abdominal pain	3.2
Dyspepsia	3.1
Vomiting	3.1
Sweating	2.9
Chest pain (CV)	2.8
Asthenia	2.7
Chest pain (non CV)	2.6
Nervousness	2.5
VT	2.5
Paresthesia	2.4
Cardiac failure	2.4
Musculoskeletal	2.2
Diarrhea	2.2
Dry mouth	2.1
Death	2.1
Sleep disorder	2.1

Source: From Reference 65.

Table 10 Noncardiac Adverse Effects During CAPS at 1 Year

	Patients with Adverse effects	
Adverse effects	Moricizine ($n = 77$)	Placebo ($n = 87$)
Dizziness	10	0
Respiratory	8	5
Cutaneous	6	3
Gastrointestinal	26	21
Genitourinary	18	11
Neurologic	34	38
Other	44	43

Only dizziness was a statistically important side effect of moricizine.

SUMMARY

Moricizine is a new antiarrhythmic agent with wide efficacy in a variety of clinical arrhythmias. It has efficacy against premature ventricular contractions that are nonmalignant. It has modest efficacy in arrhythmias that are life threatening. Extensive clinical trials have shown that the drug is well tolerated with minimal long-term toxic effects. The greatest advantage of moricizine appears to be in its minimal cardiodepressant and hemodynamic effects.

Moricizine has been reported to be effective in treating patients with a variety of supraventricular arrhythmias. It appears to be most efficacious in the reentry type tachyarrhythmias.

The long-term efficacy and safely of moricizine now appears to be tied to the results of the Cardiac Arrhythmia Suppression Trial. The class Ic agents, flecainide and encainide, have been shown to increase mortality when given to patients with asymptomatic ventricular arrhythmias and assessed with Holter monitoring techniques. The effects of moricizine on the treatment of ventricular arrhythmias in patients after myocardial infarction remain to be determined.

ACKNOWLEDGMENT

Supported in part by NIH Grant HL 24354.

REFERENCES

1. Gritsenko A N, Ermakova Z I, Zhuravlev S V. The synthesis of ethmozine—a new preparation with antiarrhythmic action. Khim Farmat Zh 1972; 6:17–9.

2. Kaverina N V, Senova Z P, Vikhlyaev Y I, et al. On the antiarrhythmic properties of ethmozine. Farmakol Toksikol 1970; 33:693–7.

3. Mahler S A, Borland R M. Clinical development of moricizine as an antiarrhythmic agent. Am J Cardiol 1990; 65:11D–14D.

4. Kaverina N V, Senova Z P, Mitrofanov V, et al. On the pharmacology of ethmosine—a new antiarrhythmic drug. Farmakol Toksikol 1972; 35:182–5.

5. Senova Z P, Lvov M V. On the mode of antiarrhythmic action of aetmozine. Farmakol Toksikol 1973; 36:703–6.

6. Ostapyuk F E. The effect of ethmozine on cardiac arrhythmias in patients with coronary insufficiency, myocardial infarction, and cardiosclerosis. Terep Arkh 1969; 41:73–7.

7. Zaslavskaya R M, Skorobogatora I F, Kulbanovskaya E Y. Ethmosine medication of patients with deranged rhythm of the cardiac activity. Soretskaya Mcd 1969; 32:59–62.

8. Gomzyakova T G. Results of clinical studies of the antiarrhythmic drug carbazin (ethmozin). Vrach Delo 1970; 4:62–4.

9. Votchal B E, Lozinskii L G. Effectiveness of the new antiarrhythmic compound ethmozine. Klin Med 1971; 10:16–21.

10. Seňova Z P. Antiarrhythmic properties of phenothiazine derivatives. Success in creating new medicinal substances. Kharkevich (Moscow) 1974; 288–300.

11. Zakusov V V. Principles of studies of pharmacological substances. Vestn Akad Med Nauk SSSR 1976; 9:7–14.

12. Morganroth J, Pearlman A J, Dunkman W B, et al. Ethmozine: a new antiarrhythmic agent developed in the USSR: efficacy and tolerance. Am Heart J 1979; 98:621–8.

13. Podrid P J, Lyakishev A, Lown B, et al. Ethmozine, a new antiarrhythmic drug for suppressing ventricular premature complexes. Circulation 1980; 61:450–7.

14. Chazov E I, Shugushev K K, Rozenshtraukh L V. Ethmozine. I. Effects of intravenous drug administration of paroxysmal supraventricular tachycardia in the ventricular preexcitation syndrome. Am Heart J 1984; 108:475–82.

15. Chazov E I, Rozenshtraukh L V, Shugushev K K. Ethmozine. II. Effects of intravenous drug administration on atrioventricular nodal reentrant tachycardia. Am Heart J 1984; 108:483–9.

16. Pratt C M, Young J B, Francis M L, et al. Comparative effect of disopyramide and ethmozine in suppressing complex ventricular arrhythmias by use of a double-blind, placebo-controlled, longitudinal crossover design. Circulation 1984; 69:288–97.

17. Pratt C M, Yepsen S C, Taylor A A, et al. Ethmozine suppression of single and repetitive ventricular premature depolarization during therapy: documentation of efficacy and long term safety. Am Heart J 1983; 106:85–91.

18. Butman S M, Knoll M L, Gardin J M. Comparison of ethmozine to propranolol and combination for ventricular arrhythmias. Am J Cardiol 1987; 60:603–7.

19. Kennedy H L, DeMaria A N, Sprague M K, et al. Comparative efficacy of moricizine and quinidine for benign and potentially lethal ventricular arrhythmias. Am J Noninvasive Cardiol 1988; 2:98–105.

20. Miura D S, Wynn J, Torres V, et al. Antiarrhythmic efficacy of ethmozine in patients with ventricular tachycardia as determined by programmed electrical stimulation. Am Heart J 1986; 111:661–6.

21. Danilo P, Langan W B, Rosen M R, et al. Effects of the phenothiazine derivative analog EN-313 on ventricular arrhythmias in dogs. Eur J Pharmacol 1977; 45:127–39.

22. Dangman K H, Hoffman B F. Antiarrhythmic effects of ethmozine in cardiac Purkinje fibers: suppression of antomaticity and abolition of triggering. J. Pharmacol Exp Ther 1983; 227:578–86.

23. Tsuji Y, Nishimura M, Osada M, et al. Membrane action of ethmozin on normoxic and hypoxic canine Purkinje fibers. J Cardiovasc Pharmacol 1983; 5:961–7.

24. Makielski J C, Undrovinas A I, Hanck D A, et al. Use-dependent block of sodium current by ethmozin in voltage-clamped internally perfused canine cardiac Purkinje cells. J Mol Cell Cardiol 1988; 20:255–65.

25. Rozenshtraukh L V, Ruffy R, Elharrar V, et al. Electrophysiologic effects of ethmozine on the dog's myocardium. Kardiologiia 1979; 19:63–72.

26. Arnsdorf M F, Sawicki G J. Effects of ethmozine on excitability in sheep Purkinje fi-

bers: the balance among active and passive cellular properties which comprise the electrophysiologic matrix. J Pharmacol Exp Ther 1989; 248:1158–66.

27. Dremin S A, Aniukhovskii E P, Rozenshtraukh L V, et al. Action of ethacizin on normal and anomalous forms of Purkinje fiber automaticity in the dog. Kardiologiia 1986; 26:10–5.

28. Smetner A S, Shugushev K K, Rosenshtraukh L V. Clinical electrophysiologic and antiarrhythmic efficacy of moricizine HCl. Am J Cardiol 1987; 60:40F–44F.

29. Wyndham C R C, Pratt C M, Mann D E, et al. Electrophysiology of ethmozine (moricizine HCl) for ventricular tachycardia. Am J Cardiol 1987; 60:67F–72F.

30. Bigger J T. Cardiac electrophysiologic effects of moricizine hydrochloride. Am J Cardiol 1990; 65:15D–20D.

31. Rozenshtraukh L V. Effect of ethmozine on the autonomic function of the sinoatrial node and sinoatrial conduction in patients with normal and impaired function of the sinoatrial node. Kardiologiia 1983; 23:47–50.

32. Rakovec P, Jakopin J, Rode P, et al. Electrophysiological effects of ethmozin on sinus nodal function in patients with and without sinus node dysfunction. Eur Heart J 1984; 5:243–6.

33. Woolsley R L, Morganroth J, Forgoros R N, et al. Pharmacokinetics of moricizine HCl. Am J Cardiol 1987; 60:35F–39F.

34. Siddoway L A, Schwartz S L, Barbey J T, et al. Clinical pharmacokinetics of moricizine. Am J Cardiol 1990; 65:21D–25D.

35. Ethmozine package insert. DuPont Pharmaceuticals, 1990.

36. Kennedy H L, Sprague M K, Redd R M, et al. Serium digoxin concentrations during ethmozine therapy. Am Heart J 1986; 111:667–72.

37. Antman E M, Arnold J M O, Friedman P L, et al. Drug interactions with cardiac glycosides: evaluation of a possible digoxin-ethmozine pharmacokinetic interaction. J Cardiovasc Pharmacol 1987; 9:622–7.

38. Biollaz J, Shaheen O, Wood A J J. Cimetidine inhibition of ethmozine metabolism. Clin Pharmacol Ther 1985; 37:665–8.

39. Pratt C M, Podrid P J, Seals A A, et al. Effects of ethmozine (moricizine HCl) on ventricular function using echocardiographic hemodynamic and radionuclide assessment. Am J Cardiol 1987; 60:73F–78F.

40. Podrid P J, Bean S L. Antiarrhythmic drug therapy for congestive heart failure with focus on moricizine. Am J Cardiol 1990; 65:56D–64D.

41. Ethmozine (moricizine HCl) product monograph, DuPont Pharmaceuticals, p. 19.

42. Morganroth J. Dose effect of moricizine on suppression of ventricular arrhythmias. Am J Cardiol 1990; 65:26D–31D.

43. The CAPS Investigators. The Cardiac Arrhythmia Pilot Study. Am J Cardiol 1984; 54:31–6.

44. The Cardiac Arrhythmia Suppression Trial (CAST) Investigators. Preliminary report: effect of encainide and flecainide on mortality in a randomized trial of arrhythmia suppression after myocardial infarction. N Engl J Med 1989; 321:406–12.

45. Fitton A, Buckley M M T. Moricizine. A review of its pharmacological properties, and therapeutic efficacy in cardiac arrhythmias. Drugs 1990; 40:138–67.

46. Baker B J, Dinh H, Franciosa J A. Moricizine (ethmozine): dose titration and long term efficacy (abstract). Clin Pharmacol Ther 1985; 37:181.

47. Gear K, Marcus F I, Huang S K, et al. Ethmozine for ventricular premature conmplexes. Am J Cardiol 1986; 57:947–9.

48. Kennedy H L, Pescarmona J E, Joyner V, et al. The efficacy and tolerance of ethmozin for chronic ventricular ectopy (abstract). Circulation 1978; 58(Suppl.II):177.

49. Kurbanov R D, Mazur N A. Results of the long-term treatment with ethmozine of patients with ventricular cardiac arrhythmias. Kardiologiia 1983; 23:51–5.

50. Pratt C M, Young J B, Wierman A M, et al. Complex ventricular arrhythmias associated with the mitral valve prolapse syndrome. Effectiveness of moricizine (ethmozine) in patients resistant to conventional antiarrhythmics. Am J Med 1986; 80:626–32.

51. Salerno D M, Sharkey P J, Granrud G A, et al. Efficacy, safety, hemodynamic effects, and pharmacokinetics of high-dose moricizine during short- and long-term therapy. Clin Pharmacol Ther 1987; 42:201–9.

52. Singh S N, DiBianco R, Gottdiener J S, et al. Effect of moricizine hydrochloride in reducing chronic high-frequency ventricular arrhythmia: results of a prospective, controlled trial. Am J Cardiol 1984; 53:745–50.

53. Yepsen S C, Pratt C M, English L J, et al. Ethmozine: a unique antiarrhythmic drug with

combined efficacy and excellent tolerance (abstract). Clin Res 1982; 30:836A.

54. Hession M J, Lampert S, Podrid P J, et al. Ethmozine (moricizine HCl) therapy for complex ventricular arrhythmias. Am J Cardiol 1987; 60:59F–66F.

55. Calvo R, Saksena S, Barr M J. Electrophysiologic effects, efficacy, and safety of oral moricizine hydrochloride in sustained ventricular tachycardia (abstract). Clin Pharmacol Ther 1985; 37:186.

56. Doherty J U, Rogers D P, Waxman H L, et al. Electrophysiologic properties and efficacy of ethmozine in sustained ventricular tachycardia (abstract). Circulation 1984; 70(Suppl. II):1758.

57. Mann D E, Luck J C, Pratt C M, et al. Electrophysiologic evaluation of the efficacy of ethmozine in patients with ventricular tachycardia (abstract) J Am Coll Cardiol 1984; 3:537.

58. Wyndham C R C, Pratt C M, Mann D E, et al. Electrophysiology of ethmozine (moricizine HCl) for ventricular tachycardia. Am J Cardiol 1987; 60:67F–72F.

59. Evans V L, Garson A, Smith R T, et al. Ethmozine (moricizine HCl): a promising drug for "automatic" atrial ectopic tachycardia. Am J Cardiol 1987; 60:83F–86F.

60. Zhivoderov V M, Zakhorov V N, Doschitsin VL, et al. The antiarrhythmic efficacy of ethmozine, cordarone and rhythmodan in the treatment of patients with ischaemic heart disease. Kardiologiia 1981; 21:41–4.

61. Korkushko O V, Butenko A G, Kaukenas Y K. Efficacy and characteristic of action of ethmozine in the treatment of extrasystole in middle-aged and elderly patients. Terap Arkh 1986; 58:65–70.

62. Mazur N A, Lyakishev A A, Kurbanov R D. Experience in the clinical use of ethmozine in various disturbances of cardiac rhythm. Kardiologiia 1980; 20:44–9.

63. Shugushev K K, Rozenstraukh L V, Smetnev A S. Electrophysiological study of the antiarrhythmic activity of ethmozine and its diethylamine analogue in patients with Wolff-Parkinson-White syndrome. Terap Arkh 1982; 54:84–91.

64. Shugushev K K, Smetnev A S, Rozenshtraukh L V. Action of ethmozine in patients with paroxysmal atrioventricular nodal tachycardia. Kardiologiia 1982; 22:72–7.

65. Kennedy H L. Noncardiac adverse effects and organ toxicity of moricizine during short- and long-term studies. Am J Cardiol 1990; 65:47D–50D.

32

Class II Drugs

Dennis S. Miura and William H. Frishman

*Albert Einstein College of Medicine
Bronx, New York*

Kenneth H. Dangman

*College of Physicians and Surgeons, Columbia University
New York, New York*

INTRODUCTION

β-Adrenergic receptor blocking agents have been introduced to medicine for a variety of clinical applications. These agents as a group have defined our knowledge of the adrenergic receptor. Variations in the properties of these β-adrenoceptor blocking drugs have been used to classify these receptors as well as the adrenoceptor agonists. When Ahlquist used catecholamines to stimulate a number of physiologic responses in 1948, he used this as the basis of the initial subtypes, termed α- and β-receptors (1). Subsequent investigators found that the β-receptors can be further differentiated into subtypes called $β_1$ and $β_2$ and found that some agents specific to the β-adrenergic receptor may also have excitatory as well as inhibitory effects. In addition, some β-blocking agents may have membrane-stabilizing or antiarrhythmic effects. See Table 1, which shows various agents and their relative effects, including presence or absence of intrinsic sympathomimetic activity (ISA) or partial β-adrenoceptor agonist activity and membrane-stabilizing activity (MSA).

β-Blockers are approved for use in a variety of clinical conditions. These include propra-

nolol for angina pectoris, arrhythmias, hypertension, benign essential tremors, prevention of migraine headaches, and in survivors of myocardial infarction to reduce mortality; timolol for hypertension, patients after a myocardial infarction, and open-angle glaucoma; atenolol and metoprolol for hypertension, angina, reducing risk of mortality and reinfarction in survivors of myocardial infarction; nadolol for hypertension and angina; acebutol for hypertension and ventricular arrhythmias; and pindolol and penbutolol for hypertension (3–7).

Extensive clinical experience has shown that there appears to be no significant advantage of one agent over another. Therefore, when any given agent is carefully titrated for the treatment arrhythmias, hypertension, or angina, it can be effective in any given patient. The limitations of clinical use continue to be side effects and adverse reactions.

BASIC PHARMACOLOGY AND ELECTROPHYSIOLOGY OF β-BLOCKING AGENTS

Antiarrhythmic drugs are thought to work by directly altering the electrophysiology of

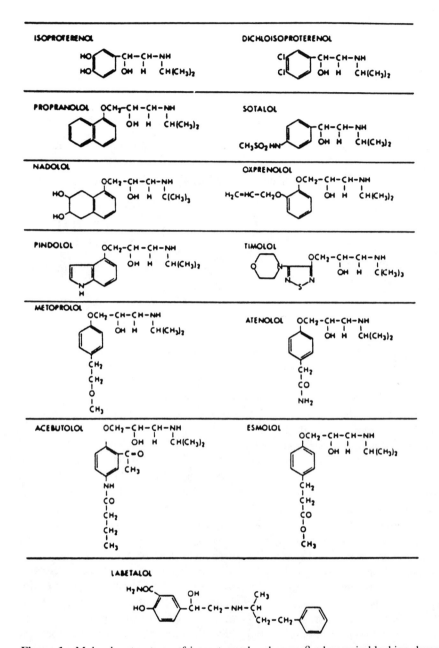

Figure 1 Molecular structures of isoproterenol and some β-adrenergic blocking drugs.

abnormal myocardial cells. The important cellular actions of these drugs are identified as class I effects, inhibition of the fast inward (sodium) current; class II effects, inhibition of the arrhythmogenic effects of the sympathetic nervous system and circulatory catecholamines; class III effects, increasing action potential duration; and class IV effects, inhibition of slow inward (calcium) current (8–10).

This chapter focuses on the electrophysiologic and antiarrhythmic properties of class II drugs. A "pure" class II drug is expected to be able to reduce or prevent arrhythmias provoked by catecholamine administration or increased sympathetic tone (11). The arrhythmogenic effects of epinephrine or norepinephrine can be mediated by either α- or β-receptor activation, and thus the original

Table 1 Classification Scheme of β-Adrenoceptor Blocking Agents

β-blockade	Partial Agonist Effect	Membrane-stabilizing effect
Nonselective		
Propranolol	−	+
Oxprenolol	+	+
Pindolol	+	
Alprenolol		
Sotalol	−	+
Timolol		
Esmolol		
Nadolol		
Carteolol		
Penbutolol		
Selective		
Acebutolol	+	+
Practolol	+	−
Atenolol	−	−
Metoprolol		

definition of the class II agents enunciated by Vaughan Williams encompassed blockers of both types of receptor. However, α-blockers are not used for antiarrhythmic actions in the clinic and so the class II drugs today effectively consist only of the β-adrenergic blockers (3,9–12).

Many of the drugs that are classed as class II β-blockers also exert class I or class II antiarrhythmic effects. Some authors have suggested that the class I and/or III effects of β-blockers are much less important than their class II effects for reduction of arrhythmias (13–16). These direct effects of β-adrenergic blockers can be significant factors for the in vivo actions of these drugs. For example, the class I antiarrhythmic effects of some β-blockers (e.g., propranolol, alprenolol, and metoprolol) may help to reduce arrhythmias caused by digitalis intoxication or myocardial infarction or help synergistically to elevate ventricular fibrillation thresholds (1–18). Propranolol plasma concentrations > 1 mg/L (3×10^{-6} M) are often required for antiarrhythmic effects, and a "substantial" β-blockade occurs at 0.1–0.3 mg/L ($<10^{-6}$ M) (19). Likewise, the class III effects of sotalol (20,21) may help reduce arrhythmias provoked

by programmed extrastimulus (PES) techniques (22). Some antiarrhythmic effects of β-blockers can be better explained by class III effects than class II effects (22,23). Thus combining class II with class I or III antiarrhythmic drug effects may enhance the efficacy of the drug on ventricular ectopic activity in the in situ heart.

CELLULAR ELECTROPHYSIOLOGY OF β-ADRENERGIC BLOCKING DRUGS

The cellular electrophysiologic effects of several of the β-adrenergic blocking drugs have been studied in isolated cardiac tissues.

Propranolol is the prototypical class II antiarrhythmic drug (8). It was shown to be a β-receptor blocking drug in 1964 (24). Propranolol is a "nonspecific" blocker. That is, it blocks both β_1- and β_2-receptors (25).

Transmembrane action potentials recorded from cardiac tissues can be significantly affected by propranolol in two ways. The drug can work "directly," by blocking ionic channels (e.g., sodium channels) in the sarcolemma, or it may work "indirectly," by blocking the effects of sympathetic or sympathomimetic stimulation of the β-receptors. In the literature, the direct effects are often referred to as "membrane-stabilizing effects" or "quinidinelike effects" (25). According to Davis and Temte (26), the indirect and direct effects of propranolol on cardiac tissue are dose dependent. Low concentrations of the drug (less than 1 μg/ml, or about 3 μM) produce significant β-receptor blockade, but this does not exert direct effects on transmembrane potentials of Purkinje fibers or myocardial cells. At higher concentrations propranolol is a local anesthetic drug; that is, it reduces the fast inward current carried by sodium (27,28). At concentrations above 1 μg/ml propranolol decreases dV/dt_{max} action potential amplitude, action potential duration, and conduction velocity in Purkinje tissue and myocardium (10,26–30). Recently it has been found that propranolol (10 μM) exerts use-dependent effects on dV/dt_{max} of cardiac action potentials (30).

Additionally propranolol may alter cardiac cellular electrophysiology by blocking the effects of catecholamines. These effects may be antiarrhythmic. For instance, diseased regions of the myocardium may contain partially depolarized cells with resting membrance potentials of -55 mV or less. These cells may be quiescent in the absence of catecholamines. If sympathetic tone is increased, slow-response action potentials may be induced in these zones of depolarized cells. Depending on the geometry of the diseased zone and the degree of coupling that exists to the more normal zones of the heart, different sorts of arrhythmias may result. These zones may produce ectopic activity if they develop (1) abnormal automaticity, (2) delayed afterdepolarizations and triggered activity, or (3) unidirectional conduction block, slow conduction, and reentrant excitation. It is likely that β-receptor blockade by propranolol could reduce arrhythmias if they depend on sympathetic tone to circulatory catecholamines (11–30).

Sotalol, or MJ-1999, was introduced in the mid-1960s as a β-adrenergic blocking compound (31). It is a "nonspecific" blocker in that it inhibits stimulation of both β_1- and β_2-adrenergic receptors (25). Sotalol does not exert intrinsic sympathomimetic actions, and most studies report that it does not have significant membrane-stablizing (local anesthetic) effects (32–37). It does, however, have significant class III antiarrhythmic effects on action potential duration (21–38). This class III effect is mediated through a reduction in the time-dependent outward potassium current $i_{K.2}$, as well as a small reduction in background potassium conductance, $i_{K.1}$ (36).

Labetalol is an antihypertensive drug with combined α- and β-adrenergic receptor blocking activity. It is devoid of intrinsic sympathometic activity (25). Labetalol has significant antiarrhythmic and antifibrillatory effects during myocardial ischemia and reperfusion (39). In isolated cardiac tissue labetalol produces electrophysiologic effects on transmembrane action potentials. Vaughan Williams et al. (8) studied rabbit ventricular muscle preparations and reported that labetalol at concentrations of 3–5 μM exerts significant local anesthetic effects on Purkinje fibers and working ventricular myocardial cells. They also reported that labetalol increases action potential duration ($APD_{50\%}$) of both types of cells. Thus labetalol has both class I and class III antiarrhythmic effects (10) in addition to class II activity.

Dilevalol is the R,R stereoisomer of labetalol. It has β-blocking activity equivalent to that of propranolol (30) but does not produce α-block (40,42). Dilevalol at 1 μM produces near maximal β-blockade but does not alter transmembrane action potentials or normal automaticity in Purkinje fibers (30). In concentrations of 10 μM dilevalol produced rate-dependent decreases in dV/dt_{max} and prolonged action potential duration of the Purkinje fibers. In contrast, low concentrations of dilevalol (10 nM to 0.1 μM) increased action potential duraction in ventricular muscle cells (30). This effect is consistent with the QT prolongation that occurs in vivo (43,44) after treatment with this drug.

Alprenolol is a nonselective β-blocking drug (i.e., it inhibits stimulation of both β_1- and β_2-receptors) that has some intrinsic sympathomimetic activity (25). Alprenolol exerts significant membrane-stabilizing effects. It reduces dV/dt_{max} in the rabbit atrium (38) and canine Purkinje fibers (45). These effects are use dependent (46). In addition, depolarized and ischemic myocardium appears to be more sensitive to alprenolol. Thus the drug's membrane depressant actions may contribute significantly to preventing or terminating arrhythmias in ischemic tissues (45).

Nadolol is a nonselective β-blocking drug that is devoid of intrinsic sympathomimetic activity and membrane-stabilizing effects (25). Nadolol at 1 μM has little effect on transmembrane action potentials recorded from normal canine Purkinje fibers (47,48). It does, however, appear to have relatively selective effects on partially depolarized cells studied under "ischemic" conditions (8).

CLINICAL ARRHYTHMIAS

β-Adrenoceptor blocking agents are competitive inhibitors of catecholamine binding at the β-adrenoceptor sites. A dose-response curve of the physiologic effects of catecholamine is shifted to the right by β-adrenoceptor blocking agents; that is, a higher concentration of catecholamines is required to elicit the same response in the presence of a β-receptor blocking agent.

Catecholamines increase the rate of phase 4 depolarization in pacemaker tissues. These effects are clinically manifest by an increase in the rate of impulse initiation and of conduction through the AV node and by shortened refractory periods. The effects of catecholamines on cardiac myocardial tissues additionally predispose the tissue to reentry arrhythmias and to lower ventricular fibrillation threshold (49–51). β-Adrenoceptor blocking agents inhibit the effects of catecholamines on myocardial tissues. These effects may inhibit the initiation of arrhythmias and, in addition, may modify other processes that may predispose ventricular muscle to arrhythmias, for example, ischemia and thyrotoxicosis. Most evidence suggests that these antiarrhythmic effects are mediated directly via β-blockade (52). When conditions of high sympathetic tone or high circulating catecholamines are present, β-blockers with and without ISA appear to have similar antiarrhythmic effects, and direct antiarrhythmic membrane-stabilizing actions appear to occur only at high dosages (53,54). Most direct membrane-stabilizing properties of β-adrenoceptor agents are quinidinelike in action. There is a suppression of rapid depolarization of phase 0 resulting in slowing of conduction velocity of the depolarization sequence in the heart. One β-blocker, sotalol, differs in this regard. It appears to have Vaughan Williams class III activity; that is, there is a prolongation of the action potential duration with prolongation of refractoriness (54). On the surface electrocardiogram a lengthening of the QT interval is seen.

The potency of the β-blocker is related to the quantity of drug that must be administered to inhibit the effects of the catecholamine agonist. Potency can be assessed by noting the dose of the drug that must be given to inhibit a tachycardia produced by an agonist or exercise (55,56). Potency varies from agent to agent, which in turn leads to differing doses. This, however, has no therapeutic relevance except on changing a given patient from one drug to another (55,56).

VENTRICULAR TACHYARRHYTHMIAS

Arrhythmias that originate in ventricular myocardial tissues in response to ischemia, stress, emotion, or exercise may often respond to β-adrenergic receptor blockade (57–59). Ventricular tachycardia is frequently seen in patients after a myocardial infarction (59–61). If sufficiently high sympathetic tone is present as one of the initiating factors, suppression of ventricular arrhythmias may occur with β-adrenergic blocking agents (56–62). Recently investigators have shifted their therapy of ventricular arrhythmias away from the use of antiarrhythmic agents (63–65). These concepts of treatment of ventricular tachyarrhythmias are a result of a multicenter study called the Cardiac Arrhythmia Suppression Trial (CAST) (65). The CAST study was based upon two previous trials: (1) the Multicenter Post Infarction Program (MPIP) (63) and (2) the Cardiac Arrhythmia Pilot Study (CAPS) (67). MPIP was a study of patients with a myocardial infarction and their prognosis. A 2 year survival following a myocardial infarction was best seen in patients who did not have low ejection fraction or runs of nonsustained ventricular tachycardia. An intermediate risk occurred in patients with one of these conditions, and the worst prognosis occurred in patients in whom both conditions were present. A clinical judgment was made in the past that used the logic that suppression of the ventricular tachyarrhythmias present in these patients would improve the outcome. Studies were presented showing the efficacy of various antiarrhythmic agents in suppressing ventricular arrhythmias after myocardial infarction.

However, a large-scale randomized control study was not available until the CAPS data were presented (67). These showed antiarrhythmic drug efficacy in suppressing ventricular arrhythmias in patients following myocardial infarction. The efficacy of these agents in suppressing ventricular arrhythmias ranged from 66 to 83%, and they were more effective than placebo (37%). The results further suggested that a large-scale trial (CAST) should be attempted since there were an insufficient number of patients in the trial to conclude that antiarrhythmic therapy was more effective than placebo in terms of long-term mortality. The CAST data, however, provided a surprising announcement in April 1989, in that the overall mortality associated with therapy using class Ic antiarrhythmic agents had a higher mortality (7.7 versus 3.3%) than placebo (65). The CAST criteria for drug efficacy included 80% suppression of ventricular premature contractions and 90–100% suppression of ventricular tachycardia. The incidence of sudden death was 4.5% in the encainide and flecainide group compared to a 1.2% rate in the placebo group. The moricizine arm of therapy is still continuing, however. These results of CAST II should be available within the next few years. Treatment of patients with ventricular arrhythmias following myocardial infarction has therefore shifted back to the early 1980s therapy, which demonstrated the efficacy of β-adrenoceptor blocking agents (55–58).

SUPRAVENTRICULAR TACHYCARDIAS

Arrhythmias that originate in the atria often respond clinically to β-adrenoceptor blocking agents (50,52,55). The exception to this therapy in supraventricular arrhythmias is multifocal atrial tachycardia associated with chronic pulmonary diseases. Use of β-blocking agents may in addition be useful in the diagnosis as well as therapy of these types of arrhythmias.

Sinus Tachycardia

This arrhythmia is usually associated with an underlying clinical cause, for example fever, anemia, thyrotoxicosis, or congestive heart failure. Therapy should be addressed at correcting the underlying condition. If the sinus tachycardia is complicating the clinical setting, such as angina in a patient with coronary artery disease, then treatment with a β-adrenoceptor blocking agent to slow the heart rate may be effective. Patients with pulmonary disease or congestive heart failure should generally not be treated with these agents since suppression of sympathetic tone may exacerbate these conditions. The exception may occur in some patients with cardiomyopathy that may respond to low-dose β-blocker therapy (59).

Supraventricular Ectopic Beats

These types of ectopic activity are similar to sinus tachycardia, in which therapy is directed at treating the underlying cause. There is no evidence that prophylactic β-blocker therapy may prevent the development of chronic atrial arrhythmias from occasional ectopic beats. Therefore treatment is directed only at symptomatic relief.

Paroxysmal Supraventricular Tachycardia

These arrhythmias, which are not associated with bypass tracts, may often respond to β-blockade therapy. β-blockers are known to increase conduction times through the AV node, prolonging refractoriness (60). Treatment with intravenous β-blockers is often more successful than vagal maneuvers (61). Chronic oral therapy is often successful in patients with frequent episodes of paroxysmal supraventricular tachycardia, particularly when the arrhythmia is associated with exercise, emotion, or stress (55–68).

Propranolol, when given at doses 50–100 times the catecholamine blocking dose, exhibits class Ia antiarrhythmic properties (60). This property may provide additional benefit in the treatment of supraventricular arrhythmias or in controlling ventricular response rates in chronic atrial fibrillation. The limitation of this approach to therapy is in patients with chronic lung disease or in hearts with depressed left ventricular function that depends on increased levels of adrenergic tone.

Sotalol is a β-blocking agent with additional class III properties that may often benefit patients with supraventricular tachycardias (69). When given acutely this agent prolongs atrial and ventricular refractory periods and the refractoriness of accessory pathways (70,71). This latter property suggest some efficacy in arrhythmias involving bypass tracts, which are unaffected by other β-blockers.

Chronic atrial fibrillation or atrial flutter may respond to β-blocker therapy in slowing AV nodal conduction and limiting ventricular response rates. These agents may be used concomitantly with digitalis to control ventricular response rates. The clinical limitations, however, are in patients with sick sinus or brady-tachy syndrome, in whom β-blockade may exacerbate the underlying clinical condition (56–58,61).

USE IN PATIENTS AFTER A MYOCARDIAL INFARCTION

β-Adrenergic receptor blocking agents have been demonstrated to be useful in patients after a myocardial infarction (56,57,72,73). These placebo-controlled long-term treatment trials have demonstrated a favorable effect of β-adrenergic blocking agents on total mortality and cardiovascular mortality, including sudden and nonsudden cardiac deaths, as well as the incidence of nonfatal reinfarction. These effects of the β-adrenergic blocking agents have provoked considerable interest in their mechanism of action. There is speculation about β-blocker effects on the reduction in oxygen demand of the heart, particularly on exercise and under sympathetic nervous system stress. Therefore there appears to be a decrease in resting heart rate, systolic blood pressure, and oxygen consumption. In addition there may be decreased episodes of silent ischemia (53–56). β-Adrenergic blocking agents appear to be effective in reducing these episodes, not necessarily associated with an increase in heart rate. Propranolol and timolol have been approved by the U.S. Food and Drug Administration for reducing the risk of mortality in

myocardial infarction survivors when drug therapy is initiated 5–28 days after a myocardial infarction. Two additional β-selective adrenergic blocking agents, metoprolol and atenolol, are approved for the same indications in both intravenous and oral forms. There is additional evidence that β-adrenergic blocking agents decrease the incidence of ventricular premature contractions associated with the high sympathetic nervous system tone after a myocardial infarction. The decrease in the frequency of arrhythmias following infarction may contribute to the decrease in sudden death and cardiovascular mortality (52–55,72,73).

OTHER CARDIOVASCULAR APPLICATIONS
Mitral Valve Prolapse

With the advent of echocardiography into clinical medicine, a finding of prolapse of the mitral valve has been described with increasing frequency in the cardiac literature. This has also been termed Barlow's syndrome, billowing mitral syndrome, floppy valve syndrome, click-murmur syndrome, and redundant cusp syndrome (74–78). This condition has been recognized as one of the most prevalent cardiac abnormalities, affecting as much as 5–10% of the population. It has also been associated with an increase in episodes of atypical chest pain and malignant arrhythmias (74,75). The palpitations that the patient generally feels in this condition are associated in an increased frequency of sudden death. It has been suggested that many of the symptoms are related to a dysfunction of the autonomic nervous system, which is frequently associated with this syndrome (74,75). Current therapy is directed at symptomatic relief of this condition. Propranolol appears to be the drug of choice for many of the ventricular arrhythmias, especially in those patients with a prolongation of the QT interval (79).

QT Interval Prolongation Syndrome

Two clinical syndromes associated with a prolonged QT interval have been described extensively in the literature. The Romano-

Table 2 Adverse Effects Associated with β-Adrenoceptor
Blocking Agents

Adverse cardiac effects related to β-adrenergic blockade
  1. Congestive heart failure: inhibition of sympathetic nervous system
  2. Sinus node dysfunction: inhibition of sinus node function, especially
      in patients with sick sinus syndrome
  3. Atrioventricular conduction delay: slowing of conduction through the
      AV node
  4. Abrupt withdrawal syndrome

Adverse noncardiac effects related to β-adrenergic blockade
  1. Blockade of bronchodilator effects of catecholamines: contraindicated
      in patients with lung disease
  2. Peripheral vascular disease: contraindicated in patients with Ray-
      naud's phenomenon
  3. Glucose metabolism: muscle glycogen is a β-receptor-mediated func-
      tion; β-blockers blunts sympathetic responses to hypoglycemia
  4. Central nervous system effects: insomnia, dreams, hallucinations,
      and depression, among other CNS effects commonly seen

Ward syndrome and the Jervell and Lange-Nielsen syndrome have been demonstrated as predisposing individuals to ventricular fibrillation and sudden death (80,82). These two syndromes are clinically distinct since they are associated with syncope and sudden death, the latter syndrome in individuals with congential deafness. Deafness, however, is not a feature of the Romano-Ward syndrome. Generally, patients who present with these problems have an abnormality in the activation of the adrenergic sympathetic nervous system, possibly accounting for the QT prolongation noted on the surface electrocardiogram (83,84). These are individuals who are at great risk for paroxysmal ventricular tachyarrhythmias and sudden death. The most effective agent currently is propranolol. This agent appears to decrease the frequency of syncopal episodes and may prevent sudden death.

ADVERSE EFFECTS OF β-ADRENERGIC BLOCKING AGENTS

The limitations to the use of β-adrenergic blocking agents are primarily due to the side effects. Commonly described side effects are difficult to assess since many of these are dose related. The profiles of these agents are summarized in Table 2 and are primarily divided into two categories: those that result from the the known pharmacologic consequences of β-adrenergic receptor blockade and those that do not appear to result from β-adrenergic receptor blockade.

The side effects of the first type are generally due to the fact that the sympathetic nervous system is important in the control of many physiologic and metabolic activities. These effects include congestive heart failure, hypoglycemia, pulmonary function effects, such as asthma, bradycardia and heart block, intermittent claudication, and Raynaud's phenomenon. The incidence of frequency of these adverse effects varies with the specific type of β-adrenergic blocking agents and dose used.

ACKNOWLEDGMENT

Supported in part by NIH Grant HL 24354.

REFERENCES

  1. Ahlquist R P. Study of the adrenotropic receptors. Am J Physiol 1948; 153:586–600.

2. Land A M, Luduena F P, Buzzo H J. Differentiation of receptor systems responsive to isoproterenol. Life Sci 1967; 6:2241.

3. Frishman W H. Beta adrenergic blockers. Med Clin North Am 1988; 72:37–81.

4. Koch-Weser J. Metroprolol. N Engl J Med 1979; 301:698–703.

5. Frishman W H. Atenolol and timolol, two new systemic adrenoceptor antagonists. N Engl J Med 1982; 306:1456–62.

6. Frishman W H. Nadolol: a new beta-adrenoceptor antagonist. N Engl J Med 1981; 305:678–82.

7. Frishman W H. Pindolol: a new beta adrenoceptor antagonist with partial agonist activity. N Engl J Med 1983; 308:940–4.

8. Vaughan Williams E M, Miller J S, Campbell T J. Electrophysiological effects of labetalol on rabbit atrial, ventricular and Purkinje cells, in normoxia and hypoxia. Cardiovasc Res 1982; 16:233–9.

9. Vaughan William E M. A classification of antiarrhythmic actions reassessed after a decade of new drugs. J Clin Pharmacol 1984; 24:129–47.

10. Harrison D C. Current classification of antiarrhythmic drugs as a guide to their rational clinical use. Drug 1986; 31:93–5.

11. Frishman W H. Beta adrenoceptor antagonists: new drugs and new indications. N Engl J Med 1980; 305:500–6.

12. Anderson J L, Rodier H E, Green L S. Comparative effects of beta-adrenergic blocking drugs on experimental ventricular fibrillation threshold. Am J Cardiol 1983; 51:1196–202.

13. Aberg G, Adler G, Duker G, Ek B, Telemo E. Effects of adrenergic beta blockers and a membrane stabilizing agent on ouabain-induced cardiac arrhythmias in anaesthetized guinea pigs. Acta Pharmacol Toxicol 1979; 45:102–96.

14. Pratt C, Lichstein E. Ventricular antiarrhythmic effects of beta-adrenergic blocking drugs: a review of mechanism and clinical studies. J Clin Pharmacol 1982; 22:335–47.

15. Hirsowitz, G. The role of beta blocking agents as adjunct therapy to membrane stabilizing drugs in malignant ventricular arrhythmia. Am Heart J 1986; 111:852–60.

16. Campbell T J. Antiarrhythmic drugs. In: Eckert G M, Gutmann F, Keyzer H, eds. Electropharmacology. Boca Raton, FL: CRC Press 1990.

17. Sivam S P, Seth S D. Metoprolol—a new cardioselective beta adrenoceptor antagonist in experimental cardiac arrhythmias. Indian J Med Res 1978; 68:176–82.

18. Coram W M, Olson R W, Beil M E, Cabot C F, Weiss G B. Effects of metoprolol, alone and in combination with lidocaine, on ventricular fibrillation threshold: comparison with atenolol, propranolol and pindolol. J Cardiovasc Pharmacol 1987; 9:611–21.

19. Bigger J T, Hoffman B F. Antiarrhythmic drugs. In: Gilman A G, Goodman L S, Tall T W, Murad F, eds. The pharmacological basis of therapeutics, 7th ed. New York: Macmillan 1985.

20. Singh B N, Vaughan Williams E M. A third class of antiarrhythmic action. Effects on atrial and ventricular intracellular potentials and other pharmacological actions on cardiac of MJ 1999 and AH 34/4. Br J Pharmacol 1970; 39:675–87.

21. Strauss H C, Bigger J T, Hoffman B F. Electrophysiological and beta blocking effects of MJ-1999 on dog and rabbit cardiac tissues. Circ Res 1970; 26:661–78.

22. Nademanee K, Feld G, Hendrickson J A, Singh P N, Singh B N. Electrophysiologic and antiarrhythmic effects of sotalol in patients with life threatening ventricular tachyarrhythmias. Circulation 1985; 72:555–64.

23. Feld G K, Venkatesh N, Singh B N. Pharmacologic conversion and suppression of experimental canine atrial flutter; differing effects of d-sotalol, quinidine, and lidocaine and significance of changes in refractoriness and conduction. Circulation 1986; 74:197–204.

24. Black J W, Crowther A F, Shaks R G, Smith L H, Dornhurst A C. A new beta receptor antagonist. Lancet 1964; 1:1080–1.

25. Pritchard B N C. Beta adrenoceptor blocking drugs. In: Hornbach V, Hilger H, Kennedy H L, eds. Electrocardiography and cardiac drug therapy. Dordrecht: Kluwer, 1989: 298–322.

26. Davis L D, Temte J V. Effects of propranolol on the transmembrane potentials of ventricular muscle and Purkinje fibers in the dog. Circ Res 1968; 22:661–77.

27. Pitt C A, Cox A R. The effects of the beta-adrenergic antagonist propranolol on rabbit atrial cells. Am Heart J 1968; 76:242–7.

28. Papp J, Vaughan Williams E M. A Comparison of the antiarrhythmic actions of ICI

501772 and propranolol and their effects on intracellular cardiac action potentials and other features of cardiac function. Br J Pharmacol 1969; 36:391–8.

29. Spinelli W, Danilo P, Buchthal S D, Rosen M R. Developmental changes in the effects of beta-adrenergic blocking concentrations of propranolol on canine Purkinje fibers. Dev Pharmacol Ther 1986; 9:412–26.

30. Zaim S, Dangman K H. Cellular electrophysiology and beta-adrenergic blocking activity of dilevalol, the R,R-isomer of labetalol, on isolated canine cardiac tissues. J Cardiovasc Pharmacol 1989; 14:496–501.

31. Lish P, Weikal J, Dugan K. Pharmacological and toxicological properties of two new beta-receptor antagonists. J Phamacol Exp Ther 1965; 149:161–8.

32. Singh B N, Nademanee K. Sotalol: a beta blocker with unique antiarrhythmic properties. Am Heart J 1987, 144:121–39.

33. Cobble S N, Manley B S. Effects of elevated extracellular potassium concentrations on the class III antiarrhythmic action of sotalol. Cardiovasc Res 1985; 19:69–75.

34. Yabek S, Kato R, Ikeda N, Singh B N. Cellular electrophysiologic responses of isolated neonatal and adult cardiac fibers to d-sotalol. J Am Coll Cardiol 1988; 11:1094–9.

35. Lathrop D A. Electromechanical characterization of the effects of sotalol on isolated canine ventricular muscle and Purkinje strands. Can J Physiol Pharmacol 1985; 63:1506–12.

36. Carmeliet E. Electrophysiologic and voltage clamp analysis of the effects of sotalol on isolated cardiac muscle and Purkinje fibers. J Pharmacol Exp Ther 1985; 232:817–25.

37. Berman N D, Loukides J E. A comparison of the cellular electrophysiology of mexiletine and sotalol in canine Purkinje fibers. J Cardiovasc Pharmacol 1988; 12:286–92.

38. Singh B N, Vaughan William E M. Local anesthetic and antiarrhythmic actions of alprenolol relative to its effect on intracellular potentials and other properties of isolated cardiac muscle. Br J Pharmacol 1970; 38: 749–57.

39. Pogwizd S M, Sharma A D, Corr P B. Influence of labetalol on a combined alpha- and beta-adrenergic blocking agent on the dysrhythmias induced by coronary occlusion and reperfusion. Cardiovasc Res 1982; 16: 398–407.

40. Brittain R T, Drew G M, Levy G P. The alpha- and beta-adrenoceptor blocking poten-

cies of labetalol and its individual steroisomers in anesthetized dogs and in isolated tissues. Br J Pharmacol 1982; 77:195–14.

41. Sybertz E J, Sabin C S, Pula K K, et al. Alpha and beta adrenoceptor blocking properties of labetalol and its R,R-isomer, SCH 19927. J Pharmacol Exp Ther 1981; 218:435–43.

42. Monopoli A, Bamonte F, Forlani A, et al. Effects of the R,R-isomer of labetalol, SCH 19927, in isolated tissues and in spontaneouly hypertensive rats during a repeated treatment. Arch Int Pharmacodyn 1984; 272:256–63.

43. Lynch J J, Montgomery D G, Luchesi B R. Cardiac electrophysiologic actions of SCH 19927 (Dilevalol), the R,R-isomer of labetalol. J Pharmacol Exp Ther 1986; 239: 719–23.

44. Lynch J J, Nelson S D, MacEwen S A, et al. Antifibrillatory efficacy of concomitant beta adrenergic receptor blockade with dilevalol, the R,R-isomer of labetalol, and muscarinic receptor blockade with methylscopolamine. J Pharmacol Exp Ther 1987; 241:741–9.

45. Guse P, Gaide M, Myerburg R J, et al. Electrophysiological effects of alprenolol on depressed canine myocardiaum. Cardiovasc Res 1980; 14:654–60.

46. Sada H. Effect of phentolamine, alprenolol and prenylamine on maximum rate of rise of the action potential in guinea pig papillary muscle. Naunyn Schmiedebergs Arch Pharmacol 1978; 304:191–201.

47. Gibson J K, Gelband H, Bassett A L. Direct and beta-adrenergic blocking actions of nadalol in electrophysiologic properties of isolated canine myocardium. J Pharmacol Exp Ther 1977; 202:702–10.

48. Hamra M, Danilo P, Rosen M R. Developmental changes in the effects of nadolol on adult and neonatal canine Purkinje fibers. Dev Pharmacol Ther 1988; 11:155–65.

49. Gibson D, Sowton E. The use of beta adrenergic receptor blocking drugs in dysrhythmias. Prog Cardiovasc Dis 1969; 12:16–39.

50. Singh B N. Clinical aspects of the antiarrhythmic actions of beta-receptor blocking drugs. Part I. Pattern of response of common arrhythmias. N Z Med J 1973; 78:482–6.

51. Hombach V, Braun V, Hopp H W, et al. Electrophysiology effects of cardioselective and non-cardioselective beta-adrenoceptor blockers with and without ISA at rest and during exercise. Br J Clin Pharmacol 1982; 13:285S–293S.

52. Cruickshank J M, Richard B N C. Beta blockers in clinical practice. London: Churchill Livingston, 1988.

53. Coltart D J, Gibson D G, Shand D G. Plasma propranolol levels associated with suppression of ventricular ectopic beats. Br Med J 1971; 1:490–1.

54. Creamer J E, Nathan A W, Shennan A, et al. Acute and chronic effects of sotalol and propranolol on ventricular repolarization using constant rate pacing. Am J Cardiol 1986; 57:1092–6.

55. Frishman W H. Clinical pharmacology of the beta-adrenoceptor blocking drugs, 2nd ed. Norwalk, CT: Appleton-Crofts, 1984.

56. Pratt C M, Yepsim S C, Bloom M G K, et al. Evaluation of metroprolol in suppressing complex ventricular arrhythmias. Am J Cardiol 1983; 52:73–8.

57. Beta blocker heart attack study group. The beta blocker heart attack trial. JAMA 1981: 246:2073–4.

58. Hjalmarson A. Myocardial metabolic changes related to ventricular fibrillation. Cardiology 1980; 65:226–47.

59. Waagstein F, Hjalmarson A, Swedeberg K, et al. Beta blockers in dilated cardiomyopathies: they work. Eur Heart J 1983; 4(Suppl.A):173

60. Wit A L, Hoffman B F, Rosen M R. Electrophysiology and pharmacology of cardiac arrhythmias. IX. Cardiac electrophysiology effects of beta blockade. Part C. Am Heart J 1975; 90:795–803.

61. Singh B N, Jewitt D E. Beta adrenoreceptor blocking drugs in cardiac arrhythmias. Cardiovasc Drugs 1977; 2:119–59.

62. Ruberman W. Weinblatt E, Goldberg J D, et al. Ventricular premature complexes and sudden death after myocardial infarction. Circulation 1981; 64:297–305.

63. The Multicenter Post Infarction Research Group. Risk stratification and survival after myocardial infarction. N Engl J Med 1983; 309:331–6.

64. Pratt C M, Brater D C, Harrell F E, et al. Clinical and regulatory implications of the cardiac arrhythmia suppression trial. Am J Cardiol 1990; 65:103–5.

65. The Cardiac Arrhythmia Suppression Trial (CAST) Investigators. Preliminary report: Effect of encainide and flecainide on mortality in a randomized trial of arrhythmia suppression after myocardial infarction. N Engl J Med 1989; 321:406–12.

66. Bigger J T, Fleiss J L, Kleiger R, et al. The relationships among ventricular arrhythmias, left ventricular dysfunction, and mortality in the 2 years after myocardial infaction. Circulation 1984; 69:250–8.

67. The CAPS Investigators. The Cardiac Arrhythmia Pilot Study. Am J Cardiol 1984; 54:31–6.

68. Gibson D, Sowton E. The use of beta adrenergic receptors blocking drugs in dysrhythmias. Prog Cardiovasc Dis 1969; 12:16–39.

69. Schofield P M, Bennett D H. A comparison of atenolol and sotalol in the treatment of patients with paroxysmal supraventricular tachycardia. J Am Coll Cardiol 1987; 9:247A.

70. Echt D S, Berte L E, Clusin W T, et al. Prolongation of the human cardiac monophasic action potential by sotalol. Am J Cardiol 1982; 50:1082–6.

71. Creamer J E, Nathan A W, Shennan A, et al. Acute and chronic effects of sotalol and propranolol on ventricular repolarization using constant-rate pacing. Am J Cardiol 1986; 57:1092–1.

72. Hjalmarson A, Hulitz J, Malek I, et al. Effect on mortality of metoprolol in acute myocardial infarction. Lancet 1981; 2:823–7.

73. Norwegian Multicenter Study Group. Timolol-induced reduction in morality and reinfarction in patients surviving acute myocardial infarction. N Engl J Med 1981; 304:801–7.

74. Winkle R A, Lopes M G, Fitzgerald J W, et al. Arrhythmias in patients with mitral valve prolapse. Circulation 1975; 52:73.

75. Leichtman D, Nelson R, Gobel F L, et al. Bradycardia with mitral valve prolapse: a potential mechanism of sudden death. Ann Intern Med 1976; 85:453.

76. Barlow J B, Pocock W A. Mitral valve prolapse, the specific billowing mitral leaflet syndrome, or an insignificant non-ejection systolic click. Am Heart J 1979; 97:277.

77. Devereaux R B, Perloff J K, Reichek N, et al. Mitral valve prolapse. Circulation 1976; 54:3.

78. Procacci P M, Savran S V, Schreiter S L, et al. Prevalence of clinical mitral valve prolapse in 1,169 young women. N Engl J Med 1976; 294:1086.

79. Winkle R A, Harrison D. Propranolol for patients with mitral valve prolapse. Am Heart J 1977; 93:422.

80. Romano C, Gemme G, Pongiglione R. Aritmie cardiache rare dell'eta pediatrica. Clin Paediatr 1963; 45:656.

81. Ward O C. A new familial cardiac syndrome in children. J Irish Med Assoc 1964; 54:103.

82. Jervell A, Lange-Nielsen F. Congential deaf mutism, functional heart disease with prolongation of QT interval and sudden death. Am Heart J 1957; 54:59.

83. Schwartz P J, Periti M, Malliani A. The long QT syndrome. Am Heart J 1975; 89:378–90.

84. Denes P. Congenital and acquired syndrome of a long QT interval. Chest 1977; 71:126–7.

33

Class III Antiarrhythmic Agents

Thomas M. Argentieri, Mark E. Sullivan and Jay R. Wiggins

Berlex Laboratories, Inc.
Cedar Knolls, New Jersey

INTRODUCTION

In his original classification of antiarrhythmic drugs by electrophysiologic profile, Vaughan Williams (1) defined class III agents as those whose *predominant* effect was to increase the duration of the cardiac action potential (Table 1).* Since this original definition the concept of class III antiarrhythmic agents has been refined to incude only those agents whose sole action (in pharmacologically relevant doses) is to increase action potential duration, with no effect on maximum upstroke velocity or on other cellular processes, such as adrenergic function. Such selective agents are rare in experimental medicine, and none of these agents are yet approved (in the United States) as antiarrhythmic drugs.

In theory an agent can prolong action potential duration by increasing inward current or by decreasing outward current during the action potential plateau. Compounds that increase inward sodium current, such as the sea

anemone toxin anthopleurin A and the cardiotonic agent DPI 201-106, have not been studied extensively as antiarrhythmic agents, but isolated reports suggest a proarrhythmic effect of such compounds, at least under certain well-defined circumstances (2). Therefore this review addresses only those agents that have selective class III actions and have shown antiarrhythmic efficacy either in animal models or in humans. We include discussions on acecainide (*N*-acetylprocainamide), clofilium, sematilide, and *d*-sotalol (Fig. 1). These compounds differ widely in potency (Fig. 2), but all selectively and significantly increase action potential duration at concentrations that have little or no effect on the maximum rate of depolarization $(dV/dt)_{max}$ or on conduction velocity. The effect of class III agents on action potential duration are use dependent; the effect is *decreased* as stimulation rate increases. This is in marked contrast to the familiar use dependence of the class I agents, in

---

*Bretylium was described as a class III agent, but in hindsight it probably does not deserve this classification, as the extent of increase in action potential duration of the canine cardiac Purkinje fiber action potential is quite modest compared to newer agents in this class.

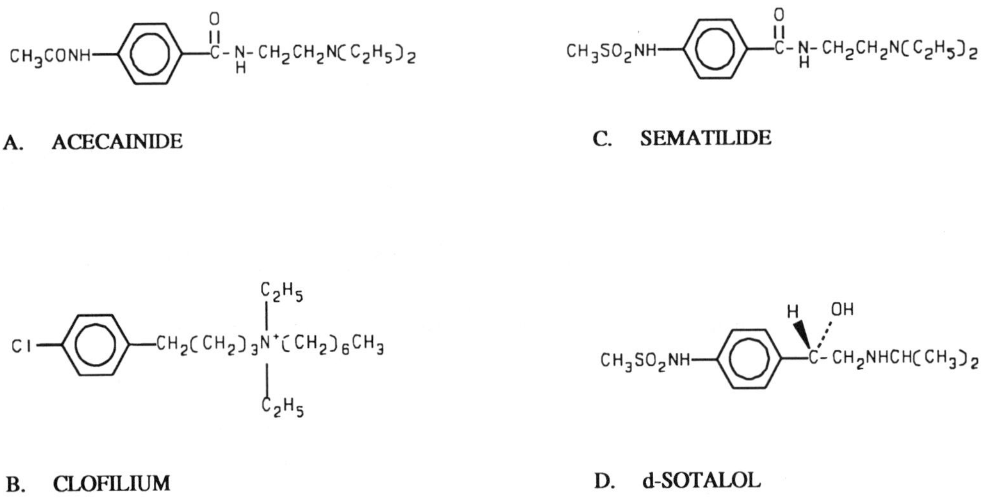

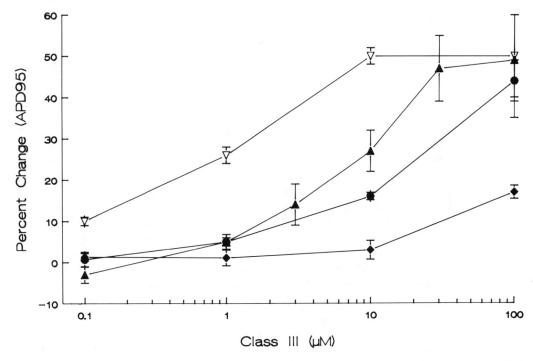

A. ACECAINIDE

C. SEMATILIDE

B. CLOFILIUM

D. d-SOTALOL

Figure 1 Chemical structures of class III drugs.

which the class I activity increases as stimulation rate increases.

Class I agents are readily identified in the laboratory, as they are effective against a variety of experimental arrhythmias, including those evoked by aconitine, cardiac glycosides, coronary artery ligation, and so on. All these experimental arrhythmias, however, are disorders of automaticity. It is generally accepted that the most important arrhythmias clinically

Figure 2 Effect of class III drugs on action potential duration at 95% of repolarization (APD95) of canine cardiac Purkinje fibers. The effects of a 30 min exposure to acecainide (◆), d-sotalol (●), sematilide (▲), and clofilium (▽) are shown. Fibers were studied at 37°C and stimulated at 1 Hz. Data for each point are expressed as the mean ± SEM.

Table 1 Effects of Agents that Prolong Action Potential Duration:[a]

Agent	$(dV/dt)_{max}$	APD	Other actions
Acecainide	→	↑ ↑	
Amiodarone	↓	↑ ↑	Thyrotoxic, antiadrenergic, calcium antagonist, pneumotoxic
Bepridil	→	↑ ↑	Calcium antagonist
Bretylium	→	↑	Releases then blocks release of catecholamines
Clofilium	→	↑ ↑ ↑	
DPI 201–106	↓	↑ ↑ [b]	Na channel agonist, positive inotropic agent
Melperone	↓ →	↑	Neuroleptic
Quinidine	↓	↑	Vagolytic, inhibits Na-Ca exchange, α-adrenergic blocking agent, smooth muscle relaxant
Sematilide	→	↑ ↑ ↑	
d-Sotalol	→	↑ ↑	
d,l-Sotalol	→	↑ ↑	β-Adrenergic blocking agent

[a]$(dV/dt)_{max}$ maximum rate of depolarization; APD, action potential duration.
[b]In ventricular tissue only; shortens atrial refractoriness.

are those that are reentrant in origin. Experimentally, reentrant arrhythmias are evoked by programmed electrical stimulation; in this model the class I drugs are generally ineffective. In contrast, class III agents are generally ineffective against automatic arrhythmias but are quite effective in preventing arrhythmias evoked by programmed electrical stimulation. In addition, the class III drugs appear to be free of hemodynamic and central nervous system (CNS) side effects and thus have a wider margin of safety than do the class I drugs.

ACECAINIDE

Acecainide (4-(acetylamino)-N-[2-(diethylamino)ethyl]benzamide; Fig. 1) is the official U.S. Adopted Name (USAN) for N-acetylprocainamide, the major metabolite of procainamide. Acecainide was first described as an active antiarrhythmic agent in its own right in 1974 (3). Because it has a longer half-life than procainamide, acecainide can accumulate during procainamide therapy. This review considers acecainide independently of procainamide, which is considered elsewhere in this text. Several recent reviews have directly compared the two agents (4). NAPA, widely used as an abbreviation for N-acetylprocainamide, has become a registered trademark for acecainide and is not used in this review.

Animal Studies

Basic Pharmacology

In isolated rabbit atria acecainide causes a concentration-dependent (30–1000 μM) increase in the maximum follow-frequency without significantly affecting threshold voltage (5). In contrast, in isolated rat atria acecainide has relatively little effect on atrial refractoriness; maximum follow-frequency is reduced to only 75% of control in the presence of 3 mM acecainide (6). This high concentration of acecainide has, however, no effect on excitability.

In canine cardiac Purkinje fibers and ventricular muscle, acecainide (10–40 mg/L, 32–128 μM) increases action potential duration in a concentration-dependent manner without significantly affecting (in Purkinje fibers) the rate of spontaneous depolarization, resting membrane potential, action potential amplitude, or $(dV/dt)_{max}$ (7). In higher concentrations and in preparations driven at slow stimulation rates, acecainide can cause failure of repolarization, with maintained depolarization at about -55 mV, and the appearance of early afterdepolarizations and spontaneous action potentials. This is a common property of class III antiarrhythmics and may predispose to spontaneous ectopy in vivo and, perhaps, to proarrhythmic actions in the human.

In pentobarbital-anesthetized dogs acecainide causes a dose-dependent negative chronotropic effect (8), a finding not seen in conscious animals (9) or in dogs anesthetized with chloralose (10). Acecainide (8.5–68 mg/kg IV) does not significantly affect sinus node recovery time in dogs, but it does produce a dose-dependent increase in atrial refractory period (8,10). Intraatrial conduction time is either unchanged (10) or slowed (8). Atrial conduction may be preferentially slowed at faster heart rates (11). In the atrioventricular node only high doses of acecainide effectively prolong refractory period, and AV conduction is not affected (8,10).

In the dog ventricle acecainide increases QTc, Wenckebach cycle length, monophasic action potential duration, and refractory period in a dose-dependent manner (10,12). The increase in duration of the monophasic action potential is greater at slower heart rates than at faster heart rates (Fig. 3) (12).

Intraventricular conduction is slowed by acecainide (8), but His-ventricular conduction is not affected (8,10). In dogs with chronic atrioventricular block a high dose (35.7 mg/kg IV) of acecainide slows the intrinsic ventricular rate (9). The increase in intraventricular conduction time and a rate-dependent increase in ventricular refractoriness led Amlie and Landmark (12) to suggest that acecainide is more properly categorized as a class I than a class III drug. It is, however, not clear whether the slowing of conduction is a direct effect of acecainide on the sodium channel or an indirect effect, secondary to an increase in action potential duration and, thus, refractoriness. The overall electrophysiologic profile suggests that it is best categorized as a class III agent.

Antiarrhythmic Efficacy

Acecainide (16–64 mg/kg IV) effectively terminates or prevents atrial flutter in a variety of dog models, including both excitable gap (11,13) and leading circle (14) models. Acecainide slows the flutter rate, lengthens the excitable gap (when present) and, in the majority of the animals in these three studies, terminates the arrhythmia and prevents the re-

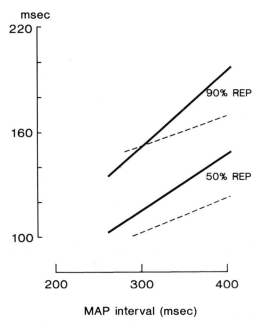

Figure 3 Effect of acecainide on monophasic action potential duration of the in situ dog heart. The times for 50 and 90% repolarization of the right ventricle are shown for six dogs. Repolarization times were measured at the spontaneous heart rate before (dotted line) and after (solid line) acecainide (50 mg/kg, IV). The lines were calculated from linear regression; correlation coefficient $r = 0.79$ for each group. Similar results were obtained when each heart was paced at different cycle lengths. Note that the extent of acton potential prolongation was greater at longer MAP intervals (slower heart rates). (Redrawn from Ref. 12.)

induction of atrial flutter. Acecainide is significantly more effective than the class I agent recainam in terminating and preventing reinduction of this arrhythmia (15).

The efficacy of acecainide against ventricular arrhythmias is less clear. Class III drugs are most effective against reentrant arrhythmias, but acecainide has been most thoroughly studied in models of ventricular arrhythmias that respond best to class I agents. At a high dose (130 mg/kg) acecainide prevents chloroform-induced ventricular fibrillation in mice (3,16). Acecainide also prolongs the time to ouabain-induced ventricular fibrillation in rabbits (75 mg/kg IV) (5) and reverses ouabain-induced ventricular tachycardia in dogs (140–220 mg/kg IV) (17). In dogs acecainide (60 mg/kg IV) reduces the incidence of ventricular fibrillation following acute coronary artery ligation, perhaps as a consequence of its bradycardic action (18). Higher doses (140–220 mg/kg IV), suppress ventricular arrhythmias which occur 4–7 hr following acute coronary artery ligation (17), and in doses up to 100 mg/kg IV acecainide has limited efficacy against ventricular arrhythmias that arise 24 hr after a two-stage coronry artery ligation (7). In contrast to the high doses needed to show efficacy against these automatic arrhythmias, lower doses (1–60 mg/kg IV) of acecainide are effective in preventing ventricular tachycardia induced by programmed electrical stimulation in dogs (unpublished observations). Thus the efficacy of acecainide against reentrant ventricular arrhythmias is seen in the same dose range as its efficacy against reentrant atrial arrhythmias.

Clinical Studies

Electrophysiology

In patients (without arrhythmias) undergoing cardiac catheterization, acecainide (10.5–21 mg/kg IV) increases atrial and ventricular refractory periods and QTc without significantly affecting sinus cycle length, sinus node recovery time, conduction intervals, or functional refractory period of the atrioventricular node (19). In patients with syptomatic ventricular arrhythmias acecainide (18–20 mg/kg IV) has no significant effect on sinus rate or atrioventricular conduction but prolongs the QTc interval (20,21). Conduction in the His-Purkinje system is slowed during atrial pacing, but not at normal heart rates, leading to aberrant ventricular conduction or bundle branch block in some patients (20). On oral dosing acecainide does not significantly affect the PR interval or QRS duration but does significantly prolong QTc (22).

Efficacy

The clinical efficacy of acecainide has been studied only in ventricular arrhythmias. Overall acecainide is not as effective in suppressing ventricular premature depolarizations (VPD) as are the class IC antiarrhythmic agents; efficacy in all these studies was defined as 70–75% suppression of VPD. In long-term treatment acecainide appears to effectively suppress arrhythmias in approximately one-half to two-thirds of patients.

In doses of 10–20 mg/kg, sufficient to achieve blood levels of 16–36 µg/ml, the acute intravenous administration of acecainide is effective in approximately half of patients with ventricular tachycardia induced by programmed electrical stimulation (PES), either slowing rate or preventing inducibility. Acecainide has no significant effect on malignant arrhythmias provoked by exercise (20,23–26) but reduces the incidence of spontaneous or exercise-induced extrasystoles in approximately half the patients. Lee et al. (27) showed that a single oral dose of acecainide (1.5 g) was effective in 6 of 9 patients with stable premature ventricular depolarizations. The 6 responders all had coupled VPD, whereas the nonresponders did not. In a separate trial from the same study site (28), acecainide was effective in 8 of 10 patients given 0.5 g every 6 hr for 3 days. At blood levels of 10–24 µg/ml acecainide reduced the frequency of ventricular arrhythmia by at least 75% in 9 of 16 patients (29) but caused significant side effects, including light-headedness, insomnia, nausea, and diarrhea, in 6 patients. The blood level associated with adverse reactions was in the same range (11–22 µg/ml) as that associated with efficacy.

Long-term trials of acecainide have been reported in those patients in whom it was effective acutely. In selected patients acecainide has been effective for up to 4 years (29a). Somberg et al. (25) reported that of 6 patients in whom acecainide was shown to be effective by PES, 3 continued in long-term (>6 months) therapy and 2 other patients had breakthrough tachycardia. Kluger et al. (30) reported that of 19 patients whose arrhythmias were initially suppressed by acecainide, 11 were still controlled after 12 months of treatment; however, 6 patients had died, 4 from sudden cardiac death. In these trials the effective plasma concentration ranged from approximately 10 to 35 µg/ml; side effects, which were common, appeared at plasma concentrations from 10 to 38 µg/ml.

Pharmacokinetics

Animal Studies

The pharmacokinetics of acecainide have been described in rat and dog. In the rat the time course of acecainide elimination can best be described by a pseudo-three-compartment model, with a terminal half-life of 2.1 hr (31), the elimination half-life increases with age (32). Acecainide reaches equilibrium with tissues in approximately 5 min and is present in greater concentration in heart, kidney, and liver than in plasma (33). Acecainide is cleared primarily by the kidney, with a significant increase in plasma half-life following acute renal failure in the rat (34).

In the dog the biologic half-life is approximately 4 hr and the apparent volume of distribution is 2 L/kg (35). Coronary artery ligation does not affect the biologic half-life, apparent volume of distribution, or total clearance of acecainide, but it does cause an increase in the initial plasma concentration, suggesting a decrease in the apparent volume of the central compartment.

Clinical Studies

Following intravenous administration acecainide has an elimination half-life of approximately 6–8 hr and a total volume of distribution of approximately 1.38 L/kg (26, 36). Of the administered dose of acecainide 80% is eliminated unchanged in the urine; a small fraction is deacetylated to form procainamide (36).

Safety

In isolated rat atria acecainide (300–3000 μM) has a modest positive inotropic action (6). In the globally ischemic rabbit heart acecainide has a slight positive inotropic effect that is blocked by previous treatment with reserpine; a negative inotropic effect is seen only following concentrations 50 times greater than the usually effective antiarrhythmic concentration (37).

The lack of significant negative inotropic actions is also evident in studies of the hemodynamic effects of acecainide. Myocardial contractility, measured either by strain gauge or estimated from changes in left ventricular dp/dt or internal diameter, is increased by acecainide (38,39). The positive inotropic effect of acecainide appears to depend on the release of endogenous catecholamines, since it is not seen in dogs pretreated with reserpine or hexamethonium (39) and is blocked by propranolol (40). In high doses (60 mg/kg IV) acecainide has a negative inotropic effect that is apparent only after blockade of cardiac β-adrenoceptors with propranolol (40). Acecainide has no effect on left ventricular end-diastolic pressure (41). Mean arterial pressure is usually decreased (38,42). The hemodynamic actions of acecainide are proportional to its plasma concentration (41,43), but the effects on heart rate appear to be somewhat delayed and longer lasting than the effects on blood pressure and cardiac contractility (41). Vagolytic and ganglionic blocking actions complicate the hemodynamic actions of acecainide (42,44).

In patients undergoing diagnostic cardiac catheterization intravenous acecainide (18 mg/kg) exerts mild but significant dilating effects on both the arterial and venous sides of the circulation, accompanied by a slight reduction in contractility and cardiac output; heart rate is increased (45). Oral acecainide (to 6 g/day) has no effect on heart rate, blood pressure, or echocardiographic indices of left ventricular function (24).

In normal conscious dogs acecainide (50–100 mg/kg IV) can provoke ventricular extrasystoles with constant coupling intervals, which can degenerate into ventricular fibrillation (7). In the human, the proarrhythmic effects of acecainide include torsades de pointes (26,46,47), polymorphic ventricular tachycardia, and ventricular fibrillation (48), as well as an increase in the frequency of VPD (28). The overall incidence of the proarrhythmic effects of acecainide has not been defined because of the relatively low number of patients who have received this drug.

Drug-induced lupus erythematosus is much less of a problem with acecainide than with procainamide; there is no crossover hypersensitivity, allowing patients with procainamide-induced lupus syndrome to safely receive acecainide (49,50). It has recently been shown that acecainide is a less potent inducer of T cell autoreactivity than is procainamide (51).

Other side effects include nausea and vomiting, diarrhea, nervousness, insomnia, fatigue, and blurred vision.

CLOFILIUM

Clofilium (4-chloro-N,N-diethyl-N-heptylbenzenebutanaminium; Fig. 1) was the first prospectively developed class III antiarrhythmic agent. As such, its pure class III action makes it different from many currently used antiarrhythmic agents, which were found to increase action potential duration only after they were developed and in clinical practice for other indications (e.g., amiodarone, d, l-sotalol, or bretylium). Clofilium has often been referred to as a congener of bretylium; however, the drug is devoid of adrenergic neuronal blocking activity, is approximately 1000 times more potent than bretylium for increasing action potential duration, and exhibits reasonably strict chemical structure-activity relationships, indicating that slight structural modifications can completely abolish activity (52).

Animal Studies

Basic Pharmacology

Clofilium produces a concentration-dependent prolongation of action potential duration in isolated tissue preparations from rabbit sinoatrial (SA) node and atria (53) and from canine ventricular muscle and the specialized conduction network (54,55). In rabbit atrial tissues 3 μM clofilium increases action potential duration 14% in SA nodal cells and 21% in atrial muscle cells (53). In canine ventricular tissues 1 μM clofilium increases action potential duration 32% in Purkinje fibers and 11% in ventricular muscle preparations (unpublished observations).

Prolongation of action potential in these isolated preparations is accompanied by a concomitant increase in cellular refractoriness without a significant effect on indices of cellular conduction (dV/dt_{max}). The class III effect is most pronounced in cardiac Purkinje fibers, occurs at concentrations as low as 10 nM,

and is not reversible upon superfusion with drug-free media for up to 2 hr. Class I agents (lidocaine, quinidine, and procainamide), α-antagonists (phentolamine and phenoxybenzamine), and adrenergic agonists (norepinephrine) signifcantly reduce the ability of clofilium to prolong action potential duration; however, the class III activity of clofilium in canine cardiac Purkinje fibers is not inhibited by superfusion with either propranolol or atropine (56).

The cellular mechanism of action of clofilium has been studied in enzymatically isolated single-cell preparations obtained from guinea pig hearts using patch clamp techniques (57,58). These studies indicate that clofilium significantly inhibits the delayed rectifier potassium channel without affecting other plateau currents. However, these enzymatically dissociated cells are much less sensitive to clofilium than is intact tissue.

In tissues taken from dogs 48 hr following an acute myocardial infarction, the class III activity of clofilium is greater in free-running false tendons from the non-infarcted area than in surviving subendocardial Purkinje fibers from the infarcted zone (55). The authors concluded that the resulting decrease in dispersion of action potential duration was responsible for the antiarrhythmic effect of the drug. In contrast, we demonstrated (59) that clofilium preferentially prolongs action potential duration from surviving epicardial ventricular muscle cells and subendocardial Purkinje fiber preparations taken from the ischemic zone. This preferential action on ischemic tissues leads to a decrease in dispersion of action potential duration and refractoriness for ventricular muscle tissue and an increase in dispersion of action potential duration and refractoriness in subendocardial Purkinje fibers. We concluded that (1) clofilium preferentially prolongs action potential duration of surviving subendocardial Purkinje fibers from the ischemic zone compared to similar fibers from an adjacent normal zone, and (2) this increase in dispersion of action potential duration is responsible for the appearance of early afterdepolarizations (EAD) seen in our studies and previously reported by Gough et al. (60).

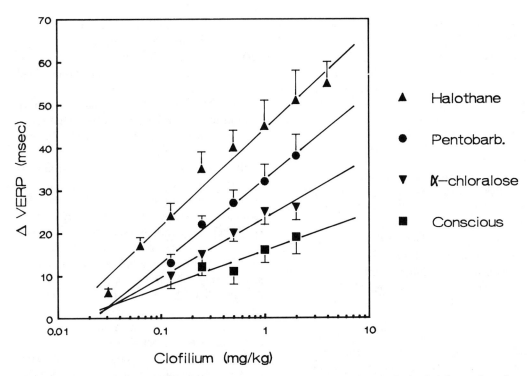

Figure 4 Effect of clofilium on ventricular effective refractory period in anesthetized and conscious dogs. Ordinate: increase in ventricular effective refractory period (VERP) from baseline values. Abscissa: intravenous dose of clofilium. Baseline values (mean ± SEM) were 178 ± 3, 174 ± 4, 178 ± 3, and 174 ± 6 msec for halothane-, pentobarbital-, and α-chloralose-anesthetized and for conscious dogs, respectively.

Consistent with its selective class III properties in isolated cardiac tissue preparations, clofilium produces a significant prolongation of atrial and ventricular refractoriness in intact anesthetized or conscious animals without affecting intracardiac (AH or HV) conduction intervals (14,52,61–65). On the surface electrocardiogram clofilium has no effect on the PR interval or QRS duration but produces a dose-dependent increase in QT and QTc intervals.

Anesthesia alters the ability of clofilium to prolong ventricular refractoriness in intact dogs (61). For a given dose of clofilium refractoriness is most prolonged in animals under halothane anesthesia and least in animals in the conscious state, with effects under pentobarbital and chloralose anesthesia intermediate (Fig. 4). The class III action of clofilium is potentiated in intact dogs pretreated with propranolol (66). These data suggest that the ability of clofilium to prolong ventricular refractoriness may be significantly modified by the level of adrenergic tone.

In infarcted anesthetized dogs clofilium prolongs the refractory period of ischemic myocardium to a greater degree than it prolongs refractoriness in the normal zone (67). Although Kopia et al. (63) reported that clofilium has no significant effect on the ventricular effective refractory period of ischemic myocardium, the preponderance of the data suggests that ischemic tissue is more sensitive to the class III action of clofilium than is normal ventricular myocardium. The physiologic significance of a differential sensitivity of clofilium for normal versus ischemic tissues remains unclear but could have a significant impact on understanding the antiarrhythmic and proarrhythmic activity of clofilium and other class III drugs.

Antiarrhythmic Efficacy

In a model of atrial reentrant arrhythmias produced by PES techniques in dogs following surgery to produce tricuspid insufficiency, clofilium (0.34 mg/kg IV) converts sustained atrial flutter to normal sinus rhythm (14).

Clofilium prevents PES-induced reentrant ventricular arrhythmias in dogs with chronic myocardial ischemia (63,67,68), but it is ineffective against ouabain-induced ventricular tachyarrhythmias or ventricular ectopic activity 24 hr after coronary artery occlusion (56). Despite its efficacy against PES-induced reentrant atrial or ventricular tachyarrhythmias, clofilium was effective in preventing mortality in only 3 of 10 animals subjected to a second ischemic event produced by an electrically induced intimal lesion of the circumflex coronary artery (63).

The effect of clofilium on the ventricular fibrillation threshold (VFT) appears to be model dependent. Steinberg and Molloy (54), using the technique of a train of impulses applied during the vulnerable period, reported that clofilium produces a dose-dependent increase in VFT (200% at a dose of 0.5 mg/kg IV). In addition they reported the occurrence of spontaneous defibrillation in animals receiving clofilium. Using a similar technique Kopia et al (63) also showed a dose-dependent increase in VFT with clofilium in both the normal and infarcted canine heart. However, only the highest dose tested (2 mg/kg IV) produced a statistically significant increase in VFT (350%), whereas the effective refractory period was significantly and maximally increased at 0.5 mg/kg IV. This observation led Kopia et al. (63) to conclude that the class III actions of clofilium were not necessarily involved in its ability to increase VFT. Euler and Scanlon (65), using the single-pulse technique, demonstrated that clofilium had no significant effect on VFT at doses up to 3 mg/kg IV, despite significant increases in ventricular refractoriness. In contrast, Kowey et al. (62), also using the single stimulus technique, demonstrated that clofilium increased VFT in cats before and during acute coronary artery occlusion. The increase in VFT produced by clofilium is less pronounced during coronary occlusion. In cats, decreases in the dispersion of refractoriness produced by clofilium are correlated with an increase in VFT (62).

Clinical Studies

The electrophysiologic effects of intravenous clofilium in patients parallels the effects seen in animal models. It produces a significant increase in both atrial and ventricular refractoriness and QT interval without affecting PR interval, QRS duration, or intracardiac conduction intervals (66,69,70). Overall the drug has been effective in preventing PES-induced sustained ventricular tachycardia in 42% of the patients tested (66), but it has no significant effect on VPD (56).

Pharmacokinetics

Animal Studies

Following intravenous administration of [^{14}C]-clofilium to rats and dogs, 10% of the compound is excreted in the urine and 55% excreted in the feces within 72 hr (71). These data indicate a significant biliary pathway for elimination of the drug. The plasma elimination half-life of a 5 mg/kg IV dose administered to either rats or dogs is between 2.5 and 3.0 hr. In contrast, the half-life of elimination from cardiac tissues is 5 days in the rat and 14 days in the dog, suggesting that the drug is sequestered by cardiac tissues. Correlation of the pharmacokinetics obtained in dogs was also related to the cellular electrophysiologic effects of clofilium by measuring action potential duration in Purkinje fibers of dogs sacrificed at different time intervals following intravenous administration (71). The half-life of action potential prolongation is approximately 10 days, which correlates favorably with pharmacokinetic data obtained with radiolabeled compound.

Clinical Studies

Pharmacokinetic studies in normal healthy volunteers with intravenously administered [^{14}C]-clofilium suggest a three-compartment model, with peak plasma levels occurring 5 min following administration (56). The average half-life of radioactivity is 39 hr. Approximately 58% of the radioactivity is recovered

CONTROL   **CLOFILIUM**

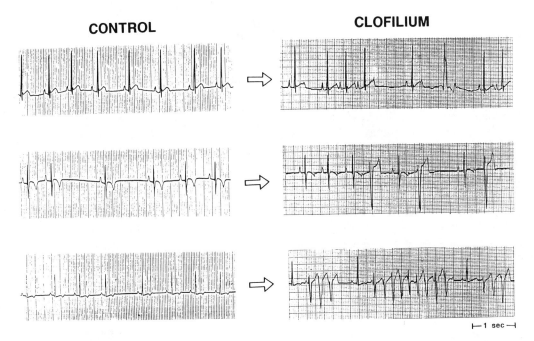

⊢ 1 sec ⊣

Figure 5 Examples of the types of proarrhythmic responses produced by clofilium (1–2 mg/kg IV) in dogs 4–7 days after permanent coronary artery ligation. Ventricular ectopic beats, often with fixed coupling intervals, and runs of nonsustained ventricular tachycardia were seen in 29 of 49 animals studied.

in the urine after 5 days and 31% recovered in the feces after 3 days. In subjects given oral [14C]-clofilium, peak plasma levels occur 2–4 hr following administration. Only 5% of the administered oral dose is excreted in the urine. Thus the absolute bioavailability of clofilium is approximately 9%. To date there is no information available regarding the potential metabolism of the drug.

Safety

Clofilium has no significant effects in either the isolated field-stimulated guinea pig vas deferens model or the positive chronotropic response to isoproterenol in isolated guinea pig atria, indicating that clofilium lacks any significant effects on α-receptors, β_1-receptors, or norepinephrine release mechanisms (66). In anesthetized dogs clofilium has no effect on right ventricular contractile tension measured using a strain gauge (56) but produces a slight increase in left ventricular $(dP/dt)_{max}$ (approximately 30–40%) measured using a left ventricular catheter (52). In conscious dogs

clofilium increases $(dP/dt)_{max}$ only slightly (about 10%). Blood pressure was unaffected in either anesthetized or conscious dogs at doses up to 4 mg/kg IV.

In contrast to the variable results on fibrillation threshold, studies on defibrillation threshold have consistently shown that clofilium lowers the energy required to defibrillate the nonischemic heart (72,73).

In dogs 4–7 days following permanent coronary artery occlusion the administration of clofilium (1–2 mg/kg IV) produced spontaneous ectopic activity, ranging from simple VPD to runs of nonsustained ventricular tachycardia (Fig. 5) in 29 of 49 animals studied (74). Other investigators have previously reported proarrhythmic responses to clofilium in experimental animals (56,60,63). EAD, dispersion of refractoriness, and differential tissue sensitivity have all been implicated as potential mechanisms for this proarrhythmic effect. In the human a proarrhythmic response has been seen in 6 of the 75 patients studied (8%) at a mean dose of 0.2 mg/kg IV (66). No other side effects have been reported to date.

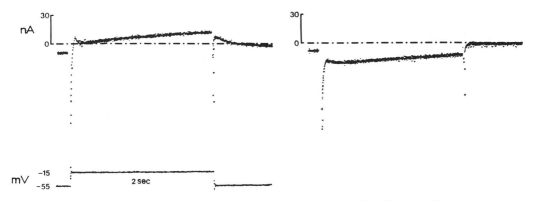

Figure 6   Effect of sematilite on outward current in isolated ferret cardiac Purkinje fiber. A representative, digitized voltage clamp record from an isolated ferret Purkinje fiber before (left) and after (right) a 10 min exposure to 10 μM sematilide. After sematilide the magnitude of outward (repolarizing) current during the test potential of and delayed rectifier tail current amplitude is significantly reduced. Fibers were held at a holding potential of -55 mV, and currents were evoked at a test potential of -15 mV for 2 sec. The dashed line indicates 0 current in each record.

SEMATILIDE

Sematilide (N-[2-(diethylamino)ethyl]-4-[(methylsulfonyl)amino]benzamide hydrochloride; Fig. 1) was prospectively developed as a class III antiarrhythmic agent. Although structurally similar to procainamide, sematilide is devoid of local anesthetic (class I) activity.

Animal Studies

Basic Pharmacology

The electrophysiologic effects of sematilide have been evaluated in rabbit atrial tissues (53). In the sinoatrial node sematilide produces a concentration-dependent (1–100 μM) increase in sinus cycle length and APD_{95} (16 and 42%, respectively, at 30 μM sematilide). In atrial muscle sematilide (30 μM) increases APD_{95} 20% and effective refractory period 36%. Action potential amplitude, maximum diastolic potential, and $(dV/dt)_{max}$ are unchanged.

In canine cardiac Purkinje fibers sematilide produces a parallel, concentration-dependent increase in APD_{50} and APD_{95} (Fig. 2) (75). Similar changes are observed in the effective refractory period. As with the other class III agents the increase in action potential duration is less pronounced at faster rates of stimulation.

Parallel findings were made in ventricular muscle. Action potential recordings from canine ventricular muscle show a significant increase in action potential duration; 10 μM sematilide increases APD_{50} and APD_{95} by 29 ± 7 and $29 \pm 5\%$, respectively, at a stimulation rate of 1 Hz, with no change in other action potential parameters. The effective refractory period also increases in a concentration-dependent manner, using either intracellular or extracellular recording techniques, with no change in conduction velocity.

The mechanism of class III action has been investigated in ferret Purkinje fibers. Voltage clamp studies using the two-microelectrode technique have shown that 10 μM sematilide decreases outward current during plateau potentials and decreases the delayed rectifier current by approximately 50% (Fig. 6).

The in vivo profile of sematilide is consistent with the cellular electrophysiologic findings. Intravenous administration of sematilide (up to 3 mg/kg) significantly increases both right atrial and right ventricular refractoriness in a dose-dependent manner (50 ± 4 and $18 \pm 4\%$, respectively, at the 3 mg/kg dose). There are no effects on intracardiac conduction intervals (AH or HV). QTc increases in a dose-dependent manner (20% at the 3 mg/kg IV dose); the PR interval and QRS duration are unchanged. There was also a dose-dependent decrease in heart rate, which was most likely due to the increase in action potential duration.

Sematilide is effective against reentrant arrhythmias in dogs (76). Sematilide (mean dose 1 mg/kg IV) prevented tachyarrhythmias induced by PES in 8 of 9 dogs tested 3–4 days following an occlusion-reperfusion infarct. Oral administration of sematilide was effective in 7 of 10 animals at a mean dose of 3.6 mg/kg. The effective protective dose in these animals correlated with plasma levels >0.5 µg/ml. There were no significant changes in heart rate, blood pressure, or diastolic pacing threshold. From these studies sematilide appears to be an effective antiarrhythmic agent, preventing PES-induced ventricular tachycardia in conscious dogs with no adverse central nervous system or hemodynamic effects.

Sematilide (1–10 mg/kg IV) is ineffective in abolishing ouabain-induced arrhythmias in dogs. However, at 3 mg/kg sematilide can significantly decrease the rate of the tachycardia and improve hemodynamic stability. Sematilide (1–10 mg/kg IV) had no significant effect on spontaneous arrhythmias arising in dogs studied 24 hr following myocardial infarction.

Administration of sematilide (1–5 mg/kg IV) has no significant effect on VFT using the extrastimulus technique (Euler, personal communication). In contrast to the hemodynamic depression seen after treatment with bretylium (77) or β-adrenergic blocking drugs, no biologically significant effects have been observed on hemodynamic recovery following termination of 1 min of ventricular fibrillation.

Clinical Studies

The effects of sematilide on normal healthy human subjects has been evaluated in placebo-controlled studies. Oral doses of 20–120 mg were studied in a sequential manner, with no clinically significant observed changes in vital signs or clinical laboratory tests. A dose-related prolongation of the QTc interval was observed that was consistent with the class III properties of the drug. The maximum change

in QTc was 30% at the highest dose, and the degree of QTc prolongation correlated with plasma drug concentrations. At this time, no human antiarrhythmic efficacy date are available.

Pharmacokinetics

In dogs the intravenous plasma level profile of sematilide fits predictions for a two-compartment open model with an elimination half-life of 3.2 hr. The absolute bioavailability, which was determined by comparison of the area under the curve for intravenous and oral doses, is 71%. The kinetics appear to be linear, following ascending oral doses over the pharmacologic dose range. Examination of urine and plasma for metabolites indicated that procainamide, N-acetylprocainamide, and n-desethylsematilide were not present. This indicates a lack of metabolism to a free aromatic amine, which greatly reduces the potential for induction of lupus syndrome.

In 12 normal subjects the mean individual time to reach apparent peak plasma concentrations was approximately 2 hr and the mean individual plasma elimination half-life was 2.8 hr.

Safety

In guinea pig papillary muscle 100 µM sematilide produces a modest, positive inotropic effect associated with a decrease in the time to peak force and in the relative rate of relaxation. Lower concentrations have no significant effects.

Defibrillation threshold was studied in 16 dogs; half received sematilide and the others received saline. The defibrillation threshold did not increase, and tended to decrease, after sematilide (3 mg/kg IV) (Ideker, personal communication).

In pentobarbital-anesthetized dogs sematilide (1–30 mg/kg IV) produces a dose-dependent decrease in heart rate and increases stroke index. Left ventricular dp/dt is transiently depressed only following doses of 10 and 30 mg/kg IV in anesthetized animals and is not significantly affected in conscious dogs (Wiggins, unpublished observations). There are no significant effects on mean arterial pressure or left ventricular end-diastolic pressure. A similar lack of hemodynamic effects is seen in animals with acute, ischemia-induced heart failure. No CNS actions of sematilide have been reported.

In one limited series of 10 dogs 4 days after permanent coronary artery ligation sematilide (1–10 mg/kg IV) did not significantly increase the degree of ventricular ectopy compared to saline-treated control animals.

SOTALOL

Sotalol was originally developed in the mid-1960s as an antihypertensive agent. In 1966 Somani and coworkers (78) reported that sotalol inhibited epinephrine-induced arrhythmias in dogs. In 1968 Somani and Watson (79) performed studies to evaluate and compare the antiarrhythmic properties of racemic sotalol and its two optical isomers l- and d-sotalol. Using the same adrenergically induced ventricular tachycardia model they found that d-sotalol was ineffective in preventing arrhythmias. They concluded that the antiarrhythmic effect of racemic sotalol resides in its β-adrenergic blocking property. However, 2 years later Singh and Vaughan Williams (80) identified the action potential-prolonging effect of sotalol as a mechanism for preventing tachycardia and fibrillation induced by cardiac glycosides. This type of action was not typical of other β-adrenergic blocking agents and led to the conclusion that sotalol had additional electrophysiologic properties. In 1985 Carmeliet (81) demonstrated that sotalol inhibits the delayed rectifier potassium current in rabbit Purkinje fibers, thus producing an increase in action potential duration. Since d-sotalol is virtualy devoid of β-adrenergic blocking activity (82) the discussions here are limited to the d-isomer only.

Animal Studies

Basic Pharmacology

d-Sotalol increases action potential duration and refractory periods in artrial and ventricular tissues. In rabbit sinoatrial node d-sotalol produces a significant dose-dependent increase in action potential duration (83–85). This re-sults in a concentration-dependent increase in sinus cycle length (from 473 to 609 msec at 100 μM). The decrease in firing frequency occurs without significant changes in $(dV/dt)_{max}$ or in the slope of phase 4 depolarization. The increase in sinus cycle length was attributed to the increase in action potential duration. Concentration-dependent increases in atrial muscle were also observed by Kato et al. (84); APD_{90} increased 16% in the presence of 10 μM d-sotalol. Thus in atrial tissue d-sotalol exhibits only class III effects, producing no significant changes in action potential amplitude, overshoot, or $(dV/dt)_{max}$ even at higher (100 μM) concentrations.

The effects of d-sotalol on ventricular myocardium and Purkinje fibers are consistent with the class III properties seen in atrial tissue. In the canine ventricle d-sotalol produces a concentration-dependent increase in action potential duration in both Purkinje fiber and ventricular muscle (82,84,86). d-Sotalol (10 μM) increased APD_{90} by 51 and 25% in Purkinje fiber and ventricular muscle, respectively (86). The effective refractory period increased in parallel. Lathrop (86) also reported that in Purkinje fibers d-sotalol exhibits rate dependency; as the stimulation rate is increased, the increase in action potential duration is proportionally decreased. In these fibers early afterdepolarizations were often observed after returning to slower stimulation rates, and this activity occasionally became repetitive. Early afterdepolarizations have also been described in canine Purkinje fibers by Gough and El-Sherif (87).

The effects of d-sotalol on canine atrial and ventricular tissues were described by Gomoll and Bartek (88). In anesthetized dogs, using the extrastimulus technique, d-sotalol (4 mg/kg IV) increased atrial and ventricular refractoriness by 61 and 38 msec, respectively. In addition, AV nodal conduction time is increased.

In anesthetized, open-chest dogs d-sotalol increases ventricular monophasic action potential duration in a dose-dependent manner (89).

Antiarrhythmic Efficacy

In a canine model of atrial flutter intravenous administration of d-sotalol (2 mg/kg) restored sinus rhythm in 14 of 15 dogs and prevented reinduction in 8 dogs (90). This effect occurred simultaneously with a significant increase in atrial effective and function refractory periods (32 and 30%, respectively). Rensma et al. (91) examined the effect of several antiarrhythmic agents on the wavelength (92) of the atrial impulse in conscious dogs by measuring the conduction velocity and the refractory period (wavelength = conduction velocity × refractory period). At short wavelengths (<7.8 cm; induced by premature stimuli) the atria are prone to fibrillation, but an increase in the wavelength protects against repetitive responses, flutter, and fibrillation. All the class I antiarrhythmic agents increase refractoriness but depress conduction, thus having little effect on wavelength or arrhythmia suppression. d-Sotalol (8 mg/kg), however, significantly increases wavelength by increasing refractoriness without depressing conduction, protecting the atria from fibrillation.

Lynch et al. (93) demonstrated that d-sotalol prevents fibrillation in a canine sudden death model. In their study d-sotalol (8 mg/kg IV) suppressed PES-induced ventricular tachycardia in six of nine dogs tested. d-Sotalol also provided protection (in five of eight dogs tested) against the development of ventricular fibrillation in response to ischemia produced by an electrically induced intimal lesion of the circumflex coronary artery. At the same time these authors observed an increase in ventricular refractoriness and QTc interval, suggesting that the antiarrhythmic effects were due to the class III properties of the drug.

Clinical Studies

The class III property of d-sotalol has also been demonstrated in humans (94). In this study each patient ($n = 20$) was given 1, 1.5, or 2 mg/kg of the drug by intravenous infusion. d-Sotalol significantly increased the QT and QTc intervals and the refractory periods of the atrium, atrioventricular node, His-Purkinje system, and right ventricle in a dose-dependent manner. The degree of increase correlated closely with plasma levels of d-sotalol.

Table 2   Average Pharmacokinetic Values for d-Sotalol[a]

$T_{1/2}e$, hr	3.67 ± 0.72
MRT, hr	4.94 ± 0.85
Vd_{ss}, ml/kg	1345 ± 381
Cl_t, ml/min per kg	1.71 ± 0.67

[a]$T_{1/2}e$, elimination half-life;
MRT, mean residence time;
Vd_{ss}, volume of distribution at steady state;
Cl_t, total clearance.
Source: Data from Reference 84.

Schwartz et al. (95) reported similar results in 38 patients undergoing electrophysiologic studies. All patients were off antiarrhythmic drugs and had inducible ventricular tachycardia. d-Sotalol (2 mg/kg IV) infused over a 15 min period did not significantly change the PR, QRS, or QTc intervals from baseline values in the group as a whole. However, in the patients protected from ventricular tachycardia ($n = 18$) by d-sotalol, there was a significant increase in the QTc interval, as well as in ventricular refractoriness. d-Sotalol also significantly reduced heart rate. In the patients who remained inducible d-sotalol significantly slowed the rate of the tachycardia. After the study 11 patients were discharged on oral d-sotalol (100–400 mg twice a day). The authors reported that during the following month 1 patient died from acute myocardial infarction and 1 patient had a cardiac arrest, survived, and was switched to amiodarone. After a 14 month period the remaining 9 patients were alive and well.

Pharmacokinetics

In dogs d-sotalol disappears from the plasma in a biexponential (second-order) manner with a mean α-phase half-life of 12 min (84). The pharmacokinetics of d-sotalol in dogs are summarized in Table 2.

Studies on the pharmacokinetics of d-sotalol in the human have not been reported. Since stereoisomerism can influence pharmacokinetics as well as pharmacodynamics, one cannot reliably estimate the pharmacokinetics of d-sotalol from the data reported for the racemate.

Safety

In rats d-sotalol has no effects on $(dP/dt)_{max}$ heart rate, or mean arterial pressure (96).

d-Sotalol (5 mg/kg IV) reduces the amount of energy necessary for defibrillation of anesthetized dogs with internal patch electrodes (73). The current and energy required for defibrillation was reduced by 14 and 29%, respectively.

In contrast to the high incidence of adverse reactions that have been reported for racemic sotalol (97), few if any adverse effects have been reported to date for d-sotalol. However, the clinical experience with d-sotalol is very limited.

CONCLUSIONS

Class III antiarrhythmic agents hold great promise in the prevention of life-threatening ventricular arrhythmias. As a group they have significantly greater efficacy in preventing the appearance of ventricular and atrial tachyarrhythmias and fibrillation, evoked by programmed electrical stimulation, than the class I compounds, including the class IA group. In general, efficacy against these arrhythmias appears to be associated with an increase in refractoriness. Class III agents are relatively ineffective, however, against the simpler, and perhaps clinically less significant, forms of ventricular ectopy.

As a group the class III compounds are devoid of adverse cardiac and central nervous system actions, holding the promise of improved efficacy with greater safety than the currently available agents. The absence of any cardiovascular depression may allow their use in patients with impaired ventricular function, a patient group at high risk of sudden cardiac death. Although their effect on fibrillation threshold remains undefined, the class III drugs do not significantly increase, and may decrease, the defibrillation threshold, a significant advantage in patients in whom antiarrhythmic therapy fails. In addition their improved safety may allow treatment of atrial arrhythmias that now are left untreated because the risk of therapy exceeds the risk of the arrhythmia itself.

It must be recognized, however, that the class III agents are a new therapeutic class and their potential limitations have not yet been fully explored. Of great concern is their potential to induce arrhythmic episodes. The proarrhythmic effects of the class I antiarrhythmic compounds are well-known, occurring in approximately 10–15% of patients. Occasional proarrhythmic effects have been described for acecainide and clofilium. It is unclear, however, that the prolongation of the QT interval, which is the hallmark of the class III agents, and proarrhythmia are linked. It seems probable that local inhomogeneities in refractoriness, rather than the global increase in QT, is responsible for this action. Clofilium, sotalol, and sematilide all preferentially increase action potential duration in ischemic tissue, an action that undoubtedly contributes to their efficacy but may also lead to local inhomogeneities in refractoriness, which in turn may predispose to coupled beats and other reentrant tachyarrhythmias. Although devoid of direct hemodynamic effects the electrophysiologic safety of class III agents needs to be proven in patients with myocardial dysfunction.

In summary, the evolving data for class III agents suggest that these drugs will have a significant impact in preventing reentrant ventricular and atrial tachyarrhythmias. Their favorable safety profile may allow for the treatment of patients who are intolerant of traditional antiarrhythmic drug therapies.

REFERENCES

1. Vaughan Williams E M. Classification of antiarrhythmic drugs. In: Sandoz E, Flensted-Jensen E, Olesen K H, eds. Symposium on cardiac arrhythmics. Sweden: AB Astra 1970PR:449–69.

2. Butrous G S, Debbas N M, Erwin J, Davies D W, Keller H P, Lunnon M W, Nathan A W, Camm A J. Clinical cardiac electrophysiologic evaluation of the positive inotropic agent, DPI 201–106. Eur Heart J 1988; 9:489–97.

3. Drayer D E, Reidenberg M M, Sevy R W. N-acetylprocainamide: an active metabolite of procainamide. Proc Soc Exp Biol Med 1974; 146:358–63

4. Atkins A J Jr, Ruo T I, Piergies A A. Comparison of the pharmacokinetic and pharmacodynamic properties of procainamide and N-acetylprocainamide. Angiology 1988; 39:655–67.

5. Minchin R F, Ilett K F, Paterson J W. Antiarrhythmic potency of procainamide and N-acetylprocainamide in rabbits. Eur J Pharmacol 1978; 47:51–6.

6. Refsum H, Frislid K, Lunde P K M, Landmark K H. Effects of N-acetyprocainamide as compared with procainamide in isolated rat atria. Eur J Pharmacol 1975; 33:47–52.

7. Dangman K H, Hoffman B F. In vivo and in vitro antiarrhythmic and arrhythmogenic effects of N-acetyl procainamide. J Pharmacol Exp Ther 1981; 217:851–62.

8. Amlie J P, Nesje O A, Frislid K, Lunde P K M, Landmark K. Serum levels and electrophysiological effects of N-acetylprocainamide as compared with procainamide in the dog heart in situ. Acta Pharmacol Toxicol (Coperh) 1978 42:280–6.

9. Boucher M, Dubray C, Paire M, Duchene-Marullaz P. Comparative effects of procainamide and its N-acetylated metabolite in conscious dogs with atrioventricular block: plasma concentration-response relationships. J Cardiovasc Pharmacol 1987; 10:562–7.

10. Jaillon P, Winkle R A. Electrophysiologic comparative study of procainamide and N-acetylprocainamide in anesthetized dogs: concentration-response relationships. Circulation 1979; 60:1385–94.

11. Okamura K, Waldo A L. Effects of N-acetylprocainamide on experimental atrial flutter and atrial electrophysiologic properties in conscious dogs with sterile pericarditis: comparison with the effects of quinidine. J Am Coll Cardiol 1987; 9:1332–8.

12. Amlie J P, Landmark K. N-acetylprocainamide induced changes in refractoriness and monophasic action potentials of the dog heart in situ. Cardiovasc Res 1981; 15:159–63.

13. Wu K M, Hoffman B F. Effect of procainamide and N-acetylprocainamide on atrial flutter: studies in vivo and in vitro. Circulation 1987; 76:1397–408.

14. Boyden P A. Effects of pharmacologic agents on induced atrial flutter in dogs with right atrial enlargement. J Cardiovasc Pharmacol 1986; 8:170–7.

15. Feld G K, Venkatesh N, Singh B N. Effects of N-acetylprocainamide and recainam in the pharmacologic conversion and suppression of experimental canine atrial flutter: significance of changes in refractoriness and conduction. J Cardiovasc Pharmacol 1988; 11:573–80.

16. Elson J, Strong J M, Lee W-K, Atkinson A J Jr. Antiarrhythmic potency of N-acetylprocainamide. Clin Pharmacol Ther 1975; 17:134–40.

17. Bagwell E E, Walle T, Drayer D E, Reidenberg M M, Pruett J K. Correlation of the electrophysiological and antiarrhythmic properties of the N-acetyl metabolite of procainamide with plasma and tissue drug concentrations in the dog. J Pharmacol Exp Ther 1976; 197:38–48.

18. Reynolds R D, Kamath B L. N-acetylprocainamide and ischemia-induced ventricular fibrillation in the dog. Eur J Pharmacol 1979; 59:115–9.

19. Jaillon P, Rubenson D, Peters F, Mason J W, Winkle R A. Electrophysiologic effects of N-acetylprocainamide in human beings. Am J Cardiol 1981; 47:1134–40.

20. Sung R J, Juma Z, Saksena S. Electrophysiologic properties and antiarrhythmic mechanisms of intravenous N-acetylprocainamide in patients with ventricular dysrhythmias. Am Heart J 1983; 105:811–9.

21. Wynn J, Miura D S, Torres V, et al. Electrophysiologic evaluation of the antiarrhythmic effect of N-acctylprocainamide for ventricular tachycardia, secondry to coronary artery disease. Am J Cardiol 1985; 56:877–81.

22. Winkle R A, Jaillon P, Kates R E, Peters F. Clinical pharmacology and antiarrhythmic efficacy of N-acetylprocainamide. Am J Cardiol 1981; 947:123–30.

23. Sonnhag C, Karlsson E. Comparative antiarrhythmic efficacy of intravenous N-acetylprocainamide and procainamide. Eur J Clin Pharmacol 1979; 15:311–7.

24. Crawford M H, Ludden T M, Kennedy G T, Sodums M T, O'Rourke R A, Amon K W. Hemodynamic effects of N-acetylprocainamide in heart disease. Clin Pharmacol Ther 1982; 31:459–65.

25. Somberg J, Wynn J, Miura D, Torres V, Williams S, Keefe D. N-acetylprocainamide's antiarrhythmic action in patients with ventricular tachycardia. Angiology 1986; 37:972–81.

26. Piergies A A, Ruo T I, Jansyn E M, Belknap S M, Atkinson A J Jr. Effect kinetics of N-acetylprocainamide-induced QT interval prolongation. Clin Pharmacol Ther 1987; 42:107–12.

27. Lee W K, Strong J M, Kehoe R F, Dutcher J S, Atkinson A J Jr. Antiarrhythmic efficacy of N-acetylprocainamide in patients with premature ventricular contractions. Clin Pharmacol Ther 1976; 19:508–14.

28. Atkinson A J Jr, Lee W-K, Quinn M L, Kushner W, Nevin M J, Strong J M. Dose-ranging trial of N-acetylprocainamide in patients with premature ventricular contractions. Clin Pharmacol Ther 1977; 21:575–87.

29. Kluger J, Drayer D, Reidenberg M, Ellis G, Lloyd V, Tyberg T, Hayes J. The clinical pharmacology and antiarrhythmic efficacy of acetylprocainamide in patients with arrhythmias. Am J Cardiol 1980; 45:1250–7.

29a. Atkinson A J Jr, Lertora J J, Kushner W, Chao G C, Nevin M J. Efficacy and safety of N-acetylprocainamide in long-term treatment of ventricular arrhythmias. Clin Pharmacol Ther 1983; 33:565–76.

30. Kluger J, Leech S, Reidenberg M M, Lloyd V, Drayer D E. Long-term antiarrhythmic therapy with acetylprocainamide. Am J Cardiol 1981; 48:1124–32.

31. Kamath B L, Lai C M, Gupta S D, Durrani M J, Yacobi A. Pharmacokinetics of procainamide and N-acetylprocainamide in rats. J Pharm Sci 1981; 70:299–302.

32. Yacobi A, Kamath B L, Stampfli H F, Look Z M, Lai C M. Age-related pharmacokinetics of N-acetylprocainamide in rats. J Pharm Sci 1983; 72:789–92.

33. Yacobi A, Stampfli H F, Lai C M, Kamath B L. Tissue distribution of N-acetylprocainamide in rats. Drug Metab Dispos 1981; 9:193–5

34. Silberstein D J, Bowmer C J, Yates M S, Dean H G. Effect of acute renal failure on the disposition and elimination of [^{3}H]N-acetyl procainamide ethobromide in the rat. J Pham Pharmacol 1986; 38:679–85.

35. Lai C M, Reynolds R D, Kamath B L, Calzadilla S, Gupta S D, Look Z M, Yacobi A. Effect of coronary artery ligation on the pharmacokinetics of N-acetylprocainamide in dogs. Res Commun Chem Pathol Pharmacol 1980; 29:369–72.

36. Strong J M, Dutcher J S, Lee W K, Atkinson AJ Jr. Pharmacokinetics in man of the N-acetylated metabolite of procainamide. J Pharmacokinet Biopharm 1975; 3:223–35.

37. Kluger J, Horner H, Reidenberg M M. Effects of procainamide and N-acetylprocainamide on myocardial contractility in ischemic isolated rabbit hearts. Proc Soc Exp Biol Med 1981; 168:350–5.

38. Lertora J J L, Glock D, Stec G P, Atkinson A J Jr, Goldberg L I. Effects of N-acetylprocainamide and procainamide on myocardial contractile force, heart rate, and blood pressure. Proc Soc Exp Biol Med 1979; 161:332–6.

39. Badke F R, Walsh R A, Crawford M H, Ludden T, ORourke T A. Hemodynamic effects of N-acetylprocainamide compared with procainamide in conscious dogs. Circulation 1981; 64:1142–50.

40. Lertora J J, King L W, Donkor K A. The inotropic actions of N-acetylprocainamide: blockage and reversal by propranolol. Angiology 1986; 37:939–49.

41. Lertora J J, Stec G P, Kushner W, Eudeikis J R. The hemodynamic actions of N-acetylprocainamide in dogs: kinetics of effects and plasma concentration-response relationships. Proc Soc Exp Biol Med 1980; 164:128–36.

42. Pearle D L, Souza J D, Gillis R A. Comparative vagolytic effects of procainamide and N-acetylprocainamide in the dog. J Cardiovasc Pharmacol 1983; 5:450–3.

43. Eudeikis J R, Henthorn T K, Lertora J J, Atkinson A J Jr, Chao G C, Kushner W. Kinetic analysis of the vasodilator and ganglionic blocking actions of N-acetylprocainamide. J Cardiovasc Pharmacol 1982; 4:303–9.

44. Reynolds R D, Gorczynski R J. Comparison of the autonomic efects of procainamide and N-acetylprocainamide in the dog. J Pharmacol Exp Ther 1980; 212:579–83.

45. Josephson M A, Schwab M, Coyle K, Singh B N. Effects of intravenous N-acetylprocainamide on hemodynamics and left ventricular function in man. Am Heart J 1987; 113:952–7.

46. Chow M J, Piergies A A, Bowsher D J, Murphy J J, Kushner W, Ruo T I, Asada A, Talano J V, Atkinson A J Jr. Torsades de pointes induced by N-acetylprocainamide. J Am Coll Cardiol 1984; 4:621–24.

47. Stratmann H G, Walter K E, Kennedy H L. Torsades de pointes associated with elevated N-acetylprocainamide levels. Am Heart J 1985; 109:375–7.

48. Herre J M, Thompson J A. Polymorphic ventricular tachycardia and ventricular fibrillation due to N-acetyl procainamide. Am J Cardiol 1985; 55:227–8.

49. Roden D M, Reele S B, Higgins S B, Wilkinson G R, Smith R F, Oates J A, Woosley R L. Antiarrhythmic efficacy, pharmacokinetics and safety of N-acetylprocainamide in human subjects: comparison with procainamide. Am J Cardiol 1980; 46:463–8.

50. Kluger J, Drayer D E, Reidenberg M M, Lahita R. Acetylprocainamide therapy in patients with previous procainamide-induced lupus syndrome. Ann Intern Med 1981; 95:18–23.

51. Richardson B, Cornacchia E, Golbus J, Maybaum J, Strahler J, Hanash S. N-acetylprocainamide is a less potent inducer of T cell autoreactivity than procainamide. Arthritis Rheum 1988; 31:995–9.

52. Steinberg M I, Michelson E L. Cardiac electrophysiologic effects of specific class III substances. In: Reiser H J, Horowitz L N, eds. Mechanisms and treatment of cardiac arrhythmias; relevance of basic studies to clinical management. Baltimore: Urban and Schwarzenberg 1985:263–81.

53. Carroll M S, Argentieri T M. The in vitro electrophysiological effects of clofilium and sematilide on rabbit atrial tissues (abstract). Pharmacologist 1989; 31:387.

54. Steinberg M I, Molloy B B. Clofilium—a new antifibrillatory agent that selectively increases cellular refractoriness. Life Sci 1979; 25:1397–406.

55. Steinberg M I, Sullivan M E, Wiest S A, Rockhold F W, Molloy B B. Cellular electrophysiology of clofilium, a new antifibrillatory agent, in normal and ischemic canine Purkinje fibers. J Cardiovasc Pharmacol 1981; 3:881–95.

56. Steinberg M I, Lindstrom T D, Fasola A F. Clofilium. In: Scriabine A, ed. New drugs annual: cardiovascular drugs, Vol. 2. New York: Raven Press 1984:103–21.

57. Snyders D J, Katzung B G. Clofilium reduces the plateau potassium current in isolated cardiac myocytes (abstract). Circulation 1985; 72(III):III-233.

58. Arena J P, Kass R S. Block of heart potassium channels by clofilium and its tertiary analogs: relationship between drug structure and type of channel blocked. Mol Pharmacol 1988; 34:60–6.

59. Argentieri T M, Sullivan M E, Ambelas E, Wiggins J. Proarrhythmic effects of clofilium in dogs with acute myocardial infarction (abstract). J Mol Cell Cardiol 1987; 19:S.68.

60. Gough W B, Hu D, El-Sherif N. Effects of clofilium on ischemic subendocardial Purkinje fibers 1 day postinfarction. J Am Coll Cardiol 1988; 11:431–7.

61. Sullivan M E, Steinberg M I. Cardiovascular and electrocardiographic effects of clofilium in conscious or anesthetized dogs (abstract). Pharmacologist 1981; 23:209.

62. Kowey P R, Friehling T D, O'Connor K M, Wetstein L, Kelliher G J. The effect of bretylium and clofilium on dispersion of refractoriness and vulnerability to ventricular fibrillation in the ischemic feline heart. Am Heart J 1985; 110:363–70.

63. Kopia G A, Eller B T, Patterson E, Shea M J, Lucchesi B R. Antiarrhythmic and electrophysiologic actions of clofilium in experimental canine models. Eur J Pharmacol 1985; 116:49–61.

65. Euler D E, Scanlon P J. Comparative effects of antiarrhythmic drugs on the ventricular fibrillation threshold. J Cardiovasc Pharmacol 1988; 11:291–8.

66. Steinberg M I, Smallwood J K. Clofilium and other class III agents. In: Vaughan Williams E M, ed. Handbook of experimental pharmacology, Vol. 89, Antiarrhythmic drugs. Berlin: Springer-Verlag 1989:389–412.

67. Michelson E L, Naito M, David D, Dreifus L S, Moore E N. Antiarrhythmic efficacy and electropharmacology of clofilium in a chronic canine ventricular tachyarrhythmia model. Circulation 1981; 64:IV-124.

68. Morgan T K, Lis R, Marisca A J, Argentieri T M, Sullivan M E, Wong S S. Synthesis and cardiac electrophysiological activity of 2- and 3- [(substituted phenyl) alkyl] quinuclidines. Structure-activity relationships. J Med Chem 1987; 30:2259–69.

69. Greene H L, Werner J A, Gross B W, Sears G K, Trobaugh G B, Cobb L A. Prolongation of cardiac refractory times in man by clofilium phosphate, a new antiarrhythmic agent. Am Heart J 1983; 106:492–501.

70. Platia E V, Reid P R. Dose-ranging studies of clofilium, an antiarrhythmic quarternary ammonium. Clin Pharmacol Ther 1984; 35:193–202.

71. Lindstrom T D, Murphy P J, Smallwood J K, Wiest S A, Steinberg M I. Correlation be-

tween the dispostion of [14C]-clofilium and its cardiac electrophysiological effect. J Pharmacol Exp Ther 1982; 221:584–9.

72. Tacker W A. Niebauer M J, Babbs C F, Combs W J, Hahn B M, Barker M A, Seipel J F, Bourland J D, Geddes L A. The effect of newer antiarrhythmic drugs on defibrillation threshold. Crit Care Med 1980; 8:177–80.

73. Dawson A K, Steinberg M I, Shapland J E. Effect of class I and class III drugs on current and energy required for internal defibrillation (abstract). Circulation 1985; 72:III-384.

74. Sansone K J, Sullivan M E. The effects of propatenone, propranolol, and verapamil on clofilium-induced proarrhythmic responses in conscious dogs (abstract). Pharmacologist 1988; 30:A177.

75. Sullivan M E, Argentieri T M, Stoner S, Wiggins J, Reiser H J. Electrophysiologic properties of CK-1752A, a new specific class III agent (abstract). Cardiovasc Drugs Ther 1987; 1:294.

76. Wiggins J, Sullivan M E, Doroshuk C M, Reiser H J. Antiarrhythmic and hemodynamic properties of CK-1752A, a new class III agent, in experimental myocardial infarction (abstract). Cardiovasc Drugs Ther 1987; 1:302.

77. Euler D E, Zeeman T W, Wallock, ME, Scanlon P J. Deleterious effects of bretylium on hemodynamic recovery from ventricular fibrillation. Am Heart J 1986; 112:25–32.

78. Somani P, Fleming J G, Chan G K, Lum B K B. Antagonism of epinephrine-induced cardiac arrhythmias by 4-(2-isopropyl-amino-1hydroxyethyl) methanesulfonanilide (MJ 1999). J Pharmacol Exp Ther 1966; 151:32–37.

79. Somani P, Watson D L. Antiarrhythmic activity of the *dextro-* and *levo*-rotary isomers of 4-(2-isopropylamino-1-hydroxyethyl) methanesulfonanilide (MJ 1999). J Pharmacol Exp Ther 1968; 164:317–25.

80. Singh B N, Vaughan Williams E M. A third class of antiarrhythmic action. Effect on atrial and ventricular intracellular potentials, and other pharmacological actions on cardiac muscle. Br J Pharmacol 1970; 39:675–87.

81. Carmeliet E. Electrophysiologic and voltage clamp analysis of the effects of sotalol on isolated cardiac muscle and Purkinje fibers. J Pharmacol Exp Ther 1985; 232:817–25.

82. Manley B S, Alexopoulos D, Robinson G J, Cobbe S M. Subsidiary class III effects of

beta blocker? A comparison of atenolol, metoprolol, nadolol, oxprenolol and sotalol. Cardiovasc Res 1986; 20:705–9.

83. McComb J M, McGowan J B, McGovern B A, Ruskin G H. Comparison of the electrophysiologic properties of d- and dl- sotalol (abstract). J Am Coll Cardiol 1985; 5:438.

84. Kato R, Ikeda N, Yabek S M, Kannan R, Singh B N. Electrophysiologic effects of the levo and dextrortotatory isomers of sotalol in isolated cardiac muscle and their in vivo pharmacokinetics. J Am Coll Cardiol 1986; 7:116–25.

85. Beyer T, Brachmann J, Aidonidis I, Rizos I, Kübler W. Effects of *d*-sotalol on electrophysiological parameters in rabbit AV-nodal preparations: demonstration of acute class II actions (abstract). J Mol Cell Cardiol 1986; 18(Suppl.):279.

86. Lathrop D A. Electromechanical characterization of the effects of racemic sotalol and its optical isomers in isolated canine ventricular trabecular muscles and Purkinje strands. Can J Physiol Pharmacol 1985; 63:1506–12.

87. Gough W B, El-Sherif N. The differential response of ischemic endocardium to type III antiarrhythmics: early afterpolarizations (abstract). Circulation 1986; 74(Suppl. II):253.

88. Gomoll A W, Bartek M J. Comparative β-blocking activities and electrophysiologic actions of racemic sotalol and its optical isomers in anesthetized dogs. Eur J Pharmacol. 1986; 132:123–35.

89. Taggart P, Sutton P, Donaldson R. *d*-Sotalol: a new potent class III anti-arrhythmic agent. Clin Sci 1985;69:631–6.

90. Feld G K, Venkatesh N, Singh B N. Pharmacologic conversion and suppresion of experimental canine atrial flutter: differing effects of *d*-sotalol, quinidine, and lidocaine and significance of changes in refractoriness and conduction. Circulation 1986; 74-1:197–204.

91. Rensma P L, Allessie M A, Lammers W J E P, Bonke F I M, Schanlij M J. Length of excitation wave and susceptibility to reentrant atrial arrhythmias in normal conscious dogs. Circ Res 1988; 62:395–410.

92. Méndez C, Mueller W J, Merideth J, Moe G K. Interaction of transmembrane potentials in canine Purkinje fibers and at Purkinje fiber-muscle junction. Circ Res 1969; 24:361–72.

93. Lynch J J, Coskey L A, Montgomery D G, Lucchesi B R. Prevention of ventricular

fibrillation by dextrorotatory sotalol in a conscious canine model of sudden coronary death. Am Heart J 1985; 109:949–58.

94. McComb J M, McGovern B, McGowan J B, Ruskin J N, Garan H. Electrophysiologic effects of *d*-sotalol in humans. J Am Coll Cardiol 1987; 10:211–7.

95. Schwartz J, Crocker K, Wynn J, Somberg J C. The antiarrhythmic effects of *d*-sotalol. Am Heart J 1987; 114(3):539–44.

96. Hoffmeister H M, Seipel L. Comparison of the hemodynamic effects of *d*-sotalol and *dl*-sotalol. Klin Wochenschr 1988; 66(10):451–4.

97. Anastasiou-Nana M I, Anderson J L, Askins J C, Gilbert E M, Nanas J N, Menlove R L. Long-term experience with sotalol in the treatment of complex ventricular arrhythmias. Am Heart J 1987; 114:288–96.

34

Class IV Antiarrhythmic Drugs

Elliott M. Antman and James D. Marsh

Brigham and Women's Hospital and Harvard Medical School
Boston, Massachusetts

INTRODUCTION

Observations by Singh and Vaughan Williams in 1972 suggested that the electrophysiologic effects of the then new compound verapamil were markedly different from those exhibited by local anesthetic type of antiarrhythmic agents (class I drugs) and β-adrenoceptor blocking agents (class II drugs) (1). Since verapamil did not appear to prolong the action potential duration of myocardial cells it also seemed different from drugs like amiodarone (class III drugs), and therefore a new class of antiarrhythmic drugs was proposed (class IV drugs). Considerable investigation by basic scientists and clinical electrophysiologists confirmed that this new class of pharmacotherapeutic agents constituted an important "breakthrough" with exciting research and therapeutic potential.

Since class IV drugs act principally by inhibiting the inward movement of calcium ions into myocardial and vascular cells a variety of terms have been put forth, including "calcium channel blockers", "calcium entry blockers", and "calcium antagonists". Although none of these terms is ideal, we are inclined to agree with the recent arguments by Nayler, that for the present the most suitable term appears to be "calcium antagonists," and this term is utilized for the remainder of this chapter (2). Class IV calcium antagonist drugs include compounds from three structurally and pharmacologically distinct classes: phenylalkylamines, exemplified by verapamil; dihydropyridines, with nifedipine a representative compound; and benzothiazepines, represented by diltiazem. There are additional class IV drugs that do not belong to these three groups. Compounds in these groups have been classified as organic calcium antagonists. There are a number of inorganic species, such as the polyvalent cations Co^{2+}, Ni^{2+}, La^{3+}, and Mn^{2+}, which also inhibit calcium entry into cells. The inorganic calcium antagonists inhibit calcium entry by mechanisms distinct from those of organic calcium antagonists and display different selectivity for types of calcium channels. The inorganic calcium antagonists represent useful research tools, but they are not applied clinically because of their generalized systemic effects and toxicity. Therefore the major emphasis in this chapter is on the organic calcium antagonists.

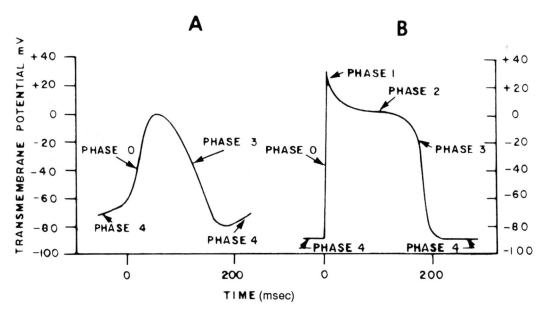

Figure 1 Typical action potentials recorded from cells in the sinoatrial node (A) and ventricular myocardium (B). Note the slower rate of rise and smaller amplitude of the sinoatrial node action potential since it is dependent on the slow inward current for depolarization. (Reproduced from Ref. 48 and reprinted by permission of Ann. Intern. Med.)

OVERVIEW OF SLOW INWARD CURRENT

Electrophysiology of the Slow Inward Current

Appreciation of the pivotal role of Ca^{2+} fluxes in cardiac cellular electrophysiology requires an understanding of the electrical activity of cardiac cells (Table 1). The shape of the action potential varies among different types of cardiac cells (3,4). Cells in the sinoatrial (SA) and atrioventricular (AV) nodes (Fig. 1A) depolarize considerable more slowly than do cells in Purkinje fibers or atrial or ventricular contractile fibers (Fig. 1B). Upon depolarization from a resting transmembrane voltage of -90 mV the membrane conductance for Na^+ rapidly increases. This fast inward current can be described in terms of activation (m) and inactivation gates (h) in a model of the Na^+ channel (3,5,6). As Na^+ ions rush into the cell through open m gates, the transmembrane potential becomes less negative (inside with respect to outside) and the h gates close, thereby terminating the fast inward current.

When the cell has been depolarized from -90 to about -40 mV, a second inward current, termed the slow inward current, develops (5,7–10). The kinetics of the slow inward current are several orders of magnitude slower than those of the fast inward current (Table 1) (8,11,12). It can be activated at levels of membrane voltage that would ordinarily inactivate the fast inward Na^+ current (7,12–15), and it reaches its maximum value when membrane potential is in the range of -20 to 0 mV (12). The major but not exclusive ionic species traversing the cell membrane during the slow current is Ca^{2+} (7,16). Since the "slow channels" as estimated by Reuter are 100 times more selective for Ca^{2+} than for Na^+ or K^+, the use of the term "calcium channel" is justified (7,13).

Action potentials from contractile cells in atrium and myocardium, specialized intracardiac conduction system, and distal AV nodal regions depend on both the fast and slow inward currents. Pacemaker cells of the SA node and cells in the proximal regions of the AV node have slowly rising action potentials and a reduced rate of conduction and are activated largely by the slow inward current. Such "slow responses" may also be observed in

Table 1 Characteristics of Fast and Slow Inward Currents of Cardiac Action Potential

Property	Fast	Slow
Ionic selectivity	$Na^+ > Li^+ > K^+ > Rb^+ > Cs^+$	$Ca^{2+} > Ba^{2+} > Sr^{2+} > Na^+$
Ion-carrying capacity of channel, ions/sec per channel	$5 \times 10^5\ Na^+$	$3 \times 10^6\ Ca^{2+}$
Threshold of activation, mV	-60 to -70	-40 to -50
Maximal rate of depolarization, V/sec	Rapid (100–1000)	Slow (1–20)
Overshoot potential, mV	20–35	0–15
Action potential amplitude, mV	100–130	35–75
Conduction velocity, m/sec	0.5–2.0	0.01–0.1
Safety factor for conduction	High	Low
Initiation of current flow	IK_2 pacemaker current, normally conducted impulses	Depolarization
Type of response to stimulus	All or none	Variable
Stimulators of current flow	Veratridine	Cyclic AMP
Time constant of inactivation, msec	Rapid (1–2)	Slow (50–200)
Time course of refractoriness	Ends with repolarization (voltage dependent)	Ends after repolarization (time dependent)
Inhibitors of current flow	TTX, local anesthetics	Calcium antagonists
Current inactivated by voltage clamp to -50 mV	+	–
Cellular localization		
SA node	–	+
Atrial myocardium	+	+
AV node		
Proximal	–	+
Distal	+	+
His-Purkinje system	+	+
Ventricular myocardium	+	+
Other		Mitral and tricuspid valves, coronary sinus, under pathologic conditions

Source: Modified from References 16, 48, and 92.

other cardiac cells under abnormal conditions, such as ischemia, hypoxia, and exposure to catecholamines (4).

In addition to spontaneous phase 4 depolarization there is another mechanism whereby electrical impulses can be rhythmically generated in cardiac cells. This repetitive activity requires triggering by a preceding depolarization and is referred to as triggered repetitive activity (17). Impulses arising through this mechanism are generated by delayed afterdepolarizations of sufficient magnitude to depolarize the cell membrane to the threshold for activation. Delayed afterdepolarizations have been recorded in normal simian mitral valve leaflet tissue (18), in a human anterior mitral valve leaflet obtained from the heart of a recipient of a cardiac transplant (19), in fibers of rat atrial pectinate muscle and crista terminalis (20), in the coronary sinus of dogs (21), in ouabain-poisoned fibers (22–23,25) and in mitral valve tissue exposed to epinephrine (17,26). The precise ionic currents underlying delayed afterdepolarizations have not been completely elucidated, but it appears that class IV antiarrhythmic drugs, which reduce the slow inward current, can prevent the development of triggered activity (17). It does not appear, however, that the slow inward current is directly responsible for triggered activity but may lead to the oscillatory release of calcium ions from other intracellular sources (27).

Structure of the Calcium Channel

Calcium channels have been identified in virtually all electrically excitable tissue. There are three types of calcium channels that are defined by voltage dependence, inactivation kinetics, and sensitivity to organic and inorganic channel blockers (28). The channel types have been termed L, T, and N, depending on the kinetics of inactivation of the calcium current. All three types of calcium channel are present in neurons, whereas only the L and T types are present in cardiac atrial and ventricular tissue. A considerable amount is known about the structure and pharmacology of the L-type channel, whereas considerably less is known about the T-type channel. Organic calcium channel blockers specifically interact with the L channel, and it is the L channel that is commonly described as the "cardiac calcium channel." Thus the L channel is the channel discussed throughout this chapter.

Understanding of the structure of the cardiac calcium channel is relatively limited, but a great deal can be inferred from its similarity to the structure of the skeletal muscle calcium channel, about which a great deal is known. By far the highest concentration of calcium channels is found in t-tubules of skeletal muscle, where they appear to primarily play the role of a voltage transducer. Work on purification and structural analysis of the calcium channel has therefore been based largely on skeletal muscle (29–32). The skeletal muscle calcium channel comprises a tightly bound α_1-β-γ structure with an additional α_2-δ subunit that is less tightly associated. The α_1 and β subunits contain phosphorylation sites for cyclic AMP dependent protein kinase (30,33). The γ, α_2, and δ subunits contain glycosylation sites whereas the α_1 subunit is not a glycoprotein (29). The entire calcium channel complex is a large structure with an apparent mass of approximately 370 kilodaltons (kD). The α_1 subunit has an apparent mass of about 175 kD, the α_2 has a mass of 143 kD, and the δ subunit has a mass of 27 kD (see Fig. 2). The α_1 subunit contains the binding site for organic calcium channel blockers. In 1987 the complete amino acid sequence of the α_1 subunit from rabbit skeletal muscle was deduced by cloning and sequence analysis of the cDNA for the subunit (32). The α_1 subunit has four membrane spanning domains assumed to surround the ionic channel. A striking finding was that there is a very high degree of similarity between amino acid sequences of the calcium channel and sodium channel (55%) (32). This observation strongly suggests that the genes coding for the α_1 subunit of the calcium channel and for the sodium channel arose from a common ancestor and furthermore suggests that voltage-dependent ionic channels represent a family of evolutionarily and structurally related gene products (30,32). The sequence of the α_2 subunit of calcium channel has recently been de-

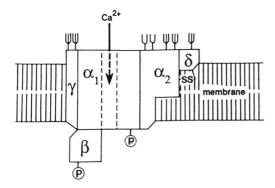

Figure 2 Proposed model for calcium channel structure. Sites for phosphorylation (P) are indicated. Forked structures indicate points for glycosylation. It is proposed that calcium enters through a pore formed by membrane-spanning domains of the α_1 subunit. (Reproduced with permission from Takahashi M, Seagar MJ, Jones JF, Reber BFX, Catterall WA. Subunit structure of dihydropyridine-sensitive calcium channels from skeletal muscle. Proc Natl Acad Sci USA 1987; 84:5478–82.

termined (31) and does not show homology with other known protein sequences.

The organic calcium channel antagonists, including the dihydropyridines, the phenylalkylamines, and the benzothiazepines, all bind to the α_1 subunit. The dihydropyridine (DHP) binding site is distinct but allosterically related to the phenylalkylamine and benzothiazepine binding site. Not only can the organic calcium channel blockers block the L-type channel in skeletal muscle and in heart tissue, but elevated concentrations of intracellular calcium can also block the channel (34).

Although examination of the structure of the cardiac calcium channel is less advanced than that for the skeletal muscle calcium channel, it appears that there are very substantial similarities and that the primary and secondary structures of the channels are quite similar (35,36). Importantly, the α_1 subunit of the cardiac calcium channel appears to be very similar to that of the skeletal muscle calcium channel (35).

Modulation of Slow Inward Current

β-Adrenergic agonists, methylxanthines, histamine, angiotensin II, cyclic AMP, and dibu-

tyryl cyclic AMP all increase the magnitude of the slow inward current (8,11,13,37–41); β-adrenergic blocking agents reduce Ca^{2+} influx (37,42,43). Compounds that increase the concentration of cyclic AMP cells share a common mode of action in modulating calcium entry through the calcium channel in cardiac tissue. Elevated cAMP concentration activates cAMP-dependent protein kinase, which in turn phosphorylates the α_1 subunit of the L-type calcium channel (33). Single-channel recordings of mammalian heart cells utilizing the patch clamp technique (44) have revealed the following sequence of events (45). The average Ca channel current I_{Ca} can be described as $I_{Ca} = N \times P_o \times i$, where N is the number of calcium channels, P_o is the overall probability of opening of the channel, and i is the current flowing through individual channels when they are open. The unitary conductance i is almost always constant. Phosphorylation of the calcium channel increases the probability that a channel will open with depolarization (P_o) and thus increases the calcium current I_{Ca} (33). Conversely, pharmacologic interventions, such as exposure to muscarinic agonists (e.g., acetylcholine), reduces cAMP concentration and leads to less phosphorylation of calcium channels, thus reducing the probability of channel opening and reducing the calcium current. The net slow inward calcium current for a cell is therefore determined by the number of calcium channels in the cell membrane and the probability that they will open. It should be noted that the foregoing discussion has dealt with only a limited aspect of the many components of the cell responsible for maintaining calcium homeostasis. A more detailed summary of these components is shown in Figure 3, and the reader is referred to a recent review on this topic (46).

A distinct mechanism of modulating calcium channel function has been described recently by Brown and Birnbaumer (47). It appears that G proteins coupled to stimulatory and inhibitory membrane receptors (such as G_s coupled to the β-adrenergic receptor) can directly modulate the cardiac calcium channel independently of cAMP-dependent pathways.

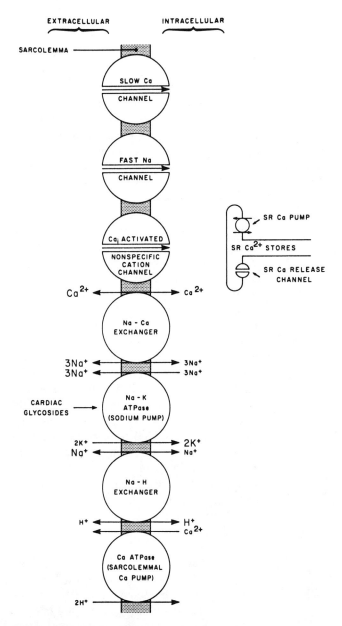

Figure 3 Selected components regulating cellular calcium homeostasis in the membrane of cardiac cells. The slow calcium channel selectivity permits entry of calcium ions into the cell upon depolarization. It is to the slow calcium channel that calcium antagonists bind. The fast sodium channel permits sodium entry during the upstroke of the action potential. Class I antiarrhythmic drugs bind to the sodium channel. The nonspecific cation channel is inactivated by intracellular calcium ions and permits entry of sodium as well as calcium under some conditions. The sodium-calcium exchanger facilitates bidirectional exchange of calcium and sodium in and out of the cell. The direction of ion flux is dependent upon membrane potential. The Na^+, K^+-ATPase is the cardiac glycoside binding site and mediates the active pumping of sodium out of the cell and pumping potassium into the cell. The sodium-hydrogen exchanger facilitates the electroneutral exchange of sodium for hydrogen ions. The sarcolemmal calcium ATPase extrudes calcium from cells and is energy dependent. Within the cell, in the sarcoplasmic reticulum membrane, is an ATP-dependent sarcoplasmic reticulum calcium pump responsible for sequestration of calcium within the sarcoplasmic reticulum. The sacroplasmic reticulum calcium release channel accounts for most calcium release within the cell during depolarization. (Reproduced from Ref. 46 and reprinted with permission from N Engl J Med.)

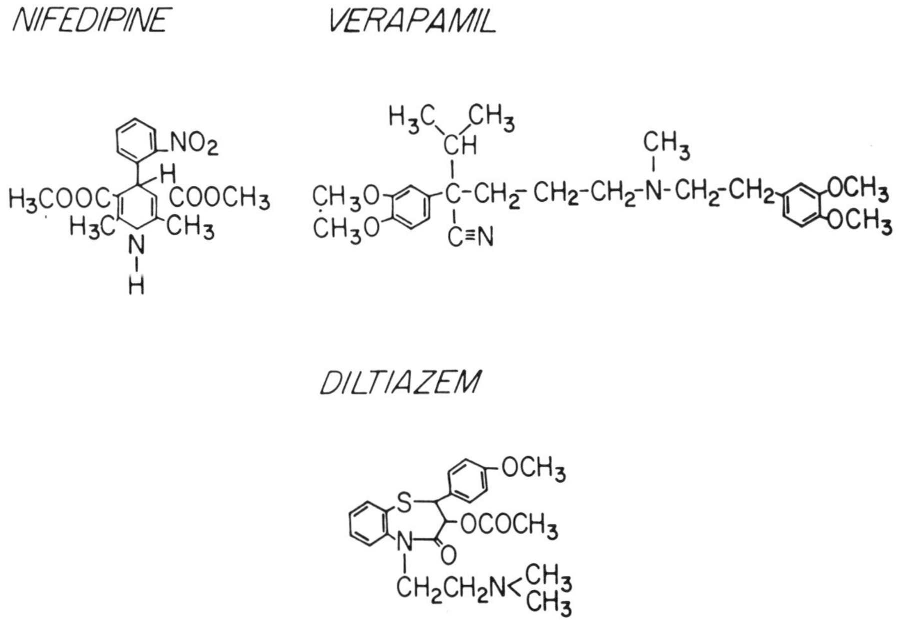

NIFEDIPINE   VERAPAMIL

DILTIAZEM

Figure 4 Structures of the prototypical calcium antagonists. Nifedipine is representative of the dihydropyridine class of calcium antagonists, verapamil is representative of the phenylalkylamine calcium antagonists, and diltiazem is representative of the benzothiazepine calcium antagonists. The three classes of calcium antagonists show great structural diversity that underlies their markedly different pharmacology.

The physiologic role for this direct coupling mechanism remains to be determined.

A number of organic calcium antagonists with very diverse chemical structures are clinically available and are of great potential value in the treatment of numerous cardiovascular disorders (Fig.4). The structural classification system includes the dihydrophyridines, phenylalkylamines, and benzothiazepines. Organic calcium antagonists decrease calcium channel-dependent calcium influx into a myocardial cell by decreasing the probability P_o that a channel will open when the cell is depolarized. The binding affinity of calcium channel antagonists is increased by membrane depolarization (45) so that one expects calcium channel blockers to be bound more tightly to depolarized or partly depolarized cardiac tissue.

It is evident from the structure of the calcium antagonists (Fig.4) that the three classes of compounds are structurally unrelated. It is therefore not surprising that they bind to pharmacologically distinct sites on the α_1 subunit of the cardiac calcium channel. It appears that binding sites for DHP, phenylalkylamines, and benzothiazepines exist in 1:1:1 stoichiometry. In some preparations diltiazem binding appears to enhance DHP binding, although the clinical significance of this remains uncertain. Because the calcium channel blockers of different classes bind to distinct binding sites on the α_1 subunit of the cardiac calcium channel, there is a rationale for the clinical use simultaneously of two calcium antagonists. One anticipates additive and possibly synergistic effects.

The impact of the organic calcium antagonists on cardiovascular physiology extends well beyond their use as antiarrhythmic agents and includes important roles for the treatment of myocardial, cerebral and peripheral isch-

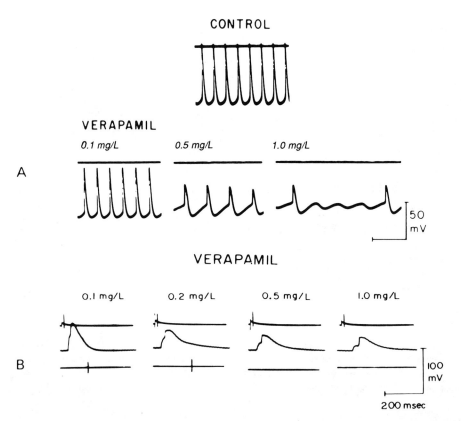

Figure 5 (A) Action potentials recorded from fibers in the periphery of the sinus node. Increasing concentrations of verapamil cause progressive decrease in the rate, amplitude, and maximum diastolic potential of the sinus node action potentials. The sharp angles of phase 4 and phase 0 indicate that these recordings were not made in pacemaker fibers in the sinus node. (B) The effects of increasing concentrations of verapamil on action potentials recorded from the upper region of the atrioventricular node of the rabbit. The atrial electrogram is above the action potential, and the His bundle electrogram is below. (Reproduced from Ref. 66 and reprinted with permission of the American Heart Association.)

emia, hypertension, and possibly for cardiomyopathy, as well as for a number of noncardiovascular disorders (e.g., esophageal spasm). Several exhaustive reviews are available that should be consulted for information on these related topics (48–50).

The prototypic antiarrhythmic compound is verapamil. Clinically relevant antiarrhythmic effects have been reported with gallopamil (D600), a methoxy derivative of verapamil, tiapamil, an analog of verapamil, diltiazem, and the less specific calcium antagonist bepridil, which has complex electrophysiologic effects including inhibition of the fast inward current (51). Nifedipine does not have an important role as an antiarrhythmic agent in view of the reflex sympathetic activation that

accompanies its hypotensive effects. Also, the dose-response curve for inhibition of AV nodal conduction is farther to the right than that for vasorelaxation, compared to verapamil or diltiazem (see later). Moreover, nifedipine displays little use dependence in its action on the calcium channel, as opposed to the prominent use dependence exhibited by verapamil and diltiazem (52). Verapamil, but not nifedipine, is also capable of blocking an outward current carried by K^+ that occurs during repolarization (53–55), although the role of this in clinical arrhythmia management is unclear.

Another interesting aspect of the pharmacology of verapamil and D-600 has also been described (56–58). The (−)-enantiomers possess potent Ca^{2+} blocking and negative

Table 2 Relative Potencies of Calcium Antagonists on Various Cardiovascular Functions Determined with the Excised Blood-Perfused Preparations of the Dog[a]

Agent	Negative chronotropic action	Negative dromotropic action	Negative inotropic action	Vasodilator action
Nifedipine	1	1	1	1
Verapamil	1	1/2	1/13	1/12
Diltiazem	1/3	1/2	1/40	1/26

[a]The effects listed are for the direct calcium antagonist actions exhibited by direct intraarterial injection into the tissues being investigated. However, in clinical practice the vasodilating effect of nifedipine predominates and no significant direct negative chronotropic or dromotropic actions are encountered. In the case of verapamil and to a lesser extent for diltiazem the dose-response curves for vasodilator action, negative chronotropic, negative dromotropic, and negative inotropic actions are closer together than they are for nifedipine. Therefore SA node, AV node, and myocardial depression are more commonly encountered with verapamil and diltiazem.
Source: Adapted from Reference 61.

inotropic properties, whereas the (+)-enantiomers are much less potent Ca^{2+} channel blockers. The (+)-enantiomers may also block the fast inward current (20,58). The majority of the laboratory and clinical studies with verapamil used a racemic mixture. The potential clinical utility of pure enantiomers remains to be determined.

ELECTROPHYSIOLOGIC EFFECTS IN ISOLATED CARDIAC TISSUES

Calcium antagonists cause a depressant effect on the rate of sinus node discharge (negative chronotropic effect) and inhibit conduction through the AV node (negative dromotropic effect) (Fig. 5) (59). These effects are easily demonstrated in experimental preparations by injection of the agents directly into the arteries supplying the SA and AV nodes (60–64). These effects, which can also be demonstrated in isolated tissue preparations in which the perfusing medium contains varying concentrations of the drug (65,66) do not appear to be mediated via the autonomic nervous system because they occur in the presence of autonomic blockade with atropine and propranolol (59). Upon exposure to verapamil action potentials of the upper and middle sections of the AV node develop diminished amplitude and upstroke velocity (66), the effective re-

fractory period of the AV node is prolonged, and conduction velocity is suppressed.

The relative potencies of the negative chronotropic and negative dromotropic properties of the calcium blockers depend on the dose and route of administration (Table 2). When equal doses of nifedipine and verapamil were administered via intraarterial injections into blood-perfused isolated SA and AV node preparations equivalent negative chronotropic effects were seen (60–64). Verapamil was only one-half as potent as nifedipine in slowing AV nodal conduction. However, different results were obtained in an in vivo model in which autonomic nervous system influences remained intact. Verapamil (0.1–0.4 mg/kg body weight) and nifedipine (0.01–0.04 mg/kg body weight) administered intravenously to chronically instrumented conscious dogs caused equal reductions in blood pressure and similar increases in heart rate (67). Only the verapamil-treated dogs had prolongation of AV conduction provoking second-degree AV block in some cases. Nifedipine in this dose range had no detectable effect on AV conduction.

The excitability of atrial fibers is depressed by 2×10^{-5} M verapamil but not by 1×10^{-6} M nifedipine (67). Both (±)-verapamil (3 × 10^{-5} M) and diltiazem (2.2×10^{-5} M) lengthen the duration and slow the maximal rate of rise

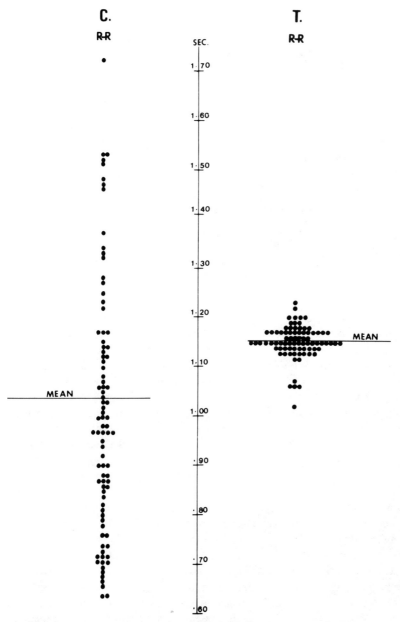

Figure 6 Scattergrams of cardiac cycles (RR intervals) from ECG recordings in a patient with atrial fibrillation. Control (C) or intravenous verapamil (T). Note the reduction in the scatter of RR intervals and the tendency to cluster in a narrower range, an example of the regularization of the ventricular rate that may be seen following both intravenous and oral verapamil. (Reproduced from Ref. 85 and reprinted with permission of Cardiovasc Res.)

of the atrial action potential; nifedipine (2.9×10^{-6} M) has no effect on these variables (68). The dose-response curve for prolongation of the atrial refractory period is much less steep for nifedipine than for verapamil (67), and the (−)-enantiomer of verapamil is nearly 10 times more potent than the (+)-enantiomer in this regard (69).

Pronounced differences between nifedipine and verapamil are apparent when simultaneous effects on coronary blood flow and atrioventricular conduction are ascertained (70). Verapamil increases blood flow through the AV node and prolongs the AV nodal conduction time in the same dose range, whereas nifedipine causes a greater increase in AV nodal artery flow than in AV nodal conduction time. In hearts deprived of sympathetic nervous system influences, however, nifedipine has been shown to prolong AV nodal conduction as well as increase coronary blood flow (70).

Neither nifedipine nor verapamil injected directly into the artery supplying isolated blood-perfused preparations of canine papillary muscles affect the automaticity of these ventricular fibers (71). Kohlhardt et al. (72) eliminated the fast inward Na^+ current in isolated trabeculae from the right ventricle of cats by depolarizing the cell membrane and then showed that the second inward current was dependent on the extracellular Ca^{2+} concentration. This current could be markedly inhibited by 4.4×10^{-6} M verapamil, and the inhibitory effects of verapamil were completely neutralized by a fourfold increase in extracellular Ca^{2+} concentration from 2.2 to 8.8 mM. Purkinje fibers exposed to Na^+-free Tyrode's solution develop action potentials that are Ca^{2+} dependent. Verapamil depresses excitability in such fibers and suppresses spontaneous and electrically stimulated rhythmic activity (65).

obtained during cardiac surgery. Fibers removed from dilated atria with a propensity to atrial arrhythmias and prolonged P wave durations had resting membrane potentials in the range of-50 mV. These were of low amplitude and slowly rising and appeared to be slow channel responses (26). They differed from action potentials recorded in fibers obtained from less diseased atria that had a rapid upstroke indicative of fast channel responses. Verapamil markedly inhibited the slow channel-dependent action potentials but affected only the plateau phase of the fast channel-dependent action potentials. Since slowly conducting action potentials can increase the propensity to reentry, their depression by verapamil provides further rationale for the use of phenylalkylamine-type calcium antagonists in reentrant paroxysmal supraventricular arrhythmias.

The direct electrophysiologic effects of calcium antagonists on ventricular muscle are probably of little potential use for the treatment of ventricular arrhythmias. However, the antiischemic action of these drugs produces an indirect antiarrhythmic action that may be helpful in combating ventricular dysrhythmias arising from myocardial ischemia. Pretreatment with verapamil has been shown to favorably affect the tendency to ventricular fibrillation in several animal preparations of myocardial ischemia (74,75).

ANTIARRHYTHMIC EFFECTS IN EXPERIMENTAL PREPARATIONS

Prolongation of AV nodal refractoriness and slowing of conduction by verapamil prevents the experimental induction of reentrant AV nodal tachycardia in isolated rabbit atrial preparations, an action in vitro that is likely the basis for its clinical effectiveness in controlling supraventricular rhythm disturbances dependent on reentry involving the AV node (66).

In an attempt to elucidate the role of slow response in atrial arrhythmias in humans, Hordoff and colleagues (73) recorded action potentials of diseased human right atrial fibers

CLINICAL USE OF CLASS IV ANTIARRHYTHMIC DRUGS: ELECTROPHYSIOLOGIC EFFECTS IN THE HUMAN

The clinical electrophysiologic effects show an excellent correlation with the findings already discussed for isolated tissues and experimental preparations (Table 3) (51,76,77). The net effect of these drugs in the human represents a balance of direct electrophysiologic actions and reflex activation of sympathetic tone provoked by their potent vasodilatory actions. Thus the more prominent hypotensive effects of nifedipine are usually associated with an increase in heart rate (↓ RR interval), and ver-

Table 3 Clinical Electrophysiologic Effects of Calcium Antagonists[a]

Effect	Verapamil	Diltiazem	Nifedipine
Intracardiac recordings			
SNRT	↑ in SSS	↑ in SSS	0
Atrial ERP	0	0	0
AV Node ERP	↑ ↑	↑	0
A-H	↑	↑	0
His-Purkinje ERP	0	0	0
H-V	0	0	0
Accessory pathway ERP	↑ ↓	?	0
Ventricular automaticity	0	0	0
ECG			
RR interval	↑ ↓	↓	↑ ↓
PR	↑ ↑	↑	0
QRS	0	0	0
QTc	0	0	0
Antiarrhythmic action			
Atrial fibrillation			
Control ventricular rate	+ +	+	−
Maintain NSR	0	0	0
PSVT			
Acute termination (intravenous)	+ + + +	+ +	0
Prophylaxis against recurrences	+ +	+	0
VT (direct action)	[b]	0	0

[a]Electrophysiologic properties of gallopamil (D600) and tiapamil are similar to those of verapamil.
↑, Increase; ↓, decrease; ↑ ↓, variable effect; SNRT, sinus node recovery time; SSS, sick sinus syndrome.
[b]In selected clinical subsets (see text).

apamil and diltiazem have more variable effects, with many patients exhibiting considerable slowing of the sinus rate, particularly in the presence of sick sinus syndrome. Both verapamil and diltiazem slow conduction through the AV node increased (↑ AH interval and PR interval) and prolong the AV nodal effective and functional refractory periods (78,79). Little effect is seen in tissues dependent on the fast inward current, and therefore the effective refractory periods of atrial, ventricular, and accessory pathway fibers are usually unchanged. Since conduction velocity in the His-Purkinje system and myocardium is not affected, intracardiac measurements of HV intervals and surface ECG measurements of QRS and QT duration are unchanged.

Antiarrhythmic Therapy: Supraventricular Arrhythmias

Atrial Fibrillation and Atrial Flutter
In the absence of antiarrhythmic drugs the re-

sponse of the normal AV node to the development of atrial fibrillation is the transmission of a large number of fibrillatory impulses resulting in a rapid ventricular rate. Determinants of the speed of the ventricular response include the atrial electrical input (400–800 impulses/min; the rate may be augmented by an increase in vagal tone, which shortens the action potential duration in atrial fibers), the AV nodal conduction of fibrillatory impulses, and the effects of modulating factors on the AV node, such as the increase in sympathetic tone that accompanies exercise (Table 4). Digitalis glycosides may actually increase the rate of the fibrillating atria through a central vagomimetic action but through the same mechanism also decrease the amount of fibrillatory impulses transmitted through the AV node. However, the rate-reducing property of digitalis decreases during suppression of vagal tone by exercise, and it is a common clinical observation that digitalis-treated patients with atrial fibrillation develop poor control of the ventricular rate upon exertion. β-Adrenoceptor

Table 4 Atrial Fibrillation: Response to Therapy[a]

Determinants of ventricular rate in AF	Drug effects on ventricular rate		
	Verapamil	Digoxin	β-Adrenoceptor blockers
Atrial electrical input, 400–800 impulses/min	↓ ↑	↑ (vagal)	0
AV nodal conduction	↓ ↓	↓	↓
ANS tone in response to exercise: Vagal ↓ Sympathetic ↑	Use dependence increases effects at high drive rates through AV node	Rate-reducing potential decreases with exercise	Blunt effects of increased sympathetic tone

[a] ↑, increase; ↓, decrease; ↑ ↓, variable effect; ANS, autonomic nervous system.

blocking agents have no significant effect on the rate of the fibrillating atria but reduce AV nodal transmission of supraventricular impulses via inhibition of sympathetic tone and for this reason retain their efficacy as ventricular rate-controlling agents during exercise, albeit in some patients at the cost of a decreased exercise capacity (80).

Verapamil has a negligible direct effect on the rate of the fibrillating atria, but in the event that vasodilation evokes a reflex sympathetic response there may be a slight increase in the atrial fibrillatory rate. Since verapamil (and diltiazem) is an ionized calcium antagonist, according to the modulated receptor hypothesis it may gain access to the calcium channel via the channel lumen as opposed to movement laterally in the membrane lipid bilayer as occurs with a lipophilic drug like nifedipine (52). It therefore exhibits its electrophysiologic effects most prominently when the calcium channel is in the open state. Consequently, rapid repetitive depolarizations of the AV node as occurs in atrial fibrillation (particularly upon exercise) are particularly well treated by verapamil in view of its use dependence properties, as noted earlier. Therefore, although digitalis and β-adrenoceptor blockers decrease the ventricular rate at rest, verapamil and drugs with similar actions (gallopamil and tiapamil) are emerging as the drugs of choice for blunting the exercise-induced increases in ventricular rate in patients without congestive heart failure (51,81–83). The effects of digitalis, β-blockers, and verapamil for slowing

the ventricular rate are additive, allowing carefully titrated drug combinations. No large-scale comparisons of verapamil, digitalis glycosides, and β-adrenoceptor blockers have been reported to date.

Clinical trials with intravenous verapamil indicate that the onset of slowing of the ventricular rate is extremely rapid, but the rate begins to accelerate again within 30 min of a bolus injection (5–10 mg), necessitating repeated boluses or initiation of a continuous infusion (2.5–5.0 µg/kg per min). Composite results from several trials indicate that slowing of the ventricular rate can be achieved in about 90% of patients, whereas conversion to sinus rhythm occurs in less than 10% of cases (84–91). The slowing of the ventricular rate appears to be greatest in those individuals who have the highest pretreatment ventricular rates. Schamroth et al. emphasized that some patients develop a partial "regularization" of the ventricular rate that has a superficial appearance of AV junctional rhythm but can be differentiated from that disorder by the still discernible cycle-to-cycle variability (86). The precise mechanism of this regularization response remains unclear, but it has also been reported after large doses of verapamil (Fig. 6).

In cases of atrial flutter the administration of intravenous verapamil causes a prompt reduction in the ventricular rate in about 50% of cases, conversion to sinus rhythm in about 30% of cases, and a change in the rhythm to atrial fibrillation in about 20% of cases

(84,92). As noted by Singh and coworkers intravenous doses of verapamil may be of diagnostic value in differentiating atrial flutter with 2:1 AV conduction from paroxysmal supraventricular tachycardia since higher grade AV block is likely to develop with the former rhythm and abrupt restoration of sinus rhythm is likely to be seen with the latter rhythm (51,76,86).

Long-term oral therapy with verapamil for control of the ventricular rate in atrial fibrillation has been reported by several investigators (76,81,93). Doses between 160 and 240 mg/day and occasionally as high as 480–720 mg/day have been reported, with a clear increase in the rate of adverse effects as the dose is increased. These trials have shown a consistent verapamil-induced slowing of the ventricular rate at rest and impressive control of the ventricular rate with exercise as would be predicted from the foregoing discussion. In addition the effects of verapamil were found to be additive to those of digoxin. Klein and Kaplinsky have proposed that verapamil replace digitalis as the drug of choice for such patients, provided ventricular function is not depressed (81,83). The absence of bronchospastic or vasoconstrictor effects of calcium antagonists also makes them attractive alternatives to β-adrenoceptor blockers in patients with chronic obstructive pulmonary disease or peripheral vascular disease. Insufficient data are available to determine whether verapamil would be a useful agent for the maintenance of sinus rhythm following direct current (DC) cardioversion, but the electrophysiologic effects of the drug do not lead one to believe that it would be particularly effective in that regard (94).

Paroxysmal Supraventricular Tachycardia

It is estimated that about 60% of cases of paroxysmal supraventricular tachycardia (PSVT) are caused by AV nodal reentry, about 30% are due to atrioventricular reentry involving an accessory pathway, and the remaining 10% are due to sinus node reentry tachycardia, intraatrial reentry tachycardia, or ectopic automatic atrial tachycardia (e.g., paroxysmal atrial tachycardia) (95). Conversion to sinus rhythm

can be seen in 90% of cases of reentrant PSVT involving the AV node as part of the circuit when intravenous verapamil is administered (Fig. 7) (51,76,84–90,92,96–99). Responses of a similar nature have been reported for intravenous diltiazem (0.15–0.25 mg/kg) (100–102), tiapamil (1–2 mg/kg) (103–107), gallopamil (0.03–0.05 mg/kg) (51), and an oral combination of diltiazem (108). The nearly pathognomonic observation of restoration of sinus rhythm, excellent response rate in all age groups, and the improved rate of conversion compared with intravenous digitalis glycosides and conventional β-adrenoceptor blockers led many investigators to propose that verapamil and related compounds should be considered drugs of choice for reentrant-type PSVT (Fig. 7). However, recent reports of high conversion rates with intravenous infusions of the ultra-short-acting β-blocker esmolol or boluses of intravenous adenosine must be taken into consideration, and the therapeutic armamentarium therefore appears to be broadening (109,110).

In a review of the results of intravenous verapamil trials for reentrant, narrow-complex PSVT, Singh et al. summarized the various types of responses that may be observed clinically (51,76,111,112): (1) abrupt termination of the arrhythmia as might be seen with carotid sinus massage, (2) a reduction in the cycle length of the tachycardia followed by a short pause before the restoration of sinus rhythm, (3) AV dissociation followed by a junctional escape rhythm and ultimately restoration of sinus rhythm, (4) transient atrial fibrillation followed by sinus rhythm, (5) isolated ventricular premature depolarizations or short paroxysms of nonsustained ventricular tachycardia followed by sinus rhythm, and (6) alternation of the cycle length of the tachycardia (due to unclear mechanisms) before restoration of sinus rhythm. In contrast to the dramatic response noted with intravenous verapamil or related drugs the long-term prophylaxis against PSVT with chronic oral administration is somewhat less encouraging as a result of recurrence of arrhythmia, appearance of bothersome side effects (113), and less significant electrophysiologic effects on

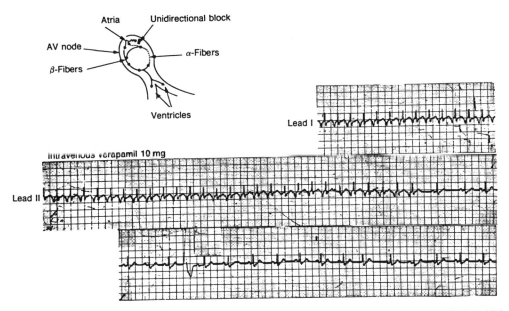

Figure 7 An unusual form of AV nodal reentrant paroxysmal supraventricular tachycardia in which the antegrade limb of circuit is the "fast" pathway and the retrograde limb of the circuit is the "slow" pathway. This produces retrograde P waves appearing approximately 310 msec after the preceding QRS. Treatment with intravenous verapamil provokes block in the retrograde limb and the tachycardia is terminated. (Reproduced from Ref. 76 and reprinted with permission of Drugs.)

the tachycardia circuit (78). The precise predictive accuracy of a beneficial response to verapamil during acute electrophysiologic testing as regards long-term suppression of PSVT recurrences remains unclear at the present time (114).

Cases of PSVT due to an ectopic automatic atrial tachycardia appear to be much less responsive to verapamil like drugs (113), perhaps with the exception of digitalis toxic-related arrhythmias in which triggered automaticity may play a pivotal pathogenic role. Limited clinical data also suggest a beneficial role of verapamil in multifocal atrial tachycardia, but this requires further clinical examination (115).

Preexcitation Syndromes

The role of verapamil in patients with arrhythmias related to the preexcitation syndromes deserves special comment. The most common type of arrhythmia encountered in such patients is the atrioventricular reentry tachy-cardia form of PSVT, with antegrade conduction over the AV node and retrograde conduction over the accessory pathway (orthodromic tachycardia). In some cases the accessory pathway does not conduct in the antegrade direction and is said to be "concealed" since no delta wave is seen on the ECG. Less frequently a tachycardia circuit develops with antegrade conduction over the accessory pathway and retrograde conduction over the AV node (antidromic tachycardia). Since verapamil has little effect on the accessory pathway it terminates the tachycardia by interrupting the AV nodal limb of the reentrant circuit. Therefore its effects may be more variable than in cases of reentry confined exclusively to the AV node (51,76).

When atrial fibrillation or atrial flutter develops in patients with preexcitation and antegrade conduction occurs over the accessory pathway, the ventricular rate may be quite rapid. Interventions that shorten the antegrade refractory period of the accessory pathway, as reported with digitalis [and possibly verapamil (113,116,117)], and/or lengthen the antegrade refractory period of the AV node are to be avoided because of the potential for acceleration of the ventricular rate since more conduction may occur over the accessory pathway. More preferable treatments include cardioversion or administration of a drug known to have more direct depressant effects on the accessory pathway, such as class I agents. When there is clinical uncertainty about whether antegrade conduction occurs over an accessory pathway in the presence of atrial fibrillation most authorities recommend avoiding both digitalis and verapamil.

Ventricular Arrthymias

From the foregoing discussion of the electrophysiologic effects of verapamil it seems unlikely that it has any significant clinical role in the management of ventricular arrhythmias since ventricular tachycardia in the setting of structural organic heart disease is usually not related to abnormalities of the slow inward current. However, recent reports (118) raise the intriguing notion that verapamil may be effective for ventricular tachyarrhythmias in certain infrequent, carefully defined circumstances, including (1) the acute phase of myocardial infarction (as opposed to the healed phase of myocardial infarction), (2) idiopathic VT with a right bundle branch block and left axis deviation pattern in young patients, (3) exercise-induced VT with a left bundle branch block and right axis deviation pattern, and (4) "torsades de pointes" with a normal QT and short coupling intervals. The precise electrophysiologic substrate responsible for these arrhythmias is unclear, but the possibilities of a reentrant circuit involving a slow channel mechanism or triggered activity have been considered (118).

CLINICAL PHARMACOLOGY

Since verapamil is the calcium antagonist that has been used most extensively for the management of cardiac arrhythmias, this review predominantly focuses on the pharmacology of this compound. The details of the clinical pharmacology of diltiazem and nifedipine are summarized in Table 5. Fortunately, considerable pharmacokinetic information is available for verapamil since it has been thoroughly investigated in a variety of clinical settings (50,119–121). Although early assay methods used fluorometric techniques (122) for determination of blood levels of verapamil, these were supplanted by gas chromatographic (123) and high-performance liquid chromatographic methods (124,125), which more accurately distinguish verapamil from its metabolites.

Studies in normal subjects given intravenous doses of verapamil suggest that a two-compartment model can be used to describe the pharmacokinetics (126–129). The α-phase lasts approximately 15–30 min, and the β-phase ranges from 170 to 440 min. The apparent volume of distribution is reported to be between 2.5 and 5.0 L/kg and total plasma clearance is 800–1500 ml/min. However, in patients with severe hepatic dysfunction due to cirrhosis or individuals with a reduced hepatic blood flow the clearance of verapamil is markedly prolonged, with extension of the half-life of elimination to approximately 14 hr (130,131).

Verapamil is about 90% absorbed following oral administration, and peak plasma levels may be seen after 1 hr (132). Because of extensive first-pass hepatic metabolism the bioavailability of the tablet form may only be 20–40% in some patients (126,127). Single-dose oral pharmacokinetic studies are also consistent with a pattern of first-order kinetics, which can be suitably analyzed by a two-compartment model. Studies of long-term chronic oral administration of verapamil have suggested that nonlinear clearance of the drug may develop, with prolongation of the apparent half-life to 10–12 hr (133). As proposed by Shand (134) this may be due to a high-affinity, low-capacity hepatic clearance mechanism that may become saturated during chronic drug administration.

Verapamil is extensively bound to plasma proteins (90%), and this does not appear to be altered in postsurgical patients or in persons with chronic renal failure who are on dialysis (135). A number of studies have examined

Table 5 Clinical Pharmacology of Calcium Antagonists[a]

	Verapamil[b]	Diltiazem[b]	Nifedipine[b]
Dose	75–150 µg/kg IV bolus 2.5–5.0 µg/kg per min IV infusion 160–480 mg/day PO	150–250 µg/kg IV bolus 90–360 mg/day PO	30–120 mg/day PO
Absorption	90%	90%	90%
Onset of action	1–3 min IV 1–2 hr PO	1–3 min IV 15–30 min PO	2–3 min SL 20 min PO
Peak effect	10–15 min IV 5 hr PO	30–60 min PO	1–2 hr PO
Plasma half-life	3–7 hr (↑ in hepatic failure)	4–6 hr	4 hr
Protein binding	90%	90%	90%
Metabolism	Hepatic (first pass, saturable)	Hepatic (saturable)	Hepatic
Excretion	Renal	Renal	Renal
Active metabolites	Norverapamil	Desacetyldiltiazem	None
Adverse effects	Constipation, headache, flushing, hypotension, conduction disturbances, CHF	Headache, dizziness, flushing, conduction disturbances, CHF, leg edema	Headache, hypotension, flushing dizziness, leg edema, tachycardia
Proprietary names	Calan, Isoptin	Cardizem	Procardia, Adalat
Therapeutic range (ng/ml)[c]	50–300	50–150	25–100

[a] IV, Intravenous; PO, orally; SL, sublingually
[b] Sustained-release preparations are available.
[c] The precise therapeutic range for each drug under different clinical circumstances is still under investigation.

correlations between the pharmacokinetics and electrophysiologic effects of verapamil both following single intravenous doses and during steady state following prolonged drug administration. The data are inconclusive, but it appears that it is unlikely to see prolongation of the PR interval with plasma verapamil concentrations < 30 ng/ml (136); slowing of the ventricular rate in atrial fibrillation is associated with levels of at least 50 ng/ml (137); termination of PSVT may require somewhat higher plasma levels (99). Such side effects as constipation may be seen more frequently with levels of 500 ng/ml, and significant hemodynamic derangements and AV dissociation have been reported with levels in the range of 1000 ng/ml (138). It should be emphasized, however, that measurement of plasma verapamil levels is not currently a usual clinical practice, and it remains to be shown whether patients can be treated more effectively and safely if such measurements were more readily available (76).

Metabolism

Verapamil undergoes extensive hepatic metabolism, and at least 12 separate metabolites have been identified. However, only one of these, norverapamil, an N-demethylated product of verapamil, appears to have biologic activity (about one-fifth that of verapamil in dog studies) and it accounts for about 6% of urinary metabolites collected in 48 hr (139).

Drug Interactions

Clinically significant pharmacodynamic and pharmacokinetic drug interactions have been reported between verapamil and β-adrenoceptor blockers and digoxin (140). The depressant electrophysiologic effects of verapamil and both β-blockers and digitalis glycosides on SA nodal and AV nodal function are additive (141). This may have adverse consequences in patients with intrinsic abnormalities of the conduction system (e.g., sick sinus syndrome) (142). It is also important to note that the coadministration of verapamil and a β-blocker must be undertaken with extreme caution because of the potential risk of addi-

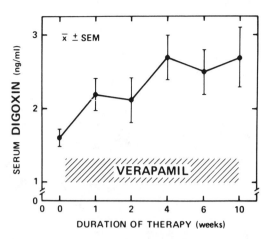

Figure 8 Mean serum digoxin concentrations for 10 patients before verapamil (week 0) and after 1, 2, 4, 6, and 10 weeks of combined digoxin and verapamil. The increase in serum digoxin concentration was significant (p < .0001) after only 1 week of verapamil administration. This elevation was maintained during combined verapamil and digoxin administration. (Reproduced from Ref. 146 and reprinted with permission of the American Heart Association.)

tive depression of myocardial contractile function (143). This may be due to interference with excitation-contraction coupling by verapamil and/or blunting of reflex sympathetic responses by β-blockers. Verapamil also attenuates the positive inotropic effects of digitalis glycosides, possibly resulting in exacerbation of congestive heart failure for those patients in a clinically precarious state. Clinical experience suggests that the majority of such adverse hemodynamic responses is detectable in the first week after initiation of combination therapy, indicating a particular need for careful observation of the patient during that time.

Coadministration of verapamil to patients chronically receiving digoxin has been reported to result in an increase in serum digoxin concentration (Fig. 8) (144–146). This appears to be a result of initial reductions in both renal and nonrenal clearance of digoxin, although with chronic administration of verapamil the extent of the interaction appears to diminish, probably due to a return of renal clearance of digoxin to normal (145). In a summary of pharmacokinetic drug interactions with digoxin, Marcus indicates that as much as a 70–100% increase in serum digoxin concentrations may be seen acutely with initiation of verapamil (147). It has also been reported that tiapamil and gallopamil may produce somewhat less prominent elevations of digoxin concentrations than verapamil. Diltiazem and nifedipine were also described as producing slight elevations in serum digoxin levels (in the range of 20%), but the accuracy and clinical significance of such findings remains unclear because of a number of methodologic concerns (148).

Adverse Reactions

The overall frequency of side effects during verapamil treatment is approximately 10% (140). Following the intravenous use of verapamil the most frequently reported adverse reactions include hypotension, sinus node depression, and AV block. Clinicians can usually predict which patients are a greatest risk for such events since the majority of cases in whom such responses occur are in persons receiving β-blockers or those who have a history of left ventricular dysfunction or conduction system disease (143,149). Such acute reactions to verapamil can be reversed with intravenous isoproterenol, atropine, glucagon, or calcium gluconate (150); on occasion dopamine and temporary transvenous pacing are required (151).

Chronic oral therapy with verapamil is usually well tolerated, although a minority of patients complain of gastrointestinal intolerance and constipation, headache, dizziness, and facial flushing (140). Exacerbation of congestive heart failure and progression of AV block may also develop during chronic treatment.

SUMMARY OF ROLE OF CLASS IV DRUGS IN THERAPY OF ARRHYTHMIAS

Verapamil has emerged as the prototype phenylalkylamine calcium antagonist and is an important therapeutic agent for the treatment of cardiac arrhythmias arising from mechanisms involving the slow inward current. Intravenous verapamil is an important treatment for reentrant PSVT and should be strongly considered for slowing the ventricular rate in atrial fibrillation and flutter, especially in patients with well-preserved left ventricular function. The efficacy of long-term oral verapamil for prophylaxis against PSVT is less clear, and its role must be reassessed in the face of newer class IC antiarrhythmics, such as propafenone, encainide, and flecainide, which are particularly efficacious in reentrant PSVT. However, long-term oral verapamil seems superior to digitalis for control of the ventricular rate during exercise in patients with chronic atrial fibrillation.

Oral administration of the benzothiazepine calcium antagonist diltiazem is also a possible adjunct to digitalis for ventricular rate control in chronic atrial fibrillation. It has less potent effects on AV conduction than verapamil but also has substantially less negative inotropic effect in the doses utilized so it may be better tolerated in patients with impaired ventricular function.

Except for preliminary evidence in selected subsets of patients, no substantial clinical role has been defined for calcium antagonists as ventricular antiarrhythmic agents. It remains to be determined whether their antiischemic properties contribute to a reduction in ventricular arrhythmias and possibly sudden cardiac death in the coronary heart disease patient.

FUTURE DIRECTIONS

Over the short term there are three major directions of development of calcium channel blockers. First, sustained-release preparations of dihydropyridines have become clinically available, along with sustained-release formulations of diltiazem and verapamil. These preparations afford the patient greater convenience and permit once or twice a day dosing of all the major calcium channel blocker drugs. Because of the considerable interpatient variation in drug clearance, clinical monitoring of therapeutic end points and side effects continues to be necessary.

A second new direction for calcium channel drugs is development of dihydropyridine calcium channel agonists that have effects opposite to those of calcium antagonists. By rather minor structural alterations in the nifedipine prototype molecular structure, such compounds as BAYK 8644 have been synthesized. These drugs increase the average time the calcium channel remains open and increase calcium influx through the calcium channel. The myocardial effects are those expected for a compound with effects opposite to those of a calcium antagonist. There is a potent positive inotropic effect from such calcium channel agonists. Moreover, the specialized conduction tissue of the heart responds in a manner opposite to that of a calcium antagonist. Thus AV conduction is enhanced by a calcium channel agonist instead of inhibited. Desirable and undesirable therapeutic effects are considerable. Efforts are underway to increase the tissue selectivity of these calcium channel agonist compounds.

The third new direction is development of compounds that have greater specificity for binding to either vascular tissue or myocardial tissue. The goal is to create compounds with desired effects on impulse formation or conduction, or the myocardium, with minimal peripheral vascular or coronary effects, or conversely to develop drugs with coronary or peripheral vascular effects and minimal myocardial and electrophysiologic modulating properties. Prospects for development of compounds with a high degree of selectivity appear bright.

REFERENCES

1. Singh B N, Vaughan-Williams E M. A fourth class of antidysrhythmic action? Effect of verapamil on ouabain toxicity on atrial and ventricular potentials and on other features of cardiac function. Cardiovasc Res 1972; 6:109–19.
2. Nayler W G. Identification, mode of action and nomenclature of calcium antagonists. In: Calcium antagonists. London: Academic Press 1988:69–85.
3. Coraboeuf E. Ionic basis of electrical activity in cardiac tissues. Am J Physiol 1976; 234:H101–16.
4. Cranefield P F. Conduction of the cardiac impulse. New York: Futura 1975.
5. Noble D. The initiation of the heartbeat. Oxford: Clarendon Press 1975.
6. Hodgkin A L, Huxley A F. A quantitative description of membrane current and its application to conduction and excitation in nerve. J Physiol (Lond) 1952; 117:500–44.
7. Reuter H. Properties of two inward membrane currents in the heart. Annu Rev Physiol 1979; 26:413–24.
8. Reuter H. Divalent cations as charge carriers in excitable membranes. Prog Biophys Mol Biol 1973; 26:1–43.
9. Vitek M, Trautwein W. Slow inward current and action potential in cardiac Purkinje fibers of Mn^{2+} ions. Pfluegers Arch 1971; 323:204–18.
10. Mascher D and Peper K. Two components of inward current in myocardial muscle fibers. Pflugers Arch 1969; 307:190–203.
11. Reuter, H, Scholtz H. The regulation of the Ca conductance of cardiac muscle by adrenaline. J Physiol (Lond) 1977; 264:49–62.
12. Beeler G W, Reuter H. Reconstruction of the action potential of ventricular myocardial fibres. J Physiol (Lond) 1977; 268:177–210.
13. Reuter H, Scholz H. A study of the ion selectivity and the kinetic properties of the calcium dependent slow inward current in mammalian cardiac muscle. J Physiol (Lond) 1977; 264: 17–47.
14. McDonald T F, Trautwein W. Membrane currents in cat myocardium: separation of inward and outward components. J Physiol (Lond) 1978; 274:193–216.
15. Trautwein W, McDonald T F, Tripathi O. Calcium conductance and tension in mammalian ventricular muscle. Pflugers Arch 1975; 354:55–74.
16. Nayler W G. Ion-conducting channels: sodium and potassium. In: Calcium antagonists. London: Academic Press 1988:5–21.
17. Cranefield P F. Action potentials, after potentials and arrhythmias. Circ Res 1977; 41:415–23.
18. Wit A L, Cranefield P F. Triggered activity in cardiac muscle fibers of the simian mitral valve. Circ Res 1976; 38:85–98.
19. Wit A L, Fenoglio J J, Hordof A J, Reemtsma K. Ultrastructure and transmembrane potentials of cardiac muscle in the human anterior mitral valve leaflet. Circulation 1979; 59:1284–92.

20. Saito T, Otoguro M, Matsubara T. Electrophysiological studies on the mechanism of electrically induced sustained rhythmic activity in the rabbit right atrium. Circ Res 1978; 42:199–206.

21. Wit A L, Cranefield P F. Triggered and automatic activity in the canine coronary sinus. Circ Res 1977; 41:435–45.

22. Cranefield P F, Aronson R S. Initiation of sustained rhythmic activity by single propagated action potentials in canine cardiac Purkinje fibers exposed to sodium-free solution or to ouabain. Circ Res 1974; 34:477–81.

23. Ferrier G R, Saunders J H, Mendez C. A cellular mechanism for the generation of ventricular arrhythmias by acetylstrophanthidin. Circ Res 1973; 32:600–9.

24. Ferrier G R, Moe G K. Effect of calcium on acetylstrophanthidin-induced transient depolarization in canine Purkinje tissue. Circ Res 1973; 33:508–15.

25. Wit A L, Cranefield P F, Hoffman B F. Slow conduction and reentry in the ventricular conducting system: II. Single and sustained circus movement in networks of canine and bovine Purkinje fibers. Circ Res 1972; 30:11–22.

26. Carmeliet E, Vereecke J. Adrenaline and the plateau phase of the cardiac action potential: importance of Ca^{++}, Na^+ and K^+ conductance. Pflugers Arch 1969; 313:300–15.

27. Kass R S, Lederer W J, Tsien R W, Weingart R. Role of calcium ions in transient inward currents and after contractions induced by strophanthidin in cardiac Purkinje fibers. J Physiol (Lond) 1978; 281:187–208.

28. Nowycky M C, Fox A P, Tsien R W. Three types of neuronal calcium channels with different calcium agonist sensitivity. Nature 1985; 316:440–3.

29. Catterall W A, Seagar M J, Takahashi M. Molecular properties of dihydrophyridine-sensitive calcium channels in skeletal muscle. J Biol Chem 1988; 263:3535–8.

30. Catterall W A. Structure and function of voltage-sensitive ion channels. Science 1988; 242:50–61.

31. Ellis S B, William M E, Ways N R, Brenner R, Sharp A H, Leung A T, Campbell K P, McKenna E, Koch W J, Hui A, Schwartz A, Harpold M M. Sequence and expression of NRNAS encoding the alpha1 and alpha2 subunits of a DHP-sensitive calcium channel. Science 1988; 241:1661–4.

32. Tanabe T, Takeshima H, Mikami A, Flockerzi V, Takahashi H, Kangawa K, Kojima M, Matsuo H, Hirose T, Numa S. Primary structure of the receptor for calcium blockers from skeletal muscle. Nature 1987; 328:323–8.

33. Tsien R W, Bean B P, Hess P, Lansmann J B, Nilius B, Nowycky MC. Mechanism of calcium channel modulation by beta-adrenergic agents and dihydropyridine calcium channel agonists. J Moll Cell Cardiol 1986; 18:691–710.

34. Lee K S, Tsien R W. Mechanism of calcium channel blockade by verapamil, D600, diltiazem and nitrendipine in single dialysed heart cells. Nature 1983; 302:790–4.

35. Cooper C L, Vandaele S, Barhanin J, Fosset M, Lazdunski M, Hosey M M. Purification and characterization of the dihydropyridine-sensitive voltage-dependent calcium channel from cardiac tissue. J Biol Chem 1987; 262:509–12.

36. Horne W A, Weiland G A, Oswald R E. Solubilization and hydrodynamic characterization of the dihydropyridine receptor from rat ventricular muscle. J Biol Chem 1986; 261:3588–94.

37. Carmeliet E, Vereecke J. Electrogenesis of the action potential and automaticity. In: Bern R M, Sperelakis N, Geiger S R, eds. Handbook of physiology. Section 2. The cardiovascular system. Vol. 1. The heart. Bethesda: American Physiological Society 1979:269–334.

38. Sperelakis N, Schneider J A. A metabolic control mechanism for calcium ion influx that may protect the ventricular myocardial cell. Am J Cardiol 1976; 37:1079–85.

39. Reuter H. The dependence of slow inward current in Purkinje fibers on the extracellular calcium-concentration. J Physiol (Lond) 1967; 192:479–92.

40. Brown H F, McNaughton P A, Noble D, Noble S J. Adrenergic control of pacemaker currents. Philos Trans R Soc Lond [Biol] 1975; 270:527–37.

41. Tsien R W. Cyclic AMP and contractile activity in heart. Adv Cyclic Nucleotide Res 1977; 8:363–420.

42. Fleckenstein A. Specific pharmacology of calcium in myocardium, cardiac pacemakers, and vascular smooth muscle. Annu Rev Pharmacol Toxicol 1977; 17:149–66.

43. Schneider J A, Sperelakis N. Slow Ca^{++} and Na^+ responses induced by isoproterenol

and methylxanthines in isolated perfused guinea pig hearts exposed to elevated K$^+$. J Moll Cell Cardiol 1975; 7:249–73.

44. Sakmann B, Neher E. Single channel recordings. New York: Plenum Press 1983.

45. Reuter H, Kokubun S, Prodhom B. Properties and modulation of cardiac calcium channels. J Exp Biol 1986; 124:191–201.

46. Smith T W. Digitalis. Mechanisms of action and clinical use. N Engl J Med 1988; 318:358–65.

47. Brown A M, Birnbaumer L. Direct G protein gating of ion channels. Am J Physiol 1988; 254:H401–10.

48. Antman E M, Stone P H, Muller J E, Braunwald E. Calcium channel blocking agents in the treatment of cardiovascular disorders. Part I. Basic and clinical electrophysiologic effects. Ann Intern Med 1980; 93:875–85.

49. Stone P H, Antman E M, Muller J E, Braunwald E. Calcium channel blocking agents in the treatment of cardiovascular disorders. Part II. Hemodynamic effects and clinical applications. Ann Intern Med 1980; 93:886–904.

50. Nayler W G, Horowitz J D. Calcium antagonists: a new class of drugs. Pharmacol Ther 1983; 20:203–62.

51. Singh B N, Nademanee K. Use of calcium antagonists for cardiac arrhythmias. Am J Cardiol 1987; 1987:153B–62B.

52. Nayler W G. Tissue-selectivity. In: Calcium antagonists. London: Academic Press 1988:113–29.

53. Henry P D. Calcium ion (Ca^{++} antagonists: mechanisms of action and clinical applications. Pract Cardiol 1979; 5:145–56.

54. Kass R S, Tsien R W. Multiple effects of calcium antagonists on plateau currents in cardiac Purkinje fibers. J Gen Physiol 1975; 66:169–92.

55. Chen C, Gettes L S. Effects of verapamil in premature and nonpremature sodium dependent action potentials at various potassium levels. Circulation 1977; 56(Suppl. III):III–127.

56. Bayer R, Hennekes R, Kaufman R, Mannhold R. Inotropic and electrophysiological actions of verapamil and D-600 in mammalian myocardium. I. Pattern of inotropic effects of the racemic compounds. Naunyn Schmiedebergs Arch Pharmacol 1975; 290:49–68.

57. Bayer R, Kaufman R, Mannhold R. Inotropic and electrophysiological actions of verapamil and D-600 in mammalian myocardium. II. Pattern of inotropic effects of the optical isomers. Naunyn Schmiedebergs Arch Pharmacol 1975; 290:69–80.

58. Bayer R, Kalusche D, Kaufmann R, Mannhold R. Inotropic and electrophysiological actions of verapamil and D-600 in mammalian myocardium. III. Effects of the optical isomers on transmembrane action potentials. Naunyn Schmiedebergs Arch Pharmacol 1975; 290:81–97.

59. Zipes D P, Fischer J C. Effects of agents which inhibit the slow channel on sinus node automaticity and atrioventricular conduction in the dog. Circ Res 1974;34:184–92.

60. Ono H, Hashimoto K. Ca^{2+} antagonism in various parameters of cardiac function including coronary dilation with the use of nifedipine, perhexiline, and verapamil. In: Winbury MM, Abiko Y, eds. Ischemic myocardium and antianginal drugs. New York: Raven Press 1979:77–88.

61. Ono H, Hashimoto K. In vitro effects of calcium flux inhibition. In: Stone P H, Antman E M, eds. Calcium channel blocking agents in the treatment of cardiovascular disorders. Mount Kisco, NY: Futura 1983:155–75.

62. Ono H, Himori N, Taira N. Chronotropic effects of coronary vasodilators as assessed in the isolated, blood-perfused sino-atrial preparation of the dog. Tohoku J Exp Med 1977; 121:383–90.

63. Himori N, Ono H, Taira N. Simultaneous assessment of effects of coronary vasodilators on the coronary blood flow and the myocardial contractility by using the blood perfused canine papillary muscle. Jpn J Pharmacol 1976; 26:427–35.

64. Narrimatsu A, Taira N. Effects on atrioventricular conduction of calcium-antagonistic coronary vasodilators, local anesthetics and quinidine injected into the posterior and the anterior septal artery of the atrio-ventricular node preparation of the dog. Naunyn Schmiedebergs Arch Pharmacol 1976; 294:169–77.

65. Cranefield P F, Aronson R S, Wit A L. Effect of verapamil on the normal action potential and on a calcium-dependent slow response of canine cardiac Purkinje fibers. Circ Res 1974; 34:204–13.

66. Wit A L, Cranefield P F. Effect of verapamil on the sinoatrial and atrioventricular nodes

of the rabbit and the mechanism by which it arrests reentrant atrioventricular nodal tachycardia. Circ Res 1974; 35:413–25.

67. Raschack M. Differences in the cardiac actions of the calcium antagonists verapamil and nifedipine. Arzneimittelforsch 1976; 26:1330–3.

68. Nabata H. Effects of calcium-antagonistic coronary vasodilators on myocardial conctractility and membrane potentials. Jpn J Pharmacol 1977; 27:239–49.

69. Raschack M. Relationship of antiarrhythmic to inotropic activity and antiarrhythmic qualities of the optical isomers of verapamil. Naunyn Schmiedebergs Arch Phamacol 1976; 294:285–91.

70. Taira N, Narimatsu A. Effects of nifedipine, a potent calcium antagonistic coronary vasodilator, on atrioventricular conduction and blood flow in the isolated atrioventricular node preparation of the dog. Naunyn Schmiedebergs Arch Pharmacol 1975; 290:107–12.

71. Endoh M, Yanagisawa T, Taira N. Effects of calcium-antagonistic coronary vasodilators, nifedipine and verapamil, on ventricular automaticity of the dog. Naunyn Schmiedebergs Arch Phamacol 1978: 302:235–8.

72. Kohlhardt M, Bauer B, Krause H, Fleckenstein A. Differentiation of the transmembrane Na and Ca channels in mammalian cardiac fibers by the use of specific inhibitors. Pflugers Arch 1972; 335:309–22.

73. Hordof A J, Edie R, Malm J R, Hoffman B F, Rosen M R. Electrophysiologic properties and response to pharmacologic agents of fibers from diseased human atria. Circulation 1976; 54:774–9.

74. Kaumann A J, Serur J R. Optical isomers of verapamil on canine heart: prevention of ventricular fibrillation induced by coronary artery occlusion, impaired atrioventricular conductance and negative inotropic and chronotropic effects. Naunyn Schmiedebergs Arch Pharmacol 1975; 291:347–58.

75. Brooks W W, Verrier R L, Lown B. Protective effect of verapamil on ventricular vulnerability during coronary artery occlusion and reperfusion. Am J Cardiol 1978; 41:429.

76. Singh B N, Nademanee K, Baky S. Calcium antagonists: clinical uses in treating arrhythmias. Drugs 1983; 25:125–53.

77. Singh B N. The mechanism of action of calcium antagonists relative to their clinical applications. Br J Clin Pharmacol 1986; 21:109S–121S.

78. Wellens H J J, Tan S L, Bar F W H, Durer D R, Lie K I, Dohmen H M. Effect of verapamil studied by programmed electrical stimulation of the heart in patients with paroxysmal re-entrant supraventricular tachycardia. Br Heart J 1977; 39:1058–66.

79. Kawai C, Tomotsuga K, Matsuyama E, Okazaki H. Comparative effects of three calcium antagonists, diltiazem, verapamil and nifedipine on the sinoatrial and atrioventricular nodes. Experimental and clinical studies. Circulation 1981; 63:1035–42.

80. Brown R W, Goble A J. Effect of propranolol on exercise tolerance of patients with atrial fibrillation. Br Med J 1969; 2:279–80.

81. Klein H O, Kaplinsky E. Digitalis and verapamil in atrial fibrillation and flutter. Is verapamil now the preferred agent? Drugs 1986; 31:185–97.

82. Klein H O, Kaplinsky E. Verapamil and digoxin: their respective effects on atrial fibrillation and their interaction. Am J Cardiol 1982; 50:894–902.

83. Klein H O, Pauzner H, DiSegni E, David D, Kaplinsky E. The beneficial effects of verapamil in chronic atrial fibrillation. Arch Intern Med 1979; 139:747–9.

84. Heng M K, Singh B N, Roche A H G, Norris R M, Mercer C J. Effects of intravenous verapamil on cardiac arrhythmias and on the electrocardiogram. Am Heart J 1975; 90:487–98.

85. Schamroth L. Immediate effects of intravenous verapamil on atrial fibrillation. Cardiovasc Res 1971; 5:419–24.

86. Schamroth L, Krikler D M, Garrett C. Immediate effects of intravenous verapamil in cardiac arrhythmias. Br Med 1972; 1:660–4.

87. Slome R. The use of intravenous verapamil in cardiac arrhythmias S Afr Med J 1973; 47:913–4.

88. Gotsman M S, Lewis B S, Bakst A, Mitha AS. Verapamil in life-threatening tachyarrhythmias. S Afr Med J 1972; 46:2017–9.

89. Hartel G, Haratikainen M. Comparison of verapamil and practolol in paroxysmal supraventricular tachycardia. Eur J Cardiol 1976; 4:87–90.

90. Waxman H L, Myerburg R J, Appel R, Sung R J. Verapamil for control of ventricular rate in paroxysmal supraventricular tachycardia and atrial fibrillation or flutter. Ann Intern Med 1981; 94:1–6.

91. Plumb V J, Karp R B, Kouchoukos N T, Zorn G L, James T N, Waldo A L. Verapamil therapy of atrial fibrillation and atrial flutter following cardiac operation. J Thorac Cardiovasc Surg 1982; 83:590–6.

92. Singh B N, Ellrodt G, Peter C T. Verapamil: a review of its pharmacological properties and therapeutic use. Drugs 1978; 15:169–97.

93. Panidis I P, Morganroth J, Baessler C. Effectiveness and safety of oral verapamil to control exercise-induced tachycardia in patients with atrial fibrillation receiving digitalis. Am J Cardiol 1983; 52:1197–201.

94. Rasmussen K, Wang H, Faisa D. Comparative efficacy of quinidine and verapamil in the maintenance of sinus rhythm after DC conversion of atrial fibrillation. Acta Med Scand 1981; 645:23–8.

95. Josephson M E, Kastor J A. Supraventricular tachycardia: mechanisms and management. Ann Intern Med 1977; 87:346–58.

96. Singh B N, Collett J T, Chew C Y C. New perspectives in the pharmacologic therapy of cardiac arrhythmias. Prog Cardiovasc Dis 1980; 22:243–301.

97. Krikler D M. Verapamil in cardiology. Eur J Cardiol 1974; 2:3–10.

98. Schamroth L, Antman E M. Calcium channel blocking agents in the treatment of cardiac arrhythmias. In: Stone P H, Antman E M, eds. Calcium channel blocking agents in the treatment of cardiovascular disorders. Mount Kisco, NY: Futura 1983:347–75.

99. Sung R J, Elser B, McAllister R G. Intravenous verapamil for termination of re-entrant supraventricular tachycardias. Intracardiac studies correlated with plasma verapamil concentrations. Ann Intern Med 1980; 93:682–9.

100. Rozansky J J, Zaman L, Castellanos A. Electrophysiologic effects of diltiazem hydrochloride on supraventricular tachycardia. Am J Cardiol 1982; 49:621–8.

101. Bertin A, Chaitman B R, Bourassa M G, Breuess G, Scholl J M, Bruneau P, Gague P, Chabot M. Beneficial effect of intravenous diltiazem in the acute management of supraventricular tachyarrhythmias. Circulation 1983; 67:88–94.

102. Hung J S, Yeh S J, Liu F C, Fu M, Lee Y S, Wu D. Usefulness of intravenous diltiazem in predicting subsequent electrophysiologic and clinical responses to oral diltiazem. Am J Cardiol 1984; 54:1259–62.

103. Brisse B, Bender F, Bramann H, Kuhs H, Schwippe G. Management of cardiac arrhythmias with tiapamil. Cardiology 1982; 69:144–8.

104. Fauchier J P, Elkik F, Cosnay P, Rouesnel P, Neel C, Quillet L. Effect of i.v. and oral tiapamil in the treatment of paroxysmal supraventricular tachycardia. Eur Heart J 1985; 6:525–31.

105. Gmeiner R, Ng C K. Electrophysiology of tiapamil in concealed accessory pathways. Cardiology 1982; 69:130–9.

106. Menzel T, Kirchner P. Parenteral tiapamil treatment of arrhythmias in cardiac patients. Cardiology 1982; 69:192–8.

107. Opie L H, Muller C A, Thandroyen F T, Lloyd E A, Mabin T, Commerford P J, Eichler H G. Tiapamil—a new calcium antagonist. S Afr Med J 1985; 67:881–3.

108. Yeh S H, Liu F C, Chan Y Y, Hung J S, Wu D. Termination of paroxysmal supraventricular tachycardia with a single oral dose of diltiazem and propranolol. Circulation 1985; 71:104–9.

109. Esmolol Research Group. Intravenous esmolol for the treatment of supraventricular tachyarrhythmia: results of a multicenter, baseline-controlled safety and efficacy study in 160 patients. Am Heart J 1986; 112:498–505.

110. Belhassen B, Pelleg M. Acute management of paroxysmal supraventricular tachycardia: verapamil, adenosine triphosphate or adenosine? Am J Cardiol 1984; 54:225–7.

111. Vohra J, Peter T, Hunt D, Sloman G. Verapamil induced premature ventricular beats before reversion of supraventricular tachycardia. Br Heart J 1974; 36:1186–93.

112. Vohra J, Hunt D, Stuckey J, Sloman G. Cycle length alternation in supraventricular tachycardia after administration of verapamil. Br Heart J 1974; 36:570–6.

113. Rinkenberger R L, Prystowsky E N, Heger J J, Troup P J, Jackman W M, Zipes D P. Effects of intravenous and chronic oral verapamil administration in patients with supraventricular tachyarrhythmias. Circulation 1980; 62:996–1010.

114. Klein G J, Gulamhusein S, Carruthers S G, Donner A P, Ko P T. Comparison of the electrophysiologic effects of intravenous and oral verapamil in patients with paroxysmal supraventricular tachycardia. Am J Cardiol 1982; 49:117–24.

115. Levine H J H, Guarnieri J R M. Treatment of multifocal atrial tachycardia with verapamil. N Engl J Med 1985; 312:21–5.

116. Gulamhusein S, Ko P, Carruthers S G, Klein G J. Acceleration of the ventricular response during atrial fibrillation in the Wolff-Parkinson-White syndrome after verapamil. Circulation 1982; 65:348–54.

117. Harper R W, Whitford E, Middlebrook K, Federman J, Anderson S, Pitt A. Effects of verapamil on the electrophysiologic properties of the accessory pathway in patients with the Wolff-Parkinson-White syndrome. Am J Cardiol 1982; 50:1323–30.

118. Belhassen B, Horowitz L N. Use of intravenous verapamil for ventricular tachycardia. Am J Cardiol 1984; 54:1131–3.

119. McAllister R G, Hamann S R, Blouin R A. Pharmacokinetics of calcium entry blockers. Am J Cardiol 1985; 55:30B–40B.

120. McAllister R G. Clinical pharmacology of slow channel blocking agents. Prog Cardiovasc Dis 1982; 25:83–102.

121. Abernethy D R, Schwartz J B, Todd E L, Luchi R, Snow E. Verapamil pharmacodynamics and disposition in young and elderly hypertensive patients. Ann Intern Med 1986; 105:329–36.

122. McAllister R G, Howell S M. Fluorometric assay of verapamil in biological fluids and tissues. J Pharm Sci 1976; 1976:431–2.

123. McAllister R G, Tan T G, Dourne D W A. GLC assay of verapamil in plasma: identification of fluorescent metabolites after oral drug administration. J Pharm Sci 1979; 68:574–6.

124. Harapat S R, Kates R E. High-performance liquid chromatographic analysis of verapamil. II. Simultaneous quantitation of verapamil and its active metabolite, norverapamil. J Chromatogr 1980; 181:484–9.

125. Watson E, Kapur P A. High-performance liquid chromatographic determination of verapamil in plasma by fluorescence detection. J Pharm Sci 1981; 70:800–1.

126. Schomerus M, Spiegelhalder B, Stieren B, Eichelbaum M. Physiological disposition of verapamil in man. Cardiovasc Res 1976; 10:605–12.

127. Johnston A, Burgess C D, Hamer J. Systemic availability of oral verapamil and effect on PR interval in man. Br J Clin Pharmacol 1981; 12:397–400.

128. Dominic J A, Bourne D W A, Tan T G, Kirsten E B, McAllister R G. The pharmacology of verapamil. III. Pharmacokinetics in normal subjects after intravenous drug administration. J Cardiovasc Pharmacol 1981; 3:25–38.

129. Kates R E, Keefe D L D, Schwartz J, Harapat S, Kirsten E B, Harrison D C. Verapamil disposition kinetics in chronic atrial fibrillation. Clin Pharmacol Ther 1981; 30:44–51.

130. Woodcock B G, Reitbrock I, Vohringer H F, Rietbrock N. Verapamil disposition in liver disease and intensive-care patients: kinetics, clearance, and apparent blood flow relationships. Clin Pharmacol Ther 1981; 29:27–34.

131. Somogyi A, Albrecht M, Kleims G, Schafer K, Eichelbaum M. Pharmacokinetics, bioavailability and ECG response of verapamil in patients with liver cirrhosis. Br J Clin Pharmacol 1981; 12:51–60.

132. Eichelbaum M, Somogyi A, Unruh G E V, Dengler H J. Simultaneous determination of the intravenous and oral pharmacokinetic parameters of D,L-verapamil using stable isotope labelled verapamil. Eur J Clin Pharmacol 1981; 19:133–7.

133. Woodcock B G, Hopf R, Kaltenbach M. Verapamil and norverapamil plasma concentrations during long-term therapy in patients with hypertrophic obstructive cardiomyopathy. J Cardiovasc Pharmacol 1980; 2:17–23.

134. Shand D G, Hammill S C, Aanonsen L, Pritchett L C. Reduced verapamil clearance during long-term oral administration. Clin Pharmacol Ther 1981; 30:701–3.

135. Keefe D L, Yee Y, Kates R E. Verapamil protein binding in patients and in normal subjects. Clin Pharmacol Ther 1981; 29:21–6.

136. Eichelbaum M, Birkel P, Grube E, Gutgemann U, Somogyi A. Effects of verapamil on P-R intervals in relation to verapamil plasma levels following single i.v. and oral administration and during chronic treatment. Klin Wochenschr 1980; 58:919–25.

137. Dominic J, McAllister R G, Kuo S, Reddy C P, Surawicz B. Verapamil plasma levels and ventricular rate response in patients with atrial fibrillation and flutter. Clin Pharmacol Ther 1979; 26:710–4.

138. Woie L, Storstein L. Successful treatment of suicidal verapamil poisoning with calcium gluconate. Eur Heart J 1981; 2:239–42.

139. Neugebauer G. Comparative cardiovascular actions of verapamil and its major metabo-

lites in the anaesthetised dog. Cardiovasc Res 1978; 12:247–54.

140. Lewis J G. Adverse reactions to calcium antagonists. Drugs 1983; 25:196–222.

141. Lee T H, Salomon D R, Rayment C M, Antman E M. Hypotension and sinus arrest with exercise-induced hyperkalemia and combined verapamil/propranolol therapy. Am J Med 1986; 80:1203–4.

142. Carrasco H A, Fuenmayor A, Barboza J S, Gonzalez G. Effect of verapamil on normal sinoatrial node function and on sick sinus syndrome. Am Heart J 1978; 96:760–71.

143. Denis B, Pellet J, Machecourt J, Martin-Noel P. Verapamil et beta-bloquant. Une association therapeutic dangereuse. Nouv Presse Med 1977; 6:2075.

144. Pedersen K E, Dorph-Pedersen A, Hvidt S, Klitgaard N A, Nielsen-Kudsk F. Digoxin-verapamil interaction. Clin Pharmacol Ther 1981; 30:311–6.

145. Pedersen K E, Dorph-Pedersen A, Hvidt S, Klitgaard N A, Pedersen K K. The long-term effect of verapamil on plasma digoxin concentration and renal digoxin clearance in

healthy subjects. Eur J Clin Pharmacol 1982; 22:123–7.

146. Schwartz J B, Keefe D, Kates R E, Kirsten E, Harrison D C. Acute and chronic pharmacodynamic interaction of verapamil and digoxin in atrial fibrillation. Circulation 1982; 65:1163–70.

147. Marcus F I. Pharmacokinetic interactions between digoxin and other drugs. J Am Coll Cardiol 1985; 5:82A–90A.

148. Antman E M, Arnold J M O, Friedman P L, Smith T W. Pharmocokinetic drug interactins between digoxin and antiarrhythmic agents and calcium channel blocking agents: an appraisal of study methodology. Cardiovasc Drugs Ther 1987; 1:183–9.

149. Epstein S E, Rosing D R. Verapamil: its potential for causing serious complications in patients with hypertrophic cardiomyopathy. Circulation 1981; 64:437–41.

150. Hattori V T, Mandel W J, Peter T. Calcium for myocardial depression from verapamil. N Engl J Med 1982; 306:238.

151. Immonen P, Linkola A, Waris E. Three cases of severé verapamil poisoning. Int J Cardiol 1981; 1:101–5.

35

Antifibrillatory Drugs

Andrew C. G. Uprichard* and Benedict R. Lucchesi

*The University of Michigan Medical School
Ann Arbor, Michigan*

INTRODUCTION

> From lightening and tempest; from plague,
> pestilence and famine; from battle and murder,
> and from sudden death, Good Lord, deliver us.
>
> The Litany, *Book of Common Prayer*

Despite the innumerable technological and medical advances that have occurred since the writing of the Litany, it remains clear that sudden death is as real a problem today as it appears to have been in the sixteenth century. In medical terms "sudden death" generally denotes death that is nonviolent, unexpected, witnessed, and instantaneous or occurs within a few minutes of an abrupt change in the previous clinical state (1). An idea of the magnitude of the problem can be gauged from epidemiologic data that suggest that sudden cardiac death may account for up to 30% of all deaths (2) and is further compounded by the observation that in nearly 25% of these individuals sudden cardiac death is the first manifestation of underlying heart disease (3).

The development of modern electrocardiographic monitoring, however, has at least allowed us a better understanding of the arrhythmic basis of the problem, since several reports have identified ventricular fibrillation as the most common terminal mechanism (4–7).

Since, once established, the only management of ventricular fibrillation is the application of a direct current countershock, for many years researchers and clinicians alike have looked for treatable factors that might be identified in those at risk of sudden cardiac death. As yet there appears no way initially of distinguishing these individuals from the overall population of patients with ischemic heart disease (8). However, studies of patients after myocardial infarction have been able to identify chronic ventricular ectopy as a significant risk factor for subsequent sudden death (9–14). Despite this, several studies with currently available antiarrhythmic agents have been unable to demonstrate a significant effect upon overall mortality. Reviews of 6 (15) and 14 (16) clinical trials have revealed marked discrepancies between centers, with no overall

---

*Present affiliation: Parke-Davis Clinical Research, Ann Arbor, Michigan.

effect on survival from short- or long-term studies. Conversely, however, a number of trials have provided good evidence that the use of β-adrenoceptor antagonists in the postinfarction period is associated with a reduction in both reinfarction and sudden death (17–22). The precise mechanism mediating the beneficial effect of β-adrenoceptor antagonists on sudden cardiac death, however, remains unclear; in particular there is uncertainty over whether the drugs act by a direct antifibrillatory effect or via a primary anti-ischemic influence. Thus one is faced with the paradox that, although chronic ventricular ectopy presents a significant risk for subsequent ventricular fibrillation, decreasing the frequency of ectopic complexes with antiarrhythmic agents does not appear to improve survival. A better understanding of the problem must therefore require a greater knowledge of the pathophysiologic milieu pertaining at the time of sudden death.

THE SUBSTRATE AND THE INSULT

Postmortem studies have indicated that in the majority of cases ventricular fibrillation is a primary event and not related to acute myocardial infarction (23,24), but it is known to occur most commonly in patients with previous myocardial infarction (25–27). Furthermore, the finding in many cases of intracoronary thrombus without acute infarction suggests that ischemia, per se, may be acting as the trigger for the genesis of ventricular fibrillation in a vulnerable, electrically unstable ventricular myocardium. The electrophysiologic properties of ischemic myocardium, such as increased excitability, shortening of refractoriness, slowing of conduction, and increased inhomogeneity in recovery, may be seen to provide the milieu for the emergence of reentrant rhythms in a heart critically deranged by previous infarction. The concept of distant ischemia acting as the trigger for fatal ventricular arrhythmias was first rasied by Schuster and Bulkley (28). In a study of two groups of patients with early postinfarction angina, they found that those with remote ischemia constituted a group of hemo-

dynamically stable patients who faced an unexpectedly high mortality compared with those patients whose angina arose from the periinfarction region. Schwartz and coworkers reproduced this phenomenon experimentally when they demonstrated a high incidence of ventricular fibrillation in a chronic model of myocardial infarction in which additional ischemia was initiated using a hydraulic coronary artery occluder (29,30). Also using a canine model, Kabell and coworkers (31) demonstrated a diminution in infarct collateral blood flow with distant ischemia. Since this was preceded by delayed epicardial activity within the area of preexisting infarction, it suggested that ischemia may be influencing the substrate of an infarcted area of myocardium to render it more suitable for the emergence of lethal arrhythmias.

Coronary vasospasm has also been considered a triggering mechanism for sudden death, especially since patients with atypical angina have demonstrated serious ventricular arrhythmias during episodes of spasm (32). Although the majority of survivors of cardiac arrest give no previous or subsequent history of atypical angina, in one study sudden death was observed in 17% of 114 patients with coronary vasospasm followed for a mean of 24 months (33).

Another mechanism that must be considered in the genesis of lethal arrhythmias is the role of the autonomic nervous system. Alterations in autonomic tone are well recognized in acute myocardial ischemia and may be inherently arrhythmogenic by nature of the increase in myocardial oxygen consumption and alterations in refractoriness. Inhomogenous adrenergic stimulation has been shown to precipitate arrhythmias in a number of animal models (34), and others have demonstrated a possible role of the sympathetic nervous system when acute ischemia is produced in the setting of previous myocardial infarction (29). Other factors contributing to the precipitating trigger in sudden death include those biochemical alterations (hypokalemia and hypomagnesemia, among others) known to precipitate fatal arrhythmias in individuals at risk, as well as possible proarrhythmic effects

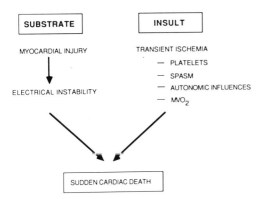

Figure 1 The potential "insults" capable of contributing to the emergence of fatal ventricular arrhythmias in a heart critically deranged from previous myocardial infarction.

from the very drugs prescribed in an effort to prevent sudden death (35,36).

Thus a variety of factors may predispose the individual at risk to the development of lethal ventricular arrhythmias; these points are summarized in Figure 1.

MODELS FOR THE EVALUATION OF POTENTIAL ANTIFIBRILLATORY DRUGS

For obvious reasons there exists no clinical model of sudden death apart from prospective studies of large numbers of postinfarction patients, the results of which (as has already been mentioned) have generally been disappointing. Even when ventricular fibrillation is induced by programmed electrical stimulation in the electrophysiology laboratory, one cannot be sure that the substrate of the arrhythmia thus generated is identical to that pertaining at the time of sudden death or that pharmacologic prevention of stimulus-induced ventricular fibrillation reflects protection against sudden death. Furthermore, these methods fail to take into account the critical ischemic event that is thought to trigger the fatal arrhythmia. It is not surprising, therefore, that recent studies have suggested that electrophysiologic techniques, per se, may not help in identifying high-risk patients, even when the study population is restricted to survivors of sudden death (37–39).

Until recently whole-animal models for the evaluation of antiarrhythmic activity have generally relied upon arrhythmogenesis by cardiotoxic agents, electrical stimuli, or arrhythmias associated with coronary artery occlusion, with or without reperfusion (40). More complicated maneuvers include arrhythmias induced by catecholamines (41) or electrical stimuli (42,43) in the subacute phase of myocardial infarction. It is apparent, however, that although each of these techniques is capable of generating reliable and reproducible arrhythmias, they fail to provide an opportunity to examine the electrophysiologic milieu at the time of ventricular fibrillation or to study pharmacologic interventions aimed at preventing sudden death.

The ventricular fibrillation threshold (VFT) has been considered a reflection of the electrical stability of the whole heart and therefore a measure of its resistance to fibrillate (44). Although used for some time as an indicator of potential antifibrillatory potential, the model has recently come under criticism for an inability to correlate alterations in fibrillation thresholds with direct electrophysiologic actions (45). Despite procedural modifications, such as determinations of VFT under normal and ischemic conditions (46), it appears that, particularly when trains of current are employed, there is a release of local stores of epinephrine, which has the effect of markedly lowering the fibrillation threshold (47). If this is the case the elevation of fibrillation thresholds seen with the β-adrenoceptor antagonists (48,49) may relate more to antagonism of the effects of stimulus-induced epinephrine release than to any direct antifibrillatory phenomenon.

THE CONSCIOUS CANINE MODEL OF SUDDEN CARDIAC DEATH

Some years ago this laboratory described a conscious canine model that was susceptible to the initiation of stimulus-induced ventricular arrhythmias in the subacute phase of anterior myocardial infarction (50). Of particular interest in this model was the finding that an additional ischemic insult (initiated by a 150 μA anodal current to the left circumflex coro-

Table 1 Characteristics of the Chronic Canine Model of Sudden Death

Features	Inducible	Non-inducible
Anterior infarct size, % left ventricular mass	24.7 ± 1.7	5.3 ± 1.1[a]
Time to ischemia, min	196 ± 39	225 ± 30
Sudden VF, < 1 hr	11/15	2/15
Delayed VF, < 24 hr	3/15	0/15
Thrombus mass, mg	7.2 ± 1.81	11.2 ± 2.3
Posterolateral infarct mass	19.0 ± 1.0 ($n = 3$)	16.7 ± 2.3 ($n = 13$)

[a] $p < 0.001$.
Source: Summarized from Wiber et al, 1985.

nary artery) served as a reliable model of acute ventricular fibrillation. The same study also demonstrated that previous myocardial damage was a prerequisite for the observed high mortality, since dogs without anterior infarctions exhibited a low risk of ventricular fibrillation (50). A subsequent study (51) further evaluated the model by looking at the relationship between inducible ventricular tachycardia and the subsequent development of ventricular fibrillation. Results suggested that inducible arrhythmias (either sustained or nonsustained) were highly predictive of spontaneous ventricular fibrillation during posterolateral ischemia. Of additional interest was the observation that the mass of previously injured myocardium was a critical determinant of both, since animals with inducible arrhythmias (24 hr mortality 93%) had much larger infarct sizes (24.7 ± 1.7% of left ventricular mass) than those that were noninducible at baseline testing (24 hr mortality 15%: infarct size 5.3 ± 1.1% of left ventricular mass); (Table 1). The use of this model therefore enabled not only the evaluation of antiarrhythmic activity against arrhythmias thought to share the same reentrant basis as ischemic arrhythmias in the human (42,52), but also a correlation of antiarrhythmic activity with antifibrillatory activity in the sudden death protocol. Experimental methods are described here and summarized in Figure 2.

Methods

Mongrel dogs of either sex are anesthetized by the intravenous administration of sodium pen-

tobarbital, intubated, and ventilated with room air. Using aseptic technique the left jugular vein is isolated and cannulated for subsequent drug administration. A left thoracotomy is performed, and the heart exposed and suspended in a pericardial cradle. The left anterior descending coronary artery (LAD) is dissected free at the tip of the left atrial appendage, and the left circumflex coronary artery (LCX) is isolated approximately 1 cm from its origin. Anterior wall infarction is achieved by a 2 hr occlusion of the LAD followed by reperfusion in the presence of a critical stenosis. An epicardial bipolar electrode is sutured to the left atrial appendage for subsequent atrial pacing. A bipolar plunge electrode is sutured onto the surface of the heart in the region of the right ventricular outflow tract (RVOT) for the subsequent introduction of extrastimuli during programmed electrical stimulation. In addition, two bipolar plunge electrodes are sutured to the left ventricular wall: one in the distribution of the LAD distal to the site of occlusion (infarct zone, IZ) and the second in the distribution of the LCX (normal zone, NZ). Finally, a 30-gauge electrode is inserted into the lumen of the LCX and secured by suturing to the heart wall.

Programmed electrical stimulation and electrophysiologic testing is performed in the conscious, unsedated animal 3–5 days after surgical preparation. After determination of the RVOT excitation threshold and refractory period, programmed stimulation continues with the introduction of double (S2 and S3) and triple (S2,S3, and S4) extrastimuli (4 msec duration at twice RVOT excitation

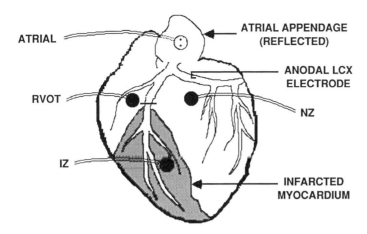

Figure 2 The conscious canine model of sudden death: surgical preparation. Anterior myocardial infarction is produced by a 2 hr occulsion of the left anterior descending coronary artery, with subsequent reperfusion in the presence of a critical stenosis. An atrial bipolar epicardial electrode is illustrated, as well as bipolar plunge electrodes in normal myocardium (normal zone, NZ), infarcted tissue (infarct zone, IZ), and the right ventricular outflow tract (RVOT). The latter is subsequently used for the introduction of extrastimuli during programmed electrical stimulation 3–5 days after surgery. A silver wire electrode is illustrated within the lumen of the left circumflex coronary artery (LCX). Ultimate introduction of a 150 μA anodal current results in acute posterolateral ischemia and a high incidence of ventricular fibrillation in the sudden death protocol.

threshold) during sinus rhythm. Previous studies from this laboratory showed that these stimulation methods do not induce arrhythmias in sham-operated animals (50). Electrophysiologic parameters from normal and infarcted myocardium are determined from the construction of strength-interval curves using data obtained from the NZ and IZ electrodes, respectively. Dogs with sustained or nonsustained VT are allocated randomly to drug or vehicle groups, and electrophysiologic testing and programmed stimulation are repeated in full after drug equilibration.

Upon completion of the posttreatment stimulation protocol a direct anodal current of 150 μA is applied to the intimal surface of the left circumflex coronary artery (LCX) using a 9 V nickel-cadmium battery and variable resistor. This has been shown to result in intimal damage, platelet aggregation, cyclic variations in blood flow, and a high incidence of acute ventricular fibrillation within 1 hr of the onset of ischemia. Lead II of the ECG is recorded at preset intervals (30 sec every 15 min) by a programmable cardiocassette recorder. After 24 hr of constant anodal current or the devel-

opment of ventricular fibrillation, the heart is excised and any thrombus in the LCX removed and weighed. The heart is sectioned transversely and incubated in a 0.4% solution of triphenyltetrazolium chloride (TTC) for 15 min. Anterior and posterolateral areas of infarction are identified by their inability to reduce TTC enzymatically to a brick-red formazan precipitate. Infarct masses in the myocardial regions are quantified gravimetrically and expressed as a percentage of total left ventricular mass. Playback of the cardiocassette provides information regarding the time of onset of ischemia (as assessed by the appearance of ventricular ectopy and/or ST segment changes), the time from ischemia to death, and the percentage change in heart rate before death.

Drug Protection Against Sudden Death

Of a total of 201 inducible, vehicle-treated dogs studied in this laboratory over the past 6 years, 188 (94%) died within 24 hr of posterolateral ischemia in the sudden death protocol. An interesting observation in many of the

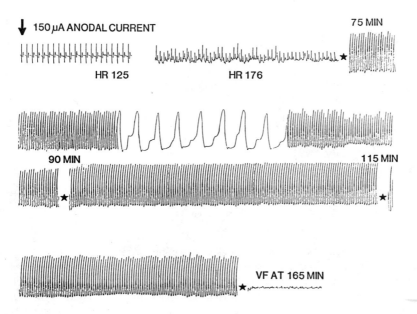

Figure 3 The conscious canine model of sudden death. An example of ischemic ventricular fibrillation preceded by a sustained ventricular tachycardia in response to acute posterolateral ischemia during the subacute phase of myocardial infarction (vehicle-treated animal). The onset of ischemia is determined by an increase in heart rate after 60 min, and the arrhythmia is apparent at 75 min. Stars refer to preprogrammed breaks (15 min) during ECG monitoring.

animals that die is the finding of variable periods of sustained monomorphic ventricular tachycardia before the onset of ventricular fibrillation (Fig. 3); in this respect the model can be seen to resemble closely the clinical situation, in which ambulatory monitoring has identified sustained ventricular arrhythmias as the most common terminal mechanism in sudden death (53–55). Drug protection in this model is apparent when animals survive the arrhythmias of acute posterolateral ischemia and ultimately develop second infarcts in the distribution of the left circumflex coronary artery (Fig. 4). The results of various pharmacologic interventions in the conscious canine model of sudden death are summarized in Table 2.

What is immediately obvious from Table 2 is the apparent dichotomy of action of several antiarrhythmic agents when tested both against the arrhythmias of programmed electrical stimulation and in their effects against ischemic ventricular fibrillation. Thus it can be seen that clinically relevant plasma concentrations of the class IA agent quinidine were ca-

pable of preventing the induction of stimulus-induced arrhythmias but were ineffective in preventing ventricular fibrillation (56). A subsequent study with flecainide (57) not only demonstrated a failure of the drug to prevent ventricular fibrillation but raised the possibility of proarrhythmia, with three of seven noninducible animals failing to survive the sudden death protocol. Although accepting that conclusions regarding an entire class of drug action cannot be based on the evaluation of two agents, these results do tend to support the clinical observation that restriction of the fast inward sodium channel with slowing of conduction velocity does not provide antifibrillatory protection. Similarly, antagonism of myocardial calcium channels did not appear to offer significant protection in studies with the class IV agents bepridil (58) and diltiazem (59). In identifying a common electrophysiologic characteristic for antifibrillatory efficacy in this model, it becomes apparent that the greatest overall protection has been seen with agents that have as part of their pharmacologic profile prolongation of the action potential du-

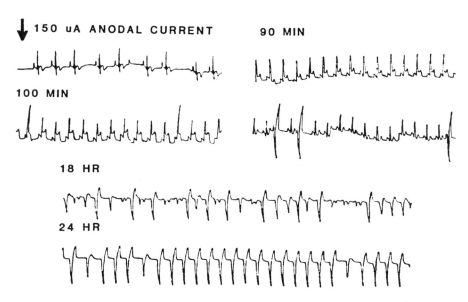

Figure 4 Drug protection in the conscious canine model of sudden death. A sinus tachycardia develops after 90 min of posterolateral ischemia, and ST segment elevation is apparent after 100 min. Shortly thereafter there is ECG confirmation of the early arrhythmias of myocardial ischemia. From 18 hr the heart rate is almost exclusively ventricular in origin, confirming the development of a second infarction (left circumflex coronary artery territory). Example of a sotalol-treated animal.

ration (class III activity). Studies with bretylium (60), amiodarone (61), and sotalol (62,63) have all demonstrated significant protection in placebo-controlled studies. The effects of clofilium, an alternative class III drug, were less clear (64).

Bretylium was introduced into clinical cardiology in the early 1980s and is currently the only drug marketed as an antifibrillatory agent. Its electrophysiologic properties include direct effects upon cardiac action potential duration and indirect effects mediated via its actions on the autonomic nervous system. The initial effect of the drug is to liberate catecholamines from nerve terminals with resultant sympathomimetic features of tachycardia and increased blood pressure, but after some 20–30 min these features dissipate with the development of chronic adrenergic blockade. Early studies with the drug demonstrated suppression of stimulus-induced ventricular tachycardia (65,66) and elevation in ventricular fibrillation thresholds (67). In our model of sudden death bretylium (10 mg/kg IV every 6 hr) resulted in significant prolongation of ven-

tricular refractoriness and the survival of 6 of the 10 animals studied ($p < 0.05$ versus placebo). The exact antifibrillatory mechanism of the drug, however, remains obscure; bretylium has been shown to exert similar electrophysiologic effects in the denervated heart (68), but the significance of the drug's autonomic effects upon the development of ventricular fibrillation are unknown. Furthermore, studies with bethanidine (69) and meobentine (70) failed to prevent sudden death in the same model, despite similar structural and electrophysicologic characteristics.

It is important at this point to distinguish between homogeneous prolongation of the action potential as occurs with the class III drugs and the heterogeneous prolongation seen in the so-called long QT syndromes that lead to spatial variations in refractoriness and subsequent arrhythmogenicity (71,72). Unlike class IA agents, which produce a time-dependent increase in refractoriness by altering sodium conductance, class III drugs exert a voltage-dependent prolongation in refractory periods by slowing repolarization (73). Fur-

Table 2 Drug Efficacy in the Conscious Canine Model of Myocardial Infarction and Sudden Death

Agent	Suppression of PVS-induced VT	24 hr Post ischemic survival (%)
Vehicle	−	6[a]
Class I		
Quinidine	+	9
Flecainide	−	14
Class II		
Nadolol	−	56–63
Dilevalol	−	20–60
Sotalol	+	63
Celiprolol	−	30
Class III		
d-Sotalol	+	65
Bretylium	+	60
Amiodarone	−	40–80
Clofilium	+	30
Class IV		
Diltiazem	−	10
Bepridil	+	30–40
Class V: Alinidine	−	60
Others		
Meobentine	−	0
Bethanidine	−	0
Prazosin	−	50
CGS 12970[b]	−	30

[a]Cumulative (11 of 172 vehicle-treated animals).
[b]Thromboxane synthetase inhibitor.
Source: Adapted from Lynch and Lucchesi, 1987.

ther, experiments with bretylium have shown a greater increase in action potential duration in periinfarcted myocytes than in those of the infarct itself, where action potential duration has already been lengthened by the ischemic process (74). This can be interpreted as resulting in a reduction in the disparity of action potentials (and refractory periods) between normal and infarcted regions, thus reducing the likelihood of reentrant arrhythmias.

Amiodarone originally was introduced as an antianginal agent but subsequently was found to have electrophysiologic features attributable to each of the four classes of antiarrhythmic action (75–77). In addition, the drug reduces the inotropic and chronotropic responses of other agents and has vasodilatory effects on the coronary and systemic vasculature (78). Its outstanding property, however, is prolongation of the cardiac action potential, prompting its

clinical use as a potential antifibrillatory agent (79). Despite the observation that alterations in action potential duration and ventricular refractoriness are usually apparent only with chronic dosing, studies in this laboratory have demonstrated significant antifibrillatory protection after long- and short-term oral therapy. Despite no differences being observed in plasma or myocardial concentrations of amiodarone between the two dosing regimens, the greater survival in those animals treated for 10 days (80 versus 60% treated acutely) suggests that long-term therapy may have additional, as yet unidentified actions contributing to greater efficacy. Although the electrophysiologic effects of amiodarone resemble closely those of hypothyroidism (80,81), that this is not due to the iodine moiety of the drug has been shown in experiments in which the administration of iodine had no effect on cardiac action potentials (82). However, the concomitant administration of amiodarone and thyroid hormone prevented the repolarization changes seen with amiodarone alone, and a recent study in this laboratory demonstrated that prior thyroidectomy can protect postinfarction animals from ischemic ventricular fibrillation in the sudden death protocol (83).

The effects of sotalol and its dextrorotatory enantiomer, *d*-sotalol, have been of particular importance in correlating the antifibrillatory potential of pharmacologic agents with their known electrophysiologic characteristics. Racemic sotalol is a noncardioselective β-adrenergic receptor antagonist that causes a dose-dependent prolongation of action potential duration without associated class I (membrane-stabilizing) properties. D-sotalol, however, although retaining the same cardiac electrophysiologic profile, does not share to the same extent the parent compound's β-blocking properties. The use of *d*-sotalol therefore allows the investigator to assess the relative antifibrillatory effect of the drug's direct electrophysiologic effects divorced from the confounding influence of β-adrenoceptor antagonism. Initial studies with racemic sotalol demonstrated a 65% survival in animals treated with the drug and entered into the sudden death protocol (62). This protective effect was associated with significant prolongation of the QT interval (an electrocardiographic parameter of action potential duration) and bridging diastolic electrical activity of the lead II ECG, a phenomenon invariably followed by ventricular fibrillation in vehicle-treated animals. In a subsequent study with the d-enantiomer, Lynch and coworkers (63) demonstrated similar electrophysiologic and antifibrillatory effects, only without the attenuation of the ischemic increase in heart rate seen with the parent compound. This suggested that the observed antifibillatory effect of *d*-sotalol was not related to any β-adrenergic receptor antagonism but stemmed directly from prolongation of action potential duration and refractoriness.

The antiarrhythmic and antifibrillatory potential of β-adrenoceptor antagonism remains unclear. Except when ancillary electro-physiologic properties are part of a particular agent's pharmacologic profile, these agents as a group are without direct effect on the heart. Despite this, several studies have reported significant antiarrhythmic effects with these drugs, in both clinical (84) and experimental (85,86) studies. This laboratory has been involved in the evaluation of four β-blocking agents. The effects of sotalol have been discussed already. Nadolol is a noncardioselective agent studied in the sudden death protocol after pretreatment with 1 (*n* = 9) and 8 (*n* = 13) mg/kg. Respective survival figures were 56 and 63% (*p* < 0.01 versus placebo) (87). *D*-Nadolol, an enantiomer devoid of β-blocking properties, was ineffective. An interesting feature in this study was the observation that the majority of nadolol-treated dogs that died did so, not from ventricular fibrillation, but as the result of complete heart block, severe bradycardia, and pump failure. This phenomenon was also observed in a subsequent study with dilevalol, the R,R-enantiomer of labetalol, in which 75% of deaths were consequent upon severe bradyarrhythmias (88,89). The administration of methylscopolamine to postinfarction animals pretreated with dilevalol, however, significantly reduced mortality (40 versus 100% vehicle-treated, *p* < 0.05), suggesting that dilevalol, like nadolol, was capable of preventing ischemic ventricular fibrillation in this model but that death was due to the unopposed effects of parasympathetic stimulation.

In a recent series of experiments (90) we evaluated the effects of celiprolol, a class II drug with intrinsic stimulant properties. In view of recent studies with sotalol, nadolol, and dilevalol, it was of significance that the drug was without effect in preventing sudden death. In particular it was apparent that ventricular fibrillation was identified as the terminal mechanism for each of the seven deaths in the drug-treated group. Although the model is not designed specifically to address the question of intrinsic cardiostimulant phenomena, it was noted that resting heart rate did not alter after celiprolol and it is possible that this feature of the drug attenuated any protection during acute posterolateral ischemia. It has been demonstrated, for example, that the propensity of sympathetic stimulation to induce arrhythmias in the late myocardial infarction period may relate primarily to heart rate (91), and previous studies have shown antagonism of the antiarrhythmic protection afforded by propanolol by overdrive atrial pacing (92). In a recent review of several large prospective double-blind trials with β-adrenoceptor antagonists, Kjekshus demonstrated an almost linear relationship between the reduction in resting heart rate and mortality and noted that drugs with intrinsic sympathomimetic activity produced small reductions in heart rate and lesser effects on mortality (93). Although it is unclear whether celiprolol's stimulant properties are due entirely to partial agonism (94), intrinsic sympathomimetic activity is cited as a possible reason the drug failed to exert a beneficial influence upon ventricular arrhythmias in a group of patients with acute myocardial infarction (95).

In an attempt to clarify the role of heart rate in the genesis of sudden death, we next evaluated the antifibrillatory effects of alinidine, the N-allyl derivative of clonidine. Alinidine is one of a number of agents, the main pharmacologic action of which appears to be a reduction in heart rate from a direct action on the sinus node (96,97). Although capable of attenuating the chronotropic response to isoproterenol, the curves are not shifted, indicating that these drugs do not operate by antagonism of β-adrenergic receptors (96,98). Similarly, there is no evidence that the specific bradycardic action involves α-adrenergic or muscarinic receptors, or calcium channels (96,98,99). However, studies in isolated tissues have shown a non-voltage-dependent decrease in the slope of the slow diastolic depolarization, indicating that the drugs' effects may be mediated by restriction of current through anion-selective channels (99). Since the demonstrated antiarrhythmic effects of these agents in experimental models (100,101) cannot be explained on the basis of the four main antiarrhythmic classes, this has prompted the suggestion that anion antagonism be included as a fifth antiarrhythmic class (102).

In our model of sudden death alinidine at a dose of 1 mg/kg produced a significant ($p <$ 0.01) decrease in resting heart rate and prevented ventricular fibrillation in 6 of 10 animals studied ($p < 0.05$ versus concurrent placebo group). In a third group of dogs in which constant atrial pacing maintained heart rates at predrug values throughout the sudden death protocol, mortality was 100% (103). Since alinidine was without significant effect on parameters of refractoriness, conduction, or action potential duration, this suggested an indirect effect of the drug, possibly by influencing the degree of posterolateral ischemia during the sudden death protocol.

Kobinger and coworkers (97) first demonstrated a reduction in the degree of ST segment elevation with alinidine during acute coronary occlusion in cats, and evidence followed of enhanced collateral flow and improvement in myocardial function in pigs with coronary artery stenosis (104). More recent studies in dogs confirmed significant reductions in infarct size with alinidine (105), as well as other related bradycardic agents (106). Further studies revealed that the bradycardic agents, like the β-adrenoceptor antagonists, are capable of increasing perfusion pressure distal to a coronary artery stenosis, but unlike the latter only the bradycardic agents were capable of enhancing flow (107). Furthermore, this effect appears to be attenuated by atrial pacing to control (predrug) heart rate values (108). Thus during posterolateral ischemia alinidine may be contributing to enhanced collateral flow in the ischemic bed secondary to prolongation of diastole and a presumed reduction in myocardial oxygen consumption. Because of the high mortality in vehicle-treated animals, our model of sudden death does not allow accurate comparison of posterolateral infarct sizes between drug- and vehicle-treated groups, but the ischemia-related increase in heart rate was attenuated in the alinidine group and the time from introduction of anodal LCX current to the onset of posterolateral ischemia tended to be prolonged, both of which may indicate a lesser degree of ischemia in alinidine-treated animals.

Another agent that demonstrated significant antifibrillatory protection in the conscious canine model of sudden death was the α-1-adrenoceptor antagonist prazosin. Despite an inability to alter electrocardiographic intervals, ventricular refractoriness, or the induction of ventricular tachycardia by programmed stimulation, pretreatment with 500 µg/kg of drug resulted in a 50% survival rate in the sudden death protocol ($p < 0.05$ versus placebo) (109). This may be of particular significance in view of the recent suggestion that α-adrenergic responsiveness may be enhanced under conditions of myocardial ischemia (110,111) and that this is correlated with an increase in α-adrenoceptor concentration (112). Although the relative contributions of α- and β-adrenergic influences in the genesis of ventricular fibrillation remain unclear, it has been suggested that α-mediated prolongation of action potential duration in ischemic areas may combine with β-mediated shortening of action potential duration in nonischemic areas to increase the disparity in refractory periods and produce the arrhythmogenic milieu suitable for the emergence of fatal reentrant pathways (113). Antagonism of either adrenergic pathway (by the respective adrenergic antagonist) could therefore be seen as reducing the electrophysiologic derangements leading to ventricular fibrillation and explain the protection afforded by both the β-blockers and prazosin in our model.

Hypokalemia has long been recognized as a risk factor in patients with ischemic heart disease, and recent interest has been focused on the role of the ionic potassium current I_K in the genesis of ventricular fibrillation (114). It has been argued that pharmacologic antagonism of I_K increases action potential duration and, by an argument similar to that employed for the class III agents, prolongs refractoriness and reduces the likelihood for reentrant pathways. Antagonism of I_K has been reported in guinea pig heart cells exposed to clofilium (115) but does not appear to have been evaluated with other class III drugs. Nevertheless, the unrelated oral hypoglycemic agent glibenclamide is known to antagonize intracellular potassium efflux and has demonstrated significant antiarrhythmic efficacy in an isolated preparation (116). The profound metabolic consequences of glibenclamide therapy are likely to influence significantly any whole-animal studies, but an alternative approach to the problem has been to investigate the potential proarrhythmic effects of agents that stimulate potassium ionic currents. Pinacidil is an antihypertensive agent that promotes intracellular potassium efflux and significantly reduces action potential duration (117). In a recent series of experiments we evaluated the drug in two groups of noninducible dogs and found a 100% mortality in pinacidil-treated animals compared with 20% mortality in a concurrent vehicle group ($p < 0.001$) (128). The evidence for a proarrhythmic effect of pinacidil appears strong, but one cannot be sure regarding the causal influence of potassium channel involvement, far less that a drug with reciprocal ionic characteristics should prevent ventricular fibrillation. Nevertheless, such experiments are likely to generate increasing research into the role of specific ionic currents in the genesis of life-threatening arrhythmias and sudden death.

CONCLUSIONS

The Evaluation of Antifibrillatory Agents

Ventricular premature depolarizations constitute a risk factor for sudden coronary death in patients after acute myocardial infaction (118,119). The Cardiac Arrhythmia Suppression Trial (CAST) was undertaken to examine the question of whether suppression of asymptomatic or mildly symptomatic ventricular arrhythmias in the postmyocardial infarction period would reduce mortality from arrhythmia. Encainide, flecainide, and moricizine were identified in the Cardiac Arrhythmia Pilot Study (120) as able to suppress ventricular premature complexes and were considered the agents of choice by the CAST. The multicenter CAST revealed that encainide and flecainide caused an excessive mortality among postmyocardial infarction patients, thereby suggesting that the suppression of premature ventricular complexes does not provide evidence that an intervention will prevent a lethal arrhythmia (121).

Encainide and flecainide are classified as class IC antiarrhythmic agents based upon their ability to slow conduction velocity without affecting the duration of the refractory period of myocardial tissue. Depending on the length of the reentrant circuit, slowing of conduction velocity without a coincident lengthening of the refractory period may result in multiple reentrant circuits (122). Quinidine and procainamide, two class IA antiarrhythmic agents, produce a prolongation of refractoriness and a rate-dependent depression of conduction velocity. The precise role of these electrophysiologic effects in mediating an antiarrhythmic action is not clear. Recent studies (123) with procainamide indicate that lesser slowing of conduction velocity and greater prolongation of refractoriness tend to abolish reentry within the reentrant circuit. Greater slowing of conduction velocity and lesser prolongation of refractoriness function to stabilize a reentrant circuit and promote the continued induction of ventricular tachycardia by programmed electrical stimulation. Class I antiarrhythmic agents produce a rate-dependent slowing of conduction due to use-dependent blockade of fast sodium channels. Drugs that prolong refractoriness may be more effective against tachycardia caused by reentry than are drugs that produce a prolongation of conduction as their major electrophysiologic effect (124). The unsettling conclusions regarding the potential of antiarrhythmic agents to be proarrhythmic are not confined to the members of class IC. Proarrhythmic actions have been reported for all drugs, including several of the more recently described agents (125). As with other antiarrhythmic agents the second-generation drugs have not been demonstrated to prevent sudden death in patients with ventricular ectopy.

The lack of truly effective and safe drugs for the prevention of lethal arrhythmias and sudden coronary death has served to stimulate renewed interest in the area of drug development and the introduction of several new candidate agents that are classified as belonging to the class III group of antiarrhythmic drugs. Equally important is the recognition that most antiarrhythmic agents have been evaluated with in vitro or in vivo models, which have little relevance to the clinical situation of sudden coronary death. As the recent CAST report (121) has emphasized, the final analysis of a drug's ultimate utility depends on appropriate clinical testing in patients who are at risk of developing sudden and unexpected life-threatening arrhythmias and/or ventricular fibrillation. We can no longer afford to employ the more expedient and less dependable approach to evaluating new agents for their ability to reduce the frequency and/or complexity of ventricular depolarizations or their ability to modify the patient's response to programmed electrical stimulation. Despite the formidable task involved in the clinical assessment of an effective therapy for the prevention of ventricular fibrillation, the challenge could be made more readily attainable by preclinical assessment of a candidate drug, based upon studies conducted in relevant animal models using meaningful electrophysiologic end points that occur spontaneously. To this end we have employed an animal model of sudden coronary death in which ventricular fibrillation develops within 1 hr from the onset of an ischemic event in a myocardial substrate that has been identified, through the use of programmed electrical stimulation, to be capable of supporting an arrhythmic mechanism. The conscious, postinfarcted canine model model has been employed by us to identify a number of antifibrillatory agents (126–129), as well as those that have potential proarrhythmic effects (130–133).

ACKNOWLEDGMENT

Published investigations cited from this laboratory were supported by the National Institutes of Health, National Institute of Heart, Lung and Blood Grant HL–05806–28.

REFERENCES

1. Roberts W C. Sudden cardiac death: Definitions and causes. Am J Cardiol 1986; 57:1410–3.

2. Madsen J K. Ischaemic heart disease and prodromes of sudden cardiac death. Br Heart J 1985; 54:27–32.

3. Kuller L. Sudden and unexpected non-traumatic deaths in adults: a review of epidemiological and clinical studies. J Chron Dis 1966; 19:1165–92.

4. Hinkle L E, Argyros D C, Hayes J C, Robinson T, Alonso D R. Pathogenesis of an unexpected sudden death: role of early cycle ventricular premature contractions. Am J Cardiol 177; 39:873–9.

5. Lown B, Graboys T B. Sudden death: an ancient problem newly perceived. Cardiovasc Med 1977; 2:219–33.

6. Gradman A H, Bell P A, De Busk R F. Sudden death during ambulatory monitoring. Clinical and electrocardiographic correlations. Report of a case. Circulation 1977; 55:210–1.

7. Nikolic G, Bishop R L, Singh J B. Sudden death recorded during holter monitoring. Circulation 1982; 66:218–25.

8. Doyle J T, Kannel W B, McNamara P M, Quickenton P, Gordon T. Factors related to sudden death from coronary disease: combined Albany-Framingham studies. Am J Cardiol 1976; 37:1073–8.

9. The Coronary Drug Project Research Group. Prognostic importance of premature beats following myocardial infarction. JAMA 1973; 223:116–24.

10. Moss A J, Davis H T, DeCamilla J, Bayer L W. Ventricular ectopic beats and their relation to sudden and nonsudden cardiac death after myocardial infarction. Circulation 1979; 60:998–1003.

11. Hinkle L E. The immediate antecedents of sudden death. Acta Med Scand 1981; 651:207–17.

12. The Multicenter Postinfarction Research Group. Risk stratification and survival after myocardial infarction. N Engl J Med 1983; 309:331–6.

13. Mukharji J, Rude R E, Poole W K, et al. Risk factors for sudden death after myocardial infarction: Two-year follow-up. Am J Cardiol 1984; 54:31–6.

14. Bigger J T, Fleiss J L, Kleiger R, Miller J P, Rolnitzky L M, Multicenter Postinfarction Research Group. The relationships among ventricular arrhythmias, left ventricular dysfunction, and mortality in the 2 years after myocardial infarction. Circulation 1984; 69:250–80.

15. Furberg C D. Effects of antiarrhythmic drugs on mortality after myocardial infarction. Am J Cardiol 1983; 52:32C–136C.

16. May G S, Furberg C D, Eberlein K A, Geraci B J. Secondary prevention after myocardial infarction: a review of short-term acute phase trials. Prog Cardiovasc Dis 1983; 25:335–59.

17. Multicentre International Study. Improvement in prognosis of myocardial infarction by long-term β-adrenoceptor blockade using practolol. Br Med J 1975; 3:735–40.

18. Norwegian Multicenter Study Group. Timolol-induced reduction in mortality and reinfarction in patients surviving acute myocardial infarction. N Engl J Med 1981; 304:801–7.

19. Beta-Blocker Heart Attack Trial Research Group. A randomized trial of propranolol in patients with acute myocardial infarction. JAMA 1982; 247:1707–14.

20. Yusuf S, Peto R, Lewis J, Collins R, Sleight P. Beta blockade during and after myocardial infarction: an overview of the randomised trials. Prog Cardiovasc Dis 1985; 27:335–71.

21. The MIAMI Trial Research Group. Metoprolol in acute myocardial infarction (MIAMI): a randomised placebo-controlled international trial. Eur Heart J 1985; 6:199–226.

22. ISIS–1 (First International Study of Infarct Survival) Collaborative Group. Randomised trial of intravenous atenolol among 16,027 cases of suspected acute myocardial infarction. Lancet 1986; 2:56–66.

23. Kuller L, Cooper M, Perper J. Epidemiology of sudden death. Arch Intern Med 1972; 129:714–9.

24. Baum R S, Alvares H, Cobb L A. Survival after resuscitation from out-of-hospital ventricular fibrillation. Circulation 1974; 50:1231–5.

25. Weaver W D, Lorch G S, Alvarez H A, Cobb L A. Angiographic findings and prognostic indicators in patients resuscitated from sudden cardiac death. Circulation 1976; 54:895–900.

26. Reichenbach D D, Moss N S, Meyer E. Pathology of the heart in sudden cardiac death. Am J Cardiol 1977; 39:865–72.

27. Goldstein S, Landis R, Leighton R, et al. Characteristics of the resuscitated out-of-hospital cardiac arrest victim with

coronary heart disease. Circulation 1981; 64:977–84.

28. Schuster E H, Bulkley B H. Ischemia at a distant site after myocardial infarction: a cause of early postinfarction angina. Circulation 1980; 62:509–15.

29. Schwartz P J, Stone H L. Left stellectomy in the prevention of ventricular fibrillation caused by acute myocardial ischemia in conscious dogs with anterior myocardial infarction. Circulation 1980; 62:1256–65.

30. Schwartz P J, Billman G E, Stone H L. Autonomic mechanism in ventricular fibrillation induced by myocardial ischemia during exercise in dogs with healed myocardial infarction. An experimental preparation for sudden death. Circulation 1984; 69:790–800.

31. Kabell G, Brachmann J, Scherlag B J, Harrison L, Lazzara R. Mechanisms of ventricular arrhythmias in multivessel coronary disease: the effects of collateral zone ischemia. Am Heart J 1984; 108:447–54.

32. Previtali M, Klersy C, Salerno J A, et al. Ventricular tachyarrhythmias in Prinzmetal's variant angina: clinical significance and relation to the degree and time course of ST segment elevation. Am J Cardiol 1983; 52:19–25.

33. Miller D D, Waters D D, Szlachcic J, Thereoux P. Clinical characteristics associated with sudden death in patients with variant angina. Circulation 1982; 66:588–92.

34. Malliani A, Schwartz P J, Zanchetti A. Neural mechanisms in life-threatening arrhythmias. Am Heart J 1980; 100:705–15.

35. Ruskin J N, McGovern B, Garan H, Dimarco J P, Kelly E. Antiarrhythmic drugs: A possible cause of out-of-hospital cardiac arrest. N Engl J Med 1983; 309:1302–6.

36. Torres V, Flowers D, Somberg J C. The arrhythmogenicity of antiarrhythmic agents. Am Heart J 1985; 109:1090–7.

37. Marchlinski R E, Buxton A E, Doherty J V, et al. Use of programmed electrical stimulation to predict sudden death after myocardial infarction. In Josephson ME, ed. Sudden cardiac death. Philadelphia: F. A. Davis 1985: 163–9.

38. Roy D, Marchlinski F E, Doherty J V, Buxton A E, Waxman H L, Josephson M E. Electrophysiologic testing of survivors of cardiac arrest. In: Josephson ME, ed. Sudden cardiac death. Philadelphia: F. A. Davis 1985:171–7.

39. Wellens H J J, Brugada P, Stevenson W G. Programmed electrical stimulation of the heart in patients with life-threatening ventricular arrhythmias: what is the significance of induced arrhythmias and what is the correct stimulation protocol? Circulation 1985; 72:1–7.

40. Lucchesi B R, Lynch J J. Preclinical assessment of antiarrhythmic drugs. Fed Proc 1986; 45:2197–205.

41. Maling H M, Moran N C. Ventricular arrhythmias induced by sympathomimetic amines in unanesthetized dogs following coronary artery occlusion. Circ Res 1957; 5:409–13.

42. El-Sherif N, Scherlag B J, Lazzara R, Hope R R. Re-entrant ventricular arrhythmias in the late myocardial infarction period. 1. Conduction characteristics in the infarction zone. Circulation 1977; 55:686–702.

43. Karagueuzian H S, Fenoglio J J, Weiss M B, Wit A L. Protracted ventricular tachycardia induced by premature stimulation of the canine heart after coronary artery occlusion and reperfusion. Circ Res 1979; 44:833–46.

44. Moore E N, Spear J F. Ventricular fibrillation threshold. Its physiological and pharmacological importance. Arch Intern Med 1975; 135:446–53.

45. Euler D E, Scanlon P J. Comparative effects of antiarrhythmic drugs on the ventricular fibrillation threshold. J Cardiovasc Pharmacol 1988; 11:291–8.

46. Axelrod P J, Verrier R L, Lown B. Vulnerability to ventricular fibrillation during acute coronary artery occlusion and release. Am J Cardiol 1975; 36:776–82.

47. Euler D E. Norepinephrine release by ventricular stimulation: Effect on fibrillation thresholds. Am J Physiol 1980; 238:H406–13.

48. Anderson J L, Rodier H E, Green L S. Comparative effects of beta-adrenergic blocking drugs on experimental ventricular fibrillation thresholds. Am J Cardiol 1983; 51:1196–202.

49. Patterson E, Lucchesi B R. Antifibrillatory properties of the beta-adrenergic receptor antagonists nadolol, sotalol, atenolol and propranolol, in the anesthitized dog. Pharmacology 1984; 28:121–9.

50. Patterson E, Holland K, Eller B T, Lucchesi BR. Ventricular fibrillation resulting from ischemia at a site remote from previous

myocardial infarction. A conscious canine model of sudden coronary death. Am J Cardiol 1982; 50:1412–23.

51. Wilber D J, Lynch J J, Montgomery D G, Lucchesi B R. Postinfarction sudden death: significance of inducible ventricular tachycardia and infarct size in a conscious canine model. Am Heart J 1985; 109:8–18.

52. Josephson M E, Horowitz L N, Farhshidi A, Kastor J A. Recurrent sustained ventricular tachycardia. 1. Mechanisms. Circulation 1978; 57:431–40.

53. Panidis J P, Morganroth J. Sudden death in hospitalized patients: Cardiac rhythm disturbances detected by ambulatory echocardiographic monitoring. J Am Coll Cardiol 1983; 2:798–805.

54. Kempf F C, Josephson M E. Cardiac arrest recorded on ambulatory electrocardiograms. Am J Cardiol 1984; 53:1577–82.

55. Milner P G, Platia E V, Reid P R, Griffith LSC. Ambulatory electrocardiographic recordings at the time of fatal cardiac arrest. Am J Cardiol 1985; 56:588–92.

56. Patterson E, Lucchesi B R. Quinidine gluconate in chronic myocardial ischemic injury—differential effects in response to programmed stimulation and acute myocardia ischemia in the dog. Circulation 1983; 68:III–155.

57. Kou W H, Nelson S D, Lynch J J, Montgomery D G, DiCarlo L, Lucchesi B R. Effect of flecainide acetate on prevention of electrical induction of ventricular tachycardia and occurence of ischemic ventricular fibrillation during the early postmyocardial periods: evaluation in a conscious canine model of sudden death. J Am Coll Cardiol 1987; 9:359–65.

58. Lynch J J, Montgomery D G, Ventura A, Lucchesi B R. Antiarrhythmic and electrophysiologic effects of bepridil in chronically infarcted conscious dogs. J Pharmacol Exp Ther 1985; 234:72–80.

59. Patterson E, Eller B T, Lucchesi B R. Effects of diltizaem upon experimental ventricular dysrhythmias. J Pharmacol Exp Ther 1983; 225:224–33.

60. Holland K, Patterson E, Lucchesi B R. Prevention of ventricular fibrillation by bretylium in a conscious canine model of sudden coronary death. Am Heart J 1983; 105:711–71.

61. Patterson E, Eller B T, Abrams G D, Vasiliades J, Lucchesi BR. Ventricular fibrillation in a conscious canine preparation of a sudden coronary death—prevention by short- and long-term amiodarone administration. Circulation 1983; 68:857–64.

62. Patterson E, Lynch J J, Lucchesi B R. Antiarrhythmic and antifibrillatory actions of the beta adrenergic receptor antagonist, dl-sotalol. J Pharmacol Exp Ther 1984; 230:519–26.

63. Lynch J J, Coskey L A, Montgomery D G, Lucchesi B R. Prevention of ventricular fibrillation by dextrorotatory sotalol in a conscious canine model of sudden coronary death. Am Heart J 1985; 109:949–58.

64. Kopia G A, Eller B T, Patterson E, Shea M J, Lucchesi B R. Antiarrhythmic and electrophysiologic actions of clofilium in experimental canine models. Eur J Pharmacol 1985; 116:49–61.

65. Patterson E, Gibson J K, Lucchesi B R. Postmyocardial infarction reentrant ventricular arrhythmias in conscious dogs: suppression by bretylium tosylate. J Pharmacol Exp Ther 1981; 216:453–8.

66. Patterson E, Gibson J K, Lucchesi B R. Prevention of chronic canine ventricular arrhythmias with bretylium tosylate. Circulation 1981; 64:1045–50.

67. Anderson J L, Patterson E, Conlon M, Pasyk S, Pitt B, Lucchesi B R. Kinetics of antifibrillatory effects of bretylium: correlation with myocardial drug concentrations. Am J Cardiol 1980; 46:583–92.

68. Namm D H, Wang C M, El-Sayad S, Copp F C, Maxwell R A. Effects of bretylium on rat cardiac muscle: the electrophysiological effect and its uptake and binding in normal and immunosympathectomized rat hearts. J Pharmacol Exp Ther 1975; 193:194–208.

69. Patterson E, Amalfitano D J, Lucchesi B R. Development of ventricular tachyarrhythmias in the conscious canine during the recovery phase of experimental ischemic injury: effect of bethanidine administration. J Cardiovasc Pharmacol 1984; 6:470–5.

70. Zimmerman J M, Patterson E, Pitt B, Lucchesi B R. Antidysrhythmic actions of meobentine. Am Heart J 1984; 107:1117–24.

71. Ward O C. A new familial cardiac syndrome in children. J Irish Med Assoc 1964; 54:103–6.

72. Khan MM, Logan KR, McComb J M, Adgey A A J. Management of recurrent ventricular arrhythmias associated with QT prolongation. Am J Cardiol 1981; 47:1301–8.

73. Singh B N, Nadamanee K. The electrophysiological classification of antiarrhythmic drugs. In: Coltart D G, Jewitt D E, eds. Recent developments in cardiovascular drugs. London: Churchill-Livingstone 1982:59–77.

74. Cardinal R, Sesyniuk B I. Electrophysiological effects of bretylium tosylate on subendocardial Purkinje fibers from infarcted canine heart. J Pharmacol Exp Ther 1978; 204:159–74.

75. Bexton R S, Camm A J. Drugs with a class III antiarrhythmic action. 1. Amiodarone. Pharmacol Ther 1982; 17:315–55.

76. Gloor H O, Urthaler F, James T N. Acute effects of amiodarone upon the canine sinus node and antrioventricular junctional region. J Clin Invest 1983; 71:1457–66.

77. Mason J W, Hondeghem L M, Katzung B G. Block of inactivated sodium channels and of depolarization-induced automaticity in guinea pig papillary muscle by amiodarone. Circ Res 1984; 55:277–85.

78. Charlier R. Cardiac actions in the dog of a new antagonist of adrenergic excitation which does not produce competitive blockade of adrenoceptors. Br J Pharmacol 1970; 39:668–74.

79. Heger J J, Prystowsky E N, Jackman W M, et al. Amiodarone: clinical efficacy and electrophysiology during long-term therapy for recurrent ventricular tachycardia. N Engl J Med 1981; 305:539–45.

80. Freedberg A S, Papp J G, Vaughan Williams E M. The effect of altered thyroid state on atrial intracellular potentials. J Physiol (Lond) 1970; 207:357–69.

81. Johnson P N, Freedberg A S, Marshall J M. Action of thyroid hormone on the transmembrane potentials from sinoatrial node cells and atrial muscle cells in isolated atria of rabbits. Cardiology 1973; 58:273–89.

82. Singh B N, Vaughan Williams E M. The effects of amiodarone, a new anti-anginal drug, on cardiac muscle. Br. J Pharmacol 1970; 39:657–67.

83. Venkatesh N, Lynch J J, Uprichard A C G, Kitzen J M, Singh B N, Lucchesi B R. Anti-arrhythmic and anti-fibrillatory effects of hypothyroidism in a conscious canine model of sudden death. Circulation 1988; 78 (4): II–639.

84. Rossi P R, Yusuf S, Ramsdale D, Furze L, Sleight P. Reduction of ventricular arrhythmias by early intravenous atenolol in suspected acute myocardial infarction. Br Med J 1983; 286:506–10.

85. Echt D S, Griffin J C, Ford A J, Knutti J W, Feldman R C, Mason J W. Nature of inducible ventricular arrhythmias in a canine chronic myocardial infarction model. Am J Cardiol 1983; 52:1127–32.

86. Gang E S, Bigger J T, Uhl E W. Effects of timolol and propranolol on inducible sustained ventricular tachyarrhythmias in dogs with subacute myocardial infarction. Am J Cardiol 1984; 53:275–81.

87. Patterson E, Lucchesi B R. Antifibrillatory actions of d,l-nadolol in a conscious canine model of sudden coronary death. J Cardiovasc Pharmacol 1983; 5:737–44.

88. Lynch J J, Nelson S D, MacEwen S A, Driscoll E M, Lucchesi BR. Antifibrillatory efficacy of concomitant beta adrenergic receptor blockade with dilevalol, the R,R-isomer of labetalol, and muscarinic receptor blockade with methylscopolamine. J Pharmacol Exp Ther 1987; 241:741–7.

89. Lynch J J, Lucchesi BR. How are animal models best for the study of antiarrhythmic drugs? In: Hearse D J, Manning A S, Janse M J, eds., Life-threatening arrhythmias and infarction. New York: Raven Press 1987: 169–96.

90. Uprichard A C G, Lynch J J, Kitzen J M, Frye J W, Lucchesi B R. Celiprolol, a β_1-selective adrenoceptor antagonist with intrinsic stimulant properties, does not protect against ventricular tachycardia or ventricular fibrillation in a conscious canine model of myocardial infarction and sudden death. J Pharmacol Exp Ther 1989; 251:571–7.

91. El-Sherif N. Re-entrant ventricular arrhythmias in the late myocardial infarction period 6. Effects of the autonomic system. Circulation 1978; 58:103–10.

92. Hope R R, Williams D O, El-Sherif N, Lazzara R, Scherlag B J. The efficacy of antiarrhythmic agents during acute myocardial ischemia and the role of heart rate. Circulation 1974; 50:507–14.

93. Kjekshus J. Comments—beta blockers: heart rate reduction—a mechanism of benefit. Eur Heart J 1985; 6:29–30.

94. Wolf P S, Smith R D, Khandwala A, et al. Celiprolol—pharmacological profile of an unconventional beta-blocker. Br J Clin Pract 1985; 39:5–11.

95. Payrhuber K, Kratzer H, Kuhn P. Celiprolol

in acute myocardial infarct. Wien Klin Wochenschr 1986; 98:171–4.

96. Kobinger W, Lillie C, Pichler L. N-allyl-derative of clonidine, a substance with specific bradycardic action at a cardiac site. Naunyn Schmiedeberms Arch Pharmacol 1979; 306:255–62.

97. Kobinger W, Lillie C, Pichler L. Cardiovascular actions of N-allyl-clonidine (ST 567), a substance with specific bradycardic action. Eur J Pharmacol 1979; 58:141–50.

98. Lillie C, Kobinger W. Actions of alinidine and AQ-A 39 on rate and contractility of guinea pig atria during β-adrenoceptor stimulation. J Cardiovasc Pharmacol 1983; 5:1048–51.

99. Millar J S, Vaughan Williams E M. Pacemaker selectivity: influence on rabbit atria of ionic environment and of alinidine, a possible anion antagonist. Cardiovasc Res 1981; 15:335–50.

100. Harron D W G, Allen J D, Wilson R, Shanks R G. Effect of alinidine on experimental cardiac arrhythmias. J Cardiovas Pharmacol 1982; 4:221–5.

101. Harron D W G, Brezina M, Lillie C, Kobinger W. Antifibrillatory properties of alinidine after coronary artery occlusion in rats. Eur J Pharmacol 1985; 110:301–8.

102. Millar J S, Vaughan Williams E M. Anion antagonism—a fifth class of antiarrhythmic action? Lancet 1981; 1:1291–3.

103. Uprichard A C G, Chi L, Lynch J J, Driscoll E M, Frye J W, Lucchesi B R. Alinidine protects against ischemic ventricular fibrillation in a conscious canine model: probable anti-ischemic mode of action. J Cardiovasc Pharmacol 1989; 14:475–482.

104. Schamhardt H C, Vedouw P D, Saxena P R. Improvement of perfusion and function of ischaemic procine myocardium after reduction of heart rate by alinidine. J Cardiovasc Pharmacol 1981; 3:728–38.

105. Keiser J, Cheung W, Falotico R, Tobia A. Effects of alinidine on infarct size in a canine model of coronary occlusion/reperfusion. FASEB J 1988; 2:A920.

106. Gross G J, Warltier D C, Daemmgen J W. Effects of AQ-AH 208, a new specific bradycardic agent, on myocardial ischemia-reperfusion injury in anesthetized dogs. J Cardiovasc Pharmacol 1985; 7:929–36.

107. Gross G J, Lamping K G, Warltier D C, Hardman H F. Effects of three bradycardic drugs on regional myocardial blood flow and function in areas distal to a total or partial coronary occlusion in dogs. Circulation 1984; 69:391–9.

108. Gross G J, Daemmgen J W. Effect of the new specific bradycardic agent AQ-A39 (falipamil) on coronary blood flow in dogs. J Cardiovasc Pharmacol 1987; 10:123–7.

109. Wilber D J, Lynch J J, Montgomery D G, Lucchesi B R. Alpha-adrenergic influences in canine ischemic sudden death: effects of alpha 1-adrenoceptor blockade with prazosin. J Cardiovasc Phamacol 1987; 10:96–106.

110. Juhasz-Nagy A, Aviado D M. Increased role of alpha-adrenoceptors in ischemic myocardial zones. Physiologist 1976; 19:245.

111. Sheridan D J, Penkoske P A, Sobel B E, Corr P B. Alpha adrenergic contributions to dysrhythmia cardiac muscle. Br J Pharmacol 1970; 39:657–67.

112. Corr P B, Shayman J A, Kramer J B, Kpnis R J. Increased alpha-adrenergic receptors in ischemic cat myocardium. J Cli Invest 1981; 67:1232–6.

113. Vaughan Williams E M. Cardiac electrophysiological effects of selective adrenoceptor stimulation and their possible roles in arrhythmias. J Cardiovasc Pharmacol 1985; 7:S61–4.

114. Bacaner M B, Clay J R, Shrier A, Brochu R M. Potassium channel blockade: a mechanism for suppressing ventricular fibrillation. Proc Natl Acad Sci USA 1986; 83:2223–7.

115. Snyders D J, Katzung B G. Clofilium reduces the plateau potassium in isolated cardiac myocytes. Circulation 1985; 72: III–223.

116. Kantor P F, Coetzee W A, Dennis S C, Opie L H. Effects of glibenclamide on ischemic arrhythmias. Circulation 1987; 76:IV–17.

117. Smallwood J K, Steinberg M I. Cardiac electrophysiological effects of pinacidil and related pyridylcyanoguanidines: relationship to antihypertensive activity. J Cardiovasc Pharmacol 1988; 12:102–9.

118. The CAPS Investigators. The Cardiac Arrhythmia Pilot Study. Am J Cardiol 1986; 57:91–5.

119. CAST Investigators. Preliminary report: effect of encainide and flecainide on mortality in a randomized trial of arrhythmia suppression after myocardial infarction. N Engl J Med 1989; 321:406–12.

120. Brugada J, Boersma L, Brugada P, Havenith M, Wellens H J J, Allessie M. Double wave

re-entry as a mechanism of ventricular tachy cardia acceleration. Circulation 1989; in press.

121. Furukawa T, Rozanski J J, Moroe K, Gossellin A J, Lister J W. Efficacy of procainamide on ventricular tachycardia: relation to prolongation of refractoriness and slowing of conduction. Am Heart J 1989; 118:702–8.

122. Sasyniuk B I, McQuillan J. Mechanisms by which antiarrhythmic drugs influence induction of reentrant responses in subendocardial Purkinje network of 1-day-old infarcted canine ventricle. In: Zipes DP, Jalife J, eds. Cardiac electrophysiology and arrhythmias. Orlando, FL: Grune & Stratton, 1983:389.

123. Horowitz L N, Mortganroth J. Second generation antiarrhythmic agents: have we reached antiarrhythmic nirvana? J Am Coll Cardiol 1987; 9:459–63.

124. Patterson E, Eller B T, Abrams G D, Vasiliades J, Lucchesi B R. Ventricular fibrillation in a conscious canine preparation of sudden coronary death—prevention by short- and long-term amiodarone administration. Circulation 1983; 68:857–64.

125. Lynch J J, Kitzen J M, Hoff P T, Lucchesi B R. Reduction in digitalis-associated postinfarction mortality with nadolol in conscious dogs. Am Heart J 1988; 115:67–76.

126. Lynch J J, Montgomery D G, Lucchesi B R. Facilitation of lethal ventricular arrhythmia by therapeutic digoxin in conscious postinfarction dogs. Am Heart J 1986; 111:883–90.

127. Lynch J J, DiCarlo L A, Montgomery D G, Lucchesi B R. Effects of flecainide acetate on ventricular tachyarrhythmia and fibrillation in dogs with recent myocardial infarction. Pharmacology 1987; 35:181–93.

128. Uprichard A C G, Chi L, Driscoll E M, Lucchesi B R. Pinacidil is proarrhythmic in a conscious canine model of sudden death. J Moll Cell Cardiol 1989; 21 (suppl II): S13.

Index

AC amplifiers, 6
Accessory AV pathway (*see* Atrioventricular by-
    pass tracts)
Acebutolol, 665,667
Acecainide (*N*-acetylprocainamide), 360, 518,
    521, 524, 525, 527–529, 677–679, 688
  antiarrhythmic efficacy, 680
  basic pharmacology, 679
  cardiotoxicity, 525
  clinical electrophysiology and efficacy, 681
  electrophysiology, 527
  pharmacokinetics and safety, 682–3
  renal clearance, 528
  toxicity, 681
Acetylation phenotype, 529
Acetylcholine, 11, 30, 42, 44, 50, 51, 60, 83,
    85, 86, 111, 113, 114, 119, 204, 277,
    435, 465, 495, 538, 541, 543
Aconitine, 450, 543, 640
Acquired chronic valvular disease, 418
Activation, channel, 62
  i_{Ca}, 63
  i_K, 63,122
  i_{Na}, 45, 116, 202, 207, 208
Activation patterns:
  atrial flutter, 240, 241, 244–246, 258
  normal sinus beat, 86
  ventricular reentry, 261–262, 333, 335–336,
    365

Activator calcium, 452
Active cellular properties, 224; 518
Acute ischemia, 354, 367–8, 523, 612
Acute myocardial ischemia, 574, 589
Adenosine, 111, 116, 126, 154, 157, 434, 461
Adenylate cyclase, 47, 446, 447, 449
Adrenaline (*see* Epinephrine)
Aequorin, 285, 286, 288, 444, 445
Aetmozine (*see* Moricizine)
Aftercontractions, 124, 285–287
Age-related changes, 127, 162, 290
Aglycones, 277
Agranulocytosis, 595
A-H interval, 11, 141, 142, 147, 498, 518, 528,
    588–589, 628, 632, 642, 656, 657
Albumin, 638
Alinidine, 730,732
Alpha-adrenergic:
  agonist effects, 182, 183, 433–440, 686
    inhibition of i_{to}, 122, 157
    inotropic effects, 122, 453, 454
    ischemia, 316, 369
    K channel activation, 50
    ouabain toxicity, 290
  blockade:
    amiodarone, 641
    phentolamine, 316, 360
    prazocin, 433–439, 471
    quinidine, 493, 497

[Alpha-adrenergic]
    yohimbine, 433
Alpha-1-acid glycoprotein, 500, 525, 546–548, 577
Alprenolol, 667
Amantadine, 224
Amiloride, 207, 288, 448, 449
p-Aminobenzoic acid, 517
4 Aminopyridine, 120–122, 126, 171, 211
Amiodarone, 483, 505, 526, 545, 618, 622, 637–648, 679, 683, 690, 697, 729–731
    antiarrhythmic effects in experimental animals, 641
        in humans, 642–644
    clinical pharmacology, 641–644
    desethylamiodarone, 638–640, 644–645
    didesethylamiodarone, 645
    electrophysiologic effects in humans, 641–42
        electrophysiologic effects in isolated tissue, 638–640
        electrophysiologic effects in vivo, 640–641
    pharmacokinetics, 644–645
    toxicology, 377, 645–647
Ammonium, 30
Amphibian sinus venosus, 61 (see also Sinus venosus)
Amphipathic properties, 225
Amrinone, 449, 467, 470
AN cells (of AV node), 146–148, 150, 151, 154
Angina pectoris, 665, 670
Angiotensin II, 701
Anion selective channels, 732
Anisotropy:
    and collagen septa in atria, 127
    epicardial, 332, 345, 487
    His-Purkinje fiber system, 163
    quinidine effects, 496
    uniform vs. nonuniform, 4, 127
    ventricular, 225
Anthracyclines, 453
Anthopleurin A, 678
Antiarrhythmic drugs (see also individual listings):
    class I drugs, 477–661
    class II drugs, 665–672
    class III drugs, 677–691
    class IV drugs, 697–716
    class V drugs, 732
Anticholinergic effects, 587, 594, 604
    acecainide, 682
    disopyramide, 537–538, 541–542, 549–551
    procainamide, 521
    quinidine, 495–498, 679
Antidromic tachycardia, 711
Antifibrillatory drugs, 668, 723–734

[Antifibrillatory drugs]
    drug protection against sudden death, 727–733
    evaluation, 725, 733–734
Antinuclear antibodies, 529,621
Aplastic anemia, 594
APP 201–533,469
Aprindine, 290
Aqueous pore, pathway, 167, 539, 562 (see also hydrophillic pathway)
Arc of conduction block, 257, 333–335, 341–343
ARL 115 BS (see Sulmazole)
Atenolol, 545, 665, 667, 671
Atrial arrhythmias, 498, 522, 542, 543, 641, 643, 660, 667, 670
    atrial fibrillation, 95, 143, 278, 419, 421, 423, 465, 497–499, 542–545, 574, 577, 618, 641, 643, 644, 708, 711, 714, 715
    atrial flutter, 241, 242, 278, 498, 542, 577, 588, 643, 680, 685, 689, 710–711, 715
    atrial premature beats, 90, 278, 423, 545
    atrial tachycardia, 257, 278, 419, 423, 588, 618, 644
Atrial depolarization sequence, 86
Atrial muscle, 62, 85, 93, 109–128, 151, 154, 493–495, 498, 517, 537, 538, 542–544, 567, 572, 586, 604, 606–607, 638–639, 668, 683, 686, 689, 698
    background potassium conductance, 71, 111–114, 214
    delayed conduction and reflection, 264
    delayed rectifier, 122, 123
    passive properties, 110, 111
    sodium-calcium exchange current, 69, 124
    sodium/potassium pump current, 123, 124
    transient outward current, 119–122, 211
    transmembrane action potentials, 109, 110, 202
    triggered activity, 127, 128, 360
    voltage-clamp studies of trabeculae, 35, 37
    voltage-dependent calcium currents, 117–119, 212
    voltage-dependent sodium current, 114–117
Atriosinus:
    block, 89, 90, 98
    conduction, 89
Atrioventricular:
    block, 175, 277, 418, 425, 521
    bypass tracts, 12, 252, 577, 589, 603, 642, 643, 671, 708, 710–712
    conduction, 465, 521, 570, 577, 628, 640, 668, 680, 704
    junctional rhythms, 175, 709

[Atrioventricular]
node, 50, 199, 202, 225, 247, 277, 278, 697, 708
activation time of nodal cells, 147
antiarrhythmic drug effects, 495, 517, 521, 538, 572, 586, 611, 618, 680
automaticity, 151
classification of nodal cells, 147
disease, 418
functional properties, 141–151
ionic currents, 151–157
background ionic currents, 151, 152
calcium current, 153, 154
pacemaker current, 156
potassium current, 154–156
sodium/potassium pump current, 152
sodium current, 152–153
transient inward current, 157
recovery curve, 142
transmembrane action potential characteristics, 146, 147, 150
Atropine, 87, 97, 98, 113, 434, 538, 544, 604–607, 614, 683, 715
Automatic implantable defibrillator, 643
Automaticity, 161, 174, 176, 178, 202, 278, 279, 284, 356, 378, 433, 435, 436, 438, 439, 524, 537, 678, 707, 708
abnormal (depolarization-induced), 127, 161, 176, 219, 221, 222, 224, 305, 311, 314, 318, 323, 357, 358, 495, 519, 542, 573, 587, 628, 629, 656, 640, 668
normal Purkinje fiber, 177–181, 184, 221, 310, 311, 495, 519, 542, 73, 587, 610, 628, 656, 668, 679
sinus Node, assessment, 87–89, 570 (see also Sinus node)
Autonomic nervous system, 60, 62, 79, 85, 87, 88, 96, 415, 537, 565, 573, 614, 641, 724, 729
parasympathetic/vagal tone, 80, 87, 97, 313, 378, 416, 418, 465, 629, 708
sympathetic tone, 87, 97, 288, 289, 303, 316, 416, 417, 434, 436, 497, 498, 629, 666, 668, 671, 707, 709, 714
transmitters, 154, 290

Bachmann's bundle, 109, 243, 247
BAPTA, 444
Barbiturates, 503
Barium, 44, 48, 64–65, 83, 84, 112, 113, 118, 119, 125, 173, 176, 177, 181, 213, 218, 224, 438, 439, 449, 610, 656, 699

Barlow's syndrome, 671
BAY K 8644, 47, 48, 213, 224, 285, 446, 468, 469, 716
Benzocaine, 564
Benzothiazepines, 47, 446, 697, 701, 703, 715 (also see diltiazem)
Bepridil, 679, 704, 728, 730
Beta-adrenergic blockade, 305, 439, 497, 498, 502, 527, 587, 594, 604, 611, 614, 621, 628, 641, 647, 665–672, 679, 688, 689, 697, 708–710, 714, 715, 725, 731
Beta-adrenergic effects, 11, 42, 47, 52, 60, 79, 85, 87, 118, 123, 128, 157, 182, 184, 212, 213, 217, 227, 290, 316, 319, 359, 379, 446–449, 454, 467, 686, 701, 725
Betaxolol, 448
Bethanechol, 549
Bethanidine, 729, 730
Bidirectional block, 364, 380, 524, 570
Bigeminal rhythm, 267, 278, 284, 285, 421
Bilayer, membrane lipid, 225
Bioavailability, 593, 657, 686, 688, 712
Bipolar recording, 5, 6, 126
Boltzmann constant, distribution, 44,67
Border zone, ischemic, 290
Boxer dogs, cardiomyopathy, 419, 420, 422
Brachycephalic breeds, 416
Bradycardia, 80, 87, 93, 95, 96, 98, 173, 277, 378, 410, 502, 504, 551, 644, 647, 672
Bradycardia-tachycardia syndrome, 95, 98, 422, 521, 551 (see also Sick sinus syndrome)
Bretylium, 327, 677, 679, 683, 688, 729, 730
Bridging diastolic electrical activity (see Fractionated electrograms)
Bullfrog sinus venosus, 61 (see also Sinus venosus)
Bundle of Kent, 418
Bupivicaine, 484, 565

Cable properties, theory, 3, 33–35, 62, 110, 111, 224–226, 487, 566, 569
Cadmium, 119, 153, 155, 212, 213
Caffeine, 120, 122, 211, 286, 449, 453, 461, 594
Calcium-binding proteins, 71, 72, 74, 75 (see also Calmodulin, Troponin)
Calcium channel:
blockers, 122, 697–716
structure, 700
types, 700
Calcium current, 43, 47, 48, 63, 65, 66, 67, 71, 73, 75, 76, 79, 117, 153, 203, 205, 212, 702

[Calcium current]
  L-type, 42, 43, 47, 52, 63, 117, 118, 119,
    124, 154, 171–172, 174–176, 181, 183,
    188, 212, 213, 446, 448, 449, 468, 700,
    701
  N-type, 700
  T-type, 47, 48, 61, 119, 154, 171, 212, 449,
    700
    and sinus node pacemaker activity, 119
  sarcolemmal pump, 69, 71, 227, 445, 451, 702
  window current, 203, 213
Calcium gluconate, 715
Calcium-induced calcium release, 212, 286, 452
Calcium (intracellular), 51, 69, 72, 74, 171,
    174, 181, 188, 206, 207, 214, 226, 287,
    290, 292, 356, 361, 363, 407, 409, 438,
    444, 445, 450, 451, 453–455, 469, 565,
    566, 570, 701, 702
Calcium overload, 286, 452
Calcium paradox, 214
Calcium release channel, 453
Calmodulin, 71, 72, 74, 75, 82, 291, 454, 467
Capacitance neutralization, 23
Capacity-coupled amplifiers, 6
Captopril, 471
Carbazin (see Moricizine)
Cardiac arrest, 591, 592
Cardiac Arrhythmia Pilot Study (CAPS), 658,
    661, 659, 670, 733
Cardiac Arrhythmia Suppression Trial (CAST),
    375, 660, 669, 670, 733, 734
Cardiac arrhythmias (see Atrial arrhythmias,
    Ventricular arrhythmias)
Cardiac glycosides, 11, 80, 128, 152, 157, 204,
    220, 227, 361, 443, 450, 451, 463–466,
    498, 520, 528, 550, 678, 689, 708–710,
    712
  acetylstrophanthidin, 280, 290
  digitoxin, 463, 464
  digoxin, 277, 285, 288, 290, 463, 464, 471,
    501, 526, 594, 621, 647, 657, 710, 714
  dihydro-ouabain, 123, 438
  ouabain, 67, 128, 154, 157, 278–280, 285,
    289, 291, 463, 466, 519, 543, 571, 588,
    637, 641, 680, 688
  strophanthidin, 67, 286
  toxicity, 161, 277–292, 379, 572, 575, 656,
    667, 711
    bradycardias, 277, 278
    cellular mechanisms for arrhythmias, 279–
    290
    negative inotropy, 452
    premature beats and tachycardias, 278, 279
    reentry, 291–292

Cardiac hypertrophy, 397–410
Cardiac pacing, 90, 504
Cardiac standstill, 290
Cardiomyopathy, 397–410, 413, 418–421, 424,
    619, 670
Cardioversion (DC), 710, 723
Carotid sinus massage, 710
Carteolol, 667
Celiprolol, 730, 731
Cell-attached patches, 41
Cell swelling, 221
Cellular electrophysiology in healed myocardial
    infarction, 353
Cellular uncoupling, 35, 226, 278, 332, 356,
    363, 399
Cesium, 30, 61, 112, 124, 178, 222, 224, 301,
    360, 571, 699
CGS 12970, 730
Channel density:
  calcium, L-type, 118
  potassium, 151
  sodium, 115–117
Channel function, 199
Chaos theory, 99
Charge threshold, 226
Chloralose, 680, 684
Chloramphenicol, 594
Chloride current, 119, 211
Chloride (intracellular), 29
Chloroform, 680, 684
Cholera toxin, 449
Chromkalim (BRL-34915), 125
Chronic heart failure, treatment, 471
Chronic obstructive pulmonary disease, 710
Cibenzoline, 627–633
  acute antiarrhythmic effects, 631–632
  adverse reactions, 632–633
  antiarrhythmic effects in animals, 629
  cellular electrophysiology, 627–629
  effects on the electrocardiogram, 630
  pharmacokinetics, 629–630
Cimetidine, 503, 527, 594, 612, 657
Cinchonism, 376, 503
Ciprilan, 627
Circus movement (see Reentry)
Cirrhosis, 712
Clofilium, 677–679, 729, 730, 733
  antiarrhythmic efficacy, 685
  basic pharmacology, 683, 684
  pharmacokinetics, 685, 686
  safety, 686
Clonidine, 732
Cobalt, 697
Cobalt-sensitive inward current, 119

Cocaine, 562
Cocker spaniel, cardiomyopathy, 420, 421
Competitive binding, 484
Complete heart block, 379
Computer simulations, 61–63, 72–83, 157, 409, 478 (*see also* Mathematical modeling)
Conductance, 201
Conduction, conduction velocity, 3, 89, 127, 143, 150, 151, 163, 165, 168, 210, 223, 224, 242, 263, 278, 291, 363, 479, 677, 734
  assessment of sinoatrial, 89–92
  block/disturbances, 377, 418
  depression by:
    amiodarone, 639
    disopyramide, 544
    propafenone, 606, 608
    quinidine, 496
Conduction system disease, 715
Congenital heart disease, 413, 593
Congestive heart failure, 277, 288, 397, 405, 426, 403, 464, 465, 497, 505, 548, 551, 577, 594, 595, 619, 620, 646, 658, 670, 672, 709, 714, 715
Continuous atrial pacing, 91, 92
Continuous/fractionated electrical activity, 13, 321, 322, 365
Contractile proteins, 453, 469
Contractility, 287, 629, 682 (*see also* Inotropic effects)
Coomb's test, 529
Corneal microdeposits, 377, 378, 647
Coronary artery disease, 631, 670
Coronary artery occlusion, 301–324, 331–347, 520, 612, 614, 615, 641, 655, 678, 682, 685, 689, 725, 732
Coronary sinus, atrial fibers, 128, 360
Coronary vasospasm, 724
Corticosteroids, 646
Countershock (*see* Cardioversion)
Coupling intervals, 283
Crista terminalis, 85, 86, 89, 93, 96, 98, 109, 120, 121, 126, 128, 151, 154, 240, 259, 266, 606–608, 700
Cross-bridge cycling, 445
Cryoablation, 338
Current rundown, 478
Cycle length–dependent changes, 121, 143, 144, 148, 150, 154, 172, 174, 186, 217, 265, 266, 234, 517, 538, 587, 606, 640
Cyclic AMP, 43, 47, 118, 119, 123, 183, 184, 188, 213, 227, 447, 449, 453, 454, 466, 467, 469, 538, 699–701
Cyclic GMP, 467

Cytochrome P-450, 502
Cytosolic (*see* Intracellular) inclusion bodies

D-600, gallopamil, methoxyverapamil, 320, 332, 704, 708–710, 715
Dapsone, 529
Deactivation, channel, 62, 208
Debrisoquin, 502, 617, 618
Decreases of contractility by drugs (*see* Negative inotropic effects)
Decremental conduction, 338, 340
Delayed afterdepolarizations, 13, 51, 124, 161, 181, 187–189, 208, 220–222, 279–291, 305, 316–318, 320, 323, 324, 359–361, 398, 401, 402, 404, 406, 407, 409, 410, 519, 570, 588, 610, 640, 656, 668, 700
Delayed conduction, 267, 271
Delta wave, 320
Deoxycorticosterone acetate, 402
Depolarization, 199
Depressed fast response, 176, 268, 332
Desacetyl-diltiazem, 713
Desethyl-N-acetylprocainamide, 525
Desmosomes, 163
Diabetic animal models, 402–410
Diacylglycerol, 437
Diastolic depolarization (*see* Phase 4 depolarization)
Dibenzamil, dichlorobenzamil, 207, 449
Dicumarol, 594
Dielectric properties, 225
Diethylaminoethanol, 517
Differential effects of drugs on repolarization of Purkinje fibers and ventricular myocardium, 382–384, 609
Digitalis (*see* Cardiac glycosides)
Digoxin-specific Fab fragments/antibodies, 291
Dihydropyridines, 47, 213, 224, 446, 697, 701, 703 (*see also* nifedipine, nitrendipine, BAY K 8644)
Dilated cardiomyopathy, 416, 619
Diltiazem, 47, 171, 291, 316, 446, 697, 703, 705, 709, 710, 712, 713, 715, 728, 730
2, 3-Dimethylnitrobenzene, 30
Dipole, 3, 4
Direct-coupled amplifiers, 6
Discontinuities in conduction, 268
Disopyramide, 290, 328, 483, 484, 494, 505, 521, 527, 529, 537–551, 567–569, 646
  antiarrhythmic effects in experimental animals, 542–543

[Disopyramide]
    clinical pharmacology, 543–549
    electrophysiologic effects on isolated cardiac
        tissues, 537–542
    mono-*N*-dealkylated (MND), 541, 542, 547,
        548, 550
    pharmacokinetics, 546–549
    supraventricular arrhythmias, 545, 546
    toxicology, 376, 549–551
    ventricular arrhythmias and tachycardia, 546
Dispersion of refractoriness (*see* Refractoriness)
Distant ischemia, 724
Divalent cations, shielding of surface charge, 210
Doberman pinscher, cardiomyopathy, 420, 421
Dobutamine, 448
Dopamine, 448, 715
Doxorubicin, 291, 316, 319
DPI 201–106, 448, 468–470, 677, 679
Drug-induced arrhythmias, 375–393
Drug protection against sudden death, 727–733
Drug-receptor interactions, 479
Drug therapy, combination, 484
dV/dt_{max} (dV/dt, $\dot{V}_{max}$), 3, 21, 45, 60, 115, 152,
        163, 168, 171, 173, 186, 202, 207, 267,
        270, 377, 380, 405, 477, 478, 494, 517,
        518, 527, 537–539, 542, 562–565, 586,
        587, 604, 606, 609, 628, 638, 639, 655,
        667, 668, 677, 679, 683, 686, 689, 699

Early afterdepolarizations, 13, 183, 202, 208,
        219, 222, 224, 281, 282, 359, 363, 398,
        401, 402, 406, 407, 408, 409, 496, 502,
        505, 541, 571, 588, 679, 683, 686, 689
Early afterhyperpolarizations, 281, 282
Ectopic activity, 277, 279
Effective refractory period (ERP), 169, 170, 173,
        342, 485, 493, 498, 517–519, 521, 542,
        544, 565, 573, 587–589, 611, 613, 631,
        655, 685, 686, 689, 708
Electrical uncoupling (*see* Cellular uncoupling)
Electrocardiogram (ECG), 6, 9,1 2, 87, 89, 90,
        93, 95, 96, 126, 199, 201, 210, 265,
        281, 285, 308, 312, 320, 322, 398, 405,
        413–426, 444, 496, 499, 520, 572, 593,
        657, 708 (*see also* PR, QRS, QT, U
        wave)
Electrocardiographic lead systems, dog and cat,
        414
Electrodes:
    endocardial catheter, 6
    extracellular, 4, 5

[Electrodes]
    needle, 6
    suction, 6
    wick, 6
Electrograms, 342
    bipolar vs. unipolar, 5, 6
Electrophysiologic testing, 680
Electrotonic effects, 149, 163, 223, 227, 259,
        263, 265, 266, 269, 341, 354, 356, 567,
        568
EN-313 (*see* Moricizine)
Enalapril, 471
Encainide, 483, 499, 502, 521, 523, 527, 529,
        660, 670, 715, 733, 734
Endogenous:
    catecholamines, 182,682
    digitalis-like substance, 289,451
Ensemble current, single-channel activity, 46,
        48, 49, 448
Entrainment, 278, 345
Entrance block:
    sinus node, 88
    variable, 321, 401, 408, 409
Enzymatically isolated myocytes, 21, 41, 60–65,
        99, 109, 110, 116, 117, 119, 121–125,
        151, 161, 168, 171, 172, 174, 178, 210,
        211, 214–217, 219, 226, 289, 538, 572,
        638, 639, 683
Epinephrine, 11, 48, 52, 85, 181, 183, 184, 186,
        267, 271, 316, 320, 359, 406, 437, 666,
        683, 700, 725
Equilibrium/reversal potential, 206
    E_{Ca}, 66, 67, 69, 70
    E_K, 70, 113, 122, 178, 200, 214, 215, 216,
        218, 219, 314
    E_{Na}, 69, 70, 166, 168
    E_{NaCa}, 69
    E_{TI}, 220, 285
Erythema multiforme, 595
Escape interval, 284
Esmolol, 667, 710
Ethanol, 527, 548, 642
Ethmozine, etmosin (*see* Moricizine)
Exacerbation of arrhythmias, 324
Excitable gap, 242, 346, 544
Excitability, 278, 519, 655
    hypothesis of altered, 561
Excitation-contraction coupling, 403, 404, 449,
        453, 454
Exercise, 669–671, 681, 708, 709, 712
Exit block, 321
Extracellular potentials, general concepts, 3, 4
    atrioventricular bypass tracts, 12
    coronary sinus ostium, 13

[Extracellular potentials, general concepts]
  delayed afterdepolarizations, 13, 14
  His bundle, 11
  sinus node, 7–11, 92
Extracellular spaces, restricted (ECS), 62, 63,
  71, 85

Facilitation, 143, 144, 147
Fatigue, AV node, 143, 144, 147
Fenoximone, 467, 470
Fibrosing alveolitis, 595
Figure 8 activation pattern (see Reentry)
Filters:
  bessel, 44
  low pass and high pass, 6, 7, 8, 11–15
  notch, 7
Flecainide, 483, 499, 521, 523, 527, 529, 545,
  591, 609, 660, 670, 715, 728, 730, 733,
  734
Flunarizine, 449
Focal necrosis, catecholamine-induced, 406
Forskolin, 47, 449
Fractionated electrical activity/electrograms, 13,
  127, 366, 731
Frank-Starling effect, 454
Frequency-dependent changes (see Cycle length–
  dependent changes)
Full recovery time, 169, 170
Functional conduction block, 338, 340, 341, 345
  (see also Arc of block)
Functional longitudinal dissociation, 243, 255,
  378, 379
Fura-2, 438

Gallopamil (see D-600)
Ganglionic transmission block:
  acecainide, 682
  procainamide, 520
Gap junctions, 33, 63, 85, 89, 225–227, 292,
  332, 566, 569
Gastrointestinal symptoms, 595
Gating processes, 35, 43, 47, 61, 62, 67, 166,
  167, 213, 449, 478, 539
Geometry, effects on impulse conduction, 271
Gigaohm seal, 41
Glass tubing:
  aluminasilicate, 20
  borosilicate, 20
Glucagon, 575, 715

Glybenclamide, 125, 733
Glycylxylidide, 484, 576, 577
Goldman-Hodgkin-Katz (GHK) formulation, 200,
  203
G proteins, 47, 48, 50, 51, 114, 119, 157, 183,
  217, 431–439, 446, 448, 449, 701
Guarded receptor hypothesis, 481, 494, 539, 564

Half-life, drug elimination:
  acecainide, 682
  amiodarone, 644, 645
  cibenzoline, 629
  clofilium, 685
  digitalis, 501
  disopyramide, 547, 548
  lidocaine, 575, 576
  moricizine, 657
  N-acetylprocainamide, 524, 528, 679
  procainamide, 524, 525
  propafenone, 618
  quinidine, 500
  sematilide, 688
  sotolol, 690
  tocainide, 594
  verapamil, 712
Halothane, 291
H cells (of AV node), 146–150
Hemodialysis, 594
Heparin, 500
Heptanol, 257
Heredity cardiomyopathy, hamsters, 405
Heterogeneity of repolarization, 505
Hexamethonium, 682
H infinity curves, 478,480
His-atrial interval, 149
His bundle, 141, 142, 161, 162, 311, 320, 628
  electrograms, 3, 6, 7, 11,13, 14, 312, 322,
    324, 325, 326, 574
Histamine, 701
Hodgkin-Huxley model, 46, 62, 63, 65, 114,
  116, 123, 165, 167, 200, 209, 478, 482,
  494 Holter monitor, 591, 593
H-V interval, 11, 498, 518, 521, 528, 544, 573,
  588, 611, 613, 615, 628, 632, 640, 656,
  657, 684, 687, 708
Hybrid voltage clamp technique, 37
Hydralizine, 529
Hydrophilic pathway, 481, 482, 539
Hydrophobic pathway, 481, 482, 484, 539, 562
Hydroxypropafenone, 502
Hydroxyquinidine, 501, 503

Hyperkalemia, 733
Hypertension, 397–399, 401, 409, 425, 665
Hyperthyroidism, 423
Hypertrophic cardiomyopathy, 397, 406, 426
Hypertrophy, 290
  induced by pressure overload, 397–401
Hypothyroidism, 684
Hypoxia, 181, 700

I_X, 172, 216
IBE 2254, 435
Idiopathic dilated cardiomyopathy, 420
Idioventricular tachycardias, 418,614
Inactivation, channel, 62
  i_{Ca}, 63,65,67,68
  i_K, 63,123
  i_{Na}, 45–47,115, 116, 170, 202, 208, 209, 215,
    478, 479, 698
Indecainide, 521, 523, 527
Inexcitable gap, 263–266, 269
Infarction, myocardial, 251, 267, 270, 301–328,
    331–347, 351–370, 572, 612–614, 632,
    658, 670, 683
Inorganic calcium antagonists, 697
Inositol triphosphate (IP_3), 437, 438, 453
Inotropic effects (see Contractility)
Inotropy:
  positive, 288, 463–471, 679, 682, 686, 688,
    691, 716
  negative, 452, 542, 550, 551, 565, 577, 595,
    682, 704, 715
Input resistance:
  sinus venosus myocytes, 64
  ventricular cell, 226
Inside-out patches, 42
Insulin, 290, 549
Intact dog heart, 86
Intercalated disks, 162
Intermittent claudication, 672
Interpolated beats, 284
Interstitial pneumonitis, 595
Intracellular inclusion bodies, 645
Intrinsic sympathomimetic activity, 665, 660,
    686
Invasive evaluation of sinus node function, 97,
    98
Ion accumulation and depletion, 37, 62, 112,
    172, 173, 217
Ion channels, 200, 201
Ion-specific microelectrodes, 314, 354
Ischemia/ischemic conditions, 13, 50, 204, 210,
    211, 219, 227, 264–266, 269, 285, 289,

[Ischemia/ischemic conditions]
    301–328, 331–347, 351–370, 439, 487,
    496, 543, 562, 564, 573, 587, 640, 655,
    656, 668, 669, 683, 684, 689, 699, 707,
    727
Ischemic heart disease, 397
Isobutylmethylxanthine (IBMX), 448
Isochronal mapping (see Activation patterns)
Isomazole, 467
Isoniazid, 519, 594
Isoproterenol, 13, 14, 47, 87, 119, 123, 184–
    188, 217, 290, 321, 359, 448, 466, 495,
    504, 541, 550, 570, 575, 628, 638, 686,
    715, 732
Isosorbide dinitrate, 622

Jervell and Lang-Nielson syndrome, 672
Junctional pacemaker, 14

Lactate, 181, 289
Lanthanum, 64, 697
Left anterior descending coronary artery, 301,
    341, 352, 629, 726
Left anterior fascicular block, 425
Left circumflex coronary artery, 726
Length constant, 567, 568
Length-tension curve, 454
Leukopenia, 595
Lidocaine, 228, 290–292, 319, 320, 328, 376,
    468, 481, 483–485, 487, 494, 495, 504,
    520, 522, 525, 527, 539, 561–577, 585,
    586, 589, 591–593, 611, 612, 614, 655,
    683
  acute effects in humans, 574
  antiarrhythmic effects:
    in experimental animals, 572, 573
    in humans, 574, 575
  effects on normal human electrocardiogram,
    573, 574
  electrophysiologic effects on isolated cardiac
    tissues, 561–572
  pharmacokinetics, 575
  toxicology, 577
Lidoflazine, 178, 179
Liminal length, 226, 567, 568
Lipoxygenase pathway, 50
Lithium, 22, 288, 438, 699
Liver disease, 594
Local anesthetics, 46, 290, 687, 697, 699
  as antiarrhythmic drugs, 477–488

Local circuit current, 223, 269, 478
Long QT syndrome, 729
Longitudinal dissociation (*see* functional longitudinal dissociation)
Longitudinal resistance, 567
Lorcainide, 483
Lupus-like syndrome, 504, 505, 528, 529, 682, 688
Lysophosphatides (lysophosphotidylcholine, lysophosphoglycerides), 216, 227, 289, 316, 332, 567, 570

Macro reentry (*see* Reentry)
Magnesium ion, 23, 29, 30, 31, 49, 72, 235, 288, 495, 504, 505, 529
Manganese ion, 207, 283, 697
Mapping, high resolution, 338 (*see also* Activation patterns)
Mathematical models (*see* Computer simulations):
    sinus venosus activity, 62, 70–83
Matrix, electrophysiologic, 201, 561, 526, 527
Maximum follow frequency, 679
Maximum rate of depolarization (*see* dV/dt)
MCI 154, 470
MDL 17043 (*see* Fenoximone)
MDL 19205 (*see* Piroximone)
Mechanoreceptors, 221
Melperone, 679
Membrane capacitance, 34–36, 110, 205, 226, 399, 567, 568
Membrane length constant, 33, 34, 111, 226
Membrane resistance, 34, 36, 110, 111, 204, 216, 226, 228, 399, 567
Membrane responsiveness, 565, 566, 586
Membrane stabilizing activity (local anesthesia by β-blockers), 665, 667–669
Meobentine, 729, 730
Methimazole, 647
Methoxy-*O*-desmethylencainide, 502
Methylscopalamine, 731
Methylxanthines, 449, 466, 699
Metoprolol, 502, 575, 594, 665, 671
Mexiletine, 280, 483, 487, 503, 505, 522, 585–596, 545, 546, 646
    antiarrhythmic effects in experimental animals, 587, 588
    clinical pharmacology, 588–594
    electrophysiologic effects on isolated tissues, 585–587
    toxicology, 594–595

Microelectrodes:
    standard intracellular, 19–23
    ion-selective, 23–31
        apparatus, 25, 26
        calibration, 29
        electrical response time, 28
        glass tubing, 26, 27
        silanization, 27
        reference electrode, 24
        capacitance neutralization, 23
        electrical, tip and taper characteristics, 20–21
        electrolyte filling solution, 21, 22
        glass tubing, 20
Microreentry (*see* Reentry)
Milrinone, 449, 467, 470
Mitral valve prolapse, 418
Mixed function oxidases, induction, 503
MJ-1999 (*see* Sotolol)
Modeling (*see* Computer simulations, Mathematical models)
Mode switching and arrhythmogenic inward current, 213
Modulated receptor hypothesis, 479, 482, 484, 485, 494, 539, 563, 564, 586, 709
Monochlorotrimethylsilane (MCTMS), 27, 28
Monoethylglycylxylidide, 576, 577
Monophasic action potentials, 6, 13, 126, 242, 243, 290, 498, 505, 543, 544, 680, 689
Moricizine (ethmozine), 290, 319, 545, 573, 655–661, 670, 733
    adverse effects, 661
    antiarrhythmic effects, 658–661
    cellular electrophysiology, 655–656
    clinical electrophysiology, 656–657
    pharmacokinetics, 657–658
Multicenter postinfarction program (MPIP), 669
Multiple sites of impulse initiation, 312, 321
Muscarinic cholinergic effects, 11, 42, 44, 50, 60, 85, 119, 126, 217, 277, 542
Myocardial:
    disease, canine, 419
    disease, feline, 425
    infarction (*see* Infarction, myocardial)
Myofibrillar sensitization, 450
Myosin light-chain kinase, 454
Myxomatous degeneration, 418

N-acetyl procainamide (NAPA) (*see* Acecainide)
Nadolol, 305, 308, 665, 667, 668, 730, 731
Narcotic analgesics, 594

N cells (of the AV node), 146–151

N-desmethylsematilide, 688

Negative inotropic effects, 376–377, 497, 528, 549, 577, 595, 620, 630–631, 714

Negative slope conductance, 112, 125

Nernst equation, equilibrium potentials, 69, 200

Nerve growth factor, 436

Neuraminidase, 449

Neuroleptic actions, melperone, 679

Neurologic side effects, 595

Neurotoxins, receptor sites in sodium channels, 478

Nicardipine, 290

Nickel ion, 119, 171, 212, 449, 697

Nifedipine, 47, 171, 213, 291, 314, 315, 446, 697, 703–707, 709, 712, 713, 716

Nitrendipine, 213, 290, 446

Nitroblue tetrazolium, 332

Nodal recovery time, 149

Nodal refractoriness, 150

Noise, electrical, 5, 7, 44, 45

Noninvasive evaluation of sinus node function, 95–97

Nonlinear dynamics theory, 99

Nonselective/nonspecific β-blockers, 667, 668

Nonspecific cation channels, currents, 51, 52, 69, 124, 125, 154, 189, 287, 288, 702

Norepinephrine, 60, 156, 181, 183, 184, 204, 210–212, 406, 438, 465, 666, 683, 686

Norverapamil, 713–714

N-shaped I-V curve, 112, 216

Nuclear magnetic resonance, 445

Nystatin, 43

O-desmethylencainide, 502

O-desmethylquinidine, 501

OPC 8212, 468, 470

Open channel blockers, 486

Open probability, 209

Orthodromic tachycardia, 711

Oscillations, voltage, 206 (*see also* Delayed afterdepolarizations)

Oscillatory afterpotentials, 280–292 (*see also* Delayed afterdepolarizations)

Ouabain (*see* Cardiac glycosides)

Outside-out patch, 44

Overdrive, 285

  hyperpolarization, 175, 176

  suppression, 87, 88, 98, 175, 176, 357, 366, 378

Oxoquinidinone, 501

Oxpranolol, 667

P wave, 7, 89, 126

Pacemaker activity, 7, 8, 35, 48, 52, 59, 61, 63, 73, 85, 92, 124, 127, 151, 183, 628

  acceleration of sinus, digitalis toxicity, 278

  and $i_{Ca, T}$, 48, 120

Pacemaker current, i_f, 37, 52, 61, 67, 82, 124, 156, 177–181, 184, 222

Pacing-induced rhythms, 316, 321, 366

Parasympathetic (*see* Autonomic nervous system)

Parasystole, 378, 379

Paroxysmal supraventricular arrhythmias, 707–708, 710–711, 714

Passive membrane properties, 110, 225, 399, 410, 495

Patch clamp technique, 41–53, 62, 99, 154, 161, 168, 450, 477, 481, 683, 701

  limitations and sources of error, 44, 45, 478, 683

Pectinate muscle, 700

Penbutolol, 665, 667

Pentobarbital, 680, 684, 726

Perforated patch technique, 43

Periodic premature stimulation of the atrium, 141

Peripheral vascular disease, 710

Peritoneal dialysis, 594

Permeability ratio, 63, 200

Pertussis toxin, 50, 51, 114, 434–439, 448, 449

pH, pH effects, 23, 29, 31, 204, 206, 210, 213–216, 226, 227, 289, 290, 454, 484, 486, 503, 525

Phase 4 (diastolic) depolarization, 280, 410, 519, 524, 527, 689, 699

  bullfrog atrial myocyte, 60, 84

  depressed human atrial tissue, 406

  extracellular recording, 7, 9, 13, 14

  Purkinje fiber, 52, 202, 222, 628, 656

    facilitates impulse reflection, 264

    enhanced by ouabain toxicity, 279

    suppressed when DADs occur, 280

  sinus node, 60, 85, 87–89, 156

  sinus venosus model, 72–73

  subsidiary atrial pacemakers, 127

Phases, transmembrane action potential, 168, 169, 200, 202, 698

Phenoxybenzamine, 683

Phentolamine, 185, 316, 360, 683

Phenylalkylamines, 47, 446, 697, 701, 703, 707, 715 (*see also* Verapamil)

Phenylephrine, 316, 359, 360, 434–436

Phenytoin, 290, 291, 376, 468, 503, 522, 527

Phorbal esters, 438

Phosphodiesterase/inhibitors, 227, 447, 449, 466–470

Phospholamban, 183, 188, 447, 453
Phospholipase, 437, 438
Phosphorylation, 47, 48, 183, 213, 447, 700, 701
Pimobendan, 467, 469, 470
Pinacidil, 733
Pindolol, 665, 667
Pirbuterol, 448
Piroximone, 467, 470
Pinacidil, 125
Plasma protein binding:
    acecainide, 524
    amiodarone, 644
    class IV drugs, 713
    disopyramide, 546–548
    mexiletine, 594
    moricizine, 657
    procainamide, 524
    propafenone, 617
    quinidine, 500, 501
    tocainide, 593
Positive inotropy, 182, 184, 214, 227, 443–455,
        463–471
Postpacing acceleration, 279
Postrepolarization refractoriness (see Refractoriness)
Postsurgical atrioventricular block, 11
Potassium currents, 48, 52, 83, 205, 214–221,
        450, 704, 733
    acetylcholine-activated K current, 42, 50, 83,
        113, 114, 172, 495
    ATP-gated K channel, 50, 125, 154, 172,
        218–220, 222, 356
    background K current ($i_{K, 1}$), 48, 49, 69, 71,
        72, 76, 83, 85, 111–113, 151, 172–174,
        178, 179, 183, 214, 439, 495, 668,
        blockade by Mg^{2+}, 49
        sodium-dependent inactivation, 215
    delayed rectifier K current (i_K), 35, 49, 63,
        72, 73, 122, 123, 154, 172–174, 178,
        181, 183, 184, 203, 216, 495, 668, 683,
        687, 689
    inward K rectifier (see Background K currents, $i_{K, 1}$)
    pacemaker channel ($i_{K, 2}$), 52, 177, 184, 699
    sodium-gated K channel, 50, 172, 220, 222
    transient outward K current (i_{to}), 49, 52, 93,
        119–122, 153–157, 171, 172, 174, 178,
        202, 203, 210, 211
    i_{to} window current, 211
    instantaneous outward plateau K current,
        218
Potassium (intracellular), 24, 29, 31, 172, 314,
        354–356
    measurement technique, 29–31

Potassium tetrakis (p-chlorophenyl) borate, 29
PR interval, 141, 520, 630–632, 656, 657, 684,
        685, 690, 708, 714
Pracizoline, 627
Practolol, 667
Prazocin, 433, 438, 439, 471, 730, 733
Premature stimulation:
    atrial, 90, 91
    ventricular, 333–337
Prenalterol, 448
Pressure overload, 347
Proarrhythmic effects of drugs, 375–393, 477,
        487, 503–505, 529, 677, 679, 682–684,
        687, 728, 733, 734
Procainamide, 228, 290, 363–365, 479, 483,
        494, 495, 505, 683, 687, 688, 734
    agranulocytosis, 528
    antiarrhythmic effects in experimental animals,
        520
    atrial arrhythmias, 522
    bioavailability, 525
    chronic antiarrhythmic therapy, 522
    clinical pharmacology, 520–528
    effects on normal ECG, 520–521
    electrophysiologic effects on isolated tissues,
        517–520
    extracardiac effects, 528
    mechanism of action, 524
    methods of administration, 525–527
    peak plasma concentrations, 525
    pharmacokinetics, 524–528, 679
    programmed extrastimulation studies, 521–522
    therapeutic concentration range, 523
    toxicity, 376, 528, 529, 682
        decreased myocardial performance, 529
    use during pregnancy, 525
    ventricular arrhythmias, 523–524
    volume of distribution, 525
    Wolff-Parkinson-White syndrome, 522, 523
Procaine hydrochloride, 30, 517
Programmed electrical stimulation, 285, 331,
        338, 352, 365, 366, 521, 522, 629, 631,
        632, 660, 667, 679, 681, 685, 688, 689,
        691, 725–727
Propafenone, 502, 603–622, 715
    cellular electrophysiologic effects, 603–611
    drug interactions, 621–622
    effects against supraventricular arrhythmias in
        humans, 618–619
    effects against ventricular arrhythmias:
        in animals, 612–614
        in humans, 619–620
    electrophysiologic effects:
        in experimental animals, 611

[Propafenone]
  in humans, 614–616
  hemodynamic effects, 612, 615, 616
  5-hydroxy propafenone, 613, 617, 618
  N-depropyl propafenone, 617
  pharmacokinetics, 616–618
  side effects, 620–621
Propagation (*see* Conduction)
Propranolol, 97, 98, 182, 185, 186, 359, 360,
    376, 379, 433, 434, 438, 439, 502, 520,
    527, 665, 667, 668, 670–672, 682, 683
Prostaglandins, 289
Protein kinase, 43, 122, 123, 173, 183, 188,
    447, 454, 700, 701
Pulmonary capillary wedge pressure, 631
Pulmonary fibrosis, 595
Pump function of the heart, 141
Purkinje fiber, 24, 26, 33–35, 37, 38, 49, 50,
    62, 75, 114–117, 119–125, 141, 146, 156,
    161–189, 202, 209, 210, 212, 216, 217,
    219, 222, 225–228, 253–256, 271, 279–
    282, 284, 288, 289, 309–312, 317, 324,
    325, 352, 353, 355–361, 363, 381, 433,
    436, 438, 439, 493–496, 501, 505, 517–
    520, 527, 628, 655, 656, 667, 668, 683,
    685, 687, 689, 698, 707

QRS duration, 165, 168, 415, 416, 423, 496,
    498, 499, 503, 518, 520–522, 525, 630–
    632, 656, 657, 684, 685, 690, 708
QT interval, 173, 199, 378, 415, 416, 423, 496–
    498, 500, 504, 518, 520, 521, 525, 527–
    528, 631, 632, 656, 657, 668, 669, 671,
    680, 684, 685, 688–690, 708, 731
Quinidine, 122, 155, 157, 224, 290, 376, 479,
    483–485, 487, 493–505, 520–522, 526,
    529, 537, 539, 541, 543, 545, 549, 550,
    590, 591, 619, 646, 647, 667, 679, 683,
    728, 730, 734
  action potential prolongation, 494–496
  basic pharmacology, 493–496
  clinical pharmacology, 496–503
  drug interactions, 501–503
  effects on electrocardiogram, 496, 497
  hemodynamic effects, 497
  local anesthetic actions, 494
  place in therapy, 505
  quinidine-*N*-oxide, 501
  quinidine syncope, 376, 550
  side effects, 503–505
  therapeutic use, 505

Quinine, 493, 495, 497, 502, 503
QX-222, 485
QX-314, 485, 562–564

Radioligand assay technique, 484
Ranitidine, 527, 575
Rate-dependent changes (*see* Cycle length-
    dependent changes)
Raynaud's phenomenon, 672
Reactivation, 173, 479
Recainam, 680
Reentry, reentrant excitation, 13, 187, 214, 227,
    239–248, 251–272, 278, 323, 324, 331–
    347, 363–369, 377, 518, 524, 570, 608,
    618, 656, 660, 668, 669, 680, 685, 687,
    691, 707, 710, 724, 733
  anatomical barrier/ring model, 240–242, 251–
    257, 378
  anatomical and electrophysiologic substrates,
    331–47
  circus movement, 251–272, 379
  clinical observations, 365, 366
  digitalis arrhythmias, 291, 292
  entrainment, termination or acceleration by
    programmed stimulation, 345–346
  epicardial activation patterns, 333–347
  functional barrier, block, 242–243, 260
    AV node, 247, 248
    Figure 8, 251, 252, 261–263, 331, 335,
      338, 339, 343, 345
    leading circle, 244–247, 257–261, 378–380
  macroreentry, 267
  microreentry, 255, 266
  pleomorphic tachycardia, 338
Reflection, 11, 227, 255, 263–270
Refractoriness, 92, 331, 340, 346, 363, 367,
    368, 496, 519, 691, 734
  atrium, 519, 521, 522, 679, 680, 684–686
  AV node, 142, 144, 145, 150, 278, 542, 544,
    669, 670
  dispersion, 187, 363, 364, 400, 683, 685,
    686, 733
  postrepolarization, 257, 259, 332, 363
  prolonged, 338
  Purkinje fiber, 169
  sinus node, 89, 92, 97
  ventricular, 519, 528, 680, 684, 685, 689
Refractory gradient, 338
Regenerative depolarization, 167, 168, 567, 568
Reinfarction, 724
Relative refractory period, 169, 170, 381, 589

Reperfusion, arrhythmias, 289, 290, 352, 439, 543, 572, 573, 588, 612, 668, 688, 725
Repetitive ventricular response (RVR), 280, 284
Repolarization:
  atrial muscle cell action potential, 109, 110, 123, 126
  Purkinje fiber action potential, 75, 170–173
  sinus node action potential, 73–76
  ventricular muscle action potential, 199, 203, 216
Reserpine, 682
Resting potential, 151, 200
Rest/resting block of sodium channels (see Tonic block)
Restrictive cardiomyopathy, 426
Return extrasystole, 255 (see also Ventricular arrhythmias, Premature ventricular depolarizations)
Rifampin/rifampicin, 503, 548
Right bundle branch block, 425
Ritmalan, 627
RO 22–796/001, 627
Romano-Ward syndrome, 671, 672
R-on-T phenomenon, 169, 379, 382, 389, 391
Rubidium, 30, 699
"Ruptured patch" voltage clamp technique, 63
Ruthenium red, 453
Ryanodine, 120, 211, 286, 438, 453

Safety factor, 571
Saltatory conduction, 269
Sarcolemmal membrane, 200
Sarcoplasmic reticulum (SR), 25, 171, 181, 183, 189, 205, 206, 211, 214, 286, 290, 702
Saterinone, 469
Schmitt-Erlanger diagram, 253, 379–381
Schnauzer dogs, sick sinus syndrome, 418
Sea anemone toxin, 450, 677
Seasonal differences, myocardial infarction, 308
Selectivity:
  calcium channels, 66, 67
  filter, 167, 481, 482, 563
Selenium deficiency, 425
Sematilide, 677–679
  basic pharmacology, 687, 688
  clinical studies, 688
  pharmacokinetics, 688
  safety, 688, 689
Shift of pacemaker site, 11, 85–87, 98
Sick sinus syndrome, 98, 99, 418, 422, 574, 588, 671, 708 (see also Bradycardia-tachycardia syndrome)

Silent ischemia, 671
Simian mitral valve (see Valve leaflet)
Single cells (see Enzymatically isolated myocytes)
Single channel currents, 41–52, 161, 209, 218
Sinoatrial block, 544, 621, 657
Sinoatrial conduction, 538, 586
Sinoatrial conduction time (SACT), 89, 91, 92, 97, 98, 614, 657
Sinoventricular conduction, 425
Sinus arrest, 278
Sinus arrhythmia, 11, 277, 303, 306, 423
Sinus bradycardia, 416, 423, 426, 621, 642, 647
Sinus node, 49, 50, 52, 59–100, 119, 122, 124, 127, 151, 153, 156, 175, 199, 202, 277, 439, 527, 528, 537, 538, 542, 572, 585, 586, 588, 603, 604, 614, 627, 638, 683, 686, 689, 697, 698
  action potential, 59, 73–76, 605, 697
  dysfunction, 59, 93, 95, 97, 278, 521, 544, 657
  evaluation of function, 95–98
  exit block, 95, 97, 98, 278, 594
  extracellular recording, electrograms, 7–11, 92, 97
  functional and morphologic organization, 83–87
  function in multicellular preparations, 85
  human, evaluation of function, 93–98
  interpolation of premature impulses, 92–95
  recovery time (SNRT), 88–89, 97–98, 518, 574, 588, 589, 611, 613, 614, 657, 660, 680, 708
  refractoriness, 92, 93, 97
  reset, 92, 94, 95
Sinus tachycardia, 173, 309, 416, 419, 421–423, 497
Sinus venosus (SV), 59, 61, 71, 122
  mathematical model of pacemaker activity, 61, 71
  SV myocytes, 62
Site of earliest activation, 13, 320, 323, 338, 366, 367
Skinned cardiac fibers, 452, 453, 469
Slow conduction, 157, 210, 214, 255, 260, 268, 332, 333, 380
Slow inward current, i_{si} (see calcium current), 168, 172, 281, 538, 541, 604, 701–705
Slow response action potentials, 164, 586, 611, 641, 668
Sodium bicarbonate, 503
Sodium-calcium exchange, 43, 51, 60, 67–69, 71, 72, 74, 75, 80, 82, 88, 124, 125, 154, 189, 204–207, 220, 222, 286–288, 314, 356, 363, 445, 450, 451, 565, 702
inhibitors, 207, 679

Sodium channels/current, 43, 52, 152, 165, 168, 175, 183, 202, 205, 267, 268, 450, 468, 477–488, 494, 503, 538, 542, 562–564, 572, 586, 637–639, 641, 655, 666, 667, 678–680, 698, 702, 728
  atrial muscle, 114–117
  atrioventricular node, 152, 153
  availability (H infinity) curve, 478
  background Na current, 63, 71–73, 80, 152, 184
  multiple types, 209
  patch clamp, 45–47
  Purkinje fiber, 167
  sinus node, 69, 71, 73
    background current, I_B, 63, 71–73, 78, 80, 82, 83
  subconductance states, 209
  ventricular muscle, 207–210
  window (slowly inactivating, late) Na current, 117, 171, 184, 203, 209, 656
Sodium (intracellular), 29, 31, 206, 286, 290, 314, 355, 356, 361, 363, 438, 450–452, 564
Sodium lactate, 503
Sodium-potassium (Na/K) pump, 35, 43, 60, 67, 71, 72, 75, 80, 81, 88, 123, 152, 170, 171, 174–176, 178, 183, 184, 204–206, 216, 217, 220, 227, 278, 285, 286, 288, 314, 332, 361, 438, 451, 465, 469
Sodium-proton exchange, 206, 207, 215, 702
Sotalol, 224, 360, 445, 464, 667, 668, 677–679, 683, 729–731
  antiarrhythmic efficacy, 689, 690
  basic pharmacology, 689
  clinical studies, 690
  pharmacokinetics, 690
  safety, 691
Springer spaniel, atrial standstill, 418
Specialized atrial conduction tracts, 109, 126, 175
Specific bradycardic agents, 732 (*see also* Alinidine)
Spontaneous arrhythmias:
  cats, 422
  dogs, 414
Spontaneous defibrillation, 685
Spontaneous diastolic depolarization (*see* Phase 4 depolarization)
Stellate ganglion, 290
Stereospecificity, 484, 541, 690, 705, 706
Stevens-Johnson syndrome, 595
Stomatitis, 595
Streptozotocin, 290, 402–405
Strength-interval curve, 611

Stretch:
  activated channels, 221
  effects on conduction, 570
Strontium, 65, 122, 699
Subconductance states, 209
Subsidiary atrial pacemaker cells, 127
Subthreshold response, 259
Sucrose gap voltage clamp, 35–37
Sudden death, 303, 306–308, 351, 397, 589, 590, 595, 641, 643, 660, 670–672, 723, 724, 731, 733, 734
  conscious canine model, 690, 727–729
Sulfamethazine, 529
Sulmazole, 467, 469, 470
Supernormal period, 169, 381
Supraventricular premature complexes and tachycardia, 416, 419
Surface charge, membrane, 209, 210, 485
Surgical resection, 11, 366
Sustained-release preparations, 715
Sympathectomy, 290
Sympathetic tone (*see* Autonomic nervous system)
Syncope, 422, 504, 544, 589, 591, 592, 672

Tachycardia (*see* Atrial arrhythmias, Ventricular arrhythmias)
Tachyphylaxis, 186
Taurine, 425, 426
T-cell autoreactivity, 683
Terminal cisternae, 452
Termination of arrhythmias by pacing, 544
Tetrabutylammonium, 30
Tetraethylammonium chloride, 401, 450
Tetralogy of Fallot, 593
Tetramethylammonium, 30
Tetrodotoxin (TTX), 8, 46, 63, 64, 69, 117, 153, 154, 171, 209, 224, 264, 290, 314, 332, 334, 468, 487, 540, 562, 565, 572, 587, 609, 699
Theobromine, 466
Theophylline, 113, 449, 466, 657
Threshold potential/voltage, 166, 167, 184, 187, 202, 207, 222, 225, 226, 284, 316, 361, 610, 679
Thrombocytopenia, 503
Thyroidectomy, 685
Thyroid-stimulating hormone (TSH), 646
Thyrotoxicosis, 422, 425, 426, 669
Thyroxin (T_4, thyroid hormone), 640, 646, 647, 731
Tiapamil, 704, 709, 710, 715
Timolol, 502, 665, 667, 671

Tip potential, 22

Tocainide, 483, 485, 488, 545

Tolbutamide, 125

Tonic block, sodium channels, 479–481, 484, 485, 518, 539, 564, 606, 638

Torsade-des-pointes, 224, 496, 497, 501, 503–505, 528, 541, 542, 550, 571, 593, 619, 620, 646, 682, 712

Transducin, 114

Transient depolarization (*see* Delayed afterdepolarizations)

Transient inward current, 51, 124, 154, 189, 220, 222, 281, 285–288, 290

Transient outward current (*see* Potassium currents)

Transitional cells, 162, 169

Transplanted hearts, 277

Tricuspid insufficiency, 685

Tricyclic antidepressants, 527

Trigeminy, 278

Trigger calcium (*see* Calcium-induced calcium release)

Triggered activity/rhythms, 14, 127, 183, 187, 220–222, 284, 289–291, 359–363, 366, 378, 401, 404, 406, 409, 410, 496, 505, 519, 541, 565, 568, 588, 610, 640, 656, 668, 700, 711, 712

Triiodothyronine, 640, 646, 647

Triphenyltetrazolium chloride, 725

Troponin, 70–72, 74, 75, 82, 447, 453

Two levels of resting potential, 216

Two-microelectrode voltage clamp technique, 33–35

UD-CG 115 (*see* Pimobendan)

Unblock, channel kinetics, 483

Uncoupling (*see* Cellular uncoupling)

Unidirectional block, 252, 272, 337, 363, 364, 380, 524, 570

Unipolar recording, 5, 6, 126

Unitary conductance, 168, 701

UP 339.01, 627

Use-dependent block:
  calcium channel, 699, 709
  sodium channel, 378, 479, 480, 485, 494, 517, 518, 539, 570, 572, 586, 587, 606, 638, 639, 611, 642, 667, 668, 734

U wave, 497, 504, 642

Vagal afferent fibers, 468

Vagal efferent fibers/effects (*see* Autonomic tone)

Vagolytic effects (*see* Anticholinergic effects)

Valve leaflet, atrial myocardial cells, 127, 128, 360

Vectorcardiograms, 422

Ventricular arrhythmias, 351, 517, 521, 656, 681, 685, 707
  delayed phase (24 hr) in infarcted dog heart, 303
  effects of drugs, 523, 524, 543, 619, 620, 641–644
  ventricular fibrillation, 187, 277, 278, 301, 306, 322, 346, 367, 379, 503, 521, 590–592, 595, 672, 680–682, 689, 707, 723, 727, 734
  ventricular flutter, 278
  ventricular premature depolarizations, 15, 277, 278, 352, 365, 417, 419, 423, 502, 523, 524, 550, 585, 589, 595, 619, 621, 629, 643, 670, 681, 685, 733
    coupled: 253, 682
  ventricular tachycardia, 141, 260, 277, 278, 301, 306, 321, 352, 363, 365–367, 409, 417, 499, 503, 521, 524, 525, 528, 545, 546, 550, 585, 589, 591–593, 595, 612, 631, 632, 642–644, 647, 657, 659, 668, 670, 672, 681, 685, 689, 690, 708, 734
    monomorphic, 303–307, 334, 615, 728
    multiform, 322, 525, 629, 682

Ventricular defibrillation, energy requirements, 589, 686, 688, 691

Ventricular fibrillation threshold, 520, 570, 573, 588, 629, 641, 667, 669, 685, 688, 725, 729

Ventricular myocardium, cells, 26, 37, 41, 62, 71, 110, 112–114, 117, 119, 122, 124, 125, 154, 169, 199–228, 352, 381, 628, 668, 683, 687, 697
  abnormal automaticity, 221–224
  antiarrhythmic drug effects, 227, 228, 494, 517–520, 538, 540–542, 564–565, 567, 586–588, 606, 608, 639
  ATP-sensitive K current, 218–220
  cable properties, 224–226
  delayed outward rectifying K current, 216–218
  factors influencing impulse conduction, 226, 227
  instantaneous outward plateau K current, 218
  inward rectifying K current, 214–216
  normal transmembrane action potential, 201–207
  resting potential, 200, 201
  sodium current, 207–210
  sodium-sensitive K current, 220
  stretch-activated channels, 221

[Ventricular myocardium, cells]
  transient inward current, 220, 221
  transient outward current, 210–212
Ventricular pacing, 303, 309, 313
Ventricular preexcitation, 418, 423, 425
Verapamil, 47, 154, 171, 264, 291, 316, 334,
      377, 379, 438, 446, 498, 503, 697, 703–
      707, 709, 710, 712, 713, 715
Veratridine, 450, 468, 699
Voltage clamp, 33–39, 165, 168, 285, 603
  hybrid gap technique, 37
  modeling of results from bullfrog sinus veno-
      sus myocytes, 62–83
  ruptured patch technique, 63
  sucrose gap technique, 35, 37
  suction microelectrode technique, 151
  terminology, 61
    gating, 61
    gating states, 539
      activated/open, 61, 62, 539, 563, 586
      deactivation, 62
      inactivated, 61, 62, 539, 563, 586
      resting, 61, 62, 539, 563, 586
    recovery, 62
  two-microelectrode technique, 33–35
Voltage-dependent conductance changes, 48, 49,
      203, 484, 700
Voltage sensor, sodium channel, 563

Warfarin, 621, 647
Wavelength, circus movement, 242, 690
Wenkebach periodicity, 332, 333, 337, 640, 680
Whole animal models of arrhythmia:
  accelerated idioventricular arrhythmia, 614
  atrial fibrillation, 543, 641
  atrial flutter, 245–246, 572, 588, 680, 685, 689
  digitalis tocicity:
    atrial/supraventricular rhythms, 278, 572
    ventricular rhythms, 277–278, 520, 572–
      573, 588, 641, 680, 688
  paroxysmal atrial tachycardia, 240–243
  ventricular tachycardia:
    bradycardia dependent triggered rhythms, 389
    diabetes and hypertension, 403
    myocardial ischemia/infarction, 13, 261–
      263, 288, 301–324, 331–346, 351–369,
      386, 520, 543, 572, 588, 612–614, 629,
      641, 681, 685, 688, 690, 707
  reperfusion, 572
Whole cell patch clamp, 37, 43, 207, 210, 438
Win 40680 (see Amrinone)
Win 47203 (see Milrinone)
Wolff-Parkinson-White syndrome, 11, 271, 425,
      498, 522, 523, 603, 619, 643

Yohimbine, 433

About the Editors

KENNETH H. DANGMAN is a Research Scientist in the Department of Pharmacology, College of Physicians and Surgeons, Columbia University, New York, New York. The author or coauthor of over 70 scientific reports, book chapters, and review articles, he is a member of the American Society for Pharmacology and Experimental Therapeutics and the American Heart Association, Basic Science Council. Dr. Dangman received the B.Sci. degree in biology (1971) from Bucknell University, Lewisburg, Pennsylvania, and the M.S. (1974) and Ph.D. (1977) degrees in pharmacology from Columbia University, New York, New York.

DENNIS S. MIURA is Assistant Professor of Medicine, Division of Cardiology, and Director of the Clinical Arrhythmia and Electrophysiology Service, Albert Einstein College of Medicine, Bronx, New York. The author or coauthor of over 90 journal articles and book chapters, he is a Fellow of the American College of Cardiology, American College of Chest Physicians, American College of Clinical Pharmacology, and American College of Physicians, as well as a member of several other societies. Dr. Miura received the B.S. (1965) and M.S. (1967) degrees in chemical engineering; and M.Phil degree (1976), M.D. degree (1976), and Ph.D. degree (1976) in pharmacology from Columbia University, New York, New York.